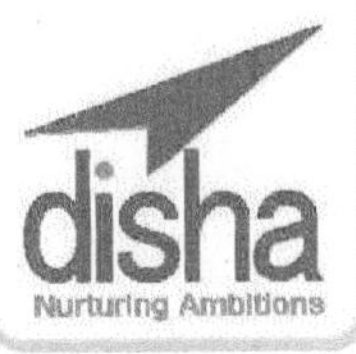

NTA
NEET
101 Speed Tests

(96 Chapter-wise + 3 Subject-wise + 2 Full Tests)

• **Corporate Office :** 45, 2nd Floor, Maharishi Dayanand Marg, Corner Market, Malviya Nagar, New Delhi-110017
Tel. : 011-49842349 / 49842350

Typeset by Disha DTP Team

DISHA PUBLICATION

For further information about books from DISHA,
Log on to **www.dishapublication.com** or **www.aiets.co.in** or email to **info@aiets.co.in**

CONTENTS

PHYSICS – Chapter-wise Tests

CHEMISTRY – Chapter-wise Tests

BIOLOGY – Chapter-wise Tests

PHYSICS – Subject-wise Test

CHEMISTRY – Subject-wise Test

BIOLOGY – Subject-wise Test

FULL TESTS

HINTS & SOLUTIONS

101 SPEED TESTS						
Speed Test	Time	Max. Marks	Cut-off Marks	Qualifying Marks	Marks Scored = Correct Answers × 4 - (1 × Incorrect Answers)	Success Gap = Qualifying Marks - Marks Scored
1	60	180	50	70		
2	60	180	50	70		
3	60	180	50	70		
4	60	180	45	60		
5	60	180	50	70		
6	60	180	45	60		
7	60	180	45	60		
8	60	180	50	70		
9	60	180	45	60		
10	60	180	45	60		
11	60	180	45	60		
12	60	180	50	70		
13	60	180	45	60		
14	60	180	50	70		
15	60	180	50	70		
16	60	180	50	70		
17	60	180	45	60		
18	60	180	45	60		
19	60	180	50	70		
20	60	180	50	70		
21	60	180	50	70		
22	60	180	50	70		
23	60	180	45	60		
24	60	180	45	60		
25	60	180	45	60		
26	60	180	50	70		
27	60	180	50	70		
28	60	180	50	70		
29	60	180	35	55		
30	60	180	35	52		
31	60	180	40	65		
32	60	180	38	60		
33	60	180	36	58		
34	60	180	34	55		
35	60	180	39	57		

101 SPEED TESTS						
Speed Test	Time	Max. Marks	Cut-off Marks	Qualifying Marks	Marks Scored = Correct Answers × 4 - (1 × Incorrect Answers)	Success Gap = Qualifying Marks - Marks Scored
36	60	180	45	65		
37	60	180	42	66		
38	60	180	36	58		
39	60	180	38	65		
40	60	180	35	60		
41	60	180	37	62		
42	60	180	45	68		
43	60	180	40	58		
44	60	180	42	63		
45	60	180	36	65		
46	60	180	38	64		
47	60	180	46	68		
48	60	180	43	63		
49	60	180	37	58		
50	60	180	42	65		
51	60	180	39	64		
52	60	180	37	59		
53	60	180	38	62		
54	60	180	35	57		
55	60	180	34	55		
56	60	180	38	58		
57	60	180	46	65		
58	60	180	46	68		
59	60	180	45	60		
60	60	180	45	60		
61	60	180	35	50		
62	60	180	40	65		
63	60	180	45	60		
64	60	180	45	60		
65	60	180	40	55		
66	60	180	45	60		
67	60	180	45	55		
68	60	180	40	50		
69	60	180	40	55		
70	60	180	40	55		

101 SPEED TESTS						
Speed Test	Time	Max. Marks	Cut-off Marks	Qualifying Marks	Marks Scored = Correct Answers × 4 - (1 × Incorrect Answers)	Success Gap = Qualifying Marks - Marks Scored
71	60	180	45	60		
72	60	180	45	60		
73	60	180	45	60		
74	60	180	45	60		
75	60	180	50	65		
76	60	180	50	60		
77	60	180	45	60		
78	60	180	45	60		
79	60	180	45	60		
80	60	180	40	50		
81	60	180	55	65		
82	60	180	40	55		
83	60	180	55	60		
84	60	180	48	55		
85	60	180	45	60		
86	60	180	55	65		
87	60	180	45	60		
88	60	180	48	55		
89	60	180	55	60		
90	60	180	45	60		
91	60	180	48	60		
92	60	180	40	55		
93	60	180	40	55		
94	60	180	50	70		
95	60	180	50	60		
96	60	180	40	60		
97	60	180	30	45		
98	60	180	30	40		
99	60	360	55	85		
100	180	720	135	100		
101	180	720	140	190		

PHYSICS

Physical World, Units & Measurements

Speed TEST 1 Chapter-wise

No. of Questions	Maximum Marks	Time
45	180	1 Hour

GENERAL INSTRUCTIONS

- This test contains 45 MCQ's. For each question only one option is correct. Darken the correct circle/ bubble in the Response Grid provided on each page.
- You have to evaluate your Response Grids yourself with the help of solutions provided at the end of this book.
- Each correct answer will get you 4 marks and 1 mark shall be deduced for each incorrect answer. No mark will be given/ deducted if no bubble is filled. Keep a timer in front of you and stop immediately at the end of 60 min.
- The sheet follows a particular syllabus. Do not attempt the sheet before you have completed your preparation for that syllabus.
- After completing the sheet check your answers with the solution booklet and complete the Result Grid. Finally spend time to analyse your performance and revise the areas which emerge out as weak in your evaluation.

1. The density of material in CGS system of units is $4 g/cm^3$. In a system of units in which unit of length is 10 cm and unit of mass is 100 g, the value of density of material will be
   (a) 0.4 unit (b) 40 unit
   (c) 400 unit (d) 0.04 unit
2. The time period of a body under S.H.M. is represented by: $T = P^a D^b S^c$ where P is pressure, D is density and S is surface tension, then values of a, b and c are
   (a) $-\frac{3}{2}, \frac{1}{2}, 1$ (b) $-1, -2, 3$
   (c) $\frac{1}{2}, -\frac{3}{2}, -\frac{1}{2}$ (d) $1, 2, \frac{1}{3}$
3. The respective number of significant figures for the numbers 23.023, 0.0003 and 2.1×10^{-3} are
   (a) 5, 1, 2 (b) 5, 1, 5 (c) 5, 5, 2 (d) 4, 4, 2
4. Young's modulus of a material has the same unit as that of
   (a) pressure (b) strain
   (c) compressibility (d) force
5. Of the following quantities, which one has dimensions different from the remaining three?
   (a) Energy per unit volume
   (b) Force per unit area
   (c) Product of voltage and charge per unit volume
   (d) Angular momentum
6. The pressure on a square plate is measured by measuring the force on the plate and length of the sides of the plate by using the formula $P = \frac{F}{\ell^2}$. If the maximum errors in the measurement of force and length are 4% and 2% respectively, then the maximum error in the measurement of pressure is
   (a) 1% (b) 2% (c) 8% (d) 10%

RESPONSE GRID	
	1. ⓐⓑⓒⓓ 2. ⓐⓑⓒⓓ 3. ⓐⓑⓒⓓ 4. ⓐⓑⓒⓓ 5. ⓐⓑⓒⓓ
	6. ⓐⓑⓒⓓ

Space for Rough Work

7. The siemen is the SI unit of
(a) resistivity (b) resistance
(c) conductivity (d) conductance

8. An object is moving through the liquid. The viscous damping force acting on it is proportional to the velocity. Then dimensions of constant of proportionality are
(a) $[ML^{-1}T^{-1}]$ (b) $[MLT^{-1}]$
(c) $[M^0LT^{-1}]$ (d) $[ML^0T^{-1}]$

9. The least count of a stop watch is 0.2 second. The time of 20 oscillations of a pendulum is measured to be 25 second. The percentage error in the measurement of time will be
(a) 8% (b) 1.8% (c) 0.8% (d) 0.1%

10. Weber is the unit of
(a) magnetic susceptibility
(b) intensity of magnetisation
(c) magnetic flux
(d) magnetic permeability

11. The physical quantity which has the dimensional formula $[M^1T^{-3}]$ is
(a) surface tension (b) solar constant
(c) density (d) compressibility

12. The dimensions of Wien's constant are
(a) $[ML^0TK]$ (b) $[M^0LT^0K]$
(c) $[M^0L^0TK]$ (d) [MLTK]

13. If the capacitance of a nanocapacitor is measured in terms of a unit '*u*' made by combining the electric charge '*e*', Bohr radius 'a_0', Planck's constant 'h' and speed of light '*c*' then

(a) $u=\frac{e^2h}{a_0}$ (b) $u=\frac{hc}{e^2a_0}$

(c) $u=\frac{e^2c}{ha_0}$ (d) $u=\frac{e^2a_0}{hc}$

14. The dimensions of $\frac{1}{\epsilon_0}\frac{e^2}{hc}$ are
(a) $M^{-1}L^{-3}T^4A^2$ (b) $ML^3T^{-4}A^{-2}$
(c) $M^0L^0T^0A^0$ (d) $M^{-1}L^{-3}T^2A$

15. The density of a cube is measured by measuring its mass and length of its sides. If the maximum error in the measurement of mass and length are 4% and 3% respectively, the maximum error in the measurement of density will be
(a) 7% (b) 9% (c) 12% (d) 13%

16. Which is different from others by units ?
(a) Phase difference (b) Mechanical equivalent
(c) Loudness of sound (d) Poisson's ratio

17. A quantity X is given by $\varepsilon_0 L\frac{\Delta V}{\Delta t}$ where ϵ_0 is the permittivity of the free space, L is a length, DV is a potential difference and Dt is a time interval. The dimensional formula for X is the same as that of
(a) resistance (b) charge
(c) voltage (d) current

18. If the error in the measurement of the volume of sphere is 6%, then the error in the measurement of its surface area will be
(a) 2% (b) 3% (c) 4% (d) 7.5%

19. If velocity (V), force (F) and energy (E) are taken as fundamental units, then dimensional formula for mass will be
(a) $V^{-2}F^0E$ (b) V^0FE^2 (c) $VF^{-2}E^0$ (d) $V^{-2}F^0E$

20. Multiply 107.88 by 0.610 and express the result with correct number of significant figures.
(a) 65.8068 (b) 65.807 (c) 65.81 (d) 65.8

21. Which of the following is a dimensional constant?
(a) Refractive index (b) Poissons ratio
(c) Strain (d) Gravitational constant

22. If E, m, J and G represent energy, mass, angular momentum and gravitational constant respectively, then the dimensional formula of EJ^2/m^5G^2 is same as that of the
(a) angle (b) length (c) mass (d) time

23. The refractive index of water measured by the relation $m=\frac{\text{real depth}}{\text{apparent depth}}$ is found to have values of 1.34, 1.38, 1.32 and 1.36; the mean value of refractive index with percentage error is
(a) $1.35 \pm 1.48\%$ (b) $1.35 \pm 0\%$
(c) $1.36 \pm 6\%$ (d) $1.36 \pm 0\%$

RESPONSE GRID					
	7. ⓐⓑⓒⓓ	8. ⓐⓑⓒⓓ	9. ⓐⓑⓒⓓ	10. ⓐⓑⓒⓓ	11. ⓐⓑⓒⓓ
	12. ⓐⓑⓒⓓ	13. ⓐⓑⓒⓓ	14. ⓐⓑⓒⓓ	15. ⓐⓑⓒⓓ	16. ⓐⓑⓒⓓ
	17. ⓐⓑⓒⓓ	18. ⓐⓑⓒⓓ	19. ⓐⓑⓒⓓ	20. ⓐⓑⓒⓓ	21. ⓐⓑⓒⓓ
	22. ⓐⓑⓒⓓ	23. ⓐⓑⓒⓓ			

Space for Rough Work

24. If e is the charge, V the potential difference, T the temperature, then the units of $\frac{eV}{T}$ are the same as that of
(a) Planck's constant (b) Stefan's constant
(c) Boltzmann's constant (d) gravitational constant

25. The dimensions of mobility are
(a) $M^{-2}T^2A$ (b) $M^{-1}T^2A$
(c) $M^{-2}T^3A$ (d) $M^{-1}T^3A$

26. Two quantities A and B have different dimensions which mathematical operation given below is physically meaningful?
(a) A/B (b) A+B (c) A–B (d) A=B

27. The velocity of water waves (v) may depend on their wavelength l, the density of water r and the acceleration due to gravity, g. The method of dimensions gives the relation between these quantities is
(a) v (b) $v^2 \propto g\lambda$
(c) $v^2 \propto g\lambda^2$ (d) $v^2 \propto g^{-1}\lambda^2$

28. The physical quantities not having same dimensions are
(a) torque and work
(b) momentum and Planck's constant
(c) stress and Young's modulus
(d) speed and $(m_0e_0)^{-1/2}$

29. A physical quantity of the dimensions of length that can be formed out of c, G and $\frac{e^2}{4\pi\varepsilon_0}$ is [c is velocity of light, G is universal constant of gravitation and e is charge]
(a) $c^2\left[G\frac{e^2}{4\pi\varepsilon_0}\right]^{1/2}$ (b) $\frac{1}{c^2}\left[\frac{e^2}{G4\pi\varepsilon_0}\right]^{1/2}$
(c) $\frac{1}{c}G\frac{e^2}{4\pi\varepsilon_0}$ (d) $\frac{1}{c^2}\left[G\frac{e^2}{4\pi\varepsilon_0}\right]^{1/2}$

30. The unit of impulse is the same as that of
(a) energy (b) power
(c) momentum (d) velocity

31. If Q denote the charge on the plate of a capacitor of capacitance C then the dimensional formula for $\frac{Q^2}{C}$ is
(a) $[L^2M^2T]$ (b) $[LMT^2]$
(c) $[L^2MT^{-2}]$ (d) $[L^2M^2T^2]$

32. The mass of the liquid flowing per second per unit area of cross-section of the tube is proportional to (pressure difference across the ends)^n and (average velocity of the liquid)^m. Which of the following relations between m and n is correct?
(a) m=n (b) m=–n (c) m^2=n (d) m=–n^2

33. The Richardson equation is given by $I = AT^2e^{-B/kT}$. The dimensional formula for AB^2 is same as that for
(a) IT^2 (b) kT (c) Ik^2 (d) Ik^2/T

34. Turpentine oil is flowing through a capillary tube of length ℓ and radius r. The pressure difference between the two ends of the tube is p. The viscosity of oil is given by : $\eta = \frac{p(r^2-x^2)}{4v\ell}$. Here v is velocity of oil at a distance x from the axis of the tube. From this relation, the dimensional formula of η is
(a) $[ML^{-1}T^{-1}]$ (b) $[MLT^{-1}]$
(c) $[ML^2T^{-2}]$ (d) $[M^0L^0T^0]$

35. Given that $y = A\sin\left[\left(\frac{2\pi}{\lambda}(ct-x)\right)\right]$, where y and x are measured in metre. Which of the following statements is true?
(a) The unit of λ is same as that of x and A
(b) The unit of λ is same as that of x but not of A
(c) The unit of c is same as that of $\frac{2\pi}{\lambda}$
(d) The unit of (ct – x) is same as that of $\frac{2\pi}{\lambda}$

36. If L = 2.331 cm, B = 2.1 cm, then L + B =
(a) 4.431 cm (b) 4.43 cm (c) 4.4 cm (d) 4 cm

37. In the relation x = cos (ωt + kx), the dimension(s) of ω is/are
(a) $[M^0LT]$ (b) $[M^0L^{-1}T^0]$
(c) $[M^0L^0T^{-1}]$ (d) $[M^0LT^{-1}]$

RESPONSE GRID					
	24. ⓐⓑⓒⓓ	25. ⓐⓑⓒⓓ	26. ⓐⓑⓒⓓ	27. ⓐⓑⓒⓓ	28. ⓐⓑⓒⓓ
	29. ⓐⓑⓒⓓ	30. ⓐⓑⓒⓓ	31. ⓐⓑⓒⓓ	32. ⓐⓑⓒⓓ	33. ⓐⓑⓒⓓ
	34. ⓐⓑⓒⓓ	35. ⓐⓑⓒⓓ	36. ⓐⓑⓒⓓ	37. ⓐⓑⓒⓓ	

Space for Rough Work

38. In a vernier callipers, ten smallest divisions of the vernier scale are equal to nine smallest division on the main scale. If the smallest division on the main scale is half millimeter, then the vernier constant is
(a) 0.5 mm (b) 0.1 mm (c) 0.05 mm (d) 0.005 mm

39. Which two of the following five physical parameters have the same dimensions?
(A) Energy density (B) Refractive index
(C) Dielectric constant (D) Young's modulus
(E) Magnetic field
(a) (B) and (D) (b) (C) and (E)
(c) (A) and (D) (d) (A) and (E)

40. In the eqn. $\left(P+\frac{a}{V^2}\right)(V-b)$ = constant, the unit of a is
(a) dyne cm^5 (b) dyne cm^4
(c) dyne/cm^3 (d) dyne cm^2

41. The dimensions of Reynold's constant are
(a) $[M^0L^0T^0]$ (b) $[ML^{-1}T^{-1}]$
(c) $[ML^{-1}T^{-2}]$ (d) $[ML^{-2}T^{-2}]$

42. Which of the following do not have the same dimensional formula as the velocity?
Given that m_0 = permeability of free space, e_0 = permittivity of free space, n = frequency, l = wavelength, P = pressure, r = density, w = angular frequency, k = wave number,
(a) $1/\sqrt{\mu_0 \varepsilon_0}$ (b) n l (c) $\sqrt{P/\rho}$ (d) ωk

43. Unit of magnetic moment is
(a) ampere–metre^2 (b) ampere–metre
(c) weber–metre^2 (d) weber/metre

44. An experiment is performed to obtain the value of acceleration due to gravity g by using a simple pendulum of length L. In this experiment time for 100 oscillations is measured by using a watch of 1 second least count and the value is 90.0 seconds. The length L is measured by using a meter scale of least count 1 mm and the value is 20.0 cm. The error in the determination of g would be:
(a) 1.7% (b) 2.7% (c) 4.4% (d) 2.27%

45. The dimensional formula for magnetic flux is
(a) $[ML^2T^{-2}A^{-1}]$ (b) $[ML^3T^{-2}A^{-2}]$
(c) $[M^0L^{-2}T^2A^{-2}]$ (d) $[ML^2T^{-1}A^2]$

RESPONSE GRID					
	38. ⓐⓑⓒⓓ	39. ⓐⓑⓒⓓ	40. ⓐⓑⓒⓓ	41. ⓐⓑⓒⓓ	42. ⓐⓑⓒⓓ
	43. ⓐⓑⓒⓓ	44. ⓐⓑⓒⓓ	45. ⓐⓑⓒⓓ		

PHYSICS CHAPTERWISE SPEED TEST-1			
Total Questions	45	Total Marks	180
Attempted		Correct	
Incorrect		Net Score	
Cut-off Score	50	Qualifying Score	70
Success Gap = Net Score – Qualifying Score			
Net Score = (Correct × 4) – (Incorrect × 1)			

Space for Rough Work

PHYSICS

Motion in a Straight Line

Speed TEST 2

Chapter-wise

No. of Questions	Maximum Marks	Time
45	180	1 Hour

GENERAL INSTRUCTIONS

- This test contains 45 MCQ's. For each question only one option is correct. Darken the correct circle/ bubble in the Response Grid provided on each page.
- You have to evaluate your Response Grids yourself with the help of solutions provided at the end of this book.
- Each correct answer will get you 4 marks and 1 mark shall be deduced for each incorrect answer. No mark will be given/ deducted if no bubble is filled. Keep a timer in front of you and stop immediately at the end of 60 min.
- The sheet follows a particular syllabus. Do not attempt the sheet before you have completed your preparation for that syllabus.
- After completing the sheet check your answers with the solution booklet and complete the Result Grid. Finally spend time to analyse your performance and revise the areas which emerge out as weak in your evaluation.

1. A particle starts moving rectilinearly at time t = 0 such that its velocity v changes with time t according to the equation $v = t^2 - t$ where t is in seconds and v is in m/s. Find the time interval for which the particle retards.

   (a) $\frac{1}{2} < t < 1$ (b) $\frac{1}{2} > t > 1$

   (c) $\frac{1}{4} < t < 1$ (d) $\frac{1}{2} < t < \frac{3}{4}$

2. The co-ordinates of a moving particle at any time '*t*' are given by $x = \alpha t^3$ and $y = \beta t^3$. The speed of the particle at time '*t*' is given by

   (a) $3t\sqrt{\alpha^2 + \beta^2}$ (b) $3t^2\sqrt{\alpha^2 + \beta^2}$

   (c) $t^2\sqrt{\alpha^2 + \beta^2}$ (d) $\sqrt{\alpha^2 + \beta^2}$

3. If a car covers $2/5^{th}$ of the total distance with v_1 speed and $3/5^{th}$ distance with v_2 then average speed is

   (a) $\frac{1}{2}\sqrt{v_1 v_2}$ (b) $\frac{v_1 + v_2}{2}$ (c) $\frac{2v_1 v_2}{v_1 + v_2}$ (d) $\frac{5v_1 v_2}{3v_1 + 2v_2}$

4. Choose the correct statements from the following.
   (a) The magnitude of instantaneous velocity of a particle is equal to its instantaneous speed
   (b) The magnitude of the average velocity in an interval is equal to its average speed in that interval.
   (c) It is possible to have a situation in which the speed of the particle is never zero but the average speed in an interval is zero.
   (d) It is possible to have a situation in which the speed of particle is zero but the average speed is not zero.

5. A particle located at $x = 0$ at time $t = 0$, starts moving along with the positive x-direction with a velocity 'v' that varies as $v = \alpha\sqrt{x}$. The displacement of the particle varies with time as

   (a) t^2 (b) t (c) $t^{1/2}$ (d) t^3

6. Figure here gives the speed-time graph for a body. The displacement travelled between t = 1.0 second and t = 7.0 second is nearest to

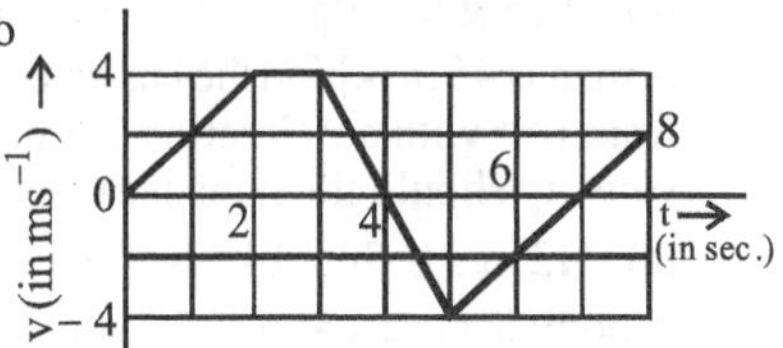

   (a) 1.5m
   (b) 2m
   (c) 3m
   (d) 4m

7. A particle is moving in a straight line with initial velocity and uniform acceleration *a*. If the sum of the distance travelled in t^{th} and $(t + 1)^{th}$ seconds is 100 cm, then its velocity after *t* seconds, in cm/s, is

   (a) 80 (b) 50 (c) 20 (d) 30

RESPONSE GRID					
	1. ⓐⓑⓒⓓ	2. ⓐⓑⓒⓓ	3. ⓐⓑⓒⓓ	4. ⓐⓑⓒⓓ	5. ⓐⓑⓒⓓ
	6. ⓐⓑⓒⓓ	7. ⓐⓑⓒⓓ			

Space for Rough Work

8. A thief is running away on a straight road on a jeep moving with a speed of 9 m/s. A police man chases him on a motor cycle moving at a speed of 10 m/s. If the instantaneous separation of jeep from the motor cycle is 100 m, how long will it take for the police man to catch the thief?
(a) 1 second (b) 19 second
(c) 90 second (d) 100 second

9. The displacement x of a particle varies with time according to the relation $x = \frac{a}{b}(1 - e^{-bt})$. Then select the false alternative.
(a) At $t = \frac{1}{b}$, the displacement of the particle is nearly $\frac{2}{3}\left(\frac{a}{b}\right)$
(b) The velocity and acceleration of the particle at t = 0 are a and –ab respectively
(c) The particle cannot go beyond $x = \frac{a}{b}$
(d) The particle will not come back to its starting point at $t \to \infty$

10. A metro train starts from rest and in five seconds achieves a speed 108 km/h. After that it moves with constant velocity and comes to rest after travelling 45m with uniform retardation. If total distance travelled is 395 m, find total time of travelling.
(a) 12.2 s (b) 15.3 s (c) 9 s (d) 17.2 s

11. The deceleration experienced by a moving motor boat after its engine is cut off, is given by $dv/dt = -kv^3$ where k is a constant. If v_0 is the magnitude of the velocity at cut-off, the magnitude of the velocity at a time *t* after the cut-off is
(a) $\frac{v_0}{\sqrt{(2v_0^2 kt + 1)}}$ (b) $v_0 e^{-kt}$
(c) $v_0 / 2$ (d) v_0

12. The velocity of a particle is $v = v_0 + gt + ft^2$. If its position is $x = 0$ at $t = 0$, then its displacement after unit time ($t = 1$) is
(a) $v_0 + g/2 + f$ (b) $v_0 + 2g + 3f$
(c) $v_0 + g/2 + f/3$ (d) $v_0 + g + f$

13. A man is 45 m behind the bus when the bus starts accelerating from rest with acceleration 2.5 m/s². With what minimum velocity should the man start running to catch the bus?
(a) 12 m/s (b) 14 m/s (c) 15 m/s (d) 16 m/s

14. A body is at rest at $x = 0$. At $t = 0$, it starts moving in the positive x-direction with a constant acceleration. At the same instant another body passes through $x = 0$ moving in the positive x-direction with a constant speed. The position of the first body is given by $x_1(t)$ after time '*t*'; and that of the second body by $x_2(t)$ after the same time interval. Which of the following graphs correctly describes $(x_1 - x_2)$ as a function of time '*t*'?

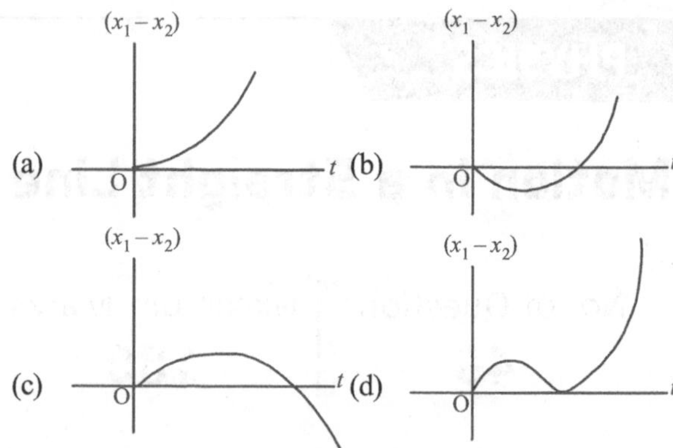

15. From the top of a building 40 m tall, a boy projects a stone vertically upwards with an initial velocity 10 m/s such that it eventually falls to the ground. After how long will the stone strike the ground ? Take g = 10 m/s².
(a) 1 s (b) 2 s (c) 3 s (d) 4 s

16. Two bodies begin to fall freely from the same height but the second falls T second after the first. The time (after which the first body begins to fall) when the distance between the bodies equals L is
(a) $\frac{1}{2}T$ (b) $\frac{T}{2} + \frac{L}{gT}$ (c) $\frac{L}{gT}$ (d) $T + \frac{2L}{gT}$

17. Let A, B, C, D be points on a vertical line such that AB = BC = CD. If a body is released from position A, the times of descent through AB, BC and CD are in the ratio.
(a) $1 : \sqrt{3} - \sqrt{2} : \sqrt{3} + \sqrt{2}$ (b) $1 : \sqrt{2} - 1 : \sqrt{3} - \sqrt{2}$
(c) $1 : \sqrt{2} - 1 : \sqrt{3}$ (d) $1 : \sqrt{2} : \sqrt{3} - 1$

18. The water drops fall at regular intervals from a tap 5 m above the ground. The third drop is leaving the tap at an instant when the first drop touches the ground. How far above the ground is the second drop at that instant? (Take g = 10 m/s²)
(a) 1.25m (b) 2.50m (c) 3.75m (d) 5.00m

19. The displacement '*x*' (in meter) of a particle of mass '*m*' (in kg) moving in one dimension under the action of a force, is related to time '*t*' (in sec) by $t = \sqrt{x} + 3$. The displacement of the particle when its velocity is zero, will be
(a) 2m (b) 4m (c) zero (d) 6m

20. A body moving with a uniform acceleration crosses a distance of 65 m in the 5 th second and 105 m in 9th second. How far will it go in 20 s?
(a) 2040m (b) 240m (c) 2400m (d) 2004m

21. An automobile travelling with a speed of 60 km/h, can brake to stop within a distance of 20m. If the car is going twice as fast i.e., 120 km/h, the stopping distance will be
(a) 60m (b) 40m (c) 20m (d) 80m

RESPONSE GRID					
	8. ⓐⓑⓒⓓ	9. ⓐⓑⓒⓓ	10. ⓐⓑⓒⓓ	11. ⓐⓑⓒⓓ	12. ⓐⓑⓒⓓ
	13. ⓐⓑⓒⓓ	14. ⓐⓑⓒⓓ	15. ⓐⓑⓒⓓ	16. ⓐⓑⓒⓓ	17. ⓐⓑⓒⓓ
	18. ⓐⓑⓒⓓ	19. ⓐⓑⓒⓓ	20. ⓐⓑⓒⓓ	21. ⓐⓑⓒⓓ	

Space for Rough Work

22. A particle accelerates from rest at a constant rate for some time and attains a velocity of 8 m/sec. Afterwards it decelerates with the constant rate and comes to rest. If the total time taken is 4 sec, the distance travelled is
(a) 32m (b) 16m
(c) 4m (d) None of the above

23. The equation represented by the graph below is :
(a) $y = \frac{1}{2} gt$
(b) $y = \frac{-1}{2} gt$
(c) $y = \frac{1}{2} gt^2$
(d) $y = \frac{-1}{2} gt^2$

24. A particle moves a distance x in time t according to equation $x = (t + 5)^{-1}$. The acceleration of particle is proportional to:
(a) $(velocity)^{3/2}$ (b) $(distance)^2$
(c) $(distance)^{-2}$ (d) $(velocity)^{2/3}$

25. A particle when thrown, moves such that it passes from same height at 2 and 10 seconds, then this height h is :
(a) 5g (b) g (c) 8g (d) 10g

26. The distance through which a body falls in the nth second is h. The distance through which it falls in the next second is
(a) h (b) $h + \frac{g}{2}$ (c) h – g (d) h + g

27. A stone thrown upward with a speed u from the top of the tower reaches the ground with a velocity 3u. The height of the tower is
(a) $3u^2/g$ (b) $4u^2/g$ (c) $6u^2/g$ (d) $9u^2/g$

28. A particle moves along a straight line OX. At a time t (in seconds) the distance x (in metres) of the particle from O is given by $x = 40 + 12t - t^3$. How long would the particle travel before coming to rest?
(a) 40m (b) 56m (c) 16m (d) 24m

29. The graph shown in figure shows the velocity v versus time t for a body.
Which of the graphs represents the corresponding acceleration versus time graphs?

(a) 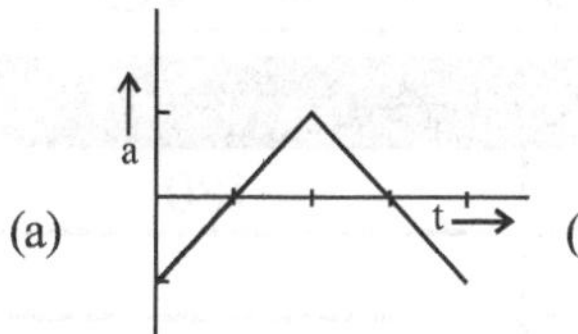
(b) 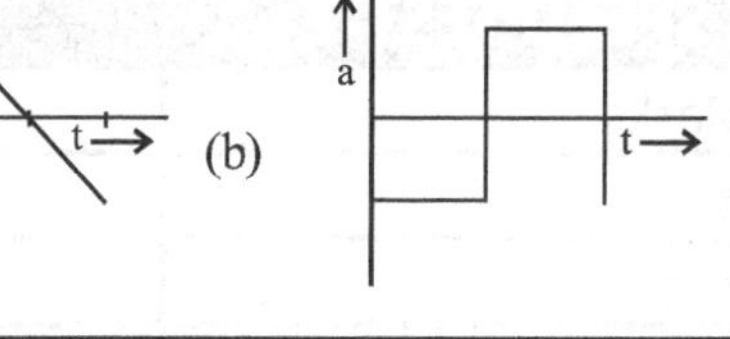
(c) (d) 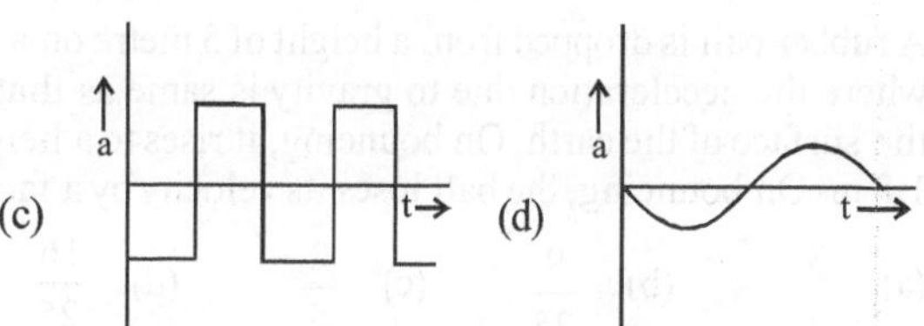

30. A particle moving along x-axis has acceleration f, at time t, given by $f = f_0\left(1 - \frac{t}{T}\right)$, where f_0 and T are constants. The particle at t = 0 has zero velocity. In the time interval between $t = 0$ and the instant when f = 0, the particle's velocity (v_x) is
(a) $\frac{1}{2} f_0 T^2$ (b) $f_0 T^2$ (c) $\frac{1}{2} f_0 T$ (d) $f_0 T$

31. A body is thrown vertically up with a velocity u. It passes three points A, B and C in its upward journey with velocities $\frac{u}{2}, \frac{u}{3}$ and $\frac{u}{4}$ respectively. The ratio of AB and BC is
(a) 20 : 7 (b) 2 (c) 10 : 7 (d) 1

32. A boat takes 2 hours to travel 8 km and back in still water lake. With water velocity of 4 km h^{-1}, the time taken for going upstream of 8 km and coming back is
(a) 160 minutes (b) 80 minutes
(c) 100 minutes (d) 120 minutes

33. A body starts from rest and travels a distance x with uniform acceleration, then it travels a distance 2x with uniform speed, finally it travels a distance 3x with uniform retardation and comes to rest. If the complete motion of the particle is along a straight line, then the ratio of its average velocity to maximum velocity is
(a) 2/5 (b) 3/5 (c) 4/5 (d) 6/7

34. A man of 50 kg mass is standing in a gravity free space at a height of 10 m above the floor. He throws a stone of 0.5 kg mass downwards with a speed 2 m/s. When the stone reaches the floor, the distance of the man above the floor will be:
(a) 9.9m (b) 10.1m (c) 10m (d) 20m

35. A boy moving with a velocity of 20 km h^{-1} along a straight line joining two stationary objects. According to him both objects
(a) move in the same direction with the same speed of 20 km h^{-1}
(b) move in different direction with the same speed of 20 km h^{-1}
(c) move towards him
(d) remain stationary

RESPONSE GRID					
	22. ⓐⓑⓒⓓ	23. ⓐⓑⓒⓓ	24. ⓐⓑⓒⓓ	25. ⓐⓑⓒⓓ	26. ⓐⓑⓒⓓ
	27. ⓐⓑⓒⓓ	28. ⓐⓑⓒⓓ	29. ⓐⓑⓒⓓ	30. ⓐⓑⓒⓓ	31. ⓐⓑⓒⓓ
	32. ⓐⓑⓒⓓ	33. ⓐⓑⓒⓓ	34. ⓐⓑⓒⓓ	35. ⓐⓑⓒⓓ	

Space for Rough Work

36. A rubber ball is dropped from a height of 5 metre on a plane where the acceleration due to gravity is same as that onto the surface of the earth. On bouncing, it rises to a height of 1.8 m. On bouncing, the ball loses its velocity by a factor of

(a) $\frac{3}{5}$ (b) $\frac{9}{25}$ (c) $\frac{2}{5}$ (d) $\frac{16}{25}$

37. A stone falls freely from rest from a height h and it travels a distance $\frac{9h}{25}$ in the last second. The value of h is

(a) 145 m (b) 100 m (c) 122.5 m (d) 200 m

38. Which one of the following equations represents the motion of a body with finite constant acceleration ? In these equations, y denotes the displacement of the body at time t and a, b and c are constants of motion.

(a) $y = at$ (b) $y = at + bt^2$
(b) $y = at + bt^2 + ct^3$ (d) $y = \frac{a}{t} + bt$

39. A particle travels half the distance with a velocity of 6 ms^{-1}. The remaining half distance is covered with a velocity of 4 ms^{-1} for half the time and with a velocity of 8 ms^{-1} for the rest of the half time. What is the velocity of the particle averaged over the whole time of motion ?

(a) 9 ms^{-1} (b) 6 ms^{-1} (c) 5.35 ms^{-1} (d) 5 ms^{-1}

40. A bullet is fired with a speed of 1000 m/sec in order to penetrate a target situated at 100 m away. If g = 10 m/s^2, the gun should be aimed

(a) directly towards the target
(b) 5 cm above the target
(c) 10 cm above the target
(d) 15 cm above the target

41. A body covers 26, 28, 30, 32 meters in 10th, 11th, 12th and 13th seconds respectively. The body starts

(a) from rest and moves with uniform velocity
(b) from rest and moves with uniform acceleration
(c) with an initial velocity and moves with uniform acceleration
(d) with an initial velocity and moves with uniform velocity

42. A particle is moving with uniform acceleration along a straight line. The average velocity of the particle from P to Q is 8ms^{-1} and that Q to S is 12ms^{-1}. If QS = PQ, then the average velocity from P to S is

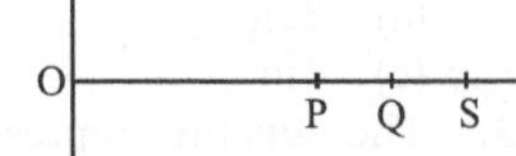

(a) 9.6 ms^{-1} (b) 12.87 ms^{-1}
(c) 64 ms^{-1} (d) 327 ms^{-1}

43. The variation of velocity of a particle with time moving along a straight line is illustrated in the figure. The distance travelled by the particle in four seconds is

(a) 60m
(b) 55m
(c) 25m
(d) 30m

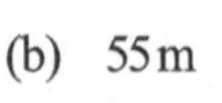

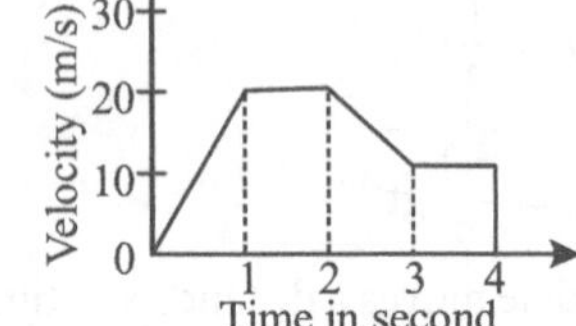

44. A stone falls freely under gravity. It covers distances h_1, h_2 and h_3 in the first 5 seconds, the next 5 seconds and the next 5 seconds respectively. The relation between h_1, h_2 and h_3 is

(a) $h_1 = \frac{h_2}{3} = \frac{h_3}{5}$ (b) $h_2 = 3h_1$ and $h_3 = 3h_2$
(c) $h_1 = h_2 = h_3$ (d) $h_1 = 2h_2 = 3h_3$

45. A car, starting from rest, accelerates at the rate f through a distance S, then continues at constant speed for time t and then decelerates at the rate $\frac{f}{2}$ to come to rest. If the total distance traversed is 15 S, then

(a) $S = \frac{1}{6}ft^2$ (b) $S = ft$
(c) $S = \frac{1}{4}ft^2$ (d) $S = \frac{1}{72}ft^2$

RESPONSE GRID					
	36. ⓐⓑⓒⓓ	37. ⓐⓑⓒⓓ	38. ⓐⓑⓒⓓ	39. ⓐⓑⓒⓓ	40. ⓐⓑⓒⓓ
	41. ⓐⓑⓒⓓ	42. ⓐⓑⓒⓓ	43. ⓐⓑⓒⓓ	44. ⓐⓑⓒⓓ	45. ⓐⓑⓒⓓ

PHYSICS CHAPTERWISE SPEED TEST-2			
Total Questions	45	Total Marks	180
Attempted		Correct	
Incorrect		Net Score	
Cut-off Score	50	Qualifying Score	70
Success Gap = Net Score – Qualifying Score			
Net Score = (Correct × 4) – (Incorrect × 1)			

Space for Rough Work

PHYSICS

Speed TEST 3

Chapter-wise

Motion in a Plane

No. of Questions	Maximum Marks	Time
45	180	1 Hour

GENERAL INSTRUCTIONS

- This test contains 45 MCQ's. For each question only one option is correct. Darken the correct circle/ bubble in the Response Grid provided on each page.
- You have to evaluate your Response Grids yourself with the help of solutions provided at the end of this book.
- Each correct answer will get you 4 marks and 1 mark shall be deduced for each incorrect answer. No mark will be given/ deducted if no bubble is filled. Keep a timer in front of you and stop immediately at the end of 60 min.
- The sheet follows a particular syllabus. Do not attempt the sheet before you have completed your preparation for that syllabus.
- After completing the sheet check your answers with the solution booklet and complete the Result Grid. Finally spend time to analyse your performance and revise the areas which emerge out as weak in your evaluation.

1. A projectile is given an initial velocity of $(\hat{i}+2\hat{j})$ m/s, where $\hat{i}$ is along the ground and $\hat{j}$ is along the vertical. If g = 10 m/s^2, the equation of its trajectory is :
   (a) $y = x - 5x^2$ (b) $y = 2x - 5x^2$
   (c) $4y = 2x - 5x^2$ (d) $4y = 2x - 25x^2$

2. An aircraft moving with a speed of 250 m/s is at a height of 6000 m, just overhead of an anti aircraft–gun. If the muzzle velocity is 500 m/s, the firing angle θ should be:
   (a) 30°
   (b) 45°
   (c) 60°
   (d) 75°

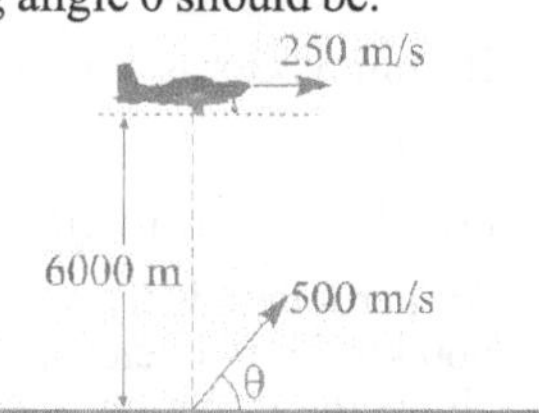

3. Two racing cars of masses m_1 and m_2 are moving in circles of radii r_1 and r_2 respectively. Their speeds are such that each makes a complete circle in the same duration of time t. The ratio of the angular speed of the first to the second car is
   (a) $m_1 : m_2$ (b) $r_1 : r_2$
   (c) 1 : 1 (d) $m_1r_1 : m_2r_2$

4. A boy playing on the roof of a 10 m high building throws a ball with a speed of 10m/s at an angle of 30° with the horizontal. How far from the throwing point will the ball be at the height of 10 m from the ground ?
   $[g = 10\text{m/s}^2,\ \sin 30^o = \frac{1}{2},\ \cos 30^o = \frac{\sqrt{3}}{2}]$
   (a) 5.20m (b) 4.33m (c) 2.60m (d) 8.66m

5. A bomber plane moves horizontally with a speed of 500 m/s and a bomb released from it, strikes the ground in 10 sec. Angle at which it strikes the ground wil be (g = 10 m/s^2)
   (a) $\tan^{-1}\left(\frac{1}{5}\right)$ (b) $\tan\left(\frac{1}{5}\right)$
   (c) $\tan^{-1}(1)$ (d) $\tan^{-1}(5)$

6. Two particles start simultaneously from the same point and move along two straight lines, one with uniform velocity v and other with a uniform acceleration a. If α is the angle between the lines of motion of two particles then the least value of relative velocity will be at time given by
   (a) $\frac{v}{a}\sin\alpha$ (b) $\frac{v}{a}\cos\alpha$ (c) $\frac{v}{a}\tan\alpha$ (d) $\frac{v}{a}\cot\alpha$

7. Initial velocity with which a body is projected is 10 m/sec and angle of projection is 60°. Find the range R
   (a) $\frac{15\sqrt{3}\text{m}}{2}$
   (b) $\frac{40}{3}$m
   (c) $5\sqrt{3}$m
   (d) $\frac{20}{3}$m

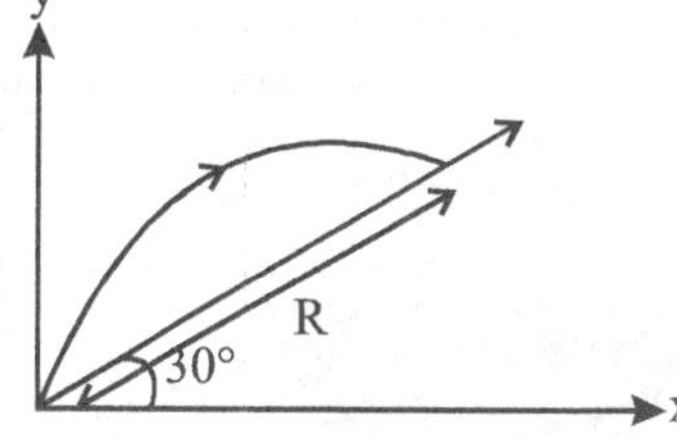

RESPONSE GRID					
	1. ⓐⓑⓒⓓ	2. ⓐⓑⓒⓓ	3. ⓐⓑⓒⓓ	4. ⓐⓑⓒⓓ	5. ⓐⓑⓒⓓ
	6. ⓐⓑⓒⓓ	7. ⓐⓑⓒⓓ			

Space for Rough Work

8. The position vectors of points A, B, C and D are $A = 3\hat{i}+4\hat{j}+5\hat{k}, B = 4\hat{i}+5\hat{j}+6\hat{k}, C = 7\hat{i}+9\hat{j}+3\hat{k}$ and $D = 4\hat{i}+6\hat{j}$ then the displacement vectors $\overrightarrow{AB}$ and $\overrightarrow{CD}$ are
(a) perpendicular (b) parallel
(c) antiparallel (d) inclined at an angle of 60°

9. A person swims in a river aiming to reach exactly on the opposite point on the bank of a river. His speed of swimming is 0.5 m/s at an angle of 120° with the direction of flow of water. The speed of water is
(a) 1.0 m/s (b) 0.5 m/s (c) 0.25 m/s (d) 0.43 m/s

10. A projectile thrown with velocity v making angle θ with vertical gains maximum height H in the time for which the projectile remains in air, the time period is
(a) $\sqrt{H\cos\theta/g}$ (b) $\sqrt{2H\cos\theta/g}$
(c) $\sqrt{4H/g}$ (d) $\sqrt{8H/g}$

11. A ball is thrown from a point with a speed 'v_0' at an elevation angle of θ. From the same point and at the same instant, a person starts running with a constant speed $\frac{'v_0'}{2}$ to catch the ball. Will the person be able to catch the ball? If yes, what should be the angle of projection θ ?
(a) No, 0° (b) Yes, 30° (c) Yes, 60° (d) Yes, 45°

12. If vectors $\vec{A} = \cos\omega t\hat{i} + \sin\omega t\hat{j}$ and $\vec{B} = \cos\frac{\omega t}{2}\hat{i} + \sin\frac{\omega t}{2}\hat{j}$ are functions of time, then the value of t at which they are orthogonal to each other is :
(a) $t = \frac{\pi}{2\omega}$ (b) $t = \frac{\pi}{\omega}$ (c) $t = 0$ (d) $t = \frac{\pi}{4\omega}$

13. A bus is moving on a straight road towards north with a uniform speed of 50 km/hour turns through 90°. If the speed remains unchanged after turning, the increase in the velocity of bus in the turning process is
(a) 70.7 km/hour along south-west direction
(b) 70.7 km/hour along north-west direction.
(c) 50 km/hour along west
(d) zero

14. The velocity of projection of oblique projectile is $(6\hat{i}+8\hat{j})\,ms^{-1}$. The horizontal range of the projectile is
(a) 4.9 m (b) 9.6 m (c) 19.6 m (d) 14 m

15. A point P moves in counter-clockwise direction on a circular path as shown in the figure. The movement of 'P' is such that it sweeps out a length $s = t^3 + 5$, where s is in metres and t is in seconds. The radius of the path is 20 m. The acceleration of 'P' when t = 2 s is nearly

y, B, P(x,y), 20m, O, A, x

(a) 13 m/s² (b) 12 m/s² (c) 7.2 ms² (d) 14 m/s²

16. The resultant of two vectors $\vec{A}$ and $\vec{B}$ is perpendicular to the vector $\vec{A}$ and its magnitude is equal to half the magnitude of vector $\vec{B}$. The angle between $\vec{A}$ and $\vec{B}$ is
(a) 120° (b) 150° (c) 135° (d) 180°

17. A man running along a straight road with uniform velocity $\vec{u} = u\hat{i}$ feels that the rain is falling vertically down along $-\hat{j}$. If he doubles his speed, he finds that the rain is coming at an angle θ with the vertical. The velocity of the rain with respect to the ground is
(a) $ui - uj$ (b) $ui - \frac{u}{\tan\theta}\hat{j}$
(c) $2u\hat{i} + u\cot\theta\hat{j}$ (d) $ui + u\sin\theta\hat{j}$

18. Two projectiles A and B thrown with speeds in the ratio $1:\sqrt{2}$ acquired the same heights. If A is thrown at an angle of 45° with the horizontal, the angle of projection of B will be
(a) 0° (b) 60° (c) 30° (d) 45°

19. A projectile can have the same range 'R' for two angles of projection. If 'T_1' and 'T_2' be time of flights in the two cases, then the product of the two time of flights is directly proportional to
(a) R (b) $\frac{1}{R}$ (c) $\frac{1}{R^2}$ (d) R^2

20. A man standing on the roof of a house of height h throws one particle vertically downwards and another particle horizontally with the same velocity u. The ratio of their velocities when they reach the earth's surface will be
(a) $\sqrt{2gh+u^2} : u$ (b) 1 : 2
(c) 1 : 1 (d) $\sqrt{2gh+u^2} : \sqrt{2gh}$

21. If a unit vector is represented by $0.5\hat{i} + 0.8\hat{j} + c\hat{k}$, the value of c is
(a) 1 (b) $\sqrt{0.11}$ (c) $\sqrt{0.01}$ (d) 0.39

22. An aeroplane is flying at a constant horizontal velocity of 600 km/hr at an elevation of 6 km towards a point directly above the target on the earth's surface. At an appropriate time, the pilot releases a ball so that it strikes the target at the earth. The ball will appear to be falling
(a) on a parabolic path as seen by pilot in the plane
(b) vertically along a straight path as seen by an observer on the ground near the target
(c) on a parabolic path as seen by an observer on the ground near the target
(d) on a zig-zag path as seen by pilot in the plane

RESPONSE GRID					
	8. ⓐⓑⓒⓓ	9. ⓐⓑⓒⓓ	10. ⓐⓑⓒⓓ	11. ⓐⓑⓒⓓ	12. ⓐⓑⓒⓓ
	13. ⓐⓑⓒⓓ	14. ⓐⓑⓒⓓ	15. ⓐⓑⓒⓓ	16. ⓐⓑⓒⓓ	17. ⓐⓑⓒⓓ
	18. ⓐⓑⓒⓓ	19. ⓐⓑⓒⓓ	20. ⓐⓑⓒⓓ	21. ⓐⓑⓒⓓ	22. ⓐⓑⓒⓓ

Space for Rough Work

23. A particle is projected with a velocity v such that its range on the horizontal plane is twice the greatest height attained by it. The range of the projectile is (where g is acceleration due to gravity)
(a) $\frac{4v^2}{5g}$ (b) $\frac{4g}{5v^2}$ (c) $\frac{v^2}{g}$ (d) $\frac{4v^2}{\sqrt{5}g}$

24. Two stones are projected from the same point with same speed making angles $(45° + \theta)$ and $(45° - \theta)$ with the horizontal respectively. If $\theta \leq 45°$, then the horizontal ranges of the two stones are in the ratio of
(a) 1 : 1 (b) 1 : 2 (c) 1 : 3 (d) 1 : 4

25. Three forces acting on a body are shown in the figure. To have the resultant force only along the y-direction, the magnitude of the minimum additional force needed is:
(a) 0.5 N
(b) 1.5 N
(c) 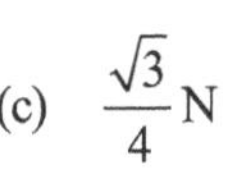
$\frac{\sqrt{3}}{4}$ N
(d) $\sqrt{3}$N

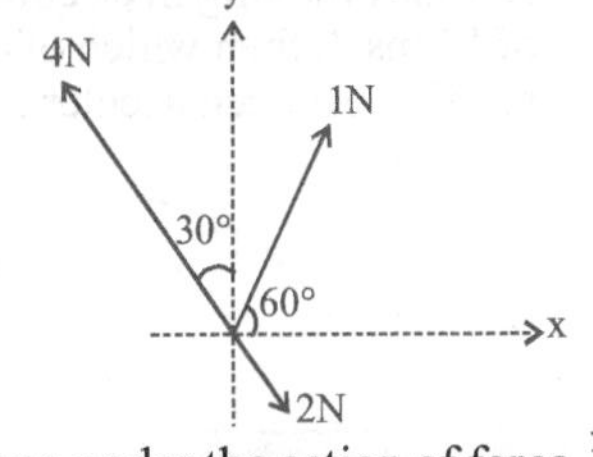

26. A particle moves in x-y plane under the action of force $\vec{F}$ and $\vec{p}$ at a given time t $p_x = 2\cos\theta$, $p_y = 2\sin\theta$. Then the angle θ between $\vec{F}$ and $\vec{p}$ at a given time t is :
(a) $\theta = 30°$ (b) $\theta = 180°$ (c) $\theta = 0°$ (d) $\theta = 90°$

27. A person sitting in the rear end of the compartment throws a ball towards the front end. The ball follows a parabolic path. The train is moving with velocity of 20 m/s. A person standing outside on the ground also observes the ball. How will the maximum heights (y_m) attained and the ranges (R) seen by the thrower and the outside observer compare with each other?
(a) Same y_m different R (b) Same y_m and R
(c) Different y_m same R (d) Different y_m and R

28. A car moves on a circular road. It describes equal angles about the centre in equal intervals of time. Which of the following statement about the velocity of the car is true ?
(a) Magnitude of velocity is not constant
(b) Both magnitude and direction of velocity change
(c) Velocity is directed towards the centre of the circle
(d) Magnitude of velocity is constant but direction changes

29. Three particles A, B and C are thrown from the top of a tower with the same speed. A is thrown up, B is thrown down and C is horizontally. They hit the ground with speeds v_A, v_B and v_C respectively then,
(a) $v_A = v_B = v_C$ (b) $v_A = v_B > v_C$
(c) $v_B > v_C > v_A$ (d) $v_A > v_B = v_C$

30. A particle is moving such that its position coordinate (x, y) are
(2m, 3m) at time t = 0
(6m, 7m) at time t = 2 s and
(13m, 14m) at time t = 5s.
Average velocity vector $(\vec{V}_{av})$ from t = 0 to t = 5s is :
(a) $\frac{1}{5}(13\hat{i} + 14\hat{j})$ (b) $\frac{7}{3}(\hat{i} + \hat{j})$
(c) $2(\hat{i} + \hat{j})$ (d) $\frac{11}{5}(\hat{i} + \hat{j})$

31. A particle moves so that its position vector is given by $\vec{r} = \cos\omega t\hat{x} + \sin\omega t\hat{y}$. Where ω is a constant. Which of the following is true ?
(a) Velocity and acceleration both are perpendicular to $\vec{r}$
(b) Velocity and acceleration both are parallel to $\vec{r}$
(c) Velocity is perpendicular to $\vec{r}$ and acceleration is directed towards the origin
(d) Velocity is perpendicular to $\vec{r}$ and acceleration is directed away from the origin

32. Two boys are standing at the ends A and B of a ground where $AB = a$. The boy at B starts running in a direction perpendicular to AB with velocity v_1. The boy at A starts running simultaneously with velocity v and catches the other boy in a time t, where t is
(a) $a/\sqrt{v^2 + v_1^2}$ (b) $a/(v + v_1)$
(c) $a/(v - v_1)$ (d) $\sqrt{a^2/(v^2 - v_1^2)}$

33. A projectile is fired at an angle of 45° with the horizontal. Elevation angle of the projectile at its highest point as seen from the point of projection is
(a) 60° (b) $\tan^{-1}\left(\frac{1}{2}\right)$ (c) $\tan^{-1}\left(\frac{\sqrt{3}}{2}\right)$ (d) 45°

34. The position vector of a particle $\vec{R}$ as a function of time is given by $\vec{R} = 4\sin(2\pi t)\hat{i} + 4\cos(2\pi t)\hat{j}$
where R is in meter, t in seconds and $\hat{i}$ and $\hat{j}$ denote unit vectors along x-and y-directions, respectively.
Which one of the following statements is wrong for the motion of particle?
(a) Magnitude of acceleration vector is $\frac{v^2}{R}$, where v is the velocity of particle
(b) Magnitude of the velocity of particle is 8 meter/second
(c) Path of the particle is a circle of radius 4 meter.
(d) Acceleration vector is along - $\vec{R}$

35. The vectors $\vec{A}$ and $\vec{B}$ are such that $|\vec{A} + \vec{B}| = |\vec{A} - \vec{B}|$
The angle between the two vectors is
(a) 60° (b) 75° (c) 45° (d) 90°

RESPONSE GRID					
	23. ⓐⓑⓒⓓ	24. ⓐⓑⓒⓓ	25. ⓐⓑⓒⓓ	26. ⓐⓑⓒⓓ	27. ⓐⓑⓒⓓ
	28. ⓐⓑⓒⓓ	29. ⓐⓑⓒⓓ	30. ⓐⓑⓒⓓ	31. ⓐⓑⓒⓓ	32. ⓐⓑⓒⓓ
	33. ⓐⓑⓒⓓ	34. ⓐⓑⓒⓓ	35. ⓐⓑⓒⓓ		

Space for Rough Work

36. The velocity of projection of oblique projectile is $(6\hat{i}+8\hat{j})\,ms^{-1}$. The horizontal range of the projectile is
(a) 4.9m (b) 9.6m (c) 19.6m (d) 14m

37. An artillary piece which consistently shoots its shells with the same muzzle speed has a maximum range R. To hit a target which is R/2 from the gun and on the same level, the elevation angle of the gun should be
(a) 15° (b) 45° (c) 30° (d) 60°

38. A car runs at a constant speed on a circular track of radius 100 m, taking 62.8 seconds in every circular loop. The average velocity and average speed for each circular loop respectively, is
(a) 0, 10 m/s (b) 10 m/s, 10 m/s
(c) 10 m/s, 0 (d) 0,0

39. A vector of magnitude b is rotated through angle θ. What is the change in magnitude of the vector?
(a) $2b\sin\frac{\theta}{2}$ (b) $2b\cos\frac{\theta}{2}$ (c) $2b\sin\theta$ (d) $2b\cos\theta$

40. A stone projected with a velocity u at an angle θ with the horizontal reaches maximum height H_1. When it is projected with velocity u at an angle $\left(\frac{\pi}{2}-\theta\right)$ with the horizontal, it reaches maximum height H_2. The relation between the horizontal range R of the projectile, heights H_1 and H_2 is
(a) $R=4\sqrt{H_1H_2}$ (b) $R=4(H_1-H_2)$
(c) $R=4(H_1+H_2)$ (d) $R=\frac{H_1^2}{H_2^2}$

41. The vector sum of two forces is perpendicular to their vector differences. In that case, the forces
(a) cannot be predicted
(b) are equal to each other
(c) are equal to each other in magnitude
(d) are not equal to each other in magnitude

42. A particle crossing the origin of co-ordinates at time t = 0, moves in the xy-plane with a constant acceleration a in the y-direction. If its equation of motion is $y = bx^2$ (b is a constant), its velocity component in the x-direction is
(a) $\sqrt{\frac{2b}{a}}$ (b) $\sqrt{\frac{a}{2b}}$ (c) $\sqrt{\frac{a}{b}}$ (d) $\sqrt{\frac{b}{a}}$

43. A vector $\vec{A}$ is rotated by a small angle Δθ radian (Δθ << 1) to get a new vector $\vec{B}$ In that case $|\vec{B}-\vec{A}|$ is :
(a) $|\vec{A}|\Delta\theta$ (b) $|\vec{B}|\Delta\theta-|\vec{A}|$
(c) $|\vec{A}|\left(1-\frac{\Delta\theta^2}{2}\right)$ (d) 0

44. If a body moving in circular path maintains constant speed of 10 ms^{-1}, then which of the following correctly describes relation between acceleration and radius ?

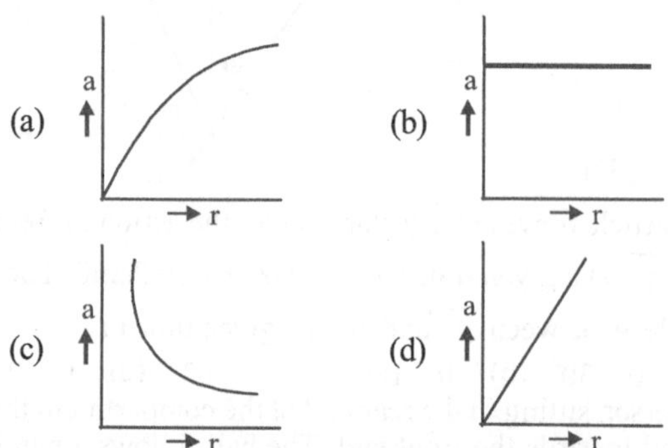

45. The position of a projectile launched from the origin at $t=0$ is given by $\vec{r}=(40\hat{i}+50\hat{j})$ m at $t=2$s. If the projectile was launched at an angle θ from the horizontal, then θ is (take g = 10 ms^{-2})
(a) $\tan^{-1}\frac{2}{3}$ (b) $\tan^{-1}\frac{3}{2}$ (c) $\tan^{-1}\frac{7}{4}$ (d) $\tan^{-1}\frac{4}{5}$

RESPONSE GRID					
	36. ⓐⓑⓒⓓ	37. ⓐⓑⓒⓓ	38. ⓐⓑⓒⓓ	39. ⓐⓑⓒⓓ	40. ⓐⓑⓒⓓ
	41. ⓐⓑⓒⓓ	42. ⓐⓑⓒⓓ	43. ⓐⓑⓒⓓ	44. ⓐⓑⓒⓓ	45. ⓐⓑⓒⓓ

PHYSICS CHAPTERWISE SPEED TEST-3

Total Questions	45	Total Marks	180
Attempted		Correct	
Incorrect		Net Score	
Cut-off Score	50	Qualifying Score	70
Success Gap = Net Score – Qualifying Score			
Net Score = (Correct × 4) – (Incorrect × 1)			

Space for Rough Work

PHYSICS

Laws of Motion

Speed TEST 4

Chapter-wise

No. of Questions	Maximum Marks	Time
45	180	1 Hour

GENERAL INSTRUCTIONS

- This test contains 45 MCQ's. For each question only one option is correct. Darken the correct circle/ bubble in the Response Grid provided on each page.
- You have to evaluate your Response Grids yourself with the help of solutions provided at the end of this book.
- Each correct answer will get you 4 marks and 1 mark shall be deduced for each incorrect answer. No mark will be given/ deducted if no bubble is filled. Keep a timer in front of you and stop immediately at the end of 60 min.
- The sheet follows a particular syllabus. Do not attempt the sheet before you have completed your preparation for that syllabus.
- After completing the sheet check your answers with the solution booklet and complete the Result Grid. Finally spend time to analyse your performance and revise the areas which emerge out as weak in your evaluation.

1. A player stops a football weighing 0.5 kg which comes flying towards him with a velocity of 10m/s. If the impact lasts for 1/50th sec. and the ball bounces back with a velocity of 15 m/s, then the average force involved is
   (a) 250 N (b) 1250 N (c) 500 N (d) 625 N
2. For the given situation as shown in the figure, the value of θ to keep the system in equilibrium will be

T_1, 2 m, θ, 60N, 2 m, T_2, W = 60N

   (a) 30° (b) 45° (c) 0° (d) 90°
3. A 5000 kg rocket is set for vertical firing. The exhaust speed is 800 m/s. To give an initial upward acceleration of 20 m/s^2, the amount of gas ejected per second to supply the needed thrust will be (Take g = 10 m/s^2)
   (a) 127.5 kg/s (b) 137.5 kg/s
   (c) 155.5 kg/s (d) 187.5 kg/s
4. Which one of the following statements is correct?
   (a) If there were no friction, work need to be done to move a body up an inclined plane is zero.
   (b) If there were no friction, moving vehicles could not be stopped even by locking the brakes.
   (c) As the angle of inclination is increased, the normal reaction on the body placed on it increases.
   (d) A duster weighing 0.5 kg is pressed against a vertical board with force of 11 N. If the coefficient of friction is 0.5, the work done in rubbing it upward through a distance of 10 cm is 0.55 J.
5. A stone is dropped from a height h. It hits the ground with a certain momentum P. If the same stone is dropped from a height 100% more than the previous height, the momentum when it hits the ground will change by :
   (a) 68% (b) 41% (c) 200% (d) 100%
6. A 3 kg ball strikes a heavy rigid wall with a speed of 10 m/s at an angle of 60°. It gets reflected with the same speed and angle as shown here. If the ball is in contact with the wall for 0.20s, what is the average force exerted on the ball by the wall?

60°, 60°

   (a) 150N (b) zero
   (c) $150\sqrt{3}$N (d) 300N

RESPONSE GRID	
	1. ⓐⓑⓒⓓ 2. ⓐⓑⓒⓓ 3. ⓐⓑⓒⓓ 4. ⓐⓑⓒⓓ 5. ⓐⓑⓒⓓ
	6. ⓐⓑⓒⓓ

Space for Rough Work

7. The upper half of an inclined plane of inclination θ is perfectly smooth while lower half is rough. A block starting from rest at the top of the plane will again come to rest at the bottom, if the coefficient of friction between the block and lower half of the plane is given by

(a) $\mu = \frac{2}{\tan\theta}$ (b) $\mu = 2\tan\theta$

(c) $\mu = \tan\theta$ (d) $\mu = \frac{1}{\tan\theta}$

8. A block of mass m is in contact with the cart C as shown in the figure.

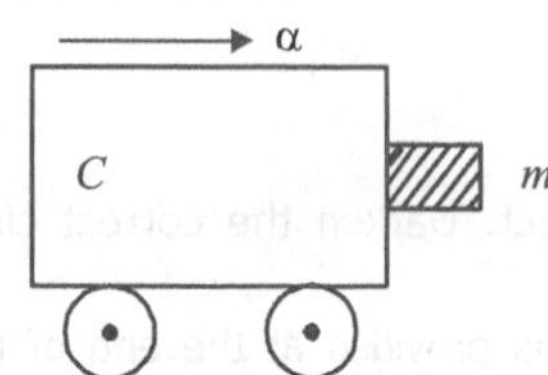

The coefficient of static friction between the block and the cart is μ. The acceleration α of the cart that will prevent the block from falling satisfies:

(a) $\alpha > \frac{mg}{\mu}$ (b) $\alpha > \frac{g}{\mu m}$ (c) $\alpha \geq \frac{g}{\mu}$ (d) $\alpha < \frac{g}{\mu}$

9. A bridge is in the from of a semi-circle of radius 40m. The greatest speed with which a motor cycle can cross the bridge without leaving the ground at the highest point is ($g = 10\ m\ s^{-2}$) (frictional force is negligibly small)

(a) $40\ m\ s^{-1}$ (b) $20\ m\ s^{-1}$
(c) $30\ m\ s^{-1}$ (d) $15\ m\ s^{-1}$

10. An explosion blows a rock into three parts. Two parts go off at right angles to each other. These two are, 1 kg first part moving with a velocity of $12\ ms^{-1}$ and 2 kg second part moving with a velocity of $8\ ms^{-1}$. If the third part flies off with a velocity of $4\ ms^{-1}$, its mass would be

(a) 5 kg (b) 7 kg (c) 17 kg (d) 3 kg

11. A monkey is decending from the branch of a tree with constant acceleration. If the breaking strength is 75% of the weight of the monkey, the minimum acceleration with which monkey can slide down without breaking the branch is

(a) g (b) $\frac{3g}{4}$ (c) $\frac{g}{4}$ (d) $\frac{g}{2}$

12. A car having a mass of 1000 kg is moving at a speed of 30 metres/sec. Brakes are applied to bring the car to rest. If the frictional force between the tyres and the road surface is 5000 newtons, the car will come to rest in

(a) 5 seconds (b) 10 seconds
(c) 12 seconds (d) 6 seconds

13. A spring is compressed between two toy carts of mass m_1 and m_2. When the toy carts are released, the springs exert equal and opposite average forces for the same time on each toy cart. If v_1 and v_2 are the velocities of the toy carts and there is no friction between the toy carts and the ground, then :

(a) $v_1/v_2 = m_1/m_2$ (b) $v_1/v_2 = m_2/m_1$
(c) $v_1/v_2 = -m_2/m_1$ (d) $v_1/v_2 = -m_1/m_2$

14. A plate of mass M is placed on a horizontal frictionless surface (see figure), and a body of mass m is placed on this plate. The coefficient of dynamic friction between this body and the plate is μ. If a force 2μ mg is applied to the body of mass m along the horizontal, the acceleration of the plate will be

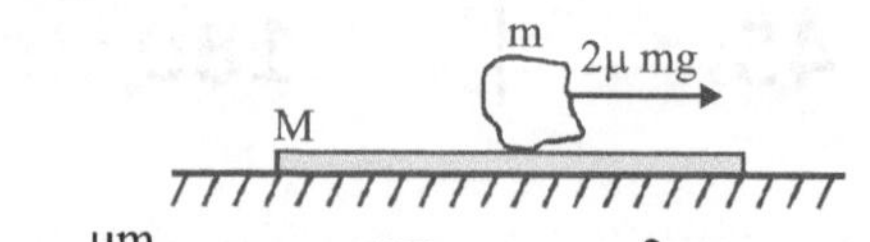

(a) $\frac{\mu m}{M}g$ (b) $\frac{\mu m}{(M+m)}g$ (c) $\frac{2\mu m}{M}g$ (d) $\frac{2\mu m}{(M+m)}g$

15. The rate of mass of the gas emitted from rear of a rocket is initially 0.1 kg/sec. If the speed of the gas relative to the rocket is 50 m/sec and mass of the rocket is 2 kg, then the acceleration of the rocket in m/sec^2 is

(a) 5 (b) 5.2 (c) 2.5 (d) 25

16. A plank with a box on it at one end is gradually raised about the other end. As the angle of inclination with the horizontal reaches 30º the box starts to slip and slides 4.0 m down the plank in 4.0s. The coefficients of static and kinetic friction between the box and the plank will be, respectively :

(a) 0.6 and 0.5 (b) 0.5 and 0.6
(c) 0.4 and 0.3 (d) 0.6 and 0.6

17. Four blocks of same mass connected by cords are pulled by a force F on a smooth horizontal surface, as shown in fig. The tensions T_1, T_2 and T_3 will be

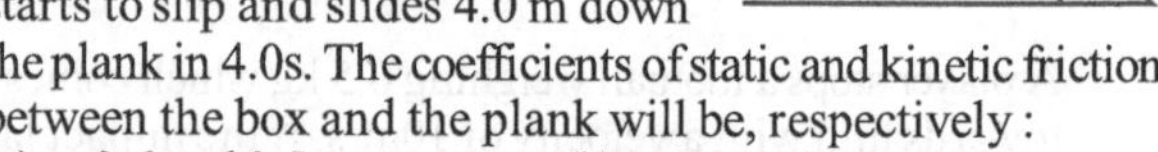

(a) $T_1 = \frac{1}{4}F, T_2 = \frac{3}{2}F, T_3 = \frac{1}{4}F$

(b) $T_1 = \frac{1}{4}F, T_2 = \frac{1}{2}F, T_3 = \frac{1}{2}F$

(c) $T_1 = \frac{3}{4}F, T_2 = \frac{1}{2}F, T_3 = \frac{1}{4}F$

(d) $T_1 = \frac{3}{4}F, T_2 = \frac{1}{2}F, T_3 = \frac{1}{2}F$

18. A body of mass M is kept on a rough horizontal surface (friction coefficient μ). A person is trying to pull the body by applying a horizontal force but the body is not moving. The force by the surface on the body is F, then

(a) F = Mg (b) F = μMg

(c) $Mg \leq F \leq Mg\sqrt{1+\mu^2}$ (d) $Mg \geq F \geq Mg\sqrt{1+\mu^2}$

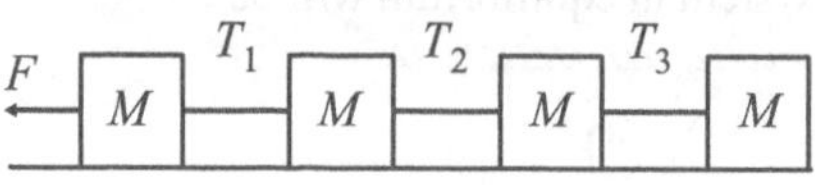

RESPONSE GRID					
	7. ⓐⓑⓒⓓ	8. ⓐⓑⓒⓓ	9. ⓐⓑⓒⓓ	10. ⓐⓑⓒⓓ	11. ⓐⓑⓒⓓ
	12. ⓐⓑⓒⓓ	13. ⓐⓑⓒⓓ	14. ⓐⓑⓒⓓ	15. ⓐⓑⓒⓓ	16. ⓐⓑⓒⓓ
	17. ⓐⓑⓒⓓ	18. ⓐⓑⓒⓓ			

Space for Rough Work

19. Which one of the following motions on a smooth plane surface does not involve force?
(a) Accelerated motion in a straight line
(b) Retarded motion in a straight line
(c) Motion with constant momentum along a straight line
(d) Motion along a straight line with varying velocity

20. A block A of mass m_1 rests on a horizontal table. A light string connected to it passes over a frictionless pulley at the edge of table and from its other end another block B of mass m_2 is suspended. The coefficient of kinetic friction between the block and the table is μ_k. When the block A is sliding on the table, the tension in the string is
(a) $\frac{(m_2 - \mu_k m_1)g}{(m_1 + m_2)}$ (b) $\frac{m_1 m_2 (1 + \mu_k)g}{(m_1 + m_2)}$
(c) $\frac{m_1 m_2 (1 - \mu_k)g}{(m_1 + m_2)}$ (d) $\frac{(m_2 + \mu_k m_1)g}{(m_1 + m_2)}$

21. The upper half of an inclined plane with inclination f is perfectly smooth while the lower half is rough. A body starting from rest at the top will again come to rest at the bottom if the coefficient of friction for the lower half is given by
(a) $2 \cos \phi$ (b) $2 \sin \phi$ (c) $\tan \phi$ (d) $2 \tan \phi$

22. A particle describes a horizontal circle in a conical funnel whose inner surface is smooth with speed of 0.5 m/s. What is the height of the plane of circle from vertex of the funnel?
(a) 0.25 cm (b) 2 cm (c) 4 cm (d) 2.5 cm

23. You are on a frictionless horizontal plane. How can you get off if no horizontal force is exerted by pushing against the surface?
(a) By jumping
(b) By spitting or sneezing
(c) by rolling your body on the surface
(d) By running on the plane

24. The coefficient of static and dynamic friction between a body and the surface are 0.75 and 0.5 respectively. A force is applied to the body to make it just slide with a constant acceleration which is
(a) $\frac{g}{4}$ (b) $\frac{g}{2}$ (c) $\frac{3g}{2}$ (d) g

25. In the system shown in figure, the pulley is smooth and massless, the string has a total mass 5g, and the two suspended blocks have masses 25 g and 15 g. The system is released from state $\ell = 0$ and is studied upto stage $\ell' = 0$. During the process, the acceleration of block A will be
(a) constant at $\frac{g}{9}$
(b) constant at $\frac{g}{4}$
(c) increasing by factor of 3
(d) increasing by factor of 2

26. The minimum force required to start pushing a body up rough (frictional coefficient μ) inclined plane is F_1 while the minimum force needed to prevent it from sliding down is F_2. If the inclined plane makes an angle θ from the horizontal such that $\tan \theta = 2\mu$ then the ratio $\frac{F_1}{F_2}$ is
(a) 1 (b) 2 (c) 3 (d) 4

27. Two blocks are connected over a massless pulley as shown in fig. The mass of block A is 10 kg and the coefficient of kinetic friction is 0.2. Block A slides down the incline at constant speed. The mass of block B in kg is
(a) 3.5 (b) 3.3 (c) 3.0 (d) 2.5

28. Tension in the cable supporting an elevator, is equal to the weight of the elevator. From this, we can conclude that the elevator is going up or down with a
(a) uniform velocity (b) uniform acceleration
(c) variable acceleration (d) either (b) or (c)

29. A particle tied to a string describes a vertical circular motion of radius r continually. If it has a velocity $\sqrt{3\,gr}$ at the highest point, then the ratio of the respective tensions in the string holding it at the highest and lowest points is
(a) 4 : 3 (b) 5 : 4 (c) 1 : 4 (d) 3 : 2

30. It is difficult to move a cycle with brakes on because
(a) rolling friction opposes motion on road
(b) sliding friction opposes motion on road
(c) rolling friction is more than sliding friction
(d) sliding friction is more than rolling friction

31. A plumb line is suspended from a celling of a car moving with horizontal acceleration of a. What will be the angle of inclination with vertical?
(a) $\tan^{-1}(a/g)$ (b) $\tan^{-1}(g/a)$
(c) $\cos^{-1}(a/g)$ (d) $\cos^{-1}(g/a)$

32. A cart of mass M has a block of mass m attached to it as shown in fig. The coefficient of friction between the block and the cart is μ. What is the minimum acceleration of the cart so that the block m does not fall?

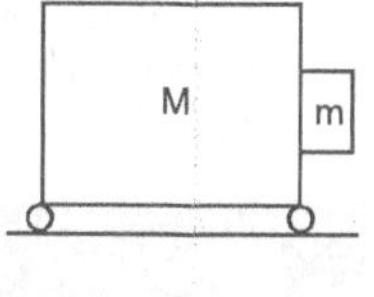

(a) μg (b) g/μ
(c) μ/g (d) $M \mu g/m$

RESPONSE GRID					
	19. ⓐⓑⓒⓓ	20. ⓐⓑⓒⓓ	21. ⓐⓑⓒⓓ	22. ⓐⓑⓒⓓ	23. ⓐⓑⓒⓓ
	24. ⓐⓑⓒⓓ	25. ⓐⓑⓒⓓ	26. ⓐⓑⓒⓓ	27. ⓐⓑⓒⓓ	28. ⓐⓑⓒⓓ
	29. ⓐⓑⓒⓓ	30. ⓐⓑⓒⓓ	31. ⓐⓑⓒⓓ	32. ⓐⓑⓒⓓ	

Space for Rough Work

33. What is the maximum value of the force F such that the block shown in the arrangement, does not move?

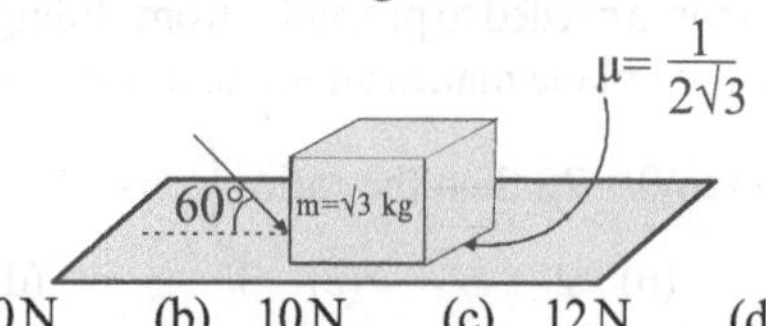

(a) 20 N (b) 10 N (c) 12 N (d) 15 N

34. A block has been placed on an inclined plane with the slope angle θ, block slides down the plane at constant speed. The coefficient of kinetic friction is equal to

(a) sin θ (b) cos θ (c) g (d) tan θ

35. A block of mass *m* is connected to another block of mass *M* by a spring (massless) of spring constant *k*. The block are kept on a smooth horizontal plane. Initially the blocks are at rest and the spring is unstretched. Then a constant force *F* starts acting on the block of mass *M* to pull it. Find the force of the block of mass *m*.

(a) $\frac{MF}{(m+M)}$ (b) $\frac{mF}{M}$ (c) $\frac{(M+m)F}{m}$ (d) $\frac{mF}{(m+M)}$

36. A block of mass m is placed on a surface with a vertical cross section given by $y = \frac{x^3}{6}$. If the coefficient of friction is 0.5, the maximum height above the ground at which the block can be placed without slipping is:

(a) $\frac{1}{6}$m (b) $\frac{2}{3}$m (c) $\frac{1}{3}$m (d) $\frac{1}{2}$m

37. A ball of mass 10 g moving perpendicular to the plane of the wall strikes it and rebounds in the same line with the same velocity. If the impulse experienced by the wall is 0.54 Ns, the velocity of the ball is

(a) 27 ms^{-1} (b) 3.7 ms^{-1} (c) 54 ms^{-1} (d) 37 ms^{-1}

38. A block is kept on a inclined plane of inclination θ of length ℓ. The velocity of particle at the bottom of inclined is (the coefficient of friction is μ)

(a) $[2g\ell(\mu\cos\theta - \sin\theta)]^{1/2}$ (b) $\sqrt{2g\ell(\sin\theta - \mu\cos\theta)}$

(c) $\sqrt{2g\ell(\sin\theta + \mu\cos\theta)}$ (d) $\sqrt{2g\ell(\cos\theta + \mu\sin\theta)}$

39. A 100 g iron ball having velocity 10 m/s collides with a wall at an angle 30° and rebounds with the same angle. If the period of contact between the ball and wall is 0.1 second, then the force experienced by the wall is

(a) 10 N (b) 100 N (c) 1.0 N (d) 0.1 N

40. A bullet is fired from a gun. The force on the bullet is given by $F = 600 - 2 \times 10^5\, t$ where, F is in newton and t in second. The force on the bullet becomes zero as soon as it leaves the barrel. What is the average impulse imparted to the bullet?

(a) 1.8 N-s (b) zero (c) 9 N-s (d) 0.9 N-s

41. Two stones of masses m and 2 m are whirled in horizontal circles, the heavier one in radius $\frac{r}{2}$ and the lighter one in radius r. The tangential speed of lighter stone is n times that of the value of heavier stone when they experience same centripetal forces. The value of n is :

(a) 3 (b) 4 (c) 1 (d) 2

42. A 0.1 kg block suspended from a massless string is moved first vertically up with an acceleration of $5ms^{-2}$ and then moved vertically down with an acceleration of $5ms^{-2}$. If T_1 and T_2 are the respective tensions in the two cases, then

(a) $T_2 > T_1$
(b) $T_1 - T_2 = 1$ N, if g = $10ms^{-2}$
(c) $T_1 - T_2 = 1$ kg f
(d) $T_1 - T_2 = 9.8$ N, if g = 9.8 ms^{-2}

43. Three forces start acting simultaneously on a particle moving with velocity, $\vec{v}$. These forces are represented in magnitude and direction by the three sides of a triangle ABC. The particle will now move with velocity

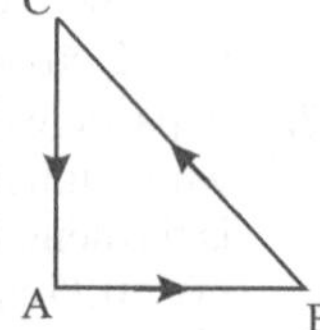

(a) less than $\vec{v}$
(b) greater than $\vec{v}$
(c) |v| in the direction of the largest force BC
(d) $\vec{v}$, remaining unchanged

44. If in a stationary lift, a man is standing with a bucket full of water, having a hole at its bottom. The rate of flow of water through this hole is R_0. If the lift starts to move up and down with same acceleration and then the rates of flow of water are R_u and R_d, then

(a) $R_0 > R_u > R_d$ (b) $R_u > R_0 > R_d$
(c) $R_d > R_0 > R_u$ (d) $R_u > R_d > R_0$

45. A stationary body of mass 3 kg explodes into three equal pieces. Two of the pieces fly off in two mutually perpendicular directions, one with a velocity of $3\hat{i}$ ms^{-1} and the other with a velocity of $4\hat{j}$ ms^{-1}. If the explosion occurs in 10^{-4} s, the average force acting on the third piece in newton is

(a) $(3\hat{i} + 4\hat{j}) \times 10^{-4}$ (b) $(3\hat{i} - 4\hat{j}) \times 10^{-4}$
(c) $(3\hat{i} - 4\hat{j}) \times 10^{4}$ (d) $-(3\hat{i} + 4\hat{j}) \times 10^{4}$

RESPONSE GRID					
	33. ⓐⓑⓒⓓ	34. ⓐⓑⓒⓓ	35. ⓐⓑⓒⓓ	36. ⓐⓑⓒⓓ	
	37. ⓐⓑⓒⓓ	38. ⓐⓑⓒⓓ	39. ⓐⓑⓒⓓ	40. ⓐⓑⓒⓓ	41. ⓐⓑⓒⓓ
	42. ⓐⓑⓒⓓ	43. ⓐⓑⓒⓓ	44. ⓐⓑⓒⓓ	45. ⓐⓑⓒⓓ	

PHYSICS CHAPTERWISE SPEED TEST-4

Total Questions	45	Total Marks	180
Attempted		Correct	
Incorrect		Net Score	
Cut-off Score	45	Qualifying Score	60
Success Gap = Net Score – Qualifying Score			
Net Score = (Correct × 4) – (Incorrect × 1)			

Space for Rough Work

PHYSICS

Work, Energy and Power

Speed TEST 5

Chapter-wise

No. of Questions	Maximum Marks	Time
45	180	1 Hour

GENERAL INSTRUCTIONS

- This test contains 45 MCQ's. For each question only one option is correct. Darken the correct circle/ bubble in the Response Grid provided on each page.
- You have to evaluate your Response Grids yourself with the help of solutions provided at the end of this book.
- Each correct answer will get you 4 marks and 1 mark shall be deduced for each incorrect answer. No mark will be given/ deducted if no bubble is filled. Keep a timer in front of you and stop immediately at the end of 60 min.
- The sheet follows a particular syllabus. Do not attempt the sheet before you have completed your preparation for that syllabus.
- After completing the sheet check your answers with the solution booklet and complete the Result Grid. Finally spend time to analyse your performance and revise the areas which emerge out as weak in your evaluation.

1. A spring of spring constant 5×10^3 N/m is stretched initially by 5cm from the unstretched position. Then the work required to stretch it further by another 5 cm is

(a) 12.50 Nm (b) 18.75 Nm
(c) 25.00 Nm (d) 6.25 Nm

2. A particle of mass 10 g moves along a circle of radius 6.4 cm with a constant tangential acceleration. What is the magnitude of this acceleration if the kinetic energy of the particle becomes equal to 8×10^{-4} J by the end of the second revolution after the beginning of the motion ?

(a) 0.1 m/s^2 (b) 0.15 m/s^2 (c) 0.18 m/s^2 (d) 0.2 m/s^2

3. A body is moved along a straight line by a machine delivering a constant power. The distance moved by the body in time 't' is proportional to

(a) $t^{3/4}$ (b) $t^{3/2}$ (c) $t^{1/4}$ (d) $t^{1/2}$

4. A ball is thrown vertically downwards from a height of 20 m with an initial velocity v_0. It collides with the ground and loses 50% of its energy in collision and rebounds to the same height. The initial velocity v_0 is : (Take g = 10 ms^{-2})

(a) 20 ms^{-1} (b) 28 ms^{-1}
(c) 10 ms^{-1} (d) 14 ms^{-1}

5. A cord is used to lower vertically a block of mass M, a distance d at a constant downward acceleration of g/4. The work done by the cord on the block is

(a) $Mg\frac{d}{4}$ (b) $3Mg\frac{d}{4}$ (c) $-3Mg\frac{d}{4}$ (d) Mg d

6. A rubber ball is dropped from a height of 5m on a plane, where the acceleration due to gravity is not shown. On bouncing it rises to 1.8 m. The ball loses its velocity on bouncing by a factor of

(a) $\frac{16}{25}$ (b) $\frac{2}{5}$ (c) $\frac{3}{5}$ (d) $\frac{9}{25}$

7. A ball of mass m moving with a constant velocity strikes against a ball of same mass at rest. If e = coefficient of restitution, then what will be the ratio of velocity of two balls after collision?

(a) $\frac{1-e}{1+e}$ (b) $\frac{e-1}{e+1}$ (c) $\frac{1+e}{1-e}$ (d) $\frac{2+e}{e-1}$

8. A particle of mass m is driven by a machine that delivers a constant power of k watts. If the particle starts from rest the force on the particle at time t is

(a) $\sqrt{mk}\, t^{-1/2}$ (b) $\sqrt{2mk}\, t^{-1/2}$
(c) $\frac{1}{2}\sqrt{mk}\, t^{-1/2}$ (d) $\sqrt{\frac{mk}{2}}\, t^{-1/2}$

RESPONSE GRID					
	1. ⓐⓑⓒⓓ	2. ⓐⓑⓒⓓ	3. ⓐⓑⓒⓓ	4. ⓐⓑⓒⓓ	5. ⓐⓑⓒⓓ
	6. ⓐⓑⓒⓓ	7. ⓐⓑⓒⓓ	8. ⓐⓑⓒⓓ		

Space for Rough Work

9. A body of mass 2 kg moving under a force has relation between displacement x and time t as $x = \frac{t^3}{3}$ where x is in metre and t is in sec. The work done by the body in first two second will be
(a) 1.6 joule (b) 16 joule
(c) 160 joule (d) 1600 joule

10. A sphere of mass 8m collides elastically (in one dimension) with a block of mass 2m. If the initial energy of sphere is E. What is the final energy of sphere?
(a) 0.8 E (b) 0.36 E
(c) 0.08 E (d) 0.64 E

11. Two similar springs P and Q have spring constants K_P and K_Q, such that $K_P > K_Q$. They are stretched, first by the same amount (case a,) then by the same force (case b). The work done by the springs W_P and W_Q are related as, in case (a) and case (b), respectively
(a) $W_P = W_Q$; $W_P = W_Q$ (b) $W_P > W_Q$; $W_Q > W_P$
(c) $W_P < W_Q$; $W_Q < W_P$ (d) $W_P = W_Q$; $W_P > W_Q$

12. In the figure, the variation of potential energy of a particle of mass m = 2 kg is represented w.r.t. its x-coordinate. The particle moves under the effect of this conservative force along the x-axis.

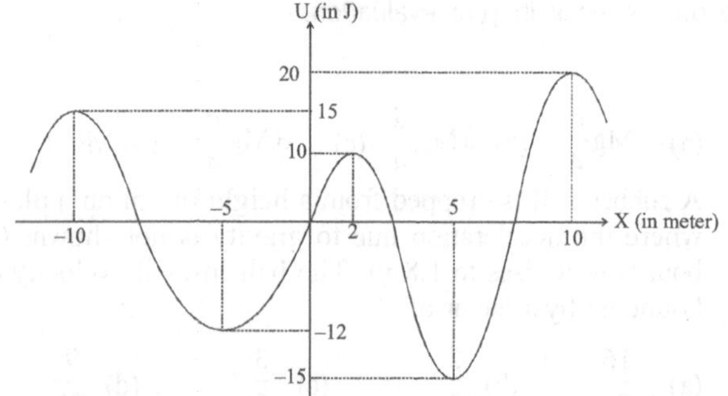

If the particle is released at the origin then
(a) it will move towards positive x-axis
(b) it will move towards negative x-axis
(c) it will remain stationary at the origin
(d) its subsequent motion cannot be decided due to lack of information

13. The potential energy of a certain spring when stretched through distance S is 10 joule. The amount of work done (in joule) that must be done on this spring to stretch it through an additional distance s, will be
(a) 20 (b) 10 (c) 30 (d) 40

14. A force applied by an engine of a train of mass 2.05×10^6 kg changes its velocity from 5m/s to 25 m/s in 5 minutes. The power of the engine is
(a) 1.025 MW (b) 2.05 MW
(c) 5 MW (d) 6 MW

15. The relationship between the force F and position x of a body is as shown in figure. The work done in displacing the body form x = 1 m to x = 5 m will be

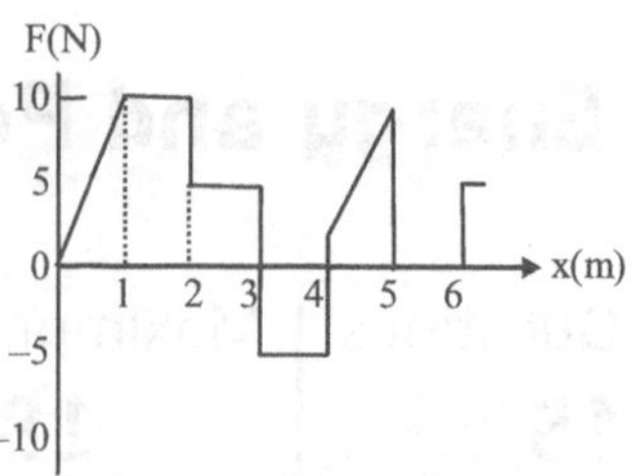

(a) 30 J (b) 15 J (c) 25 J (d) 20 J

16. A body is allowed to fall freely under gravity from a height of 10m. If it looses 25% of its energy due to impact with the ground, then the maximum height it rises after one impact is
(a) 2.5m (b) 5.0m (c) 7.5m (d) 8.2m

17. A block C of mass m is moving with velocity v_0 and collides elastically with block A of mass m and connected to another block B of mass 2m through spring constant k. What is k if x_0 is compression of spring when velocity of A and B is same?

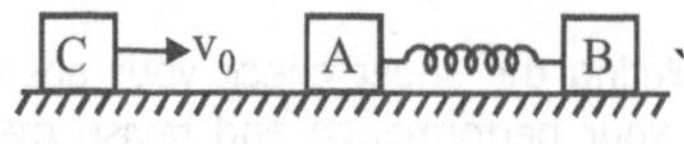

(a) $\frac{mv_0^2}{x_0^2}$ (b) $\frac{mv_0^2}{2x_0^2}$
(c) $\frac{3}{2}\frac{mv_0^2}{x_0^2}$ (d) $\frac{2}{3}\frac{mv_0^2}{x_0^2}$

18. Two springs of force constants 300 N/m (Spring A) and 400 N/m (Spring B) are joined together in series. The combination is compressed by 8.75 cm. The ratio of energy stored in A and B is $\frac{E_A}{E_B}$. Then $\frac{E_A}{E_B}$ is equal to :
(a) $\frac{4}{3}$ (b) $\frac{16}{9}$ (c) $\frac{3}{4}$ (d) $\frac{9}{16}$

19. A body of mass 1 kg begins to move under the action of a time dependent force $\vec{F} = (2t\hat{i} + 3t^2\hat{j})$ N, where $\hat{i}$ and $\hat{j}$ are unit vectors alogn x and y axis. What power will be developed by the force at the time t?
(a) $(2t^2 + 3t^3)$W (b) $(2t^2 + 4t^4)$W
(c) $(2t^3 + 3t^4)$ W (d) $(2t^3 + 3t^5)$W

20. A bullet of mass 20 g and moving with 600 m/s collides with a block of mass 4 kg hanging with the string. What is the velocity of bullet when it comes out of block, if block rises to height 0.2 m after collision?
(a) 200 m/s (b) 150 m/s (c) 400 m/s (d) 300 m/s

RESPONSE GRID					
	9. ⓐⓑⓒⓓ	10. ⓐⓑⓒⓓ	11. ⓐⓑⓒⓓ	12. ⓐⓑⓒⓓ	13. ⓐⓑⓒⓓ
	14. ⓐⓑⓒⓓ	15. ⓐⓑⓒⓓ	16. ⓐⓑⓒⓓ	17. ⓐⓑⓒⓓ	18. ⓐⓑⓒⓓ
	19. ⓐⓑⓒⓓ	20. ⓐⓑⓒⓓ			

Space for Rough Work

21. A body of mass m kg is ascending on a smooth inclined plane of inclination θ $\left(\sin\theta = \frac{1}{x}\right)$ with constant acceleration of a m/s^2. The final velocity of the body is v m/s. The work done by the body during this motion is
(Initial velocity of the body = 0)

(a) $\frac{1}{2}mv^2(g+xa)$ (b) $\frac{mv^2}{2}\left(\frac{g}{2}+a\right)$

(c) $\frac{2mv^2x}{a}(a+gx)$ (d) $\frac{mv^2}{2ax}(g+xa)$

22. A glass marble dropped from a certain height above the horizontal surface reaches the surface in time t and then continues to bounce up and down. The time in which the marble finally comes to rest is

(a) $e^n t$ (b) $e^2 t$ (c) $t\left[\frac{1+e}{1-e}\right]$ (d) $t\left[\frac{1-e}{1+e}\right]$

23. The potential energy of a 1 kg particle free to move along the x-axis is given by $V(x) = \left(\frac{x^4}{4} - \frac{x^2}{2}\right)$ J.
The total mechanical energy of the particle is 2 J. Then, the maximum speed (in m/s) is

(a) $\frac{3}{\sqrt{2}}$ (b) $\sqrt{2}$ (c) $\frac{1}{\sqrt{2}}$ (d) 2

24. Water falls from a height of 60 m at the rate of 15 kg/s to operate a turbine. The losses due to frictional force are 10% of energy. How much power is generated by the turbine?(g = 10 m/s^2)
(a) 8.1 kW (b) 10.2 kW (c) 12.3 kW (d) 7.0 kW

24. A car of mass m starts from rest and accelerates so that the instantaneous power delivered to the car has a constant magnitude P_0. The instantaneous velocity of this car is proportional to :

(a) t^2P_0 (b) $t^{1/2}$ (c) $t^{-1/2}$ (d) $\frac{t}{\sqrt{m}}$

25. When a 1.0kg mass hangs attached to a spring of length 50 cm, the spring stretches by 2 cm. The mass is pulled down until the length of the spring becomes 60 cm. What is the amount of elastic energy stored in the spring in this condition. if g = 10 m/s^2.
(a) 1.5 joule (b) 2.0 joule (c) 2.5 joule (d) 3.0 joule

26. A block of mass m rests on a rough horizontal surface (Coefficient of friction is μ). When a bullet of mass m/2 strikes horizontally, and get embedded in it, the block moves a distance d before coming to rest. The initial velocity of the bullet is $k\sqrt{2\mu gd}$, then the value of k is

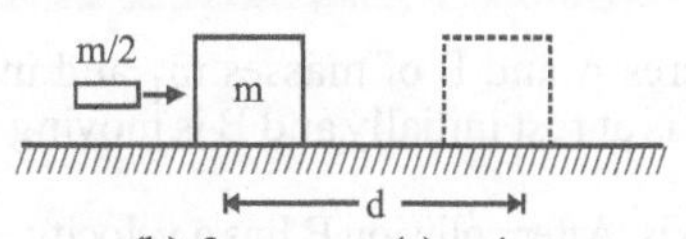

(a) 2 (b) 3 (c) 4 (d) 5

27. A force acts on a 30 gm particle in such a way that the position of the particle as a function of time is given by $x = 3t - 4t^2 + t^3$, where x is in metres and t is in seconds. The work done during the first 4 seconds is
(a) 576mJ (b) 450mJ (c) 490mJ (d) 530mJ

28. A particle of mass m_1 moving with velocity v strikes with a mass m_2 at rest, then the condition for maximum transfer of kinetic energy is
(a) $m_1 >> m_2$ (b) $m_2 >> m_2$ (c) $m_1 = m_2$ (d) $m_1 = 2m_2$

29. A mass *m* is moving with velocity v collides inelastically with a bob of simple pendulum of mass m and gets embedded into it. The total height to which the masses will rise after collision is

(a) $\frac{v^2}{8g}$ (b) $\frac{v^2}{4g}$ (c) $\frac{v^2}{2g}$ (d) $\frac{2v^2}{g}$

30. A 10 H.P. motor pumps out water from a well of depth 20 m and fills a water tank of volume 22380 litres at a height of 10 m from the ground. The running time of the motor to fill the empty water tank is (g = 10ms^{-2})
(a) 5 minutes (b) 10 minutes
(c) 15 minutes (d) 20 minutes

31. A particle of mass m_1 is moving with a velocity v_1 and another particle of mass m_2 is moving with a velocity v_2. Both of them have the same momentum but their different kinetic energies are E_1 and E_2 respectively. If $m_1 > m_2$ then

(a) $E_1 = E_2$ (b) $E_1 < E_2$ (c) $\frac{E_1}{E_2} = \frac{m_1}{m_2}$ (d) $E_1 > E_2$

32. A block of mass 10 kg, moving in x direction with a constant speed of 10 ms^{-1}, is subject to a retarding force F = 0.1 × J m during its travel from x = 20 m to 30 m. Its final KE will be :
(a) 450 J (b) 275 J (c) 250 J (d) 475 J

33. Identify the false statement from the following
(a) Work-energy theorem is not independent of Newton's second law.
(b) Work-energy theorem holds in all inertial frames.
(c) Work done by friction over a closed path is zero.
(d) No potential energy can be associated with friction.

34. A one-ton car moves with a constant velocity of 15 ms^{-1} on a rough horizontal road. The total resistance to the motion of the car is 12% of the weight of the car. The power required to keep the car moving with the same constant velocity of 15ms^{-1} is [Take g = 10 ms^{-2}]
(a) 9 kW (b) 18 kW (c) 24 kW (d) 36 kW

35. A ball is released from the top of a tower. The ratio of work done by force of gravity in first, second and third second of the motion of the ball is
(a) 1 : 2 : 3 (b) 1 : 4 : 9 (c) 1 : 3 : 5 (d) 1 : 5 : 3

RESPONSE GRID					
	21. ⓐⓑⓒⓓ	22. ⓐⓑⓒⓓ	23. ⓐⓑⓒⓓ	24. ⓐⓑⓒⓓ	25. ⓐⓑⓒⓓ
	26. ⓐⓑⓒⓓ	27. ⓐⓑⓒⓓ	28. ⓐⓑⓒⓓ	29. ⓐⓑⓒⓓ	30. ⓐⓑⓒⓓ
	31. ⓐⓑⓒⓓ	32. ⓐⓑⓒⓓ	33. ⓐⓑⓒⓓ	34. ⓐⓑⓒⓓ	35. ⓐⓑⓒⓓ

Space for Rough Work

36. Two spheres A and B of masses m_1 and m_2 respectively collide. A is at rest initially and B is moving with velocity v along x-axis. After collision B has a velocity $\frac{v}{2}$ in a direction perpendicular to the original direction. The mass A moves after collision in the direction.
(a) Same as that of B
(b) Opposite to that of B
(c) $\theta = \tan^{-1}(1/2)$ to the x-axis
(d) $\theta = \tan^{-1}(-1/2)$ to the x-axis

37. A 2 kg block slides on a horizontal floor with a speed of 4m/s. It strikes a uncompressed spring, and compresses it till the block is motionless. The kinetic friction force is 15N and spring constant is 10,000 N/m. The spring compresses by
(a) 8.5 cm (b) 5.5 cm (c) 2.5 cm (d) 11.0 cm

38. An engine pumps water through a hose pipe. Water passes through the pipe and leaves it with a velocity of 2 m/s. The mass per unit length of water in the pipe is 100 kg/m. What is the power of the engine?
(a) 400 W (b) 200 W (c) 100 W (d) 800 W

39. A uniform chain of length 2 m is kept on a table such that a length of 60 cm hangs freely from the edge of the table. The total mass of the chain is 4 kg. What is the work done in pulling the entire chain on the table ?
(a) 12 J (b) 3.6 J (c) 7.2 J (d) 1200 J

40. A mass 'm' moves with a velocity 'v' and collides inelastically with another identical mass. After collision the 1st mass moves with velocity $\frac{v}{\sqrt{3}}$ in a direction perpendicular to the initial direction of motion. Find the speed of the 2nd mass after collision.

$v/\sqrt{3}$ after collision; m m before collision

(a) $\sqrt{3}v$ (b) v (c) $\frac{v}{\sqrt{3}}$ (d) $\frac{2}{\sqrt{3}}v$

41. A spherical ball of mass 20 kg is stationary at the top of a hill of height 100 m. It rolls down a smooth surface to the ground, then climbs up another hill of height 30 m and finally rolls down to a horizontal base at a height of 20 m above the ground. The velocity attained by the ball is
(a) 20 m/s (b) 40 m/s (c) $10\sqrt{30}$ m/s (d) 10 m/s

42. A block of mass M is kept on a platform which is accelerated upward with a constant acceleration 'a' during the time interval T. The work done by normal reaction between the block and platform is

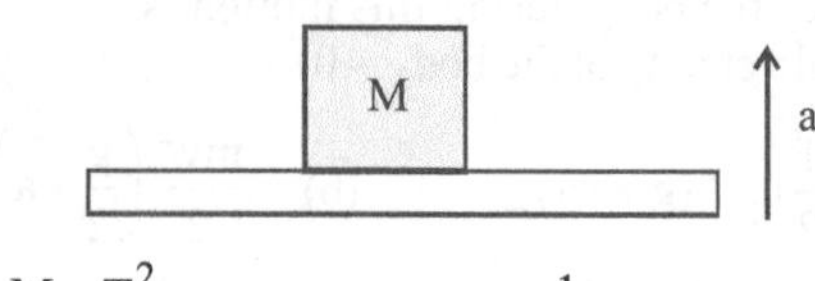

(a) $-\frac{MgaT^2}{2}$ (b) $\frac{1}{2}M(g+a)aT^2$
(c) $\frac{1}{2}Ma^2T$ (d) Zero

43. A spring lies along an x axis attached to a wall at one end and a block at the other end. The block rests on a frictionless surface at x = 0. A force of constant magnitude F is applied to the block that begins to compress the spring, until the block comes to a maximum displacement x_{max}.

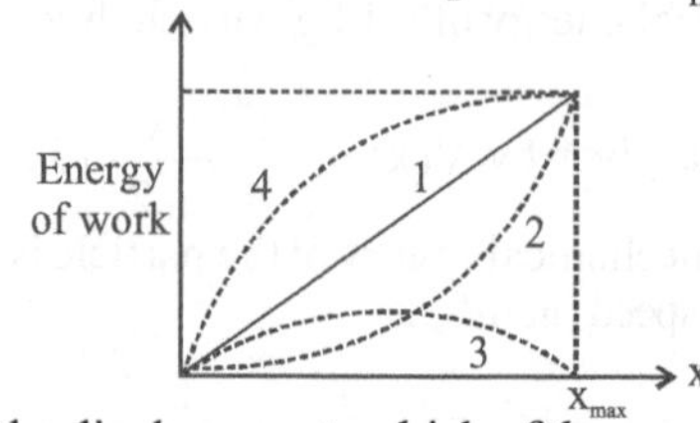

During the displacement, which of the curves shown in the graph best represents the kinetic energy of the block ?
(a) 1 (b) 2 (c) 3 (d) 4

44. The K.E. acquired by a mass m in travelling a certain distance d, starting form rest, under the action of a constant force is directly proportional to
(a) m (b) $\sqrt{m}$
(c) $\frac{1}{\sqrt{m}}$ (d) independent of m

45. A vertical spring with force constant k is fixed on a table. A ball of mass m at a height h above the free upper end of the spring falls vertically on the spring so that the spring is compressed by a distance d. The net work done in the process is
(a) $mg(h+d)-\frac{1}{2}kd^2$ (b) $mg(h-d)-\frac{1}{2}kd^2$
(c) $mg(h-d)+\frac{1}{2}kd^2$ (d) $mg(h+d)+\frac{1}{2}kd^2$

RESPONSE GRID					
	36. ⓐⓑⓒⓓ	37. ⓐⓑⓒⓓ	38. ⓐⓑⓒⓓ	39. ⓐⓑⓒⓓ	40. ⓐⓑⓒⓓ
	41. ⓐⓑⓒⓓ	42. ⓐⓑⓒⓓ	43. ⓐⓑⓒⓓ	44. ⓐⓑⓒⓓ	45. ⓐⓑⓒⓓ

PHYSICS CHAPTERWISE SPEED TEST-5

Total Questions	45	Total Marks	180
Attempted		Correct	
Incorrect		Net Score	
Cut-off Score	50	Qualifying Score	70
Success Gap = Net Score – Qualifying Score			
Net Score = (Correct × 4) – (Incorrect × 1)			

Space for Rough Work

PHYSICS

System of Particles and Rotational Motion

Speed TEST 6

Chapter-wise

No. of Questions	Maximum Marks	Time
45	180	1 Hour

GENERAL INSTRUCTIONS

- This test contains 45 MCQ's. For each question only one option is correct. Darken the correct circle/ bubble in the Response Grid provided on each page.
- You have to evaluate your Response Grids yourself with the help of solutions provided at the end of this book.
- Each correct answer will get you 4 marks and 1 mark shall be deduced for each incorrect answer. No mark will be given/ deducted if no bubble is filled. Keep a timer in front of you and stop immediately at the end of 60 min.
- The sheet follows a particular syllabus. Do not attempt the sheet before you have completed your preparation for that syllabus.
- After completing the sheet check your answers with the solution booklet and complete the Result Grid. Finally spend time to analyse your performance and revise the areas which emerge out as weak in your evaluation.

1. From a solid sphere of mass M and radius R, a cube of maximum possible volume is cut. Moment of inertia of cube about an axis passing through its center and perpendicular to one of its faces is :

(a) $\frac{4MR^2}{9\sqrt{3}\pi}$ (b) $\frac{4MR^2}{3\sqrt{3}\pi}$ (c) $\frac{MR^2}{32\sqrt{2}\pi}$ (d) $\frac{MR^2}{16\sqrt{2}\pi}$

2. A hollow sphere is held suspended. Sand is now poured into it in stages.
The centre of mass of the sphere with the sand

SAND

(a) rises continuously
(b) remains unchanged in the process
(c) first rises and then falls to the original position
(d) first falls and then rises to the original position

3. A body A of mass M while falling vertically downwards under gravity breaks into two parts; a body B of mass $\frac{1}{3}M$ and a body C of mass $\frac{2}{3}M$. The centre of mass of bodies B and C taken together shifts compared to that of body A towards

(a) does not shift
(b) depends on height of breaking
(c) body B (d) body C

4. From a uniform wire, two circular loops are made (i) P of radius r and (ii) Q of radius nr. If the moment of inertia of Q about an axis passing through its centre and perpendicular to its plane is 8 times that of P about a similar axis, the value of n is (diameter of the wire is very much smaller than r or nr)

(a) 8 (b) 6 (c) 4 (d) 2

5. A billiard ball of mass m and radius r, when hit in a horizontal direction by a cue at a height h above its centre, acquired a linear velocity v_0. The angular velocity ω_0 acquired by the ball is

(a) $\frac{5v_0r^2}{2h}$ (b) $\frac{2v_0r^2}{5h}$ (c) $\frac{2v_0h}{5r^2}$ (d) $\frac{5v_0h}{2r^2}$

6. Three bricks each of length L and mass M are arranged as shown from the wall. The distance of the centre of mass of the system from the wall is

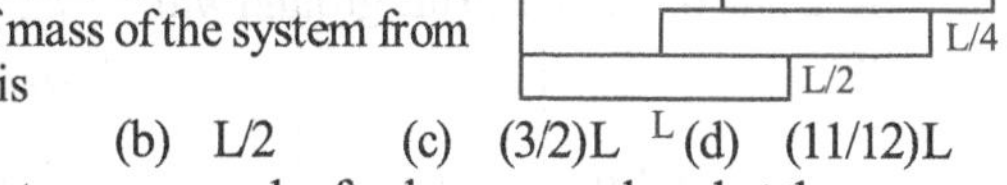

(a) L/4 (b) L/2 (c) (3/2)L (d) (11/12)L

7. Four point masses, each of value m, are placed at the corners of a square $ABCD$ of side ℓ. The moment of inertia of this system about an axis passing through A and parallel to BD is

(a) $2m\ell^2$ (b) $\sqrt{3}m\ell^2$ (c) $3m\ell^2$ (d) $m\ell^2$

8. A loop of radius r and mass m rotating with an angular velocity ω_0 is placed on a rough horizontal surface. The initial velocity of the centre of the hoop is zero. What will be the velocity of the centre of the hoop when it ceases to slip?

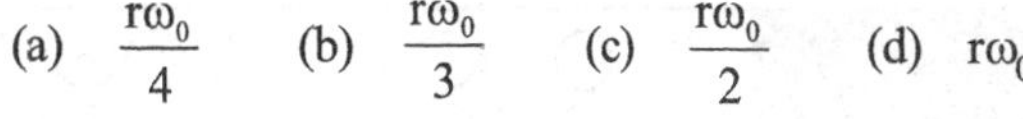

(a) $\frac{r\omega_0}{4}$ (b) $\frac{r\omega_0}{3}$ (c) $\frac{r\omega_0}{2}$ (d) $r\omega_0$

RESPONSE GRID

1. ⓐⓑⓒⓓ	2. ⓐⓑⓒⓓ	3. ⓐⓑⓒⓓ	4. ⓐⓑⓒⓓ	5. ⓐⓑⓒⓓ
6. ⓐⓑⓒⓓ	7. ⓐⓑⓒⓓ	8. ⓐⓑⓒⓓ		

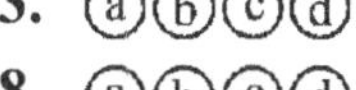
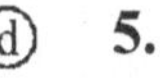
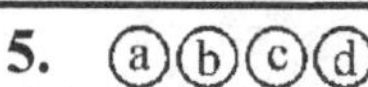

Space for Rough Work

9. Two masses m_1 and m_2 are connected by a massless spring of spring constant k and unstretched length ℓ. The masses are placed on a frictionless straight channel, which are consider our x-axis. They are initially at $x = 0$ and $x = \ell$ respectively. At $t = 0$, a velocity v_0 is suddenly imparted to the first particle. At a later time t, the centre of mass of the two masses is at :

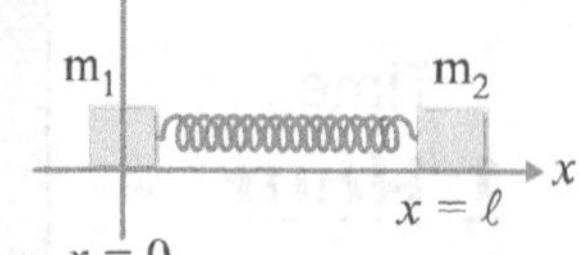

(a) $x = \frac{m_2 \ell}{m_1 + m_2}$

(b) $x = \frac{m_1 \ell}{m_1 + m_2} + \frac{m_2 v_0 t}{m_1 + m_2}$

(c) $x = \frac{m_2 \ell}{m_1 + m_1} + \frac{m_2 v_0 t}{m_1 + m_2}$ (d) $x = \frac{m_2 \ell}{m_1 + m_2} + \frac{m_1 v_0 t}{m_1 + m_2}$

10. A body of mass 1.5 kg rotating about an axis with angular velocity of 0.3 rad s^{-1} has the angular momentum of 1.8 kg m^2s^{-1}. The radius of gyration of the body about an axis is

(a) 2m (b) 1.2m (c) 0.2m (d) 1.6m

11. If $\vec{F}$ is the force acting on a particle having position vector $\vec{r}$ and $\vec{\tau}$ be the torque of this force about the origin, then:

(a) $\vec{r} \cdot \vec{\tau} > 0$ and $\vec{F} \cdot \vec{\tau} < 0$

(b) $\vec{r} \cdot \vec{\tau} = 0$ and $\vec{F} \cdot \vec{\tau} = 0$

(c) $\vec{r} \cdot \vec{\tau} = 0$ and $\vec{F} \cdot \vec{\tau} \neq 0$

(d) $\vec{r} \cdot \vec{\tau} \neq 0$ and $\vec{F} \cdot \vec{\tau} = 0$

12. A thin uniform rod of length l and mass m is swinging freely about a horizontal axis passing through its end. Its maximum angular speed is ω. Its centre of mass rises to a maximum height of

(a) $\frac{1}{6}\frac{l\omega}{g}$ (b) $\frac{1}{2}\frac{l^2\omega^2}{g}$ (c) $\frac{1}{6}\frac{l^2\omega^2}{g}$ (d) $\frac{1}{3}\frac{l^2\omega^2}{g}$

13. A wheel is rolling straight on ground without slipping. If the axis of the wheel has speed v, the instantenous velocity of a point P on the rim, defined by angle θ, relative to the ground will be

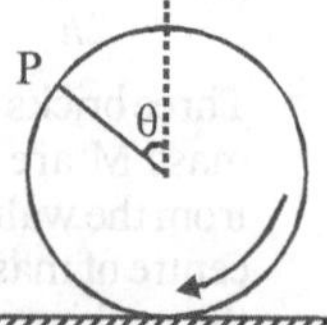

(a) $v\cos\left(\frac{1}{2}\theta\right)$ (b) $2v\cos\left(\frac{1}{2}\theta\right)$

(c) $v(1+\sin\theta)$ (d) $v(1+\cos\theta)$

14. A solid sphere having mass m and radius r rolls down an inclined plane. Then its kinetic energy is

(a) $\frac{5}{7}$ rotational and $\frac{2}{7}$ translational

(b) $\frac{2}{7}$ rotational and $\frac{5}{7}$ translational

(c) $\frac{2}{5}$ rotational and $\frac{3}{5}$ translational

(d) $\frac{1}{2}$ rotational and $\frac{1}{2}$ translational

15. A ring of mass M and radius R is rotating about its axis with angular velocity ω. Two identical bodies each of mass m are now gently attached at the two ends of a diameter of the ring. Because of this, the kinetic energy loss will be :

(a) $\frac{m(M+2m)}{M}\omega^2R^2$ (b) $\frac{Mm}{(M+m)}\omega^2R^2$

(c) $\frac{Mm}{(M+2m)}\omega^2R^2$ (d) $\frac{(M+m)M}{(M+2m)}\omega^2R^2$

16. A certain bicycle can go up a gentle incline with constant speed when the frictional force of ground pushing the rear wheel is $F_2 = 4$ N. With what force F_1 must the chain pull on the sprocket wheel if $R_1 = 5$ cm and $R_2 = 30$ cm?

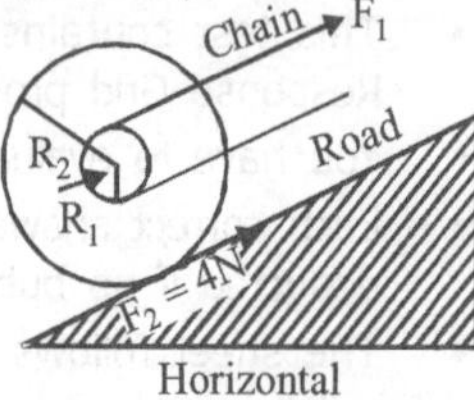

(a) 4N (b) 24N (c) 140N (d) $\frac{35}{4}$ N

17. A wooden cube is placed on a rough horizontal table, a force is applied to the cube. Gradually the force is increased. Whether the cube slides before toppling or topples before sliding is independent of :

(a) the position of point of application of the force
(b) the length of the edge of the cube
(c) mass of the cube
(d) Coefficient of friction between the cube and the table

18. From a circular ring of mass M and radius R, an arc corresponding to a 90° sector is removed. The moment of inertia of the ramaining part of the ring about an axis passing through the centre of the ring and perpendicular to the plane of the ring is k times MR^2. Then the value of k is

(a) 3/4 (b) 7/8 (c) 1/4 (d) 1

19. A mass m moves in a circle on a smooth horizontal plane with velocity v_0 at a radius R_0. The mass is attached to string which passes through a smooth hole in the plane as shown.

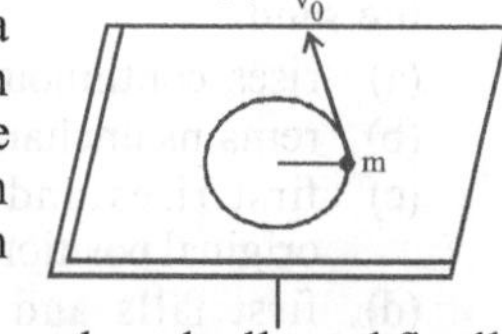

The tension in the string is increased gradually and finally m moves in a circle of radius $\frac{R_0}{2}$. The final value of the kinetic energy is

(a) $\frac{1}{4}mv_0^2$ (b) $2mv_0^2$ (c) $\frac{1}{2}mv_0^2$ (d) mv_0^2

20. A rod PQ of length L revolves in a horizontal plane about the axis YY′. The angular velocity of the rod is ω. If A is the area of cross-section of the rod and ρ be its density, its rotational kinetic energy is

RESPONSE GRID					
	9. ⓐⓑⓒⓓ	10. ⓐⓑⓒⓓ	11. ⓐⓑⓒⓓ	12. ⓐⓑⓒⓓ	13. ⓐⓑⓒⓓ
	14. ⓐⓑⓒⓓ	15. ⓐⓑⓒⓓ	16. ⓐⓑⓒⓓ	17. ⓐⓑⓒⓓ	18. ⓐⓑⓒⓓ
	19. ⓐⓑⓒⓓ				

Space for Rough Work

(a) $\frac{1}{3}AL^3\rho\omega^2$ (b) $\frac{1}{2}AL^3\rho\omega^2$

(c) $\frac{1}{24}AL^3\rho\omega^2$ (d) $\frac{1}{18}AL^3\rho\omega^2$

21. A solid sphere of mass 2 kg rolls on a smooth horizontal surface at 10 m/s. It then rolls up a smooth inclined plane of inclination 30° with the horizontal. The height attained by the sphere before it stops is

(a) 700 cm (b) 701 cm (c) 7.1 m (d) 70 m

22. A hollow smooth uniform sphere *A* of mass m rolls without sliding on a smooth horizontal surface. It collides head on elastically with another stationary smooth solid sphere *B* of the same mass m and same radius. The ratio of kinetic energy of *B* to that of *A* just after the collision is

(a) 1 : 1
(b) 2 : 3
(c) 3 : 2
(d) 4 : 3

23. Two discs of same thickness but of different radii are made of two different materials such that their masses are same. The densities of the materials are in the ratio of 1 : 3. The moments of inertia of these discs about the respective axes passing through their centres and perpendicular to their planes will be in the ratio of

(a) 1 : 3 (b) 3 : 1 (c) 1 : 9 (d) 9 : 1

24. A pulley fixed to the ceiling carries a string with blocks of mass m and 3 m attached to its ends. The masses of string and pulley are negligible. When the system is released, its centre of mass moves with what acceleration ?

(a) 0 (b) – g/4 (c) g/2 (d) – g/2

25. A ring of mass m and radius *R* has four particles each of mass m attached to the ring as shown in figure. The centre of ring has a speed v_0. The kinetic energy of the system is

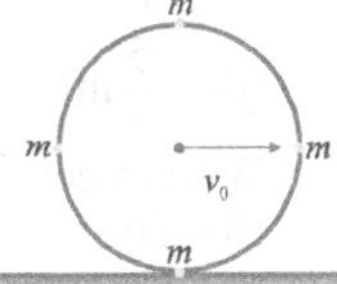

(a) mv_0^2 (b) $3mv_0^2$ (c) $5mv_0^2$ (d) $6mv_0^2$

26. Consider a uniform square plate of side '*a*' and mass '*M*'. The moment of inertia of this plate about an axis perpendicular to its plane and passing through one of its corners is

(a) $\frac{5}{6}Ma^2$ (b) $\frac{1}{12}Ma^2$ (c) $\frac{7}{12}Ma^2$ (d) $\frac{2}{3}Ma^2$

27. A dancer is standing on a stool rotating about the vertical axis passing through its centre. She pulls her arms towards the body reducing her moment of inertia by a factor of n. The new angular speed of turn table is proportional to

(a) n (b) n^{-1} (c) n^0 (d) n^2

28. A uniform square plate has a small piece Q of an irregular shape removed and glued to the centre of the plate leaving a hole behind. Then the moment of inertia about the z-axis

(a) increases
(b) decreases
(c) remains same
(d) changed in unpredicted manner.

29. A circular turn table has a block of ice placed at its centre. The system rotates with an angular speed ω about an axis passing through the centre of the table. If the ice melts on its own without any evaporation, the speed of rotation of the system

(a) becomes zero
(b) remains constant at the same value ω
(c) increases to a value greater than ω
(d) decreases to a value less than ω

30. Seven identical coins are rigidly arranged on a flat table in the pattern shown below so that each coin touches it neighbors. Each coin is a thin disc of mass *m* and radius *r*. The moment of inertia of the system of seven coins about an axis that passes through point *P* and perpendicular to the plane of the coin is :

(a) $\frac{55}{2}mr^2$ (b) $\frac{127}{2}mr^2$ (c) $\frac{111}{2}mr^2$ (d) $55\,mr^2$

31. In a two-particle system with particle masses m_1 and m_2, the first particle is pushed towards the centre of mass through a distance d, the distance through which second particle must be moved to keep the centre of mass at the same position is

(a) $\frac{m_2 d}{m_1}$ (b) d (c) $\frac{m_1 d}{(m_1+m_2)}$ (d) $\frac{m_1 d}{m_2}$

32. A uniform bar of mass M and length L is horizontally suspended from the ceiling by two vertical light cables as shown. Cable A is connected 1/4th distance from the left end of the bar. Cable B is attached at the far right end of the bar. What is the tension in cable A?

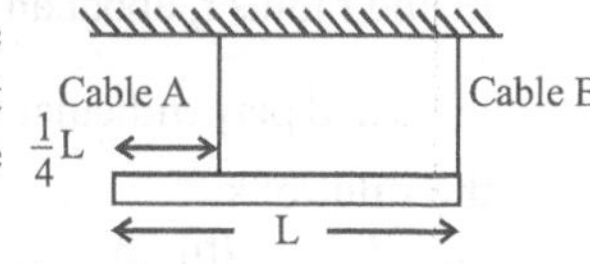

(a) 1/4 Mg (b) 1/3 Mg (c) 2/3 Mg (d) 3/4 Mg

33. A couple produces

(a) purely linear motion
(b) purely rotational motion
(c) linear and rotational motion
(d) no motion

34. Point masses 1, 2, 3 and 4 kg are lying at the point (0, 0, 0), (2, 0, 0), (0, 3, 0) and (–2, –2, 0) respectively. The moment of inertia of this system about x-axis will be

(a) 43 kgm² (b) 34 kgm² (c) 27 kgm² (d) 72 kgm²

RESPONSE GRID				
20. ⓐⓑⓒⓓ	21. ⓐⓑⓒⓓ	22. ⓐⓑⓒⓓ	23. ⓐⓑⓒⓓ	24. ⓐⓑⓒⓓ
25. ⓐⓑⓒⓓ	26. ⓐⓑⓒⓓ	27. ⓐⓑⓒⓓ	28. ⓐⓑⓒⓓ	29. ⓐⓑⓒⓓ
30. ⓐⓑⓒⓓ	31. ⓐⓑⓒⓓ	32. ⓐⓑⓒⓓ	33. ⓐⓑⓒⓓ	34. ⓐⓑⓒⓓ

Space for Rough Work

35. A solid sphere of mass M and radius R is pulled horizontally on a sufficiently rough surface as shown in the figure.

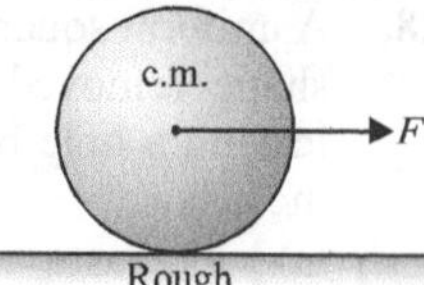

Choose the correct alternative.

(a) The acceleration of the centre of mass is F/M

(b) The acceleration of the centre of mass is $\frac{2}{3}\frac{F}{M}$

(c) The friction force on the sphere acts forward

(d) The magnitude of the friction force is F/3

36. The moment of inertia of a body about a given axis is 1.2 kg m^2. Initially, the body is at rest. In order to produce a rotational kinetic energy of 1500 joule, an angular acceleration of 25 radian/sec^2 must be applied about that axis for a duration of

(a) 4 sec (b) 2 sec (c) 8 sec (d) 10 sec

37. A gymnast takes turns with her arms and legs stretched. When she pulls her arms and legs in

(a) the angular velocity decreases

(b) the moment of inertia decreases

(c) the angular velocity stays constant

(d) the angular momentum increases

38. An equilateral triangle *ABC* formed from a uniform wire has two small identical beads initially located at *A*. The triangle is set rotating about the vertical axis *AO*. Then the beads are released from rest simultaneously and allowed to slide down, one along *AB* and the other along *AC* as shown. Neglecting frictional effects, the quantities that are conserved as the beads slide down, are

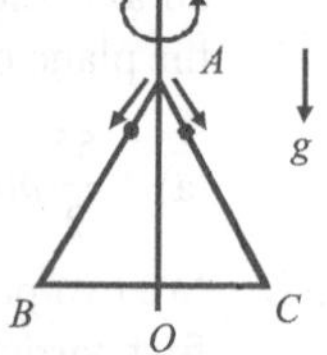

(a) angular velocity and total energy (kinetic and potential)

(b) total angular momentum and total energy

(c) angular velocity and moment of inertia about the axis of rotation

(d) total angular momentum and moment of inertia about the axis of rotation

39. The moment of inertia of a uniform semicircular wire of mass m and radius r, about an axis passing through its centre of mass and perpendicular to its plane is $mr^2\left(1-\frac{k}{\pi^2}\right)$. Find the value of k.

(a) 2 (b) 3 (c) 4 (d) 5

40. Initial angular velocity of a circular disc of mass *M* is ω_1. Then two small spheres of mass *m* are attached gently to diametrically opposite points on the edge of the disc. What is the final angular velocity of the disc?

(a) $\left(\frac{M+m}{M}\right)\omega_1$ (b) $\left(\frac{M+m}{m}\right)\omega_1$

(c) $\left(\frac{M}{M+4m}\right)\omega_1$ (d) $\left(\frac{M}{M+2m}\right)\omega_1$.

41. Two identical discs of mass m and radius r are arranged as shown in the figure. If α is the angular acceleration of the lower disc and a_{cm} is acceleration of centre of mass of the lower disc, then relation between a_{cm}, α and r is

(a) $a_{cm} = \alpha/r$ (b) $a_{cm} = 2\alpha r$

(c) $a_{cm} = \alpha r$ (d) None of these

42. Five masses are placed in a plane as shown in figure. The coordinates of the centre of mass are nearest to

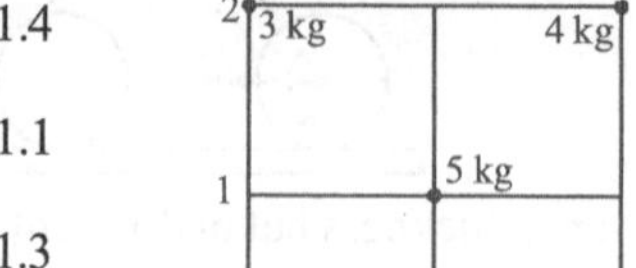

(a) 1.2, 1.4

(b) 1.3, 1.1

(c) 1.1, 1.3

(d) 1.0, 1.0

43. Three particles, each of mass *m* gram, are situated at the vertices of an equilateral triangle ABC of side ℓ cm (as shown in the figure). The moment of inertia of the system about a line AX perpendicular to AB and in the plane of ABC, in gram-cm^2 units will be

(a) $\frac{3}{2}m\ell^2$

(b) $\frac{3}{4}m\ell^2$

(c) $2m\ell^2$

(d) $\frac{5}{4}m\ell^2$

44. When a ceiling fan is switched on, it makes 10 rotations in the first 3 seconds. Assuming a uniform angular acceleration, how many rotation it will make in the next 3 seconds?

(a) 10 (b) 20 (c) 30 (d) 40

45. A solid sphere spinning about a horizontal axis with an angular velocity ω is placed on a horizontal surface. Subsequently it rolls without slipping with an angular velocity of :

(a) $\frac{2\omega}{5}$ (b) $\frac{7\omega}{5}$ (c) $\frac{2\omega}{7}$ (d) ω

RESPONSE GRID					
	35. ⓐⓑⓒⓓ	36. ⓐⓑⓒⓓ	37. ⓐⓑⓒⓓ	38. ⓐⓑⓒⓓ	39. ⓐⓑⓒⓓ
	40. ⓐⓑⓒⓓ	41. ⓐⓑⓒⓓ	42. ⓐⓑⓒⓓ	43. ⓐⓑⓒⓓ	44. ⓐⓑⓒⓓ
	45. ⓐⓑⓒⓓ				

PHYSICS CHAPTERWISE SPEED TEST-6

Total Questions	45	Total Marks	180
Attempted		Correct	
Incorrect		Net Score	
Cut-off Score	45	Qualifying Score	60
Success Gap = Net Score – Qualifying Score			
Net Score = (Correct × 4) – (Incorrect × 1)			

Space for Rough Work

PHYSICS

Gravitation

Speed TEST 7

Chapter-wise

No. of Questions	Maximum Marks	Time
45	180	1 Hour

GENERAL INSTRUCTIONS

- This test contains 45 MCQ's. For each question only one option is correct. Darken the correct circle/ bubble in the Response Grid provided on each page.
- You have to evaluate your Response Grids yourself with the help of solutions provided at the end of this book.
- Each correct answer will get you 4 marks and 1 mark shall be deduced for each incorrect answer. No mark will be given/ deducted if no bubble is filled. Keep a timer in front of you and stop immediately at the end of 60 min.
- The sheet follows a particular syllabus. Do not attempt the sheet before you have completed your preparation for that syllabus.
- After completing the sheet check your answers with the solution booklet and complete the Result Grid. Finally spend time to analyse your performance and revise the areas which emerge out as weak in your evaluation.

1. The radius of a planet is 1/4th of R_e and its acc. due to gravity is 2g. What would be the value of escape velocity on the planet, if escape velocity on earth is v_e.

   (a) $\frac{v_e}{\sqrt{2}}$ (b) $v_e\sqrt{2}$ (c) $2\,v_e$ (d) $\frac{v_e}{2}$

2. A projectile is fired vertically from the Earth with a velocity kv_e where v_e is the escape velocity and k is a constant less than unity. The maximum height to which projectile rises, as measured from the centre of Earth, is

   (a) $\frac{R}{k}$ (b) $\frac{R}{k-1}$ (c) $\frac{R}{1-k^2}$ (d) $\frac{R}{1+k^2}$

3. A solid sphere of uniform density and radius R applies a gravitational force of attraction equal to F_1 on a particle placed at A, distance 2R from the centre of the sphere.

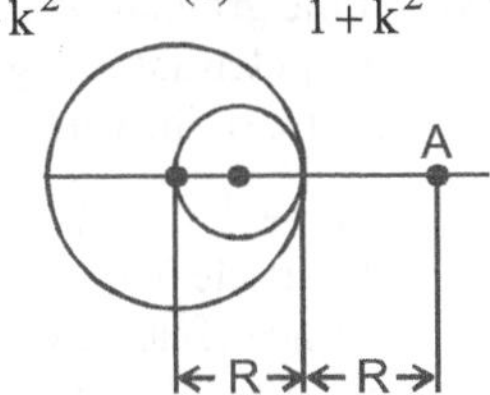

   A spherical cavity of radius R/2 is now made in the sphere as shown in the figure. The sphere with cavity now applies a gravitational force F_2 on the same particle placed at A. The ratio F_2/F_1 will be

   (a) 1/2 (b) 3 (c) 7 (d) 1/9

4. A geostationary satellite is orbiting the earth at a height of 5R above that surface of the earth, R being the radius of the earth. The time period of another satellite in hours at a height of 2R from the surface of the earth is :

   (a) 5 (b) 10 (c) $6\sqrt{2}$ (d) $\frac{6}{\sqrt{2}}$

5. A satellite of mass m is orbiting around the earth in a circular orbit with a velocity v. What will be its total energy?

   (a) $(3/4)\,mv^2$ (b) $(1/2)\,mv^2$
   (c) mv^2 (d) $-(1/2)m\,v^2$

RESPONSE GRID	1. ⓐⓑⓒⓓ	2. ⓐⓑⓒⓓ	3. ⓐⓑⓒⓓ	4. ⓐⓑⓒⓓ	5. ⓐⓑⓒⓓ

Space for Rough Work

6. The gravitational force of attraction between a uniform sphere of mass M and a uniform rod of length l and mass m oriented as shown is

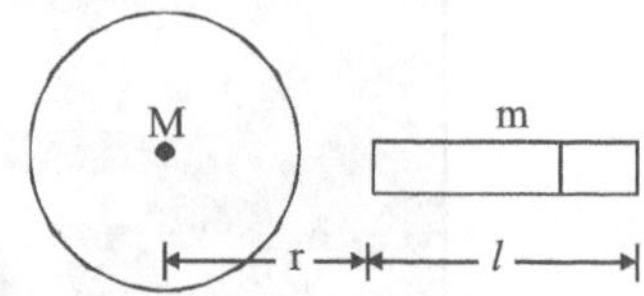

(a) $\frac{GMm}{r(r+l)}$ (b) $\frac{GM}{r^2}$ (c) $Mmr^2 + l$ (d) $(r^2 + l)mM$

7. If the gravitational force between two objects were proportional to $1/R$ (and not as $1/R^2$) where R is separation between them, then a particle in circular orbit under such a force would have its orbital speed v proportional to

(a) $1/R^2$ (b) R^0 (c) R^1 (d) $1/R$

8. A satellite of mass m revolves around the earth of radius R at a height 'x' from its surface. If g is the acceleration due to gravity on the surface of the earth, the orbital speed of the satellite is

(a) $\frac{gR^2}{R+x}$ (b) $\frac{gR}{R-x}$ (c) gx (d) $\left(\frac{gR^2}{R+x}\right)^{1/2}$

9. A body is projected up with a velocity equal to 3/4th of the escape velocity from the surface of the earth. The height it reaches from the centre of the earth is (Radius of the earth = R)

(a) $\frac{10R}{9}$ (b) $\frac{16R}{7}$ (c) $\frac{9R}{8}$ (d) $\frac{10R}{3}$

10. A Planet is revolving around the sun.

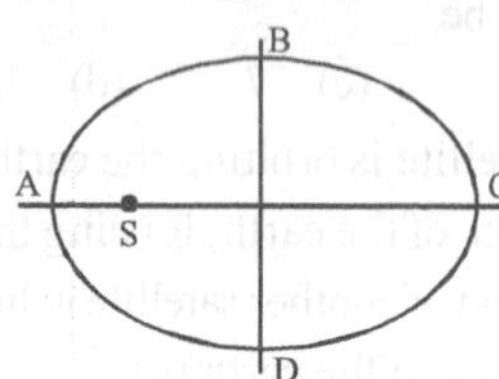

Which of the following is correct option?

(a) The time taken in travelling DAB is less than that for BCD

(b) The time taken in travelling DAB is greater than that for BCD

(c) The time taken in travelling CDA is less than that for ABC

(d) The time taken in travelling CDA is greater than that for ABC

11. The acceleration due to gravity on the planet A is 9 times the acceleration due to gravity on planet B. A man jumps to a height of 2m on the surface of A. What is the height of jump by the same person on the planet B?

(a) $\frac{2}{3}$m (b) $\frac{2}{9}$m (c) 18m (d) 6m

12. If suddenly the gravitational force of attraction between the earth and a satellite revolving around it becomes zero, then the satellite will

(a) continue to move in its orbit with same speed

(b) move tangentially to the original orbit with same speed

(c) become stationary in its orbit

(d) move towards the earth

13. Mass M is divided into two parts xM and (1 – x)M. For a given separation, the value of x for which the gravitational attraction between the two pieces becomes maximum is

(a) $\frac{1}{2}$ (b) $\frac{3}{5}$ (c) 1 (d) 2

14. The potential energy of a satellite, having mass m and rotating at a height of 6.4×10^6 m from the earth surface, is

(a) $-mgR_e$ (b) $-0.67\ mgR_e$

(c) $-0.5\ mgR_e$ (d) $-0.33\ mgR_e$

15. If the radius of the earth were to shrink by 1%, with its mass remaining the same, the acceleration due to gravity on the earth's surface would

(a) decrease by 1% (b) decrease by 2%

(c) increase by 1% (d) increase by 2%

16. Suppose the law of gravitational attraction suddenly changes and becomes an inverse cube law i.e. $F \propto \frac{1}{r^3}$, but still remaining a central force. Then

(a) Kepler's law of area still holds

(b) Kepler's law of period still holds

(c) Kepler's law of area and period still holds

(d) neither the law of area nor the law of period still holds

17. Four equal masses (each of mass M) are placed at the corners of a square of side a. The escape velocity of a body from the centre O of the square is

(a) $4\sqrt{\frac{2GM}{a}}$ (b) $\sqrt{\frac{8\sqrt{2}GM}{a}}$ (c) $\frac{4GM}{a}$ (d) $\sqrt{\frac{4\sqrt{2}GM}{a}}$

18. If the gravitational force had varied as $r^{-5/2}$ instead of r^{-2}; the potential energy of a particle at a distance 'r' from the centre of the earth would be directly proportional to

(a) r^{-1} (b) r^{-2} (c) $r^{-3/2}$ (d) $r^{-5/2}$

19. A particle of mass 'm' is kept at rest at a height 3R from the surface of earth, where 'R' is radius of earth and 'M' is mass of earth. The minimum speed with which it should be projected, so that it does not return back, is (g is acceleration due to gravity on the surface of earth)

(a) $\left(\frac{GM}{R}\right)^{\frac{1}{2}}$ (b) $\left(\frac{GM}{2R}\right)^{\frac{1}{2}}$ (c) $\left(\frac{gR}{4}\right)^{\frac{1}{2}}$ (d) $\left(\frac{2g}{4}\right)^{\frac{1}{2}}$

RESPONSE GRID					
	6. ⓐⓑⓒⓓ	7. ⓐⓑⓒⓓ	8. ⓐⓑⓒⓓ	9. ⓐⓑⓒⓓ	10. ⓐⓑⓒⓓ
	11. ⓐⓑⓒⓓ	12. ⓐⓑⓒⓓ	13. ⓐⓑⓒⓓ	14. ⓐⓑⓒⓓ	15. ⓐⓑⓒⓓ
	16. ⓐⓑⓒⓓ	17. ⓐⓑⓒⓓ	18. ⓐⓑⓒⓓ	19. ⓐⓑⓒⓓ	

Space for Rough Work

20. The ratio between the values of acceleration due to gravity at a height 1 km above and at a depth of 1 km below the Earth's surface is (radius of Earth is R)

(a) $\frac{R-2}{R-1}$ (b) $\frac{R}{R-1}$ (c) $\frac{R-2}{R}$ (d) 1

21. The weight of an object in the coal mine, sea level and at the top of the mountain, are respectively W_1, W_2 and W_3 then

(a) $W_1 < W_2 > W_3$ (b) $W_1 = W_2 = W_3$
(c) $W_1 < W_2 < W_3$ (d) $W_1 > W_2 > W_3$

22. The period of moon's rotation around the earth is nearly 29 days. If moon's mass were 2 fold its present value and all other things remain unchanged, the period of moon's rotation would be nearly

(a) $29\sqrt{2}$ days (b) $29/\sqrt{2}$ days
(c) 29×2 days (d) 29 days

23. The mean radius of earth is R, its angular speed on its own axis is ω and the acceleration due to gravity at earth's surface is g. What will be the radius of the orbit of a geostationary satellite?

(a) $(R^2g/\omega^2)^{1/3}$ (b) $(Rg/\omega^2)^{1/3}$
(c) $(R^2\omega^2/g)^{1/3}$ (d) $(R^2g/\omega)^{1/3}$

24. In order to make the effective acceleration due to gravity equal to zero at the equator, the angular velocity of rotation of the earth about its axis should be ($g = 10\ ms^{-2}$ and radius of earth is 64000 km)

(a) Zero (b) $\frac{1}{800}$ rad sec^{-1}
(c) $\frac{1}{80}$ rad sec^{-1} (d) $\frac{1}{8}$ rad sec^{-1}

25. A body weighs 72 N on the surface of the earth. What is the gravitational force on it due to earth at a height equal to half the radius of the earth from the surface?

(a) 32 N (b) 28 N (c) 16 N (d) 72 N

26. A body weighs W newton at the surface of the earth. Its weight at a height equal to half the radius of the earth, will be

(a) $\frac{W}{2}$ (b) $\frac{2W}{3}$ (c) $\frac{4W}{9}$ (d) $\frac{8W}{27}$

27. A shell of mass M and radius R has a point mass m placed at a distance r from its centre. The graph of gravitational potential energy U(r) vs distance r will be

(a)
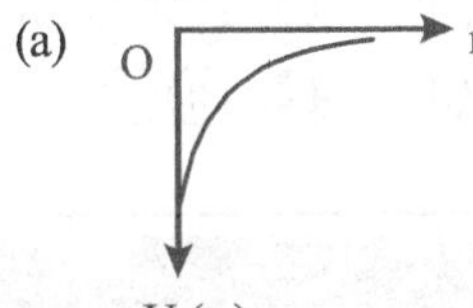

(b)
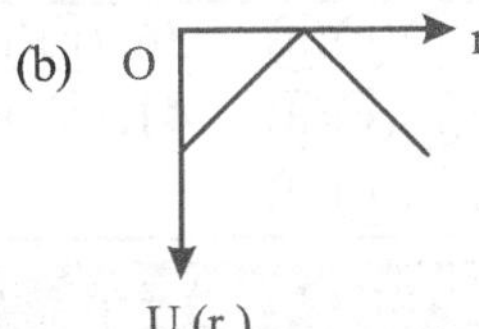

(c) O r $-\frac{GMm}{R}$ U (r)

(d) O r U (r)

28. The largest and the shortest distance of the earth from the sun are r_1 and r_2. Its distance from the sun when it is at perpendicular to the major-axis of the orbit drawn from the sun

(a) $(r_1+r_2)/4$ (b) $(r_1+r_2)/(r_1-r_2)$
(c) $2r_1r_2/(r_1+r_2)$ (d) $(r_1+r_2)/3$

29. A planet is moving in an elliptical orbit around the sun. If T, V, E and L stand respectively for its kinetic energy, gravitational potential energy, total energy and magnitude of angular momentum about the centre of force, then which of the following is correct?

(a) T is conserved
(b) V is always positive
(c) E is always negative
(d) L is conserved but direction of vector L changes continuously

30. The earth is assumed to be sphere of radius R. A platform is arranged at a height R from the surface of Earth. The escape velocity of a body from this platform is kv, where v is its escape velocity from the surface of the earth. The value of k is

(a) $\frac{1}{\sqrt{2}}$ (b) $\frac{1}{3}$ (c) $\frac{1}{2}$ (d) $\sqrt{2}$

31. A solid sphere of mass M and radius R is surrounded by a spherical shell of same mass M and radius 2R as shown. A small particle of mass m is released from rest from a height h [<< R] above the shell. There is a hole in the shell. What time will it enter the hole at A?

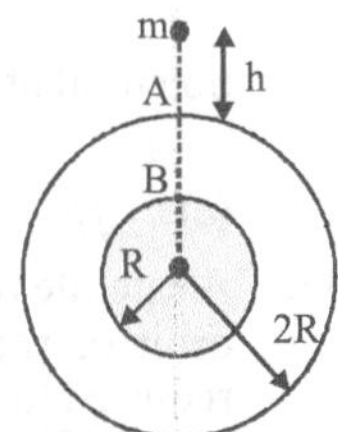

(a) $2\sqrt{\frac{hR^2}{GM}}$ (b) $\sqrt{\frac{2hR^2}{GM}}$
(c) $\sqrt{\frac{hR^2}{GM}}$ (d) $\sqrt{\frac{3hR^2}{GM}}$

32. A body starts from rest from a point distance R_0 from the centre of the earth. The velocity acquired by the body when it reaches the surface of the earth will be (R represents radius of the earth).

(a) $2GM\left(\frac{1}{R}-\frac{1}{R_0}\right)$ (b) $\sqrt{2GM\left(\frac{1}{R_0}-\frac{1}{R}\right)}$
(c) $GM\left(\frac{1}{R}-\frac{1}{R_0}\right)$ (d) $2GM\sqrt{\left(\frac{1}{R}-\frac{1}{R_0}\right)}$

RESPONSE GRID					
	20. ⓐⓑⓒⓓ	21. ⓐⓑⓒⓓ	22. ⓐⓑⓒⓓ	23. ⓐⓑⓒⓓ	24. ⓐⓑⓒⓓ
	25. ⓐⓑⓒⓓ	26. ⓐⓑⓒⓓ	27. ⓐⓑⓒⓓ	28. ⓐⓑⓒⓓ	29. ⓐⓑⓒⓓ
	30. ⓐⓑⓒⓓ	31. ⓐⓑⓒⓓ	32. ⓐⓑⓒⓓ		

Space for Rough Work

33. A satellite of mass M is moving in a circle of radius R under a centripetal force given by $(-k/R^2)$, where k is a constant. Then

(a) The kinetic energy of the particle is $\frac{k}{12}R$

(b) The total energy of the particle is $\left(-\frac{k}{2R}\right)$

(c) The kinetic energy of the particle is $\left(-\frac{k}{R}\right)$

(d) The potential energy of the particle is $\left(\frac{k}{2R}\right)$

34. The change in the value of 'g' at a height 'h' above the surface of the earth is the same as at a depth 'd' below the surface of earth. When both 'd' and 'h' are much smaller than the radius of earth, then which one of the following is correct?

(a) $d=\frac{3h}{2}$ (b) $d=\frac{h}{2}$ (c) $d=h$ (d) $d=2h$

35. Two identical geostationary satellites are moving with equal speeds in the same orbit but their sense of rotation brings them on a collision course. The debris will

(a) fall down
(b) move up
(c) begin to move from east to west in the same orbit
(d) begin to move from west to east in the same orbit

36. A diametrical tunnel is dug across the Earth. A ball is dropped into the tunnel from one side. The velocity of the ball when it reaches the centre of the Earth is .... (Given : gravitational potential at the centre of Earth $= -\frac{3}{2}\frac{GM}{R}$)

(a) $\sqrt{R}$ (b) $\sqrt{gR}$ (c) $\sqrt{2.5gR}$ (d) $\sqrt{7.1gR}$

37. A satellite revolves around the earth of radius R in a circular orbit of radius 3R. The percentage increase in energy required to lift it to an orbit of radius 5R is

(a) 10% (b) 20% (c) 30% (d) 40%

38. A (nonrotating) star collapses onto itself from an initial radius R_i with its mass remaining unchanged. Which curve in figure best gives the gravitational acceleration a_g on the surface of the star as a function of the radius of the star during the collapse

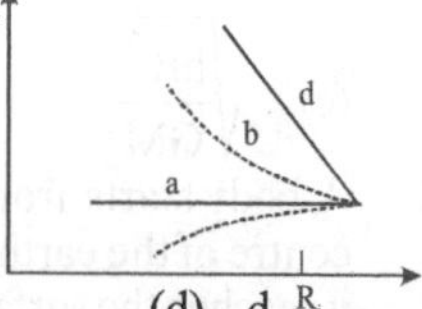

(a) a (b) b (c) c (d) d

39. If the earth is treated as a sphere of radius R and mass M; its angular momentum about the axis of its rotation with period T, is

(a) $\frac{\pi MR^3}{T}$ (b) $\frac{MR^2\pi}{T}$ (c) $\frac{2\pi MR^2}{5T}$ (d) $\frac{4\pi MR^2}{5T}$

40. A satellite is launched into a circular orbit of radius R around the earth. A second satellite is launched into an orbit of radius 1.01 R. The period of second satellite is larger than the first one by approximately

(a) 0.5% (b) 1.0% (c) 1.5% (d) 3.0%

41. A uniform spherical shell gradually shrinks maintaining its shape. The gravitational potential at the centre

(a) increases (b) decreases
(c) remains constant (d) cannot say

42. The depth d at which the value of acceleration due to gravity becomes $\frac{1}{n}$ times the value at the surface of the earth, is [R = radius of the earth]

(a) $\frac{R}{n}$ (b) $R\left(\frac{n-1}{n}\right)$ (c) $\frac{R}{n^2}$ (d) $R\left(\frac{n}{n+1}\right)$

43. Radius of moon is 1/4 times that of earth and mass is 1/81 times that of earth. The point at which gravitational field due to earth becomes equal and opposite to that of moon, is (Distance between centres of earth and moon is 60R, where R is radius of earth)

(a) 5.75 R from centre of moon
(b) 16 R from surface of moon
(c) 53 R from centre of earth
(d) 54 R from centre of earth

44. If earth is supposed to be a sphere of radius R, if g_{30} is value of acceleration due to gravity at lattitude of 30° and g at the equator, the value of $g - g_{30}$ is

(a) $\frac{1}{4}\omega^2R$ (b) $\frac{3}{4}\omega^2R$ (c) ω^2R (d) $\frac{1}{2}\omega^2R$

45. What is the minimum energy required to launch a satellite of mass m from the surface of a planet of mass M and radius R in a circular orbit at an altitude of 2R?

(a) $\frac{5GmM}{6R}$ (b) $\frac{2GmM}{3R}$ (c) $\frac{GmM}{2R}$ (d) $\frac{GmM}{2R}$

RESPONSE GRID					
	33. ⓐⓑⓒⓓ	34. ⓐⓑⓒⓓ	35. ⓐⓑⓒⓓ	36. ⓐⓑⓒⓓ	37. ⓐⓑⓒⓓ
	38. ⓐⓑⓒⓓ	39. ⓐⓑⓒⓓ	40. ⓐⓑⓒⓓ	41. ⓐⓑⓒⓓ	42. ⓐⓑⓒⓓ
	43. ⓐⓑⓒⓓ	44. ⓐⓑⓒⓓ	45. ⓐⓑⓒⓓ		

PHYSICS CHAPTERWISE SPEED TEST-7			
Total Questions	45	Total Marks	180
Attempted		Correct	
Incorrect		Net Score	
Cut-off Score	45	Qualifying Score	60
Success Gap = Net Score – Qualifying Score			
Net Score = (Correct × 4) – (Incorrect × 1)			

Space for Rough Work

PHYSICS

Mechanical Properties of Solids

Speed TEST 8

Chapter-wise

No. of Questions	Maximum Marks	Time
45	180	1 Hour

GENERAL INSTRUCTIONS

- This test contains 45 MCQ's. For each question only one option is correct. Darken the correct circle/ bubble in the Response Grid provided on each page.
- You have to evaluate your Response Grids yourself with the help of solutions provided at the end of this book.
- Each correct answer will get you 4 marks and 1 mark shall be deduced for each incorrect answer. No mark will be given/ deducted if no bubble is filled. Keep a timer in front of you and stop immediately at the end of 60 min.
- The sheet follows a particular syllabus. Do not attempt the sheet before you have completed your preparation for that syllabus.
- After completing the sheet check your answers with the solution booklet and complete the Result Grid. Finally spend time to analyse your performance and revise the areas which emerge out as weak in your evaluation.

1. Two wires A and B are of the same material. Their lengths are in the ratio 1 : 2 and the diameter are in the ratio 2 : 1. If they are pulled by the same force, then increase in length will be in the ratio

(a) 2 : 1 (b) 1 : 4 (c) 1 : 8 (d) 8 : 1

2. The load versus elongation graphs for four wires of same length and made of the same material are shown in the figure. The thinnest wire is represented by the line

(a) OA

(b) OC

(c) OD

(d) OB

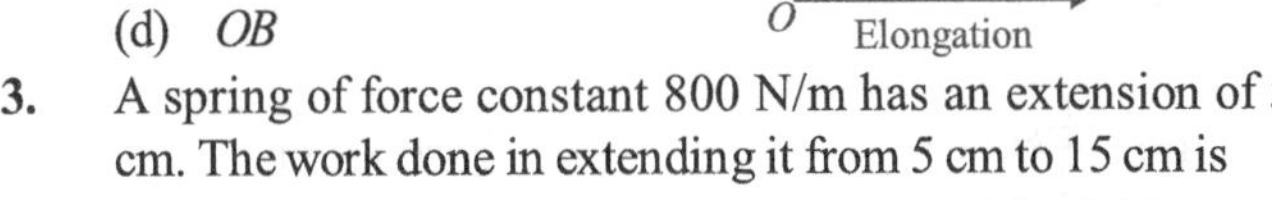

3. A spring of force constant 800 N/m has an extension of 5 cm. The work done in extending it from 5 cm to 15 cm is

(a) 16 J (b) 8 J (c) 32 J (d) 24 J

4. A metal wire of length L_1 and area of cross-section A is attached to a rigid support. Another metal wire of length L_2 and of the same cross-sectional area is attached to the free end of the first wire. A body of mass M is then suspended from the free end of the second wire. If Y_1 and Y_2 are the Young's moduli of the wires respectively, the effective force constant of the system of two wires is

(a) $\frac{(Y_1Y_2)A}{2(Y_1L_2+Y_2L_1)}$ (b) $\frac{(Y_1Y_2)A}{(L_1L_2)^{1/2}}$

(c) $\frac{(Y_1Y_2)A}{Y_1L_2+Y_2L_1}$ (d) $\frac{(Y_1Y_2)^{1/2}A}{(L_2L_1)^{1/2}}$

5. The approximate depth of an ocean is 2700 m. The compressibility of water is 45.4×10^{-11} Pa^{-1} and density of water is 10^3 kg/m^3. What fractional compression of water will be obtained at the bottom of the ocean ?

(a) 1.0×10^{-2} (b) 1.2×10^{-2}

(c) 1.4×10^{-2} (d) 0.8×10^{-2}

6. The Young's modulus of steel is twice that of brass. Two wires of same length and of same area of cross section, one of steel and another of brass are suspended from the same roof. If we want the lower ends of the wires to be at the same level, then the weights added to the steel and brass wires must be in the ratio of :

(a) 2 : 1 (b) 4 : 1 (c) 1 : 1 (d) 1 : 2

7. Choose the wrong statement.

(a) The bulk modulus for solids is much larger than for liquids.

(b) Gases are least compressible.

(c) The incompressibility of the solids is due to the tight coupling between neighbouring atoms.

(d) The reciprocal of the bulk modulus is called compressibility.

RESPONSE GRID					
	1. ⓐⓑⓒⓓ	2. ⓐⓑⓒⓓ	3. ⓐⓑⓒⓓ	4. ⓐⓑⓒⓓ	5. ⓐⓑⓒⓓ
	6. ⓐⓑⓒⓓ	7. ⓐⓑⓒⓓ			

Space for Rough Work

8. A copper wire of length 1.0 m and a steel wire of length 0.5 m having equal cross-sectional areas are joined end to end. The composite wire is stretched by a certain load which stretches the copper wire by 1 mm. If the Young's modulii of copper and steel are respectively 1.0×10^{11} Nm^{-2} and 2.0×10^{11} Nm^{-2}, the total extension of the composite wire is :

(a) 1.75 mm (b) 2.0 mm (c) 1.50 mm (d) 1.25 mm

9. A cube at temperature 0ºC is compressed equally from all sides by an external pressure P. By what amount should its temperature be raised to bring it back to the size it had before the external pressure was applied. The bulk modulus of the material of the cube is B and the coefficient of linear expansion is a.

(a) $P/B\alpha$ (b) $P/3B\alpha$ (c) $3\pi\alpha/B$ (d) $3B/P$

10. The diagram below shows the change in the length X of a thin uniform wire caused by the application of stress F at two different temperatures T_1 and T_2. The variation shown suggests that

(a) $T_1 > T_2$

(b) $T_1 < T_2$

(c) $T_2 > T_1$

(d) $T_1 \geq T_2$

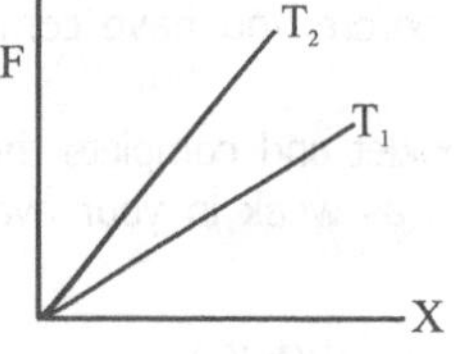

11. If the ratio of lengths, radii and Young's moduli of steel and brass wires in the figure are *a*, *b* and *c* respectively, then the corresponding ratio of increase in their lengths is :

Steel
M
Brass
2M

(a) $\frac{3c}{2ab^2}$

(b) $\frac{2a^2c}{b}$

(c) $\frac{3a}{2b^2c}$

(d) $\frac{2ac}{b^2}$

12. The Young's modulus of brass and steel are respectively 10^{10} N/m^2. and 2×10^{10} N/m^2. A brass wire and a steel wire of the same length are extended by 1 mm under the same force, the radii of brass and steel wires are R_B and R_S respectively. Then

(a) $R_S = \sqrt{2}\, R_B$ (b) $R_S = R_B/\sqrt{2}$

(c) $R_S = 4R_B$ (d) $R_S = R_B/4$

13. Steel ruptures when a shear of 3.5×10^8 N m^{-2} is applied. The force needed to punch a 1 cm diameter hole in a steel sheet 0.3 cm thick is nearly:

(a) 1.4×10^4 N (b) 2.7×10^4 N

(c) 3.3×10^4 N (d) 1.1×10^4 N

14. A ball falling in a lake of depth 400 m has a decrease of 0.2% in its volume at the bottom. The bulk modulus of the material of the ball is (in N m^{-2})

(a) 9.8×10^9 (b) 9.8×10^{10}

(c) 1.96×10^{10} (d) 1.96×10^9

15. A circular tube of mean radius 8 cm and thickness 0.04 cm is melted up and recast into a solid rod of the same length. The ratio of the torsional rigidities of the circular tube and the solid rod is

(a) $\frac{(8.02)^4 - (7.98)^4}{(0.8)^4}$ (b) $\frac{(8.02)^2 - (7.98)^2}{(0.8)^2}$

(c) $\frac{(0.8)^2}{(8.02)^4 - (7.98)^4}$ (d) $\frac{(0.8)^2}{(8.02)^3 - (7.98)^2}$

16. Two wires are made of the same material and have the same volume. However wire 1 has cross-sectional area *A* and wire 2 has cross-sectional area 3*A*. If the length of wire 1 increases by Δx on applying force *F*, how much force is needed to stretch wire 2 by the same amount?

(a) 4*F* (b) 6*F* (c) 9*F* (d) *F*

17. In materials like aluminium and copper, the correct order of magnitude of various elastic modului is:

(a) Young's modulus < shear modulus < bulk modulus.

(b) Bulk modulus < shear modulus < Young's modulus

(c) Shear modulus < Young's modulus < bulk modulus.

(d) Bulk modulus < Young's modulus < shear modulus.

18. What per cent of length of wire increases by applying a stress of 1 kg weight/mm^2 on it?
($Y = 1 \times 10^{11}$ N/m^2 and 1 kg weight = 9.8 newton)

(a) 0.0067% (b) 0.0098%

(c) 0.0088% (d) 0.0078%

19. An elastic string of unstretched length *L* and force constant *k* is stretched by a small length *x*. It is further stretched by another small length *y*. The work done in the second stretching is :

(a) $\frac{1}{2}ky^2$ (b) $\frac{1}{2}k(x^2+y^2)$

(c) $\frac{1}{2}k(x+y)^2$ (d) $\frac{1}{2}ky(2x+y)$

20. Two, spring *P* and *Q* of force constants k_p and $k_Q\left(k_Q = \frac{k_p}{2}\right)$ are stretched by applying forces of equal magnitude. If the energy stored in *Q* is E, then the energy stored in *P* is

(a) E (b) 2E (c) E/2 (d) E/4

RESPONSE GRID					
	8. ⓐⓑⓒⓓ	9. ⓐⓑⓒⓓ	10. ⓐⓑⓒⓓ	11. ⓐⓑⓒⓓ	12. ⓐⓑⓒⓓ
	13. ⓐⓑⓒⓓ	14. ⓐⓑⓒⓓ	15. ⓐⓑⓒⓓ	16. ⓐⓑⓒⓓ	17. ⓐⓑⓒⓓ
	18. ⓐⓑⓒⓓ	19. ⓐⓑⓒⓓ	20. ⓐⓑⓒⓓ		

Space for Rough Work

21. The pressure that has to be applied to the ends of a steel wire of length 10 cm to keep its length constant when its temperature is raised by 100°C is:

(For steel Young's modulus is $2\times10^{11}\,Nm^{-2}$ and coefficient of thermal expansion is $1.1\times10^{-5}\,K^{-1}$)

(a) 2.2×10^{8} Pa (b) 2.2×10^{9} Pa
(c) 2.2×10^{7} Pa (d) 2.2×10^{6} Pa

22. A steel ring of radius r and cross sectional area A is fitted onto a wooden disc of radius R (R > r). If the Young's modulus of steel is Y, then the force with which the steel ring is expanded is
(a) AY (R/r) (b) AY (R – r)/r
(c) (Y/A)[(R – r)/r] (d) Yr/AR

23. Two wires A and B of same material and of equal length with the radii in the ratio 1 : 2 are subjected to identical loads. If the length of A increases by 8 mm, then the increase in length of B is
(a) 2 mm (b) 4 mm (c) 8 mm (d) 16 mm

24. A material has poisson's ratio 0.50. If a uniform rod of it suffers a longitudinal strain of 2×10^{-3}, then the percentage change in volume is
(a) 0.6 (b) 0.4 (c) 0.2 (d) Zero

25. The upper end of a wire of diameter 12mm and length 1m is clamped and its other end is twisted through an angle of 30°. The angle of shear is
(a) 18° (b) 0.18° (c) 36° (d) 0.36°

26. The pressure on an object of bulk modulus B undergoing hydraulic compression due to a stress exerted by surrounding fluid having volume strain $\left(\frac{\Delta V}{V}\right)^2$ is

(a) $B^2\left(\frac{\Delta V}{V}\right)$ (b) $B\left(\frac{\Delta V}{V}\right)^2$
(c) $\frac{1}{B}\left(\frac{\Delta V}{V}\right)$ (d) $B\left(\frac{\Delta V}{V}\right)$

27. A structural steel rod has a radius of 10 mm and length of 1.0 m. A 100 kN force stretches it along its length. Young's modulus of structural steel is $2\times10^{11}\,Nm^{-2}$. The percentage strain is about
(a) 0.16% (b) 0.32% (c) 0.08% (d) 0.24%

28. A beam of metal supported at the two edges is loaded at the centre. The depression at the centre is proportional to

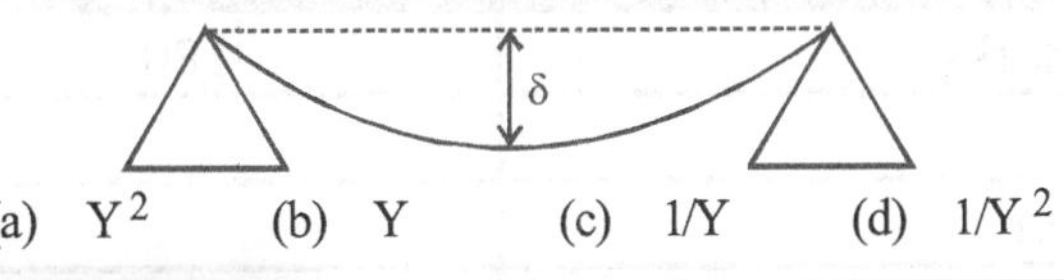

(a) Y^2 (b) Y (c) 1/Y (d) $1/Y^2$

29. When a 4 kg mass is hung vertically on a light spring that obeys Hooke's law, the spring stretches by 2 cms. The work required to be done by an external agent in stretching this spring by 5 cms will be ($g = 9.8\ m/sec^2$)
(a) 4.900 joule (b) 2.450 joule
(c) 0.495 joule (d) 0.245 joule

30. The length of a metal is ℓ_1 when the tension in it is T_1 and is ℓ_2 when the tension is T_2. The original length of the wire is

(a) $\frac{\ell_1+\ell_2}{2}$ (b) $\frac{\ell_1T_2+\ell_2T_1}{T_1+T_2}$

(c) $\frac{\ell_1T_2-\ell_2T_1}{T_2-T_1}$ (d) $\sqrt{T_1T_2\ell_1\ell_2}$

31. For the same cross-sectional area and for a given load, the ratio of depressions for the beam of a square cross-section and circular cross-section is
(a) $3:\pi$ (b) $\pi:3$ (c) $1:\pi$ (d) $\pi:1$

32. The bulk moduli of ethanol, mercury and water are given as 0.9, 25 and 2.2 respectively in units of $10^9\,Nm^{-2}$. For a given value of pressure, the fractional compression in volume is $\frac{\Delta V}{V}$. Which of the following statements about $\frac{\Delta V}{V}$ for these three liquids is correct ?
(a) Ethanol > Water > Mercury
(b) Water > Ethanol > Mercury
(c) Mercury > Ethanol > Water
(d) Ethanol > Mercury > Water

33. The graph given is a stress-strain curve for

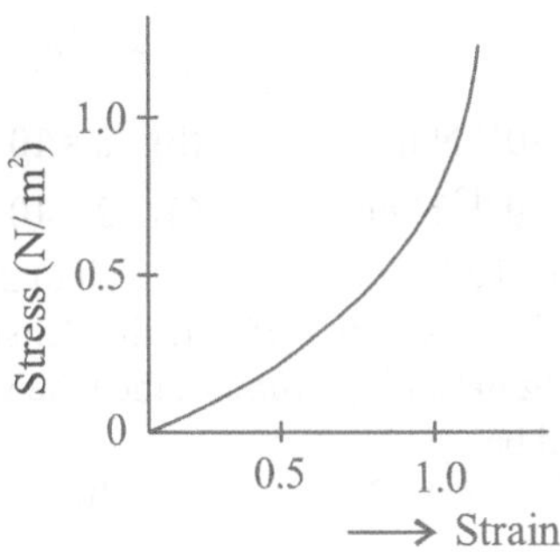

(a) elastic objects (b) plastics
(c) elastomers (d) None of these

34. A metal rod of Young's modulus $2\times10^{10}\,N\,m^{-2}$ undergoes an elastic strain of 0.06%. The energy per unit volume stored in $J\,m^{-3}$ is
(a) 3600 (b) 7200 (c) 10800 (d) 14400

35. Two wires of the same material and same length but diameters in the ratio 1 : 2 are stretched by the same force. The potential energy per unit volume of the two wires will be in the ratio
(a) 1 : 2 (b) 4 : 1 (c) 2 : 1 (d) 16 : 1

RESPONSE GRID				
21. ⓐⓑⓒⓓ	22. ⓐⓑⓒⓓ	23. ⓐⓑⓒⓓ	24. ⓐⓑⓒⓓ	25. ⓐⓑⓒⓓ
26. ⓐⓑⓒⓓ	27. ⓐⓑⓒⓓ	28. ⓐⓑⓒⓓ	29. ⓐⓑⓒⓓ	30. ⓐⓑⓒⓓ
31. ⓐⓑⓒⓓ	32. ⓐⓑⓒⓓ	33. ⓐⓑⓒⓓ	34. ⓐⓑⓒⓓ	35. ⓐⓑⓒⓓ

Space for Rough Work

36. The length of an elastic string is a metre when the longitudinal tension is 4 N and b metre when the longitudinal tension is 5 N. The length of the string in metre when the longitudinal tension is 9 N is

(a) $a-b$ (b) $5b-4a$ (c) $2b-\frac{1}{4}a$ (d) $4a-3b$

37. A force of 10^3 newton, stretches the length of a hanging wire by 1 millimetre. The force required to stretch a wire of same material and length but having four times the diameter by 1 millimetre is

(a) 4×10^3 N (b) 16×10^3 N

(c) $\frac{1}{4}\times10^3$ N (d) $\frac{1}{16}\times10^3$ N

38. A steel wire of length l and cross sectional area A is stretched by 1 cm under a given load. When the same load is applied to another steel wire of double its length and half of its cross section area, the amount of stretching (extension) is

(a) 0.5 cm (b) 2 cm (c) 4 cm (d) 1.5 cm

39. The adjacent graph shows the extension (Δl) of a wire of length 1 m suspended from the top of a roof at one end with a load W connected to the other end. If the cross-sectional area of the wire is 10^{-6} m^2, calculate the Young's modulus of the material of the wire :

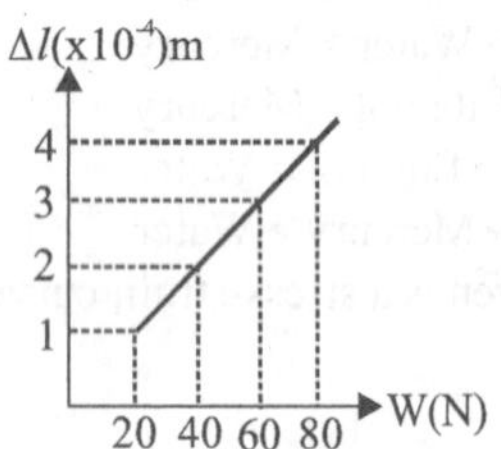

(a) 2×10^{11} N/m^2 (b) 2×10^{-11} N/m^2

(c) 3×10^{-12} N/m^2 (d) 2×10^{-13} N/m^2

40. If a rubber ball is taken at the depth of 200 m in a pool, its volume decreases by 0.1%. If the density of the water is 1×10^3 kg/m^3 and g = 10m/s^2, then the volume elasticity in N/m^2 will be

(a) 10^8 (b) 2×10^8 (c) 10^9 (d) 2×10^9

41. A ball is falling in a lake of depth 200 m creates a decrease 0.1 % in its volume at the bottom. The bulk modulus of the material of the ball will be

(a) 19.6×10^{-8} N/m^2 (b) 19.6×10^{10} N/m^2

(c) 19.6×10^{-10} N/m^2 (d) 19.6×10^{8} N/m^2

42. The diagram shows a force-extension graph for a rubber band. Consider the following statements :

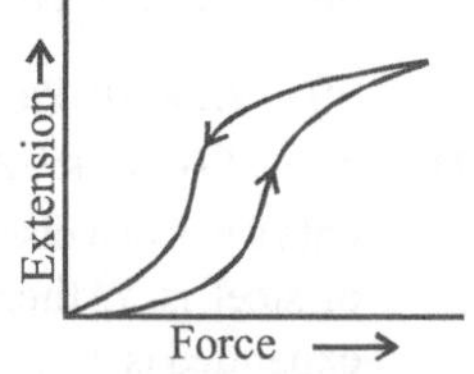

I. It will be easier to compress this rubber than expand it

II. Rubber does not return to its original length after it is stretched

III. The rubber band will get heated if it is stretched and released

Which of these can be deduced from the graph:

(a) III only (b) II and III (c) I and III (d) I only

43. The Poisson's ratio of a material is 0.5. If a force is applied to a wire of this material, there is a decrease in the cross-sectional area by 4%. The percentage increase in the length is:

(a) 1% (b) 2% (c) 2.5% (d) 4%

44. Copper of fixed volume 'V; is drawn into wire of length 'l'. When this wire is subjected to a constant force 'F', the extension produced in the wire is 'Δl'. Which of the following graphs is a straight line?

(a) Δl versus $\frac{1}{l}$ (b) Δl versus l^2

(c) Δl versus $\frac{1}{l^2}$ (d) Δl versus l

45. When a 4 kg mass is hung vertically on a light spring that obeys Hooke's law, the spring stretches by 2 cms. The work required to be done by an external agent in stretching this spring by 5 cm will be (g = 9.8 m/sec^2)

(a) 4.900 joule (b) 2.450 joule

(c) 0.495 joule (d) 0.245 joule

RESPONSE GRID					
	36. ⓐⓑⓒⓓ	37. ⓐⓑⓒⓓ	38. ⓐⓑⓒⓓ	39. ⓐⓑⓒⓓ	40. ⓐⓑⓒⓓ
	41. ⓐⓑⓒⓓ	42. ⓐⓑⓒⓓ	43. ⓐⓑⓒⓓ	44. ⓐⓑⓒⓓ	45. ⓐⓑⓒⓓ

PHYSICS CHAPTERWISE SPEED TEST-8			
Total Questions	45	Total Marks	180
Attempted		Correct	
Incorrect		Net Score	
Cut-off Score	50	Qualifying Score	70
Success Gap = Net Score – Qualifying Score			
Net Score = (Correct × 4) – (Incorrect × 1)			

Space for Rough Work

PHYSICS

Mechanical Properties of Fluids

Speed TEST 9

Chapter-wise

No. of Questions	Maximum Marks	Time
45	180	1 Hour

GENERAL INSTRUCTIONS

- This test contains 45 MCQ's. For each question only one option is correct. Darken the correct circle/ bubble in the Response Grid provided on each page.
- You have to evaluate your Response Grids yourself with the help of solutions provided at the end of this book.
- Each correct answer will get you 4 marks and 1 mark shall be deduced for each incorrect answer. No mark will be given/ deducted if no bubble is filled. Keep a timer in front of you and stop immediately at the end of 60 min.
- The sheet follows a particular syllabus. Do not attempt the sheet before you have completed your preparation for that syllabus.
- After completing the sheet check your answers with the solution booklet and complete the Result Grid. Finally spend time to analyse your performance and revise the areas which emerge out as weak in your evaluation.

1. The density of water at the surface of ocean is ρ. If the bulk modulus of water is B, what is the density of ocean water at a depth where the pressure is nP_0, where P_0 is the atmospheric pressure ?

(a) $\frac{\rho B}{B-(n-1)P_0}$ (b) $\frac{\rho B}{B+(n-1)P_0}$

(c) $\frac{\rho B}{B-nP_0}$ (d) $\frac{\rho B}{B+nP_0}$

2. A ball of radius r and density ρ falls freely under gravity through a distance *h* before entering water. Velocity of ball does not change even on entering water. If viscosity of water is η the value of h is given by

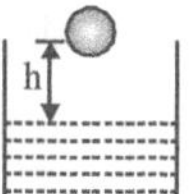

(a) $\frac{2}{9}r^2\left(\frac{1-\rho}{\eta}\right)g$ (b) $\frac{2}{81}r^2\left(\frac{\rho-1}{\eta}\right)g$

(c) $\frac{2}{81}r^4\left(\frac{\rho-1}{\eta}\right)^2 g$ (d) $\frac{2}{9}r^4\left(\frac{\rho-1}{\eta}\right)^2 g$

3. Two parallel glass plates are dipped partly in the liquid of density 'd' keeping them vertical . If the distance between the plates is 'x', surface tension for liquids is *T* and angle of contact is θ, then rise of liquid between the plates due to capillary will be

(a) $\frac{T\cos\theta}{xd}$ (b) $\frac{2T\cos\theta}{xdg}$ (c) $\frac{2T}{xdg\cos\theta}$ (d) $\frac{T\cos\theta}{xdg}$

4. A liquid is allowed to flow into a tube of truncated cone shape. Identify the correct statement from the following

(a) The speed is high at the wider end and high at the narrow end
(b) The speed is low at the wider end and high at the narrow end
(c) The speed is same at both ends in a streamline flow
(d) The liquid flows with uniform velocity in the tube

5. A wide vessel with a small hole at the bottom is filled with water (density ρ_1, height h_1) and kerosene (density ρ_2, height h_2). Neglecting viscosity effects, the speed with which water flows out is :

(a) $[2g(h_1+h_2)]^{1/2}$ (b) $[2g(h_1\rho_1+h_2\rho_2)]^{1/2}$
(c) $[2g(h_1+h_2(\rho_2/\rho_1))]^{1/2}$ (d) $[2g(h_1+h_2(\rho_1/\rho_2))]^{1/2}$

RESPONSE GRID 1. ⓐⓑⓒⓓ 2. ⓐⓑⓒⓓ 3. ⓐⓑⓒⓓ 4. ⓐⓑⓒⓓ 5. ⓐⓑⓒⓓ

Space for Rough Work

6. A capillary tube of radius r is immersed vertically in a liquid such that liquid rises in it to height h (less than the length of the tube). Mass of liquid in the capillary tube is m. If radius of the capillary tube is increased by 50%, then mass of liquid that will rise in the tube, is

(a) $\frac{2}{3}m$ (b) $\frac{4}{9}m$ (c) $\frac{3}{2}m$ (d) $\frac{9}{4}m$

7. A lead shot of 1 mm diameter falls through a long column of glycerine. The variation of its velocity v with distance covered is represented by

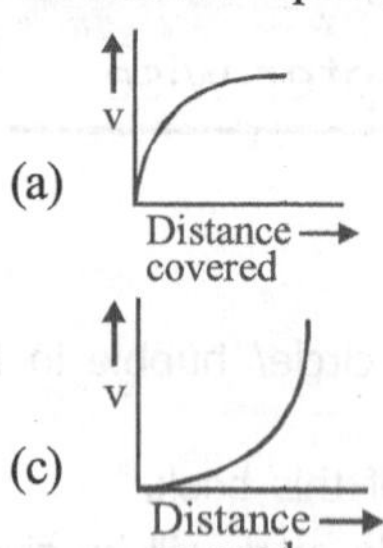

(a) [v vs Distance covered] (b) [v vs Distance covered]

(c) [v vs Distance covered] (d) [v vs Distance covered]

8. Two mercury drops (each of radius 'r') merge to form bigger drop. The surface energy of the bigger drop, if T is the surface tension, is :

(a) $4\pi r^2 T$ (b) $2\pi r^2 T$

(c) $2^{8/3}\pi r^2 T$ (d) $2^{5/3}\pi r^2 T$

9. Wax is coated on the inner wall of a capillary tube and the tube is then dipped in water. Then, compared to the unwaxed capillary, the angle of contact θ and the height h upto which water rises change. These changes are :

(a) θ increases and h also increases
(b) θ decreases and h also decreases
(c) θ increases and h decreases
(d) θ decreases and h increases

10. A rain drop of radius 0.3 mm has a terminal velocity in air = 1 m/s. The viscosity of air is 8×10^{-5} poise. The viscous force on it is

(a) 45.2×10^{-4} dyne (b) 101.73×10^{-5} dyne
(c) 16.95×10^{-4} dyne (d) 16.95×10^{-5} dyne

11. A water tank of height 10m, completely filled with water is placed on a level ground. It has two holes one at 3 m and the other at 7 m from its base. The water ejecting from

(a) both the holes will fall at the same spot
(b) upper hole will fall farther than that from the lower hole
(c) upper hole will fall closer than that from the lower hole
(d) more information is required

12. Two capillary of length L and 2L and of radius R and 2R are connected in series. The net rate of flow of fluid through them will be (given rate to the flow through single capillary, $X = \frac{\pi P R^4}{8\eta L}$)

(a) $\frac{8}{9}X$ (b) $\frac{9}{8}X$ (c) $\frac{5}{7}X$ (d) $\frac{7}{5}X$

13. A candle of diameter d is floating on a liquid in a cylindrical container of diameter D (D >> d) as shown in figure. If it is burning at the rate of 2 cm/hour then the top of the candle will

(a) remain at the same height
(b) fall at the rate of 1 cm/hour
(c) fall at the rate of 2 cm/hour
(d) go up at the rate of 1 cm/hour

14. An isolated and charged spherical soap bubble has a radius r and the pressure inside is atmospheric. T is the surface tension of soap solution. If charge on drop is $X\pi r\sqrt{2rT\varepsilon_0}$ then find the value of X.

(a) 8 (b) 9 (c) 7 (d) 2

15. A thread is tied slightly loose to a wire frame as in figure and the frame is dipped into a soap solution and taken out. The frame is completely covered with the film. When the portion A is punctured with a pin, the thread

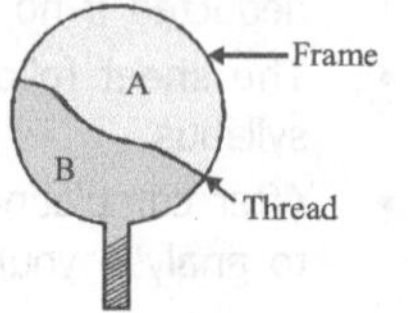

(a) becomes concave towards A
(b) becomes convex towards A
(c) remains in the initial position
(d) either (a) or (b) depending on the size of A w.r.t. B

16. Which of the following expressions represents the excess of pressure inside the soap bubble?

(a) $P_i - P_o = \frac{s}{r}$ (b) $P_i - P_o = \frac{2s}{r}$

(c) $P_i - P_o = \frac{2s}{r} + h\rho g$ (d) $P_i - P_o = \frac{4s}{r}$

17. A spherical solid ball of volume V is made of a material of density ρ_1. It is falling through a liquid of density ρ_1 $(\rho_2 < \rho_1)$. Assume that the liquid applies a viscous force on the ball that is proportional to the square of its speed v, i.e., $F_{viscous} = -kv^2$ $(k > 0)$. The terminal speed of the ball is

(a) $\sqrt{\frac{Vg(\rho_1 - \rho_2)}{k}}$ (b) $\frac{Vg\rho_1}{k}$

(c) $\sqrt{\frac{Vg\rho_1}{k}}$ (d) $\frac{Vg(\rho_1 - \rho_2)}{k}$

18. Select the correct statements from the following.

(a) Bunsen burner and sprayers work on Bernoulli's principle
(b) Blood flow in arteries is explained by Bernoulli's principle
(c) A siphon works on account of atmospheric pressure.
(d) All are correct

RESPONSE GRID					
	6. ⓐⓑⓒⓓ	7. ⓐⓑⓒⓓ	8. ⓐⓑⓒⓓ	9. ⓐⓑⓒⓓ	10. ⓐⓑⓒⓓ
	11. ⓐⓑⓒⓓ	12. ⓐⓑⓒⓓ	13. ⓐⓑⓒⓓ	14. ⓐⓑⓒⓓ	15. ⓐⓑⓒⓓ
	16. ⓐⓑⓒⓓ	17. ⓐⓑⓒⓓ	18. ⓐⓑⓒⓓ		

Space for Rough Work

19. The wetability of a surface by a liquid depends primarily on
(a) surface tension
(b) density
(c) angle of contact between the surface and the liquid
(d) viscosity

20. The relative velocity of two parallel layers of water is 8 cm/sec. If the perpendicular distance between the layers is 0.1 cm, then velocity gradient will be
(a) 80/sec (b) 60 /sec (c) 50/sec (d) 40/sec

21. Choose the correct statement
(a) Terminal velocities of rain drops are proportional to square of their radii
(b) Water proof agents decrease the angle of contact between water and fibres
(c) Detergents increase the surface tension of water
(d) Hydraulic machines work on the principle of Torricelli's law

22. When a ball is released from rest in a very long column of viscous liquid, its downward acceleration is 'a' (just after release). Its acceleration when it has acquired two third of the maximum velocity is a/X. Find the value of X.
(a) 2 (b) 3 (c) 4 (d) 5

23. A ring is cut from a platinum tube 8.5 cm internal and 8.7 cm external diameter. It is supported horizontally from the pan of a balance, so that it comes in contact with the water in a glass vessel. If an extra 3.97. If is required to pull it away from water, the surface tension of water is
(a) 72 dyne cm^{-1} (b) 70.80 dyne cm^{-1}
(c) 63.35 dyne cm^{-1} (d) 60 dyne cm^{-1}

24. Which of the following graph represents the variation of surface tension with temperature over small temperature ranges for water?

(a) 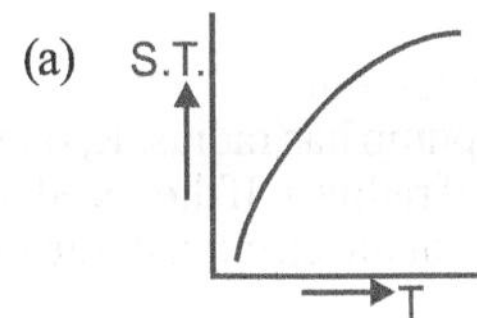

(b) 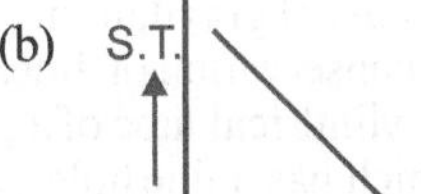

(c) 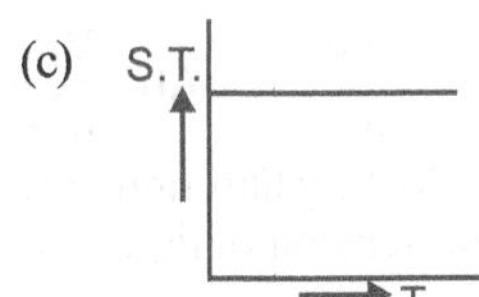

(d) 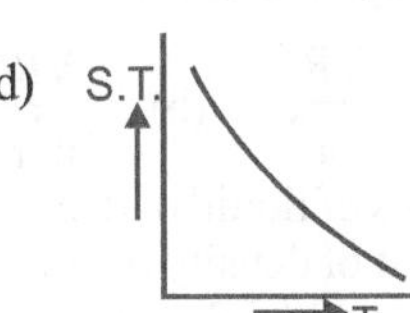

25. When a large air bubble rises from the bottom of a lake to the surface, its radius doubles. If the atmospheric pressure is equal to that of a column of water of height H, then depth of the lake is
(a) H (b) 2H (c) 7H (d) 8H

26. What is the velocity v of a metallic ball of radius r falling in a tank of liquid at the instant when its acceleration is one -half that of a freely falling body ? (The densities of metal and of liquid are ρ and σ respectively, and the viscosity of the liquid is η).
(a) $\frac{r^2 g}{9\eta}(\rho-2\sigma)$ (b) $\frac{r^2 g}{9\eta}(2\rho-\sigma)$
(c) $\frac{r^2 g}{9\eta}(\rho-\sigma)$ (d) $\frac{2r^2 g}{9\eta}(\rho-\sigma)$

27. Two pieces of metals are suspended from the arms of a balance and are found to be in equilibrium when kept immersed in water. The mass of one piece is 32 g and its density 8 g cm^{-3}. The density of the other is 5 g per cm^3. Then the mass of the other is
(a) 28 g (b) 35 g (c) 21 g (d) 33.6 g

28. A block of material of specific gravity 0.4 is held submerged at a depth of 1m in a vessel filled with water. The vessel is accelerated upwards with acceleration of $a_o = g/5$. If the block is released at $t = 0$, neglecting viscous effects, it will reach the water surface at t equal to ($g = 10$ m/s^2) :
(a) 0.60 s (b) 0.33 s (c) 3.3 s (d) 1.2 s

29. Figure shows a capillary rise H. If the air is blown through the horizontal tube in the direction as shown then rise in capillary tube will be
(a) =H
(b) >H
(c) <H
(d) zero

30. A small spherical ball falling through a viscous medium of negligible density has terminal velocity v. Another ball of the same mass but of radius twice that of the earlier falling through the same viscous medium will have terminal velocity
(a) v (b) v/4 (c) v/2 (d) 2v

31. Two non-mixing liquids of densities ρ and nρ (n > 1) are put in a container. The height of each liquid is h. A solid cylinder of length L and density d is put in this container. The cylinder floats with its axis vertical and length pL(p < 1) in the denser liquid. The density d is equal to :
(a) $\{1+(n+1)p\}\rho$ (b) $\{2+(n+1)p\}\rho$
(c) $\{2+(n-1)p\}\rho$ (d) $\{1+(n-1)p\}\rho$

32. A thin liquid film formed between a U-shaped wire and a light slider supports a weight of 1.5×10^{-2} N (see figure). The length of the slider is 30 cm and its weight negligible. The surface tension of the liquid film is

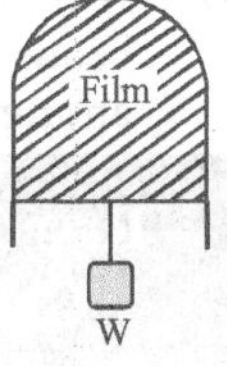

(a) 0.0125 Nm^{-1} (b) 0.1 Nm^{-1}
(c) 0.05 Nm^{-1} (d) 0.025 Nm^{-1}

RESPONSE GRID					
	19. ⓐⓑⓒⓓ	20. ⓐⓑⓒⓓ	21. ⓐⓑⓒⓓ	22. ⓐⓑⓒⓓ	23. ⓐⓑⓒⓓ
	24. ⓐⓑⓒⓓ	25. ⓐⓑⓒⓓ	26. ⓐⓑⓒⓓ	27. ⓐⓑⓒⓓ	28. ⓐⓑⓒⓓ
	29. ⓐⓑⓒⓓ	30. ⓐⓑⓒⓓ	31. ⓐⓑⓒⓓ	32. ⓐⓑⓒⓓ	

Space for Rough Work

33. Two liquids of densities d_1 and d_2 are flowing in identical capillary tubes uder the same pressure difference. If t_1 and t_2 are time taken for the flow of equal quantities (mass) of liquids, then the ratio of coefficient of viscosity of liquids must be

(a) $\frac{d_1 t_1}{d_2 t_2}$ (b) $\frac{t_1}{t_2}$ (c) $\frac{d_2}{d_1}\frac{t_2}{t_1}$ (d) $\sqrt{\frac{d_1 t_1}{d_2 t_2}}$

34. Let T_1 be surface tension between solid and air, T_2 be the surface tension between solid and liquid and T be the surface tension between liquid and air. Then in equilibrium, for a drop of liquid on a clean glass plate, the correct relation is (θ is angle of contact)

(a) $\cos\theta = \frac{T}{T_1 + T_2}$ (b) $\cos\theta = \frac{T}{T_1 - T_2}$

(c) $\cos\theta = \frac{T_1 + T_2}{T}$ (d) $\cos\theta = \frac{T_1 - T_2}{T}$

35. A uniform rod of density ρ is placed in a wide tank containing a liquid of density $\rho_0 (\rho_0 > \rho)$. The depth of liquid in the tank is half the length of the rod. The rod is in equilibrium, with its lower end resting on the bottom of the tank. In this position the rod makes an angle θ with the horizontal

(a) $\sin\theta = \frac{1}{2}\sqrt{\rho_0/\rho}$ (b) $\sin\theta = \frac{1}{2}.\frac{\rho_0}{\rho}$

(c) $\sin\theta = \sqrt{\rho/\rho_0}$ (d) $\sin\theta = \rho_0/\rho$

36. A spherical ball of iron of radius 2 mm is falling through a column of glycerine. If densities of glycerine and iron are respectively 1.3×10^3 kg/m^3 and 8×10^3 kg/m^3. η for glycerine = 0.83 Nm^{-2} sec, then the terminal velocity is

(a) 0.7 m/s (b) 0.07 m/s (c) 0.007 m/s (d) 0.0007 m/s

37. A water film is formed between two straight parallel wires of 10 cm length 0.5 cm apart. If the distance between wires is increased by 1 mm. What will be the work done ? (surface tension of water = 72 dyne/cm)

(a) 36 erg (b) 288 erg (c) 144 erg (d) 72 erg

38. A waterproofing agent changes the angle of contact
(a) from obtuse to acute.
(b) from acute to obtuse.
(c) from obtuse to π/2.
(d) from acute to π/ 2.

39. A thin metal disc of radius r floats on water surface and bends the surface downwards along the perimeter making an angle θ with vertical edge of the disc. If the disc displaces a weight of water W and surface tension of water is T, then the weight of metal disc is:

(a) $2\pi rT + W$ (b) $2\pi rT\cos\theta - W$
(c) $2\pi rT\cos\theta + W$ (d) $W - 2\pi rT\cos\theta$

40. A tank has a small hole at its botom of area of cross-section a. Liquid is being poured in the tank at the rate Vm^3/s, the maximum level of liquid in the container will be (Area of tank = A)

(a) $\frac{V}{gaA}$ (b) $\frac{V^2}{2gAa}$ (c) $\frac{V^2}{gAa}$ (d) $\frac{V}{2gaA}$

41. A jar is filled with two non-mixing liquids 1 and 2 having densities ρ_1 and, ρ_2 respectively. A solid ball, made of a material of density ρ_3, is dropped in the jar. It comes to equilibrium in the position shown in the figure. Which of the following is true for ρ_1, ρ_2 and ρ_3?

(a) $\rho_3 < \rho_1 < \rho_2$ (b) $\rho_1 > \rho_3 > \rho_2$
(c) $\rho_1 < \rho_2 < \rho_3$ (d) $\rho_1 < \rho_3 < \rho_2$

42. On heating water, bubbles being formed at the bottom of the vessel detach and rise. Take the bubbles to be spheres of radius R and making a circular contact of radius r with the bottom of the vessel. If r ≪ R and the surface tension of water is T, value of r just before bubbles detach is: (density of water is ρ_w)

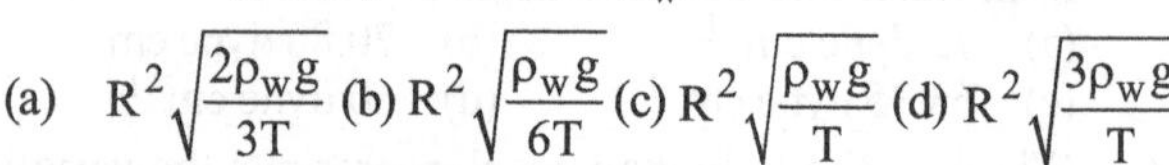

(a) $R^2\sqrt{\frac{2\rho_w g}{3T}}$ (b) $R^2\sqrt{\frac{\rho_w g}{6T}}$ (c) $R^2\sqrt{\frac{\rho_w g}{T}}$ (d) $R^2\sqrt{\frac{3\rho_w g}{T}}$

43. The lift of an air plane is based on
(a) Torricelli's theorem
(b) Bernoulli's theorem
(c) Law of gravitation
(d) conservation of linear momentum

44. The cylindrical tube of a spray pump has radius, R, one end of which has n fine holes, each of radius r. If the speed of the liquid in the tube is V, the speed of the ejection of the liquid through the holes is :

(a) $\frac{VR^2}{nr^2}$ (b) $\frac{VR^2}{n^3r^2}$ (c) $\frac{V^2R}{nr}$ (d) $\frac{VR^2}{n^2r^2}$

45. Drops of liquid of density ρ are floating half immersed in a liquid of density σ. If the surface tension of liquid is T, the radius of the drop will be

(a) $\sqrt{\frac{3T}{g(3\rho-\sigma)}}$ (b) $\sqrt{\frac{6T}{g(2\rho-\sigma)}}$ (c) $\sqrt{\frac{3T}{g(2\rho-\sigma)}}$ (d) $\sqrt{\frac{3T}{g(4\rho-3\sigma)}}$

RESPONSE GRID					
	33. ⓐⓑⓒⓓ	34. ⓐⓑⓒⓓ	35. ⓐⓑⓒⓓ	36. ⓐⓑⓒⓓ	37. ⓐⓑⓒⓓ
	38. ⓐⓑⓒⓓ	39. ⓐⓑⓒⓓ	40. ⓐⓑⓒⓓ	41. ⓐⓑⓒⓓ	42. ⓐⓑⓒⓓ
	43. ⓐⓑⓒⓓ	44. ⓐⓑⓒⓓ	45. ⓐⓑⓒⓓ		

PHYSICS CHAPTERWISE SPEED TEST-9

Total Questions	45	Total Marks	180
Attempted		Correct	
Incorrect		Net Score	
Cut-off Score	45	Qualifying Score	60
Success Gap = Net Score – Qualifying Score			
Net Score = (Correct × 4) – (Incorrect × 1)			

Space for Rough Work

PHYSICS

Thermal Properties of Matter

Speed TEST 10

Chapter-wise

No. of Questions	Maximum Marks	Time
45	180	1 Hour

GENERAL INSTRUCTIONS

- This test contains 45 MCQ's. For each question only one option is correct. Darken the correct circle/ bubble in the Response Grid provided on each page.
- You have to evaluate your Response Grids yourself with the help of solutions provided at the end of this book.
- Each correct answer will get you 4 marks and 1 mark shall be deduced for each incorrect answer. No mark will be given/ deducted if no bubble is filled. Keep a timer in front of you and stop immediately at the end of 60 min.
- The sheet follows a particular syllabus. Do not attempt the sheet before you have completed your preparation for that syllabus.
- After completing the sheet check your answers with the solution booklet and complete the Result Grid. Finally spend time to analyse your performance and revise the areas which emerge out as weak in your evaluation.

1. The total radiant energy per unit area, normal to the direction of incidence, received at a distance R from the centre of a star of radius r, whose outer surface radiates as a black body at a temperature T K is given by: (σ is Stefan's constant)

   (a) $\frac{\sigma r^2 T^4}{R^2}$ (b) $\frac{\sigma r^2 T^4}{4\pi r^2}$

   (c) $\frac{\sigma r^4 T^4}{r^4}$ (d) $\frac{4\pi\sigma r^2 T^4}{R^2}$

2. Three rods of same dimensions are arranged as shown in figure, have thermal conductivities K_1, K_2 and K_3. The points P and Q are maintained at different temeratures for the heat to flow at the same rate along PRQ and PQ. Then which of the following option is correct?

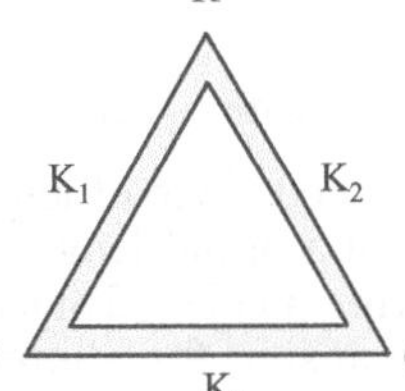

   (a) $K_3 = \frac{1}{2}(K_1 + K_2)$
   (b) $K_3 = K_1 + K_2$
   (c) $K_3 = \frac{K_1 K_2}{K_1 + K_2}$
   (d) $K_3 = -2(K_1 + K_2)$

3. The sprinkling of water slightly reduces the temperature of a closed room because
   (a) temperature of water is less than that of the room
   (b) specific heat of water is high
   (c) water has large latent heat of vaporisation
   (d) water is a bad conductor of heat

4. The value of molar heat capacity at constant temperature is
   (a) zero (b) infinity
   (c) unity (d) 4.2

5. The specific heat capacity of a metal at low temperature (T) is given as

$$C_p(kJK^{-1}kg^{-1}) = 32\left(\frac{T}{400}\right)^3$$

A 100 gram vessel of this metal is to be cooled from 20°K to 4°K by a special refrigerator operating at room temperature (27°C). The amount of work required to cool the vessel is
   (a) greater than 0.148 kJ
   (b) between 0.148 kJ and 0.028 kJ
   (c) less than 0.028 kJ
   (d) equal to 0.002 kJ

RESPONSE GRID	1. ⓐⓑⓒⓓ	2. ⓐⓑⓒⓓ	3. ⓐⓑⓒⓓ	4. ⓐⓑⓒⓓ	5. ⓐⓑⓒⓓ 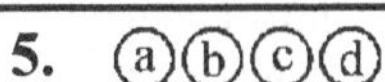

6. The emissive power of a black body at T = 300K is 100 Watt/m^2. Consider a body B of area A = $10m^2$ coefficient of reflectivity r = 0.3 and coefficient of transmission t = 0.5. Its temperature is 300K. Then which of the following is incorrect?
   (a) The emissive power of B is 20 W/m^2
   (b) The emissive power of B is 200 W/m^2
   (c) The power emitted by B is 200 Watts
   (d) The emissivity of B is 0.2

7. A solid cube and a solid sphere of the same material have equal surface area. Both are at the same temperture 120°C, then
   (a) both the cube and the sphere cool down at the same rate
   (b) the cube cools down faster than the sphere
   (c) the sphere cools down faster than the cube
   (d) whichever is having more mass will cool down faster

8. The density of water at 20°C is 998 kg/m^3 and at 40°C 992 kg/m^3. The coefficient of volume expansion of water is
   (a) 10^{-4}/°C (b) 3×10^{-4}/°C
   (c) 2×10^{-4}/°C (d) 6×10^{-4}/°C

9. A metallic rod ℓ cm long, A square cm in cross-section is heated through t°C. If Young's modulus of elasticity of the metal is E and the mean coefficient of linear expansion is α per degree celsius, then the compressional force required to prevent the rod from expanding along its length is
   (a) $EA\alpha t$ (b) $EA\alpha t/(1+\alpha t)$
   (c) $EA\alpha t/(1-\alpha t)$ (d) $E\ell\alpha t$

10. If liquefied oxygen at 1 atmospheric pressure is heated from 50 K to 300 K by supplying heat at constant rate. The graph of temperature vs time will be

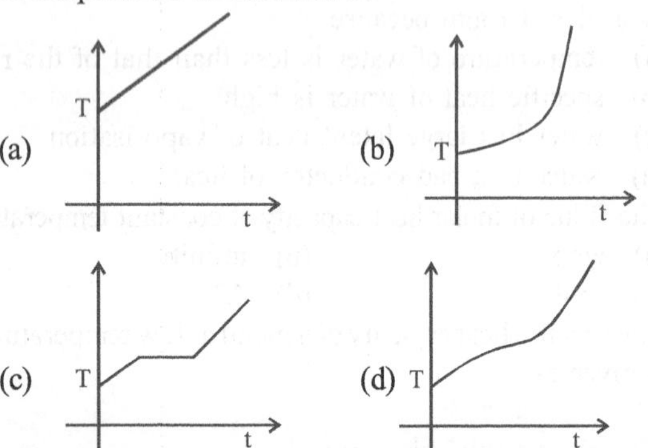

11. If a bar is made of copper whose coefficient of linear expansion is one and a half times that of iron, the ratio of force developed in the copper bar to the iron bar of identical lengths and cross-sections, when heated through the same temperature range (Young's modulus of copper may be taken to be equal to that of iron) is
   (a) 3/2 (b) 2/3 (c) 9/4 (d) 4/9

12. A piece of ice falls from a height h so that it melts completely. Only one-quarter of the heat produced is absorbed by the ice and all energy of ice gets converted into heat during its fall. The value of h is :
   [Latent heat of ice is 3.4×10^5 J/kg and g = 10 N/kg]
   (a) 34 km (b) 544 km (c) 136 km (d) 68 km

13. A body of mass 5 kg falls from a height of 20 metres on the ground and it rebounds to a height of 0.2 m. If the loss in potential energy is used up by the body, then what will be the temperature rise?
   (specific heat of material = 0.09 cal gm^{-1} °C^{-1})
   (a) 0°C (b) 4°C (c) 8°C (d) None of these

14. Two straight metallic strips each of thickness t and length ℓ are rivetted together. Their coefficients of linear expansions are α_1 and α_2. If they are heated through temperature ΔT, the bimetallic strip will bend to form an arc of radius
   (a) $t/\{\alpha_1+\alpha_2)\Delta T\}$ (b) $t/\{(\alpha_2-\alpha_1)\Delta T\}$
   (c) $t(\alpha_1-\alpha_2)\Delta T$ (d) $t(\alpha_2-\alpha_1)\Delta T$

15. The figure shows a system of two concentric spheres of radii r_1 and r_2 are kept at temperatures T_1 and T_2, respectively. The radial rate of flow of heat in a substance between the two concentric spheres is proportional to

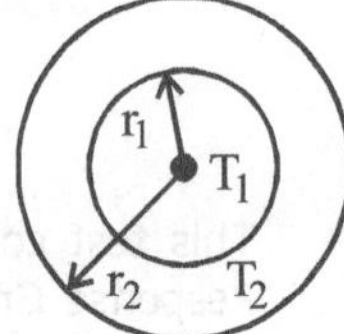

   (a) $\ell n\left(\frac{r_2}{r_1}\right)$ (b) $\frac{(r_2-r_1)}{(r_1 r_2)}$
   (c) (r_2-r_1) (d) $\frac{r_1 r_2}{(r_2-r_1)}$

16. A block of steel heated to 100°C is left in a room to cool. Which of the curves shown in fig., represents the correct behaviour?

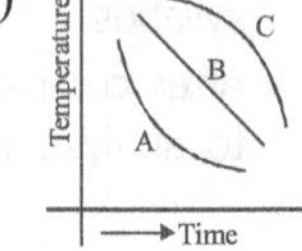

   (a) A (b) B (c) C (d) None of these

17. Which of the following will expand the most for same rise in temperature?
   (a) Aluminium (b) Glass
   (c) Wood (d) All will expand same

18. The plots of intensity versus wavelength for three black bodies at temperatures T_1, T_2 and T_3 respectively are as shown. Their temperature are such that

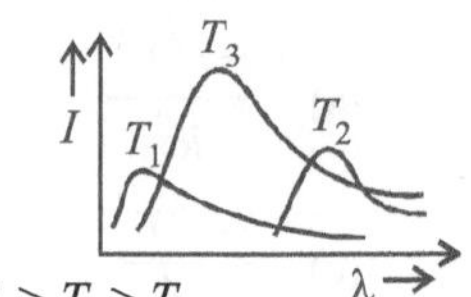

   (a) $T_1 > T_2 > T_3$ (b) $T_1 > T_3 > T_2$
   (c) $T_2 > T_3 > T_1$ (d) $T_3 > T_2 > T_1$

19. When the temperature of a rod increases from t to t + Δt, its moment of inertia increases from I to I + ΔI. If α be the coefficient of linear expansion of the rod, then the value of $\frac{\Delta I}{I}$ is
   (a) $2\alpha\Delta t$ (b) $\alpha\Delta T$ (c) $\frac{\alpha\Delta t}{2}$ (d) $\frac{\Delta t}{\alpha}$

20. Two rods, one of aluminum and the other made of steel, having initial length ℓ_1 and ℓ_2 are connected together to form a single rod of length $\ell_1+\ell_2$. The coefficients of linear expansion for aluminum and steel are α_a and α_s and respectively. If the length of each rod increases by the same amount when their temperature are raised by t°C, then find the ratio $\ell_1/(\ell_1+\ell_2)$
   (a) α_s/α_a (b) α_a/α_s (c) $\alpha_s/(\alpha_a+\alpha_s)$ (d) $\alpha_a/(\alpha_a+\alpha_s)$

RESPONSE GRID					
	6. ⓐⓑⓒⓓ	7. ⓐⓑⓒⓓ	8. ⓐⓑⓒⓓ	9. ⓐⓑⓒⓓ	10. ⓐⓑⓒⓓ
	11. ⓐⓑⓒⓓ	12. ⓐⓑⓒⓓ	13. ⓐⓑⓒⓓ	14. ⓐⓑⓒⓓ	15. ⓐⓑⓒⓓ
	16. ⓐⓑⓒⓓ	17. ⓐⓑⓒⓓ	18. ⓐⓑⓒⓓ	19. ⓐⓑⓒⓓ	20. ⓐⓑⓒⓓ

Space for Rough Work

21. A polished metal plate with a rough black spot on it is heated to about 1400 K and quickly taken into a dark room. Which one of the following statements will be true?
(a) The spot will appear brighter than the plate
(b) The spot will appear darker than the plate
(c) The spot and plate will appear equally bright
(d) The spot and the plate will not be visible in the dark room

22. On observing light from three different stars P, Q and R, it was found that intensity of violet colour is maximum in the spectrum of P, the intensity of green colour is maximum in the spectrum of R and the intensity of red colour is maximum in the spectrum of Q. If T_P, T_Q and T_R are the respective absolute temperature of P, Q and R, then it can be concluded from the above observations that
(a) $T_P > T_R > T_Q$ (b) $T_P < T_R < T_Q$
(c) $T_P < T_Q < T_R$ (d) $T_P > T_Q > T_R$

23. A partition wall has two layers of different materials A and B in contact with each other. They have the same thickness but the thermal conductivity of layer A is twice that of layer B. At steady state the temperature difference across the layer B is 50 K, then the corresponding difference across the layer A is
(a) 50 K (b) 12.5 K (c) 25 K (d) 60 K

24. Which of the following statements is/are false about mode of heat transfer?
(a) In radiation, heat is transfered from one medium to another without affecting the intervening medium
(b) Radiation and convection are possible in vaccum while conduction requires material medium.
(c) Conduction is possible in solids while convection occurs in liquids and gases.
(d) All are correct

25. In a vertical U-tube containing a liquid, the two arms are maintained at different temperatures t_1 and t_2. The liquid columns in the two arms have heights l_1 and l_2 respectively. The coefficient of volume expansion of the liquid is equal to

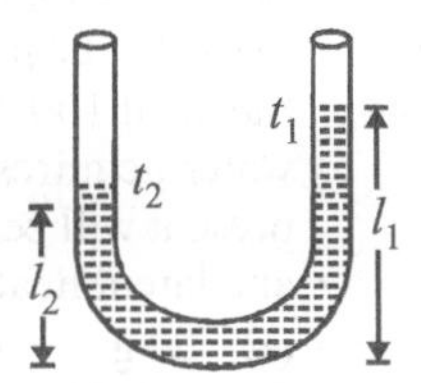

(a) $\frac{l_1 - l_2}{l_2 t_1 - l_1 t_2}$ (b) $\frac{l_1 - l_2}{l_1 t_1 - l_2 t_2}$ (c) $\frac{l_1 + l_2}{l_2 t_1 + l_1 t_2}$ (d) $\frac{l_1 + l_2}{l_1 t_1 + l_2 t_2}$

26. The top of an insulated cylindrical container is covered by a disc having emissivity 0.6 and conductivity 0.167 $WK^{-1}m^{-1}$ and thickness 1 cm. The temperature is maintained by circulating oil as shown in figure.
Find the radiation loss to the surrounding in $Jm^{-2}s^{-1}$ if temperature of the upper surface of the disc is 27°C and temperature of the surrounding is 27°C.

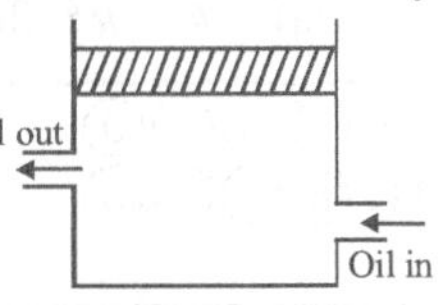

(a) 595 $Jm^{-2}s^{-1}$ (b) 545 $Jm^{-2}s^{-1}$
(c) 495 $Jm^{-2}s^{-1}$ (d) None of these

27. Wien's law is concerned with
(a) relation between emissivity and absorptivity of a radiating surface
(b) total radiation, emitted by a hot surface
(c) an expression for spectral distribution of energy of a radiation from any source
(d) a relation between the temperature of a black body and the wavelength at which there is maximum radiant energy per unit wavelength

28. If a piece of metal is heated to temperature θ and then allowed to cool in a room which is at temperature θ_0, the graph between the temperature T of the metal and time t will be closest to

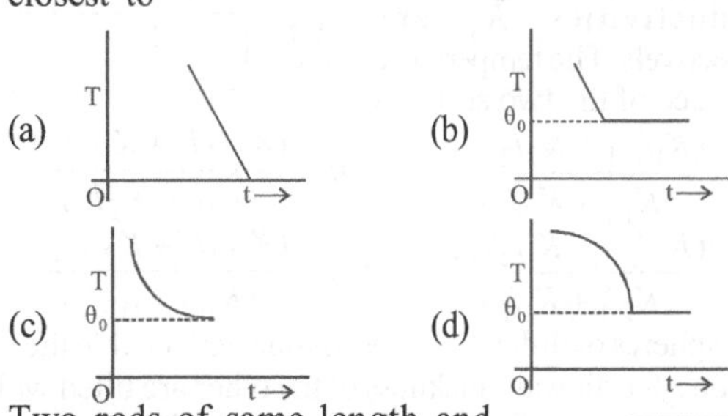

29. Two rods of same length and transfer a given amount of heat 12 second, when they are joined as shown in figure (i). But when they are joined as shwon in figure (ii), then they will transfer same heat in same conditions in

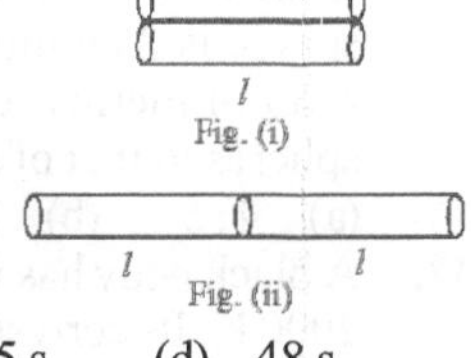

(a) 24 s (b) 13 s (c) 15 s (d) 48 s

30. Consider a compound slab consisting of two different materials having equal thicknesses and thermal conductivities *K* and 2*K*, respectively. The equivalent thermal conductivity of the slab is
(a) $\frac{4}{3}K$ (b) $\frac{2}{3}K$ (c) $\sqrt{3}\,K$ (d) $3K$

31. The coefficient of thermal conductivity of copper, mercury and glass are respectively K_c, K_m and K_g such that $K_c > K_m > K_g$. If the same quantity of heat is to flow per sec per unit area of each and corresponding temperature gradients are X_c, X_m and X_g then
(a) $X_c = X_m = X_g$ (b) $X_c > X_m > X_g$
(c) $X_c < X_m < X_g$ (d) $X_m < X_c < X_g$

32. The radiation energy density per unit wavelength at a temperature T has a maximum at a wavelength λ_0. At temperature 2T, it will have a maximum wavelength
(a) $4\lambda_0$ (b) $2\lambda_0$ (c) $\frac{\lambda_0}{2}$ (d) $\frac{\lambda_0}{4}$

33. Assuming the Sun to be a spherical body of radius *R* at a temperature of *TK*, evaluate the total radiant powerd incident of Earth at a distance *r* from the Sun
(a) $4\pi r_0^2 R^2 \sigma \frac{T^4}{r^2}$ (b) $\pi r_0^2 R^2 \sigma \frac{T^4}{r^2}$
(c) $r_0^2 R^2 \sigma \frac{T^4}{4\pi r^2}$ (d) $R^2 \sigma \frac{T^4}{r^2}$

RESPONSE GRID					
	21. ⓐⓑⓒⓓ	22. ⓐⓑⓒⓓ	23. ⓐⓑⓒⓓ	24. ⓐⓑⓒⓓ	25. ⓐⓑⓒⓓ
	26. ⓐⓑⓒⓓ	27. ⓐⓑⓒⓓ	28. ⓐⓑⓒⓓ	29. ⓐⓑⓒⓓ	30. ⓐⓑⓒⓓ
	31. ⓐⓑⓒⓓ	32. ⓐⓑⓒⓓ	33. ⓐⓑⓒⓓ		

Space for Rough Work

34. A metal ball immersed in alcohol weighs W_1 at 0°C and W_2 at 59°C. The coefficient of cubical expansion of the metal is less than that of alcohol. Assuming that the density of the metal is large compared to that of alcohol, it can be shown that

(a) $W_1 > W_2$ (b) $W_1 = W_2$
(c) $W_1 < W_2$ (d) $W_1 = (W_2/2)$

35. One end of a thermally insulated rod is kept at a temperature T_1 and the other at T_2. The rod is composed of two sections of length l_1 and l_2 and thermal conductivities K_1 and K_2 respectively. The temperature at the interface of the two sections is

(a) $\dfrac{(K_1l_1T_1 + K_2l_2T_2)}{(K_1l_1 + K_2l_2)}$ (b) $\dfrac{(K_2l_2T_1 + K_1l_1T_2)}{(K_1l_1 + K_2l_2)}$

(c) $\dfrac{(K_2l_1T_1 + K_1l_2T_2)}{(K_2l_1 + K_1l_2)}$ (d) $\dfrac{(K_1l_2T_1 + K_2l_1T_2)}{(K_1l_2 + K_2l_1)}$

36. Two spheres of different materials one with double the radius and one-fourth wall thickness of the other are filled with ice. If the time taken for complete melting of ice in the larger sphere is 25 minute and for smaller one is 16 minute, the ratio of thermal conductivities of the materials of larger spheres to that of smaller sphere is

(a) 4 : 5 (b) 5 : 4 (c) 25 : 8 (d) 8 : 25

37. A black body has maximum wavelength λ_m at temperature 2000 K. Its corresponding wavelength at temperature 3000 K will be

(a) $\frac{3}{2}\lambda_m$ (b) $\frac{2}{3}\lambda_m$ (c) $\frac{4}{9}\lambda_m$ (d) $\frac{9}{4}\lambda_m$

38. A solid material is supplied with heat at constant rate and the temperature of the material changes as shown. From the graph, the FALSE conclusion drawn is

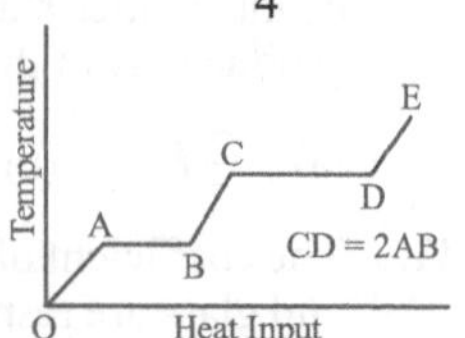

(a) AB and CD of the graph represent phase changes
(b) AB represents the change of state from solid to liquid
(c) latent heat of fusion is twice the latent heat of vaporization
(d) CD represents change of state from liquid to vapour

39. 10 gm of ice cubes at 0°C are released in a tumbler (water equivalent 55 g) at 40°C. Assuming that negligible heat is taken from the surroundings, the temperature of water in the tumbler becomes nearly (L = 80 cal/g)

(a) 31°C (b) 22°C (c) 19°C (d) 15°C

40. In a surrounding medium of temperature 10°C, a body takes 7 min for a fall of temperature from 60°C to 40°C. In what time the temperature of the body will fall from 40°C to 28°C?

(a) 7 min (b) 11 min (c) 14 min (d) 21 min

41. Two rods of same length and area of cross-section A_1 and A_2 have their ends at the same temperature. If K_1 and K_2 are their thermal conductivities, c_1 and c_2 are their specific heats and d_1 and d_2 are their densities, then the rate of flow of heat is the same in both the rods if

(a) $\dfrac{A_1}{A_2} = \dfrac{-k_1}{k_2}$ (b) $\dfrac{A_1}{A_2} = \dfrac{k_1c_1d_1}{k_2c_2d_2}$

(c) $\dfrac{A_1}{A_2} = \dfrac{k_2c_1d_1}{c_2d_2k_1}$ (d) $\dfrac{A_1}{A_2} = \dfrac{k_2}{k_1}$

42. A student takes 50gm wax (specific heat = 0.6 kcal/kg°C) and heats it till it boils. The graph between temperature and time is as follows. Heat supplied to the wax per minute and boiling point are respectively

(a) 500 cal, 50°C (b) 1000 cal, 100°C
(c) 1500 cal, 200°C (d) 1000 cal, 200°C

43. Consider two identical iron spheres, one which lie on a thermally insulating plate, while the other hangs from an insulatory thread. Equal amount of heat is supplied to the two spheres, then

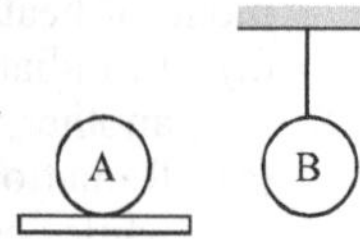

(a) temperature of A will be greater than B
(b) temperature of B will be greater than A
(c) their temperature will be equal
(d) can't be predicted

44. Steam at 100°C is passed into 20 g of water at 10°C. When water acquires a temperature of 80°C, the mass of water present will be: [Take specific heat of water = 1 cal g^{-1} °C^{-1} and latent heat of steam = 540 cal g^{-1}]

(a) 24 g (b) 31.5 g (c) 42.5 g (d) 22.5 g

45. Two solid spheres, of radii R_1 and R_2 are made of the same material and have similar surfaces. The spheres are raised to the same temperature and then allowed to cool under identical conditions. Assuming spheres to be perfect conductors of heat, their initial rates of loss of heat are

(a) R_1^2 / R_2^2 (b) R_1 / R_2 (c) R_2 / R_1 (d) R_2^2 / R_1^2

RESPONSE GRID					
	34. ⓐⓑⓒⓓ	35. ⓐⓑⓒⓓ	36. ⓐⓑⓒⓓ	37. ⓐⓑⓒⓓ	38. ⓐⓑⓒⓓ
	39. ⓐⓑⓒⓓ	40. ⓐⓑⓒⓓ	41. ⓐⓑⓒⓓ	42. ⓐⓑⓒⓓ	43. ⓐⓑⓒⓓ
	44. ⓐⓑⓒⓓ	45. ⓐⓑⓒⓓ			

PHYSICS CHAPTERWISE SPEED TEST-10

Total Questions	45	Total Marks	180
Attempted		Correct	
Incorrect		Net Score	
Cut-off Score	45	Qualifying Score	60
Success Gap = Net Score – Qualifying Score			
Net Score = (Correct × 4) – (Incorrect × 1)			

Space for Rough Work

PHYSICS

Thermodynamics

Speed TEST 11

Chapter-wise

No. of Questions	Maximum Marks	Time
45	180	1 Hour

GENERAL INSTRUCTIONS

- This test contains 45 MCQ's. For each question only one option is correct. Darken the correct circle/ bubble in the Response Grid provided on each page.
- You have to evaluate your Response Grids yourself with the help of solutions provided at the end of this book.
- Each correct answer will get you 4 marks and 1 mark shall be deduced for each incorrect answer. No mark will be given/ deducted if no bubble is filled. Keep a timer in front of you and stop immediately at the end of 60 min.
- The sheet follows a particular syllabus. Do not attempt the sheet before you have completed your preparation for that syllabus.
- After completing the sheet check your answers with the solution booklet and complete the Result Grid. Finally spend time to analyse your performance and revise the areas which emerge out as weak in your evaluation.

1. The relation between U, P and V for an ideal gas in an adiabatic process is given by relation $U = a + bPV$. Find the value of adiabatic exponent (γ) of this gas

(a) $\frac{b+1}{b}$ (b) $\frac{b+1}{a}$ (c) $\frac{a+1}{b}$ (d) $\frac{a}{a+b}$

2. Carbon monoxide is carried around a closed cycle abc in which bc is an isothermal process as shown in the figure. The gas absorbs 7000 J of heat as its temperture increases from 300 K to 1000 K in going from a to b. The quantity of heat rejected by the gas during the process ca is

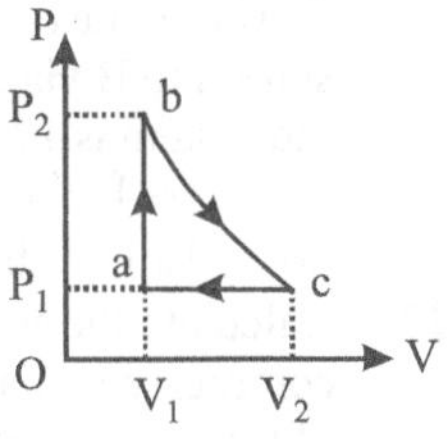

(a) 4200 J (b) 5000 J (c) 9000 J (d) 9800 J

3. A Carnot engine, having an efficiency of $\eta = 1/10$ as heat engine, is used as a refrigerator. If the work done on the system is 10 J, the amount of energy absorbed from the reservoir at lower temperature is

(a) 100 J (b) 99 J (c) 90 J (d) 1 J

4. In a thermodynamic process, fixed mass of a gas is changed in such a manner that the gas release 20 J of heat and 8 J of work was done on the gas. If the initial internal energy of the gas was 30 J. Then the final internal energy will be

(a) 2 joule (b) 18 joule (c) 42 joule (d) 58 joule

5. A closed gas cylinder is divided into two parts by a piston held tight. The pressure and volume of gas in two parts respectively are (P, 5V) and (10P, V). If now the piston is left free and the system undergoes isothermal process, then the volumes of the gas in two parts respectively are

(a) 2V,4V (b) 3V,3V (c) 5V,V (d) $\frac{10}{11}V, \frac{20}{11}V$

6. The efficiency of an ideal gas with adiabatic exponent 'γ' for the shown cyclic process would be

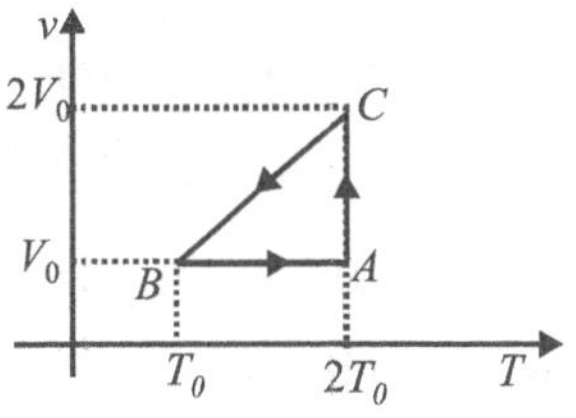

(a) $\frac{(2\ln 2-1)}{\gamma/(\gamma-1)}$

(b) $\frac{(1-2\ln 2)}{\gamma/(\gamma-1)}$

(c) $\frac{(2\ln 2+1)}{\gamma/(\gamma-1)}$

(d) $\frac{(2\ln 2-1)}{\gamma/(\gamma+1)}$

7. A mass of diatomic gas (γ = 1.4) at a pressure of 2 atmospheres is compressed adiabatically so that its temperature rises from 27°C to 927°C. The pressure of the gas in final state is

(a) 28 atm (b) 68.7 atm (c) 256 atm (d) 8 atm

RESPONSE GRID					
	1. ⓐⓑⓒⓓ	2. ⓐⓑⓒⓓ	3. ⓐⓑⓒⓓ	4. ⓐⓑⓒⓓ	5. ⓐⓑⓒⓓ
	6. ⓐⓑⓒⓓ	7. ⓐⓑⓒⓓ			

Space for Rough Work

8. A diatomic ideal gas is used in a Carnot engine as the working substance. If during the adiabatic expansion part of the cycle the volume of the gas increases from V to 32 V, the efficiency of the engine is
(a) 0.5 (b) 0.75 (c) 0.99 (d) 0.25

9. The P-V diagram of a gas system undergoing cyclic process is shown here. The work done during isobaric compression is

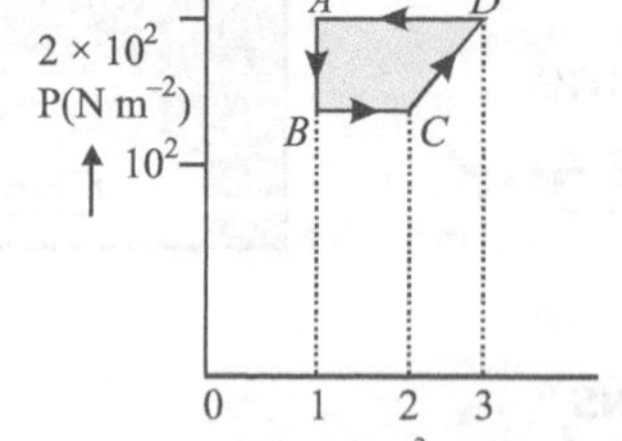

(a) 100 J
(b) 200 J
(c) 600 J
(d) 400 J

10. During an adiabatic process of an ideal gas, if P is proportional to $\frac{1}{V^{1.5}}$, then the ratio of specific heat capacities at constant pressure to that at constant volume for the gas is
(a) 1.5 (b) 0.25 (c) 0.75 (d) 0.4

11. The work of 146 kJ is performed in order to compress one kilo mole of gas adiabatically and in this process the temperature of the gas increases by 7°C. The gas is ($R = 8.3\ \text{J mol}^{-1}\text{K}^{-1}$)
(a) diatomic
(b) triatomic
(c) a mixture of monoatomic and diatomic
(d) monoatomic

12. Consider a spherical shell of radius R at temperature T. The black body radiation inside it can be considered as an ideal gas of photons with internal energy per unit volume $u = \frac{U}{V} \propto T^4$ and pressure $p = \frac{1}{3}\left(\frac{U}{V}\right)$. If the shell now undergoes an adiabatic expansion the relation between T and R is :
(a) $T \propto \frac{1}{R}$ (b) $T \propto \frac{1}{R^3}$ (c) $T \propto e^{-R}$ (d) $T \propto e^{-3R}$

13. The specific heat capacity of a metal at low temperature (T) is given as $C(\text{kJK}^{-1}\text{kg}^{-1}) = 32\left(\frac{T}{400}\right)^3$. A 100 g vessel of this metal is to be cooled from 20 K to 4 K by a special refrigerator operating at room temperature (27°C). The amount of work required to cool in vessel is
(a) equal to 0.002 kJ
(b) greater than 0.148 kJ
(c) between 0.148 kJ and 0.028 kJ
(d) less than 0.028 kJ

14. 5.6 litre of helium gas at STP is adiabatically compressed to 0.7 litre. Taking the initial temperature to be T_1, the work done in the process is
(a) $\frac{9}{8}RT_1$ (b) $\frac{3}{2}RT_1$ (c) $\frac{15}{8}RT_1$ (d) $\frac{9}{2}RT_1$

15. Four curves A, B, C and D are drawn in the figure for a given amount of a gas. The curves which represent adiabatic and isothermal changes are
(a) C and D respectively
(b) D and C respectively
(c) A and B respectively
(d) B and A respectively

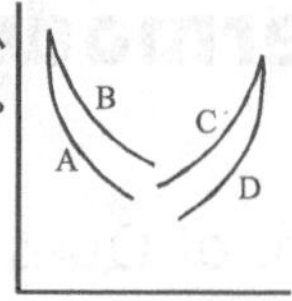

16. In an adiabatic process, the pressure is increased by $\frac{2}{3}\%$. If $\gamma = \frac{3}{2}$, then the volume decreases by nearly
(a) $\frac{4}{9}\%$ (b) $\frac{2}{3}\%$ (c) 1% (d) $\frac{9}{4}\%$

17. A reversible engine converts one-sixth of the heat input into work. When the temperature of the sink is reduced by 62°C, the efficiency of the engine is doubled. The temperatures of the source and sink are
(a) 99°C, 37°C (b) 80°C, 37°C
(c) 95°C, 37°C (d) 90°C, 37°C

18. A diatomic ideal gas is compressed adiabatically to $\frac{1}{32}$ of its initial volume. If the initial temperature of the gas is T_i (in Kelvin) and the final temperature is aT_i, the value of a is
(a) 8 (b) 4 (c) 3 (d) 5

19. When the state of a gas adiabatically changed from an equilibrium state A to another equilibrium state B an amount of work done on the stystem is 35 J. If the gas is taken from state A to B via process in which the net heat absorbed by the system is 12 cal, then the net work done by the system is (1 cal = 4.19 J)
(a) 13.2 J (b) 15.4 J (c) 12.6 J (d) 16.8 J

20. Calculate the work done when 1 mole of a perfect gas is compressed adiabatically. The initial pressure and volume of the gas are 10^5 N/m² and 6 litre respectively. The final volume of the gas is 2 litres. Molar specific heat of the gas at constant volume is 3R/2. [Given $(3)^{5/3} = 6.19$]
(a) –957 J (b) +957 J (c) – 805 J (d) + 805 J

21. A Carnot engine whose efficiency is 40%, receives heat at 500K. If the efficiency is to be 50%, the source temperature for the same exhaust temperature is
(a) 900 K (b) 600 K (c) 700 K (d) 800 K

22. 1 gm of water at a pressure of 1.01×10^5 Pa is converted into steam without any change of temperature. The volume of 1 g of steam is 1671 cc and the latent heat of evaporation is 540 cal. The change in internal energy due to evaporation of 1 gm of water is
(a) ≈ 167 cal (b) 500 cal (c) 540 cal (d) 581 cal

RESPONSE GRID					
	8. ⓐⓑⓒⓓ	9. ⓐⓑⓒⓓ	10. ⓐⓑⓒⓓ	11. ⓐⓑⓒⓓ	12. ⓐⓑⓒⓓ
	13. ⓐⓑⓒⓓ	14. ⓐⓑⓒⓓ	15. ⓐⓑⓒⓓ	16. ⓐⓑⓒⓓ	17. ⓐⓑⓒⓓ
	18. ⓐⓑⓒⓓ	19. ⓐⓑⓒⓓ	20. ⓐⓑⓒⓓ	21. ⓐⓑⓒⓓ	22. ⓐⓑⓒⓓ

Space for Rough Work

23. One mole of an ideal gas at temperature T was cooled isochorically till the gas pressure fell from P to $\frac{P}{n}$. Then, by an isobaric process, the gas was restored to the initial temperature. The net amount of heat absorbed by the gas in the process is

(a) nRT (b) $\frac{RT}{n}$

(c) $RT(1-n^{-1})$ (d) $RT(n-1)$

24. A Carnot engine, having an efficiency of $\eta = \frac{1}{10}$ as heat engine, is used as a refrigerator. If the work done on the system is 10 J, the amount of energy absorbed from the reservoir at lower temperature is

(a) 99 J (b) 90 J (c) 1 J (d) 100 J

25. The volume of an ideal gas is 1 litre and its pressure is equal to 72 cm of mercury column. The volume of gas is made 900 cm^3 by compressing it isothermally. The stress of the gas will be

(a) 8 cm of Hg (b) 7 cm of Hg
(c) 6 cm of Hg (d) 4 cm of Hg

26. An ideal gas is taken through the cycle $A \rightarrow B \rightarrow C \rightarrow A$, as shown in figure. If the net heat supplied to the gas in the cycle is 5 J, the work done by the gas in the process $C \rightarrow A$ is

(a) -5 J

(b) -10 J

(c) -15 J

(d) -20 J

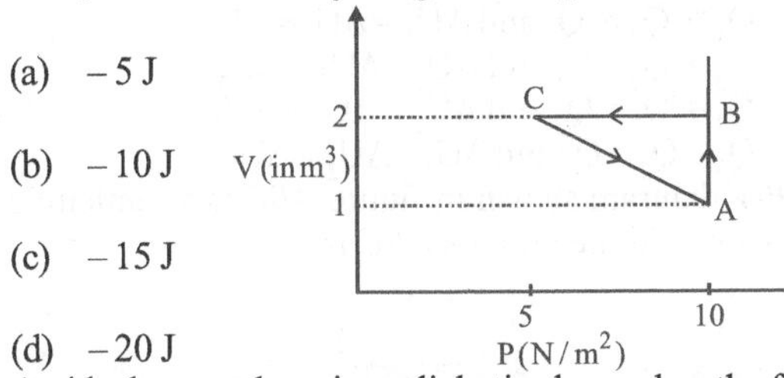

27. An ideal gas undergoing adiabatic change has the following pressure-temperature relationship

(a) $P^{\gamma-1}T^{\gamma}$ = constant (b) $P^{\gamma}T^{\gamma-1}$ = constant
(c) $P^{\gamma}T^{1-\gamma}$ = constant (d) $P^{1-\gamma}T^{\gamma}$ = constant

28. In a thermodynamic process, fixed mass of a gas is changed in such a manner that the gas release 20 J of heat and 8 J of work was done on the gas. If the initial internal energy of the gas was 30 J, the final internal energy will be

(a) 2 joule (b) 18 joule (c) 42 joule (d) 58 joule

29. The coefficient of performance of a refrigerator is 5. If the inside temperature of freezer is –20°C, then the temperature of the surroundings to which it rejects heat is

(a) 41°C (b) 11°C (c) 21°C (d) 31°C

30. Monatomic, diatomic and polyatomic ideal gases each undergo slow adiabatic expansions from the same initial volume and same initial pressure to the same final volume. The magnitude of the work done by the environment on the gas is

(a) the greatest for the polyatomic gas
(b) the greatest for the monatomic gas
(c) the greatest for the diatomic gas
(d) the question is irrelevant, there is no meaning of slow adiabatic expansion

31. The given p-v diagram represents the thermodynamic cycle of an engine, operating with an ideal monatomic gas. The amount of heat, extracted from the source in a single cycle is

(a) p_0v_0

(b) $\left(\frac{13}{2}\right)p_0v_0$

(c) $\left(\frac{11}{2}\right)p_0v_0$

(d) $4p_0v_0$

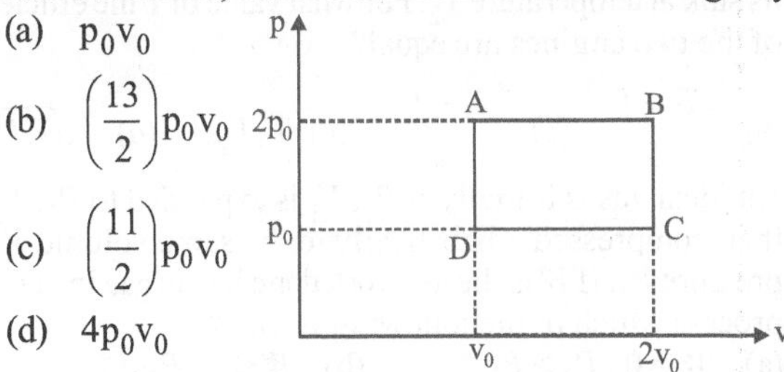

32. For an ideal gas graph is shown for three processes. Process 1, 2 and 3 are respectively.

(a) Isobaric, adiabatic, isochoric
(b) Adiabatic, isobaric, isochoric
(c) Isochoric, adiabatic, isobaric
(d) Isochoric, isobaric, adiabatic

Work done (magnitude) — graph with lines 3, 2, 1 — ΔT Temperature change

33. During an adiabatic process an object does 100J of work and its temperature decreases by 5K. During another process it does 25J of work and its temperature decreases by 5K. Its heat capacity for 2nd process is

(a) 20 J/K (b) 24 J/K (c) 15 J/K (d) 100 J/K

34. A refrigerator works between 4°C and 30°C. It is required to remove 600 calories of heat every second in order to keep the temperature of the refrigerated space constant. The power required is: (Take 1 cal = 4.2 joule)

(a) 2.365 W (b) 23.65 W (c) 236.5 W (d) 2365 W

35. A perfect gas goes from a state A to another state B by absorbing 8×10^5 J of heat and doing 6.5×10^5 J of external work. It is now transferred between the same two states in another process in which it absorbs 10^5 J of heat. In the second process

(a) work done by gas is 10^5 J
(b) work done on gas is 10^5 J
(c) work done by gas is 0.5×10^5 J
(d) work done on the gas is 0.5×10^5 J

36. One mole of a diatomic ideal gas undergoes a cyclic process ABC as shown in figure. The process BC is adiabatic. The temperatures at A, B and C are 400 K, 800 K and 600 K respectively. Choose the correct statement:

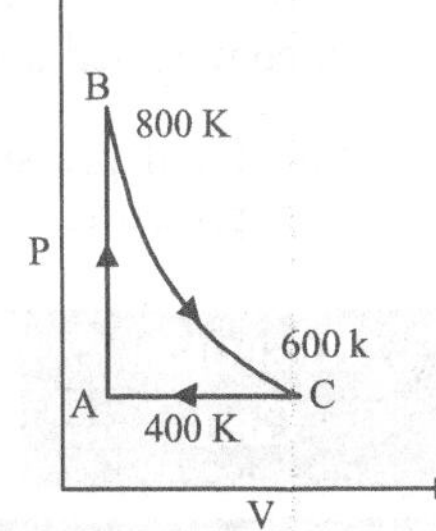

(a) The change in internal energy in whole cyclic process is 250 R.
(b) The change in internal energy in the process CA is 700 R.
(c) The change in internal energy in the process AB is -350 R.
(d) The change in internal energy in the process BC is – 500 R.

RESPONSE GRID					
	23. ⓐⓑⓒⓓ	24. ⓐⓑⓒⓓ	25. ⓐⓑⓒⓓ	26. ⓐⓑⓒⓓ	27. ⓐⓑⓒⓓ
	28. ⓐⓑⓒⓓ	29. ⓐⓑⓒⓓ	30. ⓐⓑⓒⓓ	31. ⓐⓑⓒⓓ	32. ⓐⓑⓒⓓ
	33. ⓐⓑⓒⓓ	34. ⓐⓑⓒⓓ	35. ⓐⓑⓒⓓ	36. ⓐⓑⓒⓓ	

Space for Rough Work

37. Two Carnot engines A and B are operated in series. The engine A receives heat from the source at temperature T_1 and rejects the heat to the sink at temperature T. The second engine B receives the heat at temperature T and rejects to its sink at temperature T_2. For what value of T the efficiencies of the two engines are equal?

(a) $\frac{T_1+T_2}{2}$ (b) $\frac{T_1-T_2}{2}$ (c) T_1T_2 (d) $\sqrt{T_1T_2}$

38. An ideal gas is initially at P_1, V_1 is expanded to P_2, V_2 and then compressed adiabatically to the same volume V_1 and pressure P_3. If W is the net work done by the gas in complete process which of the following is true ?

(a) $W>0; P_3>P_1$ (b) $W<0; P_3>P_1$
(c) $W>0; P_3<P_1$ (d) $W<0; P_3<P_1$

39. Which of the following statements is correct for any thermodynamic system ?

(a) The change in entropy can never be zero
(b) Internal energy and entropy are state functions
(c) The internal energy changes in all processes
(d) The work done in an adiabatic process is always zero.

40. One mole of an ideal gas goes from an initial state A to final state B via two processes : It first undergoes isothermal expansion from volume V to 3V and then its volume is reduced from 3V to V at constant pressure. The correct P-V diagram representing the two processes is :

(a) 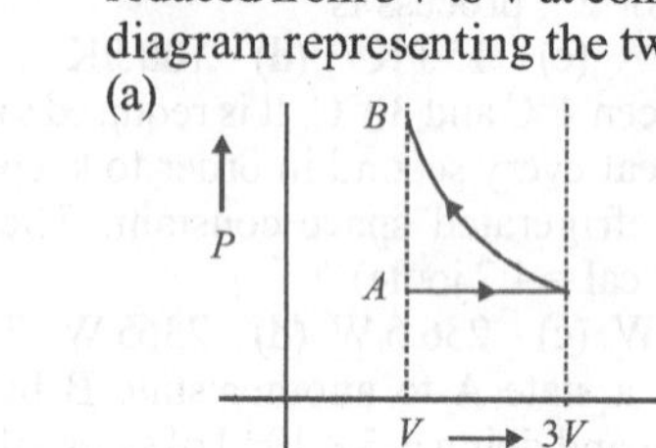

(b) 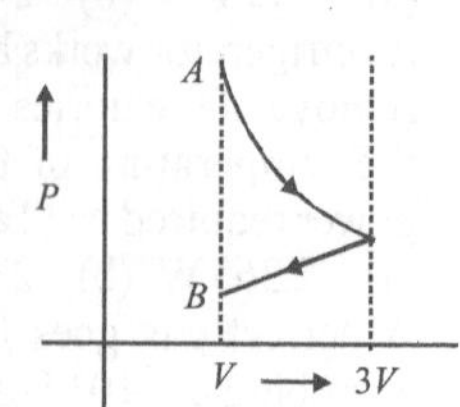

(c) 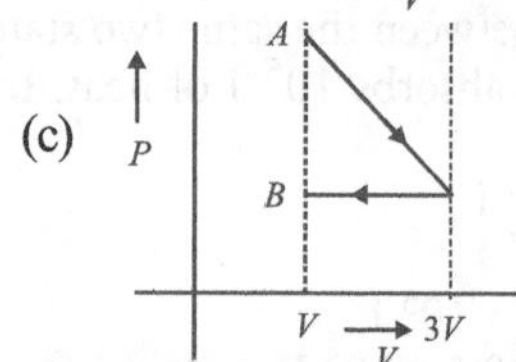

(d) 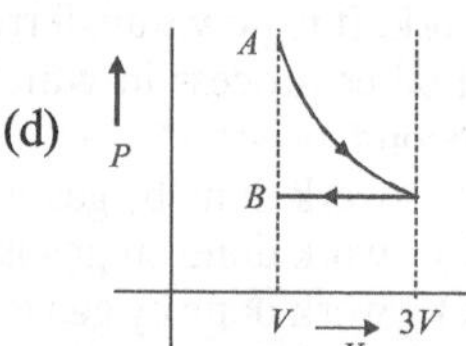

41. What will be the final pressure if an ideal gas in a cylinder is compressed adiabatically to $\frac{1}{3}$rd of its volume?

(a) Final pressure will be three times less than initial pressure.
(b) Final pressure will be three times more than initial pressure.
(c) Change in pressure will be more than three times the initial pressure.
(d) Change in pressure will be less than three times the initial pressure.

42. A gas is compressed isothermally to half its initial volume. The same gas is compressed separately through an adiabatic process until its volume is again reduced to half. Then :

(a) Compressing the gas isothermally will require more work to be done.
(b) Compressing the gas through adiabatic process will require more work to be done.
(c) Compressing the gas isothermally or adiabatically will require the same amount of work.
(d) Which of the case (whether compression through isothermal or through adiabatic process) requires more work will depend upon the atomicity of the gas.

43. An ideal gas goes from state A to state B via three different processes as indicated in the P-V diagram : If Q_1, Q_2, Q_3 indicate the heat a absorbed by the gas along the three processes and ΔU_1, ΔU_2, ΔU_3 indicate the change in internal energy along the three processes respectively, then

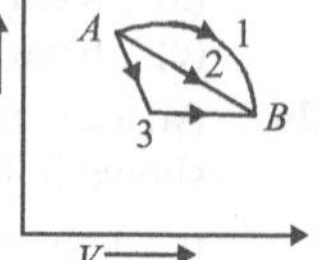

(a) $Q_1 > Q_2 > Q_3$ and $\Delta U_1 = \Delta U_2 = \Delta U_3$
(b) $Q_3 > Q_2 > Q_1$ and $\Delta U_1 = \Delta U_2 = \Delta U_3$
(c) $Q_1 = Q_2 = Q_3$ and $\Delta U_1 > \Delta U_2 > \Delta U_3$
(d) $Q_3 > Q_2 > Q_1$ and $\Delta U_1 > \Delta U_2 > \Delta U_3$

44. In *P-V* diagram shown in figure *ABC* is a semicircle. The work done in the process *ABC* is

(a) 4 J

(b) $\frac{-\pi}{2}$J 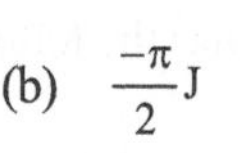

(c) $\frac{\pi}{2}$J

(d) zero

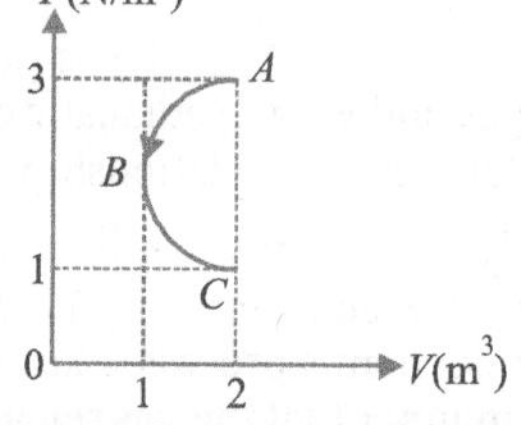

45. For an isothermal expansion of a perfect gas, the value of $\frac{\Delta P}{P}$ is equal to

(a) $-\gamma^{1/2}\frac{\Delta V}{V}$ (b) $-\frac{\Delta V}{V}$ (c) $-\gamma\frac{\Delta V}{V}$ (d) $-\gamma^2\frac{\Delta V}{V}$

RESPONSE GRID					
	37. ⓐⓑⓒⓓ	38. ⓐⓑⓒⓓ	39. ⓐⓑⓒⓓ	40. ⓐⓑⓒⓓ	41. ⓐⓑⓒⓓ
	42. ⓐⓑⓒⓓ	43. ⓐⓑⓒⓓ	44. ⓐⓑⓒⓓ	45. ⓐⓑⓒⓓ	

PHYSICS CHAPTERWISE SPEED TEST-11			
Total Questions	45	Total Marks	180
Attempted		Correct	
Incorrect		Net Score	
Cut-off Score	45	Qualifying Score	60
Success Gap = Net Score – Qualifying Score			
Net Score = (Correct × 4) – (Incorrect × 1)			

Space for Rough Work

PHYSICS

Kinetic Theory

Speed TEST 12

Chapter-wise

No. of Questions	Maximum Marks	Time
45	180	1 Hour

GENERAL INSTRUCTIONS

- This test contains 45 MCQ's. For each question only one option is correct. Darken the correct circle/ bubble in the Response Grid provided on each page.
- You have to evaluate your Response Grids yourself with the help of solutions provided at the end of this book.
- Each correct answer will get you 4 marks and 1 mark shall be deduced for each incorrect answer. No mark will be given/ deducted if no bubble is filled. Keep a timer in front of you and stop immediately at the end of 60 min.
- The sheet follows a particular syllabus. Do not attempt the sheet before you have completed your preparation for that syllabus.
- After completing the sheet check your answers with the solution booklet and complete the Result Grid. Finally spend time to analyse your performance and revise the areas which emerge out as weak in your evaluation.

1. 4.0 g of a gas occupies 22.4 litres at NTP. The specific heat capacity of the gas at constant volume is $5.0 JK^{-1}$. If the speed of any quantity x in this gas at NTP is $952 ms^{-1}$, then the heat capacity at constant pressure is (Take gas constant $R = 8.3 JK^{-1} mol^{-1}$)

   (a) $7.5 JK^{-1} mol^{-1}$ (b) $7.0 JK^{-1} mol^{-1}$
   (c) $8.5 JK^{-1} mol^{-1}$ (d) $8.0 JK^{-1} mol^{-1}$

2. A fixed mass of gas at constant pressure occupies a volume V. The gas undergoes a rise in temperature so that the root mean square velocity of its molecules is doubled. The new volume will be

   (a) V/2 (b) $V/\sqrt{2}$ (c) 2V (d) 4V

3. A gaseous mixture consists of 16 g of helium and 16 g of oxygen. The ratio $\frac{C_p}{C_v}$ of the mixture is

   (a) 1.62 (b) 1.59 (c) 1.54 (d) 1.4

4. Air is pumped into an automobile tube upto a pressure of 200 kPa in the morning when the air temperature is 22°C. During the day, temperature rises to 42°C and the tube expands by 2%. The pressure of the air in the tube at this temperature, will be approximately

   (a) 212 kPa (b) 209 kPa (c) 206 kPa (d) 200 kPa

5. The rms speed of the particles of fume of mass 5×10^{-17} kg executing Brownian motion in air at N.T.P. is ($k = 1.38 \times 10^{-23}$ J/K)

   (a) 1.5 m/s (b) 3.0 m/s (c) 1.5 cm/s (d) 3 cm/s

6. One mole of an ideal monoatomic gas requires 207 J heat to raise the temperature by 10 K when heated at constant pressure. If the same gas is heated at constant volume to raise the temperature by the same 10 K, the heat required is [Given the gas constant R = 8.3 J/ mol. K]

   (a) 198.7 J (b) 29 J (c) 215.3 J (d) 124 J

RESPONSE GRID	
	1. ⓐⓑⓒⓓ 2. ⓐⓑⓒⓓ 3. ⓐⓑⓒⓓ 4. ⓐⓑⓒⓓ 5. ⓐⓑⓒⓓ
	6. ⓐⓑⓒⓓ

Space for Rough Work

7. Figure shows the variation in temperature (ΔT) with the amount of heat supplied (Q) in an isobaric process corresponding to a monoatomic (M), diatomic (D) and a polyatomic (P) gas. The initial state of all the gases are the same and the scales for the two axes coincide. Ignoring vibrational degrees of freedom, the lines *a*, *b* and *c* respectively correspond to

(a) P, M and D
(b) M, D and P
(c) P, D and M
(d) D, M and P

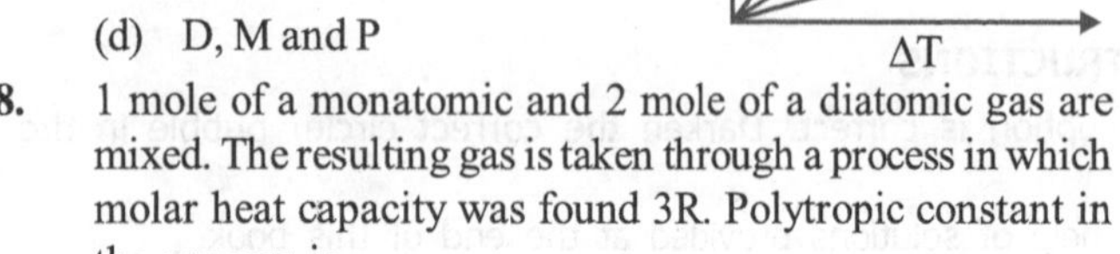

8. 1 mole of a monatomic and 2 mole of a diatomic gas are mixed. The resulting gas is taken through a process in which molar heat capacity was found 3R. Polytropic constant in the process is
(a) –1/5 (b) 1/5 (c) 2/5 (d) –2/5

9. The density of a gas is 6×10^{-2} kg/m^3 and the root mean square velocity of the gas molecules is 500 m/s. The pressure exerted by the gas on the walls of the vessel is
(a) 5×10^3 N/m^2 (b) 1.2×10^{-4} N/m^2
(c) 0.83×10^{-4} N/m^2 (d) 30 N/m^2

10. The absolute temperature of a gas is increases 3 times. The root mean square velocity of the moelcules will be
(a) 3 times (b) 9 times
(c) 1/3 times (d) √3 times

11 Consider an ideal gas confined in an isolated closed chamber. As the gas undergoes an adiabatic expansion, the average time of collision between molecules increases as V^q, where V is the volume of the gas. The value of q is : $\left(\gamma = \frac{C_p}{C_v}\right)$

(a) $\frac{\gamma+1}{2}$ (b) $\frac{\gamma-1}{2}$ (c) $\frac{3\gamma+5}{6}$ (d) $\frac{3\gamma-5}{6}$

12. One kg of a diatomic gas is at a pressure of 8×10^4 N/m^2. The density of the gas is 4kg/m^3. What is the energy of the gas due to its thermal motion?
(a) 5×10^4 J (b) 6×10^4 J
(c) 7×10^4 J (d) 3×10^4 J

13. A thermally insulated vessel contains an ideal gas of molecular mass *M* and ratio of specific heats γ. It is moving with speed *v* and it suddenly brought to rest. Assuming no heat is lost to the surroundings, its temperature increases by

(a) $\frac{(\gamma-1)}{2\gamma R}Mv^2 K$ (b) $\frac{\gamma Mv^2}{2R}K$

(c) $\frac{(\gamma-1)}{2R}Mv^2 K$ (d) $\frac{(\gamma-1)}{2(\gamma+1)R}Mv^2 K$

14. Figure shows a parabolic graph between T and 1/V for a mixture of a gases undergoing an adiabatic process. What is the ratio of V_{rms} of molecules and speed of sound in mixture?

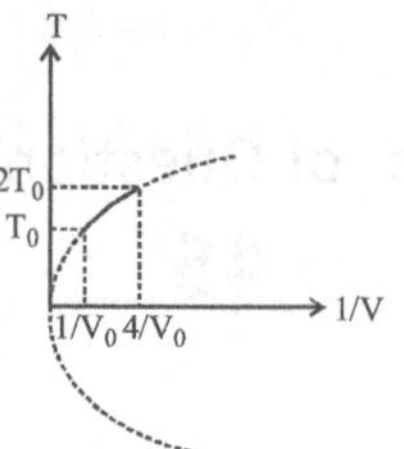

(a) $\sqrt{3/2}$
(b) $\sqrt{2}$
(c) $\sqrt{2/3}$
(d) $\sqrt{3}$

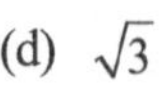

15. The work of 146 kJ is performed in order to compress one kilomole of gas adiabatically and in this process the temperature of the gas increases by 7°C. The gas is ($R = 8.3$ J mol^{-1} K^{-1})
(a) diatomic
(b) triatomic
(c) a mixture of monatomic and diatomic
(d) monatomic

16. At what temperature is root mean square velocity of gaseous hydrogen molecules equal to that of oxygen molecules at 47°C?
(a) 40K (b) 80K (c) –73K (d) 3K

17. The kinetic theory of gases states that the average squared velocity of molecules varies linearly with the mean molecular weight of the gas. If the root mean square (rms) velocity of oxygen molecules at a certain temperature is 0.5 km/sec. The rms velocity for hydrogen molecules at the same temperature will be :
(a) 2 km/sec (b) 4 km/sec (c) 8 km/sec (d) 16 km/sec

18. If 2 moles of an ideal monatomic gas at temperature T_0 is mixed with 4 moles of another ideal monatomic gas at temperature $2T_0$, then the temperature of the mixture is

(a) $\frac{5}{3}T_0$ (b) $\frac{3}{2}T_0$ (c) $\frac{4}{3}T_0$ (d) $\frac{5}{4}T_0$

19. From the following statements, concerning ideal gas at any given temperature *T*, select the incorrect one(s)
(a) The coefficient of volume expansion at constant pressure is same for all ideal gas
(b) The average translational kinetic energy per molecule of oxygen gas is 3 *KT* (*K* being Boltzmann constant)
(c) In a gaseous mixture, the average translational kinetic energy of the molecules of each component is same
(d) The mean free path of molecules increases with decrease in pressure

RESPONSE GRID					
	7. ⓐⓑⓒⓓ	8. ⓐⓑⓒⓓ	9. ⓐⓑⓒⓓ	10. ⓐⓑⓒⓓ	11. ⓐⓑⓒⓓ
	12. ⓐⓑⓒⓓ	13. ⓐⓑⓒⓓ	14. ⓐⓑⓒⓓ	15. ⓐⓑⓒⓓ	16. ⓐⓑⓒⓓ
	17. ⓐⓑⓒⓓ	18. ⓐⓑⓒⓓ	19. ⓐⓑⓒⓓ		

Space for Rough Work

20. The adjoining figure shows graph of pressure and volume of a gas at two tempertures T_1 and T_2. Which of the following inferences is correct?

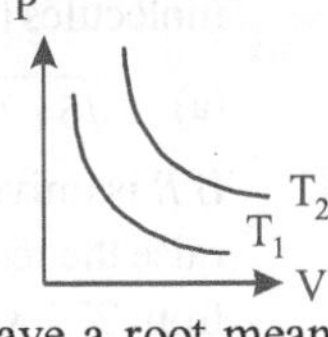

(a) $T_1 > T_2$
(b) $T_1 = T_2$
(c) $T_1 < T_2$
(d) None of these

21. The molecules of a given mass of gas have a root mean square velocity of 200m s^{-1} at 27°C and 1.0×10^5 N m^{-2} pressure. When the temperature is 127°C and the pressure 0.5×10^5 Nm^{-2}, the root mean square velocity in ms^{-1}, is

(a) $\frac{400}{\sqrt{3}}$ (b) $100\sqrt{2}$ (c) $\frac{100\sqrt{2}}{3}$ (d) $\frac{100}{3}$

22. A graph is plotted with PV/T on y-axis and mass of the gas along x-axis for different gases. The graph is

(a) a straight line parallel to x-axis for all the gases
(b) a straight line passing through origin with a slope having a constant value for all the gases
(c) a straight line passing through origin with a slope having different values for different gases
(d) a straight line parallel to y-axis for all the gases

23. At identical temperatures, the rms speed of hydrogen molecules is 4 times that for oxygen molecules. In a mixture of these in mass ratio $H_2 : O_2 = 1:8$, the rms speed of all molecules is n times the rms speed for O_2 molecules, where n is

(a) 3 (b) 4/3 (c) $(8/3)^{1/2}$ (d) $(11)^{1/2}$

24. Work done by a system under isothermal change from a volume V_1 to V_2 for a gases which obeys Vander Waal's equation $(V - \beta n)\left(P + \frac{\alpha n^2}{V}\right) = nRT$ is

(a) $nRT \log_e\left(\frac{V_2 - n\beta}{V_1 - n\beta}\right) + \alpha n^2\left(\frac{V_1 - V_2}{V_1V_2}\right)$

(b) $nRT \log_{10}\left(\frac{V_2 - n\beta}{V_1 - n\beta}\right) + \alpha n^2\left(\frac{V_1 - V_2}{V_1V_2}\right)$

(c) $nRT \log_e\left(\frac{V_2 - n\beta}{V_1 - n\beta}\right) + \beta n^2\left(\frac{V_1 - V_2}{V_1V_2}\right)$

(d) $nRT \log_e\left(\frac{V_1 - n\beta}{V_2 - n\beta}\right) + \alpha n^2\left(\frac{V_1V_2}{V_1 - V_2}\right)$

25. Two vessels separately contain two ideal gases A and B at the same temperature. The pressure of A being twice that of B. Under such conditions, the density of A is found to be 1.5 times the density of B. The ratio of molecular weight of A and B is :

(a) $\frac{3}{4}$ (b) 2 (c) $\frac{1}{2}$ (d) $\frac{2}{3}$

26. The temperature of the mixture of one mole of helium and one mole of hydrogen is increased from 0°C to 100°C at constant pressure. The amount of heat delivered will be

(a) 600 cal (b) 1200 cal (c) 1800 cal (d) 3600 cal

27. If the intermolecular forces vanish away, the volume occupied by the molecules contained in 4.5 g water at standard temperature and pressure will be

(a) 5.6 litre (b) 4.5 litre (c) 11.2 litre (d) 6.5 litre

28. A gas mixture consists of 2 moles of oxygen and 4 moles of Argon at temperature T. Neglecting all vibrational moles, the total internal energy of the system is

(a) 4 RT (b) 15 RT (c) 9 RT (d) 11RT

29. A vessel has 6g of hydrogen at pressure P and temperature 500K. A small hole is made in it so that hydrogen leaks out. How much hydrogen leaks out if the final pressure is P/2 and temperature falls to 300 K ?

(a) 2g (b) 3g (c) 4g (d) 1g

30. For a gas if ratio of specific heats at constant pressure and volume is γ then value of degrees of freedom is

(a) $\frac{3\gamma - 1}{2\gamma - 1}$ (b) $\frac{2}{\gamma - 1}$ (c) $\frac{9}{2}(\gamma - 1)$ (d) $\frac{25}{2}(\gamma - 1)$

31. The given *P-V* curve is predicted by

(a) Boyle's law
(b) Charle's law
(c) Avogadro's law
(d) Gaylussac's law

32. Three perfect gases at absolute temperatures T_1, T_2 and T_3 are mixed. The masses of molecules are m_1, m_2 and m_3 and the number of molecules are n_1, n_2 and n_3 respectively. Assuming no loss of energy, the final temperature of the mixture is :

(a) $\frac{n_1T_1 + n_2T_2 + n_3T_3}{n_1 + n_2 + n_3}$ (b) $\frac{n_1T_1^2 + n_2T_2^2 + n_3T_3^2}{n_1T_1 + n_2T_2 + n_3T_3}$

(c) $\frac{n_1^2T_1^2 + n_2^2T_2^2 + n_3^2T_3^2}{n_1T_1 + n_2T_2 + n_3T_3}$ (d) $\frac{(T_1 + T_2 + T_3)}{3}$

33. A gas is enclosed in a cube of side *l*. What will be the change in momentum of the molecule, if it suffers an elastic collision with the plane wall parallel to *yz*-plane and rebounds with the same velocity ? [(V_x, V_y & V_z) initial velocities of the gas molecules]

(a) mv_x (b) zero (c) $-mv_x$ (d) $-2mv_x$

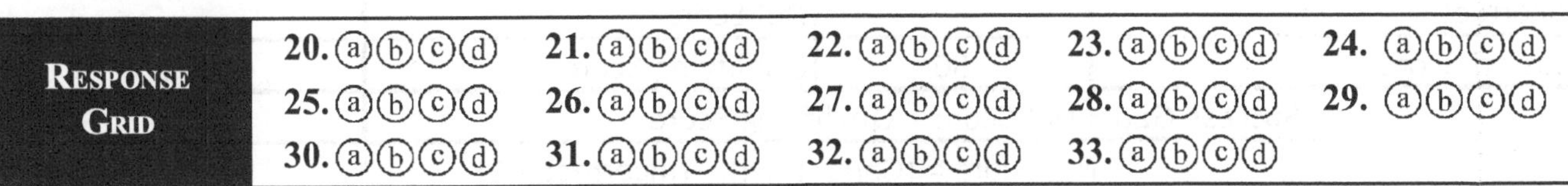

Space for Rough Work

34. What will be the ratio of number of molecules of a monoatomic and a diatomic gas in a vessel, if the ratio of their partial pressures is 5 : 3 ?

(a) 5 : 1 (b) 3 : 1 (c) 5 : 3 (d) 3 : 5

35. The average transitional energy and the rms speed of molecules in a sample of oxygen gas at 300 K are 6.21×10^{-21} J and 484 m/s respectively. The corresponding values at 600 K are nearly (assuming ideal gas behaviour)

(a) 12.42×10^{-21} J, 968 m/s (b) 8.78×10^{-21} J, 684 m/s
(c) 6.21×10^{-21} J, 968 m/s (d) 12.42×10^{-21} J, 684 m/s

36. At 10° C the value of the density of a fixed mass of an ideal gas divided by its pressure is x. At 110°C this ratio is:

(a) x (b) $\frac{383}{283}x$ (c) $\frac{10}{110}x$ (d) $\frac{283}{383}x$

37. If the potential energy of a gas molecule is $U = M/r^6 - N/r^{12}$, M and N being positive constants. Then the potential energy at equilibrium must be

(a) zero (b) $M^2/4N$ (c) $N^2/4M$ (d) $MN^2/4$

38. Consider a gas with density ρ and $\overline{c}$ as the root mean square velocity of its molecules contained in a volume. If the system moves as whole with velocity v, then the pressure exerted by the gas is

(a) $\frac{1}{3}\rho\overline{c}^2$ (b) $\frac{1}{3}\rho(c+v)^2$

(c) $\frac{1}{3}\rho(\overline{c}-v)^2$ (d) $\frac{1}{3}\rho(c^{-2}-v)^2$

39. How is the mean free path (λ) in a gas related to the interatomic distance?

(a) λ is 10 times the interatomic distance
(b) λ is 100 times the interatomic distance
(c) λ is 1000 times the interatomic distance
(d) λ is $\frac{1}{10}$ times of the interatomic distance

40. Four molecules have speeds 2 km/sec, 3 km/sec, 4 km/sec and 5 km/sec. The root mean square speed of these molecules (in km/sec) is

(a) $\sqrt{54/4}$ (b) $\sqrt{54/2}$ (c) 3.5 (d) $3\sqrt{3}$

41. If R is universal gas constant, the amount of heat needed to raise the temperature of 2 moles of an ideal monoatomic gas from 273 K to 373 K, when no work is done, is

(a) $100R$ (b) $150R$ (c) $300R$ (d) $500R$

42. N molecules, each of mass m, of gas A and 2 N molecules, each of mass 2 m, of gas B are contained in the same vessel which is maintained at a temperature T. The mean square velocity of molecules of B type is denoted by V_2 and the mean square velocity of A type is denoted by V_1, then $\frac{V_1}{V_2}$ is

(a) 2 (b) 1 (c) 1/3 (d) 2/3

43. The root mean square value of the speed of the molecules in a fixed mass of an ideal gas is increased by increasing

(a) the volume while keeping the temperature constant
(b) the pressure while keeping the volume constant
(c) the temperature while keeping the pressure constant
(d) the pressure while keeping the temperature constant

44. The P-V diagram of a diatomic gas is a straight line passing through origin. The molar heat capacity of the gas in the process will be

(a) 4R (b) 2.5R (c) 3R (d) $\frac{4R}{3}$

45. For a gas, difference between two specific heats is 5000 J/mole°C. If the ratio of specific heats is 1.6, the two specific heats in J/mole-°C are

(a) $C_P = 1.33 \times 10^4$, $C_V = 2.66 \times 10^4$
(b) $C_P = 13.3 \times 10^4$, $C_V = 8.33 \times 10^3$
(c) $C_P = 1.33 \times 10^4$, $C_V = 8.33 \times 10^3$
(d) $C_P = 2.6 \times 10^4$, $C_V = 8.33 \times 10^4$

RESPONSE GRID					
	34. ⓐⓑⓒⓓ	35. ⓐⓑⓒⓓ	36. ⓐⓑⓒⓓ	37. ⓐⓑⓒⓓ	38. ⓐⓑⓒⓓ
	39. ⓐⓑⓒⓓ	40. ⓐⓑⓒⓓ	41. ⓐⓑⓒⓓ	42. ⓐⓑⓒⓓ	43. ⓐⓑⓒⓓ
	44. ⓐⓑⓒⓓ	45. ⓐⓑⓒⓓ			

PHYSICS CHAPTERWISE SPEED TEST-12

Total Questions	45	Total Marks	180
Attempted		Correct	
Incorrect		Net Score	
Cut-off Score	50	Qualifying Score	70
Success Gap = Net Score – Qualifying Score			
Net Score = (Correct × 4) – (Incorrect × 1)			

Space for Rough Work

PHYSICS

Oscillations

Speed TEST 13 Chapter-wise

No. of Questions	Maximum Marks	Time
45	180	1 Hour

GENERAL INSTRUCTIONS

- This test contains 45 MCQ's. For each question only one option is correct. Darken the correct circle/ bubble in the Response Grid provided on each page.
- You have to evaluate your Response Grids yourself with the help of solutions provided at the end of this book.
- Each correct answer will get you 4 marks and 1 mark shall be deduced for each incorrect answer. No mark will be given/ deducted if no bubble is filled. Keep a timer in front of you and stop immediately at the end of 60 min.
- The sheet follows a particular syllabus. Do not attempt the sheet before you have completed your preparation for that syllabus.
- After completing the sheet check your answers with the solution booklet and complete the Result Grid. Finally spend time to analyse your performance and revise the areas which emerge out as weak in your evaluation.

1. If x, v and a denote the displacement, the velocity and the acceleration of a particle executing simple harmonic motion of time period T, then, which of the following does not change with time?
   (a) aT/x (b) $aT + 2\pi v$
   (c) aT/v (d) $a^2T^2 + 4\pi^2v^2$

2. A mass is suspended separately by two different springs in successive order, then time periods is t_1 and t_2 respectively. It is connected by both springs as shown in fig. then time period is t_0. The correct relation is

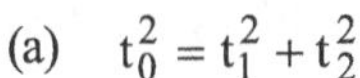

   (a) $t_0^2 = t_1^2 + t_2^2$
   (b) $t_0^{-2} = t_1^{-2} + t_2^{-2}$
   (c) $t_0^{-1} = t_1^{-1} + t_2^{-1}$
   (d) $t_0 = t_1 + t_2$

3. A rod of length ℓ is in motion such that its ends A and B are moving along x-axis and y-axis respectively. It is given that $\frac{d\theta}{dt} = 2$ rad/sec always. P is a fixed point on the rod. Let M be the projection of P on x-axis. For the time interval in which θ changes from 0 to $\frac{\pi}{2}$, the correct statement is
   (a) The acceleration of M is always directed towards right
   (b) M executes SHM
   (c) M moves with constant speed
   (d) M moves with constant acceleration

4. A particle of mass m executes simple harmonic motion with amplitude a and frequency ν. The average kinetic energy during its motion from the position of equilibrium to the end is
   (a) $2\pi^2 ma^2\nu^2$ (b) $\pi^2 ma^2\nu^2$
   (c) $\frac{1}{4}ma^2\nu^2$ (d) $4\pi^2 ma^2\nu^2$

5. A mass M attached to a spring oscillates with a period of 2s. If the mass is increased by 2 kg, then the period increases by 2s. Find the initial mass M assuming that Hooke's law is obeyed.
   (a) $\frac{2}{3}$kg (b) $\frac{1}{3}$kg (c) $\frac{1}{2}$kg (d) 1 kg

RESPONSE GRID 1. 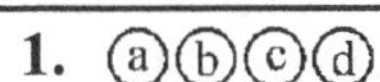 ⓐⓑⓒⓓ 2. ⓐⓑⓒⓓ 3. ⓐⓑⓒⓓ 4. ⓐⓑⓒⓓ 5. ⓐⓑⓒⓓ

Space for Rough Work

6. The amplitude of a damped oscillator becomes $\left(\frac{1}{3}\right)^{rd}$ in 2 seconds. If its amplitude after 6 seconds is $\frac{1}{n}$ times the original amplitude, the value of n is
(a) 3^2 (b) 3^3 (c) $\sqrt[3]{3}$ (d) 2^3

7. Assume the earth to be perfect sphere of uniform density. If a body is dropped at one end of a tunnel dug along a diameter of the earth (remember that inside the tunnel the force on the body is – k times the displacement from the centre, k being a constant), it (body) will
(a) reach the earth's centre and stay there
(b) go through the tunnel and comes out at the other end
(c) oscillate simple harmonically in the tunnel
(d) stay somewhere between the earth's centre and one of the ends of tunnel.

8. A particle undergoes simple harmonic motion having time period T. The time taken in 3/8th oscillation is
(a) $\frac{3}{8}$T (b) $\frac{5}{8}$T (c) $\frac{5}{12}$T (d) $\frac{7}{12}$T

9. A particle is executing simple harmonic motion with amplitude A. When the ratio of its kinetic energy to the potential energy is $\frac{1}{4}$, its displacement from its mean position is
(a) $\frac{2}{\sqrt{5}}$A (b) $\frac{\sqrt{3}}{2}$A (c) $\frac{3}{4}$A (d) $\frac{1}{4}$A

10. The length of a simple pendulum executing simple harmonic motion is increased by 21%. The percentage increase in the time period of the pendulum of increased length is
(a) 11% (b) 21% (c) 42% (d) 10%

11. The time period of a mass suspended from a spring is T. If the spring is cut into four equal parts and the same mass is suspended from one of the parts, then the new time period will be
(a) $2T$ (b) $\frac{T}{4}$ (c) 2 (d) $\frac{T}{2}$

12. Two simple harmonic motions act on a particle. These harmonic motions are $x = A\cos(\omega t + \delta)$, $y = A\cos(\omega t + \alpha)$ when $\delta = \alpha + \frac{\pi}{2}$, the resulting motion is
(a) a circle and the actual motion is clockwise
(b) an ellipse and the actual motion is counterclockwise
(c) an elllipse and the actual motion is clockwise
(d) a circle and the actual motion is counter clockwise

13. A point mass oscillates along the x-axis according to the law $x = x_0\cos(\omega t - \pi/4)$. If the acceleration of the particle is written as $a = A\cos(\omega t - \delta)$, then
(a) $A = x_0\omega^2, \delta = 3\pi/4$ (b) $A = x_0, \delta = -\pi/4$
(c) $A = x_0\omega^2, \delta = \pi/4$ (d) $A = x_0\omega^2, \delta = -\pi/4$

14. A mass M is suspended from a spring of negligible mass. The spring is pulled a little and then released so that the mass executes SHM of time period T. If the mass is increased by m, the time period becomes $\frac{5T}{3}$. Then the ratio of $\frac{m}{M}$ is
(a) $\frac{3}{5}$ (b) $\frac{25}{9}$ (c) $\frac{16}{9}$ (d) $\frac{5}{3}$

15. A body oscillates with a simple harmonic motion having amplitude 0.05 m. At a certain instant of time, its displacement is 0.01 m and acceleration is 1.0 m/s^2. The period of oscillation is
(a) 0.1 s (b) 0.2 s (c) $\frac{\pi}{10}$s (d) $\frac{\pi}{5}$s

16. The particle executing simple harmonic motion has a kinetic energy $K_0\cos^2\omega t$. The maximum values of the potential energy and the total energy are respectively
(a) $K_0/2$ and K_0 (b) K_0 and $2K_0$
(c) K_0 and K_0 (d) 0 and $2K_0$

17. A simple pendulum attached to the ceiling of a stationary lift has a time period T. The distance y covered by the lift moving upwards varies with time t as $y = t^2$ where y is in metres and t in seconds. If $g = 10$ m/s^2, the time period of pendulum will be
(a) $\sqrt{\frac{4}{5}}$T (b) $\sqrt{\frac{5}{6}}$T (c) $\sqrt{\frac{5}{4}}$T (d) $\sqrt{\frac{6}{5}}$T

18. A particle moves with simple harmonic motion in a straight line. In first τs, after starting from rest it travels a distance a, and in next τ s it travels 2a, in same direction, then:
(a) amplitude of motion is 3a
(b) time period of oscillations is 8τ
(c) amplitude of motion is 4a
(d) time period of oscillations is 6τ

19. Two simple harmonic motions are represented by the equations $y_1 = 0.1\sin\left(100\pi t + \frac{\pi}{3}\right)$ and $y_2 = 0.1\cos\pi t$. The phase difference of the velocity of particle 1 with respect to the velocity of particle 2 is
(a) $\frac{\pi}{3}$ (b) $\frac{-\pi}{6}$ (c) $\frac{\pi}{6}$ (d) $\frac{-\pi}{3}$

20. Masses M_A and M_B hanging from the ends of strings of lengths L_A and L_B are executing simple harmonic motions. If their frequencies are $f_A = 2f_B$, then
(a) $L_A = 2L_B$ and $M_A = M_B/2$
(b) $L_A = 4L_B$ regardless of masses
(c) $L_A = L_B/4$ regardless of masses
(d) $L_A = 2L_B$ and $M_A = 2M_B$

RESPONSE GRID					
	6. ⓐⓑⓒⓓ	7. ⓐⓑⓒⓓ	8. ⓐⓑⓒⓓ	9. ⓐⓑⓒⓓ	10. ⓐⓑⓒⓓ
	11. ⓐⓑⓒⓓ	12. ⓐⓑⓒⓓ	13. ⓐⓑⓒⓓ	14. ⓐⓑⓒⓓ	15. ⓐⓑⓒⓓ
	16. ⓐⓑⓒⓓ	17. ⓐⓑⓒⓓ	18. ⓐⓑⓒⓓ	19. ⓐⓑⓒⓓ	20. ⓐⓑⓒⓓ

Space for Rough Work

21. In damped oscillations, the amplitude of oscillations is reduced to one-third of its inital value a_0 at the end of 100 oscillations. When the oscillator completes 200 oscillations, its amplitude must be

(a) $a_0/2$ (b) $a_0/4$ (c) $a_0/6$ (d) $a_0/9$

22. The spring constant from the adjoining combination of springs is

(a) K
(b) 2K
(c) 4K
(d) 5K/2

23. A body executes simple harmonic motion. The potential energy (P.E), the kinetic energy (K.E) and total energy (T.E) are measured as a function of displacement x. Which of the following statements is true ?

(a) K.E. is maximum when $x=0$
(b) T.E is zero when $x=0$
(c) K.E is maximum when x is maximum
(d) P.E is maximum when $x=0$

24. A simple harmonic wave having an amplitude a and time period T is represented by the equation $y = 5\sin\pi(t+4)m$. Then the value of amplitude (a) in (m) and time period (T) in second are

(a) $a=10, T=2$ (b) $a=5, T=1$
(c) $a=10, T=1$ (d) $a=5, T=2$

25. A particle moves such that its acceleration 'a' is given by a $= -zx$ where x is the displacement from equilibrium position and z is constant. The period of oscillation is

(a) $2\pi/z$ (b) $2\pi/\sqrt{z}$ (c) $\sqrt{2\pi/z}$ (d) $2\sqrt{\pi/z}$

26. The displacement of an object attached to a spring and executing simple harmonic motion is given by $x = 2\times10^{-2}\cos\pi t$ metre. The time at which the maximum speed first occurs is

(a) 0.25 s (b) 0.5 s (c) 0.75 s (d) 0.125 s

27. A tunnel has been dug through the centre of the earth and a ball is released in it. It executes S.H.M. with time period

(a) 42 minutes (b) 1 day
(c) 1 hour (d) 84.6 minutes

28. The displacement equation of a particle is $x = 3\sin 2t + 4\cos 2t$. The amplitude and maximum velocity will be respectively

(a) 5, 10 (b) 3, 2 (c) 4, 2 (d) 3, 4

29. A body of mass 0.01 kg executes simple harmonic motion about x = 0 under the influence of a force as shown in figure. The time period of SHM is

(a) 1.05 s
(b) 0.52 s
(c) 0.25 s
(d) 0.03 s

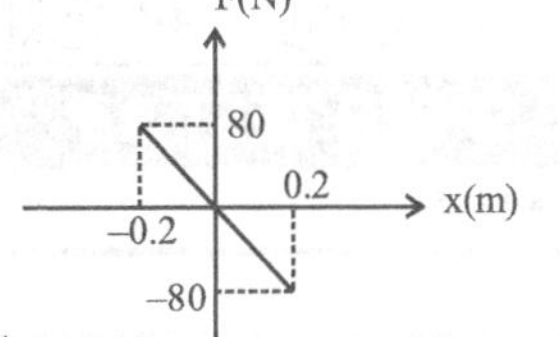

30. Two oscillators are started simultaneously in same phase. After 50 oscillations of one, they get out of phase by π, that is half oscillation. The percentage difference of frequencies of the two oscillators is nearest to

(a) 2% (b) 1% (c) 0.5% (d) 0.25%

31. The length of a second's pendulum at the surface of earth is 1 m. The length of second's pendulum at the surface of moon where g is 1/6th that at earth's surface is

(a) 1/6 m (b) 6 m (c) 1/36 m (d) 36 m

32. A simple spring has length l and force constant K. It is cut into two springs of lengths l_1 and l_2 such that $l_1 = n\,l_2$ (n = an integer). The force constant of spring of length l_1 is

(a) $K(1+n)$ (b) $(K/n)(1+n)$
(c) K (d) $K/(n+1)$

33. The displacement of a particle from its mean position (in metre) is given by $y = 0.2\sin(10\pi t + 1.5\pi)\cos(10\pi t + 1.5\pi)$. The motion of particle is

(a) periodic but not SHM
(b) non-periodic
(c) simple harmonic motion with period 0.1 s
(d) simple harmonic motion with period 0.2 *s*.

34. A point particle of mass 0.1 kg is executing S.H.M. of amplitude 0.1 m. When the particle passes through the mean position, its kinetic energy is 8×10^{-3} joule. Obtain the equation of motion of this particle, if the initial phase of oscillation is 45°.

(a) $y = 0.1\sin\left(\pm 4t + \frac{\pi}{4}\right)$ (b) $y = 0.2\sin\left(\pm 4t + \frac{\pi}{4}\right)$

(c) $y = 0.1\sin\left(\pm 2t + \frac{\pi}{4}\right)$ (d) $y = 0.2\sin\left(\pm 2t + \frac{\pi}{4}\right)$

35. For a simple pendulum, a graph is plotted between its kinetic energy (KE) and potential energy (PE) against its displacement d. Which one of the following represents these correctly? (*graphs are schematic and not drawn to scale*)

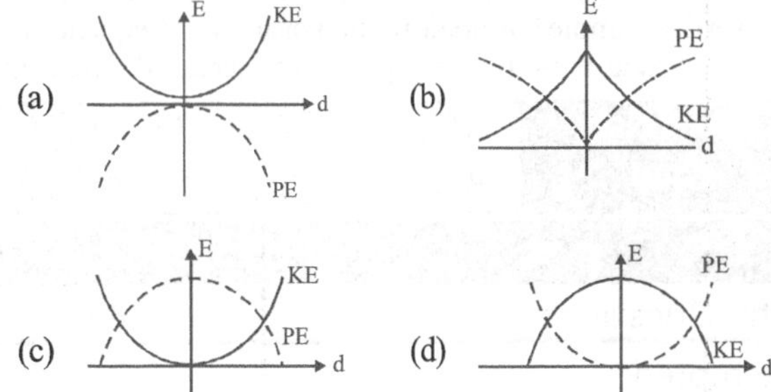

RESPONSE GRID					
	21. ⓐⓑⓒⓓ	22. ⓐⓑⓒⓓ	23. ⓐⓑⓒⓓ	24. ⓐⓑⓒⓓ	25. ⓐⓑⓒⓓ
	26. ⓐⓑⓒⓓ	27. ⓐⓑⓒⓓ	28. ⓐⓑⓒⓓ	29. ⓐⓑⓒⓓ	30. ⓐⓑⓒⓓ
	31. ⓐⓑⓒⓓ	32. ⓐⓑⓒⓓ	33. ⓐⓑⓒⓓ	34. ⓐⓑⓒⓓ	35. ⓐⓑⓒⓓ

Space for Rough Work

36. The equation of a simple harmonic wave is given by

$$y = 3\sin\frac{\pi}{2}(50t - x)$$

Where x and y are in meters and t is in seconds. The ratio of maximum particle velocity to the wave velocity is

(a) 2π (b) $\frac{3}{2}\pi$ (c) 3π (d) $\frac{2}{3}\pi$

37. If the mass shown in figure is slightly displaced and then let go, then the system shall oscillate with a time period of

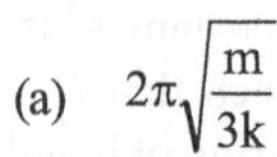

(a) $2\pi\sqrt{\frac{m}{3k}}$

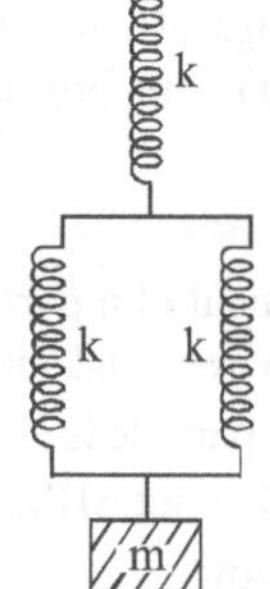

(b) $2\pi\sqrt{\frac{3m}{2k}}$

(c) $2\pi\sqrt{\frac{2m}{3k}}$

(d) $2\pi\sqrt{\frac{3k}{m}}$

38. A hollow sphere is filled with water. It is hung by a long thread. As the water flows out of a hole at the bottom, the period of oscillation will

(a) first increase and then decrease
(b) first decrease and then increase
(c) go on increasing
(d) go on decreasing

39. The figure shows a position time graph of a particle executing SHM. If the time period of SHM is 2 sec, then the equation of SHM is

(a) $x = 10\cos\pi t$

(b) $x = 5\sin\left(\pi t + \frac{\pi}{3}\right)$

(c) $x = 10\sin\left(\pi t + \frac{\pi}{3}\right)$

(d) $x = 10\sin\left(\pi t + \frac{\pi}{6}\right)$

40. A coin is placed on a horizontal platform which undergoes vertical simple harmonic motion of angular frequency ω. The amplitude of oscillation is gradually increased. The coin will leave contact with the platform for the first time

(a) at the mean position of the platform
(b) for an amplitude of $\frac{g}{\omega^2}$
(c) for an amplitude of $\frac{g^2}{\omega^2}$
(d) at the highest position of the platform

41. The bob of a simple pendulum executes simple harmonic motion in water with a period t, while the period of oscillation of the bob is t_0 in air. Neglecting frictional force of water and given that the density of the bob is (4/3) × 1000 kg/m^3. The relationship between t and t_0 is

(a) $t = 2t_0$ (b) $t = t_0/2$ (c) $t = t_0$ (d) $t = 4t_0$

42. Starting from the origin a body oscillates simple harmonically with a period of 2 s. After what time will its kinetic energy be 75% of the total energy?

(a) $\frac{1}{6}$s (b) $\frac{1}{4}$s (c) $\frac{1}{3}$s (d) $\frac{1}{12}$s

43. A body executes simple harmonic motion under the action of a force F_1 with a time period $\frac{4}{5}$ s. If the force is changed to F_2, it executes S.H.M. with time period $\frac{3}{5}$ s. If both the forces F_1 and F_2 act simultaneously in the same direction on the body, its time period in second is

(a) $\frac{12}{25}$ (b) $\frac{7}{5}$ (c) $\frac{24}{25}$ (d) $\frac{5}{7}$

44. A block connected to a spring oscillates vertically. A damping force F_d, acts on the block by the surrounding medium. Given as $F_d = -bV$, b is a positive constant which depends on :

(a) viscosity of the medium
(b) size of the block
(c) shape of the block
(d) All of these

45. If a simple pendulum of length l has maximum angular displacement θ, then the maximum K.E. of bob of mass m is

(a) $\frac{1}{2}ml/g$ (b) $mg/2l$
(c) $mgl(1 - \cos\theta)$ (d) $mgl\sin\theta/2$

RESPONSE GRID					
	36. ⓐⓑⓒⓓ	37. ⓐⓑⓒⓓ	38. ⓐⓑⓒⓓ	39. ⓐⓑⓒⓓ	40. ⓐⓑⓒⓓ
	41. ⓐⓑⓒⓓ	42. ⓐⓑⓒⓓ	43. ⓐⓑⓒⓓ	44. ⓐⓑⓒⓓ	45. ⓐⓑⓒⓓ

PHYSICS CHAPTERWISE SPEED TEST-13

Total Questions	45	Total Marks	180
Attempted		Correct	
Incorrect		Net Score	
Cut-off Score	45	Qualifying Score	60
Success Gap = Net Score – Qualifying Score			
Net Score = (Correct × 4) – (Incorrect × 1)			

Space for Rough Work

PHYSICS

Waves

Speed TEST 14

Chapter-wise

No. of Questions	Maximum Marks	Time
45	180	1 Hour

GENERAL INSTRUCTIONS

- This test contains 45 MCQ's. For each question only one option is correct. Darken the correct circle/ bubble in the Response Grid provided on each page.
- You have to evaluate your Response Grids yourself with the help of solutions provided at the end of this book.
- Each correct answer will get you 4 marks and 1 mark shall be deduced for each incorrect answer. No mark will be given/ deducted if no bubble is filled. Keep a timer in front of you and stop immediately at the end of 60 min.
- The sheet follows a particular syllabus. Do not attempt the sheet before you have completed your preparation for that syllabus.
- After completing the sheet check your answers with the solution booklet and complete the Result Grid. Finally spend time to analyse your performance and revise the areas which emerge out as weak in your evaluation.

1. Where should the two bridges be set in a 110cm long wire so that it is divided into three parts and the ratio of the frequencies are 3 : 2 : 1 ?
(a) 20cm from one end and 60cm from other end
(b) 30cm from one end and 70cm from other end
(c) 10cm from one end and 50cm from other end
(d) 50cm from one end and 40cm from other end

2. When a wave travel in a medium, the particle displacement is given by the equation y = a sin 2π (bt– cx) where a, b and c are constants. The maximum particle velocity will be twice the wave velocity if

(a) $c=\frac{1}{\pi a}$ (b) $c=\pi a$ (c) $b=ac$ (d) $b=\frac{1}{ac}$

3. The wave described by y = 0.25 sin (10πx – 2πt), where x and y are in meters and t in seconds, is a wave travelling along the:
(a) –ve x direction with frequency 1 Hz.
(b) +ve x direction with frequency π Hz and wavelength λ = 0. 2 m.
(c) +ve x direction with frequency 1 Hz and wavelength λ = 0.2 m
(d) –ve x direction with amplitude 0.25 m and wavelength λ = 0.2 m

4. The equation of a plane progressive wave is $y = 0.9 \sin 4\pi\left[t-\frac{x}{2}\right]$. When it is reflected at a rigid support, its amplitude becomes $\frac{2}{3}$ of its previous value. The equation of the reflected wave is

(a) $y = 0.6 \sin 4\pi\left[t+\frac{x}{2}\right]$

(b) $y = -0.6 \sin 4\pi\left[t+\frac{x}{2}\right]$

(c) $y = -0.9 \sin 8\pi\left[t-\frac{x}{2}\right]$

(d) $y = -0.6 \sin 4\pi\left[t+\frac{x}{2}\right]$

5. A person carrying a whistle emitting continuously a note of 272 Hz is running towards a reflecting surface with a speed of 18 km h^{-1}. The speed of sound in air is 345 m s^{-1}. The number of beats heard by him is
(a) 4 (b) 6 (c) 8 (d) zero

RESPONSE GRID	1. ⓐⓑⓒⓓ	2. ⓐⓑⓒⓓ	3. ⓐⓑⓒⓓ	4. ⓐⓑⓒⓓ	5. ⓐⓑⓒⓓ

Space for Rough Work

6. A closed organ pipe (closed at one end) is excited to support the third overtone. It is found that air in the pipe has
   (a) three nodes and three antinodes
   (b) three nodes and four antinodes
   (c) four nodes and three antinodes
   (d) four nodes and four antinodes
7. A wave disturbance in a medium is described by $y(x,t) = 0.02\cos\left(50\pi t + \frac{\pi}{2}\right)\cos(10\pi x)$ where x and y are in metre and t is in second. Which of the following is correct?
   (a) A node occurs at x = 0.15 m
   (b) An antinode occurs at x = 0.3 m
   (c) The speed wave is 5 ms^{-1}
   (d) The wavelength is 0.3 m
8. In a resonance column, first and second resonance are obtained at depths 22.7 cm and 70.2 cm. The third resonance will be obtained at a depth
   (a) 117.7 cm (b) 92.9 cm
   (c) 115.5 cm (d) 113.5 cm
9. An engine approaches a hill with a constant speed. When it is at a distance of 0.9 km, it blows a whistle whose echo is heard by the driver after 5 seconds. If the speed of sound in air is 330 m/s, then the speed of the engine is :
   (a) 32 m/s (b) 27.5 m/s (c) 60 m/s (d) 30 m/s
10. Two identical piano wires kept under the same tension T have a fundamental frequency of 600 Hz. The fractional increase in the tension of one of the wires which will lead to occurrence of 6 beats/s when both the wires oscillate together would be
   (a) 0.02 (b) 0.03 (c) 0.04 (d) 0.01
11. Two sound sources emitting sound each of wavelength λ are fixed at a given distance apart. A listener moves with a velocity u along the line joining the two sources. The number of beats heard by him per second is
   (a) $\frac{u}{2\lambda}$ (b) $\frac{2u}{\lambda}$ (c) $\frac{u}{\lambda}$ (d) $\frac{u}{3\lambda}$
12. An observer moves towards a stationary source of sound, with a velocity one-fifth of the velocity of sound. What is the percentage increase in the apparent frequency ?
   (a) 0.5% (b) zero (c) 20% (d) 5%
13. Velocity of sound in air is 320 m s^{-1}. A pipe closed at one end has a length of 1 m. Neglecting end correction, the air column in the pipe cannot resonate with sound of frequency
   (a) 80 Hz (b) 240 Hz (c) 320 Hz (d) 400 Hz
14. The driver of a car travelling with speed 30 m/sec towards a hill sounds a horn of frequency 600 Hz. If the velocity of sound in air is 330 m/s, the frequency of reflected sound as heard by driver is
   (a) 555.5 Hz (b) 720 Hz (c) 500 Hz (d) 550 Hz
15. What will be the frequency of beats formed from the superposition of two harmonic waves shown below?

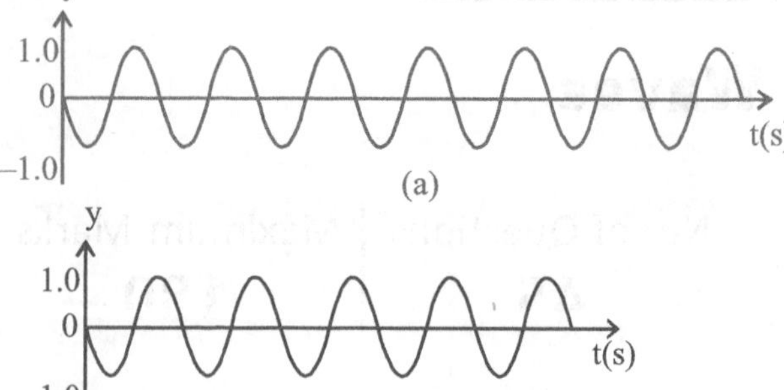

   (a) 20 Hz (b) 11 Hz (c) 9 Hz (d) 2 Hz
16. What is the effect of increase in temperature on the frequency of sound produced by an organ pipe?
   (a) increases (b) decreases
   (c) no effect (d) erratic change
17. A cylinderical tube open at both ends, has a fundamental frequency f in air. The tube is dipped vertically in water so that half of it is in water. The fundamental frequency of air column is now
   (a) f/2 (b) f (c) 3f/4 (d) 2f
18. The transverse displacement y (x, t) of a wave on a string is given by $y(x,t) = e^{-\left(ax^2 + bt^2 + 2\sqrt{ab}xt\right)}$. This represents a:
   (a) wave moving in –x direction with speed $\sqrt{\frac{b}{a}}$
   (b) standing wave of frequency $\sqrt{b}$
   (c) standing wave of frequency $\frac{1}{\sqrt{b}}$
   (d) wave moving in + x direction with speed $\sqrt{\frac{a}{b}}$
19. A longitudinal wave is represented by $x = x_0 \sin 2\pi\left(nt - \frac{x}{\lambda}\right)$
   The maximum particle velocity will be four times the wave velocity if
   (a) $\lambda = \frac{\pi x_0}{4}$ (b) $\lambda = 2\pi x_0$
   (c) $\lambda = \frac{\pi x_0}{2}$ (d) $\lambda = 4\pi x_0$
20. Two tones of frequencies n_1 and n_2 are sounded together. The beats can be heard distinctly when
   (a) $10 < (n_1 - n_2) < 20$ (b) $5 < (n_1 - n_2) > 20$
   (c) $5 < (n_1 - n_2) < 20$ (d) $0 < (n_1 - n_2) < 10$

RESPONSE GRID					
	6. ⓐⓑⓒⓓ	7. ⓐⓑⓒⓓ	8. ⓐⓑⓒⓓ	9. ⓐⓑⓒⓓ	10. ⓐⓑⓒⓓ
	11. ⓐⓑⓒⓓ	12. ⓐⓑⓒⓓ	13. ⓐⓑⓒⓓ	14. ⓐⓑⓒⓓ	15. ⓐⓑⓒⓓ
	16. ⓐⓑⓒⓓ	17. ⓐⓑⓒⓓ	18. ⓐⓑⓒⓓ	19. ⓐⓑⓒⓓ	20. ⓐⓑⓒⓓ

Space for Rough Work

21. A pipe of length 85 cm is closed from one end. Find the number of possible natural oscillations of air column in the pipe whose frequencies lie below 1250 Hz. The velocity of sound in air is 340 m/s.
(a) 12 (b) 8 (c) 6 (d) 4

22. A vehicle, with a horn of frequency n is moving with a velocity of 30 m/s in a direction perpendicular to the straight line joining the observer and the vehicle. The observer perceives the sound to have a frequency n + n_1. Then (if the sound velocity in air is 300 m/s)
(a) $n_1 = 10n$ (b) $n_1 = 0$
(c) $n_1 = 0.1n$ (d) $n_1 = -0.1n$

23. A source of sound gives 5 beats per second, when sounded with another source of frequency 100/sec. The second harmonic of the source, together with a source of frequency 205/sec gives 5 beats per second. What is the frequency of the source?
(a) 95 sec^{-1} (b) 100 sec^{-1}
(c) 105 sec^{-1} (d) 205 sec^{-1}

24. If we study the vibration of a pipe open at both ends, then which of the following statements is not true ?
(a) Odd harmonics of the fundamental frequency will be generated
(b) All harmonics of the fundamental frequency will be generated
(c) Pressure change will be maximum at both ends
(d) Antinode will be at open end

25. 41 forks are so arranged that each produces 5 beats per sec when sounded with its near fork. If the frequency of last fork is double the frequency of first fork, then the frequencies (in Hz) of the first and the last fork are respectively.
(a) 200, 400 (b) 205, 410
(c) 195, 390 (d) 100, 200

26. Two points are located at a distance of 10 m and 15 m from the source of oscillation. The period of oscillation is 0.05 sec and the velocity of the wave is 300 m/sec. What is the phase difference between the oscillations of two points?
(a) $\frac{\pi}{3}$ (b) $\frac{2\pi}{3}$ (c) π (d) $\frac{\pi}{6}$

27. A sound absorber attenuates the sound level by 20 dB. The intensity decreases by a factor of
(a) 100 (b) 1000 (c) 10000 (d) 10

28. A wave travelling along the x-axis is described by the equation $y(x, t) = 0.005 \cos(\alpha x - \beta t)$. If the wavelength and the time period of the wave are 0.08 m and 2.0s, respectively, then α and β in appropriate units are
(a) $\alpha = 25.00\pi, \beta = \pi$ (b) $\alpha = \frac{0.08}{\pi}, \beta = \frac{2.0}{\pi}$
(c) $\alpha = \frac{0.04}{\pi}, \beta = \frac{1.0}{\pi}$ (d) $\alpha = 12.50\pi, \beta = \frac{\pi}{2.0}$

29. The equation $Y = 0.02 \sin(500\pi t) \cos(4.5x)$ represents
(a) progressive wave of frequency 250 Hz along x-axis
(b) a stationary wave of wavelength 1.4 m
(c) a transverse progressive wave of amplitude 0.02 m
(d) progressive wave of speed of about 350 m s^{-1}

30. Which of the following statements is/are incorrect about waves ?
(a) Waves are patterns of disturbance which move without the actual physical transfer of flow of matter as a whole.
(b) Waves cannot transport energy.
(c) The pattern of disturbance in the form of waves carry information that propagate from one point to another.
(d) All our communications essentially depend on transmission of signals through waves.

31. An organ pipe P_1, closed at one end vibrating in its first harmonic and another pipe P_2, open at both ends vibrating in its third harmonic, are in resonance with a given tuning fork. The ratio of the lengths of P_1 and P_2 is :
(a) $\frac{8}{3}$ (b) $\frac{1}{6}$ (c) $\frac{1}{2}$ (d) $\frac{1}{3}$

32. Two vibrating tuning forks producing waves given by $y_1 = 27 \sin 600\pi t$ and $y_2 = 27 \sin 604\pi t$ are held near the ear of a person, how many beats will be heard in three seconds by him ?
(a) 4 (b) 2 (c) 6 (d) 12

33. A source of sound A emitting waves of frequency 1800 Hz is falling towards ground with a terminal speed v. The observer B on the ground directly beneath the source receives waves of frequency 2150 Hz. The source A receives waves, reflected from ground of frequency nearly: (Speed of sound = 343 m/s)
(a) 2150 Hz (b) 2500 Hz (c) 1800 Hz (d) 2400 Hz

34. Consider the three waves z_1, z_2 and z_3 as
$z_1 = A \sin(kx - \omega t)$
$z_2 = A \sin(kx + \omega t)$
$z_3 = A \sin(ky - \omega t)$
Which of the following represents a standing wave?
(a) $z_1 + z_2$ (b) $z_2 + z_3$
(c) $z_3 + z_1$ (d) $z_1 + z_2 + z_3$

35. A sonometer wire supports a 4 kg load and vibrates in fundamental mode with a tuning fork of frequency 416 Hz. The length of the wire between the bridges is now doubled. In order to maintain fundamental mode, the load should be changed to
(a) 1 kg (b) 2 kg (c) 4 kg (d) 16 kg

RESPONSE GRID					
	21. ⓐⓑⓒⓓ	22. ⓐⓑⓒⓓ	23. ⓐⓑⓒⓓ	24. ⓐⓑⓒⓓ	25. ⓐⓑⓒⓓ
	26. ⓐⓑⓒⓓ	27. ⓐⓑⓒⓓ	28. ⓐⓑⓒⓓ	29. ⓐⓑⓒⓓ	30. ⓐⓑⓒⓓ
	31. ⓐⓑⓒⓓ	32. ⓐⓑⓒⓓ	33. ⓐⓑⓒⓓ	34. ⓐⓑⓒⓓ	35. ⓐⓑⓒⓓ

Space for Rough Work

36. The vibrations of a string of length 60 cm fixed at both the ends are represented by the equation $y = 2\sin\left(\frac{4\pi x}{15}\right)\cos(96\pi t)$ where x and y are in cm. The maximum number of loops that can be formed in it is
(a) 4 (b) 16 (c) 5 (d) 15

37. If n_1, n_2 and n_3 are the fundamental frequencies of three segments into which a string is divided, then the original fundamental frequency n of the string is given by
(a) $n = n_1 + n_2 + n_3$
(b) $\frac{1}{n} = \frac{1}{n_1} + \frac{1}{n_2} + \frac{1}{n_3}$
(c) $\frac{1}{\sqrt{n}} = \frac{1}{\sqrt{n_1}} + \frac{1}{\sqrt{n_2}} + \frac{1}{\sqrt{n_3}}$
(d) $\sqrt{n} = \sqrt{n_1} + \sqrt{n_2} + \sqrt{n_3}$

38. An echo repeats two syllables. If the velocity of sound is 330 m/s, then the distance of the reflecting surface is
(a) 66.0m (b) 33.0m (c) 99.0m (d) 16.5m

39. What is the effect of humidity on sound waves when humidity increases?
(a) Speed of sound waves is more
(b) Speed of sound waves is less
(c) Speed of sound waves remains same
(d) Speed of sound waves becomes zero

40. If the ratio of maximum to minimum intensity in beats is 49, then the ratio of amplitudes of two progressive wave trains is
(a) 7 : 1 (b) 4 : 3 (c) 49 : 1 (d) 16 : 9

41. A whistle of frequency 1000 Hz is sounded on a car travelling towards a cliff with velocity of 18 m s^{-1} normal to the cliff. If velocity of sound (v) = 330 m s^{-1}, then the apparent frequency of the echo as heard by the car driver is nearly
(a) 1115 Hz (b) 115 Hz (c) 67 Hz (d) 47.2 Hz

42. The transverse wave represented by the equation $y = 4\sin\left(\frac{\pi}{6}\right)\sin(3x - 15t)$ has
(a) amplitude = 4
(b) wavelength $= \frac{4\pi}{3}$
(c) speed of propagation = 5
(d) period $= \frac{\pi}{15}$

43. If the intensities of two interfering waves be I_1 and I_2, the contrast between maximum and minimum intensity is maximum, when
(a) $I_1 >> I_2$ (b) $I_1 << I_2$
(c) $I_1 = I_2$ (d) either I_1 or I_2 is zero

44. The fundamental frequency of a closed organ pipe of length 20 cm is equal to the second overtone of an organ pipe open at both the ends. The length of organ pipe open at both the ends is
(a) 100 cm (b) 120 cm (c) 140 cm (d) 80 cm

45. The equation of a travelling wave is y = 60 cos (180 t – 6x) where y is in µm, *t* in second and x in metres. The ratio of maximum particle velocity to velocity of wave propagation is
(a) 3.6×10^{-2} (b) 3.6×10^{-4}
(c) 3.6×10^{-6} (d) 3.6×10^{-11}

RESPONSE GRID					
	36. ⓐⓑⓒⓓ	37. ⓐⓑⓒⓓ	38. ⓐⓑⓒⓓ	39. ⓐⓑⓒⓓ	40. ⓐⓑⓒⓓ
	41. ⓐⓑⓒⓓ	42. ⓐⓑⓒⓓ	43. ⓐⓑⓒⓓ	44. ⓐⓑⓒⓓ	45. ⓐⓑⓒⓓ

PHYSICS CHAPTERWISE SPEED TEST-14

Total Questions	45	Total Marks	180
Attempted		Correct	
Incorrect		Net Score	
Cut-off Score	50	Qualifying Score	70
Success Gap = Net Score – Qualifying Score			
Net Score = (Correct × 4) – (Incorrect × 1)			

Space for Rough Work

PHYSICS

Electric Charges and Fields

Speed TEST 15

Chapter-wise

No. of Questions	Maximum Marks	Time
45	180	1 Hour

GENERAL INSTRUCTIONS

- This test contains 45 MCQ's. For each question only one option is correct. Darken the correct circle/ bubble in the Response Grid provided on each page.
- You have to evaluate your Response Grids yourself with the help of solutions provided at the end of this book.
- Each correct answer will get you 4 marks and 1 mark shall be deduced for each incorrect answer. No mark will be given/ deducted if no bubble is filled. Keep a timer in front of you and stop immediately at the end of 60 min.
- The sheet follows a particular syllabus. Do not attempt the sheet before you have completed your preparation for that syllabus.
- After completing the sheet check your answers with the solution booklet and complete the Result Grid. Finally spend time to analyse your performance and revise the areas which emerge out as weak in your evaluation.

1. The surface charge density of a thin charged disc of radius R is σ. The value of the electric field at the centre of the disc is $\frac{\sigma}{2\epsilon_0}$. With respect to the field at the centre, the electric field along the axis at a distance R from the centre of the disc reduces by
   (a) 70.7% (b) 29.3% (c) 9.7% (d) 14.6%

2. A solid conducting sphere of radius a has a net positive charge 2Q. A conducting spherical shell of inner radius b and outer radius c is concentric with the solid sphere and has a net charge – Q. The surface charge density on the inner and outer surfaces of the spherical shell will be respectively

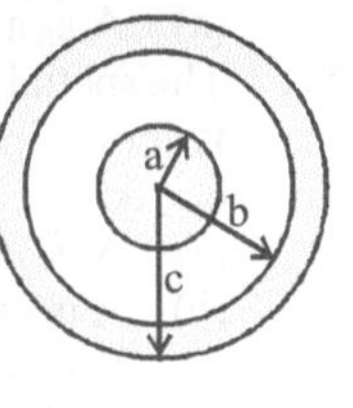

   (a) $-\frac{2Q}{4\pi b^2}, \frac{Q}{4\pi c^2}$ (b) $-\frac{Q}{4\pi b^2}, \frac{Q}{4\pi c^2}$

   (c) $0, \frac{Q}{4\pi c^2}$ (d) $\frac{Q}{4\pi c^2}, 0$

3. Two equally charged, identical metal spheres A and B repel each other with a force 'F'. The spheres are kept fixed with a distance 'r' between them. A third identical, but uncharged sphere C is brought in contact with A and then placed at the mid point of the line joining A and B. The magnitude of the net electric force on C is
   (a) F (b) $\frac{3F}{4}$ (c) $\frac{F}{2}$ (d) $\frac{F}{4}$

4. In the figure, the net electric flux through the area A is $\phi = \vec{E} \cdot \vec{A}$ when the system is in air. On immersing the system in water the net electric flux through the area

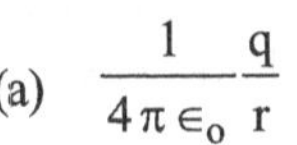

   (a) becomes zero
   (b) remains same
   (c) increases
   (d) decreases

5. ABC is an equilateral triangle. Charges +q are placed at each corner as shown in fig. The electric intensity at centre O will be

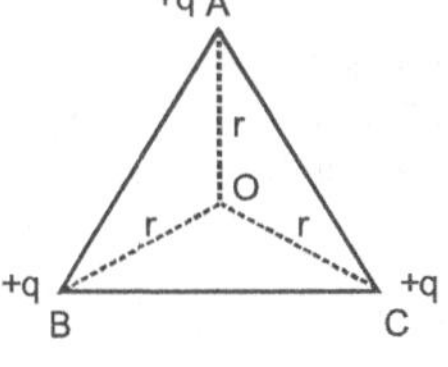

   (a) $\frac{1}{4\pi\epsilon_0}\frac{q}{r}$
   (b) $\frac{1}{4\pi\epsilon_0}\frac{q}{r^2}$
   (c) $\frac{1}{4\pi\epsilon_0}\frac{3q}{r^2}$
   (d) zero

RESPONSE GRID	1. ⓐⓑⓒⓓ	2. ⓐⓑⓒⓓ	3. ⓐⓑⓒⓓ	4. ⓐⓑⓒⓓ	5. ⓐⓑⓒⓓ

Space for Rough Work

6. An electric dipole is placed in a uniform electric field. The dipole will experience
(a) a force that will displace it in the direction of the field
(b) a force that will displace it in a direction opposite to the field.
(c) a torque which will rotate it without displacement
(d) a torque which will rotate it and a force that will displace it

7. An uniform electric field E exists along positive x-axis. The work done in moving a charge 0.5 C through a distance 2 m along a direction making an angle 60° with x-axis is 10 J. Then the magnitude of electric field is
(a) $5\,Vm^{-1}$ (b) $2\,Vm^{-1}$ (c) $\sqrt{5}\ Vm^{-1}$ (d) $20\,Vm^{-1}$

8. Which one of the following graphs represents the variation of electric field with distance r from the centre of a charged spherical conductor of radius R?

(a) 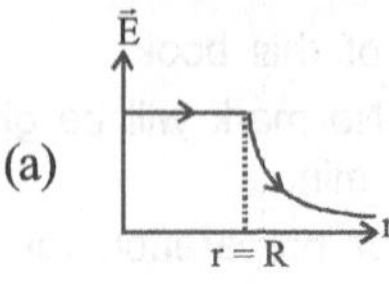

(b) 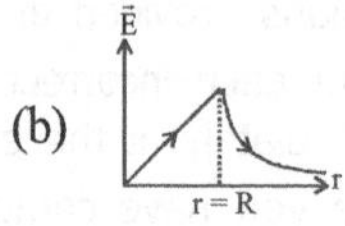

(c) 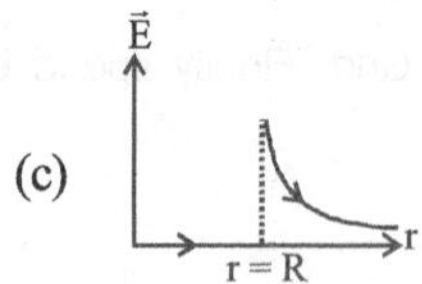

(d) 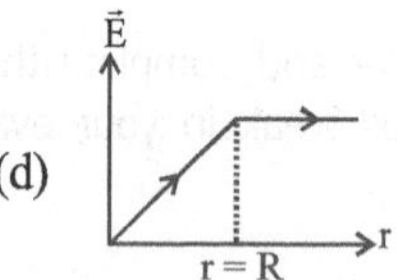

9. A hollow cylinder has a charge q coulomb within it. If ϕ is the electric flux in units of voltmeter associated with the curved surface B, the flux linked with the plane surface A in units of voltmeter will be

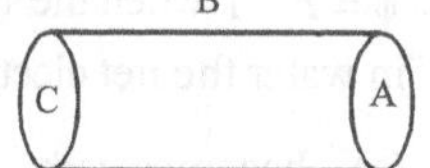

(a) $\frac{q}{2\varepsilon_0}$ (b) $\frac{\phi}{3}$

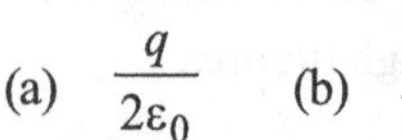

(c) $\frac{q}{\varepsilon_0}-\phi$ (d) $\frac{1}{2}\left(\frac{q}{\varepsilon_0}-\phi\right)$

10. If E_a be the electric field strength of a short dipole at a point on its axial line and E_e that on the equatorial line at the same distance, then
(a) $E_e = 2E_a$ (b) $E_a = 2E_e$
(c) $E_a = E_e$ (d) None of the above

11. Three positive charges of equal value q are placed at vertices of an equilateral triangle. The resulting lines of force should be sketched as in

(a) 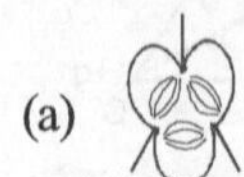 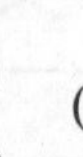 (b) 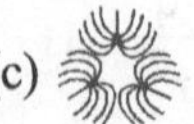 (c) (d) 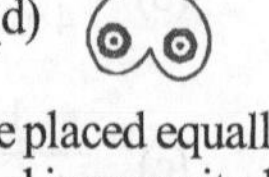

12. Three point charges Q_1, Q_2, Q_3 in the order are placed equally spaced along a straight line. Q_2 and Q_3 are equal in magnitude but opposite in sign. If the net force on Q_3 is zero. The value of Q_1 is
(a) $Q_1 = 4(Q_3)$ (b) $Q = 2(Q_3)$
(c) $Q_1 = \sqrt{2}(Q_3)$ (d) $Q_1 = |Q_3|$

13. Electric charge is uniformly distributed along a long straight wire of radius 1 mm. The charge per cm length of the wire is Q coulomb. Another cylindrical surface of radius 50 cm and length 1 m symmetrically encloses the wire. The total electric flux passing through the cylindrical surface is
(a) $\frac{Q}{\varepsilon_0}$ (b) $\frac{100Q}{\varepsilon_0}$ (c) $\frac{10Q}{\pi\varepsilon_0}$ (d) $\frac{100Q}{\pi\varepsilon_0}$

14. A small sphere carrying a charge 'q' is hanging in between two parallel plates by a string of length L. Time period of pendulum is T_0. When parallel plates are charged, the time period changes to T. The ratio T/T_0 is equal to

(a) $\left(\frac{g+\frac{qE}{m}}{g}\right)^{1/2}$ (b) $\left(\frac{g}{g+\frac{qE}{m}}\right)^{3/2}$

(c) $\left(\frac{g}{g+\frac{qE}{m}}\right)^{1/2}$ (d) $\left(\frac{g}{g+\frac{qE}{m}}\right)^{5/2}$

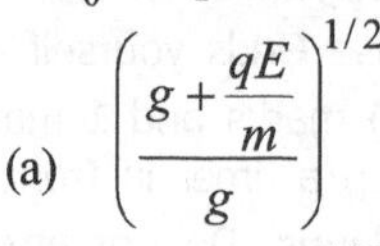
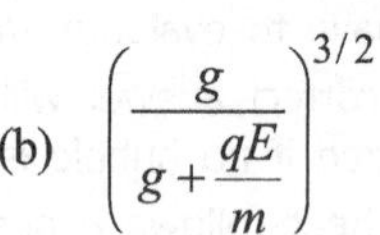
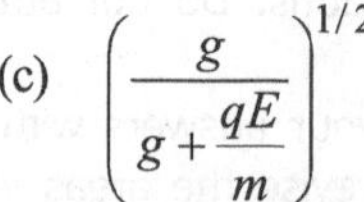

15. An electric dipole, consisting of two opposite charges of 2×10^{-6} C each separated by a distance 3 cm is placed in an electric field of 2×10^{5} N/C. Torque acting on the dipole is
(a) $12\times10^{-1}N-m$ (b) $12\times10^{-2}N-m$
(c) $12\times10^{-3}N-m$ (d) $12\times10^{-4}N-m$

16. The electric field in a certain region is acting radially outward and is given by E = Ar. A charge contained in a sphere of radius 'a' centred at the origin of the field, will be given by
(a) $A\,\varepsilon_0 a^2$ (b) $4\pi\varepsilon_0 Aa^3$ (c) $\varepsilon_0 Aa^3$ (d) $4\,\pi\varepsilon_0 Aa^2$

17. The spatial distribution of electric field due to charges (A, B) is shown in figure. Which one of the following statements is correct?

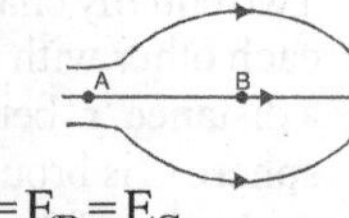

(a) A is +ve and B –ve, |A| > |B|
(b) A is –ve and B +ve, |A| = |B|
(c) Both are +ve but A > B
(d) Both are –ve but A > B

18. Point charges + $4q$, $-q$ and $+4q$ are kept on the X-axis at points $x = 0$, $x = a$ and $x = 2a$ respectively.
(a) only $-q$ is in stable equilibrium
(b) none of the charges is in equilibrium
(c) all the charges are in unstable equilibrium
(d) all the charges are in stable equilibrium.

19. Figure shows some of the electric field lines corresponding to an electric field. The figure suggests that

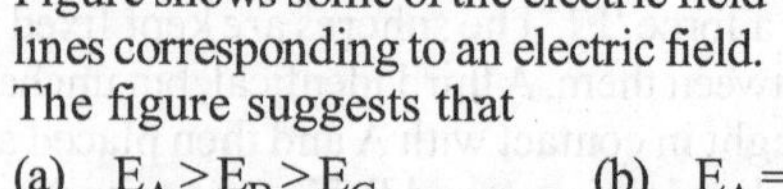

(a) $E_A > E_B > E_C$ (b) $E_A = E_B = E_C$
(c) $E_A = E_C > E_B$ (d) $E_A = E_C < E_B$

RESPONSE GRID					
	6. ⓐⓑⓒⓓ	7. ⓐⓑⓒⓓ	8. ⓐⓑⓒⓓ	9. ⓐⓑⓒⓓ	10. ⓐⓑⓒⓓ
	11. ⓐⓑⓒⓓ	12. ⓐⓑⓒⓓ	13. ⓐⓑⓒⓓ	14. ⓐⓑⓒⓓ	15. ⓐⓑⓒⓓ
	16. ⓐⓑⓒⓓ	17. ⓐⓑⓒⓓ	18. ⓐⓑⓒⓓ	19. ⓐⓑⓒⓓ	

Space for Rough Work

20. For distance far away from centre of dipole the change in magnitude of electric field with change in distance from the centre of dipole is
(a) zero.
(b) same in equatorial plane as well as axis of dipole.
(c) more in case of equatorial plane of dipole as compared to axis of dipole.
(d) more in case of axis of dipole as compared to equatorial plane of dipole.

21. Two charge q and $-3q$ are placed fixed on x–axis separated by distance d. Where should a third charge $2q$ be placed such that it will not experience any force ?

q $-3q$
A ←—— d ——→ B

(a) $\frac{d-\sqrt{3}d}{2}$ (b) $\frac{d+\sqrt{3}d}{2}$ (c) $\frac{d+3d}{2}$ (d) $\frac{d-3d}{2}$

22. A charge Q is placed at each of the opposite corners of a square. A charge q is placed at each of the other two corners. If the net electrical force on Q is zero, then Q/q equals:
(a) -1 (b) 1 (c) $-\frac{1}{\sqrt{2}}$ (d) $-2\sqrt{2}$

23. Identify the wrong statement in the following. Coulomb's law correctly describes the electric force that
(a) binds the electrons of an atom to its nucleus
(b) binds the protons and neutrons in the nucleus of an atom
(c) binds atoms together to form molecules
(d) binds atoms and molecules together to form solids

24. An oil drop of radius r and density ρ is held stationary in a uniform vertically upwards electric field 'E'. If ρ_0 ($< \rho$) is the density of air and e is quanta of charge, then the drop has–
(a) $\frac{4\pi r^3 (\rho-\rho_0) g}{3eE}$ excess electrons
(b) $\frac{4\pi r^2 (\rho-\rho_0) g}{eE}$ excess electrons
(c) deficiency of $\frac{4\pi r^3 (\rho-\rho_0) g}{3eE}$ electrons
(d) deficiency of $\frac{4\pi r^2 (\rho-\rho_0) g}{eE}$ electrons

25. A square surface of side L meter in the plane of the paper is placed in a uniform electric field E (volt/m) acting along the same plane at an angle θ with the horizontal side of the square as shown in Figure. The electric flux linked to the surface, in units of volt. m, is
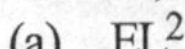
(a) EL^2 (b) $EL^2 \cos\theta$
(c) $EL^2 \sin\theta$ (d) zero

26. An electric dipole of moment $\vec{p}$ placed in a uniform electric field $\vec{E}$ has minimum potential energy when the angle between $\vec{P}$ and $\vec{E}$ is
(a) zero (b) $\frac{\pi}{2}$ (c) π (d) $\frac{3\pi}{2}$

27. Which of the following statements is incorrect?
(a) The charge q on a body is always given by q = ne, where n is any integer, positive or negative.
(b) By convention, the charge on an electron is taken to be negative.
(c) The fact that electric charge is always an integral multiple of e is termed as quantisation of charge.
(d) The quatisation of charge was experimentally demonstrated by Newton in 1912.

28. Two positive ions, each carrying a charge q, are separated by a distance d. If F is the force of repulsion between the ions, the number of electrons missing from each ion will be (e being the charge of an electron)
(a) $\frac{4\pi\varepsilon_0 Fd^2}{e^2}$ (b) $\sqrt{\frac{4\pi\varepsilon_0 Fe^2}{d^2}}$
(c) $\sqrt{\frac{4\pi\varepsilon_0 Fd^2}{e^2}}$ (d) $\frac{4\pi\varepsilon_0 Fd^2}{q^2}$

29. Two small similar metal spheres A and B having charges 4q and – 4q, when placed at a certain distance apart, exert an electric force F on each other. When another identical uncharged sphere C, first touched with A then with B and then removed to infinity, the force of interaction between A and B for the same separation will be
(a) F/2 (b) F/8 (c) F/16 (d) F/32

30. The electric field intensity just sufficient to balance the earth's gravitational attraction on an electron will be: (given mass and charge of an electron respectively are 9.1×10^{-31}kg and 1.6×10^{-19}C.)
(a) -5.6×10^{-11}N/C (b) -4.8×10^{-15}N/C
(c) -1.6×10^{-19}N/C (d) -3.2×10^{-19}N/C

31. An electric dipole is placed at an angle of 30° with an electric field of intensity 2×10^5 NC^{-1}, It experiences a torque of 4 Nm. Calculate the charge on the dipole if the dipole length is 2 cm.
(a) 8mC (b) 4mC (c) 8mC (d) 2mC

32. A particle of mass m and charge q is placed at rest in a uniform electric field E and then released. The kinetic energy attained by the particle after moving a distance y is
(a) qEy^2 (b) qE^2y (c) qEy (d) q^2Ey

33. There is an electric field E in x-direction. If the work done on moving a charge of 0.2 C through a distance of 2 m along a line making an angle 60° with x-axis is 4 J, then what is the value of E?
(a) 3 N/C (b) 4 N/C (c) 5 N/C (d) 20 N/C

RESPONSE GRID					
	20. ⓐⓑⓒⓓ	21. ⓐⓑⓒⓓ	22. ⓐⓑⓒⓓ	23. ⓐⓑⓒⓓ	24. ⓐⓑⓒⓓ
	25. ⓐⓑⓒⓓ	26. ⓐⓑⓒⓓ	27. ⓐⓑⓒⓓ	28. ⓐⓑⓒⓓ	29. ⓐⓑⓒⓓ
	30. ⓐⓑⓒⓓ	31. ⓐⓑⓒⓓ	32. ⓐⓑⓒⓓ	33. ⓐⓑⓒⓓ	

Space for Rough Work

34. A surface has the area vector $\vec{A} = \left(2\hat{i} + 3\hat{j}\right) m^2$. The flux of an electric field through it if the field is $\vec{E} = 4\hat{i}\frac{V}{m}$:

(a) 8 V-m (b) 12 V-m (c) 20 V-m (d) zero

35. There exists a non!-uniform electric field along x-axis as shown in the figure below. The field increases at a uniform rate along +ve x-axis. A dipole is placed inside the field as shown. Which one of the following is correct for the dipole?

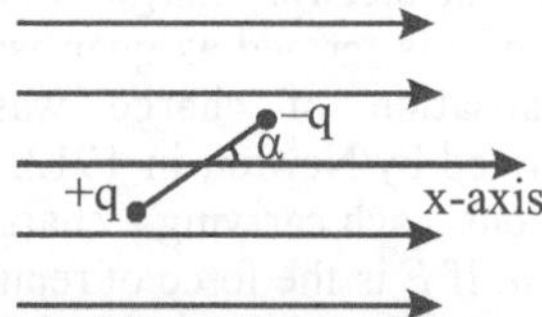

(a) Dipole moves along positive x-axis and undergoes a clockwise rotation
(b) Dipole moves along negative x-axis and undergoes a clockwise rotation
(c) Dipole moves along positive x-axis and undergoes a anticlockwise rotation
(d) Dipole moves along negative x-axis and undergoes a anticlockwise rotation

36. A square surface of side L metres is in the plane of the paper. A uniform electric field $\vec{E}$ (volt /m), also in the plane of the paper, is limited only to the lower half of the square surface (see figure). The electric flux in SI units associated with the surface is

(a) $EL^2/2$ (b) zero (c) EL^2 (d) $EL^2/(2\varepsilon_0)$

37. Among two discs A and B, first have radius 10 cm and charge 10^{-6} μC and second have radius 30 cm and charge 10^{-5} C. When they are touched, charge on both q_A and q_B respectively will, be

(a) $q_A = 2.75\mu C$, $q_B = 3.15\mu C$
(b) $q_A = 1.09\mu C$, $q_B = 1.53\mu C$
(c) $q_A = q_B = 5.5\mu C$ (d) None of these

38. The total electric flux emanating from a closed surface enclosing an α-particle (e-electronic charge) is

(a) $\frac{2e}{\varepsilon_0}$ (b) $\frac{e}{\varepsilon_0}$ (c) $e\varepsilon_0$ (d) $\frac{\varepsilon_0 e}{4}$

39. Which of the following is a wrong statement?
(a) The charge of an isolated system is conserved
(b) It is not possible to create or destroy charged particles
(c) It is possible to create or destroy charged particles
(d) It is not possible to create or destroy net charge

40. A charge q is placed at the centre of the open end of a cylindrical vessel. The flux of the electric field through the surface of the vessel is

(a) zero (b) q/ε_0
(c) $q/2\varepsilon_0$ (d) $2q/\varepsilon_0$

41. If the electric flux entering and leaving a closed surface are 6×10^6 and 9×10^6 S.I. units respectively, then the charge inside the surface of permittivity of free space ε_0 is
(a) $\varepsilon_0 \times 10^6$ (b) $-\varepsilon_0 \times 10^6$
(c) $-2\varepsilon_0 \times 10^6$ (d) $3\varepsilon_0 \times 10^6$

42. Two particle of equal mass m and charge q are placed at a distance of 16 cm. They do not experience any force. The value of $\frac{q}{m}$ is

(a) 1 (b) $\sqrt{\frac{\pi\varepsilon_0}{G}}$ (c) $\sqrt{\frac{G}{4\pi\varepsilon_0}}$ (d) $\sqrt{4\pi\varepsilon_0 G}$

43. A rod of length 2.4 *m* and radius 4.6 *mm* carries a negative charge of 4.2×10^{-7} C spread uniformly over it surface. The electric field near the mid–point of the rod, at a point on its surface is
(a) -8.6×10^5 N C^{-1} (b) 8.6×10^4 N C^{-1}
(c) -6.7×10^5 N C^{-1} (d) 6.7×10^4 N C^{-1}

44. A hollow insulated conduction sphere is given a positive charge of 10 μC. What will be the electric field at the centre of the sphere if its radius is 2 m?
(a) Zero (b) 5 μCm^{-2}
(c) 20 μCm^{-2} (d) 8 μCm^{-2}

45. A charge Q is enclosed by a Gaussian spherical surface of radius R. If the radius is doubled, then the outward electric flux will
(a) increase four times (b) be reduced to half
(c) remain the same (d) be doubled

RESPONSE GRID					
	34. ⓐⓑⓒⓓ	35. ⓐⓑⓒⓓ	36. ⓐⓑⓒⓓ	37. ⓐⓑⓒⓓ	38. ⓐⓑⓒⓓ
	39. ⓐⓑⓒⓓ	40. ⓐⓑⓒⓓ	41. ⓐⓑⓒⓓ	42. ⓐⓑⓒⓓ	43. ⓐⓑⓒⓓ
	44. ⓐⓑⓒⓓ	45. ⓐⓑⓒⓓ			

PHYSICS CHAPTERWISE SPEED TEST-15

Total Questions	45	Total Marks	180
Attempted		Correct	
Incorrect		Net Score	
Cut-off Score	50	Qualifying Score	70
Success Gap = Net Score – Qualifying Score			
Net Score = (Correct × 4) – (Incorrect × 1)			

Space for Rough Work

PHYSICS

Electrostatic Potential & Capacitance

Speed TEST 16

Chapter-wise

No. of Questions	Maximum Marks	Time
45	180	1 Hour

GENERAL INSTRUCTIONS

- This test contains 45 MCQ's. For each question only one option is correct. Darken the correct circle/ bubble in the Response Grid provided on each page.
- You have to evaluate your Response Grids yourself with the help of solutions provided at the end of this book.
- Each correct answer will get you 4 marks and 1 mark shall be deduced for each incorrect answer. No mark will be given/ deducted if no bubble is filled. Keep a timer in front of you and stop immediately at the end of 60 min.
- The sheet follows a particular syllabus. Do not attempt the sheet before you have completed your preparation for that syllabus.
- After completing the sheet check your answers with the solution booklet and complete the Result Grid. Finally spend time to analyse your performance and revise the areas which emerge out as weak in your evaluation.

1. If n drops, each charged to a potential V, coalesce to form a single drop. The potential of the big drop will be

(a) $\frac{V}{n^{2/3}}$ (b) $\frac{V}{n^{1/3}}$ (c) $Vn^{1/3}$ (d) $Vn^{2/3}$

2. The capacitance of a parallel plate capacitor is C_a (Fig. a). A dielectric of dielectric constant K is inserted as shown in fig. (b) and (c). If C_b and C_c denote the capacitances in fig. (b) and (c), then

(a) both $C_b, C_c > C_a$ (b) $C_c > C_a$ while $C_b > C_a$

(c) both $C_b, C_c < C_a$ (d) $C_a = C_b = C_c$

3. The electric potential $V(x)$ in a region around the origin is given by $V(x) = 4x^2$ volts. The electric charge enclosed in a cube of 1 m side with its centre at the origin is (in coulomb)

(a) $8\varepsilon_0$ (b) $-4\varepsilon_0$ (c) 0 (d) $-8\varepsilon_0$

4. A parallel plate condenser is immersed in an oil of dielectric constant 2. The field between the plates is

(a) increased, proportional to 2

(b) decreased, proportional to $\frac{1}{2}$

(c) increased, proportional to – 2

(d) decreased, proportional to $-\frac{1}{2}$

5. What is the effective capacitance between points *X* and *Y*?

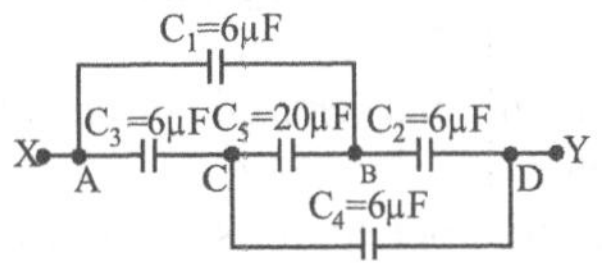

(a) 24 μ*F* (b) 18 μ*F* (c) 12 μ*F* (d) 6 μ*F*

6. Two identical particles each of mass m and having charges –q and +q are revolving in a circle of radius r under the influence of electric attraction. Kinetic energy of each particle is $\left(k = \frac{1}{4\pi\varepsilon_0}\right)$

(a) $kq^2/4r$ (b) $kq^2/2r$ (c) $kq^2/8r$ (d) kq^2/r

RESPONSE GRID					
	1. ⓐⓑⓒⓓ	2. ⓐⓑⓒⓓ	3. ⓐⓑⓒⓓ	4. ⓐⓑⓒⓓ	5. ⓐⓑⓒⓓ
	6. ⓐⓑⓒⓓ				

Space for Rough Work

7. Four metallic plates each with a surface area of one side A, are placed at a distance d from each other. The two outer plates are connected to one point A and the two other inner plates to another point B as shown in the figure. Then the capacitance of the system is

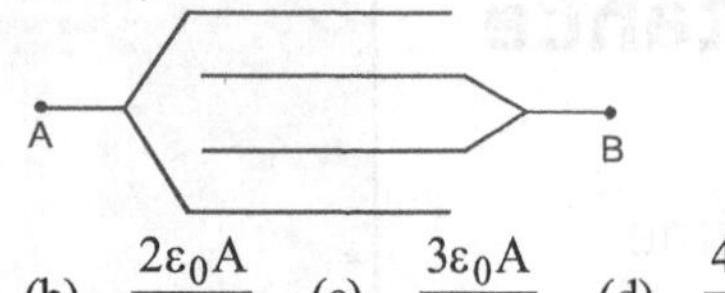

(a) $\frac{\varepsilon_0 A}{d}$ (b) $\frac{2\varepsilon_0 A}{d}$ (c) $\frac{3\varepsilon_0 A}{d}$ (d) $\frac{4\varepsilon_0 A}{d}$

8. A parallel plate condenser with a dielectric of dielectric constant K between the plates has a capacity C and is charged to a potential V volt. The dielectric slab is slowly removed from between the plates and then reinserted. The net work done by the system in this process is

(a) zero (b) $\frac{1}{2}(K-1)\,CV^2$

(c) $\frac{CV^2(K-1)}{K}$ (d) $(K-1)\,CV^2$

9. If a slab of insulating material 4×10^{-5} m thick is introduced between the plates of a parallel plate capacitor, the distance between the plates has to be increased by 3.5×10^{-5} m to restore the capacity to original value. Then the dielectric constant of the material of slab is

(a) 8 (b) 6 (c) 12 (d) 10

10. A unit charge moves on an equipotential surface from a point A to point B, then

(a) $V_A - V_B = +ve$ (b) $V_A - V_B = 0$

(c) $V_A - V_B = -ve$ (d) it is stationary

11. Identify the false statement.

(a) Inside a charged or neutral conductor, electrostatic field is zero

(b) The electrostatic field at the surface of the charged conductor must be tangential to the surface at any point

(c) There is no net charge at any point inside the conductor

(d) Electrostatic potential is constant throughout the volume of the conductor

12. In a hollow spherical shell, potential (V) changes with respect to distance (s) from centre as

(a)

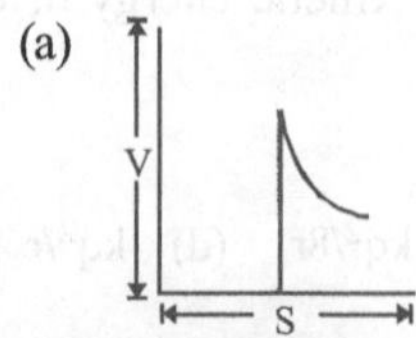

(b)

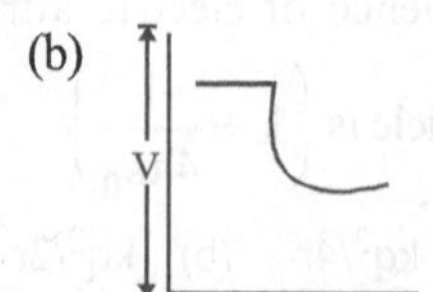

(c)

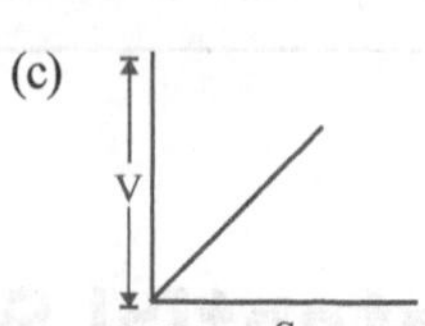

(d)

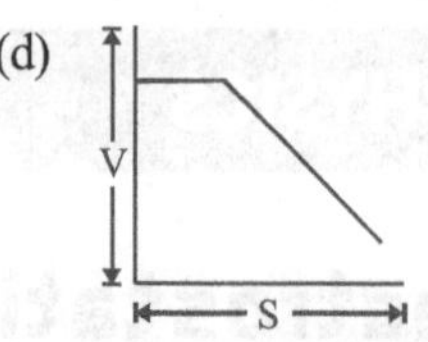

13. The 1000 small droplets of water each of radius r and charge Q, make a big drop of spherical shape. The potential of big drop is how many times the potential of one small droplet ?

(a) 1 (b) 10 (c) 100 (d) 1000

14. The work done in carrying a charge q once around a circle of radius r with a charge Q placed at the centre will be

(a) $Qq(4\pi\varepsilon_0 r^2)$ (b) $Qq/(4\pi\varepsilon_0 r)$

(c) zero (d) $Qq^2/(4\pi\varepsilon_0 r)$

15. A parallel plate condenser is filled with two dielectrics as shown. Area of each plate is A m^2 and the separation is t m. The dielectric constants are k_1 and k_2 respectively. Its capacitance in farad will be

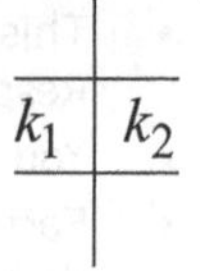

(a) $\frac{\varepsilon_0 A}{t}(k_1 + k_2)$ (b) $\frac{\varepsilon_0 A}{t}.\frac{k_1 + k_2}{2}$

(c) $\frac{2\varepsilon_0 A}{t}(k_1 + k_2)$ (d) $\frac{\varepsilon_0 A}{t}.\frac{k_1 - k_2}{2}$

16. Two metal pieces having a potential difference of 800 V are 0.02 m apart horizontally. A particle of mass 1.96×10^{-15} kg is suspended in equilibrium between the plates. If e is the elementary charge, then charge on the particle is

(a) 8 (b) 6 (c) 0.1 (d) 3

17. A one microfarad capacitor of a TV is subjected to 4000 V potential difference. The energy stored in capacitor is

(a) 8 J (b) 16 J

(c) 4×10^{-3} J (d) 2×10^{-3} J

18. An unchanged parallel plate capacitor filled with a dielectric constant K is connected to an air filled identical parallel capacitor charged to potential V_1. If the common potential is V_2, the value of K is

(a) $\frac{V_1 - V_2}{V_1}$ (b) $\frac{V_1}{V_1 - V_2}$

(c) $\frac{V_2}{V_1 - V_2}$ (d) $\frac{V_1 - V_2}{V_2}$

19. In the circuit given below, the charge in μC, on the capacitor having 5 μF is

(a) 4.5

(b) 9

(c) 7

(d) 15

RESPONSE GRID					
	7. ⓐⓑⓒⓓ	8. ⓐⓑⓒⓓ	9. ⓐⓑⓒⓓ	10. ⓐⓑⓒⓓ	11. ⓐⓑⓒⓓ
	12. ⓐⓑⓒⓓ	13. ⓐⓑⓒⓓ	14. ⓐⓑⓒⓓ	15. ⓐⓑⓒⓓ	16. ⓐⓑⓒⓓ
	17. ⓐⓑⓒⓓ	18. ⓐⓑⓒⓓ	19. ⓐⓑⓒⓓ		

Space for Rough Work

20. Two concentric, thin metallic spheres of radii R_1 and R_2 ($R_1 > R_2$) bear charges Q_1 and Q_2 respectively. Then the potential at distance r between R_1 and R_2 will be

(a) $k\left(\frac{Q_1+Q_2}{r}\right)$ (b) $k\left(\frac{Q_1}{r}+\frac{Q_2}{R_2}\right)$

(c) $k\left(\frac{Q_2}{r}+\frac{Q_1}{R_1}\right)$ (d) $k\left(\frac{Q_1}{R_1}+\frac{Q_2}{R_2}\right)$

21. Charge Q on a capacitor varies with voltage V as shown in the figure, where Q is taken along the X-axis and V along the Y-axis. The area of triangle OAB represents

(a) capacitance
(b) capacitive reactance
(c) magnetic field between the plates
(d) energy stored in the capacitor

22. An alpha particle is accelerated through a potential difference of 10^6 volt. Its kinetic energy will be

(a) 1 MeV (b) 2 MeV (c) 4 MeV (d) 8 MeV

23. Four point charges $-Q$, $-q$, $2q$ and $2Q$ are placed, one at each corner of the square. The relation between Q and q for which the potential at the centre of the square is zero is :

(a) $Q=-q$ (b) $Q=-\frac{1}{q}$ (c) $Q=q$ (d) $Q=\frac{1}{q}$

24. A parallel plate capacitor having a separation between the plates d, plate area A and material with dielectric constant K has capacitance C_0. Now one-third of the material is replaced by another material with dielectric constant 2K, so that effectively there are two capacitors one with area 1/3A, dielectric constant 2K and another with area 2/3A and dielectric constant K. If the capacitance of this new capacitor is C then $\frac{C}{C_0}$ is

(a) 1 (b) 4/3 (c) 2/3 (d) 1/3

25. Two condensers, one of capacity C and other of capacity C/2 are connected to a V-volt battery, as shown. The work done in charging fully both the condensers is

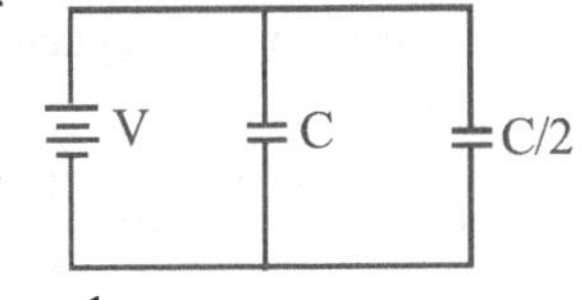

(a) $\frac{1}{4}CV^2$ (b) $\frac{3}{4}CV^2$ (c) $\frac{1}{2}CV^2$ (d) $2CV^2$.

26. A, B and C are three points in a uniform electric field. The electric potential is

(a) maximum at B
(b) maximum at C
(c) same at all the three points A, B and C
(d) maximum at A

27. Three capacitors are connected in the arms of a triangle ABC as shown in figure 5 V is applied between A and B. The voltage between B and C is

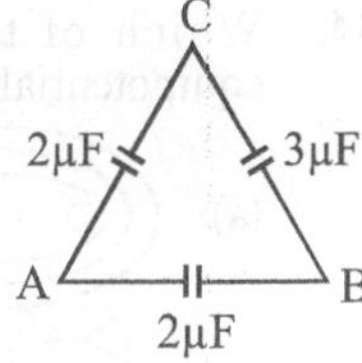

(a) 2V (b) 1V
(c) 3V (d) 1.5V

28. Two parallel metal plates having charges + Q and –Q face each other at a certain distance between them. If the plaves are now dipped in kerosene oil tank, the electric field between the plates will

(a) remain same (b) become zero
(c) increases (d) decrease

29. An air capacitor C connected to a battery of e.m.f. V acquires a charge q and energy E. The capacitor is disconnected from the battery and a dielectric slab is placed between the plates. Which of the following statements is correct ?

(a) V and q decrease but C and E increase
(b) V remains unchange, but q, E and C increase
(c) q remains unchanged, C increases, V and E decrease
(d) q and C increase but V and E decrease.

30. Choose the wrong statement about equipotential surfaces.

(a) It is a surface over which the potential is constant
(b) The electric field is parallel to the equipotential surface
(c) The electric field is perpendicular to the equipotential surface
(d) The electric field is in the direction of steepest decrease of potential

31. Two spherical conductors A and B of radii a and b (b>a) are placed concentrically in air. The two are connected by a copper wire as shown in figure. Then the equivalent capacitance of the system is

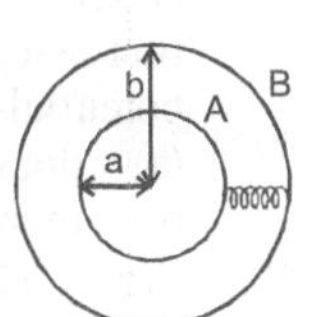

(a) $4\pi\varepsilon_0\frac{ab}{b-a}$ (b) $4\pi\varepsilon_0(a+b)$

(c) $4\pi\varepsilon_0 b$ (d) $4\pi\varepsilon_0 a$

32. A capacitor is charged to store an energy U. The charging battery is disconnected. An identical capacitor is now connected to the first capacitor in parallel. The energy in each of the capacitors is

(a) U/2 (b) 3U/2 (c) U (d) U/4

33. Equipotentials at a great distance from a collection of charges whose total sum is not zero are approximately

(a) spheres (b) planes
(c) paraboloids (d) ellipsoids

RESPONSE GRID				
20. ⓐⓑⓒⓓ	21. ⓐⓑⓒⓓ	22. ⓐⓑⓒⓓ	23. ⓐⓑⓒⓓ	24. ⓐⓑⓒⓓ
25. ⓐⓑⓒⓓ	26. ⓐⓑⓒⓓ	27. ⓐⓑⓒⓓ	28. ⓐⓑⓒⓓ	29. ⓐⓑⓒⓓ
30. ⓐⓑⓒⓓ	31. ⓐⓑⓒⓓ	32. ⓐⓑⓒⓓ	33. ⓐⓑⓒⓓ	

Space for Rough Work

34. Which of the following figure shows the correct equipotential surfaces of a system of two positive charges?

(a) 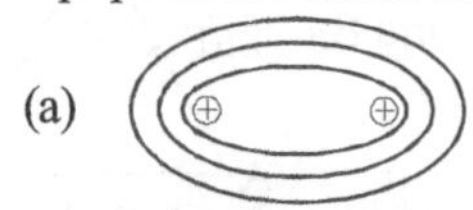
(b) 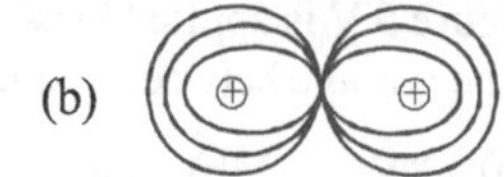
(c) 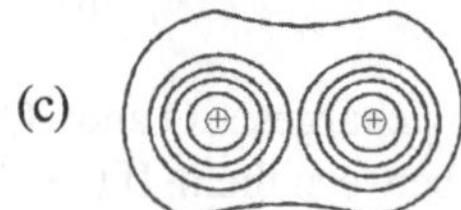
(d)

35. Two identical metal plates are given positive charges Q_1 and Q_2 ($< Q_1$) respectively. If they are now brought close together to form a parallel plate capacitor with capacitance C, the potential difference between them is

(a) $\frac{Q_1+Q_2}{2C}$ (b) $\frac{Q_1+Q_2}{C}$ (c) $\frac{Q_1-Q_2}{C}$ (d) $\frac{Q_1-Q_2}{2C}$

36. The capacitance of the capacitor of plate areas A_1 and A_2 ($A_1 < A_2$) at a distance d, as shown in figure is

(a) $\frac{\epsilon_0 (A_1+A_2)}{2d}$ (b) $\frac{\epsilon_0 A_2}{d}$

(c) $\frac{\epsilon_0 \sqrt{A_1 A_2}}{d}$ (d) $\frac{\epsilon_0 A_1}{d}$

37. In a given network the equivalent capacitance between *A* and *B* is [$C_1 = C_4 = 1\,\mu F$, $C_2 = C_3 = 2\mu F$]

(a) $3\,\mu F$ (b) $6\,\mu F$

(c) $4.5\,\mu F$ (d) $2.5\,\mu F$

38. A parallel plate air capacitor is charged to a potential difference of V volts. After disconnecting the charging battery the distance between the plates of the capacitor is increased using an insulating handle. As a result the potential difference between the plates

(a) does not change (b) becomes zero

(c) increases (d) decreases

39. Figure shows three circular arcs, each of radius R and total charge as indicated. The net electric potential at the centre of curvature is

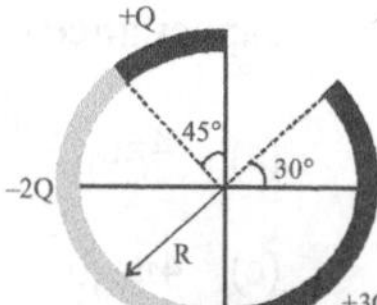

(a) $\frac{Q}{2\pi\varepsilon_0 R}$ (b) $\frac{Q}{4\pi\varepsilon_0 R}$

(c) $\frac{2Q}{\pi\varepsilon_0 R}$ (d) $\frac{Q}{\pi\varepsilon_0 R}$

40. An electric field $\vec{E} = (25\hat{i} + 30\hat{j})NC^{-1}$ exists in a region of space. If the potential at the origin is taken to be zero then the potential at $x = 2\ m$, $y = 2\ m$ is :

(a) –110 V (b) –140 V (c) –120 V (d) –130 V

41. If a unit positive charge is taken from one point to another over an equipotential surface, then

(a) work is done on the charge
(b) work is done by the charge
(c) work done is constant
(d) no work is done

42. Three large plates A, B and C are placed parallel to each other and charges are given as shown. The charge that appears on the left surface of plate B is

(a) 5C (b) 6C (c) 3C (d) –3C

43. Three charges 2 q, – q and – q are located at the vertices of an equilateral triangle. At the centre of the triangle

(a) the field is zero but potential is non-zero
(b) the field is non-zero, but potential is zero
(c) both field and potential are zero
(d) both field and potential are non-zero

44. If a charge – 150 nC is given to a concentric spherical shell and a charge +50 nC is placed at its centre then the charge on inner and outer surface of the shell is

(a) –50 nC, –100 nC (b) +50 nC, –200 nC

(c) –50 nC, –200 nC (d) 50 nC, 100 nC

45. Two capacitors of capacitances C_1 and C_2 are connected in parallel across a battery. If Q_1 and Q_2 respectively be the charges on the capacitors, then $\frac{Q_1}{Q_2}$ will be equal to

(a) $\frac{C_2}{C_1}$ (b) $\frac{C_1}{C_2}$ (c) $\frac{C_1^2}{C_2^2}$ (d) $\frac{C_2^2}{C_1^2}$

RESPONSE GRID					
	34. (a)(b)(c)(d)	35. (a)(b)(c)(d)	36. (a)(b)(c)(d)	37. (a)(b)(c)(d)	38. (a)(b)(c)(d)
	39. (a)(b)(c)(d)	40. (a)(b)(c)(d)	41. (a)(b)(c)(d)	42. (a)(b)(c)(d)	43. (a)(b)(c)(d)
	44. (a)(b)(c)(d)	45. (a)(b)(c)(d)			

PHYSICS CHAPTERWISE SPEED TEST-16

Total Questions	45	Total Marks	180
Attempted		Correct	
Incorrect		Net Score	
Cut-off Score	50	Qualifying Score	70
Success Gap = Net Score – Qualifying Score			
Net Score = (Correct × 4) – (Incorrect × 1)			

Space for Rough Work

PHYSICS

Current Electricity

Speed TEST 17

Chapter-wise

No. of Questions	Maximum Marks	Time
45	180	1 Hour

GENERAL INSTRUCTIONS

- This test contains 45 MCQ's. For each question only one option is correct. Darken the correct circle/ bubble in the Response Grid provided on each page.
- You have to evaluate your Response Grids yourself with the help of solutions provided at the end of this book.
- Each correct answer will get you 4 marks and 1 mark shall be deduced for each incorrect answer. No mark will be given/ deducted if no bubble is filled. Keep a timer in front of you and stop immediately at the end of 60 min.
- The sheet follows a particular syllabus. Do not attempt the sheet before you have completed your preparation for that syllabus.
- After completing the sheet check your answers with the solution booklet and complete the Result Grid. Finally spend time to analyse your performance and revise the areas which emerge out as weak in your evaluation.

1. When 5V potential difference is applied across a wire of length 0.1 m, the drift speed of electrons is $2.5 \times 10^{-4}\, ms^{-1}$. If the electron density in the wire is $8 \times 10^{28}\, m^{-3}$, the resistivity of the material is close to :
(a) $1.6 \times 10^{-6}\, \Omega m$ (b) $1.6 \times 10^{-5}\, \Omega m$
(c) $1.6 \times 10^{-8}\, \Omega m$ (d) $1.6 \times 10^{-7}\, \Omega m$

2. Variation of current passing through a conductor as the voltage applied across its ends is varied as shown in the adjoining diagram. If the resistance (R) is determined at the points A, B, C and D, we will find that

(V vs i graph with points A, B, C, D)

(a) $R_C = R_D$
(b) $R_B > R_A$
(c) $R_C > R_B$
(d) $R_A > R_B$

3. The length of a wire of a potentiometer is 100 cm, and the e.m.f. of its standard cell is E volt. It is employed to measure the e.m.f. of a battery whose internal resistance is 0.5Ω. If the balance point is obtained at $\ell = 30$ cm from the positive end, the e.m.f. of the battery is
(a) $\frac{30E}{100.5}$ (b) $\frac{30E}{(100-0.5)}$
(c) $\frac{30(E-0.5i)}{100}$ (d) $\frac{30E}{100}$

4. The masses of the three wires of copper are in the ratio of 1 : 3 : 5 and their lengths are in the ratio of 5 : 3 : 1. The ratio of their electrical resistance is
(a) 1 : 3 : 5 (b) 5 : 3 : 1
(c) 1 : 25 : 125 (d) 125 : 15 : 1

5. n equal resistors are first connected in series and then connected in parallel. What is the ratio of the maximum to the minimum resistance?
(a) n (b) $1/n^2$ (c) n^2 (d) $1/n$

6. A battery is charged at a potential of 15V for 8 hours when the current flowing is 10A. The battery on discharge supplies a current of 5A for 15 hours. The mean terminal voltage during discharge is 14V. The "watt-hour" efficiency of the battery is
(a) 87.5% (b) 82.5% (c) 80% (d) 90%

RESPONSE GRID	1. ⓐⓑⓒⓓ 2. ⓐⓑⓒⓓ 3. ⓐⓑⓒⓓ 4. ⓐⓑⓒⓓ 5. ⓐⓑⓒⓓ 6. ⓐⓑⓒⓓ

Space for Rough Work

7. Shown in the figure below is a meter-bridge set up with null deflection in the galvanometer.

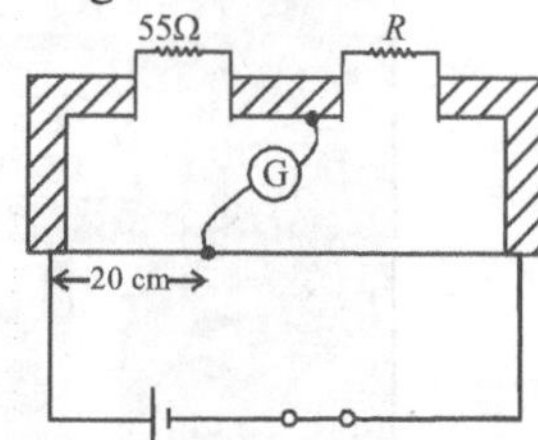

The value of the unknown resistor R is
(a) 13.75 Ω (b) 220 Ω (c) 110 Ω (d) 55 Ω

8. In the equation AB = C, A is the current density, C is the electric field, Then B is
(a) resistivity (b) conductivity
(c) potential difference (d) resistance

9. The Kirchhoff's first law ($\Sigma i = 0$) and second law ($\Sigma iR = \Sigma E$), are respectively based on
(a) conservation of charge, conservation of momentum
(b) conservation of energy, conservation of charge
(c) conservation of momentum, conservation of charge
(d) conservation of charge, conservation of energy

10. You are given a resistance coil and a battery. In which of the following cases the largest amount of heat generated ?
(a) When the coil is connected to the battery directly
(b) When the coil is divided into two equal parts and both the parts are connected to the battery in parallel
(c) When the coil is divided into four equal parts and all the four parts are connected to the battery in parallel
(d) When only half the coil is connected to the battery

11. The resistance of the coil of an ammeter is R. The shunt required to increase its range n-fold should have a resistance
(a) $\frac{R}{n}$ (b) $\frac{R}{n-1}$ (c) $\frac{R}{n+1}$ (d) nR

12. On increasing the temperature of a conductor, its resistance increases because the
(a) relaxation time increases
(b) mass of electron increases
(c) electron density decreases
(d) relaxation time decreases

13. An electric current is passed through a circuit containing two wires of the same material, connected in parallel. If the lengths and radii are in the ratio of $\frac{4}{3}$ and $\frac{2}{3}$, then the ratio of the current passing through the wires will be
(a) 8/9 (b) 1/3 (c) 3 (d) 2

14. In a meter bridge experiment null point is obtained at 20 cm. from one end of the wire when resistance X is balanced against another resistance Y. If $X < Y$, then where will be the new position of the null point from the same end, if one decides to balance a resistance of $4X$ against Y
(a) 40 cm (b) 80 cm (c) 50 cm (d) 70 cm

15. In the circuit shown, the current through 8 ohm is same before and after connecting E. The value of E is
(a) 12 V
(b) 6 V
(c) 4 V
(d) 2 V

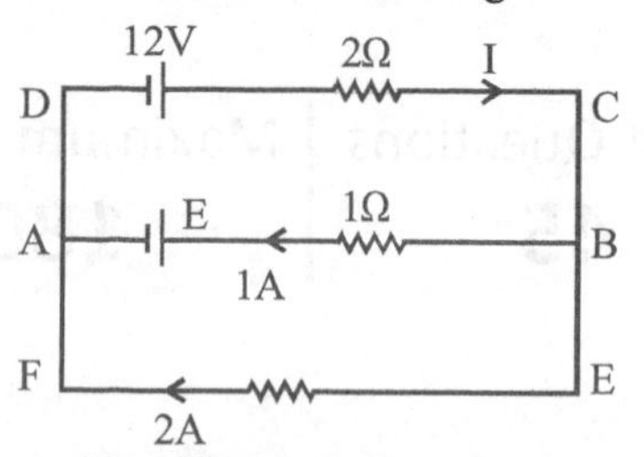

16. Find emf E of the cell as shown in figure.

12V
2Ω
I
D
C
E
1Ω
A
B
1A
F
E
2A

(a) 15V (b) 10V (c) 12V (d) 5V

17. A torch bulb rated as 4.5 W, 1.5 V is connected as shown in fig. The e.m.f. of the cell, needed to make the bulb glow at full intensity is

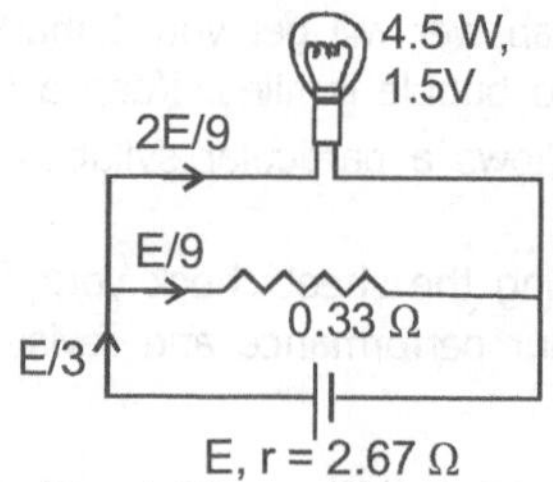

(a) 4.5 V (b) 1.5 V (c) 2.67 V (d) 13.5 V

18. In a given network, each resistance has value of 6Ω. The point X is connected to point A by a copper wire of negligible resistance and point Y is connected to point B by the same wire. The effective resistance between X and Y will be

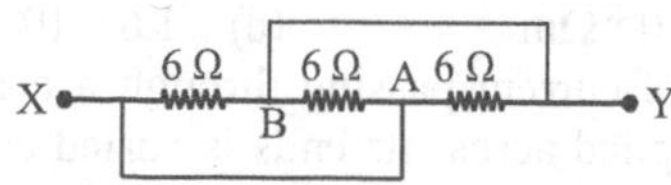

(a) 18Ω (b) 6Ω (c) 3Ω (d) 2Ω

19. If N, e, τ and m are representing electron density, charge, relaxation time and mass of an electron respectively, then the resistance of wire of length ℓ and cross-sectional area A is given by
(a) $\frac{2m\ell}{Ne^2A\tau}$ (b) $\frac{2m\tau A}{Ne^2\ell}$ (c) $\frac{Ne^2\tau A}{2m\ell}$ (d) $\frac{Ne^2A}{2m\tau\ell}$

20. Cell having an emf ε and internal resistance r is connected across a variable external resistance R. As the resistance R is increased, the plot of potential difference V across R is given by :

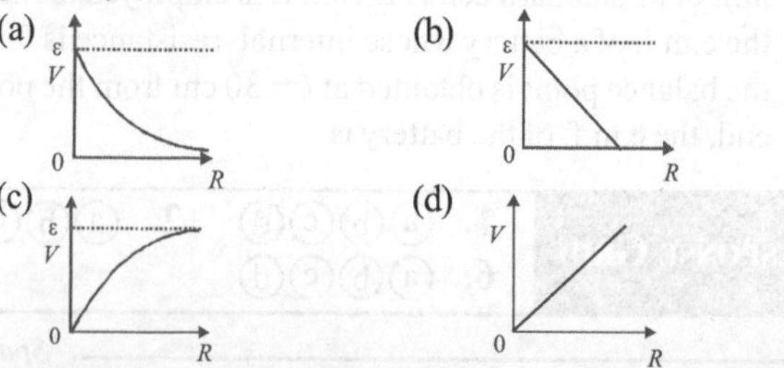

RESPONSE GRID
7. ⓐⓑⓒⓓ 8. ⓐⓑⓒⓓ 9. ⓐⓑⓒⓓ 10. ⓐⓑⓒⓓ 11. ⓐⓑⓒⓓ
12. ⓐⓑⓒⓓ 13. ⓐⓑⓒⓓ 14. ⓐⓑⓒⓓ 15. ⓐⓑⓒⓓ 16. ⓐⓑⓒⓓ
17. ⓐⓑⓒⓓ 18. ⓐⓑⓒⓓ 19. ⓐⓑⓒⓓ 20. ⓐⓑⓒⓓ

Space for Rough Work

21. If voltage across a bulb rated 220 Volt-100 Watt drops by 2.5% of its rated value, the percentage of the rated value by which the power would decrease is :
(a) 20% (b) 2.5% (c) 5% (d) 10%

22. If specific resistance of a potentiometer wire is $10^{-7}\ \Omega$m, the current flow through it is 0.1 A and the cross-sectional area of wire is $10^{-6}\ m^2$ then potential gradient will be
(a) 10^{-2} volt/m (b) 10^{-4} volt/m
(c) 10^{-6} volt/m (d) 10^{-8} volt/m

23. Two resistances R_1 and R_2 are made of different materials. The temperature coefficient of the material of R_1 is α and that of material of R_2 is $-\beta$. The resistance of the series combination of R_1 and R_2 will not change with temperature if $\frac{R_1}{R_2}$ equal to
(a) $\frac{\alpha}{\beta}$ (b) $\frac{\alpha+\beta}{\alpha-\beta}$ (c) $\frac{\alpha^2+\beta^2}{2\alpha\beta}$ (d) $\frac{\beta}{\alpha}$

24. Five cells each of emf *E* and internal resistance *r* send the same amount of current through an external resistance *R* whether the cells are connected in parallel or in series. Then the ratio $\left(\frac{R}{r}\right)$ is
(a) 2 (b) $\frac{1}{2}$ (c) $\frac{1}{5}$ (d) 1

25. The length of a given cylindrical wire is increased by 100%. Due to the consequent decrease in diameter the change in the resistance of the wire will be
(a) 200% (b) 100% (c) 50% (d) 300%

26. Potentiometer wire of length 1 m is connected in series with 490Ω resistance and 2 V battery. If 0.2 mV/cm is the potential gradient, then resistance of the potentiometer wire is
(a) 4.9 Ω (b) 7.9 Ω (c) 5.9 Ω (d) 6.9 Ω

27. See the electric circuit shown in the figure. Which of the following equations is a correct equation for it?
(a) $\varepsilon_2 - i_2 r_2 - \varepsilon_1 - i_1 r_1 = 0$
(b) $-\varepsilon_2 - (i_1 + i_2)R + i_2 r_2 = 0$
(c) $\varepsilon_1 - (i_1 + i_2)R + i_1 r_1 = 0$
(d) $\varepsilon_1 - (i_1 + i_2)R - i_1 r_1 = 0$

28. In a large building, there are 15 bulbs of 40 W, 5 bulbs of 100 W, 5 fans of 80 W and 1 heater of 1 kW. The voltage of electric mains is 220 V. The minimum capacity of the main fuse of the building will be:
(a) 8 A (b) 10 A (c) 12 A (d) 14 A

29. Two sources of equal emf are connected to an external resistance *R*. The internal resistance of the two sources are R_1 and R_2 ($R_1 > R_1$). If the potential difference across the source having internal resistance R_2 is zero, then
(a) $R = R_2 - R_1$
(b) $R = R_2 \times (R_1 + R_2)/(R_2 - R_1)$
(c) $R = R_1R_2/(R_2 - R_1)$
(d) $R = R_1R_2/(R_1 - R_2)$

30. The resistance of the series combination of two resistances is S. when they are joined in parallel the total resistance is P. If $S = nP$ then the minimum possible value of *n* is
(a) 2 (b) 3 (c) 4 (d) 1

31. If an ammeter is to be used in place of a voltmeter, then we must connect with the ammeter a
(a) low resistance in parallel
(b) high resistance in parallel
(c) high resistance in series
(d) low resistance in series.

32. A d.c. main supply of e.m.f. 220 V is connected across a storage battery of e.m.f. 200 V through a resistance of 1Ω. The battery terminals are connected to an external resistance 'R'. The minimum value of 'R', so that a current passes through the battery to charge it is:
(a) 7 Ω (b) 9 Ω (c) 11 Ω (d) Zero

33. In the given circuit diagram when the current reaches steady state in the circuit, the charge on the capacitor of capacitance C will be :
(a) $CE\frac{r_2}{(r+r_2)}$
(b) $CE\frac{r_1}{(r_1+r)}$
(c) $CE\frac{r_2}{(r+r_1)}$
(d) $CE\frac{r_1}{(r_2+r)}$

34. Suppose the drift velocity v_d in a material varied with the applied electric field E as $v_d \propto \sqrt{E}$. Then V – I graph for a wire made of such a material is best given by :

(a) 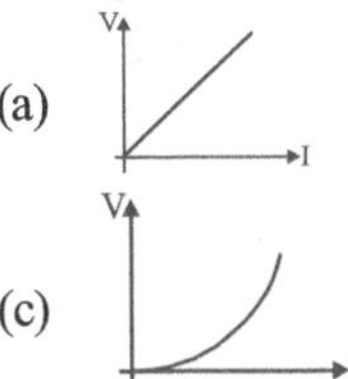

(b) 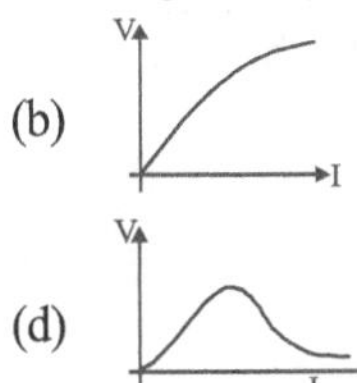

(c)

(d)

35. In a neon gas discharge tube Ne^+ ions moving through a cross-section of the tube each second to the right is 2.9×10^{18}, while 1.2×10^{18} electrons move towards left in the same time; the electronic charge being 1.6×10^{-19} C, the net electric current is
(a) 0.27 A to the right (b) 0.66 A to the right
(c) 0.66 A to the left (d) zero

36. Two rods are joined end to end, as shown. Both have a cross-sectional area of 0.01 cm^2. Each is 1 meter long. One rod is of copper with a resistivity of 1.7×10^{-6} ohm-centimeter, the other is of iron with a resistivity of 10^{-5} ohm-centimeter. How much voltage is required to produce a current of 1 ampere in the rods?
(a) 0.117V
(b) 0.00145V
(c) 0.0145V
(d) 1.7×10^{-6} V

RESPONSE GRID

21. ⓐⓑⓒⓓ 22. ⓐⓑⓒⓓ 23. ⓐⓑⓒⓓ 24. ⓐⓑⓒⓓ 25. ⓐⓑⓒⓓ
26. ⓐⓑⓒⓓ 27. ⓐⓑⓒⓓ 28. ⓐⓑⓒⓓ 29. ⓐⓑⓒⓓ 30. ⓐⓑⓒⓓ
31. ⓐⓑⓒⓓ 32. ⓐⓑⓒⓓ 33. ⓐⓑⓒⓓ 34. ⓐⓑⓒⓓ 35. ⓐⓑⓒⓓ
36. ⓐⓑⓒⓓ

Space for Rough Work

37. An energy source will supply a constant current into the load if its internal resistance is
(a) very large as compared to the load resistance
(b) equal to the resistance of the load
(c) non-zero but less than the resistance of the load
(d) zero

38. The resistance of a wire at room temperature 30°C is found to be 10 Ω. Now to increase the resistance by 10%, the temperature of the wire must be [The temperature coefficient of resistance of the material of the wire is 0.002 per °C]
(a) 36°C (b) 83°C
(c) 63°C (d) 33°C

39. If current flowing in a conductor changes by 1% then power consumed will change by
(a) 10% (b) 2% (c) 1% (d) 100%

40. In the circuit shown in figure, the 5Ω resistance develops 20.00 cal/s due to the current flowing through it. The heat developed in 2 Ω resistance (in cal/s) is

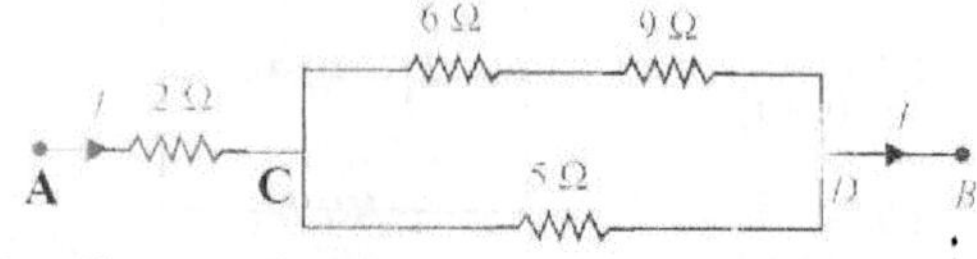

(a) 23.8 (b) 14.2 (c) 11.9 (d) 7.1

41. In a Wheatstone's bridge, three resistances P, Q and R connected in the three arms and the fourth arm is formed by two resistances S_1 and S_2 connected in parallel. The condition for the bridge to be balanced will be
(a) $\frac{P}{Q}=\frac{2R}{S_1+S_2}$ (b) $\frac{P}{Q}=\frac{R(S_1+S_2)}{S_1S_2}$
(c) $\frac{P}{Q}=\frac{R(S_1+S_2)}{2S_1S_2}$ (d) $\frac{P}{Q}=\frac{R}{S_1+S_2}$

42. The electric resistance of a certain wire of iron is R. If its length and radius are both doubled, then
(a) the resistance and the specific resistance, will both remain unchanged
(b) the resistance will be doubled and the specific resistance will be halved
(c) the resistance will be halved and the specific resistance will remain unchanged
(d) the resistance will be halved and the specific resistance will be doubled

43. A car battery has e.m.f. 12 volt and internal resistance 5×10^{-2} ohm. If it draws 60 amp current, the terminal voltage of the battery will be
(a) 15 volt (b) 3 volt (c) 5 volt (d) 9 volt

44. A conducting wire of cross-sectional area 1 cm^2 has 3×10^{23} charge carriers per m^3. If wire carries a current of 24 mA, then drift velocity of carriers is
(a) 5×10^{-2} m/s (b) 0.5 m/s
(c) 5×10^{-3} m/s (d) 5×10^{-6} m/s

45. In the series combination of *n* cells each cell having emf ε and internal resistance *r*. If three cells are wrongly connected, then total emf and internal resistance of this combination will be
(a) $n\varepsilon$, $(nr - 3r)$ (b) $(n\varepsilon - 2\varepsilon)$ nr
(c) $(n\varepsilon - 4\varepsilon)$, nr (d) $(n\varepsilon - 6\varepsilon)$, nr

RESPONSE GRID					
	37. ⓐⓑⓒⓓ	38. ⓐⓑⓒⓓ	39. ⓐⓑⓒⓓ	40. ⓐⓑⓒⓓ	41. ⓐⓑⓒⓓ
	42. ⓐⓑⓒⓓ	43. ⓐⓑⓒⓓ	44. ⓐⓑⓒⓓ	45. ⓐⓑⓒⓓ	

PHYSICS CHAPTERWISE SPEED TEST-17

Total Questions	45	Total Marks	180
Attempted		Correct	
Incorrect		Net Score	
Cut-off Score	45	Qualifying Score	60
Success Gap = Net Score – Qualifying Score			
Net Score = (Correct × 4) – (Incorrect × 1)			

Space for Rough Work

PHYSICS

Moving Charges and Magnetism

Speed TEST 18 Chapter-wise

No. of Questions	Maximum Marks	Time
45	180	1 Hour

GENERAL INSTRUCTIONS

- This test contains 45 MCQ's. For each question only one option is correct. Darken the correct circle/ bubble in the Response Grid provided on each page.
- You have to evaluate your Response Grids yourself with the help of solutions provided at the end of this book.
- Each correct answer will get you 4 marks and 1 mark shall be deduced for each incorrect answer. No mark will be given/ deducted if no bubble is filled. Keep a timer in front of you and stop immediately at the end of 60 min.
- The sheet follows a particular syllabus. Do not attempt the sheet before you have completed your preparation for that syllabus.
- After completing the sheet check your answers with the solution booklet and complete the Result Grid. Finally spend time to analyse your performance and revise the areas which emerge out as weak in your evaluation.

1. An insulating rod of length ℓ carries a charge q distributed uniformly on it. The rod is pivoted at its mid point and is rotated at a frequency f about a fixed axis perpendicular to rod and passing through the pivot. The magnetic moment of the rod system is $\frac{1}{2a}\pi q f \ell^2$. Find the value of a.
   (a) 6 (b) 4
   (c) 5 (d) 8

2. A portion of a conductive wire is bent in the form of a semicircle of radius r as shown below in fig. At the centre of semicircle, the magnetic induction will be

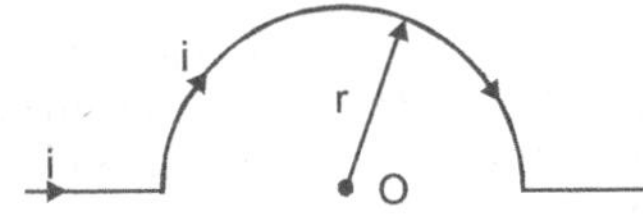

   (a) zero (b) infinite
   (c) $\frac{\mu_0}{4\pi}.\frac{2\pi i}{r}$ (d) $\frac{\mu_0}{4\pi}.\frac{\pi i}{r}$

3. A closely wound solenoid of 2000 turns and area of cross-section 1.5×10^{-4} m^2 carries a current of 2.0 *A*. It suspended through its centre and perpendicular to its length, allowing it to turn in a horizontal plane in a uniform magnetic field 5×10^{-2} tesla making an angle of 30° with the axis of the solenoid. The torque on the solenoid will be:
   (a) 3×10^{-2} N-m (b) 3×10^{-3} N-m
   (c) 1.5×10^{-3} N-m (d) 1.5×10^{-2} N-m

4. An alternating electric field, of frequency *v*, is applied across the dees (radius = *R*) of a cyclotron that is being used to accelerate protons (mass = *m*). The operating magnetic field (*B*) used in the cyclotron and the kinetic energy (*K*) of the proton beam, produced by it, are given by :
   (a) $B = \frac{mv}{e}$ and $K = 2m\pi^2 v^2 R^2$
   (b) $B = \frac{2\pi mv}{e}$ and $K = m^2 \pi v R^2$
   (c) $B = \frac{2\pi mv}{e}$ and $K = 2m\pi^2 v^2 R^2$
   (d) $B = \frac{mv}{e}$ and $K = m^2 \pi v R^2$

5. A galvanometer of 50 ohm resistance has 25 divisions. A current of 4×10^{-4} ampere gives a deflection of one per division. To convert this galvanometer into a voltmeter having a range of 25 volts, it should be connected with a resistance of
   (a) 2450 Ω in series (b) 2500 Ω in series.
   (c) 245 Ω in series. (d) 2550 Ω in series.

RESPONSE GRID	1. ⓐⓑⓒⓓ	2. ⓐⓑⓒⓓ	3. ⓐⓑⓒⓓ	4. ⓐⓑⓒⓓ	5. ⓐⓑⓒⓓ

Space for Rough Work

6. If we double the radius of a coil keeping the current through it unchanged, then the magnetic field at any point at a large distance from the centre becomes approximately
(a) double (b) three times
(c) four times (d) one-fourth

7. A particle of mass m, charge Q and kinetic energy T enters a transverse uniform magnetic field of induction $\vec{B}$. After 3 seconds, the kinetic energy of the particle will be:
(a) 3T (b) 2T
(c) T (d) 4T

8. A 10 eV electron is circulating in a plane at right angles to a uniform field at magnetic induction 10^{-4} Wb/m^2 (= 1.0 gauss). The orbital radius of the electron is
(a) 12 cm (b) 16 cm
(c) 11 cm (d) 18 cm

9. A uniform electric field and a uniform magnetic field exist in a region in the same direction. An electron is projected with velocity pointed in the same direction. The electron will
(a) turn to its right
(b) turn to its left
(c) keep moving in the same direction but its speed will increase
(d) keep moving in the same direction but its speed will decrease

10. Proton, deuteron and alpha particle of same kinetic energy are moving in circular trajectories in a constant magnetic field. The radii of proton, deuteron and alpha particle are respectively r_p, r_d and r_α. Which one of the following relation is correct?
(a) $r_\alpha = r_p = r_d$ (b) $r_\alpha = r_p < r_d$
(c) $r_\alpha > r_d > r_p$ (d) $r_\alpha = r_d > r_p$

11. A moving coil galvanometer has 150 equal divisions. Its current sensitivity is 10-divisions per milliampere and voltage sensitivity is 2 divisions per millivolt. In order that each division reads 1 volt, the resistance in ohms needed to be connected in series with the coil will be
(a) 10^5 (b) 10^3 (c) 9995 (d) 99995

12. A 2 μC charge moving around a circle with a frequency of 6.25×10^{12} Hz produces a magnetic field 6.28 tesla at the centre of the circle. The radius of the circle is
(a) 2.25 m (b) 0.25 m (c) 13.0 m (d) 1.25 m

13. A charged particle with charge q enters a region of constant, uniform and mutually orthogonal fields $\vec{E}$ and $\vec{B}$ with a velocity $\vec{v}$ perpendicular to both $\vec{E}$ and $\vec{B}$, and comes out without any change in magnitude or direction of $\vec{v}$. Then
(a) $\vec{v} = \vec{B} \times \vec{E} / E^2$ (b) $\vec{v} = \vec{E} \times \vec{B} / B^2$
(c) $\vec{v} = \vec{B} \times \vec{E} / B^2$ (d) $\vec{v} = \vec{E} \times \vec{B} / E^2$

14. A square current carrying loop is suspended in a uniform magnetic field acting in the plane of the loop. If the force on one arm of the loop is $\vec{F}$, the net force on the remaining three arms of the loop is
(a) $3\vec{F}$ (b) $-\vec{F}$
(c) $-3\vec{F}$ (d) $\vec{F}$

15. A straight section PQ of a circuit lies along the X-axis from $x = -\frac{a}{2}$ to $x = \frac{a}{2}$ and carries a steady current i. The magnetic field due to the section PQ at a point $X = +a$ will be
(a) proportional to a (b) proportional to a^2
(c) proportional to $1/a$ (d) zero

16. A and B are two conductors carrying a current i in the same direction. x and y are two electron beams moving in the same direction. Then

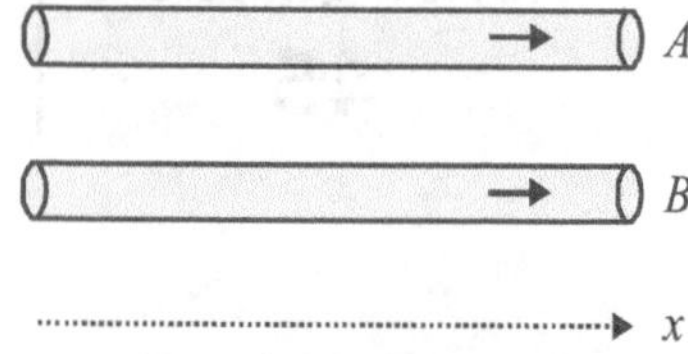

(a) there will be repulsion betwen A and B, attraction between x and y
(b) there will be attraction between A and B, repulsion between x and y
(c) there will be repulsion between A and B and also x and y
(d) there will be attraction between A and B and also x and y

17. A galvanometer of resistance, G is shunted by a resistance S ohm. To keep the main current in the circuit unchanged, the resistance to be put in series with the galvanometer is
(a) $\frac{S^2}{(S+G)}$ (b) $\frac{SG}{(S+G)}$ (c) $\frac{G^2}{(S+G)}$ (d) $\frac{G}{(S+G)}$

18. A current I flows in an infinitely long wire with cross section in the form of a semi-circular ring of radius R. The magnitude of the magnetic induction along its axis is:
(a) $\frac{\mu_0 I}{2\pi^2 R}$ (b) $\frac{\mu_0 I}{2\pi R}$ (c) $\frac{\mu_0 I}{4\pi R}$ (d) $\frac{\mu_0 I}{\pi^2 R}$

19. Two equal electric currents are flowing perpendicular to each other as shown in the figure. AB and CD are perpendicular to each other and symmetrically placed with respect to the current flow. Where do we expect the resultant magnetic field to be zero?

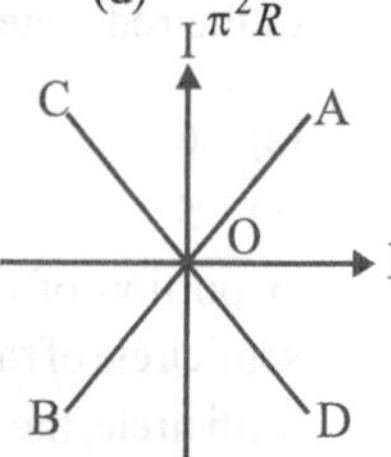

(a) On AB (b) On CD
(c) On both AB and CD (d) On both OD and BO

20. A closed loop PQRS carrying a current is placed in a uniform magnetic field.
If the magnetic forces on segments PS, SR, and RQ are F_1, F_2 and F_3 respectively and are in the plane of the paper and along the directions shown, the force on the segment QP is
(a) $F_3 - F_1 - F_2$
(b) $\sqrt{(F_3 - F_1)^2 + F_2^2}$
(c) $\sqrt{(F_3 - F_1)^2 - F_2^2}$
(d) $F_3 - F_1 + F_2$

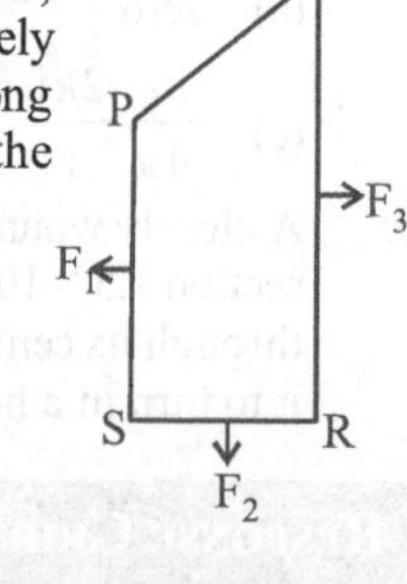

RESPONSE GRID				
6. ⓐⓑⓒⓓ	7. ⓐⓑⓒⓓ	8. ⓐⓑⓒⓓ	9. ⓐⓑⓒⓓ	10. ⓐⓑⓒⓓ
11. ⓐⓑⓒⓓ	12. ⓐⓑⓒⓓ	13. ⓐⓑⓒⓓ	14. ⓐⓑⓒⓓ	15. ⓐⓑⓒⓓ
16. ⓐⓑⓒⓓ	17. ⓐⓑⓒⓓ	18. ⓐⓑⓒⓓ	19. ⓐⓑⓒⓓ	20. ⓐⓑⓒⓓ

Space for Rough Work

21. A long solenoid carrying a current produces a magnetic field B along its axis. If the current is double and the number of turns per cm is halved, the new value of the magnetic field is

(a) $4B$ (b) $B/2$ (c) B (d) $2B$

22. A particle of charge q and mass m moves in a circular orbit of radius r with angular speed ω. The ratio of the magnitude of its magnetic moment to that of its angular momentum depends on

(a) ω and q (b) ω, q and m
(c) q and m (d) ω and m

23. A current loop in a magnetic field

(a) can be in equilibrium in one orientation
(b) can be in equilibrium in two orientations, both the equilibrium states are unstable
(c) can be in equilibrium in two orientations, one stable while the other is unstable
(d) experiences a torque whether the field is uniform or non-uniform in all orientations

24. Two long parallel wires P and Q are held perpendicular to the plane of paper with distance of 5 m between them. If P and Q carry current of 2.5 amp. and 5 amp. respectively in the same direction, then the magnetic field at a point half-way between the wires is

(a) $\mu_0/17$ (b) $\sqrt{3}\mu_0/2\pi$
(c) $\mu_0/2\pi$ (d) $3\mu_0/2\pi$

25. A very long straight wire carries a current I. At the instant when a charge $+Q$ at point P has velocity $\vec{v}$, as shown, the force on the charge is

(a) along OY (b) opposite to OY
(c) along OX (d) opposite to OX

26. Two wires with currents 2 A and 1 A are enclosed in a circular loop. Another wire with current 3 A is situated outside the loop as shown. The $\oint \vec{B}.d\vec{l}$ around the loop is

(a) μ_0
(b) $3\mu_0$
(c) $6\mu_0$
(d) $2\mu_0$

27. If in a circular coil A of radius R, current I is flowing and in another coil B of radius $2R$ a current $2I$ is flowing, then the ratio of the magnetic fields B_A and B_B, produced by them will be

(a) 1 (b) 2 (c) 1/2 (d) 4

28. A charged particle moves through a magnetic field perpendicular to its direction. Then

(a) kinetic energy changes but the momentum is constant
(b) the momentum changes but the kinetic energy is constant
(c) both momentum and kinetic energy of the particle are not constant
(d) both momentum and kinetic energy of the particle are constant

29. The deflection in a galvanometer falls from 50 division to 20 when a 12 ohm shunt is applied. The galvanometer resistance is

(a) 18 ohm (b) 36 ohm (c) 24 ohm (d) 30 ohm

30. When a long wire carrying a steady current is bent into a circular coil of one turn, the magnetic induction at its centre is B. When the same wire carrying the same current is bent to form a circular coil of n turns of a smaller radius, the magnetic induction at the centre will be

(a) B/n (b) nB (c) B/n^2 (d) n^2B

31. The magnetic field due to a current carrying circular loop of radius 3 cm at a point on the axis at a distance of 4 cm from the centre is 54 μT. What will be its value at the centre of loop ?

(a) 125 μT (b) 150 μT
(c) 250 μT (d) 75 μT

32. A charge moving with velocity v in X-direction is subjected to a field of magnetic induction in negative X-direction. As a result, the charge will

(a) remain unaffected
(b) start moving in a circular path Y–Z plane
(c) retard along X-axis
(d) move along a helical path around X-axis

33. An electron travelling with a speed u along the positive x-axis enters into a region of magnetic field where $B = -B_0\hat{k}$ $(x > 0)$. It comes out of the region with speed v then

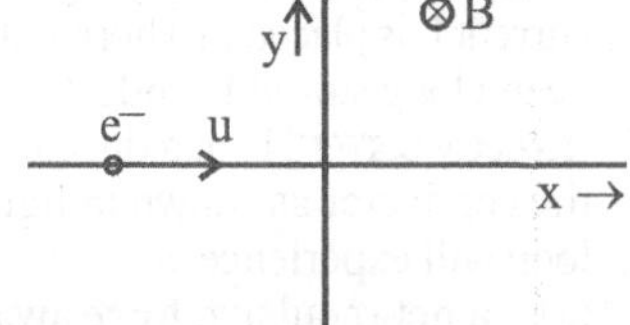

(a) $v = u$ at $y > 0$
(b) $v = u$ at $y < 0$
(c) $v > u$ at $y > 0$
(d) $v > u$ at $y < 0$

34. If an ammeter is to be used in place of a voltmeter, then we must connect with the ammeter a

(a) low resistance in parallel
(b) high resistance in parallel
(c) high resistance in series
(d) low resistance in series

35. An infinite straight conductor carrying current 2 I is split into a loop of radius r as shown in fig. The magnetic field at the centre of the coil is

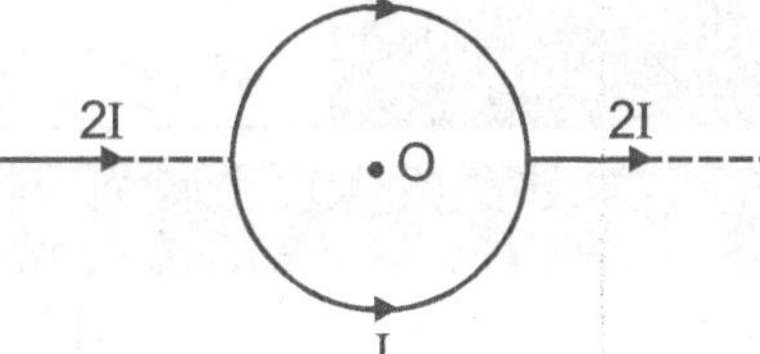

(a) $\dfrac{\mu_0}{4\pi}\dfrac{2(\pi+1)}{r}$
(b) $\dfrac{\mu_0}{4\pi}\dfrac{2(\pi-1)}{r}$
(c) $\dfrac{\mu_0}{4\pi}\dfrac{(\pi+1)}{r}$
(d) zero

RESPONSE GRID					
	21. ⓐⓑⓒⓓ	22. ⓐⓑⓒⓓ	23. ⓐⓑⓒⓓ	24. ⓐⓑⓒⓓ	25. ⓐⓑⓒⓓ
	26. ⓐⓑⓒⓓ	27. ⓐⓑⓒⓓ	28. ⓐⓑⓒⓓ	29. ⓐⓑⓒⓓ	30. ⓐⓑⓒⓓ
	31. ⓐⓑⓒⓓ	32. ⓐⓑⓒⓓ	33. ⓐⓑⓒⓓ	34. ⓐⓑⓒⓓ	35. ⓐⓑⓒⓓ

Space for Rough Work

36. A parallel plate capacitor of area 60 cm^2 and separation 3 mm is charged initially to 90 μC. If the medium between the plate gets slightly conducting and the plate loses the charge initially at the rate of 2.5×10^{-8} C/s, then what is the magnetic field between the plates ?

(a) 2.5×10^{-8} T (b) 2.0×10^{-7} T
(c) 1.63×10^{-11} T (d) Zero

37. Four wires, each of length 2.0 m, are bent into four loops P, Q, R and S and then suspended in a uniform magnetic field. If the same current is passed in each, then the torque will be maximum on the loop

(a) P (b) Q (c) R (d) S

38. A certain region has an electric field $\vec{E} = (2\hat{i} - 3\hat{j})$ N/C and a uniform magnetic field $\vec{B} = (5\hat{i} + 3\hat{j} + 4\hat{k})$ T. The force experienced by a charge 1C moving with velocity $(\hat{i} + 2\hat{j})$ ms^{-1} is

(a) $(10\hat{i} - 7\hat{j} - 7\hat{k})$ (b) $(10\hat{i} + 7\hat{j} + 7\hat{k})$
(c) $(-10\hat{i} + 7\hat{j} + 7\hat{k})$ (d) $(10\hat{i} + 7\hat{j} - 7\hat{k})$

39. A galvanometer of resistance 100 Ω gives a full scale deflection for a current of 10^{-5} A. To convert it into a ammeter capable of measuring upto 1 A, we should connect a resistance of

(a) 1 Ω in parallel (b) 10^{-3} Ω in parallel
(c) 10^5 Ω in series (d) 100 Ω in series

40. A square loop, carrying a steady current I, is placed in a horizontal plane near a long straight conductor carrying a steady current I_1 at a distance d from the conductor as shown in figure. The loop will experience

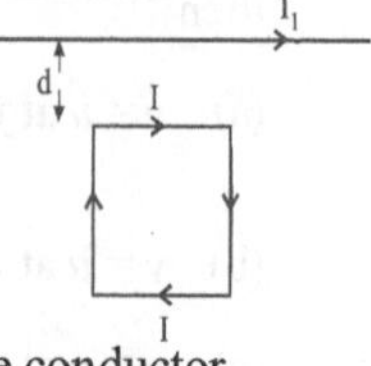

(a) a net repulsive force away from the conductor
(b) a net torque acting upward perpendicular to the horizontal plane
(c) a net torque acting downward normal to the horizontal plane
(d) a net attractive force towards the conductor

41. Two coaxial solenoids of different radius carry current I in the same direction. $\vec{F_1}$ be the magnetic force on the inner solenoid due to the outer one and $\vec{F_2}$ be the magnetic force on the outer solenoid due to the inner one. Then :

(a) $\vec{F_1}$ is radially inwards and $\vec{F_2} = 0$
(b) $\vec{F_1}$ is radially outwards and $\vec{F_2} = 0$
(c) $\vec{F_1} = \vec{F_2} = 0$
(d) $\vec{F_1}$ is radially inwards and $\vec{F_2}$ is radially outwards

42. A beam of electrons is moving with constant velocity in a region having simultaneous perpendicular electric and magnetic fields of strength 20 Vm^{-1} and 0.5 T respectively at right angles to the direction of motion of the electrons. Then the velocity of electrons must be

(a) 8 m/s (b) 20 m/s (c) 40 m/s (d) $\frac{1}{40}$ m/s

43. The magnetic flux density B at a distance r from a long straight wire carrying a steady current varies with r as

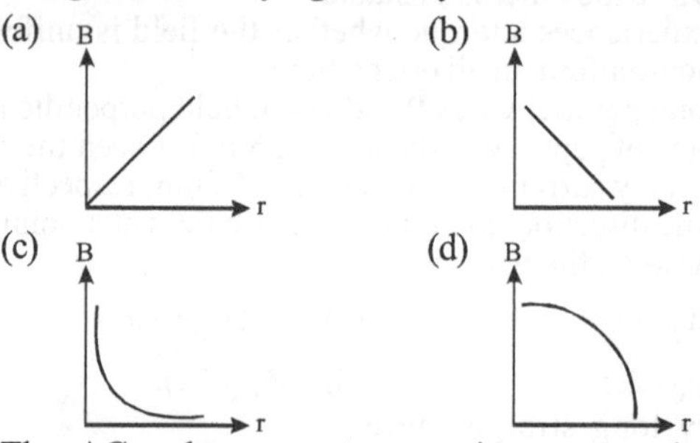

45. The AC voltage across a resistance can be measured using a :

(a) hot wire voltmeter
(b) moving coil galvanometer
(c) potential coil galvanometer
(d) moving magnet galvanometer

44. When a charged particle moving with velocity $\vec{v}$ is subjected to a magnetic field of induction $\vec{B}$, the force on it is non-zero. This implies that

(a) angle between $\vec{v}$ and $\vec{B}$ is necessarily 90°
(b) angle between $\vec{v}$ and $\vec{B}$ can have any value other than 90°
(c) angle between $\vec{v}$ and $\vec{B}$ can have any value other than zero and 180°
(d) angle between $\vec{v}$ and $\vec{B}$ is either zero or 180°

RESPONSE GRID					
	36. ⓐⓑⓒⓓ	37. ⓐⓑⓒⓓ	38. ⓐⓑⓒⓓ	39. ⓐⓑⓒⓓ	40. ⓐⓑⓒⓓ
	41. ⓐⓑⓒⓓ	42. ⓐⓑⓒⓓ	43. ⓐⓑⓒⓓ	44. ⓐⓑⓒⓓ	45. ⓐⓑⓒⓓ

PHYSICS CHAPTERWISE SPEED TEST-18

Total Questions	45	Total Marks	180
Attempted		Correct	
Incorrect		Net Score	
Cut-off Score	45	Qualifying Score	60
Success Gap = Net Score – Qualifying Score			
Net Score = (Correct × 4) – (Incorrect × 1)			

Space for Rough Work

PHYSICS

Magnetism and Matter

Speed TEST 19

Chapter-wise

No. of Questions	Maximum Marks	Time
45	180	1 Hour

GENERAL INSTRUCTIONS

- This test contains 45 MCQ's. For each question only one option is correct. Darken the correct circle/ bubble in the Response Grid provided on each page.
- You have to evaluate your Response Grids yourself with the help of solutions provided at the end of this book.
- Each correct answer will get you 4 marks and 1 mark shall be deduced for each incorrect answer. No mark will be given/ deducted if no bubble is filled. Keep a timer in front of you and stop immediately at the end of 60 min.
- The sheet follows a particular syllabus. Do not attempt the sheet before you have completed your preparation for that syllabus.
- After completing the sheet check your answers with the solution booklet and complete the Result Grid. Finally spend time to analyse your performance and revise the areas which emerge out as weak in your evaluation.

1. Two identical magnetic dipoles of magnetic moments 1.0 A-m^2 each, placed at a separation of 2 m with their axis perpendicular to each other. The resultant magnetic field at point midway between the dipole is

   (a) 5×10^{-7} T (b) $\sqrt{5} \times 10^{-7}$ T

   (c) 10^{-7} T (d) 2×10^{-7} T

2. Two identical thin bar magnets each of length ℓ and pole strength m are placed at right angles to each other, with north pole of one touching south pole of the other, then the magnetic moment of the system is

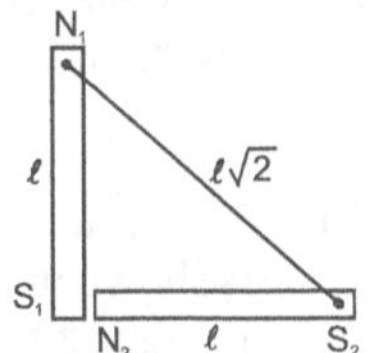

   (a) $1m\ell$ (b) $2m\ell$ (c) $\sqrt{2}\ m\ell$ (d) $m\ell/2$

3. The magnetic lines of force inside a bar magnet
   (a) are from north-pole to south-pole of the magnet
   (b) do not exist
   (c) depend upon the area of cross-section of the bar magnet
   (d) are from south-pole to north-pole of the magnet

4. Relative permittivity and permeability of a material ε_r and μ_r, respectively. Which of the following values of these quantities are allowed for a diamagnetic material?

   (a) $\varepsilon_r = 0.5, \mu_r = 1.5$ (b) $\varepsilon_r = 1.5, \mu_r = 0.5$

   (c) $\varepsilon_r = 0.5, \mu_r = 0.5$ (d) $\varepsilon_r = 1.5, \mu_r = 1.5$

5. If the period of oscillation of freely suspended bar magnet in earth's horizontal field H is 4 sec. When another magnet is brought near it, the period of oscillation is reduced to 2s. The magnetic field of second bar magnet is

   (a) 4H (b) 3H (c) 2H (d) $\sqrt{3}$ H

6. Three identical bars A, B and C are made of different magnetic materials. When kept in a uniform magnetic field, the field lines around them look as follows:

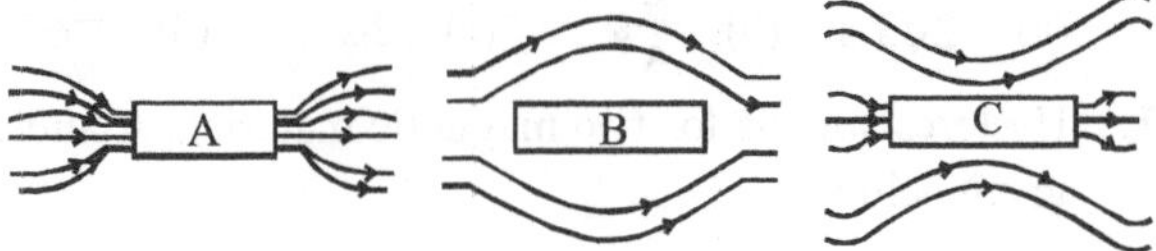

   Make the correspondence of these bars with their material being diamagnetic (D), ferromagnetic (F) and paramagnetic (P):
   (a) A ↔ D, B ↔ P, C ↔ F
   (b) A ↔ F, B ↔ D, C ↔ P
   (c) A ↔ P, B ↔ F, C ↔ D
   (d) A ↔ F, B ↔ P, C ↔ D

RESPONSE GRID	1. ⓐⓑⓒⓓ 2. ⓐⓑⓒⓓ 3. ⓐⓑⓒⓓ 4. ⓐⓑⓒⓓ 5. ⓐⓑⓒⓓ 6. ⓐⓑⓒⓓ

Space for Rough Work

7. Curie temperature is the temperature above which
(a) a ferromagnetic material becomes paramagnetic
(b) a paramagnetic material becomes diamagnetic
(c) a ferromagnetic material becomes diamagnetic
(d) a paramagnetic material becomes ferromagnetic

8. A watch glass containing some powdered substance is placed between the pole pieces of a magnet. Deep concavity is observed at the centre. The substance in the watch glass is
(a) iron (b) chromium (c) carbon (d) wood

9. A coil in the shape of an equilateral triangle of side l is suspended between the pole pieces of a permanent magnet such that $\vec{B}$ is in the plane of the coil. If due to a current i in the triangle a torque τ acts on it, the side l of the triangle is

(a) $\frac{2}{\sqrt{3}}\left(\frac{\tau}{B.i}\right)^{\frac{1}{2}}$ (b) $2\left(\frac{\tau}{\sqrt{3}B.i}\right)^{\frac{1}{2}}$

(c) $\frac{2}{\sqrt{3}}\left(\frac{\tau}{B.i}\right)$ (d) $\frac{1}{\sqrt{3}}\frac{\tau}{B.i}$

10. A compass needle whose magnetic moment is 60 Am^2, is directed towards geographical north at any place experiencing moment of force of 1.2×10^{-3} Nm. At that place the horizontal component of earth field is 40 micro W/m^2. What is the value of dip angle at that place?
(a) 30° (b) 60° (c) 45° (d) 15°

11. The materials suitable for making electromagnets should have
(a) high retentivity and low coercivity
(b) low retentivity and low coercivity
(c) high retentivity and high coercivity
(d) low retentivity and high coercivity

12. The length of a magnet is large compared to its width and breadth. The time period of its oscillation in a vibration magnetometer is 2s. The magnet is cut along its length into three equal parts and these parts are then placed on each other with their like poles together. The time period of this combination will be

(a) $2\sqrt{3}$ s (b) $\frac{2}{3}$s (c) 2 s (d) $\frac{2}{\sqrt{3}}$s

13. Hysteresis loops for two magnetic materials A and B are given below :

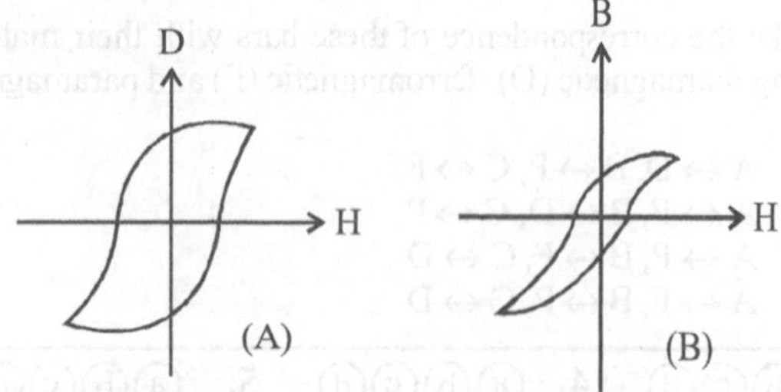

These materials are used to make magnets for elecric generators, transformer core and electromagnet core. Then it is proper to use :
(a) A for transformers and B for electric generators.
(b) B for electromagnets and transformers.
(c) A for electric generators and trasformers.
(d) A for electromagnets and B for electric generators.

14. Which of the following is responsible for the earth's magnetic field?
(a) Convective currents in earth's core.
(b) Diversive current in earth's core.
(c) Rotational motion of earth.
(d) Translational motion of earth.

15. In a vibration megnetometer, the time period of a bar magnet oscillating in horizontal component of earth's magnetic field is 2 sec. When a magnet is brought near and parallel to it, the time period reduces to 1 sec. The ratio H/F of the horizontal component H and the field F due to magnet will be
(a) 3 (b) 1/3 (c) $\sqrt{3}$ (d) $1/\sqrt{3}$

16. Let V and H be the vertical and horizontal components of earth's magnetic field at any point on earth. Near the north pole
(a) V>>H (b) V<<H (c) V=H (d) V=H=0

17. A thin circular wire carrying a current I has a magnetic moment M. The shape of the wire is changed to a square and it carries the same current. It will have a magnetic moment
(a) M (b) $\frac{4}{\pi^2}M$ (c) $\frac{4}{\pi}M$ (d) $\frac{\pi}{4}M$

18. A bar magnet of magnetic moment M is placed at right angles to a magnetic induction B. If a force F is experienced by each pole of the magnet, the length of the magnet will be
(a) F/MB (b) MB/F (c) BF/M (d) MF/B

19. If the susceptibility of dia, para and ferro magnetic materials are χ_d, χ_p, χ_f respectively, then
(a) $\chi_d < \chi_p < \chi_f$ (b) $\chi_d < \chi_f < \chi_p$
(c) $\chi_f < \chi_d < \chi_p$ (d) $\chi_f < \chi_p < \chi_d$

20. The basic magnetization curve for a ferromagnetic material is shown in figure. Then, the value of relative permeability is highest for the point

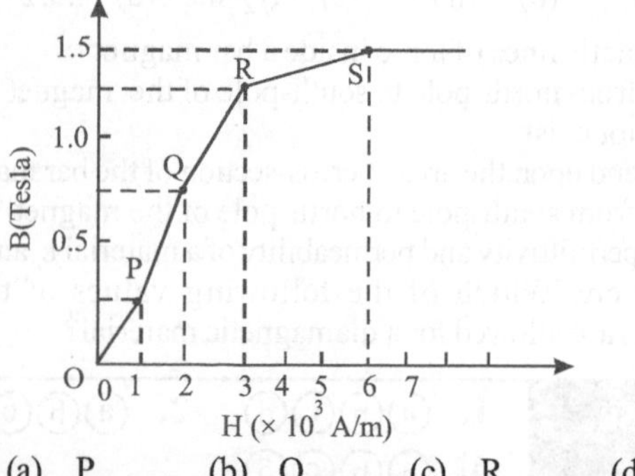

(a) P (b) Q (c) R (d) S

RESPONSE GRID

7. ⓐⓑⓒⓓ 8. ⓐⓑⓒⓓ 9. ⓐⓑⓒⓓ 10. ⓐⓑⓒⓓ 11. ⓐⓑⓒⓓ
12. ⓐⓑⓒⓓ 13. ⓐⓑⓒⓓ 14. ⓐⓑⓒⓓ 15. ⓐⓑⓒⓓ 16. ⓐⓑⓒⓓ
17. ⓐⓑⓒⓓ 18. ⓐⓑⓒⓓ 19. ⓐⓑⓒⓓ 20. ⓐⓑⓒⓓ

Space for Rough Work

21. A magnetic needle suspended by a silk thread is vibrating in the earth's magnetic field. if the temperature of the needle is increased by 700°C, then
(a) time period decreases
(b) time period increases
(c) time period remains unchanged
(d) the needle stops vibrating

22. Torques τ_1 and τ_2 are required for a magnetic needle to remain perpendicular to the magnetic fields at two different places. The magnetic fields at those places are B_1 and B_2 respectively; then ratio $\frac{B_1}{B_2}$ is
(a) $\frac{\tau_2}{\tau_1}$ (b) $\frac{\tau_1}{\tau_2}$
(c) $\frac{\tau_1+\tau_2}{\tau_1-\tau_2}$ (d) $\frac{\tau_1-\tau_2}{\tau_1+\tau_2}$

23. A bar magnet has a length 8 cm. The magnetic field at a point at a distance 3 cm from the centre in the broad side-on position is found to be 4×10^{-6} *T*. The pole strength of the magnet is.
(a) 6×10^{-5} Am (b) 5×10^{-5} Am
(c) 2×10^{-4} Am (d) 3×10^{-4} Am

24. A vibration magnetometer consists of two identical bar magnets placed one over the other such that they are perpendicular and bisect each other. The time period of oscillation in a horizontal magnetic field is $2^{5/4}$ seconds. One of the magnets is removed and if the other magnet oscillates in the same field, then the time period in seconds is
(a) $2^{1/4}$ (b) $2^{1/2}$ (c) 2 (d) $2^{3/4}$

25. A magnetic needle is kept in a non-uniform magnetic field. It experiences
(a) neither a force nor a torque
(b) a torque but not a force
(c) a force but not a torque
(d) a force and a torque

26. The angle of dip at a place is 37° and the vertical component of the earth's magnetic field is 6×10^{-5}T. The earth's magnetic field at this place is (tan 37° = 3/4)
(a) 7×10^{-5} T (b) 6×10^{-5} T
(c) 5×10^{-5} T (d) 10^{-4} T

27. Needles N_1, N_2 and N_3 are made of a ferromagnetic, a paramagnetic and a diamagnetic substance respectively. A magnet when brought close to them will
(a) attract N_1 and N_2 strongly but repel N_3
(b) attract N_1 strongly, N_2 weakly and repel N_3 weakly
(c) attract N_1 strongly, but repel N_2 and N_3 weakly
(d) attract all three of them

28. The figure shows the various positions (labelled by subscripts) of small magnetised needles P and Q. The arrows show the direction of their magnetic moment. Which configuration corresponds to the lowest potential energy among all the configurations shown ?

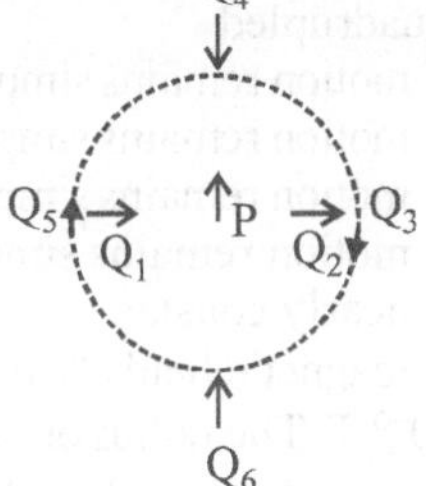

(a) PQ_3
(b) PQ_4
(c) PQ_5
(d) PQ_6

29. A dip needle lies initially in the magnetic meridian when it shows an angle of dip θ at a place. The dip circle is rotated through an angle x in the horizontal plane and then it shows an angle of dip θ′.
Then $\frac{\tan\theta'}{\tan\theta}$ is
(a) $\frac{1}{\cos x}$ (b) $\frac{1}{\sin x}$ (c) $\frac{1}{\tan x}$ (d) cos x

30. Two tangent galvanometers having coils of the same radius are connected in series. A current flowing in them produces deflections of 60° and 45° respectively. The ratio of the number of turns in the coils is
(a) 4/3 (b) $\frac{\sqrt{3}+1}{1}$ (c) $\frac{\sqrt{3}+1}{\sqrt{3}-1}$ (d) $\frac{\sqrt{3}}{1}$

31. Following figures show the arrangement of bar magnets in different configurations. Each magnet has magnet ic dipole moment $\vec{m}$. Which configuration has highest net magnetic dipole moment?

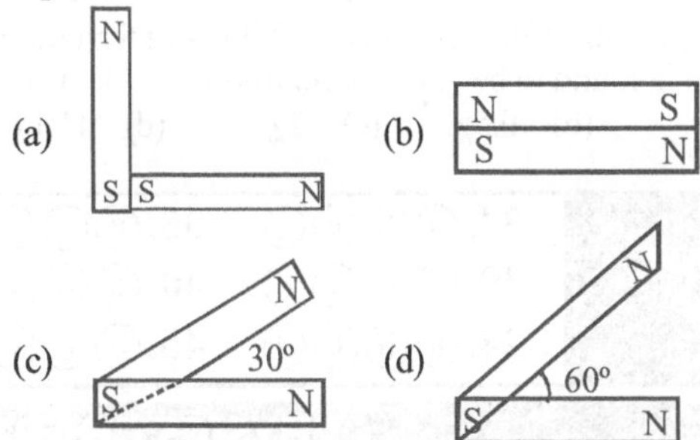

32. A compass needle which is allowed to move in a horizontal plane is taken to a geomagnetic pole. It :
(a) will become rigid showing no movement
(b) will stay in any position
(c) will stay in north-south direction only
(d) will stay in east-west direction only

33. If a magnetic dipole of moment *M* situated in the direction of a magnetic field *B* is rotated by 180°, then the amount of work done is
(a) MB (b) 2MB (c) $\frac{MB}{\sqrt{2}}$ (d) 0

RESPONSE GRID					
	21. ⓐⓑⓒⓓ	22. ⓐⓑⓒⓓ	23. ⓐⓑⓒⓓ	24. ⓐⓑⓒⓓ	25. ⓐⓑⓒⓓ
	26. ⓐⓑⓒⓓ	27. ⓐⓑⓒⓓ	28. ⓐⓑⓒⓓ	29. ⓐⓑⓒⓓ	30. ⓐⓑⓒⓓ
	31. ⓐⓑⓒⓓ	32. ⓐⓑⓒⓓ	33. ⓐⓑⓒⓓ		

Space for Rough Work

34. A bar magnet is oscillating in the earth's magnetic field with a period T. What happens to its period of motion, if its mass is quadrupled
(a) motion remains simple harmonic with new period = T/2
(b) motion remains simple harmonic with new period = 2 T
(c) motion remains simple harmonic with new period = 4T
(d) motion remains simple harmonic and the period stays nearly constant

35. The magnetic field of earth at the equator is approximately 4×10^{-5} T. The radius of earth is 6.4×10^6 m. Then the dipole moment of the earth will be nearly of the order of:
(a) 10^{23} Am^2 (b) 10^{20} Am^2 (c) 10^{16} Am^2 (d) 10^{10} Am^2

36. The relative permeability of a medium is 0.075. What is its magnetic susceptibility?
(a) 0.925 (b) –0.925 (c) 1.075 (d) –1.075

37. A dip circle is so set that its needle moves freely in the magnetic meridian. In this position, the angle of dip is 40º. Now the dip circle is rotated so that the plane in which the needle moves makes an angle of 30º with the magnetic meridian. In this position, the needle will dip by an angle
(a) 40º (b) 30º (c) more than 40º (d) less than 40º

38. The mid points of two small magnetic dipoles of length d in end-on positions, are separated by a distance x, (x > > d). The force between them is proportional to x^{-n} where n is:

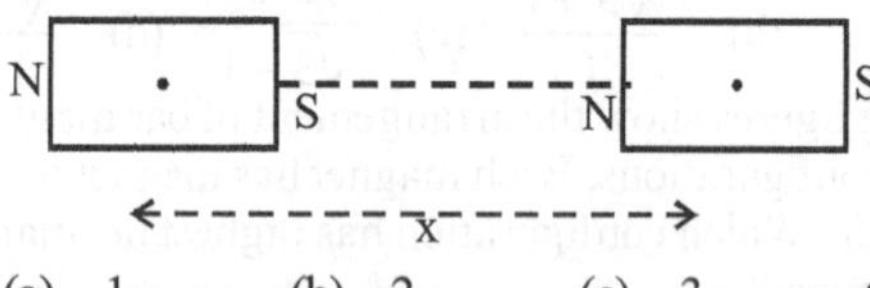

(a) 1 (b) 2 (c) 3 (d) 4

39. At a temperatur of 30°C, the susceptibility of a ferromagnetic material is found to be χ. Its susceptibility at 333°C is
(a) χ (b) 0.5χ (c) 2χ (d) 11.1χ

40. The susceptibility of annealed iron at saturation is 5500. Find the permeability of annealed iron at saturation.
(a) 6.9×10^{-3} (b) 5.1×10^{-2} (c) 5×10^2 (d) 3.2×10^{-5}

41. A short magnet oscillates in an oscillation magnetometer with a time period of 0.10s where the earth's horizontal magnetic field is 24 μT. A downward current of 18 A is established in a vertical wire placed 20 cm east of the magnet. Find the new time period.
(a) 0.076 s (b) 0.5 s (c) 0.1 s (d) 0.2 s

42. A permanent magnet in the shape of a thin cylinder of length 10 cm has magnetisation (M) = 10^6 A m^{-1}. Its magnetization current I_M is
(a) 10^5 A (b) 10^6 A (c) 10^7 A (d) 10^8 A

43. The earth's magnetic field lines resemble that of a dipole at the centre of the earth. If the magnetic moment of this dipole is close to 8×10^{22} Am^2, the value of earth's magnetic field near the equator is close to (radius of the earth = 6.4×10^6 m)
(a) 0.6 Gauss (b) 1.2 Gauss
(c) 1.8 Gauss (d) 0.32 Gauss

44. The coercivity of a small magnet where the ferromagnet gets demagnetized is 3×10^3 Am^{-1}. The current required to be passed in a solenoid of length 10 cm and number of turns 100, so that the magnet gets demagnetized when inside the solenoid, is:
(a) 30 mA (b) 60 mA (c) 3 A (d) 6 A

45. A thin bar magnet of length 2 ℓ and breadth 2 b pole strength m and magnetic moment M is divided into four equal parts with length and breadth of each part being half of original magnet.
Then, the magnetic moment of each part is
(a) M/4 (b) M (c) M/2 (d) 2 M

RESPONSE GRID					
	34. ⓐⓑⓒⓓ	35. ⓐⓑⓒⓓ	36. ⓐⓑⓒⓓ	37. ⓐⓑⓒⓓ	38. ⓐⓑⓒⓓ
	39. ⓐⓑⓒⓓ	40. ⓐⓑⓒⓓ	41. ⓐⓑⓒⓓ	42. ⓐⓑⓒⓓ	43. ⓐⓑⓒⓓ
	44. ⓐⓑⓒⓓ	45. ⓐⓑⓒⓓ			

PHYSICS CHAPTERWISE SPEED TEST-19

Total Questions	45	Total Marks	180
Attempted		Correct	
Incorrect		Net Score	
Cut-off Score	50	Qualifying Score	70
Success Gap = Net Score – Qualifying Score			
Net Score = (Correct × 4) – (Incorrect × 1)			

Space for Rough Work

PHYSICS

Electromagnetic Induction

Speed TEST 20 Chapter-wise

No. of Questions	Maximum Marks	Time
45	180	1 Hour

GENERAL INSTRUCTIONS

- This test contains 45 MCQ's. For each question only one option is correct. Darken the correct circle/ bubble in the Response Grid provided on each page.
- You have to evaluate your Response Grids yourself with the help of solutions provided at the end of this book.
- Each correct answer will get you 4 marks and 1 mark shall be deduced for each incorrect answer. No mark will be given/ deducted if no bubble is filled. Keep a timer in front of you and stop immediately at the end of 60 min.
- The sheet follows a particular syllabus. Do not attempt the sheet before you have completed your preparation for that syllabus.
- After completing the sheet check your answers with the solution booklet and complete the Result Grid. Finally spend time to analyse your performance and revise the areas which emerge out as weak in your evaluation.

1. A metal disc of radius 100 cm is rotated at a constant angular speed of 60 rad/s in a plane at right angles to an external field of magnetic induction 0.05 Wb/m^2. The emf induced between the centre and a point on the rim will be
   (a) 3V (b) 1.5V (c) 6V (d) 9V

2. In a coil of resistance $100\,\Omega$, a current is induced by changing the magnetic flux through it as shown in the figure. The magnitude of change in flux through the coil is
   (a) 250 Wb
   (b) 275 Wb
   (c) 200 Wb
   (d) 225 Wb

   10 · Current (amp.) · 0.5 s · Time

3. A 10-meter wire is kept in east-west direction. It is falling down with a speed of 5.0 meter/second, perpendicular to the horizontal component of earth's magnetic field of 0.30×10^{-4} weber/meter^2. The momentary potential difference induced between the ends of the wire will be
   (a) 0.0015V (b) 0.015V
   (c) 0.15V (d) 1.5V

4. The figure shows certain wire segments joined together to form a coplanar loop. The loop is placed in a perpendicular magnetic field in the direction going into the plane of the figure.

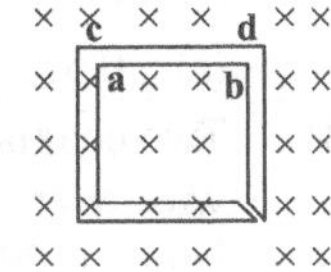

   The magnitude of the field increases with time. I_1 and I_2 are the currents in the segments ab and cd. Then,
   (a) $I_1 > I_2$ (b) $I_1 < I_2$
   (c) I_1 is in the direction ba and I_2 is in the direction cd
   (d) I_1 is in the direction ab and I_2 is in the direction dc

5. Two solenoids of equal number of turns have their lengths and the radii in the same ratio 1 : 2. The ratio of their self inductances will be
   (a) 1 : 2 (b) 2 : 1 (c) 1 : 1 (d) 1 : 4

6. A metal conductor of length 1 m rotates vertically about one of its ends at angular velocity 5 radians per second. If the horizontal component of earth's magnetic field is 0.2×10^{-4}T, then the e.m.f. developed between the two ends of the conductor is
   (a) 5mV (b) 50μV (c) 5μV (d) 50mV

7. Eddy currents do not produce
   (a) heat (b) a loss of energy
   (c) spark (d) damping of motion

RESPONSE GRID	
	1. ⓐⓑⓒⓓ 2. ⓐⓑⓒⓓ 3. ⓐⓑⓒⓓ 4. ⓐⓑⓒⓓ 5. ⓐⓑⓒⓓ
	6. ⓐⓑⓒⓓ 7. ⓐⓑⓒⓓ

Space for Rough Work

8. A conducting square frame of side 'a' and a long staight wire carrying current I are located in the same plane as shown in the figure. The frame moves to the right with a constant velocity 'V'. The emf induced in the frame will be proportional to

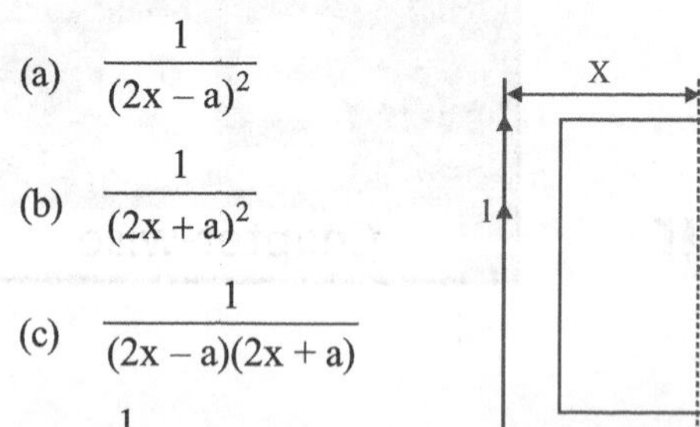

(a) $\frac{1}{(2x-a)^2}$

(b) $\frac{1}{(2x+a)^2}$

(c) $\frac{1}{(2x-a)(2x+a)}$

(d) $\frac{1}{x^2}$

9. Which of the following figure correctly depicts the Lenz's law. The arrows show the movement of the labelled pole of a bar magnet into a closed circular loop and the arrows on the circle show the direction of the induced current

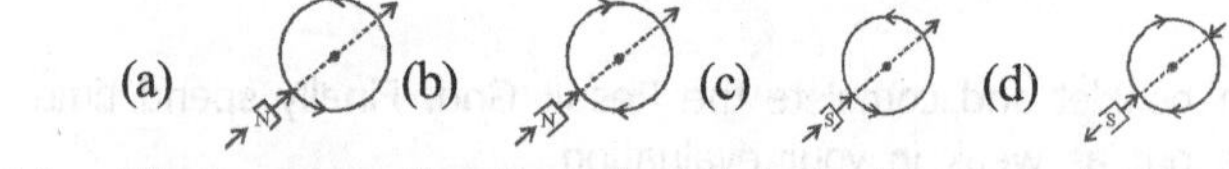

10. The magnetic flux (in weber) linked with a coil of resistance 10 Ω is varying with respect to time t as $\phi = 4t^2 + 2t + 1$. Then the current in the coil at time t = 1 second is

(a) 0.5 A (b) 2 A (c) 1.5 A (d) 1 A

11. Two coaxial solenoids are made by winding thin insulated wire over a pipe of cross-sectional area *A* = 10 cm² and length = 20 cm. If one of the solenoid has 300 turns and the other 400 turns, their mutual inductance is ($\mu_0 = 4\pi \times 10^{-7}$ Tm A^{-1})

(a) $2.4\pi \times 10^{-5}$ H (b) $4.8\pi \times 10^{-4}$ H
(c) $4.8\pi \times 10^{-5}$ H (d) $2.4\pi \times 10^{-4}$ H

12. When the current changes from +2 A to –2A in 0.05 second, an e.m.f. of 8 V is induced in a coil. The coefficient of self-induction of the coil is

(a) 0.2 H (b) 0.4 H (c) 0.8 H (d) 0.1 H

13. A long solenoid has 500 turns. When a current of 2 ampere is passed through it, the resulting magnetic flux linked with each turn of the solenoid is 4×10^{-3} Wb. The self- inductance of the solenoid is

(a) 2.5 henry (b) 2.0 henry
(c) 1.0 henry (d) 40 henry

14. A metallic square loop ABCD is moving in its own plane with velocity v in a uniform magnetic field perpendicular to its plane as shown in the figure. An electric field is induced

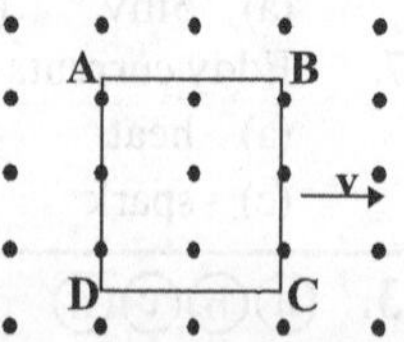

(a) in AD, but not in BC (b) in BC, but not in AD
(c) neither in AD nor in BC (d) in both AD and BC

15. In an AC generator, a coil with N turns, all of the same area A and total resistance R, rotates with frequency ω in a magnetic field B. The maximum value of emf generated in the coil is

(a) N.A.B.R.ω (b) N.A.B.
(c) N.A.B.R. (d) N.A.B.ω

16. In an inductor of self-inductance L = 2 mH, current changes with time according to relation $i = t^2 e^{-t}$. At what time emf is zero?

(a) 4s (b) 3s (c) 2s (d) 1s

17. Choke coil works on the principle of

(a) transient current (b) self induction
(c) mutual induction (d) wattless current

18. A coil having n turns and resistance R Ω is connected with a galvanometer of resistance 4R Ω. This combination is moved in time t seconds from a magnetic field W_1 weber to W_2 weber. The induced current in the circuit is

(a) $-\frac{(W_1-W_2)}{Rnt}$ (b) $-\frac{n(W_2-W_1)}{5\,Rt}$

(c) $-\frac{(W_2-W_1)}{5\,Rnt}$ (d) $-\frac{n(W_2-W_1)}{Rt}$

19. A thin circular ring of area A is held perpendicular to a uniform magnetic field of induction B. A small cut is made in the ring and a galvanometer is connected across the ends such that the total resistance of the circuit is R. When the ring is suddenly squeezed to zero area, the charge flowing through the galvanometer is

(a) $\frac{BR}{A}$ (b) $\frac{AB}{R}$ (c) ABR (d) $\frac{B^2A}{R^2}$

20. A boat is moving due east in a region where the earth's magnetic field is 5.0×10^{-5} NA^{-1}m^{-1} due north and horizontal. The boat carries a vertical aerial 2 m long. If the speed of the boat is 1.50 ms^{-1}, the magnitude of the induced emf in the wire of aerial is:

(a) 0.75 mV (b) 0.50 mV (c) 0.15 mV (d) 1 mV

21. In a coil of area 10 cm² and 10 turns with magnetic field directed perpendicular to the plane and is changing at the rate of 10^8 Gauss/second. The resistance of the coil is 20Ω. The current in the coil will be

(a) 0.5 A (b) 5 A (c) 50 A (d) 5×10^8 A

22. A horizontal straight wire 20 m long extending from east to west falling with a speed of 5.0 m/s, at right angles to the horizontal component of the earth's magnetic field 0.30×10^{-4} Wb/m². The instantaneous value of the e.m.f. induced in the wire will be

(a) 3mV (b) 4.5mV (c) 1.5mV (d) 6.0mV

RESPONSE GRID					
	8. ⓐⓑⓒⓓ	9. ⓐⓑⓒⓓ	10. ⓐⓑⓒⓓ	11. ⓐⓑⓒⓓ	12. ⓐⓑⓒⓓ
	13. ⓐⓑⓒⓓ	14. ⓐⓑⓒⓓ	15. ⓐⓑⓒⓓ	16. ⓐⓑⓒⓓ	17. ⓐⓑⓒⓓ
	18. ⓐⓑⓒⓓ	19. ⓐⓑⓒⓓ	20. ⓐⓑⓒⓓ	21. ⓐⓑⓒⓓ	22. ⓐⓑⓒⓓ

Space for Rough Work

23. The self inductance of a long solenoid cannot be increased by
(a) increasing its area of cross section
(b) increasing its length
(c) changing the medium with greater permeability
(d) increasing the current through it

24. A metallic rod of length 'ℓ' is tied to a string of length 2ℓ and made to rotate with angular speed ω on a horizontal table with one end of the string fixed. If there is a vertical magnetic field 'B' in the region, the e.m.f. induced across the ends of the rod is

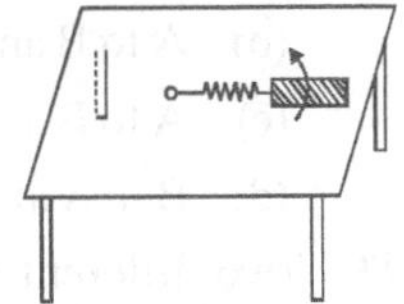

(a) $\frac{2B\omega\ell^2}{2}$ (b) $\frac{3B\omega\ell^2}{2}$ (c) $\frac{4B\omega\ell^2}{2}$ (d) $\frac{5B\omega\ell^2}{2}$

25. Lenz's law gives
(a) the magnitude of the induced e.m.f.
(b) the direction of the induced current
(c) both the magnitude and direction of the induced current
(d) the magnitude of the induced current

26. A metal ring is held horizontally and bar magnet is dropped through the ring with its length along the axis of the ring. The acceleration of the falling magnet
(a) is equal to g
(b) is less than g
(c) is more than g
(d) depends on the diameter of ring and length of magnet

27. The pointer of a dead-beat galvanometer gives a steady deflection because
(a) eddy currents are produced in the conducting frame over which the coil is wound.
(b) its magnet is very strong.
(c) its pointer is very light.
(d) its frame is made of ebonite.

28. A metal rod of length l cuts across a uniform magnetic field B with a velocity v. If the resistance of the circuit of which the rod forms a part is r, then the force required to move the rod is
(a) $\frac{B^2l^2v}{r}$ (b) $\frac{Blv}{r}$ (c) $\frac{B^2lv}{r}$ (d) $\frac{B^2l^2v^2}{r}$

29. In an A.C. generator, when the plane of the armature is perpendicular to the magnetic field
(a) both magnetic flux and emf are maximum
(b) both magnetic flux and emf are zero
(c) both magnetic flux and emf are half of their respective maximum values
(d) magnetic flux is maximum and emf is zero

30. A copper disc of radius 0.1 m rotated about its centre with 10 revolutions per second in a uniform magnetic field of 0.1 tesla with its plane perpendicular to the field. The e.m.f. induced across the radius of disc is
(a) $\frac{\pi}{10}$ volt (b) $\frac{2\pi}{10}$ volt
(c) $\pi \times 10^{-2}$ volt (d) $2\pi \times 10^{-2}$ volt

31. The mutual inductance of a pair of coils, each of N turns, is M henry. If a current of I ampere in one of the coils is brought to zero in t second, the emf induced per turn in the other coil, in volt, will be
(a) $\frac{MI}{t}$ (b) $\frac{NMI}{t}$ (c) $\frac{MN}{It}$ (d) $\frac{MI}{Nt}$

32. Consider the situation shown in figure. If the switch is closed and after some time it is opened again, the closed loop will show
(a) a clockwise current
(b) an anticlockwise current
(c) an anticlockwise current and then clockwise
(d) a clockwise current and then an anticlock wise current.

33. A magnet is moved towards a coil (i) quickly (ii) slowly, then the induced e.m.f. is
(a) larger in case (i)
(b) smaller in case (i)
(c) equal to both the cases
(d) larger or smaller depending upon the radius of the coil

34. A circular wire of radius r rotates about its own axis with angular speed ω in a magnetic field B perpendicular to its plane, then the induced e.m.f. is
(a) $\frac{1}{2}Br\omega^2$ (b) $Br\omega^2$ (c) $2Br\omega^2$ (d) zero

35. A conducting ring of radius 1 *m* kept in a uniform magnetic field *B* of 0.01 *T*, rotates uniformly with an angular velocity 100 rad s^{-1} with its axis of rotation perpendicular to *B*. The maximum induced emf in it is
(a) $1.5\pi V$ (b) πV (c) $2\pi V$ (d) $0.5\pi V$

36. A magnetic field of 2×10^{-2} T acts at right angles to a coil of area 100 cm^2, with 50 turns. The average e.m.f. induced in the coil is 0.1 V, when it is removed from the field in t sec. The value of t is
(a) 10 s (b) 0.1 s (c) 0.01 s (d) 1 s

37. The magnetic flux through a circuit of resistance R changes by an amount $\Delta\phi$ in a time Δt. Then the total quantity of electric charge Q that passes any point in the circuit during the time Δt is represented by
(a) $Q = R.\frac{\Delta\phi}{\Delta t}$ (b) $Q = \frac{1}{R}.\frac{\Delta\phi}{\Delta t}$
(c) $Q = \frac{\Delta\phi}{R}$ (d) $Q = \frac{\Delta\phi}{\Delta t}$

RESPONSE GRID					
	23. ⓐⓑⓒⓓ	24. ⓐⓑⓒⓓ	25. ⓐⓑⓒⓓ	26. ⓐⓑⓒⓓ	27. ⓐⓑⓒⓓ
	28. ⓐⓑⓒⓓ	29. ⓐⓑⓒⓓ	30. ⓐⓑⓒⓓ	31. ⓐⓑⓒⓓ	32. ⓐⓑⓒⓓ
	33. ⓐⓑⓒⓓ	34. ⓐⓑⓒⓓ	35. ⓐⓑⓒⓓ	36. ⓐⓑⓒⓓ	37. ⓐⓑⓒⓓ

Space for Rough Work

38. Fig shown below represents an area A = 0.5 m^2 situated in a uniform magnetic field B = 2.0 weber/m^2 and making an angle of 60° with respect to magnetic field.

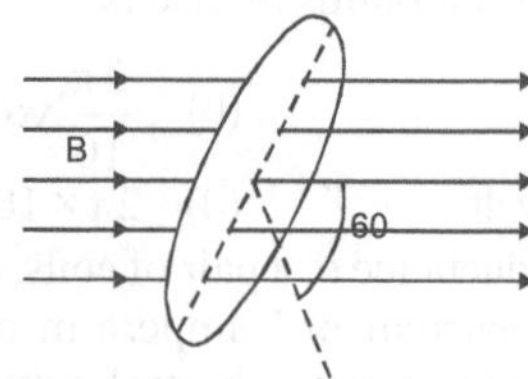

The value of the magnetic flux through the area would be equal to

(a) 2.0 weber (b) $\sqrt{3}$ weber
(c) $\sqrt{3}/2$ weber (d) 0.5 weber

39. As a result of change in the magnetic flux linked to the closed loop shown in the fig, an e.m.f. V volt is induced in the loop. The work done (joule) in taking a charge Q coulomb once along the loop is

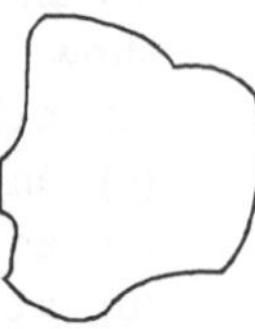

(a) QV (b) 2QV (c) QV/2 (d) Zero

40. Two coils are placed close to each other. The mutual inductance of the pair of coils depends upon
(a) the rates at which currents are changing in the two coils
(b) relative position and orientation of the two coils
(c) the materials of the wires of the coils
(d) the currents in the two coils

41. When current i passes through an inductor of self inductance L, energy stored in it is 1/2. L i^2. This is stored in the
(a) current (b) voltage
(c) magnetic field (d) electric field

42. A conducting wire frame is placed in a magnetic field which is directed into the paper. The magnetic field is increasing at a constant rate. The directions of induced current in wires AB and CD are

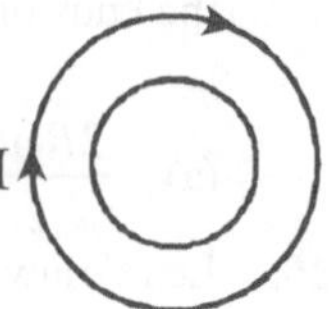

(a) B to A and D to C
(b) A to B and C to D
(c) A to B and D to C
(d) B to A and C to D

43. Two different wire loops are concentric and lie in the same plane. The current in the outer loop (I) is clockwise and increases with time. The induced current in the inner loop
(a) is clockwise
(b) is zero
(c) is counter clockwise
(d) has a direction that depends on the ratio of the loop radii.

44. When current in a coil changes from 5 A to 2 A in 0.1 s, average voltage of 50 V is produced. The self - inductance of the coil is :
(a) 6 H (b) 0.67 H (c) 3 H (d) 1.67 H

45. Two conducting circular loops of radii R_1 and R_2 are placed in the same plane with their centres coinciding. If $R_1 >> R_2$, the mutual inductance M between them will be directly proportional to
(a) R_1/R_2 (b) R_2/R_1 (c) R_1^2/R_2 (d) R_2^2/R_1

RESPONSE GRID					
	38. ⓐⓑⓒⓓ	39. ⓐⓑⓒⓓ	40. ⓐⓑⓒⓓ	41. ⓐⓑⓒⓓ	42. ⓐⓑⓒⓓ
	43. ⓐⓑⓒⓓ	44. ⓐⓑⓒⓓ	45. ⓐⓑⓒⓓ		

PHYSICS CHAPTERWISE SPEED TEST-20

Total Questions	45	Total Marks	180
Attempted		Correct	
Incorrect		Net Score	
Cut-off Score	50	Qualifying Score	70
Success Gap = Net Score – Qualifying Score			
Net Score = (Correct × 4) – (Incorrect × 1)			

Space for Rough Work

PHYSICS

Alternating Current

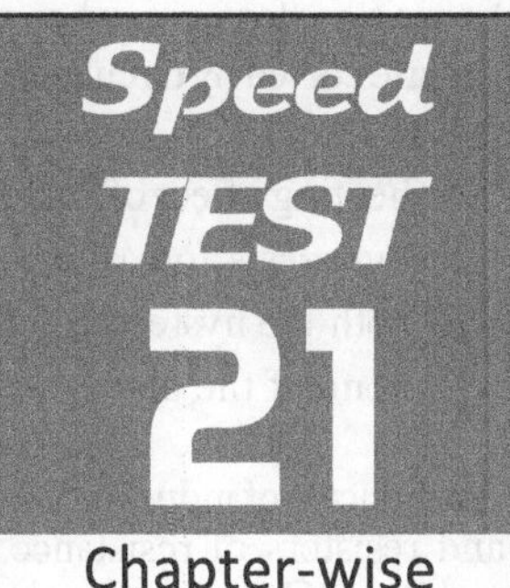

No. of Questions	Maximum Marks	Time
45	180	1 Hour

GENERAL INSTRUCTIONS

- This test contains 45 MCQ's. For each question only one option is correct. Darken the correct circle/ bubble in the Response Grid provided on each page.
- You have to evaluate your Response Grids yourself with the help of solutions provided at the end of this book.
- Each correct answer will get you 4 marks and 1 mark shall be deduced for each incorrect answer. No mark will be given/ deducted if no bubble is filled. Keep a timer in front of you and stop immediately at the end of 60 min.
- The sheet follows a particular syllabus. Do not attempt the sheet before you have completed your preparation for that syllabus.
- After completing the sheet check your answers with the solution booklet and complete the Result Grid. Finally spend time to analyse your performance and revise the areas which emerge out as weak in your evaluation.

1. In a series resonant LCR circuit, the voltage across R is 100 volts and $R = 1\ k\Omega$ with $C = 2\mu F$. The resonant frequency ω is 200 rad/s. At resonance, the voltage across L is
   (a) 2.5×10^{-2} V (b) 40 V
   (c) 250 V (d) 4×10^{-3} V

2. An alternating voltage $V = V_0 \sin \omega t$ is applied across a circuit. As a result, a current $I = I_0 \sin(\omega t - \pi/2)$ flows in it. The power consumed per cycle is
   (a) zero (b) $0.5\, V_0 I_0$
   (c) $0.707\, V_0 I_0$ (d) $1.414\, V_0 I_0$

3. For the circuit shown in the fig., the current through the inductor is 0.9 A while the current through the condenser is 0.4 A. Then

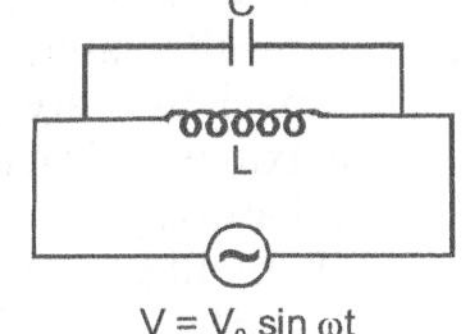

   (a) current drawn from generator I = 1.13 A
   (b) $\omega = 1/(1.5\, LC)$
   (c) I = 0.5 A
   (d) I = 0.6 A

4. A capacitor has capacity C and reactance X. If capacitance and frequency become double, then reactance will be
   (a) 4X (b) X/2 (c) X/4 (d) 2X

5. A coil of inductance 300 mH and resistance 2Ω is connected to a source of voltage 2V. The current reaches half of its steady state value in
   (a) 0.1 s (b) 0.05 s (c) 0.3 s (d) 0.15 s

6. In an A.C. circuit, a resistance of R ohm is connected in series with an inductance L. If phase angle between voltage and current be 45°, the value of inductive reactance will be
   (a) R/4 (b) R/2 (c) R (d) R/5

7. A bulb is rated at 100 V, 100 W, it can be treated as a resistor. Find out the inductance of an inductor (called choke coil) that should be connected in series with the bulb to operate the bulb at its rated power with the help of an ac source of 200 V and 50 Hz.
   (a) $\frac{\pi}{\sqrt{3}}$ H (b) 100 H (c) $\frac{\sqrt{2}}{\pi}$ H (d) $\frac{\sqrt{3}}{\pi}$ H

8. An ac source of angular frequency ω is fed across a resistor r and a capacitor C in series. The current registered is I. If now the frequency of source is changed to $\omega/3$ (but maintaining the same voltage), the current in the circuit is found to be halved. The ratio of reactance to resistance at the original frequency ω is
   (a) $\sqrt{\frac{3}{5}}$ (b) $\sqrt{\frac{2}{5}}$ (c) $\sqrt{\frac{1}{5}}$ (d) $\sqrt{\frac{4}{5}}$

RESPONSE GRID					
	1. ⓐⓑⓒⓓ	2. ⓐⓑⓒⓓ	3. ⓐⓑⓒⓓ	4. ⓐⓑⓒⓓ	5. ⓐⓑⓒⓓ
	6. ⓐⓑⓒⓓ	7. ⓐⓑⓒⓓ	8. ⓐⓑⓒⓓ		

Space for Rough Work

9. Large transformers, when used for some time, become hot and are cooled by circulating oil. The heating of transformer is due to
(a) heating effect of current alone
(b) hysteresis loss alone
(c) both the hysteresis loss and heating effect of current
(d) none of the above

10. An inductor of inductance $L = 400$ mH and resistors of resistance $R_1 = 2\Omega$ and $R_2 = 2\Omega$ are connected to a battery of emf 12 V as shown in the figure. The internal resistance of the battery is negligible. The switch S is closed at $t = 0$. The potential drop across L as a function of time is

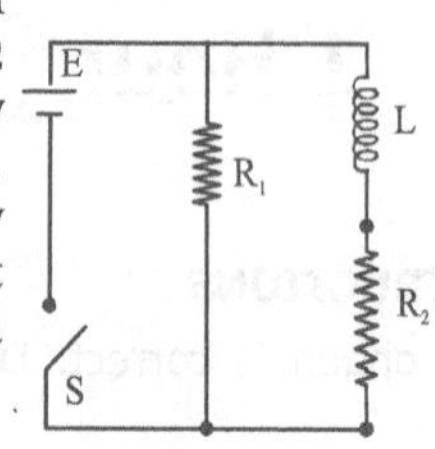

(a) $\frac{12}{t}e^{-3t}$V (b) $6(1-e^{-t/0.2})$V
(c) $12e^{-5t}$V (d) $6e^{-5t}$V

11. An ideal coil of 10H is connected in series with a resistance of 5Ω and a battery of 5V. 2second after the connection is made, the current flowing in ampere in the circuit is
(a) $(1-e^{-1})$ (b) $(1-e)$ (c) e (d) e^{-1}

12. In an A.C. circuit, the current flowing in inductance is $I = 5\sin(100t - \pi/2)$ amperes and the potential difference is $V = 200\sin(100t)$ volts. The power consumption is equal to
(a) 1000 watt (b) 40 watt
(c) 20 watt (d) Zero

13. In an oscillating LC circuit the maximum charge on the capacitor is Q. The charge on the capacitor when the energy is stored equally between the electric and magnetic field is
(a) $\frac{Q}{2}$ (b) $\frac{Q}{\sqrt{3}}$ (c) $\frac{Q}{\sqrt{2}}$ (d) Q

14. A fully charged capacitor C with initial charge q_0 is connected to a coil of self inductance L at $t = 0$. The time at which the energy is stored equally between the electric and the magnetic fields is:
(a) $\frac{\pi}{4}\sqrt{LC}$ (b) $2\pi\sqrt{LC}$ (c) $\sqrt{LC}$ (d) $\pi\sqrt{LC}$

15. For an LCR series circuit with an A.C. source of angular frequency ω
(a) circuit will be capacitive if $\omega > \frac{1}{\sqrt{LC}}$
(b) circuit will be inductive if $\omega = \frac{1}{\sqrt{LC}}$
(c) power factor of circuit will be unity if capacitive reactance equals inductive reactance
(d) current will be leading voltage if $\omega > \frac{1}{\sqrt{LC}}$

16. The r.m.s. value of potential difference V shown in the figure is

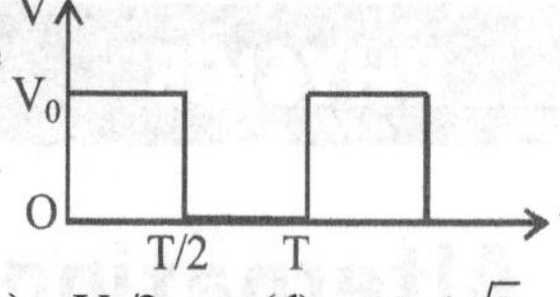

(a) V_0 (b) $V_0/\sqrt{2}$ (c) $V_0/2$ (d) $V_0/\sqrt{3}$

17. Which of the following statements is/are incorrect?
(a) If the resonance is less sharp, not only is the maximum current less, the circuit is close to resonance for a larger range Δω of frequencies and the tuning of the circuit will not be good.
(b) Less sharp the resonance less is the selectivity of the circuit or *vice–versa*.
(c) If quality factor is large, i.e., R is low or L is large, the circuit is more selective.
(d) Below resonance, voltage leads the current while above it, current leads the voltage.

18. A lamp consumes only 50% of peak power in an a.c. circuit. What is the phase difference between the applied voltage and the circuit current?
(a) $\frac{\pi}{6}$ (b) $\frac{\pi}{3}$ (c) $\frac{\pi}{4}$ (d) $\frac{\pi}{2}$

19. A step down transformer reduces 220 V to 110 V. The primary draws 5 ampere of current and secondary supplies 9 ampere. The efficiency of transformer is
(a) 20% (b) 44% (c) 90% (d) 100%

20. The voltage time (V-t) graph for triangular wave having peak value V_0 is as shown in figure. The rms value of V in time interval from t = 0 to T/4 is $\frac{V_0}{\sqrt{x}}$ then find the value of x.

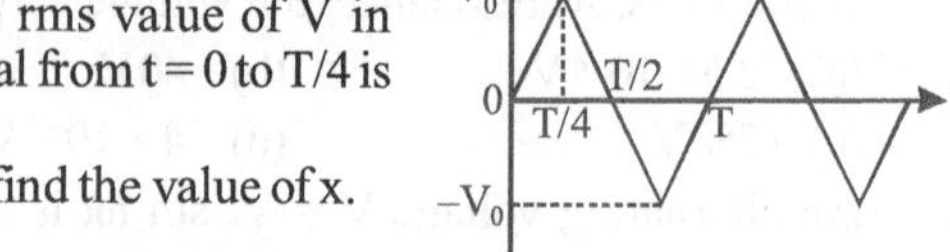

(a) 5 (b) 4 (c) 7 (d) 3

21. The tuning circuit of a radio receiver has a resistance of 50 Ω, an inductor of 10 mH and a variable capacitor. A 1 MHz radio wave produces a potential difference of 0.1 mV. The values of the capacitor to produce resonance is (Take $\pi^2 = 10$)
(a) 2.5 pF (b) 5.0 pF (c) 25 pF (d) 50 pF

22. In an alternating current circuit in which an inductance and capacitance are joined in series, current is found to be maximum when the value of inductance is 0.5 henry and the value of capacitance is 8μF. The angular frequency of applied alternating voltage will be
(a) 5000 rad/sec (b) 4000 rad/sec
(c) 2×10^5 rad/sec (d) 500 rad/sec

23. A coil has resistance 30 ohm and inductive reactance 20 ohm at 50 Hz frequency. If an ac source, of 200 volt, 100 Hz, is connected across the coil, the current in the coil will be
(a) 4.0A (b) 8.0A (c) $\frac{20}{\sqrt{13}}$A (d) 2.0A

RESPONSE GRID					
	9. ⓐⓑⓒⓓ	10. ⓐⓑⓒⓓ	11. ⓐⓑⓒⓓ	12. ⓐⓑⓒⓓ	13. ⓐⓑⓒⓓ
	14. ⓐⓑⓒⓓ	15. ⓐⓑⓒⓓ	16. ⓐⓑⓒⓓ	17. ⓐⓑⓒⓓ	18. ⓐⓑⓒⓓ
	19. ⓐⓑⓒⓓ	20. ⓐⓑⓒⓓ	21. ⓐⓑⓒⓓ	22. ⓐⓑⓒⓓ	23. ⓐⓑⓒⓓ

Space for Rough Work

24. In the figure shown, three AC voltmeters are connected. At resonance

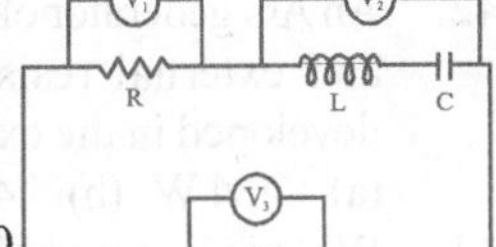

(a) $V_2 = 0$ (b) $V_1 = 0$
(c) $V_3 = 0$ (d) $V_1 = V_2 \neq 0$

25. A.C. power is transmitted from a power house at a high voltage as
(a) the rate of transmission is faster at high voltages
(b) it is more economical due to less power loss
(c) power cannot be transmitted at low voltages
(d) a precaution against theft of transmission lines

26. A transformer has an efficiency of 80%. It works at 4 kW and 100 V. If secondary voltage is 240 V, the current in primary coil is
(a) 0.4 A (b) 4 A (c) 10 A (d) 40 A

27. A 12 Ω resistor and a 0.21 henry inductor are connected in series to an a.c. source operating at 20 volt, 50 cycle. The phase angle between the current and source voltage is
(a) 30º (b) 40º (c) 80º (d) 90º

28. In LCR series circuit fed by a DC source, how does the amplitude of charge oscillations vary with time during discharge ?

(a) (b) (c) (d)

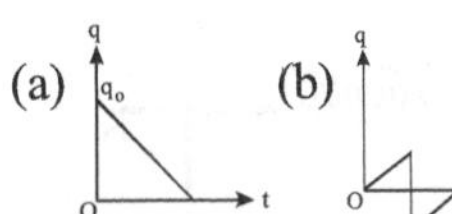

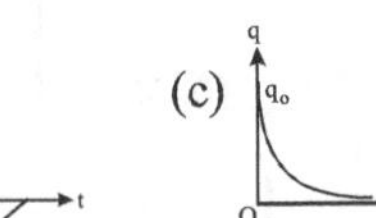

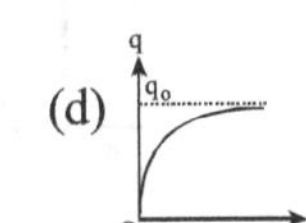

29. The primary and secondary coil of a transformer have 50 and 1500 turns respectively. If the magnetic flux ϕ linked with the primary coil is given by $\phi = \phi_0 + 4t$, where ϕ is in webers, t is time in seconds and ϕ_0 is a constant, the output voltage across the secondary coil is
(a) 120 volts (b) 220 volts
(c) 30 volts (d) 90 volts

30. The primary winding of a transformer has 100 turns and its secondary winding has 200 turns. The primary is connected to an A.C. supply of 120 V and the current flowing in it is 10 A. The voltage and the current in the secondary are
(a) 240 V, 5 A (b) 240 V, 10 A
(c) 60 V, 20 A (d) 120 V, 20 A

31. The resistance in the following circuit is increased at a particular instant. At this instant the value of resistance is 10Ω. The current in the circuit will be now

10mH, i, 5V, Rh

(a) i = 0.5 A (b) i > 0.5 A (c) i < 0.5 A (d) i = 0

32. The current in a *LR* circuit builds up to $\frac{3}{4}th$ of its steady state value in 4s. The time constant of this circuit is

(a) $\frac{1}{\ell n 2} s$ (b) $\frac{2}{\ell n 2} s$ (c) $\frac{3}{\ell n 2} s$ (d) $\frac{4}{\ell n 2} s$

33. An LCR series circuit is connected to a source of alternating current. At resonance, the applied voltage and the current flowing through the circuit will have a phase difference of

(a) π (b) $\frac{\pi}{2}$ (c) $\frac{\pi}{4}$ (d) 0

34. What is the value of inductance L for which the current is maximum in a series LCR circuit with $C = 10\mu F$ and $\omega = 1000 s^{-1}$?
(a) 1 mH
(b) cannot be calculated unless R is known
(c) 10 mH
(d) 100 mH

35. In the circuit of Fig, the bulb will become suddenly bright if

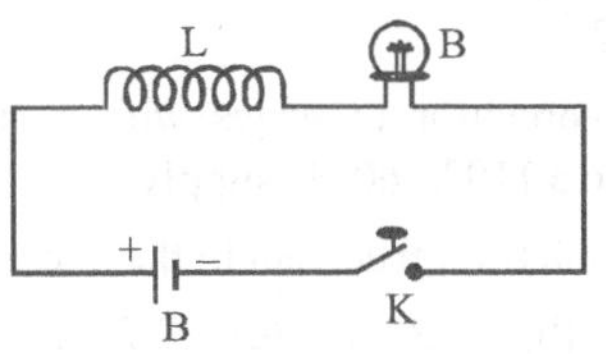

(a) contact is made or broken
(b) contact is made
(c) contact is broken
(d) won't become bright at all

36. The voltage of an ac source varies with time according to the equation $V = 100 \sin 100 \pi t \cos 100 \pi t$ where t is in seconds and V is in volt. Then
(a) the peak voltage of the source is 100 volt
(b) the peak voltage of the source is 50 volt
(c) the peak voltage of the source is $100/\sqrt{2}$ volt
(d) the frequency of the source is 50 Hz

37. The current (*I*) in the inductance is varying with time according to the plot shown in figure.

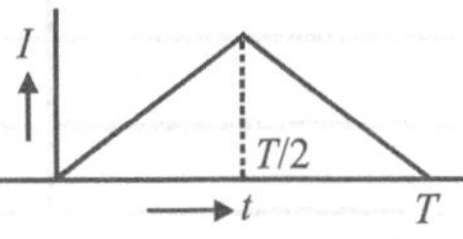

Which one of the following is the correct variation of voltage with time in the coil?

(a)

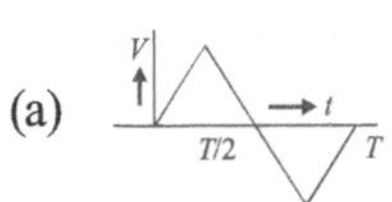

(b)

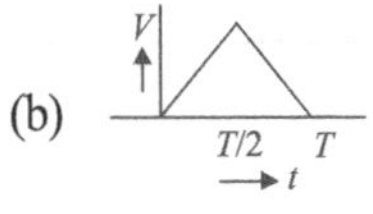

(c)

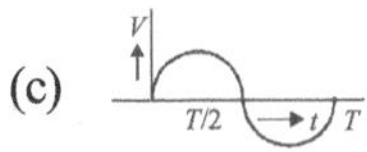

(d)

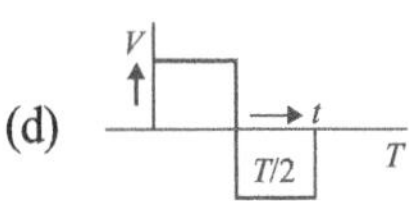

RESPONSE GRID					
	24. ⓐⓑⓒⓓ	25. ⓐⓑⓒⓓ	26. ⓐⓑⓒⓓ	27. ⓐⓑⓒⓓ	28. ⓐⓑⓒⓓ
	29. ⓐⓑⓒⓓ	30. ⓐⓑⓒⓓ	31. ⓐⓑⓒⓓ	32. ⓐⓑⓒⓓ	33. ⓐⓑⓒⓓ
	34. ⓐⓑⓒⓓ	35. ⓐⓑⓒⓓ	36. ⓐⓑⓒⓓ	37. ⓐⓑⓒⓓ	

Space for Rough Work

38. Using an A.C. voltmeter the potential difference in the electrical line in a house is read to be 234 volt. If the line frequency is known to be 50 cycles/second, the equation for the line voltage is

(a) V = 165 sin (100 πt) (b) V = 331 sin (100 πt)
(c) V = 220 sin (100 πt) (d) V = 440 sin (100 πt)

39. In the circuit shown, when the switch is closed, the capacitor charges with a time constant

(a) RC
(b) 2RC
(c) $\frac{1}{2}$RC
(d) RC ln 2

40. A 100 μF capacitor in series with a 40Ω resistance is connected to a 110 V, 60 Hz supply.

What is the maximum current in the circuit?

(a) 3.24A (b) 4.25A (c) 2.25A (d) 5.20A

41. The core of any transformer is laminated so as to

(a) reduce the energy loss due to eddy currents
(b) make it light weight
(c) make it robust and strong
(d) increase the secondary voltage

42. An AC generator of 220 V having internal resistance r = 10Ω and external resistance R = 100Ω. What is the power developed in the external circuit?

(a) 484 W (b) 400 W (c) 441 W (d) 369 W

43. What is increased in step-down transformer?

(a) Voltage (b) Current
(c) Power (d) Current density

44. In the circuit shown below, the key K is closed at t = 0. The current through the battery is

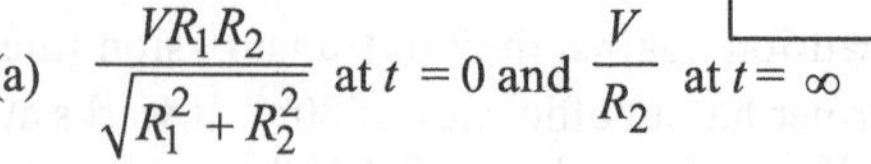

(a) $\frac{VR_1R_2}{\sqrt{R_1^2+R_2^2}}$ at $t = 0$ and $\frac{V}{R_2}$ at $t = \infty$

(b) $\frac{V}{R_2}$ at $t = 0$ and $\frac{V(R_1+R_2)}{R_1R_2}$ at $t = \infty$

(c) $\frac{V}{R_2}$ at $t = 0$ and $\frac{VR_1R_2}{\sqrt{R_1^2+R_2^2}}$ at $t = \infty$

(d) $\frac{V(R_1+R_2)}{R_1R_2}$ at $t = 0$ and $\frac{V}{R_2}$ at $t = \infty$

45. The inductance between A and D is

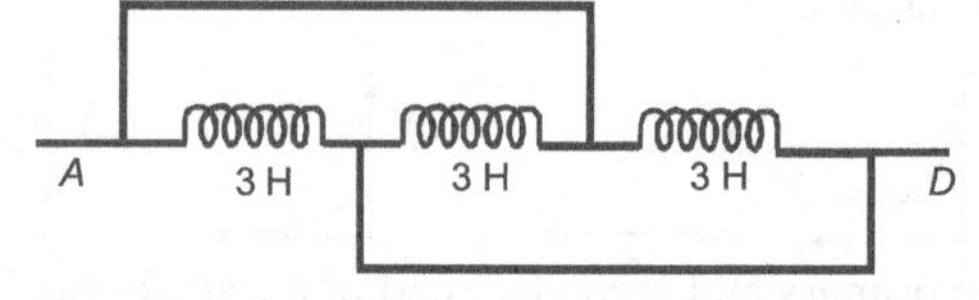

(a) 3.66 H (b) 9 H (c) 0.66 H (d) 1 H

RESPONSE GRID	38. ⓐⓑⓒⓓ	39. ⓐⓑⓒⓓ	40. ⓐⓑⓒⓓ	41. ⓐⓑⓒⓓ	42. ⓐⓑⓒⓓ
	43. ⓐⓑⓒⓓ	44. ⓐⓑⓒⓓ	45. ⓐⓑⓒⓓ		

PHYSICS CHAPTERWISE SPEED TEST-21

Total Questions	45	Total Marks	180
Attempted		Correct	
Incorrect		Net Score	
Cut-off Score	50	Qualifying Score	70

Success Gap = Net Score – Qualifying Score

Net Score = (Correct × 4) – (Incorrect × 1)

Space for Rough Work

PHYSICS

Electromagnetic Waves

Speed TEST 22

Chapter-wise

No. of Questions	Maximum Marks	Time
45	180	1 Hour

GENERAL INSTRUCTIONS

- This test contains 45 MCQ's. For each question only one option is correct. Darken the correct circle/ bubble in the Response Grid provided on each page.
- You have to evaluate your Response Grids yourself with the help of solutions provided at the end of this book.
- Each correct answer will get you 4 marks and 1 mark shall be deduced for each incorrect answer. No mark will be given/ deducted if no bubble is filled. Keep a timer in front of you and stop immediately at the end of 60 min.
- The sheet follows a particular syllabus. Do not attempt the sheet before you have completed your preparation for that syllabus.
- After completing the sheet check your answers with the solution booklet and complete the Result Grid. Finally spend time to analyse your performance and revise the areas which emerge out as weak in your evaluation.

1. An electromagnetic wave in vacuum has the electric and magnetic field $\vec{E}$ and $\vec{B}$, which are always perpendicular to each other. The direction of polarization is given by $\vec{X}$ and that of wave propagation by $\vec{k}$. Then

(a) $\vec{X} \parallel \vec{B}$ and $\vec{k} \parallel \vec{B}\times\vec{E}$ (b) $\vec{X} \parallel \vec{E}$ and $\vec{k} \parallel \vec{E}\times\vec{B}$

(c) $\vec{X} \parallel \vec{B}$ and $\vec{k} \parallel \vec{E}\times\vec{B}$ (d) $\vec{X} \parallel \vec{E}$ and $\vec{k} \parallel \vec{B}\times\vec{E}$

2. The rms value of the electric field of the light coming from the Sun is 720 N/C. The average total energy density of the electromagnetic wave is

(a) 4.58×10^{-6} J/m^3 (b) 6.37×10^{-9} J/m^3

(c) 81.35×10^{-12} J/m^3 (d) 3.3×10^{-3} J/m^3

3. In order to establish an instantaneous displacemet current of 1 mA in the space between the plates of 2μF parallel plate capacitor, the potential difference need to apply is

(a) 100 Vs^{-1} (b) 200 Vs^{-1} (c) 300 Vs^{-1} (d) 500 Vs^{-1}

4. During the propagation of electromagnetic waves in a medium:

(a) Electric energy density is double of the magnetic energy density.

(b) Electric energy density is half of the magnetic energy density.

(c) Electric energy density is equal to the magnetic energy density.

(d) Both electric and magnetic energy densities are zero.

5. An electromagnetic wave with frequency ω and wavelength λ travels in the + y direction. Its magnetic field is along + x-axis. The vector equation for the associated electric field (of amplitude E_0) is

(a) $\vec{E} = -E_0 \cos\left(\omega t + \frac{2\pi}{\lambda} y\right) \hat{x}$

(b) $\vec{E} = E_0 \cos\left(\omega t - \frac{2\pi}{\lambda} y\right) \hat{x}$

(c) $\vec{E} = E_0 \cos\left(\omega t - \frac{2\pi}{\lambda} y\right) \hat{z}$

(d) $\vec{E} = -E_0 \cos\left(\omega t + \frac{2\pi}{\lambda} y\right) \hat{z}$

RESPONSE GRID	1. ⓐⓑⓒⓓ	2. ⓐⓑⓒⓓ	3. ⓐⓑⓒⓓ	4. ⓐⓑⓒⓓ	5. ⓐⓑⓒⓓ

Space for Rough Work

6. An electromagnetic wave of frequency $\nu = 3.0$ MHz passes from vacuum into a dielectric medium with permittivity $\in = 4.0$. Then
(a) wavelength is halved and frequency remains unchanged
(b) wavelength is doubled and frequency becomes half
(c) wavelength is doubled and the frequency remains unchanged
(d) wavelength and frequency both remain unchanged.

7. The average electric field of electromagnetic waves in certain region of free space is 9×10^{-4} NC^{-1}. Then the average magnetic field in the same region is of the order of
(a) 27×10^{-4} T (b) 3×10^{-12} T
(c) $\left(\frac{1}{3}\right) \times 10^{-12}$ T (d) 3×10^{12} T

8. The electric field of an electromagnetic wave travelling through vaccum is given by the equation $E = E_0 \sin(kx - \omega t)$. The quantity that is independent of wavelength is
(a) $k\omega$ (b) $\frac{k}{\omega}$ (c) $k^2\omega$ (d) ω

9. The electric and the magnetic field associated with an E.M. wave, propagating along the +z-axis, can be represented by
(a) $\left[\vec{E} = E_0\hat{i}, \vec{B} = B_0\hat{j}\right]$ (b) $\left[\vec{E} = E_0\hat{k}, \vec{B} = B_0\hat{i}\right]$
(c) $\left[\vec{E} = E_0\hat{j}, \vec{B} = B_0\hat{i}\right]$ (d) $\left[\vec{E} = E_0\hat{j}, \vec{B} = B_0\hat{k}\right]$

10. The energy of electromagnetic wave in vacuum is given by the relation
(a) $\frac{E^2}{2\varepsilon_0} + \frac{B^2}{2\mu_0}$ (b) $\frac{1}{2}\varepsilon_0 E^2 + \frac{1}{2}\mu_0 B^2$
(c) $\frac{E^2 + B^2}{c}$ (d) $\frac{1}{2}\varepsilon_0 E^2 + \frac{B^2}{2\mu_0}$

11. A plane electromagnetic wave is incident on a plane surface of area A, normally and is perfectly reflected. If energy E strikes the surface in time t then average pressure exerted on the surface is (c = speed of light)
(a) zero (b) E/Atc (c) 2E/Atc (d) E/c

12. An electromagnetic wave travels along z-axis. Which of the following pairs of space and time varying fields would generate such a wave ?
(a) E_x, B_y (b) E_y, B_x (c) E_z, B_x (d) E_y, B_z

13. The magnetic field in a travelling electromagnetic wave has a peak value of 20 nT. The peak value of electric field strength is :
(a) 3 V/m (b) 6 V/m (c) 9 V/m (d) 12 V/m

14. Microwave oven acts on the principle of :
(a) giving rotational energy to water molecules
(b) giving translational energy to water molecules
(c) giving vibrational energy to water molecules
(d) transferring electrons from lower to higher energy levels in water molecule

15. Displacement current is
(a) continuous when electric field is changing in the circuit
(b) continuous when magnetic field is changing in the circuit
(c) continuous in both types of fields
(d) continuous through wires and resistance only

16. The electric field associated with an e.m. wave in vacuum is given by $\vec{E} = \hat{i}\, 40 \cos(kz - 6 \times 10^8 t)$, where E, z and t are in volt/m, meter and seconds respectively. The value of wave vector k is
(a) 2 m^{-1} (b) 0.5 m^{-1} (c) 6 m^{-1} (d) 3 m^{-1}

17. The charge on a parallel plate capacitor varies as $q = q_0 \cos 2\pi\upsilon t$. The plates are very large and close together (area = A, separation = d). The displacement current through the capacitor is
(a) $q_0\, 2\pi\upsilon \sin\pi\upsilon t$ (b) $-q_0\, 2\pi\upsilon \sin 2\pi\upsilon t$
(c) $q_0\, 2\pi \sin\pi\upsilon t$ (d) $q_0\, \pi\upsilon \sin 2\pi\upsilon t$

18. A radiation of energy 'E' falls normally on a perfectly reflecting surface. The momentum transferred to the surface is (C = Velocity of light)
(a) $\frac{2E}{C}$ (b) $\frac{2E}{C^2}$ (c) $\frac{E}{C^2}$ (d) $\frac{E}{C}$

19. Match List - I (Electromagnetic wave type) with List - II (Its association/application) and select the correct option from the choices given below the lists:

	List 1		List 2
1.	Infrared waves	(i)	To treat muscular strain
2.	Radio waves	(ii)	For broadcasting
3.	X-rays	(iii)	To detect fracture of bones
4.	Ultraviolet rays	(iv)	Absorbed by the ozone layer of the atmosphere

	1	2	3	4
(a)	(iv)	(iii)	(ii)	(i)
(b)	(i)	(ii)	(iv)	(iii)
(c)	(iii)	(ii)	(i)	(iv)
(d)	(i)	(ii)	(iii)	(iv)

20. A plane electromagnetic wave travels in free space along X-direction. If the value of $\vec{B}$ (in tesla) at a particular point in space and time is $1.2 \times 10^{-8}\,\hat{k}$. The value of $\vec{E}$ (in Vm^{-1}) at that point is
(a) $1.2\,\hat{j}$ (b) $3.6\,\hat{k}$ (c) $1.2\,\hat{k}$ (d) $3.6\,\hat{j}$

RESPONSE GRID					
	6. ⓐⓑⓒⓓ	7. ⓐⓑⓒⓓ	8. ⓐⓑⓒⓓ	9. ⓐⓑⓒⓓ	10. ⓐⓑⓒⓓ
	11. ⓐⓑⓒⓓ	12. ⓐⓑⓒⓓ	13. ⓐⓑⓒⓓ	14. ⓐⓑⓒⓓ	15. ⓐⓑⓒⓓ
	16. ⓐⓑⓒⓓ	17. ⓐⓑⓒⓓ	18. ⓐⓑⓒⓓ	19. ⓐⓑⓒⓓ	20. ⓐⓑⓒⓓ

Space for Rough Work

21. If v_s, v_x and v_m are the speed of soft gamma rays, X-rays and microwaves respectively in vacuum, then

(a) $v_s > v_x > v_m$ (b) $v_s < v_x < v_m$
(c) $v_s > v_x < v_m$ (d) $v_s = v_x = v_m$

22. Photons of an electromagnetic radiation has an energy 11 keV each. To which region of electromagnetic spectrum does it belong ?

(a) X-ray region (b) Ultra violet region
(c) Infrared region (d) Visible region

23. A plane electromagnetic wave travels in free space along x-axis. At a particular point in space, the electric field along y-axis is $9.3\ V\ m^{-1}$. The magnetic induction (B) along z-axis is

(a) 3.1×10^{-8} T (b) 3×10^{-5} T
(c) 3×10^{-6} T (d) 9.3×10^{-6} T

24. The ratio of amplitude of magnetic field to the amplitude of electric field for an electromagnetic wave propagating in vacuum is equal to :

(a) the speed of light in vacuum
(b) reciprocal of speed of light in vacuum
(c) the ratio of magnetic permeability to the electric susceptibility of vacuum
(d) unity

25. A plane electromagnetic wave is incident on a material surface. If the wave delivers momentum p and energy E, then

(a) $p = 0, E = 0$ (b) $p \neq 0, E \neq 0$
(c) $p \neq 0, E = 0$ (d) $p = 0, E \neq 0$

26. Intensity of electromagnetic wave will be

(a) $I = c\mu_0 B_0^2 / 2$ (b) $I = c\varepsilon_0 B_0^2 / 2$
(c) $I = B_0^2 / c\mu_0$ (d) $I = E_0^2 / 2c\varepsilon_0$

27. The decreasing order of wavelength of infrared, microwave, ultraviolet and gamma rays is

(a) microwave, infrared, ultraviolet, gamma rays
(b) gamma rays, ultraviolet, infrared, micro-waves
(c) microwaves, gamma rays, infrared, ultraviolet
(d) infrared, microwave, ultraviolet, gamma rays

28. Which radiation in sunlight, causes heating effect ?

(a) Ultraviolet (b) Infrared
(c) Visible light (d) All of these

29. The speed of electromagnetic wave in vacuum depends upon the source of radiation. It

(a) increases as we move from γ-rays to radio waves
(b) decreases as we move from γ-rays to radio waves
(c) is same for all of them
(d) None of these

30. When an electromagnetic waves enter the ionised layer of ionosphere, the motion of electron cloud produces a space current and the electric field has its own capacitative displacement current, then

(a) the space current is in phase of displacement current
(b) the space current lags behind the displacement current by a phase 180°.
(c) the space current lags behind the displacement current by a phase 90°.
(d) the space current leads the displacement current by a phase 90°.

31. The displacement current is

(a) $\varepsilon_0\, d\phi_E / dt$ (b) $\frac{\varepsilon_0}{R} d\phi_E / dt$
(c) $\varepsilon_0 E / R$ (d) $\varepsilon_0 q C / R$

32. Electromagnetic radiation of highest frequency is

(a) infrared radiations (b) visible radiation
(c) radio waves (d) γ-rays

33. A point source of electromagnetic radiation has an average power output of 1500 W. The maximum value of electric field at a distance of 3m from this sources in Vm^{-1} is

(a) 500 (b) 100 (c) $\frac{500}{3}$ (d) $\frac{250}{3}$

34. Frequency of a wave is 6×10^{15} Hz. The wave is

(a) radiowave (b) microwave
(c) x-ray (d) ultraviolet

35. The electromagnetic waves do not transport

(a) energy (b) charge
(c) momentum (d) information

36. Which of the following statement is false for the properties of electromagnetic waves?

(a) Both electric and magnetic field vectors attain the maxima and minima at the same place and same time.
(b) The energy in electromagnetic wave is divided equally between electric and magnetic vectors
(c) Both electric and magnetic field vectors are parallel to each other and perpendicular to the direction of propagation of wave
(d) These waves do not require any material medium for propagation.

RESPONSE GRID				
21. ⓐⓑⓒⓓ	22. ⓐⓑⓒⓓ	23. ⓐⓑⓒⓓ	24. ⓐⓑⓒⓓ	25. ⓐⓑⓒⓓ
26. ⓐⓑⓒⓓ	27. ⓐⓑⓒⓓ	28. ⓐⓑⓒⓓ	29. ⓐⓑⓒⓓ	30. ⓐⓑⓒⓓ
31. ⓐⓑⓒⓓ	32. ⓐⓑⓒⓓ	33. ⓐⓑⓒⓓ	34. ⓐⓑⓒⓓ	35. ⓐⓑⓒⓓ
36. ⓐⓑⓒⓓ				

Space for Rough Work

37. Which of the following electromagnetic waves has minimum frequency ?
(a) Microwaves (b) Audible waves
(c) Ultrasonic wave (d) Radiowaves

38. The wave impendance of free space is
(a) zero (b) 376.6 Ω (c) 33.66 Ω (d) 3.76 Ω

39. A plane electromagnetic wave in a non-magnetic dielectric medium is given by $\vec{E} = \vec{E}_0 (4 \times 10^{-7} x - 50t)$ with distance being in meter and time in seconds. The dielectric constant of the medium is :
(a) 2.4 (b) 5.8 (c) 8.2 (d) 4.8

40. We consider the radiation emitted by the human body. Which of the following statements is true?
(a) the radiation emitted lies in the ultraviolet region and hence is not visible.
(b) the radiation emitted is in the infra-red region.
(c) the radiation is emitted only during the day.
(d) the radiation is emitted during the summers and absorbed during the winters.

41. In a plane electromagnetic wave propagating in space has an electric field of amplitude 9×10^3 V/m, then the amplitude of the magnetic field is
(a) 2.7×10^{12} T (b) 9.0×10^{-3} T
(c) 3.0×10^{-4} T (d) 3.0×10^{-5} T

42. Out of the following options which one can be used to produce a propagating electromagnetic wave ?
(a) A charge moving at constant velocity
(b) A stationary charge
(c) A chargeless particle
(d) An accelerating charge

43. Radio waves of constant amplitude can be generated with
(a) rectifier (b) filter
(c) F.E.T. (d) oscillator

44. In an electromagnetic wave
(a) power is transmitted along the magnetic field
(b) power is transmitted along the electric field
(c) power is equally transferred along the electric and magnetic fields
(d) power is transmitted in a direction perpendicular to both the fields

45. If c is the speed of electromagnetic waves in vacuum, its speed in a medium of dielectric constant K and relative permeability μ_r is
(a) $v = \frac{1}{\sqrt{\mu_r K}}$ (b) $v = c\sqrt{\mu_r K}$
(c) $v = \frac{c}{\sqrt{\mu_r K}}$ (d) $v = \frac{K}{\sqrt{\mu_r C}}$

RESPONSE GRID					
	37. ⓐⓑⓒⓓ	38. ⓐⓑⓒⓓ	39. ⓐⓑⓒⓓ	40. ⓐⓑⓒⓓ	41. ⓐⓑⓒⓓ
	42. ⓐⓑⓒⓓ	43. ⓐⓑⓒⓓ	44. ⓐⓑⓒⓓ	45. ⓐⓑⓒⓓ	

PHYSICS CHAPTERWISE SPEED TEST-22

Total Questions	45	Total Marks	180
Attempted		Correct	
Incorrect		Net Score	
Cut-off Score	50	Qualifying Score	70

Success Gap = Net Score – Qualifying Score

Net Score = (Correct × 4) – (Incorrect × 1)

Space for Rough Work

PHYSICS

Ray Optics and Optical Instruments

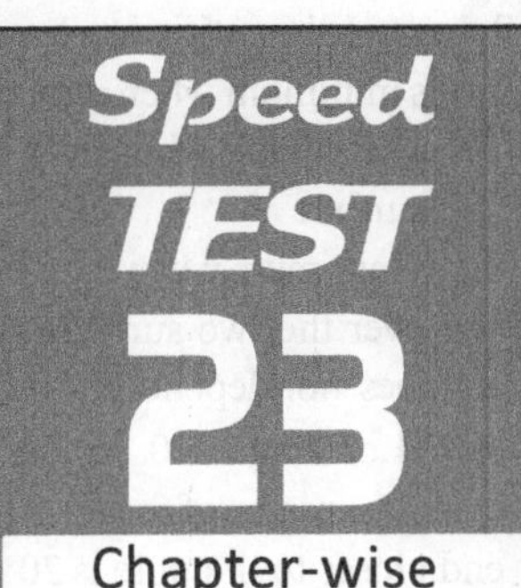

No. of Questions	Maximum Marks	Time
45	180	1 Hour

GENERAL INSTRUCTIONS

- This test contains 45 MCQ's. For each question only one option is correct. Darken the correct circle/ bubble in the Response Grid provided on each page.
- You have to evaluate your Response Grids yourself with the help of solutions provided at the end of this book.
- Each correct answer will get you 4 marks and 1 mark shall be deduced for each incorrect answer. No mark will be given/ deducted if no bubble is filled. Keep a timer in front of you and stop immediately at the end of 60 min.
- The sheet follows a particular syllabus. Do not attempt the sheet before you have completed your preparation for that syllabus.
- After completing the sheet check your answers with the solution booklet and complete the Result Grid. Finally spend time to analyse your performance and revise the areas which emerge out as weak in your evaluation.

1. A double convex lens is made of glass which has its refractive index 1.45 for violet rays and 1.50 for red rays. If the focal length for violet ray is 20cm, the focal length for red ray will be
   (a) 9 cm (b) 18 cm (c) 20 cm (d) 22 cm

2. If the refractive index of the material of a prism is $\cot\frac{A}{2}$ and the angle of prism is A, then angle of minimum deviation is
   (a) $\pi - 2A$ (b) $\pi - A$ (c) $\frac{\pi}{2} - 2A$ (d) $\frac{\pi}{2} - A$

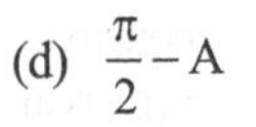

3. If two + 5 diopter lenses are mounted at some distance apart, the equivalent power will always be negative if the distance is
   (a) greater than 40 cm (b) equal to 40 cm
   (c) equal to 10 cm (d) less than 10 cm

4. Refraction of light from air to glass and from air to water are shown in figure (i) and figure (ii) below. The value of the angle θ in the case of refraction as shown in figure (iii) will be

(i) Glass, Air, 35°, 60° (ii) Air, Water, 60°, 41° (iii) Glass, Water, θ, 41°

   (a) 30° (b) 35° (c) 60° (d) 41°

5. A fish looking up through the water sees the outside world contained in a circular horizon. If the refractive index of water is $\frac{4}{3}$ and the fish is 12 cm below the surface, the radius of this circle in cm is
   (a) $36\sqrt{5}$ (b) $4\sqrt{5}$ (c) $36\sqrt{7}$ (d) $36/\sqrt{7}$

6. If f_V and f_R are the focal lengths of a convex lens for violet and red light respectively and F_V and F_R are the focal lengths of concave lens for violet and red light respectively, then we have
   (a) $f_V < f_R$ and $F_V > F_R$ (b) $f_V < f_R$ and $F_V < F_R$
   (c) $f_V > f_R$ and $F_V > F_R$ (d) $f_V > f_R$ and $F_V < F_R$

RESPONSE GRID 1. ⓐⓑⓒⓓ 2. ⓐⓑⓒⓓ 3. ⓐⓑⓒⓓ 4. ⓐⓑⓒⓓ 5. ⓐⓑⓒⓓ 6. ⓐⓑⓒⓓ

Space for Rough Work

7. Spherical aberration in a lens :
   (a) is minimum when most of the deviation is at first surface
   (b) is minimum when most of the deviation is at the second surface
   (c) is minimum when the total deviation is equally distributed over the two surfaces
   (d) does not depend on the above considerations

8. A rod of length 10 cm lies along the principal axis of a concave mirror of focal length 10 cm in such a way that its end closer to the pole is 20 cm away from the mirror. The length of the image is :
   (a) 10 cm (b) 15 cm (c) 2.5 cm (d) 5 cm

9. A telescope consists of two thin lenses of focal lengths, 0.3 m and 3 cm respectively. It is focused on moon which subtends an angle of 0.5° at the objective. Then the angle subtended at the eye by the final image will be
   (a) 5° (b) 0.25° (c) 0.5° (d) 0.35°

10. The layered lens as shown is made of two types of transparent materials-one indicated by horizontal lines and the other by vertical lines. The number of images formed of an object will be

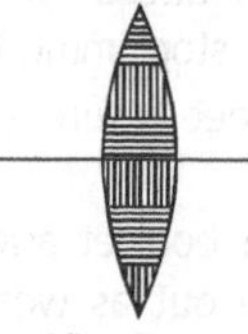

   (a) 1 (b) 2 (c) 3 (d) 6

11. A man's near point is 0.5 m and far point is 3 m. Power of spectacle lenses required for (i) reading purposes, (ii) seeing distant objects, respectively, are
   (a) –2 D and + 3 D (b) +2 D and –3 D
   (c) +2 D and –0.33 D (d) –2 D and + 0.33 D

12. A ray of light falls on a transparent glass slab of refractive index 1.62. If the reflected ray and the refracted ray are mutually perpendicular, the angle of incidence is
   (a) $\tan^{-1}(1.62)$ (b) $\tan^{-1}\left(\frac{1}{1.62}\right)$
   (c) $\tan^{-1}(1.33)$ (d) $\tan^{-1}\left(\frac{1}{1.33}\right)$

13. A telescope has an objective of focal length 100 cm and an eyepiece of focal length 5 cm. What is the magnifying power of the telescope when the final image is formed at the least distance of distinct vision ?
   (a) 20 (b) 24 (c) 28 (d) 32

14. Which light rays undergoes two internal reflection inside a raindrop, which of the rainbow is formed?
   (a) Primary rainbow (b) Secondary rainbow
   (c) Both (a) and (b) (d) Can't say

15. When a plane mirror is placed horizontally on a level ground at a distance of 60 *m* from the foot of a tower, the top of the tower and its image in the mirror subtend an angle of 90° at the eye. The height of the tower will be
   (a) 30m (b) 60m (c) 90m (d) 120m

16. A parallel beam of light is incident on the surface of a transparent hemisphere of radius *R* and refractive index 2.0 as shown in figure. The position of the image formed by refraction at the first surface is :
   (a) *R*/2
   (b) *R*
   (c) 2*R*
   (d) 3*R*

17. A lens made of glass whose index of refraction is 1.60 has a focal length of + 20 cm in air. Its focal length in water, whose refractive index is 1.33, will be
   (a) three times longer than in air
   (b) two times longer than in air
   (c) same as in air
   (d) None of these

18. A compound microscope has an eye piece of focal length 10 cm and an objective of focal length 4 cm. Calculate the magnification, if an object is kept at a distance of 5 cm from the objective so that final image is formed at the least distance vision (20 cm) :
   (a) 12 (b) 11 (c) 10 (d) 13

19. For a prism kept in air it is found that for an angle of incidence 60°, the angle of Prism A, angle of deviation δ and angle of emergence 'e' become equal. Then the refractive index of the prism is
   (a) 1.73 (b) 1.15 (c) 1.5 (d) 1.33

20. A person can see clearly only upto a distance of 30 cm. He wants to read a book placed at a distance of 50 cm from his eyes. What is the power of the lens of his spectacles ?
   (a) –1.0 D (b) –1.33 D (c) –1.67 D (d) –2.0 D

21. An object is placed at a distance of 40 cm in front of a concave mirror of focal length 20 cm. The image produced is
   (a) real, inverted and smaller in size
   (b) real, inverted and of same size
   (c) real and erect
   (d) virtual and inverted

22. A vessel of depth *x* is half filled with oil of refractive index μ_1 and the other half is filled with water of refractive index μ_2. The apparent depth of the vessel when viewed from above is
   (a) $\frac{x(\mu_1+\mu_2)}{2\mu_1\mu_2}$ (b) $\frac{x\mu_1\mu_2}{2(\mu_1+\mu_2)}$
   (c) $\frac{x\mu_1\mu_2}{(\mu_1+\mu_2)}$ (d) $\frac{2x(\mu_1+\mu_2)}{\mu_1\mu_2}$

RESPONSE GRID					
	7. ⓐⓑⓒⓓ	8. ⓐⓑⓒⓓ	9. ⓐⓑⓒⓓ	10. ⓐⓑⓒⓓ	11. ⓐⓑⓒⓓ
	12. ⓐⓑⓒⓓ	13. ⓐⓑⓒⓓ	14. ⓐⓑⓒⓓ	15. ⓐⓑⓒⓓ	16. ⓐⓑⓒⓓ
	17. ⓐⓑⓒⓓ	18. ⓐⓑⓒⓓ	19. ⓐⓑⓒⓓ	20. ⓐⓑⓒⓓ	21. ⓐⓑⓒⓓ
	22. ⓐⓑⓒⓓ				

Space for Rough Work

23. The following figure shows refraction of light at the interface of three media Correct the order of optical density (d) of the media is

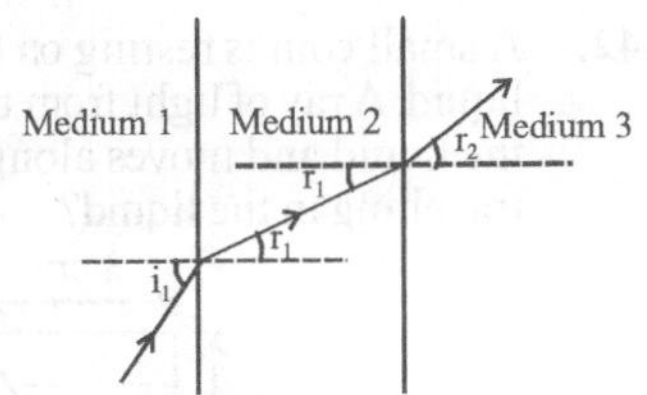

(a) $d_1 > d_2 > d_3$ (b) $d_2 > d_1 > d_3$
(c) $d_3 > d_3 > d_2$ (d) $d_2 > d_3 > d_1$

24. Light travels in two media A and B with speeds 1.8×10^8 m s^{-1} and 2.4×10^8 m s^{-1} respectively. Then the critical angle between them is
(a) $\sin^{-1}\left(\frac{2}{3}\right)$ (b) $\tan^{-1}\left(\frac{3}{4}\right)$
(c) $\tan^{-1}\left(\frac{2}{3}\right)$ (d) $\sin^{-1}\left(\frac{3}{4}\right)$

25. The refractive index of a glass is 1.520 for red light and 1.525 for blue light. Let D_1 and D_2 be angles of minimum deviation for red and blue light respectively in a prism of this glass. Then,
(a) $D_1 < D_2$ (b) $D_1 = D_2$
(c) D_1 can be less than or greater than D_2 depending upon the angle of prism
(d) $D_1 > D_2$

26. Which of the following is not due to total internal reflection?
(a) Working of optical fibre
(b) Difference between apparent and real depth of pond
(c) Mirage on hot summer days
(d) Brilliance of diamond

27. A body is located on a wall. Its image of equal size is to be obtained on a parallel wall with the help of a convex lens. The lens is placed at a distance 'd' ahead of second wall, then the required focal length will be
(a) only $\frac{d}{4}$
(b) only $\frac{d}{2}$
(c) more than $\frac{d}{4}$ but less than $\frac{d}{2}$
(d) less than $\frac{d}{4}$

28. A concave mirror forms the image of an object on a screen. If the lower half of the mirror is covered with an opaque card, the effect would be to make the
(a) image less bright.
(b) lower half of the image disappear.
(c) upper half of the image disappear.
(d) image blurred.

29. A ray of light passes through an equilateral prism such that the angle of incidence is equal to the angle of emergence and the latter is equal to $\frac{3}{4}$th of angle of prism. The angle of deviation is
(a) 25° (b) 30° (c) 45° (d) 35°

30. The power of a biconvex lens is 10 dioptre and the radius of curvature of each surface is 10 cm. Then the refractive index of the material of the lens is
(a) $\frac{3}{2}$ (b) $\frac{4}{3}$ (c) $\frac{9}{8}$ (d) $\frac{5}{3}$

31. A microscope is focussed on a mark on a piece of paper and then a slab of glass of thickness 3 cm and refractive index 1.5 is placed over the mark. How should the microscope be moved to get the mark in focus again ?
(a) 4.5 cm downward (b) 1 cm downward
(c) 2 cm upward (d) 1 cm upward

32. What causes chromatic aberration?
(a) Marginal rays
(b) Central rays
(c) Difference in radii of curvature of its surfaces
(d) Variation of focal length of lens with colour

33. The graph between angle of deviation (δ) and angle of incidence (i) for a triangular prism is represented by

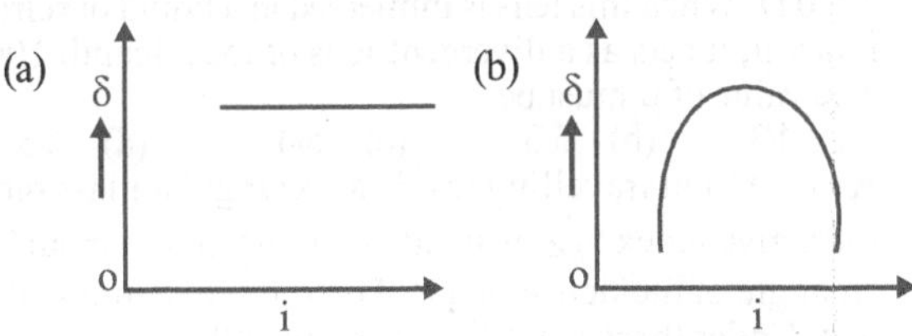

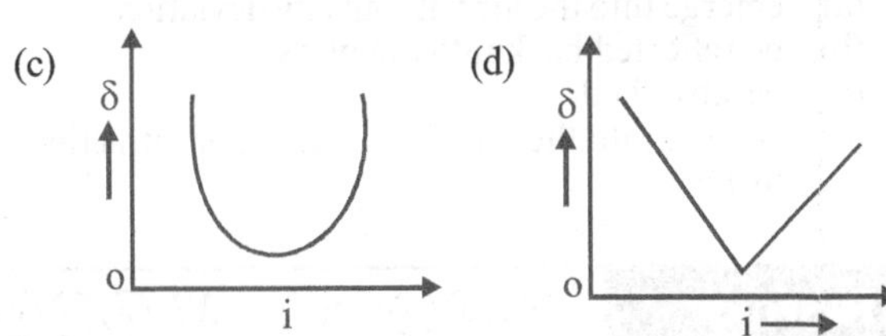

34. The ratio of thickness of plates of two transparent medium A and B is 6 : 4. If light takes equal time in passing through them, then refractive index of A with respect to B will be
(a) 1.33 (b) 1.75 (c) 1.4 (d) 1.5

35. A rectangular block of glass is placed on a mark made on the surface of the table and it is viewed from the vertical position of eye. If refractive index of glass be μ and its thickness d, then the mark will appear to be raised up by
(a) $\frac{(\mu+1)d}{\mu}$ (b) $\frac{(\mu-1)d}{\mu}$ (c) $\frac{(\mu+1)}{\mu d}$ (d) $\frac{(\mu-1)\mu}{d}$

RESPONSE GRID					
	23. ⓐⓑⓒⓓ	24. ⓐⓑⓒⓓ	25. ⓐⓑⓒⓓ	26. ⓐⓑⓒⓓ	27. ⓐⓑⓒⓓ
	28. ⓐⓑⓒⓓ	29. ⓐⓑⓒⓓ	30. ⓐⓑⓒⓓ	31. ⓐⓑⓒⓓ	32. ⓐⓑⓒⓓ
	33. ⓐⓑⓒⓓ	34. ⓐⓑⓒⓓ	35. ⓐⓑⓒⓓ		

Space for Rough Work

36. If a glass prism is dipped in water, its dispersive power
(a) increases
(b) decreases
(c) does not change
(d) may increase or decrease depending on whether the angle of the prism is less than or greater than 60°

37. A planoconcave lens is placed on a paper on which a flower is drawn. How far above its actual position does the flower appear to be?

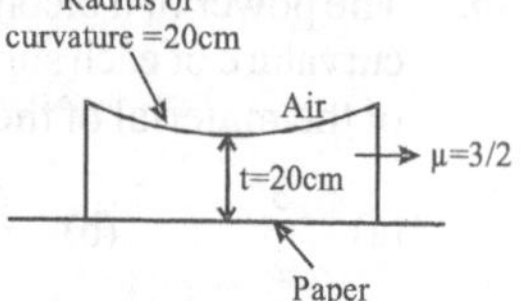

(a) 10 cm (b) 15 cm
(c) 50 cm (d) None of these

38. To get three images of a single object, one should have two plane mirrors at an angle of
(a) 60° (b) 90° (c) 120° (d) 30°

39. Light propagates with speed of 2.2×10^8 m/s and 2.4×10^8 m/s in the media P and Q respectively. The critical angle of incidence for light undergoing reflection from P and Q is
(a) $\sin^{-1}\left(\frac{1}{11}\right)$ (b) $\sin^{-1}\left(\frac{11}{12}\right)$
(c) $\sin^{-1}\left(\frac{5}{12}\right)$ (d) $\sin^{-1}\left(\frac{5}{11}\right)$

40. A thin convergent glass lens (μ_g = 1.5) has a power of + 5.0 D. When this lens is immersed in a liquid of refractive index μ, it acts as a divergent lens of focal length 100 cm. The value of μ must be
(a) 4/3 (b) 5/3 (c) 5/4 (d) 6/5

41. A ray of light travelling inside a rectangular glass block of refractive index $\sqrt{2}$ is incident on the glass-air surface at an angle of incidence of 45°. The refractive index of air is one. Under these conditions the ray will
(a) emerge into the air without any deviation
(b) be reflected back into the glass
(c) be absorbed
(d) emerge into the air with an angle of refraction equal to 90°

42. A small coin is resting on the bottom of a beaker filled with liquid. A ray of light from the coin travels upto the surface of the liquid and moves along its surface. How fast is the light travelling in the liquid?

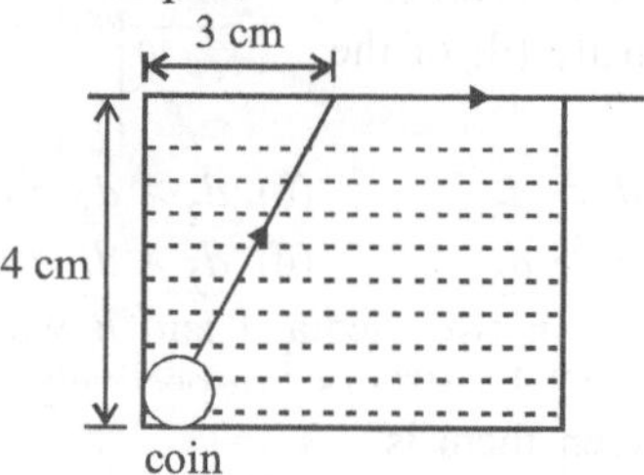

(a) 2.4×10^8 m/s (b) 3.0×10^8 m/s
(c) 1.2×10^8 m/s (d) 1.8×10^8 m/s

43. A ray PQ incident on the refracting face BA is refracted in the prism BAC as shown in the figure and emerges from the other refracting face AC as RS such that AQ = AR. If the angle of prism A = 60° and the refractive index of the material of prism is $\sqrt{3}$, then the angle of deviation of the ray is

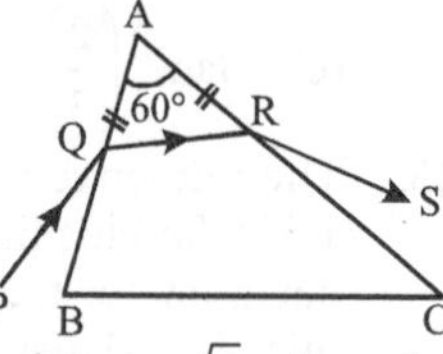

(a) 60° (b) 45°
(c) 30° (d) None of these

44. When a biconvex lens of glass having refractive index 1.47 is dipped in a liquid, it acts as a plane sheet of glass. This implies that the liquid must have refractive index.
(a) equal to that of glass
(b) less then one
(c) greater than that of glass
(d) less then that of glass

45. If a thin prism of glass is dipped in water then minimum deviation (with respect to air) of light produced by prism will be $\left({}_w\mu_g = \frac{3}{2}, {}_a\mu_w = \frac{4}{3}\right)$
(a) $\frac{1}{5}$ (b) $\frac{1}{4}$ (c) $\frac{1}{2}$ (d) $\frac{1}{3}$

RESPONSE GRID					
	36. ⓐⓑⓒⓓ	37. ⓐⓑⓒⓓ	38. ⓐⓑⓒⓓ	39. ⓐⓑⓒⓓ	40. ⓐⓑⓒⓓ
	41. ⓐⓑⓒⓓ	42. ⓐⓑⓒⓓ	43. ⓐⓑⓒⓓ	44. ⓐⓑⓒⓓ	45. ⓐⓑⓒⓓ

PHYSICS CHAPTERWISE SPEED TEST-23

Total Questions	45	Total Marks	180
Attempted		Correct	
Incorrect		Net Score	
Cut-off Score	45	Qualifying Score	60
Success Gap = Net Score – Qualifying Score			
Net Score = (Correct × 4) – (Incorrect × 1)			

Space for Rough Work

PHYSICS

Wave Optics

Speed TEST 24

Chapter-wise

No. of Questions	Maximum Marks	Time
45	180	1 Hour

GENERAL INSTRUCTIONS

- This test contains 45 MCQ's. For each question only one option is correct. Darken the correct circle/ bubble in the Response Grid provided on each page.
- You have to evaluate your Response Grids yourself with the help of solutions provided at the end of this book.
- Each correct answer will get you 4 marks and 1 mark shall be deduced for each incorrect answer. No mark will be given/ deducted if no bubble is filled. Keep a timer in front of you and stop immediately at the end of 60 min.
- The sheet follows a particular syllabus. Do not attempt the sheet before you have completed your preparation for that syllabus.
- After completing the sheet check your answers with the solution booklet and complete the Result Grid. Finally spend time to analyse your performance and revise the areas which emerge out as weak in your evaluation.

1. In young's double-slit experiment, the intensity of light at a point on the screen where the path difference is λ is I, λ being the wavelength of light used. The intensity at a point where the path difference is $\frac{\lambda}{4}$ will be

(a) $\frac{I}{4}$ (b) $\frac{I}{2}$ (c) I (d) zero

2. A beam of light is incident on a glass slab ($\mu = 1.54$) in a direction as shown in the figure. The reflected light is analysed by a polaroid prism. On rotating the polaroid, (tan 57° = 1.54)

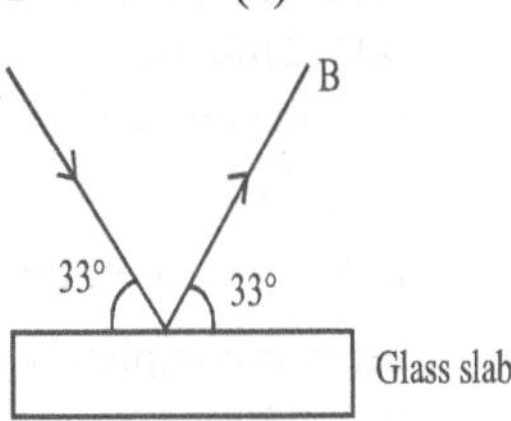

(a) the intensity remains unchanged
(b) the intensity is reduced to zero and remains at zero
(c) the intensity gradually reduces to zero and then again increase
(d) the intensity increases continuously

3. Two sources of light of wavelengths 2500 Å and 3500 Å are used in Young's double slit expt. simultaneously. Which orders of fringes of two wavelength patterns coincide?

(a) 3rd order of 1st source and 5th of the 2nd
(b) 7th order of 1st and 5th order of 2nd
(c) 5th order of 1st and 3rd order of 2nd
(d) 5th order of 1st and 7th order of 2nd

4. Figure shows behavior of a wavefront when it passes through a prism.

Which of the following statements is/are correct ?

(a) Lower portion of wavefront (*B*') is delayed resulting in a tilt.
(b) Time taken by light to reach *A*' is equal to the time taken to reach *B*' from *B*.
(c) Speed of wavefront is same everywhere.
(d) A particle on wavefront *A*' *B*' is in phase with a particle on wavefront *AB*.

5. When the angle of incidence is 60° on the surface of a glass slab, it is found that the reflected ray is completely polarised. The velocity of light in glass is

(a) $\sqrt{2} \times 10^8 \text{ms}^{-1}$ (b) $\sqrt{3} \times 10^8 \text{ms}^{-1}$
(c) $2 \times 10^8 \text{ms}^{-1}$ (d) $3 \times 10^8 \text{ms}^{-1}$

RESPONSE GRID 1. 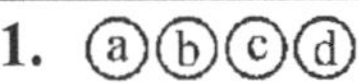 ⓐⓑⓒⓓ 2. 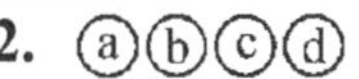 ⓐⓑⓒⓓ 3. ⓐⓑⓒⓓ 4. ⓐⓑⓒⓓ 5. ⓐⓑⓒⓓ

Space for Rough Work

6. Figure shows two coherent sources S_1 and S_2 vibrating in same phase. AB is an irregular wire lying at a far distance from the sources S_1 and S_2. Let $\frac{\lambda}{d} = 10^{-3}$ and $\angle BOA = 0.12°$. How many bright spots will be seen on the wire, including points A and B?
(a) 5
(b) 4
(c) 2
(d) 7

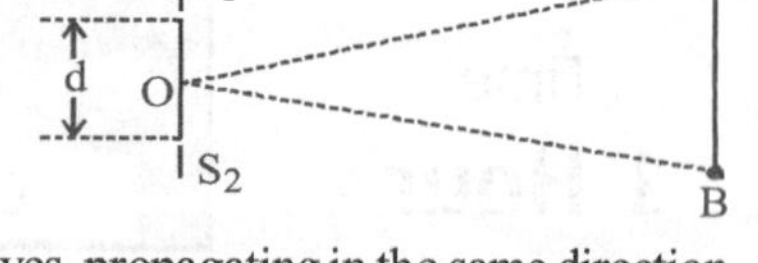

7. Two identical light waves, propagating in the same direction, have a phase difference δ. After they superpose, the intensity of the resulting wave will be proportional to
(a) $\cos \delta$ (b) $\cos (\delta/2)$
(c) $\cos^2 (\delta/2)$ (d) $\cos^2 \delta$

8. In YSDE, both slits are covered by transparent slab. Upper slit is covered by slab of R.I. 1.5 and thickness t and lower is covered by R.I. $\frac{4}{3}$ and thickness 2t, then central maxima
(a) shifts in +ve y-axis direction
(b) shifts in –ve y-axis direction
(c) remains at same position
(d) may shift in upward or downward depending upon wavelength of light

9. A beam of light of λ = 600 nm from a distant source falls on a single slit 1 mm wide and the resulting diffraction pattern is observed on a screen 2 m away. The distance between first dark fringes on either side of the central bright fringe is
(a) 1.2 cm (b) 1.2 mm
(c) 2.4 cm (d) 2.4 mm

10. A parallel beam of light of wavelength λ is incident normally on a narrow slit. A diffraction pattern is formed on a screen placed perpendicular to the direction of the incident beam. At the second minimum of the diffraction pattern, the phase difference between the rays coming from the two edges of slit is
(a) $\pi\lambda$ (b) 2π
(c) 3π (d) 4π

11. The diffraction effects in a microscopic specimen become important when the separation between two points is
(a) much greater than the wavelength of light used.
(b) much less than the wavelength of light used.
(c) comparable to the wavelength of light used.
(d) independent of the wavelength of light used.

12. On a rainy day, if there is an oil drop on tar road coloured rings are seen around this drop. This is due to
(a) total internal reflection of light
(b) polarisation
(c) diffraction pattern
(d) interference pattern produced due to oil film

13. In a Young's double slit experiment, the intensity at a point where the path difference $\frac{\lambda}{6}$ (λ – is wavelength of the light) is I. If I_0 denotes the maximum intensity, then $\frac{I}{I_0}$ is equal to
(a) $\frac{1}{2}$ (b) $\frac{\sqrt{3}}{2}$ (c) $\frac{1}{\sqrt{2}}$ (d) $\frac{3}{4}$

14. According to Huygens, medium through which light waves travel is
(a) vacuum only (b) luminiferous ether
(c) liquid only (d) solid only

15. If we observe the single slit Fraunhofer diffraction with wavelength λ and slit width b, the width of the central maxima is 2θ. On decreasing the slit width for the same λ
(a) θ increases
(b) θ remains unchanged
(c) θ decreases
(d) θ increases or decreases depending on the intensity of light

16. Aperture of the human eye is 2 mm. Assuming the mean wavelength of light to be 5000 Å, the angular resolution limit of the eye is nearly
(a) 2 minute (b) 1 minute
(c) 0.5 minute (d) 1.5 minute

17. Unpolarised light is incident on a dielectric of refractive index $\sqrt{3}$. What is the angle of incidence if the reflected beam is completely polarised?
(a) 30° (b) 45°
(c) 60° (d) 75°

18. The figure shows the interference pattern obtained in a double-slit experiment using light of wavelength 600nm. 1, 2, 3, 4 and 5 are marked on five fringes.

Central bright fringe
1 2 3 4 5

The third order bright fringe is
(a) 2 (b) 3 (c) 4 (d) 5

RESPONSE GRID

6. ⓐⓑⓒⓓ	7. ⓐⓑⓒⓓ	8. ⓐⓑⓒⓓ	9. ⓐⓑⓒⓓ	10. ⓐⓑⓒⓓ
11. ⓐⓑⓒⓓ	12. ⓐⓑⓒⓓ	13. ⓐⓑⓒⓓ	14. ⓐⓑⓒⓓ	15. ⓐⓑⓒⓓ
16. ⓐⓑⓒⓓ	17. ⓐⓑⓒⓓ	18. ⓐⓑⓒⓓ		

Space for Rough Work

19. Which of the following diagrams represent the variation of electric field vector with time for a circularly polarised light ?

(a) (b) (c) (d)

20. With a monochromatic light, the fringe-width obtained in a Young's double slit experiment is 0.133 cm. The whole set-up is immersed in water of refractive index 1.33, then the new fringe-width is

(a) 0.133 cm (b) 0.1 cm
(c) 1.33 cm (d) 0.2 cm

21. The condition for obtaining secondary maxima in the diffraction pattern due to single slit is

(a) $a \sin \theta = n\lambda$ (b) $a \sin \theta = (2n-1)\frac{\lambda}{2}$

(c) $a \sin \theta = (2n-1)\lambda$ (d) $a \sin \theta = \frac{n\lambda}{2}$

22. In double slit experiment, the angular width of the fringes is 0.20° for the sodium light ($\lambda = 5890\text{Å}$). In order to increase the angular width of the fringes by 10%, the necessary change in wavelength is

(a) zero (b) increased by 6479 Å
(c) decreased by 589 Å (d) increased by 589 Å

23. In Young's double slit experiment with sodium vapour lamp of wavelength 589 nm and the slits 0.589 mm apart, the half angular width of the central maximum is

(a) $\sin^{-1}(0.01)$ (b) $\sin^{-1}(0.0001)$
(c) $\sin^{-1}(0.001)$ (d) $\sin^{-1}(0.1)$

24. The adjacent figure shows Fraunhoffer's diffraction due to a single slit. If first minimum is obtained in the direction shown, then the path difference between rays 1 and 3 is

(a) 0
(b) $\lambda/4$
(c) $\lambda/2$
(d) λ

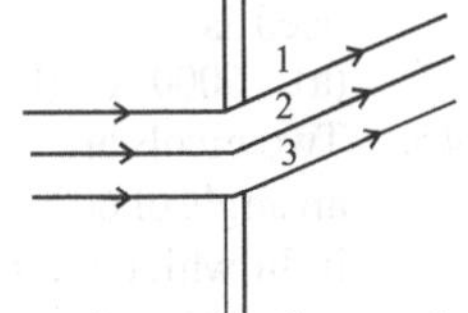

25. A YDSE is conducted in water (μ_1) as shown in figure. A glass plate of thickness t and refractive index μ_2 is placed in the path of S_2. The optical path difference at O is

(a) $(\mu_2 - 1)t$
(b) $(\mu_1 - 1)t$
(c) $\left(\frac{\mu_2}{\mu_1} - 1\right)t$
(d) $(\mu_2 - \mu_1)t$

Screen

26. In a Fresnel biprism experiment, the two positions of lens give separation between the slits as 16 cm and 9 cm respectively. What is the actual distance of separation?

(a) 12.5 cm (b) 12 cm (c) 13 cm (d) 14 cm

27. If two waves represented by $y_1 = 4 \sin \omega t$ and $y_2 = \left(\omega t + \frac{\pi}{3}\right)$ interfere at a point, then the amplitude of the resulting wave will be about

(a) 7 (b) 6 (c) 5 (d) 3.5

28. In Young's double slit experiment, the separation between the slits is halved and the distance between the slits and screen is doubled. The fringe width will

(a) be halved (b) be doubled
(c) be quadrupled (d) remain unchanged

29. At the first minimum adjacent to the central maximum of a single-slit diffraction pattern, the phase difference between the Huygen's wavelet from the edge of the slit and the wavelet from the midpoint of the slit is :

(a) $\frac{\pi}{2}$ radian (b) π radian

(c) $\frac{\pi}{8}$ radian (d) $\frac{\pi}{4}$ radian

30. The central fringe of the interference pattern produced by light of wavelength 6000Å is found to shift to the position of 4th bright fringe after a glass plate of refractive index 1.5 is introduced in front of one of slits in Young's experiment. The thickness of the glass plate will be

(a) 4.8 μm (b) 8.23 μm
(c) 14.98 μm (d) 3.78 μm

31. Sodium light ($\lambda = 6 \times 10^{-7}$ m) is used to produce interference pattern. The observed fringe width is 0.12 mm. The angle between two interfering wave trains, is

(a) 1×10^{-3} rad (b) 1×10^{-2} rad

(c) 5×10^{-3} rad (d) 5×10^{-2} rad

32. The Young's double slit experiment is performed with blue and with green light of wavelengths 4360Å and 5460Å respectively. If x is the distance of 4th maxima from the central one, then

(a) x (blue) = x (green) (b) x (blue) > x (green)

(c) x (blue) < x (green) (d) $\frac{x(\text{blue})}{x(\text{green})} = \frac{5460}{4360}$

33. If yellow light emitted by sodium lamp in Young's double slit experiment is replaced by a monochromatic blue light of the same intensity

(a) fringe width will decrease
(b) finge width will increase
(c) fringe width will remain unchanged
(d) fringes will become less intense

RESPONSE GRID					
	19. ⓐⓑⓒⓓ	20. ⓐⓑⓒⓓ	21. ⓐⓑⓒⓓ	22. ⓐⓑⓒⓓ	23. ⓐⓑⓒⓓ
	24. ⓐⓑⓒⓓ	25. ⓐⓑⓒⓓ	26. ⓐⓑⓒⓓ	27. ⓐⓑⓒⓓ	28. ⓐⓑⓒⓓ
	29. ⓐⓑⓒⓓ	30. ⓐⓑⓒⓓ	31. ⓐⓑⓒⓓ	32. ⓐⓑⓒⓓ	33. ⓐⓑⓒⓓ

Space for Rough Work

34. When unpolarised light is incident on a plane glass plate at Brewster's angle, then which of the following statements is correct?

(a) Reflected and refracted rays are completely polarised with their planes of polarization parallel to each other
(b) Reflected and refracted rays are completely polarised with their planes of polarization perpendicular to each other
(c) Reflected light is plane polarised but transmitted light is partially polarised
(d) Reflected light is partially polarised but refracted light is plane polarised

35. The maximum number of possible interference maxima for slit- separation equal to twice the wavelength in Young's double-slit experiment is

(a) infinite (b) five (c) three (d) zero

36. In the figure shown if a parallel beam of white light is incident on the plane of the slits then the distance of the nearest white spot on the screen from O is d/A. Find the value of A. (assume d << D, λ << d]

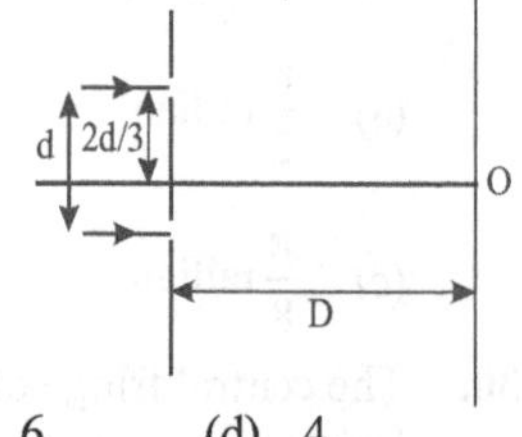

(a) 3 (b) 5 (c) 6 (d) 4

37. Two light waves superimposing at the mid-point of the screen are coming from coherent sources of light with phase difference 3π rad. Their amplitudes are 1 cm each. The resultant amplitude at the given point will be.

(a) 5 cm (b) 3 cm (c) 2 cm (d) zero

38. Spherical wavefronts, emanating from a point source, strike a plane reflecting surface. What will happen to these wave fronts, immediately after reflection?

(a) They will remain spherical with the same curvature, both in magnitude and sign.
(b) They will become plane wave fronts.
(c) They will remain spherical, with the same curvature, but sign of curvature reversed.
(d) They will remain spherical, but with different curvature, both in magnitude and sign.

39. Two coherent point sources S_1 and S_2 are separated by a small distance d as shown. The fringes obtained on the vertical screen will be :

(a) points
(b) straight bands
(c) concentric circles
(d) semicircles

d S_1 S_2 screen D

40. In the phenomena of diffraction of light, when blue light is used in the experiment in spite of red light, then

(a) fringes will become narrower
(b) fringes will become broader
(c) no change in fringe width
(d) None of these

41. On a hot summer night, the refractive index of air is smallest near the ground and increases with height from the ground. When a light beam is directed horizontally, the Huygens' principle leads us to conclude that as it travels, the light beam :

(a) bends downwards
(b) bends upwards
(c) becomes narrower
(d) goes horizontally without any deflection

42. If I_0 is the intensity of the principal maximum in the single slit diffraction pattern, then what will be its intensity when the slit width is doubled?

(a) $4I_0$ (b) $2I_0$ (c) $\frac{I_0}{2}$ (d) I_0

43. Conditions of diffraction is

(a) $\frac{a}{\lambda}=1$ (b) $\frac{a}{\lambda}>>1$ (c) $\frac{a}{\lambda}<<1$
(d) None of these

44. In Fresnel's biprism expt., a mica sheet of refractive index 1.5 and thickness 6×10^{-6} m is placed in the path of one of interfering beams as a result of which the central fringe gets shifted through 5 fringe widths. The wavelength of light used is

(a) 6000 Å (b) 8000 Å (c) 4000 Å (d) 2000 Å

45. Two nicols are oriented with their principal planes making an angle of 60°. Then the percentage of incident unpolarised light which passes through the system is

(a) 100 (b) 50 (c) 12.5 (d) 37.5

RESPONSE GRID					
	34. ⓐⓑⓒⓓ	35. ⓐⓑⓒⓓ	36. ⓐⓑⓒⓓ	37. ⓐⓑⓒⓓ	38. ⓐⓑⓒⓓ
	39. ⓐⓑⓒⓓ	40. ⓐⓑⓒⓓ	41. ⓐⓑⓒⓓ	42. ⓐⓑⓒⓓ	43. ⓐⓑⓒⓓ
	44. ⓐⓑⓒⓓ	45. ⓐⓑⓒⓓ			

PHYSICS CHAPTERWISE SPEED TEST-24			
Total Questions	45	Total Marks	180
Attempted		Correct	
Incorrect		Net Score	
Cut-off Score	45	Qualifying Score	60
Success Gap = Net Score – Qualifying Score			
Net Score = (Correct × 4) – (Incorrect × 1)			

Space for Rough Work

PHYSICS

Dual Nature of Radiation and Matter

Speed TEST 25

Chapter-wise

No. of Questions	Maximum Marks	Time
45	180	1 Hour

GENERAL INSTRUCTIONS

- This test contains 45 MCQ's. For each question only one option is correct. Darken the correct circle/ bubble in the Response Grid provided on each page.
- You have to evaluate your Response Grids yourself with the help of solutions provided at the end of this book.
- Each correct answer will get you 4 marks and 1 mark shall be deduced for each incorrect answer. No mark will be given/ deducted if no bubble is filled. Keep a timer in front of you and stop immediately at the end of 60 min.
- The sheet follows a particular syllabus. Do not attempt the sheet before you have completed your preparation for that syllabus.
- After completing the sheet check your answers with the solution booklet and complete the Result Grid. Finally spend time to analyse your performance and revise the areas which emerge out as weak in your evaluation.

1. A particle of mass 1 mg has the same wavelength as an electron moving with a velocity of $3\times10^6\ ms^{-1}$. The velocity of the particle is:

   (a) $2.7\times 10^{-18} ms^{-1}$ (b) $9\times 10^{-2} ms^{-1}$
   (c) $3\times 10^{-31} ms^{-1}$ (d) $2.7\times10^{-21} ms^{-1}$

2. An electron of mass m and a photon have same energy E. The ratio of de-Broglie wavelengths associated with them is :

   (a) $\frac{1}{c}\left(\frac{E}{2m}\right)^{\frac{1}{2}}$ (b) $\left(\frac{E}{2m}\right)^{\frac{1}{2}}$
   (c) $c(2mE)^{\frac{1}{2}}$ (d) $\frac{1}{c}\left(\frac{2m}{E}\right)^{\frac{1}{2}}$

3. All electrons ejected from a surface by incident light of wavelength 200nm can be stopped before travelling 1m in the direction of uniform electric field of 4N/C. The work function of the surface is

   (a) 4 eV (b) 6.2 eV (c) 2 eV (d) 2.2 eV

4. The maximum kinetic energy of the electrons hitting a target so as to produce X-ray of wavelength 1 Å is

   (a) 1.24 keV (b) 12.4 keV
   (c) 124 keV (d) None of these

5. An X-ray tube is operated at 15 kV. Calculate the upper limit of the speed of the electrons striking the target.

   (a) 7.26×10^7 m/s (b) 7.62×10^9 m/s
   (c) 7.62×10^7 cm/s (d) 7.26×10^9 m/s

6. A and B are two metals with threshold frequencies 1.8×10^{14} Hz and 2.2×10^{14} Hz. Two identical photons of energy 0.825 eV each are incident on them. Then photoelectrons are emitted in (Take $h = 6.6\times 10^{-34}$ Js)

   (a) B alone (b) A alone
   (c) neither A nor B (d) both A and B.

7. If E_1, E_2, E_3 are the respective kinetic energies of an electron, an alpha-particle and a proton, each having the same de-Broglie wavelength, then

   (a) $E_1 > E_3 > E_2$ (b) $E_2 > E_3 > E_1$
   (c) $E_1 > E_2 > E_3$ (d) $E_1 = E_2 = E_3$

RESPONSE GRID	1. ⓐⓑⓒⓓ	2. ⓐⓑⓒⓓ	3. ⓐⓑⓒⓓ	4. ⓐⓑⓒⓓ	5. ⓐⓑⓒⓓ
	6. ⓐⓑⓒⓓ	7. ⓐⓑⓒⓓ			

Space for Rough Work

8. Which of the following when falls on a metal will emit photoelectrons ?

(a) UV radiations (b) Infrared radiation
(c) Radio waves (d) Microwaves

9. The stopping potential (V_0) versus frequency (ν) plot of a substance is shown in figure, the threshold wavelength is

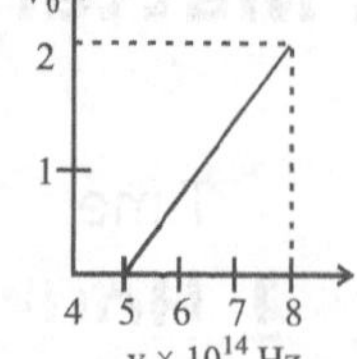

(a) 5×10^{14}m
(b) 6000 Å
(c) 5000 Å
(d) Cannot be estimated from given data

10. A material particle with a rest mass m_0 is moving with speed of light c. The de-Broglie wavelength associated is given by

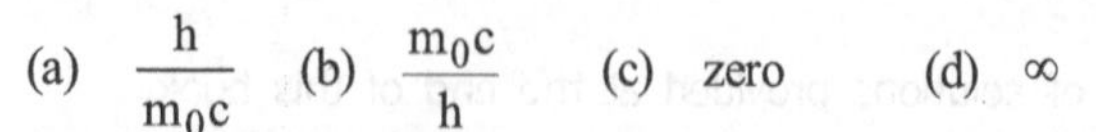

(a) $\frac{h}{m_0 c}$ (b) $\frac{m_0 c}{h}$ (c) zero (d) ∞

11. A 200 W sodium street lamp emits yellow light of wavelength 0.6 μm. Assuming it to be 25% efficient in converting electrical energy to light, the number of photons of yellow light it emits per second is

(a) 1.5×10^{20} (b) 6×10^{18}
(c) 62×10^{20} (d) 3×10^{19}

12. A proton has kinetic energy E = 100 keV which is equal to that of a photon. The wavelength of photon is λ_2 and that of proton is λ_1. The ratio of λ_2/λ_1 is proportional to

(a) E^2 (b) $E^{1/2}$ (c) E^{-1} (d) $E^{-1/2}$

13. In photoelectric effect the work function of a metal is 3.5 eV. The emitted electrons can be stopped by applying a potential of –1.2 V. Then

(a) the energy of the incident photon is 4.7 eV
(b) the energy of the incident photon is 2.3 eV
(c) if higher frequency photon be used, the photoelectric current will rise
(d) when the energy of photon is 3.5 eV, the photoelectric current will be maximum

14. The threshold frequency for a metallic surface corresponds to an energy of 6.2 eV and the stopping potential for a radiation incident on this surface is 5 V. The incident radiation lies in

(a) ultra-violet region (b) infra-red region
(c) visible region (d) X-ray region

15. When photons of energy $h\nu$ fall on an aluminium plate (of work function E_0), photoelectrons of maximum kinetic energy K are ejected. If the frequency of the radiation is doubled, the maximum kinetic energy of the ejected photoelectrons will be

(a) 2K (b) K (c) $K + h\nu$ (d) $K + E_0$

16. Which metal will be suitable for a photoelectric cell using light of wavelength 4000Å. The work functions of sodium and copper are respectively 2.0 eV and 4.0 eV.

(a) Sodium (b) Copper
(c) Both (d) None of these

17. The maximum velocity of an electron emitted by light of wavelength λ incident on the surface of a metal of work-function ϕ is

(a) $\sqrt{\frac{2(hc + \lambda\phi)}{m\lambda}}$ (b) $\frac{2(hc + \lambda\phi)}{m\lambda}$

(c) $\sqrt{\frac{2(hc - \lambda\phi)}{m\lambda}}$ (d) $\sqrt{\frac{2(h\lambda - \phi)}{m}}$

18. If the kinetic energy of a free electron doubles, it's deBroglie wavelength changes by the factor

(a) 2 (b) $\frac{1}{2}$ (c) $\sqrt{2}$ (d) $\frac{1}{\sqrt{2}}$

19. Radiations of two photon's energy, twice and ten times the work function of metal are incident on the metal surface successsively. The ratio of maximum velocities of photoelectrons emitted in two cases is

(a) 1 : 2 (b) 1 : 3 (c) 1 : 4 (d) 1 : 1

20. The cathode of a photoelectric cell is changed such that the work function changes from W_1 to W_2 ($W_2 > W_1$). If the current before and after changes are I_1 and I_2, all other conditions remaining unchanged, then (assuming $h\nu > W_2$)

(a) $I_1 = I_2$ (b) $I_1 < I_2$
(c) $I_1 > I_2$ (d) $I_1 < I_2 < 2I_1$

21. Monochromatic radiation emitted when electron on hydrogen atom jumps from first excited to the ground state irradiates a photosensitive material. The stopping potential is measured to be 3.57 V. The threshold frequency of the materials is :

(a) 4×10^{15} Hz (b) 5×10^{15} Hz
(c) 1.6×10^{15} Hz (d) 2.5×10^{15} Hz

22. Photoelectric work function of a metal is 1eV. Light of wavelength $\lambda = 3000$ Å falls on it. The photo electrons come out with velocity

(a) 10 metres/sec (b) 10^2 metres/sec
(c) 10^4 metres/sec (d) 10^6 metres/sec

23. When the energy of the incident radiation is incredased by 20%, the kinetic energy of the photoelectrons emitted from a metal surface increased from 0.5 eV to 0.8 eV. The work function of the metal is :

(a) 0.65 eV (b) 1.0 eV (c) 1.3 eV (d) 1.5 eV

24. The maximum distance between interatomic lattice planes is 15 Å. The maximum wavelength of X-rays which are diffracted by this crystal will be

(a) 15 Å (b) 20 Å (c) 30 Å (d) 45 Å

RESPONSE GRID					
	8. ⓐⓑⓒⓓ	9. ⓐⓑⓒⓓ	10. ⓐⓑⓒⓓ	11. ⓐⓑⓒⓓ	12. ⓐⓑⓒⓓ
	13. ⓐⓑⓒⓓ	14. ⓐⓑⓒⓓ	15. ⓐⓑⓒⓓ	16. ⓐⓑⓒⓓ	17. ⓐⓑⓒⓓ
	18. ⓐⓑⓒⓓ	19. ⓐⓑⓒⓓ	20. ⓐⓑⓒⓓ	21. ⓐⓑⓒⓓ	22. ⓐⓑⓒⓓ
	23. ⓐⓑⓒⓓ	24. ⓐⓑⓒⓓ			

Space for Rough Work

25. In photoelectric effect, stopping potential for a light of frequency n_1 is V_1. If light is replaced by another having a frequency n_2 then its stopping potential will be

(a) $V_1 - \frac{h}{e}(n_2 - n_1)$ (b) $V_1 + \frac{h}{e}(n_2 + n_1)$

(c) $V_1 + \frac{h}{e}(n_2 - 2n_1)$ (d) $V_1 + \frac{h}{e}(n_2 - n_1)$

26. The maximum kinetic energy of the photoelectrons ejected from a photocathode when it is irradiated with light of wavelength 440nm is 1eV. If the threshold energy of the surface is 1.9eV, then which of the following statement is/are incorrect?
(a) The threshold frequency for photo sensitive metal is 4.6×10^{14}Hz
(b) The minimum wavelength of incident light required for photoemission is 6513 Å.
(c) The maximum wavelength of incident light required for photoemission is 6513 Å.
(d) The energy of incident photon is 2.9 eV.

27. The work functions of metals A and B are in the raio 1 : 2. If light of frequencies f and 2f are incident on the surfaces of A and B respectively, the ratio of the maximum kinetic energies of photoelectrons emitted is (f is greater than threshold frequency of A, 2f is greater than threshold frequency of B)
(a) 1 : 1 (b) 1 : 2 (c) 1 : 3 (d) 1 : 4

28. Which one of the following graphs represents the variation of maximum kinetic energy (E_K) of the emitted electrons with frequency υ in photoelectric effect correctly ?

(a)
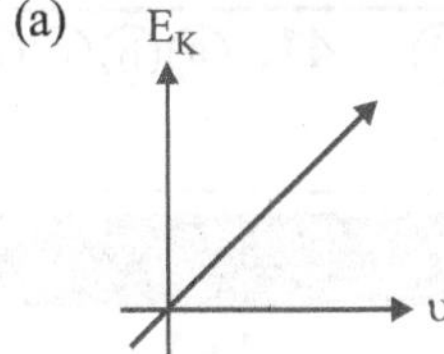

(b) E_K, υ

(c)
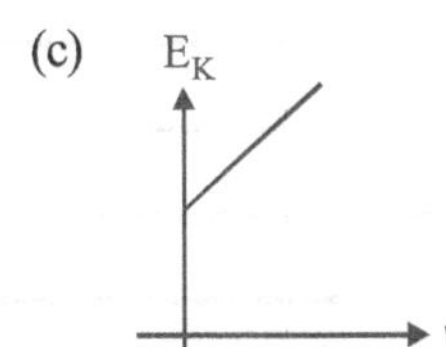

(d) E_K, $υ_0$, υ

29. The potential difference that must be applied to stop the fastest photoelectrons emitted by a nickel surface, having work function 5.01 eV, when ultraviolet light of 200 nm falls on it, must be:
(a) 2.4V (b) –1.2 V (c) –2.4 V (d) 1.2V

30. X-rays are produced in X-ray tube operating at a given accelerating voltage. The wavelength of the continuous X-rays has values from
(a) 0 to ∞
(b) λ_{min} to ∞, where $\lambda_{min} > 0$
(c) 0 to λ_{max}, where $\lambda_{max} < \infty$
(d) λ_{min} to λ_{max}, where $0 < \lambda_{min} < \lambda_{max} < \infty$

31. Electrons used in an electron microscope are accelerated by a voltage of 25 kV. If the voltage is increased to 100kV then the de–Broglie wavelength associated with the electrons would
(a) increase by 2 times (b) decrease by 2 times
(c) decrease by 4 times (d) increase by 4 times

32. In the Davisson and Germer experiment, the velocity of electrons emitted from the electron gun can be increased by
(a) increasing the potential difference between the anode and filament
(b) increasing the filament current
(c) decreasing the filament current
(d) decreasing the potential difference between the anode and filament

33. Two radiations of photons energies 1 eV and 2.5 eV, successively illuminate a photosensitive metallic surface of work function 0.5 eV. The ratio of the maximum speeds of the emitted electrons is :
(a) 1 : 4 (b) 1 : 2 (c) 1 : 1 (d) 1 : 5

34. Photoelectric emission is observed from a metallic surface for frequencies v_1 and v_2 of the incident light rays ($v_1 > v_2$). If the maximum values of kinetic energy of the photoelectrons emitted in the two cases are in the ratio of 1 : k, then the threshold frequency of the metallic surface is

(a) $\frac{v_1 - v_2}{k-1}$ (b) $\frac{kv_1 - v_2}{k-1}$

(c) $\frac{kv_2 - v_1}{k-1}$ (d) $\frac{v_2 - v_1}{k}$

35. Which of the following is/are false regarding cathode rays?
(a) They produce heating effect
(b) They don't deflect in electric field
(c) They cast shadow
(d) They produce fluorescence

36. The ratio of the respective de Broglie wavelengths associated with electrons accelerated from rest with the voltages 100 V, 200 V and 300 V is

(a) 1 : 2 : 3 (b) 1 : 4 : 9 (c) $1:\frac{1}{\sqrt{2}}:\frac{1}{\sqrt{3}}$ (d) $1:\frac{1}{2}:\frac{1}{3}$

RESPONSE GRID					
	25. ⓐⓑⓒⓓ	26. ⓐⓑⓒⓓ	27. ⓐⓑⓒⓓ	28. ⓐⓑⓒⓓ	29. ⓐⓑⓒⓓ
	30. ⓐⓑⓒⓓ	31. ⓐⓑⓒⓓ	32. ⓐⓑⓒⓓ	33. ⓐⓑⓒⓓ	34. ⓐⓑⓒⓓ
	35. ⓐⓑⓒⓓ	36. ⓐⓑⓒⓓ			

Space for Rough Work

37. A 5 watt source emits monochromatic light of wavelength 5000 Å. When placed 0.5 m away, it liberates photoelectrons from a photosensitive metallic surface. When the source is moved to a distance of 1.0 m, the number of photoelectrons liberated will be reduced by a factor of

(a) 8 (b) 16 (c) 2 (d) 4

38. In the photoeletric effect, electrons are emitted

(a) at a rate that is proportional to the amplitude of the incident radiation
(b) with a maximum velocity proportional to the frequency of the incident radiation
(c) at a rate that is independent of the emitter
(d) only if the frequency of the incident radiations is above a certain threshold value

39. The threshold frequency for a photosensitive metal is 3.3×10^{14} Hz. If light of frequency 8.2×10^{14} Hz is incident on this metal, the cut-off voltage for the photoelectric emission is nearly

(a) 2V (b) 3V (c) 5V (d) 1V

40. In an experiment on photoelectric effect, a student plots stopping potential V_0 against reciprocal of the wavelength λ of the incident light for two different metals A and B. These are shown in the figure.

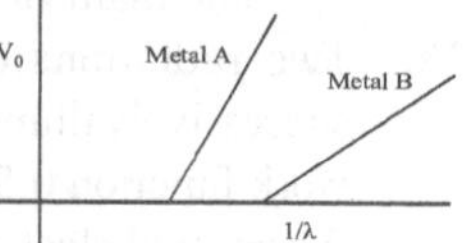

Looking at the graphs, you can most appropriately say that:

(a) Work function of metal B is greater than that of metal A
(b) For light of certain wavelength falling on both metal, maximum kinetic energy of electrons emitted from A will be greater than those emitted from B.
(c) Work function of metal A is greater than that of metal B
(d) Students data is not correct

41. White X-rays are called white due to the fact that

(a) they are electromagnetic radiations having nature same as that of white light.
(b) they are produced most abundantly in X ray tubes.
(c) they have a continuous wavelength range.
(d) they can be converted to visible light using coated screens and photographic plates are affected by them just like light.

42. The wavelength associated with an electron, accelerated through a potential difference of 100 V, is of the order of

(a) 1000 Å (b) 100 Å (c) 10.5 Å (d) 1.2 Å

43. Monochromatic light of frequency 6.0×10^{14} Hz is produced by a laser. The power emitted is 2×10^{-3} w. The number of photons emitted, on the average, by the sources per second is

(a) 5×10^{16} (b) 5×10^{17} (c) 5×10^{14} (d) 5×10^{15}

44. The de-Broglie wavelength of neutron in thermal equilibrium at temperature T is

(a) $\frac{30.8}{\sqrt{T}}$ Å (b) $\frac{3.08}{\sqrt{T}}$ Å (c) $\frac{0.308}{\sqrt{T}}$ Å (d) $\frac{0.0308}{\sqrt{T}}$ Å

45. Which of the following cannot be explained on the basis of photoelectric theory?

(a) Instantaneous emission of photoelectrons
(b) Existence of threshold frequency
(c) Sufficiently intense beam of radiation can emit photoelectrons
(d) Existence of stopping potential

RESPONSE GRID					
	37. ⓐⓑⓒⓓ	38. ⓐⓑⓒⓓ	39. ⓐⓑⓒⓓ	40. ⓐⓑⓒⓓ	41. ⓐⓑⓒⓓ
	42. ⓐⓑⓒⓓ	43. ⓐⓑⓒⓓ	44. ⓐⓑⓒⓓ	45. ⓐⓑⓒⓓ	

PHYSICS CHAPTERWISE SPEED TEST-25			
Total Questions	45	Total Marks	180
Attempted		Correct	
Incorrect		Net Score	
Cut-off Score	45	Qualifying Score	60
Success Gap = Net Score – Qualifying Score			
Net Score = (Correct × 4) – (Incorrect × 1)			

Space for Rough Work

PHYSICS

Atoms

Speed TEST 26

Chapter-wise

No. of Questions	Maximum Marks	Time
45	180	1 Hour

GENERAL INSTRUCTIONS

- This test contains 45 MCQ's. For each question only one option is correct. Darken the correct circle/ bubble in the Response Grid provided on each page.
- You have to evaluate your Response Grids yourself with the help of solutions provided at the end of this book.
- Each correct answer will get you 4 marks and 1 mark shall be deduced for each incorrect answer. No mark will be given/ deducted if no bubble is filled. Keep a timer in front of you and stop immediately at the end of 60 min.
- The sheet follows a particular syllabus. Do not attempt the sheet before you have completed your preparation for that syllabus.
- After completing the sheet check your answers with the solution booklet and complete the Result Grid. Finally spend time to analyse your performance and revise the areas which emerge out as weak in your evaluation.

1. The potential energy associated with an electron in the orbit
   (a) increases with the increases in radii of the orbit
   (b) decreases with the increase in the radii of the orbit
   (c) remains the same with the change in the radii of the orbit
   (d) None of these

2. The diagram shows the energy levels for an electron in a certain atom. Which transition shown represents the emission of a photon with the most energy?

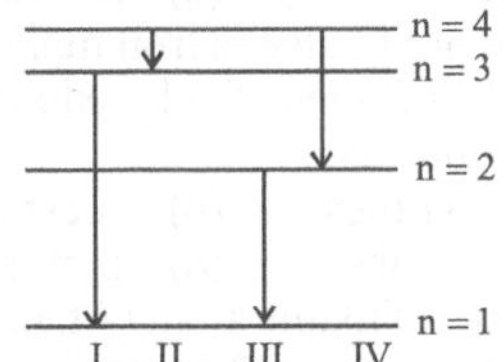

   (a) IV (b) III (c) II (d) I

3. Electrons in a certain energy level $n = n_1$, can emit 3 spectral lines. When they are in another energy level, $n = n_2$. They can emit 6 spectral lines. The orbital speed of the electrons in the two orbits are in the ratio of
   (a) 4 : 3 (b) 3 : 4 (c) 2 : 1 (d) 1 : 2

4. In Rutherford scattering experiment, the number of α-particles scattered at 60° is 5×10^6. The number of α-particles scattered at 120° will be
   (a) 15×10^6 (b) $\frac{3}{5} \times 10^6$
   (c) $\frac{5}{9} \times 10^6$ (d) None of these

5. In the Bohr model an electron moves in a circular orbit around the proton. Considering the orbiting electron to be a circular current loop, the magnetic moment of the hydrogen atom, when the electron is in n^{th} excited state, is :
   (a) $\left(\frac{e}{2m}\frac{n^2h}{2\pi}\right)$ (b) $\left(\frac{e}{m}\right)\frac{nh}{2\pi}$
   (c) $\left(\frac{e}{2m}\right)\frac{nh}{2\pi}$ (d) $\left(\frac{e}{m}\right)\frac{n^2h}{2\pi}$

RESPONSE GRID	1. ⓐⓑⓒⓓ	2. ⓐⓑⓒⓓ	3. ⓐⓑⓒⓓ	4. ⓐⓑⓒⓓ	5. ⓐⓑⓒⓓ

Space for Rough Work

6. A 12.5 eV electron beam is used to bombard gaseous hydrogen at room temperature. It will emit :
(a) 2 lines in the Lyman series and 1 line in the Balmar series
(b) 3 lines in the Lyman series
(c) 1 line in the Lyman series and 2 lines in the Balmar series
(d) 3 lines in the Balmer series

7. A Hydrogen atom and a Li^{++} ion are both in the second excited state. If ℓ_H and ℓ_{Li} are their respective electronic angular momenta, and E_H and E_{Li} their respective energies, then
(a) $\ell_H > \ell_{Li}$ and $|E_H| > |E_{Li}|$ (b) $\ell_H = \ell_{Li}$ and $|E_H| < |E_{Li}|$
(c) $\ell_H = \ell_{Li}$ and $|E_H| > |E_{Li}|$ (d) $\ell_H < \ell_{Li}$ and $|E_H| < |E_{Li}|$

8. The radius of hydrogen atom in its ground state is 5.3×10^{-11} m. After collision with an electron it is found to have a radius of 21.2×10^{-11} m. What is the principal quantum number n of the final state of the atom
(a) $n = 4$ (b) $n = 2$ (c) $n = 16$ (d) $n = 3$

9. When hydrogen atom is in its first excited level, its radius is
(a) four times its ground state radius
(b) twice
(c) same
(d) half

10. Consider 3rd orbit of He^+ (Helium), using non-relativistic approach, the speed of electron in this orbit will be [given K $= 9 \times 10^9$ constant, Z = 2 and h (Plank's Constant) $= 6.6 \times 10^{-34}$ J s]
(a) 1.46×10^6 m/s (b) 0.73×10^6 m/s
(c) 3.0×10^8 m/s (d) 2.92×10^6 m/s

11. An electron in the hydrogen atom jumps from excited state n to the ground state. The wavelength so emitted illuminates a photosensitive material having work function 2.75 eV. If the stopping potential of the photoelectron is 10 V, the value of n is
(a) 3 (b) 4 (c) 5 (d) 2

12. The electron in a hydrogen atom makes a transition from an excited state to the ground state. Which of the following statements is true?
(a) Its kinetic energy increases and its potential energy decreases.
(b) Its kinetic energy decreases, potential energy increases.
(c) Its kinetic and its potential energy increases.
(d) Its kinetic, potential energy decrease.

13. An energy of 24.6 eV is required to remove one of the electrons from a neutral helium atom. The energy in (eV) required to remove both the electrons from a neutral helium atom is
(a) 38.2 (b) 49.2 (c) 51.8 (d) 79.0

14. One of the lines in the emission spectrum of Li^{2+} has the same wavelength as that of the 2nd line of Balmer series in hydrogen spectrum. The electronic transition corresponding to this line is n = 12 → n = x. Find the value of x.
(a) 8 (b) 6 (c) 7 (c) 5

15. If the atom $_{100}Fm^{257}$ follows the Bohr model and the radius of $_{100}Fm^{257}$ is n times the Bohr radius, then find n.
(a) 100 (b) 200 (c) 4 (d) 1/4

16. The energy of He^+ in the ground state is – 54.4 eV, then the energy of Li^{++} in the first excited state will be
(a) –30.6 eV (b) 27.2 eV
(c) –13.6 eV (d) –27.2 eV

17. If the angular momentum of an electron in an orbit is J then the K.E. of the electron in that orbit is
(a) $\frac{J^2}{2mr^2}$ (b) $\frac{Jv}{r}$ (c) $\frac{J^2}{2m}$ (d) $\frac{J^2}{2\pi}$

18. Suppose an electron is attracted towards the origin by a force $\frac{k}{r}$ where 'k' is a constant and 'r' is the distance of the electron from the origin. By applying Bohr model to this system, the radius of the nth orbital of the electron is found to be 'r_n' and the kinetic energy of the electron to be 'T_n'. Then which of the following is true?
(a) $T_n \propto \frac{1}{n^2}, r_n \propto n^2$ (b) T_n independent of n, $r_n \propto n$
(c) $T_n \propto \frac{1}{n}, r_n \propto n$ (d) $T_n \propto \frac{1}{n}, r_n \propto n^2$

19. In Hydrogen spectrum, the wavelength of H_α line is 656 nm, whereas in the spectrum of a distant galaxy, H_α line wavelength is 706 nm. Estimated speed of the galaxy with respect to earth is
(a) 2×10^8 m/s (b) 2×10^7 m/s
(c) 2×10^6 m/s (d) 2×10^5 m/s

20. In the hydrogen atom, an electron makes a transition from n = 2 to n = 1. The magnetic field produced by the circulating electron at the nucleus
(a) decreases 16 times (b) increases 4 times
(c) decreases 4 times (d) increases 32 times

21. What is the radius of iodine atom (At. no. 53, mass no. 126)
(a) 2.5×10^{-11} m (b) 2.5×10^{-9} m
(c) 7×10^{-9} m (d) 7×10^{-6} m

22. When an α-particle of mass 'm' moving with velocity 'v' bombards on a heavy nucleus of charge 'Ze', its distance of closest approach from the nucleus depends on m as :
(a) $\frac{1}{m}$ (b) $\frac{1}{\sqrt{m}}$ (c) $\frac{1}{m^2}$ (d) m

RESPONSE GRID				
6. ⓐⓑⓒⓓ	7. ⓐⓑⓒⓓ	8. ⓐⓑⓒⓓ	9. ⓐⓑⓒⓓ	10. ⓐⓑⓒⓓ
11. ⓐⓑⓒⓓ	12. ⓐⓑⓒⓓ	13. ⓐⓑⓒⓓ	14. ⓐⓑⓒⓓ	15. ⓐⓑⓒⓓ
16. ⓐⓑⓒⓓ	17. ⓐⓑⓒⓓ	18. ⓐⓑⓒⓓ	19. ⓐⓑⓒⓓ	20. ⓐⓑⓒⓓ
21. ⓐⓑⓒⓓ	22. ⓐⓑⓒⓓ			

Space for Rough Work

23. The ionization energy of the electron in the hydrogen atom in its ground state is 13.6 eV. The atoms are excited to higher energy levels to emit radiations of 6 wavelengths. Maximum wavelength of emitted radiation corresponds to the transition between
(a) n = 3 to n = 1 states (b) n = 2 to n = 1 states
(c) n = 4 to n = 3 states (d) n = 3 to n = 2 states

24. The wavelengths involved in the spectrum of deuterium $\left({}_1^2D\right)$ are slightly different from that of hydrogen spectrum, because
(a) the size of the two nuclei are different
(b) the nuclear forces are different in the two cases
(c) the masses of the two nuclei are different
(d) the attraction between the electron and the nucleus is differernt in the two cases

25. An electron in hydrogen atom makes a transition $n_1 \to n_2$ where n_1 and n_2 are principal quantum numbers of the two states. Assuming Bohr's model to be valid the time period of the electron in the initial state is eight times that in the final state. The possible values of n_1 and n_2 are
(a) $n_1 = 4$ and $n_2 = 2$ (b) $n_1 = 6$ and $n_2 = 2$
(c) $n_1 = 8$ and $n_2 = 1$ (d) $n_1 = 8$ and $n_2 = 2$

26. Ina hydrogen like atom electronmake transition from an energy level with quantum number n to another with quantum number (n – 1). If n>>1, the frequency of radiation emitted is proportional to :
(a) $\frac{1}{n}$ (b) $\frac{1}{n^2}$ (c) $\frac{1}{n^{3/2}}$ (d) $\frac{1}{n^3}$

27. The spectrum obtained from a sodium vapour lamp is an example of
(a) band spectrum
(b) continuous spectrum
(c) emission spectrum
(d) absorption spectrum

28. Ionization potential of hydrogen atom is 13.6eV. Hydrogen atoms in the ground state are excited by monochromatic radiation of photon energy 12.1 eV. According to Bohr's theory, the spectral lines emitted by hydrogen will be
(a) three (b) four (c) one (d) two

29. The Bohr model of atoms
(a) predicts the same emission spectra for all types of atoms
(b) assumes that the angular momentum of electrons is quantised
(c) uses Einstein's photoelectric equation
(d) predicts continuous emission spectra for atoms

30. The largest wavelength in the ultraviolet region of the hydrogen spectrum is 122 nm. The smallest wavelength in the infrared region of the hydrogen spectrum (to the nearest integer) is
(a) 802 nm (b) 823 nm (c) 1882 nm (d) 1648 nm

31. A doubly ionised Li atom is excited from its ground state(n = 1) to n = 3 state. The wavelengths of the spectral lines are given by λ_{32}, λ_{31} and λ_{21}. The ratio $\lambda_{32}/\lambda_{31}$ and $\lambda_{21}/\lambda_{31}$ are, respectively
(a) 8.1, 0.67 (b) 8.1, 1.2
(c) 6.4, 1.2 (d) 6.4, 0.67

32. In Rutherford scattering experiment, what will be the correct angle for α-scattering for an impact parameter, $b = 0$?
(a) 90° (b) 270° (c) 0° (d) 180°

33. Consider 3rd orbit of He$^+$ (Helium), using non-relativistic approach, the speed of electron in this orbit will be [given K = 9 × 10^9 constant, Z = 2 and h (Plank's Constant) = 6.6 × 10^{-34} J s]
(a) 1.46×10^6 m/s (b) 0.73×10^6 m/s
(c) 3.0×10^8 m/s (d) 2.92×10^6 m/s

34. The ionization energy of hydrogen atom is 13.6 eV. Following Bohr's theory, the energy corresponding to a transition between 3rd and 4th orbit is
(a) 3.40 eV (b) 1.51 eV (c) 0.85 eV (d) 0.66 eV

35. The transition from the state $n = 3$ to $n = 1$ in a hydrogen like atom results in ultraviolet radiation. Infrared radiation will be obtained in the transition from :
(a) $2 \to 1$ (b) $3 \to 2$ (c) $4 \to 2$ (d) $4 \to 3$

36. Given the value of Rydberg constant is 10^7 m^{-1}, the wave number of the last line of the Balmer series in hydrogen spectrum will be :
(a) 0.025×10^4 m^{-1} (b) 0.5×10^7 m^{-1}
(c) 0.25×10^7 m^{-1} (d) 2.5×10^7 m^{-1}

37. Which of the plots shown in the figure represents speed (v_n) of the electron in a hydrogen atom as a function of the principal quantum number (n)?

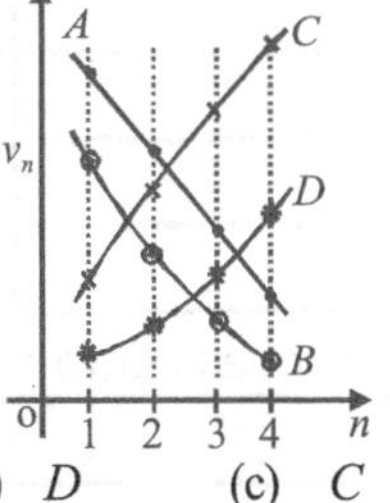

(a) B (b) D (c) C (d) A

RESPONSE GRID					
	23. ⓐⓑⓒⓓ	24. ⓐⓑⓒⓓ	25. ⓐⓑⓒⓓ	26. ⓐⓑⓒⓓ	27. ⓐⓑⓒⓓ
	28. ⓐⓑⓒⓓ	29. ⓐⓑⓒⓓ	30. ⓐⓑⓒⓓ	31. ⓐⓑⓒⓓ	32. ⓐⓑⓒⓓ
	33. ⓐⓑⓒⓓ	34. ⓐⓑⓒⓓ	35. ⓐⓑⓒⓓ	36. ⓐⓑⓒⓓ	37. ⓐⓑⓒⓓ

Space for Rough Work

38. The ionisation potential of H-atom is 13.6 V. When it is excited from ground state by monochromatic radiations of 970.6 Å, the number of emission lines will be (according to Bohr's theory)
(a) 10 (b) 8 (c) 6 (d) 4

39. The energy of hydrogen atom in nth orbit is E_n, then the energy in nth orbit of single ionised helium atom will be
(a) $4E_n$ (b) $E_n/4$ (c) $2E_n$ (d) $E_n/2$

40. In the Rutherford experiment, α-particles are scattered from a nucleus as shown. Out of the four paths, which path is not possible?

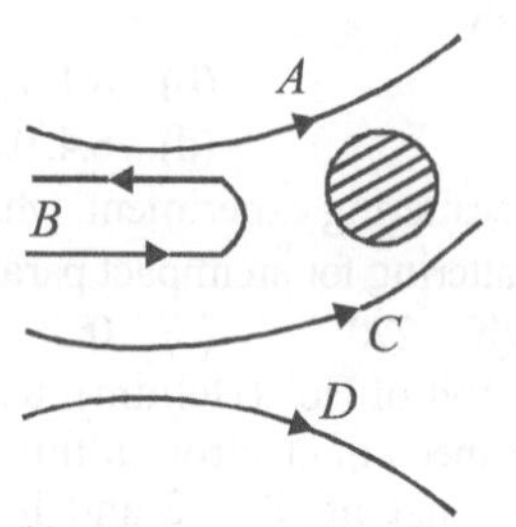

(a) D (b) B (c) C (d) A

41. An electron changes its position from orbit $n = 2$ to the orbit $n = 4$ of an atom. The wavelength of the emitted radiations is (R = Rydberg's constant)
(a) $\frac{16}{R}$ (b) $\frac{16}{3R}$ (c) $\frac{16}{5R}$ (d) $\frac{16}{7R}$

42. In a Rutherford scattering experiment when a projectile of charge Z_1 and mass M_1 approaches a target nucleus of charge Z_2 and mass M_2, the distance of closest approach is r_0. The energy of the projectile is
(a) directly proportional to $Z_1 Z_2$
(b) inversely proportional to Z_1
(c) directly proportional to mass M_1
(d) directly proportional to $M_1 \times M_2$

43. The wavelength of the first spectral line in the Balmer series of hydrogen atom is 6561 A°. The wavelength of the second spectral line in the Balmer series of singly-ionized helium atom is
(a) 1215 Å (b) 1640 Å (c) 2430 Å (d) 4687 Å

44. If υ_1 is the frequency of the series limit of Lyman series, υ_2 is the frequency of the first line of Lyman series and υ_3 is the frequency of the series limit of the Balmer series then
(a) $\upsilon_1 - \upsilon_2 = \upsilon_3$ (b) $\upsilon_1 = \upsilon_2 - \upsilon_3$
(c) $\frac{1}{\upsilon_2} = \frac{1}{\upsilon_1} + \frac{1}{\upsilon_3}$ (d) $\frac{1}{\upsilon_1} = \frac{1}{\upsilon_2} + \frac{1}{\upsilon_3}$

45. In a hypothetical Bohr hydrogen atom, the mass of the electron is doubled. The energy E'_0 and radius r'_0 of the first orbit will be (r_0 is the Bohr radius)
(a) –11.2 eV (b) –6.8 eV (c) –13.6 eV (d) –27.2 eV

RESPONSE GRID	
	38. ⓐⓑⓒⓓ 39. ⓐⓑⓒⓓ 40. ⓐⓑⓒⓓ 41. ⓐⓑⓒⓓ 42. ⓐⓑⓒⓓ
	43. ⓐⓑⓒⓓ 44. ⓐⓑⓒⓓ 45. ⓐⓑⓒⓓ

PHYSICS CHAPTERWISE SPEED TEST-26

Total Questions	45	Total Marks	180
Attempted		Correct	
Incorrect		Net Score	
Cut-off Score	50	Qualifying Score	70

Success Gap = Net Score – Qualifying Score

Net Score = (Correct × 4) – (Incorrect × 1)

Space for Rough Work

PHYSICS

Nuclei

Speed TEST 27

Chapter-wise

No. of Questions	Maximum Marks	Time
45	180	1 Hour

GENERAL INSTRUCTIONS

- This test contains 45 MCQ's. For each question only one option is correct. Darken the correct circle/ bubble in the Response Grid provided on each page.
- You have to evaluate your Response Grids yourself with the help of solutions provided at the end of this book.
- Each correct answer will get you 4 marks and 1 mark shall be deduced for each incorrect answer. No mark will be given/ deducted if no bubble is filled. Keep a timer in front of you and stop immediately at the end of 60 min.
- The sheet follows a particular syllabus. Do not attempt the sheet before you have completed your preparation for that syllabus.
- After completing the sheet check your answers with the solution booklet and complete the Result Grid. Finally spend time to analyse your performance and revise the areas which emerge out as weak in your evaluation.

1. The mass of a ^7_3Li nucleus is 0.042 u less than the sum of the masses of all its nucleons. The binding energy per nucleon of ^7_3Li nucleus is nearly
   (a) 46 MeV (b) 5.6 MeV
   (c) 3.9 MeV (d) 23 MeV
2. In the nuclear decay given below:
   $$^{A}_{Z}X \longrightarrow {}^{A}_{Z+1}Y \longrightarrow {}^{A-4}_{Z-1}B^* \longrightarrow {}^{A-4}_{Z-1}B,$$
   the particles emitted in the sequence are
   (a) γ, β, α (b) β, γ, α
   (c) α, β, γ (d) β, α, γ
3. If the nuclear radius of ^{27}Al is 3.6 Fermi, the approximate nuclear radius of ^{64}Cu in Fermi is :
   (a) 2.4 (b) 1.2 (c) 4.8 (d) 3.6
4. Which of the following statements is true for nuclear forces?
   (a) they obey the inverse square law of distance
   (b) they obey the inverse third power law of distance
   (c) they are short range forces
   (d) they are equal in strength to electromagnetic forces.
5. A radioactive sample at any instant has its disintegration rate 5000 disintegrations per minute. After 5 minutes, the rate is 1250 disintegrations per minute. Then, the decay constant (per minute) is
   (a) 0.4 ln 2 (b) 0.2 ln 2 (c) 0.1 ln 2 (d) 0.8 ln 2
6. The radioactivity of a sample is R_1 at a time T_1 and R_2 at a time T_2. If the half-life of the specimen is T, the number of atoms that have disintegrated in the time $(T_1 - T_2)$ is proportional to
   (a) $(R_1T_1 - R_2T_2)$ (b) $(R_1 - R_2)$
   (c) $(R_1 - R_2)/T$ (d) $(R_1 - R_2)\,T$
7. In the reaction, $^2_1H + {}^3_1H \longrightarrow {}^4_2He + {}^1_0n$, if the binding energies of ^2_1H, ^3_1H and ^4_2He are respectively, a, b and c (in MeV), then the energy (in MeV) released in this reaction is
   (a) $a+b+c$ (b) $a+b-c$
   (c) $c-a-b$ (d) $c+a-b$
8. If M (A; Z), M_p and M_n denote the masses of the nucleus ^A_ZX, proton and neutron respectively in units of u ($1u = 931.5\ MeV/c^2$) and BE represents its bonding energy in MeV, then
   (a) $M(A, Z) = ZM_p + (A-Z)M_n - BE/c^2$
   (b) $M(A, Z) = ZM_p + (A-Z)M_n + BE$
   (c) $M(A, Z) = ZM_p + (A-Z)M_n - BE$
   (d) $M(A, Z) = ZM_p + (A-Z)M_n + BE/c^2$

RESPONSE GRID					
	1. ⓐⓑⓒⓓ	2. ⓐⓑⓒⓓ	3. ⓐⓑⓒⓓ	4. ⓐⓑⓒⓓ	5. ⓐⓑⓒⓓ
	6. ⓐⓑⓒⓓ	7. ⓐⓑⓒⓓ	8. ⓐⓑⓒⓓ		

Space for Rough Work

9. How does the binding energy per nucleon vary with the increase in the number of nucleons?
(a) Increases continuously with mass number
(b) Decreases continuously with mass number
(c) First decreases and then increases with increase in mass number
(d) First increases and then decreases with increase in mass number

10. The energy spectrum of β-particles [Number N(E) as a function of β-energy E] emitted from a radioactive source is

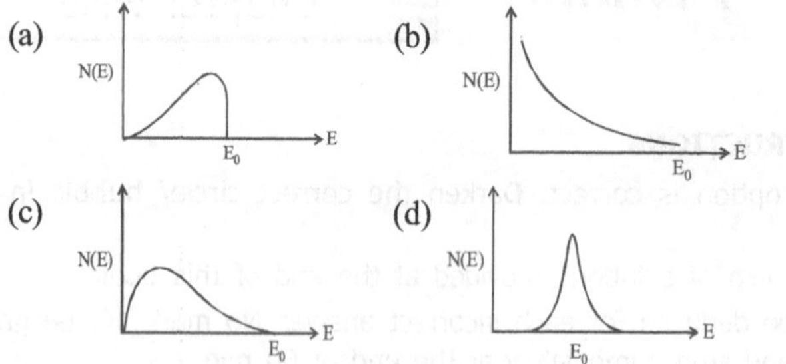

11. A radioactive nucleus undergoes a series of decay according to the scheme

$$A \xrightarrow{\alpha} A_1 \xrightarrow{\beta} A_2 \xrightarrow{\alpha} A_3 \xrightarrow{\gamma} A_4$$

If the mass number and atomic number of 'A' are 180 and 72 respectively, then what are these numbers for A_4
(a) 172 and 69 (b) 174 and 70
(c) 176 and 69 (d) 176 and 70

12. The activity of a radioactive sample is measured as 9750 counts per minute at $t = 0$ and as 975 counts per minute at $t = 5$ minutes. The decay constant is approximately
(a) 0.922 per minute (b) 0.691 per minute
(c) 0.461 per minute (d) 0.230 per minute

13. Actinium 231, $^{231}AC_{89}$, emit in succession two β particles, four α-particles, one β and one α plus several γ rays. What is the resultant isotope?
(a) $^{221}Au_{79}$ (b) $^{211}Au_{79}$
(c) $^{221}Pb_{82}$ (d) $^{211}Pb_{82}$

14. Fusion reactions take place at high temperature because
(a) atoms are ionised at high temperature
(b) molecules break up at high temperature
(c) nuclei break up at high temperature
(d) kinetic energy is high enough to overcome repulsion between nuclei

15. If M_O is the mass of an oxygen isotope $_8O^{17}$, M_P and M_N are the masses of a proton and a neutron respectively, the nuclear binding energy of the isotope is
(a) $(M_O - 17M_N)c^2$ (b) $(M_O - 8M_P)c^2$
(c) $(M_O - 8M_P - 9M_N)c^2$ (d) M_Oc^2

16. Which of the following nuclear reactions is not possible?
(a) $^{12}_{6}C + ^{12}_{6}C \longrightarrow ^{20}_{10}Ne + ^{4}_{2}He$
(b) $^{9}_{4}Be + ^{1}_{1}H \longrightarrow ^{6}_{3}Li + ^{4}_{2}He$
(c) $^{11}_{5}Be + ^{1}_{1}H \longrightarrow ^{9}_{4}Be + ^{4}_{2}He$
(d) $^{7}_{3}Li + ^{4}_{2}He \longrightarrow ^{1}_{1}H + ^{10}_{4}B$

17. The ratio of half-life times of two elements A and B is $\frac{T_A}{T_B}$. The ratio of respective decay constant $\frac{\lambda_A}{\lambda_B}$, is
(a) T_B / T_A (b) T_A / T_B
(c) $\frac{T_A + T_B}{T_A}$ (d) $\frac{T_A - T_B}{T_A}$

18. Two radioactive materials X_1 and X_2 have decay constants 10λ and λ respectively. If initially they have the same number of nuclei, then the ratio of the number of nuclei of X_1 to that of X_2 will be $1/e$ after a time
(a) $1/10\lambda$ (b) $1/11\lambda$
(c) $11/10\lambda$ (d) $1/9\lambda$

19. In a radioactive material the activity at time t_1 is R_1 and at a later time t_2, it is R_2. If the decay constant of the material is λ, then
(a) $R_1 = R_2 e^{\lambda(t_1 - t_2)}$ (b) $R_1 = R_2 e^{(t_2/t_1)}$
(c) $R_1 = R_2$ (d) $R_1 = R_2 e^{-\lambda(t_1 - t_2)}$

20. The correct relation between t_{av} = average life and $t_{1/2}$ = half life for a radioactive nuclei.
(a) $t_{av} = t_{1/2}$ (b) $t_{av} = \frac{1}{2} t_{1/2}$
(c) $0.693\, t_{av} = t_{1/2}$ (d) $t_{av} = 0.693\, t_{1/2}$

21. If the nuclear force between two protons, two neutrons and between proton and neutron is denoted by F_{pp}, F_{nn} and F_{pn} respectively, then
(a) $F_{pp} \approx F_{nn} \approx F_{pn}$ (b) $F_{pp} \neq F_{nn}$ and $F_{pp} = F_{nn}$
(c) $F_{pp} = F_{nn} = F_{pn}$ (d) $F_{pp} \neq F_{nn} \neq F_{pn}$

22. Which one is correct about fission?
(a) Approx. 0.1% mass converts into energy
(b) Most of energy of fission is in the form of heat
(c) In a fission of U^{235} about 200 eV energy is released
(d) On an average, one neutron is released per fission of U^{235}

RESPONSE GRID					
	9. ⓐⓑⓒⓓ	10. ⓐⓑⓒⓓ	11. ⓐⓑⓒⓓ	12. ⓐⓑⓒⓓ	13. ⓐⓑⓒⓓ
	14. ⓐⓑⓒⓓ	15. ⓐⓑⓒⓓ	16. ⓐⓑⓒⓓ	17. ⓐⓑⓒⓓ	18. ⓐⓑⓒⓓ
	19. ⓐⓑⓒⓓ	20. ⓐⓑⓒⓓ	21. ⓐⓑⓒⓓ	22. ⓐⓑⓒⓓ	

Space for Rough Work

23. If 200 MeV energy is released in the fission of a single U^{235} nucleus, the number of fissions required per second to produce 1 kilowatt power shall be (Given $1 eV = 1.6 \times 10^{-19}$ J)
(a) 3.125×10^{13} (b) 3.125×10^{14}
(c) 3.125×10^{15} (d) 3.125×10^{16}

24. In any fission process, the ratio of $\frac{\text{mass of fission products}}{\text{mass of parent nucleus}}$ is
(a) equal to 1
(b) greater than 1
(c) less than 1
(d) depends on the mass of the parent nucleus

25. In an α-decay the kinetic energy of α-particle is 48 MeV and Q-value of the reaction is 50 MeV. The mass number of the mother nucleus is X. Find value of X/25.
(Assume that daughter nucleus is in ground state)
(a) 2 (b) 4 (c) 6 (d) 8

26. A sample of radioactive element has a mass of 10gm at an instant t=0. The approximate mass of this element in the sample after two mean lives is
(a) 6.30 gm (b) 1.35 gm
(c) 2.50 gm (d) 3.70 gm

27. Consider a radioactive material of half-life 1.0 minute. If one of the nuclei decays now, the next one will decay
(a) after 1 minute
(b) after $\frac{1}{\log_e 2}$ minute
(c) after $\frac{1}{N}$ minute, where N is the number of nuclei present at that moment
(d) after any time

28. The mass of α-particle is
(a) less than the sum of masses of two protons and two neutrons
(b) equal to mass of four protons
(c) equal to mass of four neutrons
(d) equal to sum of masses of two protons and two neutron

29. The decay constants of a radioactive substance for α and β emission are λ_α and λ_β respectively. If the substance emits α and β simultaneously, then the average half life of the material will be
(a) $\frac{2T_\alpha T_\beta}{T_\alpha + T_\beta}$ (b) $T_\alpha + T_\beta$
(c) $\frac{T_\alpha T_\beta}{T_\alpha + T_\beta}$ (d) $\frac{1}{2}(T_\alpha + T_\beta)$

30. If the end A of a wire is irradiated with α-rays and the other end B is irradiated with β-rays. Then
(a) a current will flow from A to B
(b) a current will flow from B to A
(c) there will be no current in the wire
(d) a current will flow from each end to the mid-point of the wire

31. A radioactive nucleus of mass M emits a photon of frequency ν and the nucleus recoils. The recoil energy will be
(a) $Mc^2 - h\nu$ (b) $h^2\nu^2 / 2Mc^2$
(c) zero (d) $h\nu$

32. Radioactive element decays to form a stable nuclide. The rate of decay of reactant is correctly depicted by

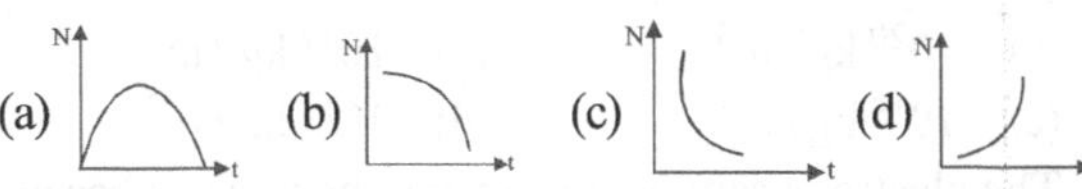

33. A nucleus of mass M + Δm is at rest and decays into two daughter nuclei of equal mass $\frac{M}{2}$ each. Speed of light is c. The speed of daughter nuclei is
(a) $c\frac{\Delta m}{M + \Delta m}$ (b) $c\sqrt{\frac{2\Delta m}{M}}$ (c) $c\sqrt{\frac{\Delta m}{M}}$ (d) $c\sqrt{\frac{\Delta m}{M + \Delta m}}$

34. Atomic weight of Boron is 10.81 and it has two isotopes ${}_5B^{10}$ and ${}_5B^{11}$. Then the ratio ${}_5B^{10} : {}_5B^{11}$ in nature would be
(a) 19 : 81 (b) 10 : 11 (c) 15 : 16 (d) 81 : 19

35. A nucleus ruptures into two nuclear parts, which have their velocity ratio equal to 2:1. What will be the ratio of their nuclear size (nuclear radius)?
(a) $2^{1/3} : 1$ (b) $1 : 2^{1/3}$ (c) $3^{1/2} : 1$ (d) $1 : 3^{1/2}$

36. A nucleus of uranium decays at rest into nuclei of thorium and helium. Then :
(a) the helium nucleus has less momentum than the thorium nucleus.
(b) the helium nucleus has more momentum than the thorium nucleus.
(c) the helium nucleus has less kinetic energy than the thorium nucleus.
(d) the helium nucleus has more kinetic energy than the thorium nucleus.

37. If radius of the ${}^{27}_{12}Al$ nucleus is taken to be R_{Al}, then the radius of ${}^{125}_{53}Te$ nucleus is nearly:
(a) $\frac{5}{3}R_{Al}$ (b) $\frac{3}{5}R_{Al}$ (c) $\left(\frac{13}{53}\right)^{1/3} R_{Al}$ (d) $\left(\frac{53}{13}\right)^{1/3} R_{Al}$

RESPONSE GRID					
	23. ⓐⓑⓒⓓ	24. ⓐⓑⓒⓓ	25. ⓐⓑⓒⓓ	26. ⓐⓑⓒⓓ	27. ⓐⓑⓒⓓ
	28. ⓐⓑⓒⓓ	28. ⓐⓑⓒⓓ	29. ⓐⓑⓒⓓ	30. ⓐⓑⓒⓓ	31. ⓐⓑⓒⓓ
	32. ⓐⓑⓒⓓ	33. ⓐⓑⓒⓓ	34. ⓐⓑⓒⓓ	35. ⓐⓑⓒⓓ	36. ⓐⓑⓒⓓ
	37. ⓐⓑⓒⓓ				

Space for Rough Work

38. M_n and M_p represent mass of neutron and proton respectively. If an element having atomic mass M has N-neutron and Z-proton, then the correct relation will be
(a) $M < [NM_n + ZM_p]$ (b) $M > [NM_n + ZM_p]$
(c) $M = [NM_n + ZM_p]$ (d) $M = N[M_n + M_p]$

39. After 300 days, the activity of a radioactive sample is 5000 dps (disintegrations per sec). The activity becomes 2500 dps after another 150 days. The initial activity of the sample in dps is
(a) 20,000 (b) 10,000
(c) 7,000 (d) 25,000

40. Order of magnitude of density of uranium nucleus is ($m_p = 1.67 \times 10^{-27}$ kg)
(a) $10^{20}\ kg/m^3$ (b) $10^{17}\ kg/m^3$
(c) $10^{14}\ kg/m^3$ (d) $10^{11}\ kg/m^3$

41. The electrons cannot exist inside the nucleus because
(a) de-Broglie wavelength associated with electron in β-decay is much less than the size of nucleus
(b) de-Broglie wavelength associated with electron in β-decay is much greater than the size of nucleus
(c) de-Broglie wavelength associated with electron in β-decay is equal to the size of nucleus
(d) negative charge cannot exist in the nucleus

42. If the total binding energies of ${}_1^2H$, ${}_2^4He$, ${}_{26}^{56}Fe$ & ${}_{92}^{235}U$ nuclei are 2.22, 28.3, 492 and 1786 MeV respectively, identify the most stable nucleus of the following.
(a) ${}_{26}^{56}Fe$ (b) ${}_1^2H$
(c) ${}_{92}^{235}U$ (d) ${}_2^4He$

43. At a specific instant emission of radioactive compound is deflected in a magnetic field. The compound cannot emit
(a) electrons (b) protons
(c) He^{2+} (d) neutrons

44. A nuclear reaction is given by
${}_Z X^A \rightarrow {}_{Z+1}Y^A + {}_{-1}e^0 + \bar{v}$, represents
(a) fission (b) β-decay
(c) ∝-decay (d) fusion

45. Radioactive material 'A' has decay constant '8 λ' and material 'B' has decay constant 'λ'. Initially they have same number of nuclei. After what time, the ratio of number of nuclei of material 'B' to that 'A' will be $\frac{1}{e}$?
(a) $\frac{1}{7\lambda}$ (b) $\frac{1}{8\lambda}$ (c) $\frac{1}{9\lambda}$ (d) $\frac{1}{\lambda}$

RESPONSE GRID					
	38. ⓐⓑⓒⓓ	39. ⓐⓑⓒⓓ	40. ⓐⓑⓒⓓ	41. ⓐⓑⓒⓓ	42. ⓐⓑⓒⓓ
	43. ⓐⓑⓒⓓ	44. ⓐⓑⓒⓓ	45. ⓐⓑⓒⓓ		

PHYSICS CHAPTERWISE SPEED TEST-27

Total Questions	45	Total Marks	180
Attempted		Correct	
Incorrect		Net Score	
Cut-off Score	50	Qualifying Score	70
Success Gap = Net Score – Qualifying Score			
Net Score = (Correct × 4) – (Incorrect × 1)			

Space for Rough Work

PHYSICS

Semiconductor Electronics: Materials, Devices and Simple Circuits

Speed TEST 28 Chapter-wise

No. of Questions	Maximum Marks	Time
45	180	1 Hour

GENERAL INSTRUCTIONS

- This test contains 45 MCQ's. For each question only one option is correct. Darken the correct circle/ bubble in the Response Grid provided on each page.
- You have to evaluate your Response Grids yourself with the help of solutions provided at the end of this book.
- Each correct answer will get you 4 marks and 1 mark shall be deduced for each incorrect answer. No mark will be given/ deducted if no bubble is filled. Keep a timer in front of you and stop immediately at the end of 60 min.
- The sheet follows a particular syllabus. Do not attempt the sheet before you have completed your preparation for that syllabus.
- After completing the sheet check your answers with the solution booklet and complete the Result Grid. Finally spend time to analyse your performance and revise the areas which emerge out as weak in your evaluation.

1. A change of 8.0 mA in the emitter current bring a change of 7.9 mA in the collector current. The values of parameters α and β are respectively
(a) 0.99,90 (b) 0.96,79 (c) 0.97,99 (d) 0.99,79

2. A pure semiconductor has equal electron and hole concentration of 10^{16} m^{-3}. Doping by indium increases number of hole concentration n_h to 5×10^{22} m^{-3}. Then, the value of number of electron concentration n_e in the doped semiconductor is
(a) $10^6/m^3$ (b) $10^{22}/m^3$
(c) $2 \times 10^6/m^3$ (d) $2 \times 10^9/m^3$

3. For LED's to emit light in visible region of electromagnetic light, it should have energy band gap in the range of:
(a) 0.1 eV to 0.4 eV (b) 0.5 eV to 0.8 eV
(c) 0.9 eV to 1.6 eV (d) 1.7 eV to 3.0 eV

4. A common emitter amplifier has a voltage gain of 50, an input impedance of 100Ω and an output impedance of 200Ω. The power gain of the amplifier is
(a) 1000 (b) 1250 (c) 100 (d) 500

5. Which logic gate with inputs A and B performs the same operation as that performed by the following circuit?

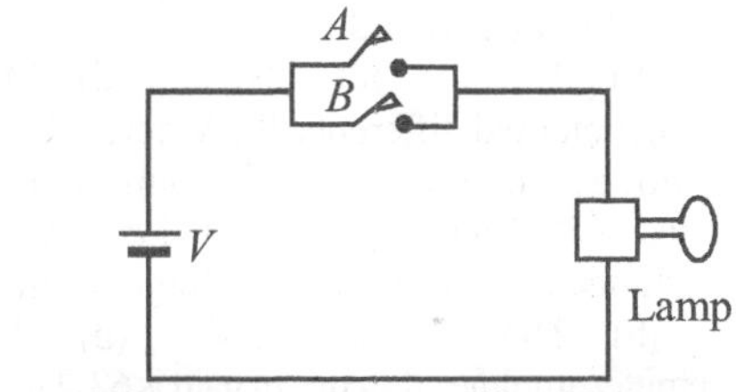

(a) NAND gate (b) OR gate
(c) NOR gate (d) AND gate

6. In an unbiased p-n junction, holes diffuse from the p-region to n-region because of
(a) the potential difference across the p-n junction
(b) the attraction of free electrons of n-region
(c) the higher hole concentration in p-region than that in n-region
(d) the higher concentration of electrons in the n-region than that in the p-region

7. A silicon diode has a threshold voltage of 0.7 V. If an input voltage given by $2 \sin(\pi t)$ is supplied to a half wave rectifier circuit using this diode, the rectified output has a peak value of
(a) 2V (b) 1.4V (c) 1.3V (d) 0.7V

RESPONSE GRID	
	1. ⓐⓑⓒⓓ 2. ⓐⓑⓒⓓ 3. ⓐⓑⓒⓓ 4. ⓐⓑⓒⓓ 5. ⓐⓑⓒⓓ
	6. ⓐⓑⓒⓓ 7. ⓐⓑⓒⓓ

Space for Rough Work

8. The current gain for a transistor working as common-base amplifier is 0.96. If the emitter current is 7.2 mA, then the base current is
(a) 0.29 mA (b) 0.35 mA (c) 0.39 mA (d) 0.43 mA

9. In a npn transistor 10^{10} electrons enter the emitter in 10^{-6} s. 4% of the electrons are lost in the base. The current transfer ratio will be
(a) 0.98 (b) 0.97 (c) 0.96 (d) 0.94

10. Assuming that the silicon diode having resistance of 20 Ω, the current through the diode is (knee voltage 0.7 V)

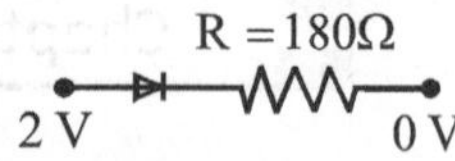

(a) 0 mA (b) 10 mA (c) 6.5 mA (d) 13.5 mA

11. Transfer characteristics [output voltage (V_0) vs input voltage (V_i)] for a base biased transistor in CE configuration is as shown in the figure. For using transistor as a switch, it is used

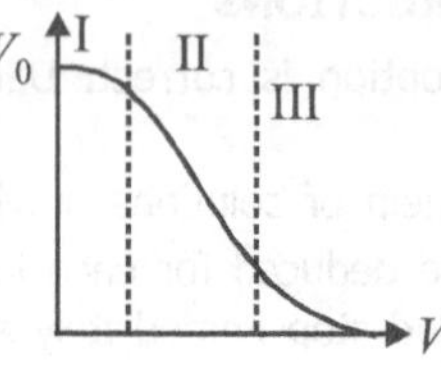

(a) in region III
(b) both in region (I) and (III)
(c) in region II
(d) in region (I)

12. A half-wave rectifier is being used to rectify an alternating voltage of frequency 50 Hz. The number of pulses of rectified current obtained in one second is
(a) 50 (b) 25 (c) 100 (d) 2000

13. A diode having potential difference 0.5 V across its junction which does not depend on current, is connected in series with resistance of 20Ω across source. If 0.1 A current passes through resistance then what is the voltage of the source?
(a) 1.5 V (b) 2.0 V (c) 2.5 V (d) 5 V

14. In common emitter amplifier, the current gain is 62. The collector resistance and input resistance are 5 kΩ an 500Ω respectively. If the input voltage is 0.01 V, the output voltage is
(a) 0.62 V (b) 6.2 V (c) 62 V (d) 620 V

15. On doping germanium with donor atoms of density 10^{17} cm^{-3} its conductivity in mho/cm will be
[Given : $\mu_e = 3800$ cm^2/V–s and $n_i = 2.5 \times 10^{13}$ cm^{-13}]
(a) 30.4 (b) 60.8 (c) 91.2 (d) 121.6

16. The voltage gain of an amplifier with 9% negative feedback is 10. The voltage gain without feedback will be
(a) 90 (b) 10 (c) 1.25 (d) 100

17. A system of four gates is set up as shown. The 'truth table' corresponding to this system is :

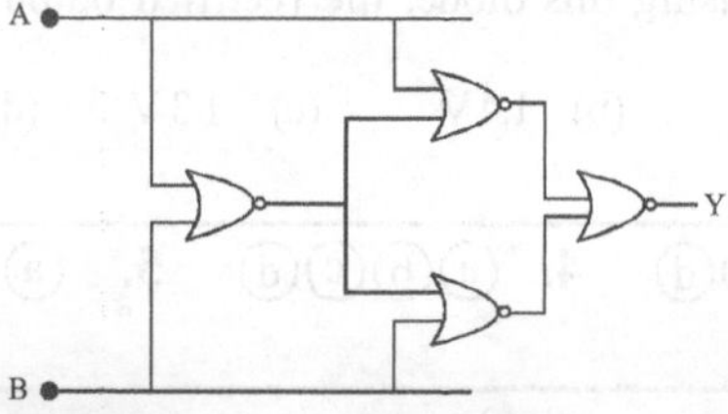

(a)

A	B	Y
0	0	1
0	1	0
1	0	0
1	1	1

(b)

A	B	Y
0	0	0
0	1	0
1	0	1
1	1	0

(c)

A	B	Y
0	0	1
0	1	0
1	0	1
1	1	0

(d)

A	B	Y
0	0	1
0	1	1
1	0	0
1	1	0

18. The intrinsic conductivity of germanium at 27° is 2.13 mho m^{-1} and mobilities of electrons and holes are 0.38 and 0.18 m^{2}V^{-1}s^{-1} respectively. The density of charge carriers is
(a) 2.37×10^{19} m^{-3} (b) 3.28×10^{19} m^{-3}
(c) 7.83×10^{19} m^{-3} (d) 8.47×10^{19} m^{-3}

19. The logic circuit shown below has the input waveforms '*A*' and '*B*' as shown. Pick out the correct output waveform

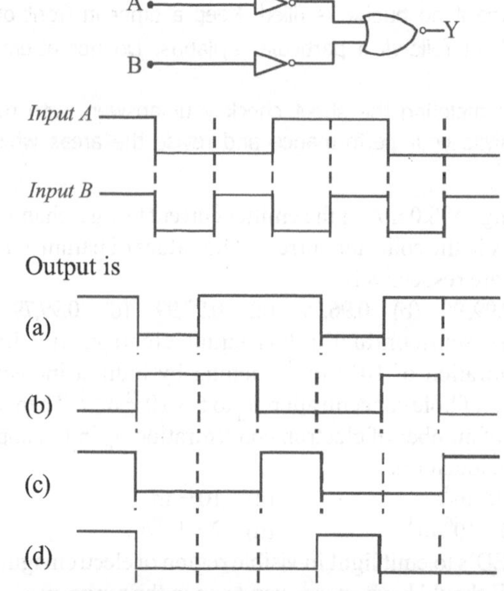

20. Pure Si at 500K has equal number of electron (n_e) and hole (n_h) concentrations of 1.5×10^{16} m^{-3}. Doping by indium increases n_h to 4.5×10^{22} m^{-3}. The doped semiconductor is of
(a) n–type with electron concentration $n_e = 5 \times 10^{22}$ m^{-3}
(b) p–type with electron concentration $n_e = 2.5 \times 10^{10}$ m^{-3}
(c) n–type with electron concentration $n_e = 2.5 \times 10^{23}$ m^{-3}
(d) p–type having electron concentration $n_e = 5 \times 10^{9}$ m^{-3}

21. Which of the following statements is incorrect?
(a) The resistance of intrinsic semiconductors decrease with increase of temperature
(b) Doping pure Si with trivalent impurities give *p*-type semiconductors
(c) The majority carriers in *n*-type semiconductors are holes
(d) A *p-n* junction can act as a semiconductor diode

RESPONSE GRID

8. ⓐⓑⓒⓓ 9. ⓐⓑⓒⓓ 10. ⓐⓑⓒⓓ 11. ⓐⓑⓒⓓ 12. ⓐⓑⓒⓓ
13. ⓐⓑⓒⓓ 14. ⓐⓑⓒⓓ 15. ⓐⓑⓒⓓ 16. ⓐⓑⓒⓓ 17. ⓐⓑⓒⓓ
18. ⓐⓑⓒⓓ 19. ⓐⓑⓒⓓ 20. ⓐⓑⓒⓓ 21. ⓐⓑⓒⓓ

Space for Rough Work

22. The relation between number of free electrons (n) in a semiconductor and temperature (T) is given by
(a) $n \propto T$ (b) $n \propto T^2$ (c) $n \propto \sqrt{T}$ (d) $n \propto T^{3/2}$

23. If a PN junction diode of depletion layer width W and barrier height V_0 is forward biased, then
(a) W increases, V_0 decreases
(b) W decreases, V_0 increases
(c) both W and V_0 increase
(d) both W and V_0 decrease

24. The circuit has two oppositively connected ideal diodes in parallel. The current flowing in the circuit is

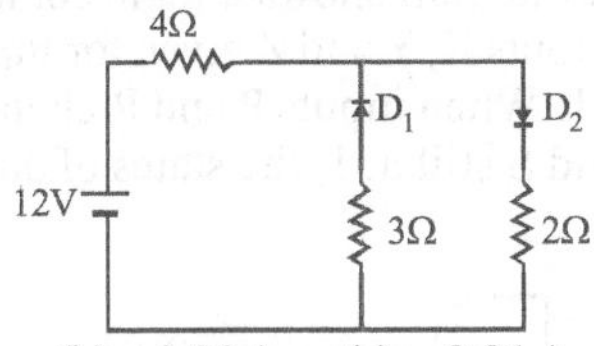

(a) 1.71 A (b) 2.00 A (c) 2.31 A (d) 1.33 A

25. For a transistor amplifier in common emitter configuration for load impedance of 1kΩ ($h_{fe} = 50$ and $h_{0e} = 25$) the current gain is
(a) −24.8 (b) −15.7 (c) −5.2 (d) −48.78

26. A PN-junction has a thickness of the order of
(a) 1 cm (b) 1 mm (c) 10^{-6} m (d) 10^{-12} cm

27. A working transistor with its three legs marked *P*, *Q* and *R* is tested using a multimeter. No conduction is found between *P* and *Q*. By connecting the common (negative) terminal of the multimeter to *R* and the other (positive) terminal to *P* or *Q*, some resistance is seen on the multimeter. Which of the following is true for the transistor?
(a) It is an npn transistor with *R* as base
(b) It is a pnp transistor with *R* as base
(c) It is a pnp transistor with *R* as emitter
(d) It is an npn transistor with *R* as collector

28. If in a p-n junction, a square input signal of 10 V is applied as shown, then the output across R_L will be

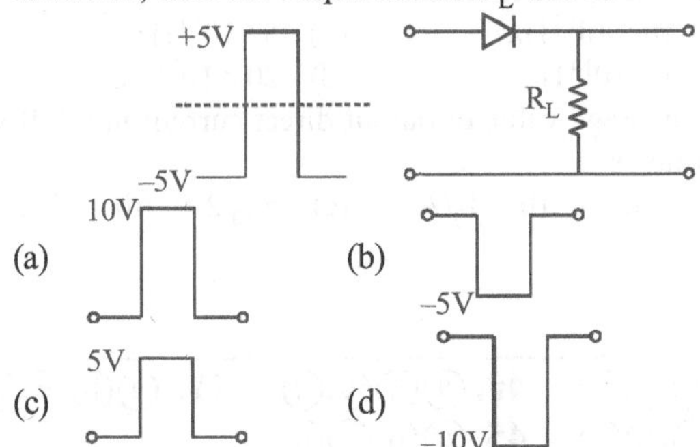

29. When *n*-type semiconductor is heated
(a) number of electrons increases while that of holes decreases
(b) number of holes increases while that of electrons decreases
(c) number of electrons and holes remain same
(d) number of electrons and holes increases equally.

30. The ratio of electron and hole currents in a semiconductor is 7/4 and the ratio of drift velocities of electrons and holes is 5/4, then the ratio of concentrations of electrons and holes will be
(a) 5/7 (b) 7/5 (c) 25/49 (d) 49/25

31. C and Si both have same lattice structure, having 4 bonding electrons in each. However, C is insulator whereas Si is intrinsic semiconductor. This is because :
(a) In case of C the valence band is not completely filled at absolute zero temperature.
(b) In case of C the conduction band is partly filled even at absolute zero temperature.
(c) The four bonding electrons in the case of C lie in the second orbit, whereas in the case of Si they lie in the third.
(d) The four bonding electrons in the case of C lie in the third orbit, whereas for Si they lie in the fourth orbit.

32. Which one of the following represents forward bias diode ?
(a) −4V —▷|— R — −3V
(b) −2V —▷|— R — +2V
(c) 3V —▷|— R — 5V
(d) 0V —▷|— R — −2V

33. An oscillator is nothing but an amplifer with
(a) positive feedback (b) negative feedback
(c) large gain (d) no feedback

34. The current gain in the common emitter mode of a transistor is 10. The input impedance is 20kΩ and load of resistance is 100kΩ. The power gain is
(a) 300 (b) 500 (c) 200 (d) 100

35. The input signal given to a CE amplifier having a voltage gain of 150 is $V_i = 2\cos\left(15t + \frac{\pi}{3}\right)$. The corresponding output signal will be :
(a) $75\cos\left(15t + \frac{2\pi}{3}\right)$ (b) $2\cos\left(15t + \frac{5\pi}{6}\right)$
(c) $300\cos\left(15t + \frac{4\pi}{3}\right)$ (d) $300\cos\left(15t + \frac{\pi}{3}\right)$

36. To use a transistor as an amplifier
(a) the emitter base junction is forward biased and the base collector junction is reverse biased
(b) no bias voltage is required
(c) both junctions are forward biased
(d) both junctions are reverse biased.

RESPONSE GRID					
	22. ⓐⓑⓒⓓ	23. ⓐⓑⓒⓓ	24. ⓐⓑⓒⓓ	25. ⓐⓑⓒⓓ	26. ⓐⓑⓒⓓ
	27. ⓐⓑⓒⓓ	28. ⓐⓑⓒⓓ	29. ⓐⓑⓒⓓ	30. ⓐⓑⓒⓓ	31. ⓐⓑⓒⓓ
	32. ⓐⓑⓒⓓ	33. ⓐⓑⓒⓓ	34. ⓐⓑⓒⓓ	35. ⓐⓑⓒⓓ	36. ⓐⓑⓒⓓ

Space for Rough Work

37. A piece of copper and another of germanium are cooled from room temperature to 77K. The resistance of
(a) copper increases and germanium decreases
(b) each of them decreases
(c) each of them increases
(d) copper decreases and germanium increases

38. A d.c. battery of V volt is connected to a series combination of a resistor R and an ideal diode D as shown in the figure below. The potential difference across R will be

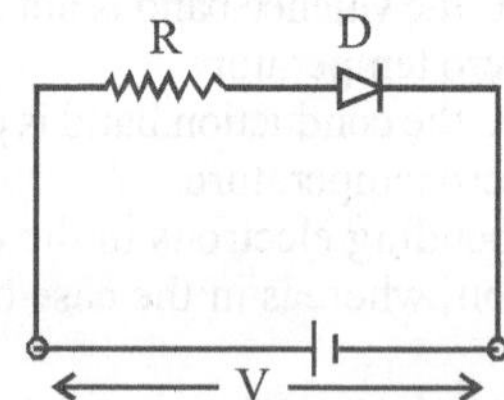

(a) 2V when diode is forward biased
(b) Zero when diode is forward biased
(c) 5V when diode is reverse biased
(d) 6V when diode is forward biased

39. The current gain for a transistor working as common-base amplifier is 0.96. If the emitter current is 7.2 mA, then the base current is
(a) 0.29 mA (b) 0.35 mA (c) 0.39 mA (d) 0.43 mA

40. In the circuit given below, *A* and *B* represent two inputs and *C* represents the output.

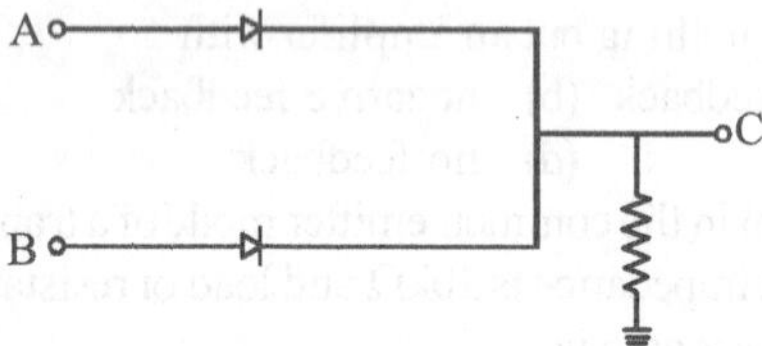

The circuit represents
(a) NOR gate (b) AND gate
(c) NAND gate (d) OR gate

41. The I-V characteristic of a P-N junction diode is shown below. The approximate dynamic resistance of the p-n junction when a forward bias voltage of 2 volt is applied is

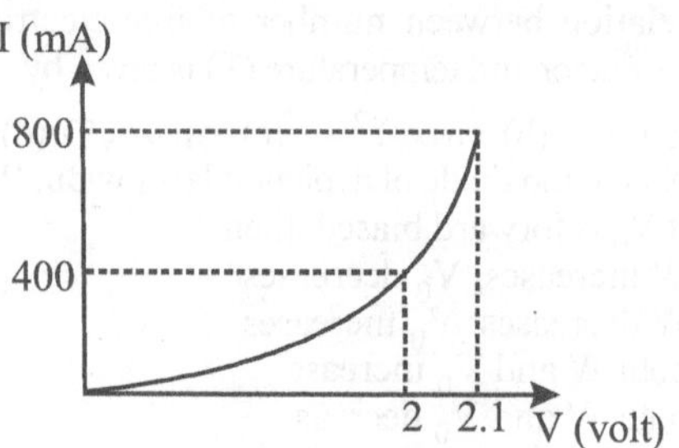

(a) 1 Ω (b) 0.25 Ω (c) 0.5 Ω (d) 5 Ω

42. The circuit diagram shows a logic combination with the states of outputs X, Y and Z given for inputs P, Q, R and S all at state 1. When inputs P and R change to state 0 with inputs Q and S still at 1, the states of outputs X, Y and Z change to

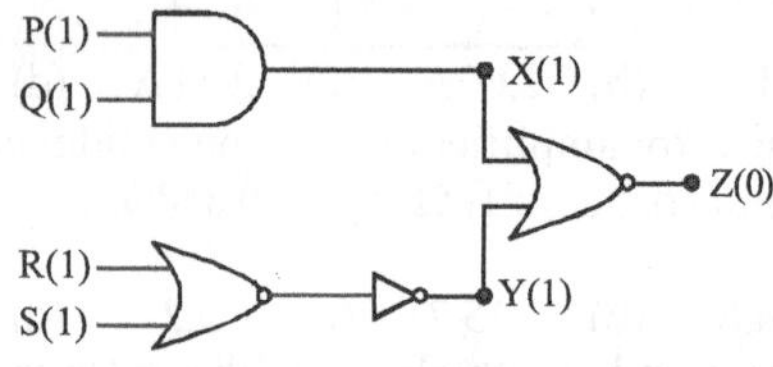

(a) 1, 0, 0 (b) 1, 1, 1 (c) 0, 1, 0 (d) 0, 0, 1

43. The following configuration of gate is equivalent to

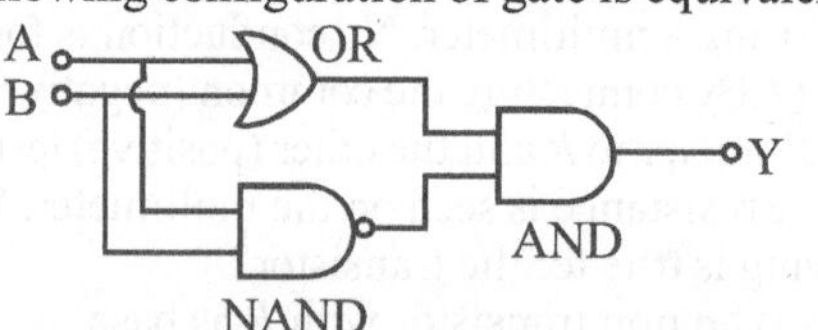

(a) NAND gate (b) XOR gate
(c) OR gate (d) NOR gate

44. A p-n photodiode is made of a material with a band gap of 2.0 eV. The minimum frequency of the radiation that can be absorbed by the material is nearly
(a) 10×10^{14} Hz (b) 5×10^{14} Hz
(c) 1×10^{14} Hz (d) 20×10^{14} Hz

45. The average value of output direct current in a full wave rectifier is
(a) I_0/π (b) $I_0/2$ (c) $\pi I_0/2$ (d) $2 I_0/\pi$

RESPONSE GRID					
	37. ⓐⓑⓒⓓ	38. ⓐⓑⓒⓓ	39. ⓐⓑⓒⓓ	40. ⓐⓑⓒⓓ	41. ⓐⓑⓒⓓ
	42. ⓐⓑⓒⓓ	43. ⓐⓑⓒⓓ	44. ⓐⓑⓒⓓ	45. ⓐⓑⓒⓓ	

PHYSICS CHAPTERWISE SPEED TEST-28			
Total Questions	45	Total Marks	180
Attempted		Correct	
Incorrect		Net Score	
Cut-off Score	50	Qualifying Score	70
Success Gap = Net Score – Qualifying Score			
Net Score = (Correct × 4) – (Incorrect × 1)			

Space for Rough Work

CHEMISTRY

Some Basic Concepts of Chemistry

Speed TEST 29

No. of Questions	Maximum Marks	Time
45	180	1 Hour

Chapter-wise

GENERAL INSTRUCTIONS

- This test contains 45 MCQ's. For each question only one option is correct. Darken the correct circle/ bubble in the Response Grid provided on each page.
- You have to evaluate your Response Grids yourself with the help of solutions provided at the end of this book.
- Each correct answer will get you 4 marks and 1 mark shall be deduced for each incorrect answer. No mark will be given/ deducted if no bubble is filled. Keep a timer in front of you and stop immediately at the end of 60 min.
- The sheet follows a particular syllabus. Do not attempt the sheet before you have completed your preparation for that syllabus.
- After completing the sheet check your answers with the solution booklet and complete the Result Grid. Finally spend time to analyse your performance and revise the areas which emerge out as weak in your evaluation.

1. Given the numbers : 161 cm, 0.161 cm, 0.0161 cm. The number of significant figures for the three numbers are

(a) 3, 4 and 5 respectively (b) 3, 3 and 4 respectively
(c) 3, 3 and 3 respectively (d) 3, 4 and 4 respectively

2. If the true value for an experimental result is 6.23 and the results reported by three students X, Y and Z are :

X: 6.18 and 6.28
Y: 6.20 and 6.023
Z: 6.22 and 6.24

Which of the following option is correct :

(a) X precise, Y accurate, Z precise and accurate.
(b) X precise and accurate, Y not precise, Z precise
(c) Both X & Z precise & accurate, Y not precise.
(d) Both X & Y neither precise nor accurate, Z both precise and accurate.

3. Number of grams of oxygen in 32.2 g $Na_2SO_4.10\,H_2O$ is

(a) 20.8 (b) 2.24
(c) 22.4 (d) 2.08

4. 3 g of an oxide of a metal is converted to chloride completely and it yielded 5 g of chloride. The equivalent weight of the metal is

(a) 3.325 (b) 33.25
(c) 12 (d) 20

5. 1 cc. N_2O at NTP contains :

(a) $\frac{1.8}{224}\times10^{22}$ atoms (b) $\frac{6.02}{22400}\times10^{23}$ molecules
(c) $\frac{1.32}{224}\times10^{23}$ electrons (d) All of the above

RESPONSE GRID	1. ⓐⓑⓒⓓ	2. ⓐⓑⓒⓓ	3. ⓐⓑⓒⓓ	4. ⓐⓑⓒⓓ	5. ⓐⓑⓒⓓ

Space for Rough Work

6. One of the following combination which illustrates the law of reciprocal proportions ?
(a) N_2O_3, N_2O_4, N_2O_5 (b) NaCl, NaBr, NaI
(c) CS_2, CO_2, SO_2 (d) PH_3, P_2O_3, P_2O_5

7. An aqueous solution of oxalic acid dihydrate contains its 6.3g in 250 mL. The volume of 0.1 N NaOH required to completely neutralize 10 mL of this solution
(a) 4 mL (b) 20 mL (c) 2 mL (d) 40 mL

8. The density of 3M solution of sodium chloride is 1.252 g mL^{-1}. The molality of the solution will be : (molar mass, NaCl = 58.5 g mol^{-1})
(a) 260 m (b) 2.18 m (c) 2.79 m (d) 3.00 m

9. The number of atoms in 0.1 mole of a triatomic gas is : ($N_A = 6.02 \times 10^{23}\ mol^{-1}$)
(a) 6.026×10^{22} (b) 1.806×10^{23}
(c) 3.600×10^{23} (d) 1.800×10^{22}

10. Match the columns.

	Column-I		Column-II
A.	88 g of CO_2	I.	0.25 mole
B.	6.022×10^{23} molecules of H_2O	II.	2 mole
C.	5.6 litres of O_2 at STP	III.	1 mole
D.	96 g of O_2	IV.	6.022×10^{23} molecules
E.	1 mol of any gas	V.	3 mole

(a) A – II; B – III; C – I; D – V; E – VI
(b) A – III; B – II; C – I; D – V; E – IV
(c) A – II; B – I; C – III; D – V; E – IV
(d) A – II; B – III; C – I; D – IV; E – V

11. The simplest formula of a compound containing 50% of element X (atomic mass 10) and 50% of element Y (atomic mass 20) is
(a) XY (b) XY_3 (c) X_2Y (d) X_2Y_3

12. Which one of the following is the lightest?
(a) 0.2 mole of hydrogen gas
(b) 6.023×10^{22} molecules of nitrogen
(c) 0.1 g of silver
(d) 0.1 mole of oxygen gas

13. If N_A is Avogadro's number then number of valence electrons in 4.2 g of nitride ions (N^{3-}) is
(a) 4.2 N_A (b) 2.4 N_A
(c) 1.6 N_A (d) 3.2 N_A

14. The set of numerical coefficients that balances the equation

$K_2CrO_4 + HCl \longrightarrow K_2Cr_2O_7 + KCl + H_2O$ is

(a) 2, 2, 1, 2, 1 (b) 2, 2, 1, 1, 1
(c) 2, 1, 1, 2, 1 (d) 1, 1, 2, 2, 1

15. Match the columns

	Column-I (Number)		Column-II (Significant figures)
A.	29900.	I.	2
B.	290	II.	1
C.	1.23 × 1.331	III.	4
D.	20.00	IV.	3
E.	2.783 – 1	V.	5

(a) A – III; B – II; C – V; D – I; E – IV
(b) A – V; B – I; C – IV; D – III; E – II
(c) A – I; B – V; C – IV; D – III; E – II
(d) A – V; B – IV; C – III; D – II; E – I

16. The maximum number of molecules are present in
(a) 15 L of H_2 gas at STP (b) 5 L of N_2 gas at STP
(c) 0.5 g of H_2 gas (d) 10 g of O_2 gas

17. The number of moles of oxygen in one litre of air containing 21% oxygen by volume, under standard conditions are
(a) 0.0093 mole (b) 0.21 mole
(c) 2.10 mole (d) 0.186 mole

18. Assuming fully decomposed, the volume of CO_2 released at STP on heating 9.85 g of $BaCO_3$ (Atomic mass, Ba = 137) will be
(a) 1.12 L (b) 2.24 L
(c) 4.06 L (d) 0.84 L

RESPONSE GRID					
	5. ⓐⓑⓒⓓ	6. ⓐⓑⓒⓓ	7. ⓐⓑⓒⓓ	8. ⓐⓑⓒⓓ	9. ⓐⓑⓒⓓ
	10. ⓐⓑⓒⓓ	11. ⓐⓑⓒⓓ	12. ⓐⓑⓒⓓ	13. ⓐⓑⓒⓓ	14. ⓐⓑⓒⓓ
	15. ⓐⓑⓒⓓ	16. ⓐⓑⓒⓓ	17. ⓐⓑⓒⓓ	18. ⓐⓑⓒⓓ	

Space for Rough Work

19. The ratio of the molar amounts of H_2S needed to precipitate the metal ions from 20 mL each of 1 M $Ca(NO_3)_2$ and 0.5M $CuSO_4$ is
(a) 1 : 1 (b) 2 : 1 (c) 1 : 2 (d) indefinite

20. Consider the following statements.
(i) Atoms of H, O, N and C have identical properties but different mass.
(ii) Matter is divisible into atoms which are further indivisible.
(iii) The ratio of N : H in NH_3 is 1 : 3 and N : O in nitric oxide is 2 : 1.
(iv) Dalton's atomic theory support law of conservation of mass.
Which of the following pairs of statements is true according to Dalton's atomic theory ?
(a) (i) and (ii) (b) (ii) and (iii)
(c) (ii) and (iv) (d) (i) and (iv)

21. How many moles of $Al_2(SO_4)_3$ would be in 50 g of the substance ?
(a) 0.083 mole (b) 0.952 mole
(c) 0.481 mole (d) 0.140 mole

22. Experimentally it was found that a metal oxide has formula $M_{0.98}O$. Metal M, present as M^{2+} and M^{3+} in its oxide. Fraction of the metal which exists as M^{3+} would be :
(a) 7.01% (b) 4.08% (c) 6.05% (d) 5.08%

23. 20.0 g of a magnesium carbonate sample decomposes on heating to give carbon dioxide and 8.0 g magnesium oxide. What will be the percentage purity of magnesium carbonate in the sample ?
(a) 75 (b) 96 (c) 60 (d) 84

24. A sample of AlF_3 contains 3.0×10^{24} F^- ions. The number of formula unit of this sample are
(a) 9×10^{24} (b) 3×10^{24}
(c) 0.75×10^{24} (d) 1.0×10^{24}

25. Read the following and choose the incorrect statements.
(i) Both weight and mass are same quantities used for measurement of amount of matter present in a substance
(ii) Mass and weight of a substance vary from one place to another due to change in gravity.
(iii) SI unit of mass is kilogram and while SI unit of weight is gram.
(a) (i) and (iii) (b) (ii) and (iii)
(c) (i) and (ii) (d) All of these

26. Number of atoms in 558.5 grams of Fe (at. wt. of Fe = 55.85 g mol^{-1}) is
(a) twice that in 60 g carbon
(b) 6.023×10^{22}
(c) half that in 8 g He
(d) $558.5 \times 6.023 \times 10^{23}$

27. What is the mass of precipitate formed when 50 mL of 16.9% solution of $AgNO_3$ is mixed with 50 mL of 5.8% NaCl solution ?
(Ag = 107.8, N = 14, O = 16, Na = 23, Cl = 35.5)
(a) 28 g (b) 3.5 g (c) 7 g (d) 14 g

28. Which of the following option represents correct limiting reagents in reactions (i), (ii) and (iii) respectively.
(i) $\underset{(26g)}{C} + \underset{(20g)}{O_2} \rightarrow CO_2$
(ii) $\underset{(60g)}{N_2} + \underset{(80g)}{3H_2} \rightarrow 2NH_3$
(iii) $\underset{(100g)}{P_4} + \underset{(200g)}{3O_2} \rightarrow P_4O_6$
(a) C, N_2, O_2 (b) C, N_2, P_4
(c) O_2, H_2, P_4 (d) O_2, N_2, P_4

29. A compound made up of two elements A and B is found to contain 25% A (atomic mass = 12.5) and 75% B (atomic mass = 37.5). The simplest formula of the compound is
(a) AB (b) AB_2 (c) AB_3 (d) A_3B

30. On analysis a certain compound was found to contain iodine and oxygen in the ratio of 254 g of iodine (atomic mass 127) and 80 g oxygen (at mass = 16). What is the formula of the compound.
(a) IO (b) I_2O
(c) I_5O_3 (d) I_2O_5

31. The following equation is a completely balanced equation :
$$3Sn + 12HCl + 4HNO_3 \longrightarrow 3SnCl_4 + 4NO + 8H_2O$$
In the above reaction, the number of equivalent per formula weight of HNO_3 is
(a) 3 (b) 4 (c) 1 (d) 2

32. In a compound C, H and N are present in 9 : 1 : 3.5 by weight. If molecular weight of the compound is 108, then the molecular formula of the compound is :
(a) $C_2H_6N_2$ (b) C_3H_4N (c) $C_6H_8N_2$ (d) $C_9H_{12}N_3$

RESPONSE GRID
19. ⓐⓑⓒⓓ 20. ⓐⓑⓒⓓ 21. ⓐⓑⓒⓓ 22. ⓐⓑⓒⓓ 23. ⓐⓑⓒⓓ
24. ⓐⓑⓒⓓ 25. ⓐⓑⓒⓓ 26. ⓐⓑⓒⓓ 27. ⓐⓑⓒⓓ 28. ⓐⓑⓒⓓ
29. ⓐⓑⓒⓓ 30. ⓐⓑⓒⓓ 31. ⓐⓑⓒⓓ 32. ⓐⓑⓒⓓ

Space for Rough Work

33. Arrange the numbers in increasing no. of significant figures. 0.002600, 2.6000, 2.6, 0.260
(a) 2.6 < 0.260 < 0.002600 < 2.6000
(b) 2.6000 < 2.6 < 0.002600 < 0.260
(c) 0.260 < 2.6 < 0.002600 < 2.6000
(d) 0.002600 < 0.260 < 2.6 < 2.6000

34. How many moles of lead (II) chloride will be formed from a reaction between 6.5 g of PbO and 3.2 g of HCl ?
(a) 0.044 (b) 0.333
(c) 0.011 (d) 0.029

35. Equal weights of NaCl and KCl are dissolved separately in equal volumes of solutions. Molarity of the two solutions will be :
(a) equal
(b) that of NaCl will be less than that of KCl
(c) that of NaCl will be more than that of KCl solution
(d) that of NaCl will be about half of that of KCl solution

36. Gastric juice contains 3.0 g of HCl per litre. If a person produces 2.5 litre of gastric juice per day. How many antacid tablets each containing 400 mg of $Al(OH)_3$ are needed to neutralize all the HCl produced in one day ?
(a) 18 (b) 14 (c) 20 (d) 17

37. Which of the following is the correct empirical and molecular formulae of a compound, if the molecular mass of a compound is 80 and compound contains 60% of C, 5% of H and 35% of N ?
(a) C_2H_2N ; $C_4H_4N_2$ (b) $C_3H_4N_2$; $C_6H_8N_4$
(c) $C_2H_4N_2$; $C_4H_8N_4$ (d) C_2H_2N ; C_2H_2N

38. A gas mixture of 3 litres of propane (C_3H_8) and butane (C_4H_{10}) on complete combustion at 25° C produced 10 litre CO_2. Find out the composition of gas mixture (Propane : Butane)
(a) 2 : 1 (b) 1 : 2
(c) 1.5 : 1.5 (d) 0.5 : 2.5

39. Arrange the following in the order of increasing mass (atomic mass: O = 16, Cu = 63, N = 14)
I. one atom of oxygen
II. one atom of nitrogen
III. 1×10^{-10} mole of oxygen
IV. 1×10^{-10} mole of copper
(a) II < I < III < IV (b) I < II < III < IV
(c) III < II < IV < I (d) IV < II < III < I

40. When 30 litres of H_2 and 30 litres of N_2 are reacted NH_3 is formed and the yield is only 50%. The composition of the gaseous mixture will be
(a) 5L of N_2, 5L of H_2 and 5 L of NH_3.
(b) 5L of N_2, 10L of H_2 and 10 L of NH_3.
(c) 10L of N_2, 15L of H_2 and 5 L of NH_3.
(d) 5L of N_2, 15L of H_2 and 10 L of NH_3.

41. How many moles of magnesium phosphate, $Mg_3(PO_4)_2$ will contain 0.25 mole of oxygen atoms?
(a) 1.25×10^{-2} (b) 2.5×10^{-2}
(c) 0.02 (d) 3.125×10^{-2}

42. 1.12 ml of a gas is produced at S.T.P. by the action of 4.12 mg of alcohol ROH with methyl magnesium Iodide. The molecular mass of alcohol is
(a) 16.0 (b) 41.2
(c) 82.4 (d) 156.0

43. If 224 mL of a triatomic gas has a mass of 1 g at 273K and 1 atmospheric pressure then the mass of one atom is
(a) 8.30×10^{-23} g (b) 2.08×10^{-23} g
(c) 5.53×10^{-23} g (d) 6.24×10^{-23} g

44. A compound contains atoms of three elements as A, B and C. If the oxidation number of A is +2, B is +5 and that of C is –2, the possible formula of the compound is
(a) $A_3(B_4C)_2$ (b) $A_3(BC_4)_2$
(d) ABC_2 (d) $A_2(BC_3)_2$

45. 5 moles of SO_2 and 5 moles of O_2 react to form SO_3. Number of moles left in total when only 60% SO_2 is used is
(a) 6.5 (b) 10
(c) 8 (d) 8.5

RESPONSE GRID					
	33. ⓐⓑⓒⓓ	34. ⓐⓑⓒⓓ	35. ⓐⓑⓒⓓ	36. ⓐⓑⓒⓓ	37. ⓐⓑⓒⓓ
	38. ⓐⓑⓒⓓ	39. ⓐⓑⓒⓓ	40. ⓐⓑⓒⓓ	41. ⓐⓑⓒⓓ	42. ⓐⓑⓒⓓ
	43. ⓐⓑⓒⓓ	44. ⓐⓑⓒⓓ	45. ⓐⓑⓒⓓ		

CHEMISTRY CHAPTERWISE SPEED TEST-29			
Total Questions	45	Total Marks	180
Attempted		Correct	
Incorrect		Net Score	
Cut-off Score	35	Qualifying Score	55
Success Gap = Net Score – Qualifying Score			
Net Score = (Correct × 4) – (Incorrect × 1)			

Space for Rough Work

CHEMISTRY

Structure of Atom

Speed TEST 30

Chapter-wise

No. of Questions	Maximum Marks	Time
45	180	1 Hour

GENERAL INSTRUCTIONS

- This test contains 45 MCQ's. For each question only one option is correct. Darken the correct circle/ bubble in the Response Grid provided on each page.
- You have to evaluate your Response Grids yourself with the help of solutions provided at the end of this book.
- Each correct answer will get you 4 marks and 1 mark shall be deduced for each incorrect answer. No mark will be given/ deducted if no bubble is filled. Keep a timer in front of you and stop immediately at the end of 60 min.
- The sheet follows a particular syllabus. Do not attempt the sheet before you have completed your preparation for that syllabus.
- After completing the sheet check your answers with the solution booklet and complete the Result Grid. Finally spend time to analyse your performance and revise the areas which emerge out as weak in your evaluation.

1. Among the following groupings which represents the collection of isoelectronic species?

(a) $NO^+, C_2^{2-}, O_2^-, CO$ (b) N_2, C_2^{2-}, CO, NO

(c) CO, NO^+, CN^-, C_2^{2-} (d) NO, CN^-, N_2, O_2^-

2. Rutherford's experiment which established the nuclear model of the atom used a beam of

(a) β-particles which impinged on a metal foil and got absorbed

(b) γ-rays which impinged on a metal foil and ejected electrons

(c) helium atoms which impinged on a metal foil and got scattered

(d) helium nuclei which impinged on a metal foil and got scattered

3. Which of the following levels of H and He^+ have same energy respectively ?

(A) 1, 2 (B) 3, 4 (C) 2, 4 (D) 3, 6

(a) A and D (b) A and B

(c) C and D (d) A, C and D

4. A 600 W mercury lamp emits monochromatic rediation of wavelength 331.3 nm. How many photons are emitted from the lamp per second ? ($h = 6.626 \times 10^{-34}$ Js; velocity of light $= 3 \times 10^8 \text{ ms}^{-1}$)

(a) 1×10^{19} (b) 1×10^{20}

(c) 1×10^{21} (d) 1×10^{23}

5. Energy of an electron is given by $E = -2.178 \times 10^{-18} \text{J}\left(\frac{Z^2}{n^2}\right)$. Wavelength of light required to excite an electron in an hydrogen atom from level n = 1 to n = 2 will be : ($h = 6.62 \times 10^{-34}$ Js and $c = 3.0 \times 10^8 \text{ ms}^{-1}$)

(a) 1.214×10^{-7} m (b) 2.816×10^{-7} m

(c) 6.500×10^{-7} m (d) 8.500×10^{-7} m

6. The energy required to break one mole of Cl – Cl bonds in Cl_2 is 242 kJ mol^{-1}. The longest wavelength of light capable of breaking a single Cl – Cl bond is ($c = 3 \times 10^8 \text{ ms}^{-1}$ and $N_A = 6.02 \times 10^{23} \text{ mol}^{-1}$).

(a) 594 nm (b) 640 nm

(c) 700 nm (d) 494 nm

7. The first emission line in the atomic spectrum of hydrogen in the Balmer series appears at

(a) $\frac{9R_H}{400} \text{cm}^{-1}$ (b) $\frac{7R_H}{144} \text{cm}^{-1}$

(c) $\frac{3R_H}{4} \text{cm}^{-1}$ (d) $\frac{5R_H}{36} \text{cm}^{-1}$

RESPONSE GRID					
	1. ⓐⓑⓒⓓ	2. ⓐⓑⓒⓓ	3. ⓐⓑⓒⓓ	4. ⓐⓑⓒⓓ	5. ⓐⓑⓒⓓ
	6. ⓐⓑⓒⓓ	7. ⓐⓑⓒⓓ			

Space for Rough Work

8. Which one of the following set of quantum numbers is not possible for 4p electron?

(a) $n=4, l=1, m=-1, m_s=+\frac{1}{2}$

(b) $n=4, l=1, m=0, m_s=+\frac{1}{2}$

(c) $n=4, l=1, m=2, m_s=+\frac{1}{2}$

(d) $n=4, l=1, m=-1, m_s=-\frac{1}{2}$

9. What will be the difference between electromagnetic radiation shown in A and B respectively ?

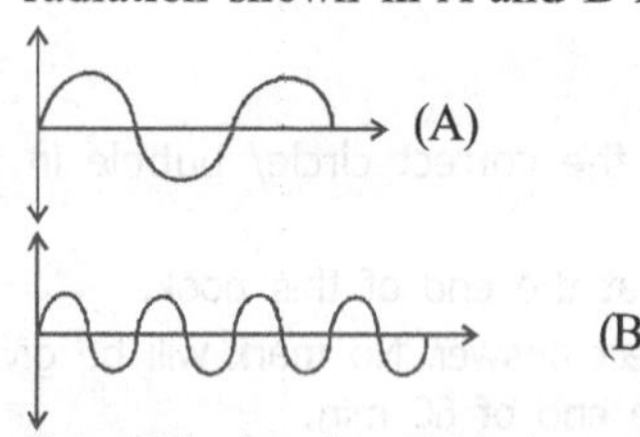

(i) Velocity (ii) Wavelength
(iii) Frequency (iv) Energy

(a) (ii) only (b) (ii) and (iv)
(c) (ii), (iii) and (iv) (d) (iv) only

10. Match the columns.

Column-I (Sub shell)	Column-II (Number of Orbitals)	Column-III (Angular/Azimuthal Quantum Number)
(A) d	(p) 1	(i) 1
(B) f	(q) 3	(ii) 2
(C) s	(r) 5	(iii) 0
(D) p	(s) 7	(iv) 3

(a) A – (r) – (ii), B – (s) – (iv), C – (p) – (iii), D – (q) – (i)
(b) A – (q) – (i), B – (s) – (iv), C – (p) – (iii), D – (r) – (ii)
(c) A – (p) – (iii), B – (s) – (iv), C – (r) – (ii), D – (q) – (i)
(d) A – (r) – (ii), B – (p) – (iii), C – (s) – (iv), D – (q) – (i)

11. The orbital angular momentum for an electron revolving in an orbit is given by $\sqrt{l(l+1)}.\frac{h}{2\pi}$. This momentum for an s-electron will be given by

(a) zero (b) $\frac{h}{2\pi}$ (c) $\sqrt{2}.\frac{h}{2\pi}$ (d) $+\frac{1}{2}.\frac{h}{2\pi}$

12. The energy of a photon is given as ΔE/atom 3.03×10^{-19} J atom^{-1}. Then the wavelength (λ) of the photon is
(a) 65.6 nm (b) 656 nm (c) 0.656 nm (d) 6.56 nm

13. The electrons, identified by quantum numbers n and l (I) n = 4, l = 1 (II) n = 4, l = 0 (III) n = 3, l = 2 (IV) n = 3, l = 1 can be placed in order of increasing energy, from the lowest to highest, as
(a) (IV) < (II) < (III) < (I) (b) (II) < (IV) < (I) < (III)
(c) (I) < (III) < (II) < (IV) (d) (III) < (I) < (IV) < (II)

14. For Balmer series in the spectrum of atomic hydrogen, the wave number of each line is given by $\bar{v} = R_H\left(\frac{1}{n_1^2}-\frac{1}{n_2^2}\right)$ where R_H is a constant and n_1 and n_2 are integers. Which of the following statement(s) is (are) correct?
(i) As wavelength decreases, the lines in the series converge.
(ii) The integer n_1 is equal to 2.
(iii) The ionization energy of hydrogen can be calculated from the wave number of these lines.
(iv) The line of longest wavelength corresponds to $n_2 = 3$.
(a) (i), (ii) and (iii) (b) (ii), (iii) and (iv)
(c) (i), (ii) and (iv) (d) (ii) and (iv)

15. The wavelength (in cm) of second line in the Lyman series of hydrogen atomic spectrum is (Rydberg constant = R cm^{-1})

(a) $\left(\frac{8R_H}{9}\right)$ (b) $\left(\frac{9}{8R_H}\right)$ (c) $\left(\frac{4}{3R_H}\right)$ (d) $\left(\frac{3R_H}{4}\right)$

16. If λ_o and λ be threshold wavelength and wavelength of incident light, the velocity of photoelectron ejected from the metal surface is:

(a) $\sqrt{\frac{2h}{m}(\lambda_o-\lambda)}$ (b) $\sqrt{\frac{2hc}{m}(\lambda_o-\lambda)}$

(c) $\sqrt{\frac{2hc}{m}\left(\frac{\lambda_o-\lambda}{\lambda\lambda_o}\right)}$ (d) $\sqrt{\frac{2h}{m}\left(\frac{1}{\lambda_o}-\frac{1}{\lambda}\right)}$

17. If wavelength of photon is 2.2×10^{-11} m, h = 6.6×10^{-34} Js, then momentum of photon is
(a) 3×10^{-23} kg/s (b) 3.33×10^{22} kg/s
(c) 1.452×10^{-44} kg/s (d) 6.89×10^{43} kg/s

18. Which of the following set of quantum numbers belong to highest energy?

(a) n = 4, l = 0, m = 0, s = $+\frac{1}{2}$

(b) n = 3, l = 0, m = 0, s = $+\frac{1}{2}$

(c) n = 3, l = 1, m = 1, s = $+\frac{1}{2}$

(d) n = 3, l = 2, m = 1, s = $+\frac{1}{2}$

RESPONSE GRID					
	8. ⓐⓑⓒⓓ	9. ⓐⓑⓒⓓ	10. ⓐⓑⓒⓓ	11. ⓐⓑⓒⓓ	12. ⓐⓑⓒⓓ
	13. ⓐⓑⓒⓓ	14. ⓐⓑⓒⓓ	15. ⓐⓑⓒⓓ	16. ⓐⓑⓒⓓ	17. ⓐⓑⓒⓓ
	18. ⓐⓑⓒⓓ				

Space for Rough Work

19. From the data given below A, B, C and D respectively are,
(A) 10 e^-, atomic no. 11 (B) 10 e^-, atomic no. 6
(C) 10 e^-, atomic no. 10 (D) 10 e^-, atomic no. 9
(a) Na^+, C^{4-}, Ne, F^- (b) C^{4-}, Ne, Na^-, F^-
(c) F^-, Na^+, Ne, C^{4-} (d) F^-, Na^+, C^{4-}, Ne

20. Suppose beam containing all three fundamental subatomic particles are allowed to pass through an electric field as shown in figure. The subatomic particles detected at three points A, B and C on the screen respectively are ?

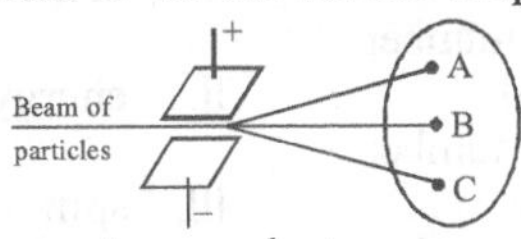

(a) Protons, neutrons, electrons
(b) Electrons, neutrons, protons
(c) Electrons, protons, neutrons
(d) Neutrons, protons, electrons

21. For a *d*-electron, the orbital angular momentum is
(a) $\sqrt{6}(h/2\pi)$ (b) $\sqrt{2}(h/2\pi)$
(c) $(h/2\pi)$ (d) $2(h/2\pi)$

22. The uncertainty in the position of an electron (mass = 9.1×10^{-28} g) moving with a velocity of 3.0×10^4 cm s^{-1} accurate upto 0.011% will be
(a) 1.92 cm (b) 7.68 cm (c) 0.175 cm (d) 3.84 cm.

23. The values of Planck's constant is 6.63×10^{-34} Js. The velocity of light is 3.0×10^8 m s^{-1}. Which value is closest to the wavelength in nanometres of a quantum of light with frequency of 8×10^{15} s^{-1}?
(a) 5×10^{-18} (b) 4×10^1
(c) 3×10^7 (d) 2×10^{-25}

24. The wavelength associated with a golf ball weighing 200 g and moving at a speed of 5 m/h is of the order
(a) 10^{-10} m (b) 10^{-20} m (c) 10^{-30} m (d) 10^{-40} m

25. Given that the abundances of isotopes ^{54}Fe, ^{56}Fe and ^{57}Fe are 5%, 90% and 5%, respectively, the atomic mass of Fe is
(a) 55.85 (b) 55.95 (c) 55.75 (d) 56.05

26. Based on the equation:
$$\Delta E = -2.0 \times 10^{-18} J\left(\frac{1}{n_2^2} - \frac{1}{n_1^2}\right)$$
the wavelength of the light that must be absorbed to excite hydrogen electron from level n = 1 to level n = 2 will be:
(h = 6.625×10^{-34} Js, C = 3×10^8 ms^{-1})
(a) 1.325×10^{-7} m (b) 1.325×10^{-10} m
(c) 2.650×10^{-7} m (d) 5.300×10^{-10} m

27. If uncertainty in position and momentum are equal, then uncertainty in velocity is :
(a) $\frac{1}{2m}\sqrt{\frac{h}{\pi}}$ (b) $\sqrt{\frac{h}{2\pi}}$
(c) $\frac{1}{m}\sqrt{\frac{h}{\pi}}$ (d) $\sqrt{\frac{h}{\pi}}$

28. The radius of an atomic nucleus is of the order of :
(a) 10^{-10} cm (b) 10^{-13} cm
(c) 10^{-15} cm (d) 10^{-8} cm

29. In Cu. (At. No. 29)
(a) 13 electrons have spin in one direction and 16 electrons in other direction
(b) 14 electrons have spin in one direction and 15 electrons in other direction
(c) one electron can have spin only in the clockwise direction
(d) None of the above is correct.

30. The correct order of increasing energy of atomic orbitals is
(a) 5p < 4f < 6s < 5d (b) 5p < 6s < 4f < 5d
(c) 5p < 5d < 4f < 6s (d) none of these

31. Match the columns.

	Column-I		Column-II
A.	X-rays	I.	$\nu = 10^0 - 10^4$ Hz
B.	UV	II.	$\nu = 10^{10}$ Hz
C.	Long radio waves	III.	$\nu = 10^{16}$ Hz
D.	Microwave	IV.	$\nu = 10^{18}$ Hz

(a) A – IV ; B – III ; C – I ; D – II
(b) A – III ; B – IV ; C – I ; D – II
(c) A – IV ; B – I ; C – III ; D – II
(d) A – IV ; B – III ; C – II ; D – I

32. What does negative sign in the electronic energy for hydrogen atom convey.
(a) Energy of electron when n = ∞
(b) The energy of electron in the atom is lower than the energy of a free electron in motion
(c) The energy of electron in the atom is lower than the energy of a free electron of rest
(d) The energy of electron decreases as it moves away from nucleus

33. If the nitrogen atom had electronic configuration $1s^7$ it would have energy lower than that of the normal ground state configuration $1s^2\ 2s^2\ 2p^3$ because the electrons would be closer to the nucleus. Yet $1s^7$ is not observed. It violates
(a) Heisenberg's uncertainty principle
(b) Hund's rule
(c) Pauli exclusion principle
(d) Bohr postulate of stationary orbits

RESPONSE GRID					
	19. ⓐⓑⓒⓓ	20. ⓐⓑⓒⓓ	21. ⓐⓑⓒⓓ	22. ⓐⓑⓒⓓ	23. ⓐⓑⓒⓓ
	24. ⓐⓑⓒⓓ	25. ⓐⓑⓒⓓ	26. ⓐⓑⓒⓓ	27. ⓐⓑⓒⓓ	28. ⓐⓑⓒⓓ
	29. ⓐⓑⓒⓓ	30. ⓐⓑⓒⓓ	31. ⓐⓑⓒⓓ	32. ⓐⓑⓒⓓ	33. ⓐⓑⓒⓓ

Space for Rough Work

34. If $n = 6$, the correct sequence for filling of electrons will be :
(a) $ns \rightarrow (n-2)f \rightarrow (n-1)d \rightarrow np$
(b) $ns \rightarrow (n-1)d \rightarrow (n-2)f \rightarrow np$
(c) $ns \rightarrow (n-2)f \rightarrow np \rightarrow (n-1)d$
(d) $ns \rightarrow np \rightarrow (n-1)d \rightarrow (n-2)f$

35. What is the expression of frequency (ν) associated with absorption spectra of the photon.

(a) $\nu = \frac{R_H}{h}\left(\frac{1}{n_i^2} - \frac{1}{n_f^2}\right) n_i > n_f$

(b) $\nu = \frac{R_H}{h}\left(\frac{1}{n_i^2} - \frac{1}{n_f^2}\right) n_f > n_i$

(c) $\nu = -\frac{R_H}{h}\left(\frac{1}{n_i^2} - \frac{1}{n_f^2}\right) n_f > n_i$

(d) All the above are correct

36. Chlorine exists in two isotopic forms, C1-37 and C1-35 but its atomic mass is 35.5. This indicates the ratio of Cl-37 and C1-35 is approximately
(a) 1 : 2 (b) 1 : 1 (c) 1 : 3 (d) 3 : 1

37. If m and e are the mass and charge of the revolving electron in the orbit of radius r for hydrogen atom, the total energy of the revolving electron will be:

(a) $\frac{1}{2}\frac{e^2}{r}$ (b) $-\frac{e^2}{r}$ (c) $\frac{me^2}{r}$ (d) $-\frac{1}{2}\frac{e^2}{r}$

38. An electron, e_1 is moving in the fifth stationary state, and another electron e_2 is moving in the fourth stationary state. The radius of orbit of electron e_1 is five times the radius of orbit of electron e_2 calculate the ratio of velocity of electron e_1 (v_1) to the velocity of electron e_2 (v_2).
(a) 5 : 1 (b) 4 : 1 (c) 1 : 5 (d) 1 : 4

39. The correct set of four quantum numbers for the valence electrons of rubidium atom ($Z = 37$) is:

(a) $5, 0, 0, \pm\frac{1}{2}$ (b) $5, 1, 0, +\frac{1}{2}$

(c) $5, 1, 1, +\frac{1}{2}$ (d) $5, 0, 1, +\frac{1}{2}$

40. Among species H, Li^{2+}, He^+, Be^{3+} and Al^{3+} Bohr's model was able to explain the spectra of
(a) all of these
(b) none of these
(c) all other species except Be^{3+}
(d) all other species except Al^{3+}

41. Match the columns.

	Column-I (Quantum number)		Column-II (Information provided)
A.	Principal quantum number	I.	orientation of the orbital
B.	Azimuthal quantum number	II.	energy and size of orbital
C.	Magnetic quantum number	III.	spin of electron
D.	Spin quantum number	IV.	shape of the orbital

(a) A – II; B – IV; C – I; D – III
(b) A – IV; B – II; C – I; D – III
(c) A – II; B – I; C – IV; D – III
(d) A – II; B – IV; C – III; D – I

42. The radius of which of the following orbit is same as that of the first Bohr's orbit of hydrogen atom?
(a) He^+ ($n = 2$) (b) Li^{2+} ($n = 2$)
(c) Li^{2+} ($n = 3$) (d) Be^{3+} ($n = 2$)

43. The average life of an excited state of hydrogen atom is of the order 10^{-8} s. The number of revolutions made by an electron when it is in state n = 2 and before it suffers a transition to state n = 9 are
(a) 8.23×10^6 (b) 2.82×10^6
(c) 22.8×10^6 (d) 2.28×10^6

44. If the kinetic energy of an electron is increased four times, the wavelength of the de-Broglie wave associated with it would become
(a) one fourth (b) half
(c) four times (d) two times

45. If the radius of first orbit of H-atom is a_0, then de-Broglie wavelength of electron in 4th orbit is

(a) $8\pi a_0$ (b) $\frac{a_0}{4}$ (c) $16a_0$ (d) $2\pi a_0$

RESPONSE GRID					
	34. ⓐⓑⓒⓓ	35. ⓐⓑⓒⓓ	36. ⓐⓑⓒⓓ	37. ⓐⓑⓒⓓ	38. ⓐⓑⓒⓓ
	39. ⓐⓑⓒⓓ	40. ⓐⓑⓒⓓ	41. ⓐⓑⓒⓓ	42. ⓐⓑⓒⓓ	43. ⓐⓑⓒⓓ
	44. ⓐⓑⓒⓓ	45. ⓐⓑⓒⓓ			

CHEMISTRY CHAPTERWISE SPEED TEST-30

Total Questions	45	Total Marks	180
Attempted		Correct	
Incorrect		Net Score	
Cut-off Score	35	Qualifying Score	52
Success Gap = Net Score – Qualifying Score			
Net Score = (Correct × 4) – (Incorrect × 1)			

Space for Rough Work

CHEMISTRY

Classification of Elements and Periodicity in Properties

Speed TEST 31 Chapter-wise

No. of Questions	Maximum Marks	Time
45	180	1 Hour

GENERAL INSTRUCTIONS

- This test contains 45 MCQ's. For each question only one option is correct. Darken the correct circle/ bubble in the Response Grid provided on each page.
- You have to evaluate your Response Grids yourself with the help of solutions provided at the end of this book.
- Each correct answer will get you 4 marks and 1 mark shall be deduced for each incorrect answer. No mark will be given/ deducted if no bubble is filled. Keep a timer in front of you and stop immediately at the end of 60 min.
- The sheet follows a particular syllabus. Do not attempt the sheet before you have completed your preparation for that syllabus.
- After completing the sheet check your answers with the solution booklet and complete the Result Grid. Finally spend time to analyse your performance and revise the areas which emerge out as weak in your evaluation.

1. Which of the following is not an actinoid ?
   (a) Curium ($Z=96$) (b) Californium ($Z=98$)
   (c) Uranium ($Z=92$) (d) Terbium ($Z=65$)
2. Which of the following species has lowest ionization potential?
   (a) O (b) O_2 (c) O_2^+ (d) O_2^-
3. On going down a main sub-group in the periodic table (example Li to Cs in IA or Be to Ra in IIA), the expected trend of changes in atomic radius is a
   (a) continuous increase
   (b) continuous decrease
   (c) periodic one, an increase followed by a decrease
   (d) decrease followed by increase
4. Match the columns

Column-I (Compounds)	Column-II (Co-ordination number, oxidation number)
A. $[BF_4]^-$	I. 7, +7
B. $[AlF_6]^{3-}$	II. 4, +4
C. OF_2	III. 6, +3
D. SiF_4	IV. 2, +2
E. IF_7	V. 4, +3

   (a) A – IV; B – II; C – V; D – III; E – I
   (b) A – V; B – III; C – IV; D – II; E – I
   (c) A – II; B – III; C – V; D – IV; E – I
   (d) A – III; B – II; C – IV; D – I; E – V
5. The decreasing order of the ionization potential of the following elements is
   (a) Ne > Cl > P > S > Al > Mg
   (b) Ne > Cl > P > S > Mg > Al
   (c) Ne > Cl > S > P > Mg > Al
   (d) Ne > Cl > S > P > Al > Mg
6. The radii of F, F^-, O and O^{2-} are in the order
   (a) $O^{2-} > F^- > F > O$ (b) $F^- > O^{2-} > F > O$
   (c) $O^{2-} > O > F^- > F$ (d) $O^{2-} > F^- > O > F$
7. Which group of the periodic table contains coinage metal ?
   (a) IIA (b) IB
   (c) IA (d) None of these

RESPONSE GRID	
	1. ⓐⓑⓒⓓ 2. ⓐⓑⓒⓓ 3. ⓐⓑⓒⓓ 4. ⓐⓑⓒⓓ 5. ⓐⓑⓒⓓ
	6. ⓐⓑⓒⓓ 7. ⓐⓑⓒⓓ

Space for Rough Work

8. Which of the following statements are correct?
   (i) The second period ($n = 2$) starts with lithium and third electron enters the $2s$ orbital. The next element, beryllium has four electrons and has the electronic configuration $1s^22s^2$. From the next element boron, the $2p$ orbitals are filled with electrons when the L shell is completed at neon ($2s^22p^6$). Thus there are 8 elements in the second period.
   (ii) Successive filling of $3s$ and $3p$ orbitals gives rise to the third period of 8 elements from sodium to argon.
   (iii) The fourth period ($n = 4$) starts at potassium and the added electron fill up the first $4s$ and $4p$ orbitals than $3d$ orbital is filled.
   (iv) Fifth period begins with rubidium with the filling of $5s$ orbital and ends at xenon with the filling up of the $5p$ orbital.
   (a) (i) and (ii) (b) (i), (ii) and (iii)
   (c) (iii) and (iv) (d) (i), (ii) and (iv)
9. Which ionisation potential (IP) in the following equations involves the greatest amount of energy ?
   (a) $Na \rightarrow Na^+ + e^-$ (b) $K^+ \rightarrow K^{2+} + e^-$
   (c) $C^{2+} \rightarrow C^{3+} + e^-$ (d) $Ca^+ \rightarrow Ca^{2+} + e^-$
10. Which of the following arrangements represents the increasing order (smallest to largest) of ionic radii of the given species O^{2-}, S^{2-}, N^{3-}, P^{3-}?
   (a) $O^{2-} < N^{3-} < S^{2-} < P^{3-}$ (b) $O^{2-} < P^{3-} < N^{3-} < S^{2-}$
   (c) $N^3 < O^{2-} < P^{3-} < S^{2-}$ (d) $N^{3-} < S^{2-} < O^{2-} < P^{3-}$
11. Which of the following series correctly represents relations between the elements from X to Y?
   $X \rightarrow Y$
   (a) $_3Li \rightarrow {}_{19}K$ Ionization enthalpy increases
   (b) $_9F \rightarrow {}_{35}Br$ Electron gain enthalpy (negative sign) increases
   (c) $_6C \rightarrow {}_{32}Ge$ Atomic radii increases
   (d) $_{18}Ar \rightarrow {}_{54}Xe$ Noble character increases
12. The formation of the oxide ion $O^{2-}(g)$, from oxygen atom requires first an exothermic and then an endothermic step as shown below :
   $O(g) + e^- \rightarrow O^-(g);\ \Delta_f H^\ominus = -141\ kJ\ mol^{-1}$
   $O^-(g) + e^- \rightarrow O^{2-}(g);\ \Delta_f H^\ominus = +780\ kJ\ mol^{-1}$
   Thus process of formation of O^{2-} in gas phase is unfavourable even though O^{2-} is isoelectronic with neon. It is due to the fact that
   (a) Electron repulsion outweighs the stability gained by achieving noble gas configuration
   (b) O^- ion has comparatively smaller size than oxygen atom
   (c) Oxygen is more electronegative
   (d) Addition of electron in oxygen results in larger size of the ion.
13. In any period the valency of an element with respect to oxygen
   (a) Increases one by one from IA to VIIA
   (b) Decreases one by one form IA to VIIA
   (c) Increases one by one from IA to IVA and then decreases from VA to VIIA one by one
   (d) Decreases one by one from IA to IVA and then increases from VA to VIIA one by one
14. An element having electronic configuration $1s^2 2s^2 2p^6 3s^2 3p^6 4s^1$ forms
   (a) Acidic oxide (b) Basic oxide
   (c) Amphoteric oxide (d) Neutral oxide
15. Which of the following order is wrong?
   (a) $NH_3 < PH_3 < AsH_3$ — Acidic
   (b) $Li < Be < B < C$ — IE_1
   (c) $Al_2O_3 < MgO < Na_2O < K_2O$ — Basic
   (d) $Li^+ < Na^+ < K^+ < Cs^+$ — Ionic radius
16. The first ionisation potential of aluminium is smaller than that of magnesium because
   (a) Atomic size of Al > Atomic size of Mg.
   (b) Atomic size of Al < Atomic size of Mg.
   (c) Al has one electron in p - orbital
   (d) None of these
17. The first ($\Delta_i H_1$) and second ($\Delta_i H_2$) ionization enthalpies (in kJ mol^{-1}) and the electron gain enthalpy ($\Delta_{eg}H$) (in kJ mol^{-1}) of the elements I, II, III, IV and V are given below

Element	$\Delta_i H_1$	$\Delta_i H_2$	$\Delta_{eg} H$
I	520	7300	−60
II	419	3051	−48
III	1681	3374	−328
IV	1008	1846	−295
V	2372	5251	+48

   The most reactive metal and the least reactive non-metal of these are respectively
   (a) I and V (b) III and II (c) II and V (d) IV and V
18. Consider the following statements:
   (i) The discovery of inert gases later on did not disturb Mendeleev's arrangement.
   (ii) In the present periodic table, periodicity in the properties of elements is related to the periodicity in their electronic configurations.
   Which of these statement(s) is/are correct ?
   (a) (i) only (b) (ii) only
   (c) Both (i) and (ii) (d) Neither (i) nor (ii)
19. Consider the following ionization enthalpies of two elements 'A' and 'B'.

Element	Ionization 1st	enthalpy 2nd	(kJ/mol) 3rd
A	899	1757	14847
B	737	1450	7731

   Which of the following statements is correct ?
   (a) Both 'A' and 'B' belong to group–1 where 'B' comes below 'A'.
   (b) Both 'A' and 'B' belong to group–1 where 'A' comes below 'B'.
   (c) Both 'A' and 'B' belong to group–2 where 'B' comes below 'A'.
   (d) Both 'A' and 'B' belong to group–2 where 'A' comes below 'B'.

RESPONSE GRID					
	8. ⓐⓑⓒⓓ	9. ⓐⓑⓒⓓ	10. ⓐⓑⓒⓓ	11. ⓐⓑⓒⓓ	12. ⓐⓑⓒⓓ
	13. ⓐⓑⓒⓓ	14. ⓐⓑⓒⓓ	15. ⓐⓑⓒⓓ	16. ⓐⓑⓒⓓ	17. ⓐⓑⓒⓓ
	17. ⓐⓑⓒⓓ	18. ⓐⓑⓒⓓ	19. ⓐⓑⓒⓓ		

Space for Rough Work

20. Sodium sulphate is soluble in water whereas barium sulphate is sparingly soluble because :
(a) the hydration energy of sodium sulphate is less than its lattice energy
(b) the lattice energy of barium sulphate is more than its hydration energy
(c) the lattice energy has no role to play in solubility
(d) the hydration energy of sodium sulphate is less than its lattice energy.

21. Which of the following is the reason for the different chemical behaviour of the first member of a group of elements in the *s*- and *p*-blocks compared to that of the subsequent members in the same group?
(i) Small size
(ii) Large charge / radius ratio
(iii) Low electronegativity of the element
(a) (i) and (iii) (b) (i), (ii) and (iii)
(c) (i) and (ii) (d) (ii) and (iii)

22. The element with outer electronic configuration $3d^6 4s^2$ is a
(a) metalloid (b) non-metal
(c) transition metal (d) noble gas

23. Which of the following statements is wrong ?
(a) van der Waal's radius of iodine is more than its covalent radius
(b) All isoelectronic ions belong to same period of the periodic table
(c) $I.E._1$ of N is higher than that of O while $I.E._2$ of O is higher than that of N
(d) The electron gain enthalpy of N is almost zero while that of P is 74.3 kJ mol^{-1}

24. Which of the following sequence correctly represents the decreasing acidic nature of oxides ?
(a) $Li_2O > BeO > B_2O_3 > CO_2 > N_2O_3$
(b) $N_2O_3 > CO_2 > B_2O_3 > BeO > Li_2O$
(c) $CO_2 > N_2O_3 > B_2O_3 > BeO > Li_2O$
(d) $B_2O_3 > CO_2 > N_2O_3 > Li_2O > BeO$

25. An atom has electronic configuration $1s^2\ 2s^2\ 2p^6\ 3s^2\ 3p^6\ 3d^3\ 4s^2$, you will place it in which group?
(a) Fifth (b) Fifteenth
(c) Second (d) Third

26. In which of the following arrangements, the sequence is not strictly according to the property written against it?
(a) $CO_2 < SiO_2 < SnO_2 < PbO_2$: increasing oxidising power
(b) $NH_3 < PH_3 < AsH_3 < SbH_3$: increasing basic strength
(c) HF < HCl < HBr < HI: increasing acid strength
(d) B < C < O < N: increasing first ionisation enthalpy.

27. Which one of the following statements is incorrect ?
(a) Greater the nuclear charge, greater is the electron affinity
(b) Nitrogen has zero electron affinity
(c) Electron affinity decreases from fluorine to iodine in 17th group
(d) Chlorine has highest electron affinity

28. An element X occurs in short period having configuration $ns^2\ np^1$. The formula and nature of its oxide is
(a) XO_3, basic (b) XO_3 acidic
(c) X_2O_3, amphoteric (d) X_2O_3 basic

29. Ionic radii of
(a) $Ti^{4+} < Mn^{2+}$ (b) $^{35}Cl^- < {}^{37}Cl^-$
(c) $K^+ > Cl^{-1}$ (d) $P^{3+} > P^{5+}$

30. The ionic radii (in Å) of N^{3-}, O^{2-} and F^- are respectively :
(a) 1.71, 1.40 and 1.36 (b) 1.71, 1.36 and 1.40
(c) 1.36, 1.40 and 1.71 (d) 1.36, 1.71 and 1.40

31. Amongst H_2O, H_2S, H_2Se and H_2Te, the one with the highest boiling point is
(a) H_2O because of hydrogen bonding
(b) H_2Te because of higher molecular weight
(c) H_2S because of hydrogen bonding
(d) H_2Se because of lower molecular weight

32. Match the Column-I and Column-II and select the correct answer by given codes.

	Column-I (Elements)		Column-II (Properties)
A.	$Li^+ < Al^{3+} < Mg^{2+} < K^+$	I.	DEA (Electron affinity)
B.	$Li^+ > Al^{3+} > Mg^{2+} > K^+$	II.	Ionic radii
C.	Cl > F > Br > I	III.	EN (Electronegativity)
D.	F > Cl > Br > I	IV.	Effective nuclear charge

(a) A – II; B – IV; C – III; D – I
(b) A – II; B – IV; C – I; D – III
(c) A – IV; B – II; C – III; D – I
(d) A – IV; B – II; C – I; D – III

33. Which of the following statement(s) is/are correct ?
(i) Aluminium react with HCl to form Al^{3+} and H_2 is liberated
(ii) Aluminium dissolve in NaOH to form $NaAl(OH)_4$ and H_2
(a) (i) and (ii) (b) Only (ii)
(c) Only (i) (d) Neither (i) nor (ii)

34. Which has most stable +2 oxidation state :
(a) Sn (b) Pb (c) Fe (d) Ag

35. Match Column-I (IUPAC nomenclature of element) with Column-II (IUPAC official name).

	Column-I		Column-II
A.	Unnilhexium	I.	Lawrencium
B.	Unniltrium	II.	Dubnium
C.	Unnilunium	III.	Seaborgium
D.	Unnilpentium	IV.	Mendelevium

(a) A – IV; B – I; C – III; D – II
(b) A – III; B – I; C – IV; D – II
(c) A – III; B – IV; C – I; D – II
(d) A – II; B – III; C – I; D – IV

RESPONSE GRID				
20. ⓐⓑⓒⓓ	21. ⓐⓑⓒⓓ	22. ⓐⓑⓒⓓ	23. ⓐⓑⓒⓓ	24. ⓐⓑⓒⓓ
25. ⓐⓑⓒⓓ	26. ⓐⓑⓒⓓ	27. ⓐⓑⓒⓓ	28. ⓐⓑⓒⓓ	29. ⓐⓑⓒⓓ
30. ⓐⓑⓒⓓ	31. ⓐⓑⓒⓓ	32. ⓐⓑⓒⓓ	33. ⓐⓑⓒⓓ	34. ⓐⓑⓒⓓ
35. ⓐⓑⓒⓓ				

Space for Rough Work

36. In the Mendeleev periodic table, which of the following element instead of having lower atomic weight was placed after the element of higher atomic weight thereby ignoring the order of increasing atomic weights.
(a) Iodine (b) Antimony
(c) Bromine (d) Molybdenum

37. The van der Waal and covalent radii of fluorine atom respectively from the following figure are.

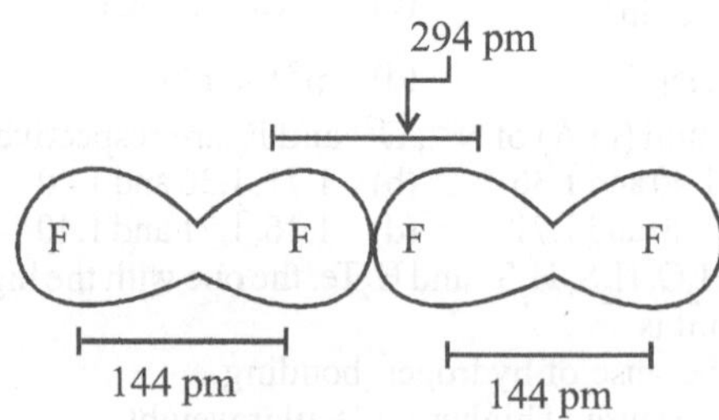

(a) 219pm, 72pm (b) 75pm, 72pm
(c) 147pm, 72pm (d) 147pm, 144pm

38. Cl, Br, I, if this is Dobereiner's triad and the atomic masses of Cl and I are 35.5 and 127 respectively the atomic mass of Br is
(a) 162.5 (b) 91.5 (c) 81.25 (d) 45.625

39. The first ionisation potential of Na is 5.1 eV. The value of electron gain enthalpy of Na^+ will be :
(a) −2.55 eV (b) −5.1 eV
(c) −10.2 eV (d) +2.55 eV

40. As we move across the second period from C to F ionisation enthalpy increases but the trend from C to F for ionisation enthalpy is C < O < N < F why it is not C < N < O < F. This is because
(a) atomic radii of O > atomic radii of N
(b) electronic configuration of N is more stable than electronic configuration of O
(c) atomic radii of N > atomic radii of O
(d) None of these

41. The electron affinity of chlorine is 3.7 eV. 1 gram of chlorine is completely converted to Cl^- ion in a gaseous state. (1 eV = 23.06 kcal mol^{-1}).
Energy released in the process is
(a) 4.8 kcal (b) 7.2 kcal (c) 8.2 kcal (d) 2.4 kcal

42. Gradual addition of electronic shells in the noble gases causes a decrease in their
(a) ionization energy (b) atomic radius
(c) boiling point (d) density

43. The formation of the oxide ion $O^{2-}_{(g)}$ requires first an exothermic and then an endothermic step as shown below

$O_{(g)} + e^- = O^-_{(g)} \quad \Delta H^\circ = -142 \text{ kJmol}^{-1}$

$O^-(g) + e^- = O^{2-}_{(g)} \quad \Delta H^\circ = 844 \text{ kJmol}^{-1}$

This is because
(a) O^- ion will tend to resist the addition of another electron
(b) Oxygen has high electron affinity
(c) Oxygen is more elecronegative
(d) O^- ion has comparatively larger size than oxygen atom

44. Which of the following is correct about Eka-Aluminium and Eka-Silicon ?
(a) Oxides of Eka-Aluminium is Al_2O_3 and Eka-Silicon is Si_2O_3
(b) Oxides of Eka-Aluminium is Ga_2O_3 and Eka-Silicon is GeO_2
(c) Melting point of Eka-Aluminium is lower than the melting point of Eka-Silicon
(d) Both (a) and (c)

45. Covalent radii of atoms varies in range of 72 pm to 133 pm from F to I while that of noble gases He to Xe varies from 120pm to 220pm. This is because in case of noble gases
(a) covalent radius is very large
(b) van der Waal radius is considered
(c) metallic radii is considered
(d) None of these

RESPONSE GRID	36. ⓐⓑⓒⓓ	37. ⓐⓑⓒⓓ	38. ⓐⓑⓒⓓ	39. ⓐⓑⓒⓓ	40. ⓐⓑⓒⓓ
	41. ⓐⓑⓒⓓ	42. ⓐⓑⓒⓓ	43. ⓐⓑⓒⓓ	44. ⓐⓑⓒⓓ	45. ⓐⓑⓒⓓ

CHEMISTRY CHAPTERWISE SPEED TEST-31

Total Questions	45	Total Marks	180
Attempted		Correct	
Incorrect		Net Score	
Cut-off Score	40	Qualifying Score	65
Success Gap = Net Score – Qualifying Score			
Net Score = (Correct × 4) – (Incorrect × 1)			

Space for Rough Work

CHEMISTRY

Chemical bonding and Molecular Structure

Speed TEST 32

Chapter-wise

No. of Questions	Maximum Marks	Time
45	180	1 Hour

GENERAL INSTRUCTIONS

- This test contains 45 MCQ's. For each question only one option is correct. Darken the correct circle/ bubble in the Response Grid provided on each page.
- You have to evaluate your Response Grids yourself with the help of solutions provided at the end of this book.
- Each correct answer will get you 4 marks and 1 mark shall be deduced for each incorrect answer. No mark will be given/ deducted if no bubble is filled. Keep a timer in front of you and stop immediately at the end of 60 min.
- The sheet follows a particular syllabus. Do not attempt the sheet before you have completed your preparation for that syllabus.
- After completing the sheet check your answers with the solution booklet and complete the Result Grid. Finally spend time to analyse your performance and revise the areas which emerge out as weak in your evaluation.

1. The electronic configuration of metal M is $1s^2\, 2s^2\, 2p^6\, 3s^1$. The formula of its oxide will be
   (a) MO (b) M_2O
   (c) SO_3 (d) All of these
2. Which of the following does not contain coordinate bond ?
   (a) BH_4^- (b) NH_4^+
   (c) CO_3^{2-} (d) H_3O^+
3. Which of the following statements is incorrect ?
   (a) The formation of ionic compounds depend upon the ease of formation of the positive and negative ions from the respective neutral atoms.
   (b) Formation of ionic compounds depend upon arrangement of the positive and negative ions in the solid.
   (c) Formation of positive ion involves addition of electron(s) while that of negative ion involves removal of electron(s).
   (d) None of these
4. Hybridisation of the underline atom changes in:
   (a) $\underline{Al}H_3$ changes to AlH_4^-
   (b) $H_2\underline{O}$ changes to H_3O^+
   (c) $\underline{N}H_3$ changes to NH_4^+
   (d) in all cases
5. The decreasing values of bond angles from NH_3 (106°) to SbH_3 (101°) down group-15 of the periodic table is due to
   (a) decreasing lp-bp repulsion
   (b) decreasing electronegativity
   (c) increasing bp-bp repulsion
   (d) increasing p-orbital character in sp^3
6. In PO_4^{3-}, the formal charge on each oxygen atom and the P – O bond order respectively are
   (a) –0.75, 0.6 (b) –0.75, 1.0
   (c) –0.75, 1.25 (d) –3, 1.25
7. KF combines with HF to form KHF_2. The compound contains the species
   (a) K^+, F^- and H^+ (b) K^+, F^- and HF
   (c) K^+, and $[HF_2]^-$ (b) $[KHF]^+$ and F_2
8. An ether is more volatile than an alcohol having the same molecular formula. This is due to
   (a) dipolar character of ethers
   (b) alcohols having resonance structures
   (c) inter-molecular hydrogen bonding in ethers
   (d) inter-molecular hydrogen bonding in alcohols
9. In which of the following ionization processes, the bond order has increased and the magnetic behaviour has changed?
   (a) $N_2 \rightarrow N_2^+$ (b) $C_2 \rightarrow C_2^+$
   (c) $NO \rightarrow NO^+$ (d) $O_2 \rightarrow O_2^+$.

RESPONSE GRID					
	1. ⓐⓑⓒⓓ	2. ⓐⓑⓒⓓ	3. ⓐⓑⓒⓓ	4. ⓐⓑⓒⓓ	5. ⓐⓑⓒⓓ
	6. ⓐⓑⓒⓓ	7. ⓐⓑⓒⓓ	8. ⓐⓑⓒⓓ	9. ⓐⓑⓒⓓ	

Space for Rough Work

10. The maximum number of 90° angles between bond pair-bond pair of electrons is observed in
(a) dsp^2 hybridization (b) sp^3d hybridization
(c) dsp^3 hybridization (d) sp^3d^2 hybridization

11. Two ice cubes are pressed over each other until they unite to form one block. Which one of the following forces dominate for holding them together?
(a) Dipole-dipole interaction
(b) Van der waals' forces
(c) Hydrogen bond formation
(d) Covalent attraction

12. In XeF_2, XeF_4 and XeF_6, the number of lone pairs on Xe are respectively
(a) 2, 3, 1 (b) 1, 2, 3
(c) 4, 1, 2 (d) 3, 2, 1

13. The hybridization of atomic orbitals of nitrogen in NO_2^+, NO_2^- and NH_4^+ are
(a) sp^2, sp^3 and sp^2 respectively
(b) sp, sp^2 and sp^3 respectively
(c) sp^2, sp and sp^3 respectively
(d) sp^2, sp^3 and sp respectively

14. Match Column-I with Column-II and Column-III and choose the correct option from the given codes.

Column-I Molecule	Column-II (No. of lone pairs and bond pairs)	Column-III (Shape of molecule)
(A) NH_3	(i) 1, 2	(p) Bent
(B) SO_2	(ii) 1, 4	(q) Trigonal pyramidal
(C) SF_4	(iii) 2, 3	(r) T-shape
(D) ClF_3	(iv) 1, 3	(s) See-Saw

(a) A – (iv, q); B – (ii, p); C – (i, r); D – (iii, s)
(b) A – (iv, q); B – (i, p); C – (ii, s); D – (iii, r)
(c) A – (i, p); B – (iii, s); C – (iv, r); D – (ii, q)
(d) A – (iv, p); B – (i, r); C – (iii, q); D – (ii, s)

15. Which of the following statements is/are not correct for combination of atomic orbitals?
(i) The combining atomic orbitals must have the same or nearly the same energy.
(ii) Greater the extent of overlap, the greater will be the electron density between the nuclei of a moleculer orbital.
(iii) $2p_z$ orbital of one atom can combine with either of $2p_x$, $2p_y$ or $2p_z$ orbital of other atom as these orbitals have same energy.
(a) (i) and (ii) (b) (iii) only
(c) (i) only (d) (ii) and (iii)

16. Which of the following is the correct increasing order of lone pair of electrons on the central atom?
(a) $IF_7 < IF_5 < ClF_3 < XeF_2$
(b) $IF_7 < XeF_2 < ClF_3 < IF_5$
(c) $IF_7 < ClF_3 < XeF_2 < IF_5$
(d) $IF_7 < XeF_2 < IF_5 < ClF_3$

17. The dipole moment of chlorobenzene (Cl-benzene) is 1.5 D.

The dipole moment of 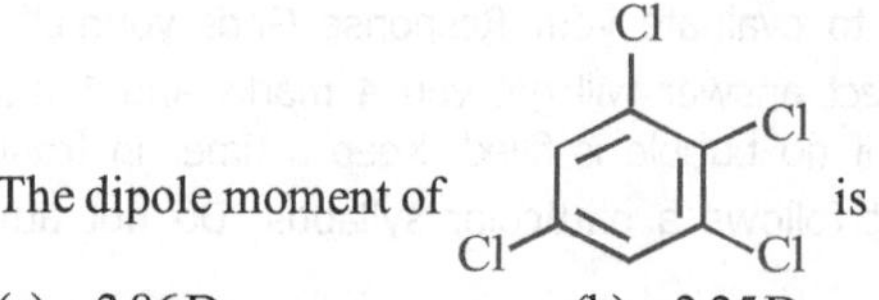 is

(a) 2.86 D (b) 2.25 D
(c) 1.5 D (d) 0 D

18. In compounds of type ECl_3, where E = B, P, As or Bi, the angles Cl - E- Cl for different E are in the order.
(a) B > P = As = Bi (b) B > P > As > Bi
(c) B < P = As = Bi (d) B < P < As < Bi

19. Which of the following substances has the greatest ionic character ?
(a) Cl_2O (b) NCl_3
(c) $PbCl_2$ (d) $BaCl_2$

20. If an organic compound contain 92.3% C and 7.7% H, then number of sp^3, sp^2 and sp hybridized carbon atoms in all possible structures of compound respectively are (molecular mass = 52 g/mol)
(a) 1, 2, 5 (b) 0, 4, 4
(c) 0, 8, 4 (d) None of these

21. Which of the following are isoelectronic and isostructural? NO_3^-, CO_3^{2-}, ClO_3^-, SO_3
(a) NO_3^-, CO_3^{2-} (b) SO_3, NO_3^-
(c) ClO_3^-, CO_3^{2-} (d) CO_3^{2-}, SO_3

RESPONSE GRID					
	10. ⓐⓑⓒⓓ	11. ⓐⓑⓒⓓ	12. ⓐⓑⓒⓓ	13. ⓐⓑⓒⓓ	14. ⓐⓑⓒⓓ
	15. ⓐⓑⓒⓓ	16. ⓐⓑⓒⓓ	17. ⓐⓑⓒⓓ	18. ⓐⓑⓒⓓ	19. ⓐⓑⓒⓓ
	20. ⓐⓑⓒⓓ	21. ⓐⓑⓒⓓ			

Space for Rough Work

22. Consider the chemical species NO_3^-, NO_2^+ and NO_2^- and point out the correct statement given below
(a) The hybrid state of N in NO_2^+ is sp^2
(b) The hybrid state of N in all the species is the same
(c) The shape of both NO_2^+ and NO_2^- is bent while NO_3^- is planar
(d) The hybrid state of N in NO_3^- and NO_2^- is the same

23. Bond order normally gives idea of stability of a molecular species. All the molecules viz. H_2, Li_2 and B_2 have the same bond order yet they are not equally stable. Their stability order is
(a) $H_2 > B_2 > Li_2$ (b) $Li_2 > H_2 > B_2$
(c) $Li_2 > B_2 > H_2$ (d) $H_2 > Li_2 > B_2$

24. ${}_1H^2 + {}_1H^2 \longrightarrow {}_2He^3 + {}_0n^1$
The above nuclear reaction is called
(a) nuclear fission
(b) nuclear fusion
(c) artificial transmutation
(d) spontaneous disintegration

25. Hydrogen chloride molecule contains
(a) polar covalent bond (b) double bond
(c) co-ordinate bond (d) electrovalent bond

26. Among the following species, identify the isostructural pairs
$NF_3, NO_3^-, BF_3, H_3O^+, HN_3$
(a) $[NF_3, NO_3^-]$ and $[BF_3, H_3O^+]$
(b) $[NF_3, HN_3]$ and $[NO_3^-, BF_3]$
(c) $[NF_3, H_3O^+]$ and $[NO_3^-, BF_3]$
(d) $[NF_3, H_3O^+]$ and $[HN_3, BF_3]$

27. In the anion $HCOO^-$ the two carbon - oxygen bonds are found to be of equal length. What is the reason for it ?
(a) Electronic orbitals of carbon atom are hybridised
(b) The C = O bond is weaker than the C – O bond
(c) The anion $HCOO^-$ has two resonating structures
(d) The anion is obtained by removal of a proton from the acid molecule

28. Which of the following is/are not essential condition(s) for hybridisation?
(i) The orbitals present in the valence shell of the atom are hybridised.
(ii) The orbitals undergoing hybridisation should have almost equal energy.
(iii) Promotion of electron is essential prior to hybridisation
(iv) Only half filled orbitals participate in hybridisation.
(a) (i) only (b) (iii) only
(c) (iv) only (d) (iii) and (iv)

29. The molecule XY_2 contains two σ and two π bonds and one lone pair of electrons in valence shell of X. The arrangement of lone pair and bond pairs is
(a) linear (b) trigonal planar
(c) square pyramidal (d) unpredictable

30. The molecules BF_3 and NF_3 are both covalent compounds, but BF_3 is non polar whereas NF_3 is polar. The reason for this is
(a) atomic size of boron is larger than nitrogen
(b) Boron is metal while nitrogen is gas
(c) B – F bonds are non-polar while N – F bonds are polar
(d) BF_3 is planar but NF_3 is pyramidal

31. Amongst LiCl, RbCl, $BeCl_2$ and $MgCl_2$ the compounds with the greatest and the least ionic character, respectively are:
(a) LiCl and RbCl (b) RbCl and $BeCl_2$
(c) $MgCl_2$ and $BeCl_2$ (d) RbCl and $MgCl_2$

32. Which of the following is the wrong statement ?
(a) ONCl and ONO^- are not isoelectronic.
(b) O_3 molecule is bent
(c) Ozone is violet-black in solid state
(d) Ozone is paramagnetic gas.

33. For which of the following molecule significant $\mu \neq 0$?

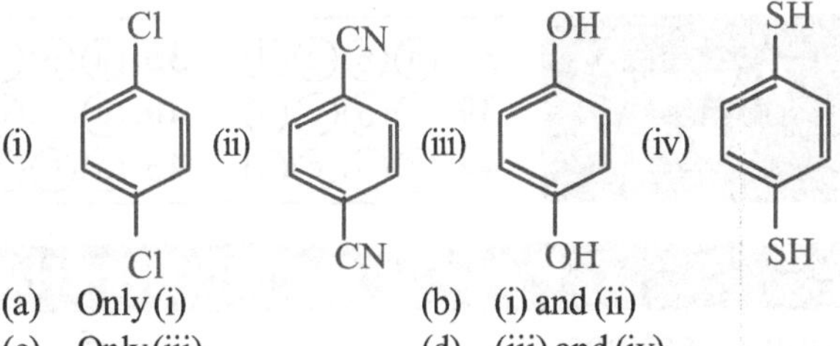

(a) Only (i) (b) (i) and (ii)
(c) Only (iii) (d) (iii) and (iv)

RESPONSE GRID					
	22. ⓐⓑⓒⓓ	23. ⓐⓑⓒⓓ	24. ⓐⓑⓒⓓ	25. ⓐⓑⓒⓓ	26. ⓐⓑⓒⓓ
	27. ⓐⓑⓒⓓ	28. ⓐⓑⓒⓓ	29. ⓐⓑⓒⓓ	30. ⓐⓑⓒⓓ	31. ⓐⓑⓒⓓ
	32. ⓐⓑⓒⓓ	33. ⓐⓑⓒⓓ			

Space for Rough Work

34. The bond dissociation energy of B – F in BF_3 is 646 kJ mol^{-1} whereas that of C – F in CF_4 is 515 kJ mol^{-1}. The correct reason for higher B – F bond dissociation energy as compared to that of C – F is
(a) stronger σ bond between B and F in BF_3 as compared to that between C and F in CF_4.
(b) significant pπ – pπ interaction between B and F in BF_3 whereas there is no possibility of such interaction between C and F in CF_4.
(c) lower degree of pπ – pπ interaction between B and F in BF_3 than that between C and F in CF_4.
(d) smaller size of B– atom as compared to that of C– atom.

35. Dipole-induced dipole interactions are present in which of the following pairs :
(a) Cl_2 and CCl_4 (b) HCl and He atoms
(c) SiF_4 and He atoms (d) H_2O and alcohol

36. The number and type of bonds in C_2^{2-} ion in CaC_2 are:
(a) One σ bond and one π-bond
(b) One σ bond and two π-bond
(c) Two σ bond and two π-bond
(d) Two σ bond and one π-bond

37. Which of the following methods is used for measuring bond length ?
(a) X-ray diffraction
(b) Electron-diffraction
(c) Spectroscopic techniques
(d) All of these

38. Which of the following molecules have same bond order ?

H_2, Cl_2, CO, Br_2, N_2
I II III IV V

Choose the correct option.
(a) I, II and IV have same bond order
(b) III and V have same bond order
(c) Both (a) and (b) are correct
(d) None of the above

39. Which of the following is/are misconception(s) associated with resonance ?
(i) The molecule exists for a certain fraction of time in one cannonical form and for other fractions of time in other cannonical forms.
(ii) The cannonical forms have no real existence.
(iii) There is no such equilibrium between the cannonical forms.
(a) (i) only (b) (ii) and (iii)
(c) (i) and (iii) (d) (iii) only.

40. A neutral molecule XF_3 has a zero dipole moment. The element X is most likely
(a) chlorine (b) boron
(c) nitrogen (d) carbon

41. The species having pyramidal shape is :
(a) SO_3 (b) BrF_3 (c) SiO_3^{2-} (d) OSF_2

42. Bond order of 1.5 is shown by :
(a) O_2^+ (b) O_2^- (c) O_2^{2-} (d) O_2

43. Which one of the following properties is **not** shown by NO?
(a) It is diamagnetic in gaseous state
(b) It is neutral oxide
(c) It combines with oxygen to form nitrogen dioxide
(d) It's bond order is 2.5

44. The charge/size ratio of a cation determines its polarizing power. Which one of the following sequences represents the increasing order of the polarizing power of the cationic species, K^+, Ca^{2+}, Mg^{2+}, Be^{2+}?
(a) $Ca^{2+} < Mg^{2+} < Be^{+} < K^{+}$
(b) $Mg^{2+} < Be^{2+} < K^{+} < Ca^{2+}$
(c) $Be^{2+} < K^{+} < Ca^{2+} < Mg^{2+}$
(d) $K^{+} < Ca^{2+} < Mg^{2+} < Be^{2+}$.

45. In which of the following pairs of molecules/ions, both the species are not likely to exist ?
(a) H_2^+, He_2^{2-} (b) H_2^-, He_2^{2-}
(c) H_2^{2+}, He_2 (d) H_2^-, He_2^{2+}

RESPONSE GRID				
34. ⓐⓑⓒⓓ	35. ⓐⓑⓒⓓ	36. ⓐⓑⓒⓓ	37. ⓐⓑⓒⓓ	38. ⓐⓑⓒⓓ
39. ⓐⓑⓒⓓ	40. ⓐⓑⓒⓓ	41. ⓐⓑⓒⓓ	42. ⓐⓑⓒⓓ	43. ⓐⓑⓒⓓ
44. ⓐⓑⓒⓓ	45. ⓐⓑⓒⓓ			

CHEMISTRY CHAPTERWISE SPEED TEST-32

Total Questions	45	Total Marks	180
Attempted		Correct	
Incorrect		Net Score	
Cut-off Score	38	Qualifying Score	60
Success Gap = Net Score – Qualifying Score			
Net Score = (Correct × 4) – (Incorrect × 1)			

Space for Rough Work

CHEMISTRY

States of Matter

Speed TEST 33

Chapter-wise

No. of Questions	Maximum Marks	Time
45	180	1 Hour

GENERAL INSTRUCTIONS

- This test contains 45 MCQ's. For each question only one option is correct. Darken the correct circle/ bubble in the Response Grid provided on each page.
- You have to evaluate your Response Grids yourself with the help of solutions provided at the end of this book.
- Each correct answer will get you 4 marks and 1 mark shall be deduced for each incorrect answer. No mark will be given/ deducted if no bubble is filled. Keep a timer in front of you and stop immediately at the end of 60 min.
- The sheet follows a particular syllabus. Do not attempt the sheet before you have completed your preparation for that syllabus.
- After completing the sheet check your answers with the solution booklet and complete the Result Grid. Finally spend time to analyse your performance and revise the areas which emerge out as weak in your evaluation.

1. A compound exists in the gaseous state both as monomer A and dimer A_2. The M. wt. of monomer is 48. In an experiment 96 g of the compound was confined in vessel of 33.6 L and heated to 273 °C. Calculate the pressure developed, if the compound exists as a dimer to the extent of 50% by weight under the conditions
(a) 0.9 atm (b) 4.0 atm (c) 2.0 atm (d) 1.0 atm

2. The molecular velocities of two gases at the same temperature are u_1 and u_2 and their masses are m_1 and m_2 respectively. Which of the following expressions are correct ?
(a) $\frac{m_1}{u_1^2}=\frac{m_2}{u_2^2}$ (b) $m_1u_1=m_2u_2$
(c) $\frac{m_1}{u_1}=\frac{m_2}{u_2}$ (d) $m_1u_1^2=m_2u_2^2$

3. A container contains certain gas of mass 'm' at high pressure. Some of the gas has been allowed to escape from the container and after some time the pressure of the gas becomes half and its absolute temperature 2/3rd. The amount of the gas escaped is
(a) 2/3 m (b) 1/2 m (c) 1/4 m (d) 1/6 m

4. Let the most probable velocity of hydrogen molecules at a temperature of t° C be V_0. When the temperature is raised to (2t + 273)°C the new rms velocity is (suppose all the molecules dissociate into atoms at latter temperature)
(a) $2\sqrt{3}V_0$ (b) $\sqrt{6}V_0$
(c) $\sqrt{3\left(2+\frac{273}{t}\right)}V_0$ (d) $\sqrt{\frac{2}{3}}V_0$

5. By what factor does the average velocity of a gaseous molecule increase when the temperature (in Kelvin) is doubled ?
(a) 2.0 (b) 2.8
(c) 4.0 (d) 1.4

6. The correct value of the gas constant 'R' is close to :
(a) 0.082 litre-atmosphere K
(b) 0.082 litre-atmosphere $K^{-1}mol^{-1}$
(c) 0.082 litre – $atmosphere^{-1}$ K mol^{-1}
(d) 0.082 $litre^{-1}$ $atmosphere^{-1}$ K mol

7. If 10^{-4} dm^3 of water is introduced into a 1.0 dm^3 flask at 300 K, how many moles of water are in the vapour phase when equilibrium is established ?
(Given : Vapour pressure of H_2O at 300 K is 3170 Pa; $R = 8.314$ J K^{-1} mol^{-1})
(a) 5.56× 10^{-3} mole (b) 1.53 × 10^{-2} mole
(c) 4.46× 10^{-2} mole (d) 1.27 × 10^{-3} mole

RESPONSE GRID	
	1. ⓐⓑⓒⓓ 2. ⓐⓑⓒⓓ 3. ⓐⓑⓒⓓ 4. ⓐⓑⓒⓓ 5. ⓐⓑⓒⓓ
	6. ⓐⓑⓒⓓ 7. ⓐⓑⓒⓓ

Space for Rough Work

8. A vessel is filled with a mixture of O_2 and N_2. At what ratio of partial pressures will be the mass of gases be identical

(a) $P_{(O_2)} = 8.75\, P_{(N_2)}$ (b) $P_{(O_2)} = 0.78\, P_{(N_2)}$

(c) $P_{(O_2)} = 0.875\, P_{(N_2)}$ (d) $P_{(O_2)} = 11.4\, P_{(N_2)}$

9. Helium has the van der Waal's constant $b = 24 \text{ mL mol}^{-1}$. The molecular diameter of helium will be

(a) 267 pm
(b) 133.5 pm
(c) 26.7 pm
(d) Data not sufficient for calculation the diameter.

10. A bubble of the gas released at the bottom of a lake increases to eight times the original volume when it reaches at the surface. Assuming that the atmospheric pressure is equivalent to pressure exerted by a column of water 10 m high, what is the depth of the lake

(a) 80 m (b) 90 m (c) 10 m (d) 70 m

11. Air at sea level is dense. This is a practical application of

(a) Boyle's law (b) Charle's law
(c) Kelvin's law (d) Brown's law

12. Which of the following represents Gay Lussac's law ?

I. $\frac{P}{T} = \text{constant}$ II. $P_1T_2 = P_2T_1$

III. $P_1V_1 = P_2V_2$

Choose the correct option.

(a) I, II and III (b) II and III
(c) I and III (d) I and II

13. A bubble of air is underwater at temperature 15°C and the pressure 1.5 bar. If the bubble rises to the surface where the temperature is 25°C and the pressure is 1.0 bar, what will happen to the volume of the bubble ?

(a) Volume will become greater by a factor of 1.6.
(b) Volume will become greater by a factor of 1.1.
(c) Volume will become smaller by a factor of 0.70.
(d) Volume will become greater by a factor of 2.5.

14. When *r*, *P* and *M* represent rate of diffusion, pressure and molecular mass, respectively, then the ratio of the rates of diffusion (r_A / r_B) of two gases *A* and *B*, is given as :

(a) $(P_A/P_B)(M_B/M_A)^{1/2}$ (b) $(P_A/P_B)^{1/2}(M_B/M_A)$

(c) $(P_A/P_B)(M_A/M_B)^{1/2}$ (d) $(P_A/P_B)^{1/2}(M_A/M_B)$

15. Longest mean free path stands for :

(a) H_2 (b) N_2 (c) O_2 (d) Cl_2

16. The root mean square velocity of an ideal gas at constant pressure varies with density (d) as

(a) d^2 (b) d (c) $\sqrt{d}$ (d) $1/\sqrt{d}$

17. The correct order of viscosity of the following liquids will be

(a) Water < methyl alcohol < dimethyl ether < glycerol
(b) methyl alcohol < glycerol < water < dimethyl ether
(c) dimethyl ether < methyl alcohol < water < glycerol
(d) glycerol < dimethyl ether < water < methyl alcohol

18. The molecular velocity of any gas is

(a) inversely proportional to absolute temperature.
(b) directly proportional to square of temperature.
(c) directly proportional to square root of temperature.
(d) inversely proportional to the square root of temperature.

19. Which of the following volume (V) - temperature (T) plots represents the behaviour of one mole of an ideal gas at one atmospheric pressure ?

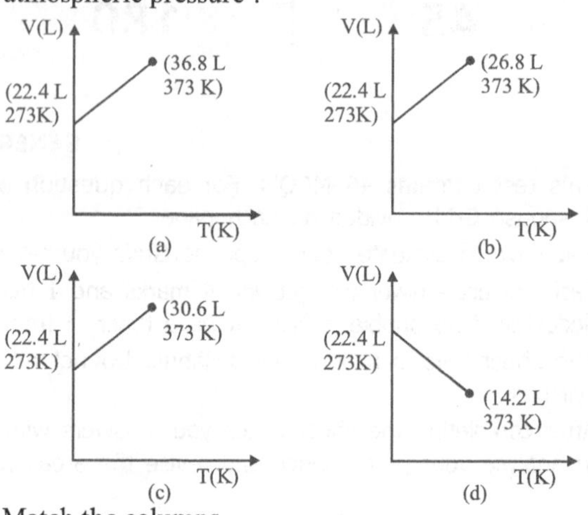

20. Match the columns

	Column-I		Column-II
A.	Boyle's law	I.	$V \propto n$ at constant T and P
B.	Charle's law	II.	$p_{total} = p_1 + p_2 + p_3 + \ldots$ at constant T, V
C.	Dalton's law	III.	$\frac{pV}{T} = \text{Constant}$
D.	Avogadro law	IV.	$V \propto T$ at constant n and p
		V.	$p \propto \frac{1}{V}$ at constant n and T

(a) A – V; B – IV; C – II; D – I
(b) A – IV; B – II; C – I; D – V
(c) A – III; B – V; C – II; D – I
(d) A – V; B – II; C – IV; D – III

21. The rms velocity of hydrogen is $\sqrt{7}$ times the rms velocity of nitrogen. If T is the temperature of the gas, then

(a) $T(H_2) = T(N_2)$ (b) $T(H_2) > T(N_2)$

(c) $T(H_2) < T(N_2)$ (d) $T(H_2) = \sqrt{7}\, T(N_2)$

22. If Z is a compressibility factor, van der Waals equation at low pressure can be written as:

(a) $Z = 1 + \frac{RT}{Pb}$ (b) $Z = 1 - \frac{a}{VRT}$

(c) $Z = 1 - \frac{Pb}{RT}$ (d) $Z = 1 + \frac{Pb}{RT}$

RESPONSE GRID					
	8. ⓐⓑⓒⓓ	9. ⓐⓑⓒⓓ	10. ⓐⓑⓒⓓ	11. ⓐⓑⓒⓓ	12. ⓐⓑⓒⓓ
	13. ⓐⓑⓒⓓ	14. ⓐⓑⓒⓓ	15. ⓐⓑⓒⓓ	16. ⓐⓑⓒⓓ	17. ⓐⓑⓒⓓ
	18. ⓐⓑⓒⓓ	19. ⓐⓑⓒⓓ	20. ⓐⓑⓒⓓ	21. ⓐⓑⓒⓓ	22. ⓐⓑⓒⓓ

Space for Rough Work

23. Refer to the figure given :
Which of the following statements is wrong?

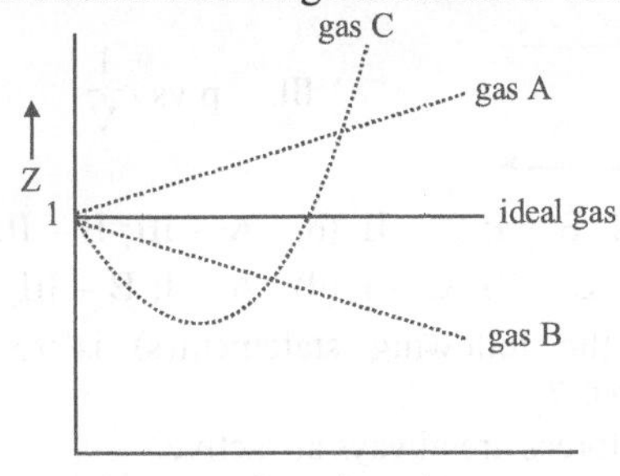

(a) For gas A, $a = 0$ and Z will linearly depend on pressure
(b) For gas B, $b = 0$ and Z will linearly depend on pressure
(c) Gas C is a real gas and we can find 'a' and 'b' if intersection data is given
(d) All van der Waal gases will behave like gas C and give positive slope at high pressure

24. Equal masses of H_2,O_2 and methane have been taken in a container of volume V at temperature 27°C in identical conditions. The ratio of the volumes of gases $H_2 : O_2$: methane would be :
(a) 8 : 16 : 1 (b) 16 : 8 : 1 (c) 16 : 1 : 2 (d) 8 : 1 : 2

25. Which one of the following statements is NOT true about the effect of an increase in temperature on the distribution of molecular speeds in a gas?
(a) The area under the distribution curve remains the same as under the lower temperature
(b) The distribution becomes broader
(c) The fraction of the molecules with the most probable speed increases
(d) The most probable speed increases

26. As the temperature is raised from 20°C to 40°C, the average kinetic energy of neon atoms changes by a factor of which of the following ?
(a) 313/293 (b) $\sqrt{(313/293)}$
(c) 1/2 (d) 2

27. The ratio between the root mean square speed of H_2 at 50 K and that of O_2 at 800 K is,
(a) 4 (b) 2 (c) 1 (d) 1/4

28. Positive deviation from ideal behaviour takes place because of
(a) Molecular interaction between atoms and $PV/nRT > 1$
(b) Molecular interaction between atoms and $PV/nRT < 1$
(c) Finite size of atoms and $PV/nRT > 1$
(d) Finite size of atoms and $PV/nRT < 1$

29. Equal masses of methane and oxygen are mixed in an empty container at 25°C. The fraction of the total pressure exerted by oxygen is
(a) 1/2 (b) 2/3 (c) $\frac{1}{3} \times \frac{273}{298}$ (d) 1/3.

30. The rate of diffusion of SO_2, CO_2, PCl_3 and SO_3 are in the following order
(a) $PCl_3 > SO_3 > SO_2 > CO_2$ (b) $CO_2 > SO_2 > PCl_3 > SO_3$
(c) $SO_2 > SO_3 > PCl_3 > CO_2$ (d) $CO_2 > SO_2 > SO_3 > PCl_3$

31. The van der Waal's equation for n = 1 mole may be expressed as $V^3 - \left(b + \frac{RT}{P}\right)V^2 + \frac{aV}{P} - \frac{ab}{P} = 0$
Where V is the molar volume of the gas. Which of the following is correct?
(a) For a temperature less than T_c, V has three real roots
(b) For a temperature more than T_c, V has one real and two imaginary roots
(c) For a temperature equal to T_c all three roots of V are real and identical
(d) All of these

32. By how many folds the temperature of a gas would increase when the root mean square velocity of the gas molecules in a container of fixed volume is increased from 5×10^4 cm/s to 10×10^4 cm/s ?
(a) Two (b) Three (c) Six (d) Four

33. The density of neon will be highest at
(a) S.T.P. (b) 0 °C, 2 atm
(c) 273 °C, 1 atm. (d) 273 °C, 2 atm.

34. Above Boyle point, real gases show ____X____ from ideality and Z values are ____Y____ than one.
(a) X = Negative deviation, Y = Less
(b) X = Negative deviation, Y = Greater
(c) X = Positive deviation, Y = Less
(d) X = Positive deviation, Y = Greater

35. Induced dipole moment depend upon the
I. dipole moment present in the permanent dipole.
II polarisability of the electrically neutral molecules.
Identify the correct option.
(a) I is correct but II is wrong
(b) I is wrong and II is correct
(c) Both I and II are wrong
(d) Both I and II are correct

36. Following table represents critical temperature of some gases. Arrange these gases in their increasing order of liquification.

Gas	T_c / K
H_2	33.2
He	5.3
N_2	126
O_2	154.3

(a) $He < N_2 < H_2 < O_2$ (b) $H_2 < He < N_2 < O_2$
(c) $He < H_2 < N_2 < O_2$ (d) $O_2 < N_2 < H_2 < He$

RESPONSE GRID					
	23. ⓐⓑⓒⓓ	24. ⓐⓑⓒⓓ	25. ⓐⓑⓒⓓ	26. ⓐⓑⓒⓓ	27. ⓐⓑⓒⓓ
	28. ⓐⓑⓒⓓ	29. ⓐⓑⓒⓓ	30. ⓐⓑⓒⓓ	31. ⓐⓑⓒⓓ	32. ⓐⓑⓒⓓ
	33. ⓐⓑⓒⓓ	34. ⓐⓑⓒⓓ	35. ⓐⓑⓒⓓ	36. ⓐⓑⓒⓓ	

Space for Rough Work

37. Which of the following liquid will exhibit highest vapour pressure?

(a) $C_2H_5OH(l)$ (b) $NH_3(l)$
(c) $HF(l)$ (d) $H_2O(l)$

38. Generally, liquid drops assume spherical shape because:

(a) a sphere has maximum surface area
(b) a sphere has minimum surface area
(c) sphere is symmetrical in shape
(d) None of these

39. Internal energy and pressure of a gas per unit volume are related as :

(a) $P=\frac{2}{3}E$ (b) $P=\frac{3}{2}E$ (c) $P=\frac{1}{2}E$ (d) $P=2E$

40. Two vessels containing gases A and B are interconected as shown in the figure. The stopper is opened, the gases are allowed to mix homogeneously. The partial pressures of A and B in the mixture will be, respectively

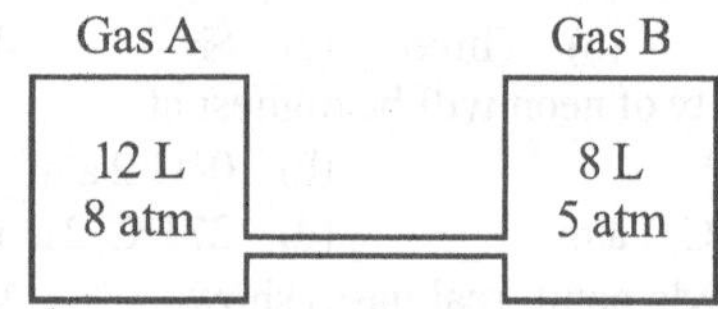

(a) 8 and 5 atom (b) 9.6 and 4 atm
(c) 4.8 and 2 atm (d) 6.4 and 4 atm

41. Match the following graphs of ideal gas (Column-I) with their co-ordinates (Column-II) :

Column-I (Graphical representation)	**Column-II (x and y co-ordinates)**
A.	I. pV vs. V
B.	II. p vs. V
C.	III. p vs. $\frac{1}{V}$

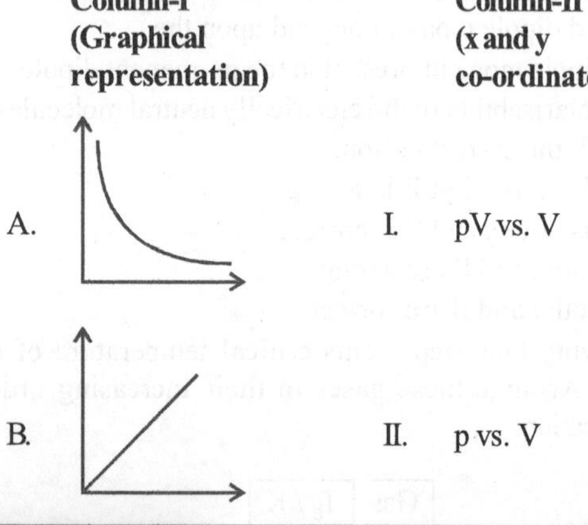

(a) A – III; B – I; C – II (b) A – III; B – II; C – I
(c) A – II; B – III; C – I (d) A – I; B – III; C – II

42. Which of the following statement(s) is/are true for London force ?

(i) These forces are always attractive.
(ii) These forces are important for long distance too.
(iii) Their magnitude depends on the polarisability of the particle.

(a) (i) and (ii) (b) (i) only
(c) (iii) only (d) (i) and (iii)

43. Kinetic theory of gases presumes that the collisions between the molecules to be perfectly elastic because

(a) the gas molecules are tiny particles and not rigid in nature
(b) the temperature remains constant irrespective of collision
(c) collision will not split the molecules
(d) the molecules are large particle and rigid in nature

44. Which of the following statements are correct ?

(i) Real gases show deviations from ideal gas law because molecules interact with each other.
(ii) Due to interaction of molecules the pressure exerted by the gas is given as :

$$p_{real} = p_{ideal} + \frac{an^2}{V^2}$$

(iii) Value of 'a' is measure of magnitude of intermolecular attractive forces within the gas and depends on temperature and pressure of gas.
(iv) At high pressure volume occupied by the molecules also becomes significant because instead of moving in volume *V*, these are now restricted to volume (*V-nb*)

(a) (i) and (iv) (b) (i), (ii) and (iii)
(c) (i), (iii) and (iv) (d) (i) and (iii)

45. The units of constant *a* in van der Waal's equation is

(a) $dm^6\,atm\,mol^{-2}$ (b) $dm^3\,atm\,mol^{-1}$
(c) $dm\,atm\,mol^{-1}$ (d) $atm\,mol^{-1}$

RESPONSE GRID					
	37. ⓐⓑⓒⓓ	38. ⓐⓑⓒⓓ	39. ⓐⓑⓒⓓ	40. ⓐⓑⓒⓓ	41. ⓐⓑⓒⓓ
	42. ⓐⓑⓒⓓ	43. ⓐⓑⓒⓓ	44. ⓐⓑⓒⓓ	45. ⓐⓑⓒⓓ	

CHEMISTRY CHAPTERWISE SPEED TEST-33			
Total Questions	45	Total Marks	180
Attempted		Correct	
Incorrect		Net Score	
Cut-off Score	36	Qualifying Score	58
Success Gap = Net Score – Qualifying Score			
Net Score = (Correct × 4) – (Incorrect × 1)			

Space for Rough Work

CHEMISTRY

Thermodynamics

Speed TEST 34

Chapter-wise

No. of Questions	Maximum Marks	Time
45	180	1 Hour

GENERAL INSTRUCTIONS

- This test contains 45 MCQ's. For each question only one option is correct. Darken the correct circle/ bubble in the Response Grid provided on each page.
- You have to evaluate your Response Grids yourself with the help of solutions provided at the end of this book.
- Each correct answer will get you 4 marks and 1 mark shall be deduced for each incorrect answer. No mark will be given/ deducted if no bubble is filled. Keep a timer in front of you and stop immediately at the end of 60 min.
- The sheet follows a particular syllabus. Do not attempt the sheet before you have completed your preparation for that syllabus.
- After completing the sheet check your answers with the solution booklet and complete the Result Grid. Finally spend time to analyse your performance and revise the areas which emerge out as weak in your evaluation.

1. In a closed insulated container a liquid is stirred with a paddle to increase the temperature. Which of the following is true?
   (a) $\Delta E = W \neq 0$ (b) $\Delta E = W, q = 0$
   (c) $\Delta E = 0, W = q \neq 0$ (d) $W = 0, \Delta W = q \neq 0$
2. One mole of a non-ideal gas undergoes a change of state (2.0 atm, 3.0 L, 95 K) $\rightarrow$ (4.0 atm, 5.0 L, 245 K) with a change in internal energy, $\Delta U = 30.0$ L atm. The change in enthalpy ΔH of the process in L atm is.
   (a) 40.0 (b) 42.3
   (c) 44.0 (d) Not defined because pressure is not constant
3. Assuming that water vapour is an ideal gas, the internal energy change (ΔU) when 1 mol of water is vapourised at 1 bar pressure and 100°C, (given : molar enthalpy of vapourisation of water at 1 bar and 373 K = 41 kJ mol^{-1} and R = 8.3 J mol^{-1} K^{-1}) will be
   (a) 41.00 kJ mol^{-1} (b) 4.100 kJ mol^{-1}
   (c) 3.7904 kJ mol^{-1} (d) 37.904 kJ mol^{-1}
4. A piston filled with 0.04 mole of an ideal gas expands reversibly from 50.0 mL to 375 mL at a constant temperature of 37.0ºC. As it does so, it absorbs 208 J of heat. The values of q and w for the process will be:
   (R = 8.314 J/mol K) (ln 7.5 = 2.01)
   (a) q = + 208 J, w = – 208 J (b) q = – 208 J, w = – 208 J
   (c) q = – 208 J, w = + 208 J (d) q = + 208 J, w = + 208 J
5. Among the following, the intensive property is (properties are)
   (a) molar conductivity (b) electromotive force
   (c) resistance (d) heat capacity
6. The variation of heat of reaction with temperature is given by:
   (a) Van't Hoff equation
   (b) Clausius- Clapeyron equation
   (c) Nernst equation
   (d) Kirchoff's equation
7. The difference between heats of reaction at constant pressure and constant volume for the reaction :
   $2\,C_6H_6(l) + 15O_2(g) \rightarrow 12CO_2(g) + 6H_2O(l)$ at 25ºC in kJ is
   (a) –7.43 (b) +3.72
   (c) –3.72 (d) +7.43
8. The enthalpy of vapourisation of water from the following two equations is.
   $$H_2(g) + \frac{1}{2}O_2(g) \longrightarrow H_2O\,(l),\ \Delta H = -286\,kJ$$
   $$H_2\,(g) + \frac{1}{2}O_2\,(g), \rightarrow H_2O\,(g),\ \Delta H = -245.5\,kJ$$
   (a) 6.02 kJ (b) 40.5 kJ (c) 62.3 kJ (d) 1.25 kJ
9. For complete combustion of ethanol,
   $C_2H_5OH(l) + 3O_2(g) \longrightarrow 2CO_2(g) + 3H_2O(l)$,
   the amount of heat produced as measured in bomb calorimeter, is 1364.47 kJ mol^{-1} at 25ºC. Assuming ideality the enthalpy of combustion, Δ_cH, for the reaction will be: (R = 8.314 kJ mol^{-1})
   (a) –1366.95 kJ mol^{-1} (b) –1361.95 kJ mol^{-1}
   (c) –1460.95 kJ mol^{-1} (d) –1350.50 kJ mol^{-1}

RESPONSE GRID					
	1. ⓐⓑⓒⓓ	2. ⓐⓑⓒⓓ	3. ⓐⓑⓒⓓ	4. ⓐⓑⓒⓓ	5. ⓐⓑⓒⓓ
	6. ⓐⓑⓒⓓ	7. ⓐⓑⓒⓓ	8. ⓐⓑⓒⓓ	9. ⓐⓑⓒⓓ	

Space for Rough Work

10. The direct conversion of A to B is difficult, hence it is carried out by the following shown path :

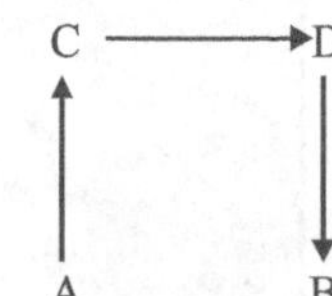

Given

$\Delta S_{(A \to C)} = 50$ e.u., $\Delta S_{(C \to D)} = 30$ e.u., $\Delta S_{(B \to D)} = 20$ e.u., where e.u. is the entropy unit, then $\Delta S_{(A \to B)}$ is

(a) +60 e.u. (b) +100 e.u. (c) –60 e.u. (d) –100 e.u.

11. The heat of combustion of CH_4(g), C (graphite), H_2(g) are –20 kcal, –40 kcal –10 kcal respectively. The heat of formation of methane is

(a) –40 kcal (b) +40 kcal (c) –80.0 kcal (d) +80 kcal

12. From the following bond energies:

H–H bond energy: 431.37 kJ mol^{-1}

C=C bond energy: 606.10 kJ mol^{-1}

C–C bond energy: 336.49 kJ mol^{-1}

C–H bond energy: 410.50 kJ mol^{-1}

Enthalpy for the reaction,

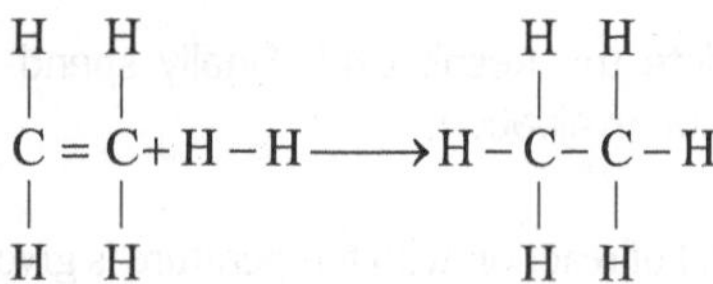

will be:

(a) –243.6 kJ mol^{-1} (b) –120.0 kJ mol^{-1}

(c) 553.0 kJ mol^{-1} (d) 1523.6 kJ mol^{-1}

13. The favourable conditions for a spontaneous reaction are

(a) $T\Delta S > \Delta H$, $\Delta H = +ve$, $\Delta S = +ve$

(b) $T\Delta S > \Delta H$, $\Delta H = +ve$, $\Delta S = -ve$

(c) $T\Delta S = \Delta H$, $\Delta H = -ve$, $\Delta S = -ve$

(d) $T\Delta S = \Delta H$, $\Delta H = +ve$, $\Delta S = +ve$

14. For which change $\Delta H \neq \Delta E$:

(a) $H_2(g) + I_2(g) \to 2HI(g)$ (b) $HCl + NaOH \to NaCl$

(c) $C(s) + O_2(g) \to CO_2(g)$ (d) $N_2(g) + 3H_2(g) \to 2NH_3(g)$

15. The species which by definition has **ZERO** standard molar enthalpy of formation at 298 K is

(a) Br_2 (g) (b) Cl_2 (g) (c) H_2O (g) (d) CH_4 (g)

16. For which of the following process, ΔS is negative?

(a) $H_2(g) \to 2H(g)$

(b) $N_2(g)(1atm) \to N_2(g)(8atm)$

(c) $2SO_3(g) \to 2SO_2(g) + O_2(g)$

(d) $C_{(diamond)} \to C_{(graphite)}$

17. Given the following entropy values (in JK^{-1} mol^{-1}) at 298 K and 1 atm :

H_2(g) : 130.6, Cl_2(g) : 223.0 and HCl (g) : 186.7. The entropy change (in JK^{-1} mol^{-1}) for the reaction

$H_2(g) + Cl_2(g) \to 2HCl(g)$ is

(a) +540.3 (b) 727.0 (c) –166.9 (d) 19.8

18. In conversion of lime-stone to lime,

$CaCO_3(s) \to CaO(s) + CO_2(g)$ the values of $\Delta H°$ and $\Delta S°$ are + 179.1 kJ mol^{-1} and 160.2 J/K respectively at 298 K and 1 bar. Assuming that $\Delta H°$ and $\Delta S°$ do not change with temperature, temperature above which conversion of lime-stone to lime will be spontaneous is

(a) 1118 K (b) 1008 K (c) 1200 K (d) 845 K.

19. $(\Delta H - \Delta U)$ for the formation of carbon monoxide (CO) from its elements at 298 K is

(R = 8.314 JK^{-1} mol^{-1})

(a) –2477.57 J mol^{-1} (b) 2477.57 J mol^{-1}

(c) –1238.78 J mol^{-1} (d) 1238.78 J mol^{-1}

20. The incorrect expression among the following is :

(a) $\dfrac{\Delta G_{system}}{\Delta S_{total}} = -T$

(b) In isothermal process, $w_{reversible} = -nRT \ \ell n \dfrac{V_f}{V_i}$

(c) $\ln K = \dfrac{\Delta H° - T\Delta S°}{RT}$

(d) $K = e^{-\Delta G°/RT}$

21. The following two reactions are known :

$Fe_2O_3(s) + 3CO(g) \longrightarrow 2Fe(s) + 3CO_2(g)$; $\Delta H = -26.8$ kJ

$FeO(s) + CO(g) \longrightarrow Fe(s) + CO_2(g)$; $\Delta H = -16.5$ kJ

The value of ΔH for the following reaction

$Fe_2O_3(s) + CO(g) \longrightarrow 2FeO(s) + CO_2(g)$ is;

(a) +6.2 kJ (b) +10.3 kJ (c) –43.3 kJ (d) –10.3 kJ

22. For a particular reversible reaction at temperature T, ΔH and ΔS were found to be both +ve. If T_e is the temperature at equilibrium, the reaction would be spontaneous when

(a) $T_e > T$ (b) $T > T_e$

(c) T_e is 5 times T (d) $T = T_e$

23. The standard enthalpy of formation of NH_3 is –46.0 kJ mol^{-1}. If the enthalpy of formation of H_2 from its atoms is –436 kJ mol^{-1} and that of N_2 is –712 kJ mol^{-1}, the average bond enthalpy of N – H bond in NH_3 is

(a) –964 kJ mol^{-1} (b) +352 kJ mol^{-1}

(c) +1056 kJ mol^{-1} (d) –1102 kJ mol^{-1}

RESPONSE GRID					
	10. ⓐⓑⓒⓓ	11. ⓐⓑⓒⓓ	12. ⓐⓑⓒⓓ	13. ⓐⓑⓒⓓ	14. ⓐⓑⓒⓓ
	15. ⓐⓑⓒⓓ	16. ⓐⓑⓒⓓ	17. ⓐⓑⓒⓓ	18. ⓐⓑⓒⓓ	19. ⓐⓑⓒⓓ
	20. ⓐⓑⓒⓓ	21. ⓐⓑⓒⓓ	22. ⓐⓑⓒⓓ	23. ⓐⓑⓒⓓ	

Space for Rough Work

24. Standard entropy of X_2, Y_2 and XY_3 are 60, 40 and 50 $J K^{-1} mol^{-1}$, respectively. For the reaction, $\frac{1}{2}X_2 + \frac{3}{2}Y_2 \rightarrow XY_3, \Delta H = -30 kJ$, to be at equilibrium, the temperature will be

(a) 1250K (b) 500K (c) 750K (d) 1000K

25. A heat engine abosrbs heat Q_1 at temperature T_1 and heat Q_2 at temperature T_2. Work done by the engine is J $(Q_1 + Q_2)$. This data

(a) violates 1st law of thermodynamics
(b) violates 1st law of themodynamics if Q_1 is –ve
(c) violates 1st law of thermodynamics of Q_2 is –ve
(d) does not violate 1st law of themodynamics.

26. The standard enthalpies of formation of $CO_2(g)$, $H_2O(l)$ and glucose(s) at 25°C are –400 kJ/mol, –300 kJ/mol and –1300 kJ/mol, respectively. The standard enthalpy of combustion per gram of glucose at 25°C is

(a) +2900 kJ (b) –2900 kJ (c) –16.11 kJ (d) +16.11 kJ

27. Using the data provided, calculate the multiple bond energy ($kJ mol^{-1}$) of a $C \equiv C$ bond in C_2H_2. That energy is (take the bond energy of a C – H bond as 350 $kJ mol^{-1}$)

$2C(s) + H_2(g) \longrightarrow HC \equiv CH(g); \quad \Delta H = 225 \, kJ \, mol^{-1}$
$2C(s) \longrightarrow 2C(g); \Delta H = 1410 \, kJ \, mol^{-1}$
$H_2(g) \longrightarrow 2H(g); \Delta H = 330 \, kJ \, mol^{-1}$

(a) 1165 (b) 837 (c) 865 (d) 815

28. The enthalpy of neutralisation of NH_4OH and CH_3COOH is – 10.5 kcal mol^{-1} and enthalpy of neutralisation of CH_3COOH with strong base is – 12.5 kcal mol^{-1}. The enthalpy of ionisation of NH_4OH will be

(a) 3.2 kcal mol^{-1} (b) 2.0 kcal mol^{-1}
(c) 3.0 kcal mol^{-1} (d) 4.0 kcal mol^{-1}

29. The enthalpy change of formation of $CO_2(g)$ is – 393 $kJmol^{-1}$ and that of H_2O (l) is – 286 $kJmol^{-1}$. The enthalpy of combustion of one mole of ethanol (C_2H_5OH) is –1360. The enthalpy change for the formation of one mole of ethanol form its constituent elements is

(a) –681 kJ (b) –284 kJ (c) +965 kJ (d) 1360 kJ

30. The lattice energy of solid NaCl is 180 kcal mol^{-1} and enthalpy of solution is 1 kcal mol^{-1}. If the hydration energies of Na^+ and Cl^- ions are in the ratio 3 : 2, what is the enthalpy of hydration of sodium ion ?

(a) – 107.4 kcal mol^{-1} (b) 107.4 kcal mol^{-1}
(c) 71.6 kcal mol^{-1} (d) – 71.6 kcal mol^{-1}

31. A certain reaction is non spontaneous at 298K. The entropy change during the reaction is 121 JK^{-1}. If the reaction is endothermic or exothermic, the minimum value of ΔH for the reaction is

(a) endothermic, ΔH = 36.06 kJ
(b) exothermic, ΔH = – 36.06 kJ
(c) endothermic, ΔH = 60.12 kJ
(d) exothermic, ΔH = – 60.12 kJ

32. Which of the following statement is incorrect ?

(a) The standard enthalpy of reaction is the enthalpy change for a reaction when all the participating substances are in their standard states.
(b) The standard state of a substance at a specified temperature is its pure form at 1 bar.
(c) The standard state of solid iron at 298 K is pure iron at 1 bar
(d) Standard conditions are denoted by adding the superscript ⦵ to the symbol ΔH e.g., –ΔH⦵

33. Match the columns

	Column-I		Column-II
A.	Exothermic	I.	ΔH = 0, ΔE = 0
B.	Spontaneous	II.	ΔG = 0
C.	Cyclic process	III.	ΔH is negative
D.	Equilibrium	IV.	ΔG is negative

(a) A – II; B – III; C – I; D – IV
(b) A – IV; B – I; C – III; D – II
(c) A – I; B – II; C – IV; D – III
(d) A – III; B – IV; C – I; D – II

34. The ΔH at 358 K for the reaction

$$Fe_2O_3(s) + 3H_2(g) \longrightarrow 2Fe(s) + 3H_2O(l)$$

given that $\Delta H_{298} = -33.29 \, kJ mol^{-1}$ and C_p for $Fe_2O_3(s)$, Fe(s), H_2O (l) and H_2 (g) and 103.8, 25.1, 75.3 and 28.8 J/K mol

(a) –28.136 kJ mol^{-1} (b) – 38.3 kJ mol^{-1}
(c) 42.5 kJ mol^{-1} (d) 56.2 kJ mol^{-1}

35. The enthalpy of neutralisation of a weak acid in 1 M solution with a strong base is – 56.1 kcal mol^{-1}. If the enthalpy of ionisation of acid is 1.5 kcal mol^{-1} and enthalpy of neutralisation of the strong acid with a strong base is –57.3 $kJ eq^{-1}$. What is the % ionisation of the weak acid in molar solution (assume the acid is monobasic)

(a) 25 (b) 20 (c) 15 (d) 10

RESPONSE GRID					
	24. ⓐⓑⓒⓓ	25. ⓐⓑⓒⓓ	26. ⓐⓑⓒⓓ	27. ⓐⓑⓒⓓ	28. ⓐⓑⓒⓓ
	29. ⓐⓑⓒⓓ	30. ⓐⓑⓒⓓ	31. ⓐⓑⓒⓓ	32. ⓐⓑⓒⓓ	33. ⓐⓑⓒⓓ
	34. ⓐⓑⓒⓓ	35. ⓐⓑⓒⓓ			

Space for Rough Work

36. ΔH_f° of NF_3 is – 113 kJ mol^{-1} and N–F bond energy is 273.0 kJ mol^{-1}. If $N \equiv N$ and F–F bond energies are in the rates 6 : 1, their magnitudes will be
(a) 780.0 kJ mol^{-1}, 130.0 kJ mol^{-1}
(b) 840 kJ mol^{-1}, 140 kJ mol^{-1}
(c) 950.0 kJ mol^{-1}, 158.3 kJ mol^{-1}
(d) 941.3 kJ mol^{-1}, 156.9 kJ mol^{-1}

37. Consider the following processes :

	ΔH (kJ/mol)
$1/2 A \rightarrow B$	+150
$3B \rightarrow 2C + D$	–125
$E + A \rightarrow 2D$	+350

For $B + D \rightarrow E + 2C$, ΔH will be :
(a) 525 kJ/mol (b) – 175 kJ/mol
(c) – 325 kJ/mol (d) 325 kJ/mol

38. For an isothermal reversible expansion process, the value of q can be calculated by the expression
(a) $q = 2.303nRT\log\frac{V_2}{V_1}$ (b) $q = -2.303nRT\log\frac{V_2}{V_1}$
(c) $q = -P_{exp}nRT\log\frac{V_1}{V_2}$ (d) None of these

39. Match the columns

	Column-I		Column-II
A.	$C_4H_{10} + \frac{13}{2}O_2 \rightarrow 4CO_2 + 5H_2O; \Delta H = -w$	I.	Enthalpy of atomisation
B.	$CH_4 \rightarrow C + 4H; \Delta H = x$	II.	Enthalpy of formation
C.	$H_2 + Br_2 \rightarrow 2HBr; \Delta H = y$	III.	Enthalpy of combustion
D.	$Na^-(s) \rightarrow Na(g); \Delta H = z$	IV.	Enthalpy of sublimation

(a) A – IV; B – I; C – II; D – III
(b) A – II; B – III; C – I; D – IV
(c) A – III; B – I; C – II; D – IV
(d) A – I; B – II; C – IV; D – III

40. From the following data ΔH of the following reactions
$C(s) + \frac{1}{2}O_2(g) \longrightarrow CO(g); \Delta H = -110$ kJ and
$C(s) + H_2O(g) \longrightarrow CO(g) + H_2(g); \Delta H = 132$ kJ
Calculate the mole composition of the mixture of steam and oxygen on being passes over coke at 1273 K, keeping the temperature constant.
(a) 1 : 0.6 (b) 0.6 : 1 (c) 2 : 3 (d) 3 : 2

41. The heats of neutralisation of CH_3COOH, HCOOH, HCN and H_2S are – 13.2, – 13.4, – 2.9 and – 3.8 kcal per equivalent respectively. Arrange the acids in increasing order of strength
(a) HCOOH > CH_3COOH > H_2S > HCN
(b) CH_3COOH > HCOOH > H_2S > HCN
(c) H_2S > HCOOH > CH_3COOH > HCN
(d) HCOOH > H_2S > CH_3COOH > HCN

42. Which of the following salts should cause maximum cooling when 1 mole of it is dissolved in the same volume of water ?
(a) NaCl; $\Delta H^\circ = 5.35$ kJ mol^{-1}
(b) KNO_3; $\Delta H^\circ = 53.5$ kJ mol^{-1}
(c) KOH; $\Delta H^\circ = -56.0$ kJ mol^{-1}
(d) HBr; $\Delta H^\circ = -83.3$ kJ mol^{-1}

43. Read the following statements carefully and choose the correct option
(i) Internal energy U of the system is a state function.
(ii) –w shows, that work is done on the system.
(iii) +w shows, that work is done by the system
(a) (i) and (ii) are correct (b) (ii) and (iii) are correct
(c) (i) and (iii) are correct (d) Only (i) is correct

44. Consider the following reaction occurring in an automobile
$2C_8H_{18}(g) + 25O_2(g) \longrightarrow 16CO_2(g) + 18H_2O(g)$
the sign of ΔH, ΔS and ΔG would be
(a) +, –, + (b) –, +, –
(c) –, +, + (d) +, +, –

45. Choose the reaction with negative ΔS value.
(a) $2NaHCO_{3(s)} \rightarrow Na_2CO_{3(s)} + CO_{2(g)} + H_2O_{(g)}$
(b) $Cl_{2(g)} \rightarrow 2Cl_{(g)}$
(c) $2SO_{2(g)} + O_{2(g)} \rightarrow 2SO_{3(g)}$
(d) $2KClO_{3(s)} \rightarrow 2KCl_{(s)} + 3O_{2(g)}$

RESPONSE GRID					
	36. ⓐⓑⓒⓓ	37. ⓐⓑⓒⓓ	38. ⓐⓑⓒⓓ	39. ⓐⓑⓒⓓ	40. ⓐⓑⓒⓓ
	41. ⓐⓑⓒⓓ	42. ⓐⓑⓒⓓ	43. ⓐⓑⓒⓓ	44. ⓐⓑⓒⓓ	45. ⓐⓑⓒⓓ

CHEMISTRY CHAPTERWISE SPEED TEST-34			
Total Questions	45	Total Marks	180
Attempted		Correct	
Incorrect		Net Score	
Cut-off Score	34	Qualifying Score	55
Success Gap = Net Score – Qualifying Score			
Net Score = (Correct × 4) – (Incorrect × 1)			

Space for Rough Work

CHEMISTRY

Equilibrium

Speed TEST 35

Chapter-wise

No. of Questions	Maximum Marks	Time
45	180	1 Hour

GENERAL INSTRUCTIONS

- This test contains 45 MCQ's. For each question only one option is correct. Darken the correct circle/ bubble in the Response Grid provided on each page.
- You have to evaluate your Response Grids yourself with the help of solutions provided at the end of this book.
- Each correct answer will get you 4 marks and 1 mark shall be deduced for each incorrect answer. No mark will be given/ deducted if no bubble is filled. Keep a timer in front of you and stop immediately at the end of 60 min.
- The sheet follows a particular syllabus. Do not attempt the sheet before you have completed your preparation for that syllabus.
- After completing the sheet check your answers with the solution booklet and complete the Result Grid. Finally spend time to analyse your performance and revise the areas which emerge out as weak in your evaluation.

1. If 1.0 mole of I_2 is introduced into 1.0 litre flask at 1000 K, at quilibrium ($K_c = 10^{-6}$), which one is correct?

(a) $[I_2(g)] > [I^-(g)]$ (b) $[I_2(g)] < [I^-(g)]$

(c) $[I_2(g)] = [I^-(g)]$ (d) $[I_2(g)] = \frac{1}{2}[I^-(g)]$

2. In a reaction, $A + 2B \rightleftharpoons 2C$, 2.0 mole of 'A', 3.0 mole of 'B' and 2.0 mole of 'C' are placed in a 2.0 L flask and the equilibrium concentration of 'C' is 0.5 mol/L. The equilibrium constant (K) for the reaction is

(a) 0.073 (b) 0.147

(c) 0.05 (d) 0.026

3. K_c for the reaction

$$N_2(g) + O_2(g) \rightleftharpoons 2NO(g)$$

at 300 K is 4.0×10^{-6}. K_p for the above reaction will be ($R = 2$ cal mol^{-1} K^{-1})

(a) 2.4×10^{-3} (b) 4×10^{-6}

(c) $4 \times 10^{-6}(RT)^2$ (d) 16×10^{-12}

4. $\Delta G°$ for the reaction $X + Y \rightleftharpoons Z$ is –4.606 kcal. The equilibrium constant for the reaction at 227°C is

(a) 100 (b) 10 (c) 2 (d) 0.01

5. The equilibrium constant for the reaction

$$SO_3(g) \rightleftharpoons SO_2(g) + \frac{1}{2}O_2(g)$$

is $K_c = 4.9 \times 10^{-2}$. The value of K_c for the reaction

$$2SO_2(g) + O_2(g) \rightleftharpoons 2SO_3(g)$$

will be

(a) 9.8×10^{-2} (b) 4.9×10^{-2}

(c) 416 (d) 2.40×10^{-3}

6. Four species are listed below:

i. HCO_3^- ii. H_3O^+ iii. HSO_4^- iv. HSO_3F

Which one of the following is the correct sequence of their acid strength?

(a) iv < ii < iii < i (b) ii < iii < i < iv

(c) i < iii < ii < iv (d) iii < i < iv < ii

7. The degree of dissociation of dinitrogen tetroxide $N_2O_4(g) \longrightarrow 2NO_2(g)$ at temperature T and total pressure P is α. Which one of the following is the correct expression for the equilibrium constant (K_p) at this temperature?

(a) $\frac{2\alpha}{(1-\alpha^2)}$ (b) $\frac{\alpha^2 P}{1-\alpha}$ (c) $\frac{4\alpha^2}{(1-\alpha^2)}$ (d) $\frac{4\alpha^2 P}{(1-\alpha^2)}$

8. The equilibrium constants K_{p_1} and K_{p_2} for the reactions $X \rightleftharpoons 2Y$ and $Z \rightleftharpoons P + Q$, respectively are in the ratio of 1 : 9. If the degree of dissociation of X and Z be equal then the ratio of total pressures at these equilibria is

(a) 1 : 1 (b) 1 : 36 (c) 1 : 3 (d) 1 : 9

RESPONSE GRID					
	1. ⓐⓑⓒⓓ	2. ⓐⓑⓒⓓ	3. ⓐⓑⓒⓓ	4. ⓐⓑⓒⓓ	5. ⓐⓑⓒⓓ
	6. ⓐⓑⓒⓓ	7. ⓐⓑⓒⓓ	8. ⓐⓑⓒⓓ		

Space for Rough Work

9. The dissociation of a gas AB_2 at equilibrium can be represented as :

$2AB_2(g) \rightleftharpoons 2AB(g) + B_2(g)$

The degree of dissociation is 'x' and is small compared to 1. The expression relating the degree of dissociation (x) with equilibrium constant K_p and total pressure P is :

(a) $(2K_p/P)$ (b) $(2K_p/P)^{1/3}$
(c) $(2K_p/P)^{1/2}$ (d) (K_p/P)

10. The exothermic formation of ClF_3 is represented by the equation :

$Cl_2(g) + 3F_2(g) \rightleftharpoons 2ClF_3(g)$; $\Delta H = -329$ kJ

Which of the following will increase the quantity of ClF_3 in an equilibrium mixture of Cl_2, F_2 and ClF_3?

(a) Adding F_2
(b) Increasing the volume of the container
(c) Removing Cl_2
(d) Increasing the temperature

11. Match the columns

	Column-I		Column-II
A.	$Q_c < K_c$,	I.	Net reaction goes from right to left.
B.	$Q_c > K_c$,	II.	Net reaction goes from left to right.
C.	$Q_c = K_c$,	III.	No net reaction occurs.

(a) A – I; B – II; C – III (b) A – III; B – II; C – I
(c) A – I; B – III; C – II (d) A – II; B – I; C – III

12. Which of the following statement(s) is/are correct ?

(i) ΔG is negative, then the reaction is spontaneous and proceeds in the forward direction.
(ii) ΔG is positive, then reaction is non-spontaneous
(iii) ΔG is 0, then reaction is at equilibrium

(a) (i), (ii) and (iii) are correct
(b) (i) and (ii)
(c) (ii) and (iii) are correct
(d) only (iii) is correct

13. On the basis of Le Chatelier's principle, predict which of the following conditions would be unfavourable for the formation of SO_3? Given that

$2SO_2 + O_2 \rightleftharpoons 2SO_3$; $\Delta H = -42$ kcal

(a) Low pressure and low temperature
(b) High pressure and low temperature
(c) High temperature and low pressure
(d) High concentration of SO_2

14. The standard Gibbs energy change at 300 K for the reaction $2A \rightleftharpoons B + C$ is 2494.2 J. At a given time, the composition of the reaction mixture is $[A] = \frac{1}{2}$, $[B] = 2$ and $[C] = \frac{1}{2}$. The reaction proceeds in the : [R = 8.314 J/K/mol, e = 2.718]

(a) forward direction because $Q < K_c$
(b) reverse direction because $Q < K_c$
(c) forward direction because $Q > K_c$
(d) reverse direction because $Q > K_c$

15. If the equilibrium constant for $N_2(g) + O_2(g) \rightleftharpoons 2NO(g)$ is K, the equilibrium constant for $\frac{1}{2}N_2(g) + \frac{1}{2}O_2(g) \rightleftharpoons NO(g)$ will be:

(a) $K^{\frac{1}{2}}$ (b) $\frac{1}{2}K$ (c) K (d) K^2

16. The following reaction is performed at 298 K.

$2NO(g) + O_2(g) \rightleftharpoons 2NO_2(g)$

The standard free energy of formation of NO(g) is 86.6 kJ/mol at 298 K. What is the standard free energy of formation of $NO_2(g)$ at 298 K? ($K_p = 1.6 \times 10^{12}$)

(a) $86600 - \dfrac{\ln(1.6 \times 10^{12})}{R(298)}$
(b) $0.5[2 \times 86{,}600 - R(298)\ln(1.6 \times 10^{12})]$
(c) $R(298)\ln(1.6 \times 10^{12}) - 86600$
(d) $86600 + R(298)\ln(1.6 \times 10^{12})$

17. Which of the following pairs constitutes a buffer?

(a) NaOH and NaCl (b) HNO_3 and NH_4NO_3
(c) HCl and KCl (d) HNO_2 and $NaNO_2$

18. For dibasic acid correct order is

(a) $K_{a_1} < K_{a_2}$ (b) $K_{a_1} > K_{a_2}$
(c) $K_{a_1} = K_{a_2}$ (d) not certain

19. Consider the expression $\Delta G = -RT\ln K_p + RT\ln Q_p$ and select the correct statement at equilibrium

(a) $\Delta G = 0, Q_p > K_p$ the equilibrium reaction will shift from left to right
(b) $\Delta G = 0, Q_p = K_p$ the equilibrium reaction will shift from left to right
(c) $\Delta G = \infty, Q_p < K_p$ the equilibrium reaction will shift from right to left
(d) $\Delta G < 0, Q_p > K_p$ the equilibrium reaction will shift from right to left

where Q_p and K_p term refer to reaction quotient and equilibrium constant at constant pressure respectively.

RESPONSE GRID				
9. ⓐⓑⓒⓓ	10. ⓐⓑⓒⓓ	11. ⓐⓑⓒⓓ	12. ⓐⓑⓒⓓ	13. ⓐⓑⓒⓓ
14. ⓐⓑⓒⓓ	15. ⓐⓑⓒⓓ	16. ⓐⓑⓒⓓ	17. ⓐⓑⓒⓓ	18. ⓐⓑⓒⓓ
19. ⓐⓑⓒⓓ				

Space for Rough Work

20. K_c for $PCl_5(g) \rightleftharpoons PCl_3(g) + Cl_2(g)$ is 0.04 at 250°C. How many moles of PCl_5 must be added to a 3 L flask to obtain a Cl_2 concentration of 0.15 M
(a) 4.2 moles (b) 2.1 moles
(c) 5.5 moles (d) 6.3 moles

21. In the following hypothetical reaction
$A + 3B \rightleftharpoons 2C + D$
initial moles of A are twice that of B. If at equilibrium moles of B and C are equal. Percentage of B reacted is
(a) 60% (b) 40% (c) 10% (d) 20%

22. Which of the following can act as both Bronsted acid and Bronsted base?
(a) Na_2CO_3 (b) OH^-
(c) HCO_3^- (d) NH_3

23. Match the columns :

	Column-I		Column-II
A.	$N_2(g) + 3H_2(g) \rightleftharpoons 2NH_3(g)$ (t = 300°C)	I.	$\Delta n > 0$
B.	$PCl_5(g) \rightleftharpoons PCl_3(g) + Cl_2(g)$ (t = 50°C)	II.	$K_P < K_C$
C.	$C(s) + H_2O(g) \rightleftharpoons CO(g) + H_2(g)$	III.	K_P not defined
D.	$CH_3COOH(l) + C_2H_5OH(l) \rightleftharpoons CH_3COOC_2H_5(l) + H_2O(l)$	IV.	$\Delta n = 1$

(a) A – II; B – I; C – IV; D – III
(b) A – I; B – II; C – III; D – IV
(c) A – III; B – I; C – IV; D – II
(d) A – IV; B – II; C – I; D – III

24. Which of the following statements are correct ?
(i) Ionic product of water $(K_w) = [H^+][OH^-] = 10^{-14} M^2$
(ii) At 298K $[H^+] = [OH^-] = 10^{-7}$
(iii) K_w does not depend upon temperature
(iv) Molarity of pure water = 55.55M
(a) (i), (ii) and (iii) (b) (i), (ii) and (iv)
(c) (i) and (iv) (d) (ii) and (iii)

25. At a certain temperature the dissociation constants of formic acid and acetic acid are 1.8×10^{-4} and 1.8×10^{-6} respectively. The concentration of acetic acid solution in which the hydrogen ion has the same concentration as in 0.001 M formic acid solution is equal to
(a) 0.001 M (b) 0.01 M
(c) 0.1 M (d) 0.0001 M

26. The first and second dissociation constants of an acid H_2A are 1.0×10^{-5} and 5.0×10^{-10} respectively. The overall dissociation constant of the acid will be
(a) 0.2×10^5 (b) 5.0×10^{-5}
(c) 5.0×10^{15} (d) 5.0×10^{-15}.

27. Equal volumes of three acid solutions of pH 3, 4 and 5 are mixed in a vessel. What will be the H^+ ion concentration in the mixture ?
(a) 1.11×10^{-4} M (b) 3.7×10^{-4} M
(c) 3.7×10^{-3} M (d) 1.11×10^{-3} M

28. The solubility product of AgCl is 4.0×10^{-10} at 298 K. The solubility of AgCl in 0.04 M $CaCl_2$ will be
(a) 2.0×10^{-5} M (b) 1.0×10^{-4} M
(c) 5.0×10^{-9} M (d) 2.2×10^{-4} M

29. The pH of a buffer containing equal molar concentrations of a weak base and its chloride
(K_b for weak base = 2×10^{-5}, log 2 = 0.3) is
(a) 5 (b) 9
(c) 4.7 (d) 9.3

30. In a saturated solution of the sparingly soluble strong electrolyte $AgIO_3$ (molecular mass = 283) the equilibrium which sets is $AgIO_3(s) \rightleftharpoons Ag^+(aq) + IO_3^-(aq)$. If the solubility product constant K_{sp} of $AgIO_3$ at a given temperature is 1.0×10^{-8}, what is the mass of $AgIO_3$ contained in 100 ml of its saturated solution?
(a) 1.0×10^{-4} g (b) 28.3×10^{-2} g
(c) 2.83×10^{-3} g (d) 1.0×10^{-7} g.

31. What is $[H^+]$ in mol/L of a solution that is 0.20 M in CH_3COONa and 0.10 M in CH_3COOH? K_a for $CH_3COOH = 1.8 \times 10^{-5}$.
(a) 3.5×10^{-4} (b) 1.1×10^{-5}
(c) 1.8×10^{-5} (d) 9.0×10^{-6}

32. The K_{sp} for $Cr(OH)_3$ is 1.6×10^{-30}. The solubility of this compound in water is :
(a) $\sqrt[4]{1.6 \times 10^{-30}}$ (b) $\sqrt[4]{1.6 \times 10^{-30} / 27}$
(c) $1.6 \times 10^{-30/27}$ (d) $\sqrt{1.6 \times 10^{-30}}$

33. For the reaction CO (g) + (1/2) O_2 (g) = CO_2 (g), K_p / K_c is
(a) RT (b) $(RT)^{-1}$
(c) $(RT)^{-1/2}$ (d) $(RT)^{1/2}$

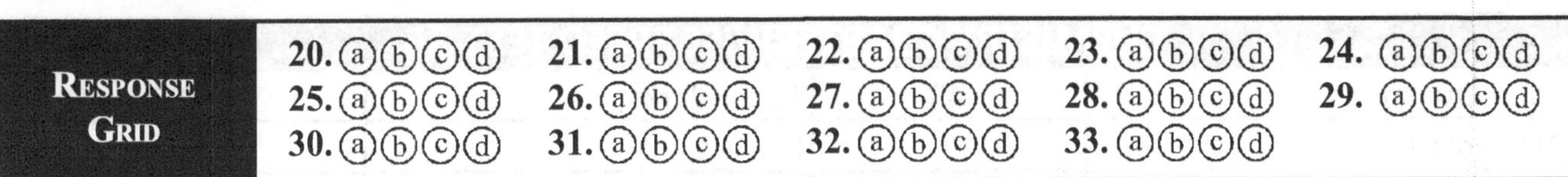

RESPONSE GRID				
20. ⓐⓑⓒⓓ	21. ⓐⓑⓒⓓ	22. ⓐⓑⓒⓓ	23. ⓐⓑⓒⓓ	24. ⓐⓑⓒⓓ
25. ⓐⓑⓒⓓ	26. ⓐⓑⓒⓓ	27. ⓐⓑⓒⓓ	28. ⓐⓑⓒⓓ	29. ⓐⓑⓒⓓ
30. ⓐⓑⓒⓓ	31. ⓐⓑⓒⓓ	32. ⓐⓑⓒⓓ	33. ⓐⓑⓒⓓ	

Space for Rough Work

34. For the reaction : $2NO_{2(g)} \rightleftharpoons 2NO_{(g)} + O_{2(g)}$,
($K_c = 1.8 \times 10^{-6}$ at 184°C) (R = 0.0831 kJ/ (mol. K))
When K_p and K_c are compared at 184°C, it is found that
(a) Whether K_p is greater than, less than or equal to K_c depends upon the total gas pressure
(b) $K_p = K_c$
(c) K_p is less than K_c
(d) K_p is greater than K_c

35. A monobasic weak acid solution has a molarity of 0.005 and pH of 5. What is the percentage ionization in this solution?
(a) 2.0 (b) 0.2 (c) 0.5 (d) 0.25

36. Values of dissociation constant, K_a are given as follows :

Acid	K_a
HCN	6.2×10^{-10}
HF	6.6×10^{-4}
HNO_2	7.2×10^{-4}

Correct order of increasing base strength of the base CN^-, F^- and NO_2^- will be :
(a) $F^- < CN^- < NO_2^-$ (b) $NO_2^- < CN^- < F^-$
(c) $F^- < NO_2^- < CN^-$ (d) $NO_2^- < F^- < CN^-$

37. How many litres of water must be added to 1 litre of an aqueous solution of HCl with a pH of 1 to create an aqueous solution with pH of 2 ?
(a) 0.1 L (b) 0.9 L (c) 2.0 L (d) 9.0 L

38. The pH of aqueous solution of 1M $HCOONH_4$, pK_a of HCOOH is 3.8 and pK_b of NH_3 is 4.8
(a) 6.5 (b) 4.8 (c) 3.8 (d) 8.6

39. Solid $Ba(NO_3)_2$ is gradually dissolved in a 1.0×10^{-4} M Na_2CO_3 solution. At what concentration of Ba^{2+} will a precipitate begin to form? (K_{SP} for for $BaCO_3 = 5.1 \times 10^{-9}$)
(a) 5.1×10^{-5} M (b) 8.1×10^{-8} M
(c) 8.1×10^{-7} M (d) 4.1×10^{-5} M

40. Solubility product of silver bromide is 5.0×10^{-13}. The quantity of potassium bromide (molar mass taken as 120g mol^{-1}) to be added to 1 litre of 0.05 M solution of silver nitrate to start the precipitation of AgBr is
(a) 1.2×10^{-10} g (b) 1.2×10^{-9} g
(c) 6.2×10^{-5} g (d) 5.0×10^{-8} g

41. Three reactions involving $H_2PO_4^-$ are given below :
(i) $H_3PO_4 + H_2O \rightarrow H_3O^+ + H_2PO_4^-$
(ii) $H_2PO_4^- + H_2O \rightarrow HPO_4^{2-} + H_3O^+$
(iii) $H_2PO_4^- + OH^- \rightarrow H_3PO_4 + O^{2-}$
In which of the above does $H_2PO_4^-$ act as an acid ?
(a) (ii) only (b) (i) and (ii)
(c) (iii) only (d) (i) only

42. Which solution has pH equal to 10 ?
(a) 10^{-4} M KOH (b) 10^{-10} M KOH
(c) 10^{-10} M HCl (d) 10^{-4} M HCl

43. Calculate the pH of 0.5 M aqueous solution of NaCN, the pK_b of CN^- is 4.70
(a) 4.70 (b) 11.5 (c) 7 (d) 6.5

44. For the following three reactions a, b and c, equilibrium constants are given:
(i) $CO(g) + H_2O(g) \rightleftharpoons CO_2(g) + H_2(g); K_1$
(ii) $CH_4(g) + H_2O(g) \rightleftharpoons CO(g) + 3H_2(g); K_2$
(iii) $CH_4(g) + 2H_2O(g) \rightleftharpoons CO_2(g) + 4H_2(g); K_3$
(a) $K_1\sqrt{K_2} = K_3$ (b) $K_2K_3 = K_1$
(c) $K_3 = K_1K_2$ (d) $K_3.K_2^3 = K_1^2$

45. A vessel at 1000 K contains CO_2 with a pressure of 0.5 atm. Some of the CO_2 is converted into CO on the addition of graphite. If the total pressure at equilibrium is 0.8 atm, the value of K is :
(a) 1.8 atm (b) 3 atm
(c) 0.3 atm (d) 0.18 atm

RESPONSE GRID					
	34. ⓐⓑⓒⓓ	35. ⓐⓑⓒⓓ	36. ⓐⓑⓒⓓ	37. ⓐⓑⓒⓓ	38. ⓐⓑⓒⓓ
	39. ⓐⓑⓒⓓ	40. ⓐⓑⓒⓓ	41. ⓐⓑⓒⓓ	42. ⓐⓑⓒⓓ	43. ⓐⓑⓒⓓ
	44. ⓐⓑⓒⓓ	45. ⓐⓑⓒⓓ			

CHEMISTRY CHAPTERWISE SPEED TEST-35			
Total Questions	45	Total Marks	180
Attempted		Correct	
Incorrect		Net Score	
Cut-off Score	39	Qualifying Score	57
Success Gap = Net Score – Qualifying Score			
Net Score = (Correct × 4) – (Incorrect × 1)			

Space for Rough Work

CHEMISTRY

Redox Reactions

Speed TEST 36

Chapter-wise

No. of Questions	Maximum Marks	Time
45	180	1 Hour

GENERAL INSTRUCTIONS

- This test contains 45 MCQ's. For each question only one option is correct. Darken the correct circle/ bubble in the Response Grid provided on each page.
- You have to evaluate your Response Grids yourself with the help of solutions provided at the end of this book.
- Each correct answer will get you 4 marks and 1 mark shall be deduced for each incorrect answer. No mark will be given/ deducted if no bubble is filled. Keep a timer in front of you and stop immediately at the end of 60 min.
- The sheet follows a particular syllabus. Do not attempt the sheet before you have completed your preparation for that syllabus.
- After completing the sheet check your answers with the solution booklet and complete the Result Grid. Finally spend time to analyse your performance and revise the areas which emerge out as weak in your evaluation.

1. The brown ring complex is formulated as $[Fe(H_2O)_5NO]SO_4$. The oxidation number of iron is
   (a) 1 (b) 2 (c) 3 (d) 0
2. In which of the following reactions, there is no change in valency ?
   (a) $4KClO_3 \rightarrow 3KClO_4 + KCl$
   (b) $SO_2 + 2H_2S \rightarrow 2H_2O + 3S$
   (c) $BaO_2 + H_2SO_4 \rightarrow BaSO_4 + H_2O_2$
   (d) $2BaO + O_2 \rightarrow 2BaO_2$
3. The oxidation state of chromium in the final product formed by the reaction between KI and acidified potassium dichromate solution is:
   (a) +3 (b) +2 (c) +6 (d) +4
4. In which of the following pairs, there is greatest difference in the oxidation number of the underlined elements ?
   (a) $\underline{N}O_2$ and $\underline{N}_2O_4$ (b) $\underline{P}_2O_5$ and $\underline{P}_4O_{10}$
   (c) $\underline{N}_2O$ and $\underline{N}O$ (d) $\underline{S}O_2$ and $\underline{S}O_3$
5. A compound of Xe and F is found to have 53.5% of Xe. What is oxidation number of Xe in this compound ?
   (a) –4 (b) 0 (c) +4 (d) +6
6. Atomic number of an element is 22. The highest O.S. exhibited by it in its compounds is
   (a) 1 (b) 2 (c) 3 (d) 4
7. The reaction in which hydrogen peroxide acts as a reducing agent is
   (a) $PbS + 4H_2O_2 \rightarrow PbSO_4 + 4H_2O$
   (b) $2KI + H_2O_2 \rightarrow 2KOH + I_2$
   (c) $2FeSO_4 + H_2SO_4 + H_2O_2 \rightarrow Fe_2(SO_4)_3 + 2H_2O$
   (d) $Ag_2O + H_2O_2 \rightarrow 2Ag + H_2O + O_2$
8. Of the following reactions, only one is a redox reaction. Identify it
   (a) $Ca(OH)_2 + 2HCl \rightarrow CaCl_2 + 2H_2O$
   (b) $BaCl_2 + MgSO_4 \rightarrow BaSO_4 + MgCl_2$
   (c) $2S_2O_7^{2-} + 2H_2O \rightarrow 4SO_4^{2-} + 4H^+$
   (d) $Cu_2S + 2FeO \rightarrow 2Cu + 2Fe + SO_2$
9. Arrange the following in the order of their decreasing electrode potentials : Mg, K, Ba and Ca
   (a) K > Ca > Ba > Mg (b) Ba > Ca > K > Mg
   (c) Ca > Mg > K > Ba (d) Mg > Ca > Ba > K

RESPONSE GRID					
	1. ⓐⓑⓒⓓ	2. ⓐⓑⓒⓓ	3. ⓐⓑⓒⓓ	4. ⓐⓑⓒⓓ	5. ⓐⓑⓒⓓ
	6. ⓐⓑⓒⓓ	7. ⓐⓑⓒⓓ	8. ⓐⓑⓒⓓ	9. ⓐⓑⓒⓓ	

Space for Rough Work

10. Which of the following statements are correct concerning redox properties?
(i) A metal M for which E° for the half life reaction $M^{n+} + ne^- \rightleftharpoons M$ is very negative will be a good reducing agent.
(ii) The oxidizing power of the halogens decreases from chlorine to iodine.
(iii) The reducing power of hydrogen halides increases from hydrogen chloride to hydrogen iodide
(a) (i), (ii) and (iii) (b) (i) and (ii)
(c) (i) only (d) (ii) and (iii)

11. A negative E° means that redox couple is a ___A___ than the H^+/H_2 couple
A positive E° means that the redox couple is a ___B___ than H^+/H_2 couple
(a) A = stronger reducing agent
B = weaker reducing agent
(b) A = stronger oxidising agent
B = weaker oxidising agent
(c) A = weaker oxidising agent
B = stronger oxidising agent
(d) Both (a) and (c)

12. If equal volume of reactants are used, then no. of moles of $KMnO_4$ (moles per litre) used in acidic medium required to completely oxidise 0.5 M $FeSO_3$?
(a) 0.3 (b) 0.1
(c) 0.2 (d) 0.4

13. If rod of a metal (x) is put in a metal ion solution which is blue in colour, solution turn colourless. The metal rod and solution respectively are?
(a) Zinc and Cu(II) (b) Zinc and Ni(II)
(c) Aluminium and Cu(II) (d) Both (a) and (c)

14. In the reaction between SO_2 and O_3 the equivalent weight of sulphur in product is
(a) the same as its molecular weight
(b) half of the molecular weight
(c) one-third of the molecular weight
(d) one-fourth of the molecular weight

15. When $KMnO_4$ reacts with acidified $FeSO_4$
(a) $FeSO_4$ is oxidised and $KMnO_4$ is reduced
(b) only $KMnO_4$ is oxidised
(c) only $FeSO_4$ is oxidised
(d) None of these

16. Consider the following reaction :

$$xMnO_4^- + yC_2O_4^{2-} + zH^+ \rightarrow xMn^{2+} + 2yCO_2 + \frac{z}{2}H_2O$$

The value's of x, y and z in the reaction are, respectively :
(a) 5, 2 and 16 (b) 2, 5 and 8
(c) 2, 5 and 16 (d) 5, 2 and 8

17. When Cl_2 gas reacts with hot and concentrated sodium hydroxide solution, the oxidation number of chlorine changes from :
(a) zero to +1 and zero to –5
(b) zero to –1 and zero to +5
(c) zero to –1 and zero to +3
(d) zero to +1 and zero to –3

18. Oxidation state for nitrogen is incorrectly given for compound oxidation state
(a) $[Co(NH_3)_5Cl]Cl_2$ 0
(b) NH_2OH –1
(c) $(N_2H_5)_2SO_4$ –2
(d) Mg_3N_2 –3

19. Standard electrode potentials of redox couples A^{2+}/A, B^{2+}/B, C^{2+}/C and D^{2+}/D are 0.3V, – 0.5V, – 0.75V and 0.9V respectively. Which of these is best oxidising agent and reducing agent respectively –
(a) D^{2+}/D and B^{2+}/B (b) B^{2+}/B and D^{2+}/D
(c) D^{2+}/D and C^{2+}/C (d) C^{2+}/C and D^{2+}/D

20. MnO_4^{2-} (1 mole) in neutral aqueous medium disproportionates to
(a) 2/3 mole of MnO_4^- and 1/3 mole of MnO_2
(b) 1/3 mole of MnO_4^- and 2/3 mole of MnO_2
(c) 1/3 mole of Mn_2O_7 and 1/3 mole of MnO_2
(d) 2/3 mole of Mn_2O_7 and 1/3 mole of MnO_2

21. In the standardization of $Na_2S_2O_3$ using $K_2Cr_2O_7$ by iodometry, the equivalent weight of $K_2Cr_2O_7$ is
(a) (molecular weight)/2 (b) (molecular weight)/6
(c) (molecular weight)/3 (d) same as molecular weight

RESPONSE GRID					
	10. ⓐⓑⓒⓓ	11. ⓐⓑⓒⓓ	12. ⓐⓑⓒⓓ	13. ⓐⓑⓒⓓ	14. ⓐⓑⓒⓓ
	15. ⓐⓑⓒⓓ	16. ⓐⓑⓒⓓ	17. ⓐⓑⓒⓓ	18. ⓐⓑⓒⓓ	19. ⓐⓑⓒⓓ
	20. ⓐⓑⓒⓓ	21. ⓐⓑⓒⓓ			

Space for Rough Work

22. The species that undergoes disproportionation in an alkaline medium are
(a) Cl_2 (b) MnO_4^{2-}
(c) NO_2 (d) All of these

23. One mole of N_2H_4 loses 10 moles of electrons to form a new compound y. Assuming that all nitrogen appear in the new compound, what is the oxidation state of nitrogen in y (There is no change in the oxidation state of hydrogen)
(a) –1 (b) –3 (c) +3 (d) +5

24. Phosphorus, sulphur and chlorine undergo disproportion in the ...A... medium.
Here, A refers to
(a) acidic (b) alkaline
(c) neutral (d) Both (a) and (b)

25. In which of the following compounds oxygen has highest oxidation state and in which it has lowest oxidation state?
OF_2, H_2O_2, KO_2, O_2F_2
(a) Highest = KO_2, lowest = H_2O_2
(b) Highest = OF_2, lowest = H_2O_2
(c) Highest = OF_2, lowest = KO_2
(d) Highest = KO_2, lowest = H_2O_2

26. The most powerful oxidizing agent from the following is
(a) H_3BO_3 (b) HPO_3 (c) H_3PO_4 (d) H_2SO_4

27. When SO_2 is passed through acidified solution of potassium dichromate, then chromium sulphate is formed. The change in valency of chromium is
(a) +4 to +2 (b) +5 to +3 (c) +6 to +3 (d) +7 to +2

28. Standard reduction potentials of the half reactions are given below :
$F_2(g) + 2e^- \rightarrow 2F^-(aq)$; $E° = +2.85$ V
$Cl_2(g) + 2e^- \rightarrow 2Cl^-(aq)$; $E° = +1.36$ V $Br_2(l) + 2e^- \rightarrow 2Br^-(aq)$; $E° = +1.06$ V $I_2(s) + 2e^- \rightarrow 2I^-(aq)$; $E° = +0.53$ V
The strongest oxidising and reducing agents respectively are :
(a) F_2 and I^- (b) Br_2 and Cl^-
(c) Cl_2 and Br^- (d) Cl_2 and I_2

29. A gas X at 1 atm is bubbled through a solution containing a mixture of 1 M Y^- and 1 M Z^- at 25°C. If the reduction potential is Z > Y > X, then
(a) Y will oxidise X and not Z
(b) Y will oxidise Z and not X
(c) Y will oxidise both X and Z
(d) Y will reduce both X and Z

30. The violent reaction between sodium and water is an example of
(a) Reduction (b) Oxidation
(c) Redox reaction (d) Neutralization reaction

31. The equivalent weight of Mohr's salt, $FeSO_4(NH_4)_2SO_4.6H_2O$ is equal to
(a) its molecular weight
(b) its atomic weight
(c) half-its molecular weight
(d) one-third its molecular weight

32. The set of numerical coefficients that balances the equation
$K_2CrO_4 + HCl \rightarrow K_2Cr_2O_7 + KCl + H_2O$
(a) 1, 1, 2, 2, 1 (b) 2, 2, 1, 1, 1
(c) 2, 1, 1, 2, 1 (d) 2, 2, 1, 2, 1

33. Thiosulphate reacts differently with iodine and bromine in the reactions given below:
$2S_2O_3^{2-} + I_2 \rightarrow S_4O_6^{2-} + 2I^-$
$S_2O_3^{2-} + Br_2 + 5H_2O \rightarrow 2SO_4^{2-} + 2Br^- + 10H^+$
Which of the following statements justifies the above dual behaviour of thiosulphate?
(a) Bromine is a stronger oxidant than iodine.
(b) Bromine is a weaker oxidant than iodine.
(c) Thiosulphate undergoes oxidation by bromine and reduction by iodine in these reactions.
(d) Bromine undergoes oxidation and iodine undergoes reduction in these reactions.

34. The chemical that undergoes self oxidation and self reduction in the same reaction is
(a) benzyl alcohol (b) acetone
(c) formaldehyde (d) acetic acid

RESPONSE GRID					
	22. ⓐⓑⓒⓓ	23. ⓐⓑⓒⓓ	24. ⓐⓑⓒⓓ	25. ⓐⓑⓒⓓ	26. ⓐⓑⓒⓓ
	27. ⓐⓑⓒⓓ	28. ⓐⓑⓒⓓ	29. ⓐⓑⓒⓓ	30. ⓐⓑⓒⓓ	31. ⓐⓑⓒⓓ
	32. ⓐⓑⓒⓓ	33. ⓐⓑⓒⓓ	34. ⓐⓑⓒⓓ		

Space for Rough Work

35. The oxidation number of an element in a compound is evaluated on the basis of certian rules. Which of the following rules is not correct in this respect?
(a) The oxidation number of hydrogen is always + 1.
(b) The algebraic sum of all the oxidation numbers in a compound is zero.
(c) An element in the free or the uncombined state bears oxidation number zero.
(d) In all its compounds, the oxidation number of fluorine is – 1.

36. Zn gives H_2 gas with H_2SO_4 and HCl but not with HNO_3 because
(a) Zn acts as an oxidising agent when it reacts with HNO_3
(b) HNO_3 is weaker acid than H_2SO_4 and HCl
(c) In electrochemical series, Zn is above hydrogen
(d) NO_3^- is reduced in preference to hydronium ion

37. Which of the following elements does not show disproportionation tendency?
(a) Cl (b) Br
(c) F (d) I

38. The oxidation number of sulphur in S_8, S_2F_2, H_2S respectively, are
(a) 0, +1 and –2 (b +2, +1 and –2
(c) 0, +1 and +2 (d) –2, +1 and –2

39. Stronger is oxidising agent, more is :
(a) standard reduction potential of that species
(b) the tendency to get it self oxidised
(c) the tendency to lose electrons by that species
(d) standard oxidation potential of that species

40. Which of the following statement(s) is/are correct for the given reaction?
$2HgCl_2\,(aq) + SnCl_2(aq) \rightarrow Hg_2Cl_2(s) + SnCl_4(aq)$
(i) Mercuric chloride is reduced to Hg_2Cl_2
(ii) Stannous chloride is oxidised to stannic chloride
(iii) $HgCl_2$ is oxidised to Hg_2Cl_2
(iv) It is an example of redox reaction
(a) (i), (ii) and (iv) (b) (i) and (ii)
(c) (iii) and (iv) (d) (iii) only

41. The standard reduction potentials for Cu^{2+}/Cu; Zn^{2+}/Zn; Li^+/Li; Ag^+/Ag and H^+/H_2 are + 0.34 V, – 0.762 V, – 3.05 V, + 0.80 V and 0.00 V respectively. Choose the strongest reducing agent among the following
(a) Zn (b) H_2
(c) Ag (d) Li

42. In the disproportionation reaction $3\,HClO_3 \rightarrow HClO_4 + Cl_2 + 2O_2 + H_2O$, the equivalent mass of the oxidizing agent is (molar mass of $HClO_3 = 84.45$)
(a) 16.89 (b) 32.22
(c) 84.45 (d) 28.15

43. Which of the following behaves as both oxidising and reducing agents ?
(a) H_2SO_4 (b) SO_2
(c) H_2O (d) HNO_3

44. Which of the following statement(s) is/are correct ?
(i) Oxidation state of carbon in C_3H_4 is –(4/3).
(ii) Electrons are never shared in fraction.
(a) (i) and (ii) (b) Only (i)
(c) Only (ii) (d) Neither (i) nor (ii)

45. In the reaction shown below, oxidation state of the carbon in reactant and product are (*i*) and (*ii*) respectively? Is the given reaction a redox reaction?
$Na_2CO_3(aq) + HCl\,(aq)$
$\longrightarrow Na^{\oplus}(aq) + Cl^-(aq) + H_2O(\ell) + CO_2(g)$
(a) (i) 6, (ii) 4, yes (b) (i) 6, (ii) 6, No
(c) (i) 4, (ii) 4, No (d) (i) 4, (ii) 4, yes

RESPONSE GRID					
	35. ⓐⓑⓒⓓ	36. ⓐⓑⓒⓓ	37. ⓐⓑⓒⓓ	38. ⓐⓑⓒⓓ	39. ⓐⓑⓒⓓ
	40. ⓐⓑⓒⓓ	41. ⓐⓑⓒⓓ	42. ⓐⓑⓒⓓ	43. ⓐⓑⓒⓓ	44. ⓐⓑⓒⓓ
	45. ⓐⓑⓒⓓ				

CHEMISTRY CHAPTERWISE SPEED TEST-36

Total Questions	45	Total Marks	180
Attempted		Correct	
Incorrect		Net Score	
Cut-off Score	45	Qualifying Score	65
Success Gap = Net Score – Qualifying Score			
Net Score = (Correct × 4) – (Incorrect × 1)			

Space for Rough Work

CHEMISTRY

Hydrogen

Speed TEST 37

Chapter-wise

No. of Questions	Maximum Marks	Time
45	180	1 Hour

GENERAL INSTRUCTIONS

- This test contains 45 MCQ's. For each question only one option is correct. Darken the correct circle/ bubble in the Response Grid provided on each page.
- You have to evaluate your Response Grids yourself with the help of solutions provided at the end of this book.
- Each correct answer will get you 4 marks and 1 mark shall be deduced for each incorrect answer. No mark will be given/ deducted if no bubble is filled. Keep a timer in front of you and stop immediately at the end of 60 min.
- The sheet follows a particular syllabus. Do not attempt the sheet before you have completed your preparation for that syllabus.
- After completing the sheet check your answers with the solution booklet and complete the Result Grid. Finally spend time to analyse your performance and revise the areas which emerge out as weak in your evaluation.

1. Which of the following will not displace hydrogen

(a) Ba (b) Pb (c) Hg (d) Sn

2. Which of the following statements is correct ?

(a) Hydrogen has same IP as alkali metals

(b) Hydrogen has same electronegativity as halogens

(c) It has oxidation number of –1 and +1

(d) It will not be liberated at anode.

3. Which one of the following pairs of substances on reaction will not evolve H_2 gas ?

(a) Iron and H_2SO_4(aq) (b) Iron and steam

(c) Copper and HCl (aq) (d) Sodium and ethanol

4. Following are some properties of hydrogen. Which of the following properties resemble with alkali metals and which with halogens

(i) Hydrogen lose one electron to form unipositive ions

(ii) Hydrogen gain one electron to form uninegative ions

(iii) Hydrogen forms oxides, halides and sulphides

(iv) Hydrogen has a very high ionization enthalpy

(v) Hydrogen forms a diatomic molecule, combines with elements to form hydrides and covalent compounds.

(a) Alkali metals resemble (i), (iii) and (iv)
Halogens resemble (ii) and (v)

(b) Alkali metals resemble (i) and (iii)
Halogens resemble (ii), (iii) and (v)

(c) Alkali metals resemble (i) and (iii)
Halogens resemble (ii), (iv) and (v)

(d) Alkali metals resemble (i) only
Halogens resemble (iv) and (v)

5. Match the columns

Column - I (Chemical property of water)	Column - II (Chemical equation)
A. Basic nature	I. $2H_2O(l) + 2Na(s) \longrightarrow 2NaOH(aq) + H_2(g)$
B. Auto-protolysis	II. $H_2O(l) + H_2O(l) \rightleftharpoons H_3O^+(aq) + OH^-(aq)$
C. Oxidising nature	III. $2F_2(g) + 2H_2O(l) \longrightarrow 4H^+(aq) + 4F^-(aq) + O_2(g)$
D. Reducing nature	IV. $H_2O(l) + H_2S(aq) \rightleftharpoons H_3O^+(aq) + HS^-(aq)$

(a) A – IV; B – II; C – III; D – I

(b) A – IV; B – II; C – I; D – III

(c) A – III; B – II; C – IV; D – I

(d) A – I; B – II; C – IV; D – III

RESPONSE GRID 1. 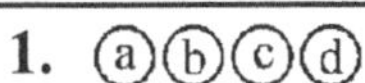 ⓐⓑⓒⓓ 2. ⓐⓑⓒⓓ 3. ⓐⓑⓒⓓ 4. ⓐⓑⓒⓓ 5. ⓐⓑⓒⓓ

Space for Rough Work

6. The unusual properties of water in the condensed phase (liquid and solid states) are due to the
   (a) presence of hydrogen and covalent bonding between the water molecules
   (b) presence of covalent bonding between the water molecules
   (c) presence of extensive hydrogen bonding between water molecules
   (d) presence of ionic bonding
7. Hydrogen bond energy is equal to :
   (a) 3-7 cals (b) 30-70 cals
   (c) 3-10 k cals (d) 30-70 k cals
8. D_2O is preferred to H_2O, as a moderator, in nuclear reactors because
   (a) D_2O slows down fast neutrons better
   (b) D_2O has high specific heat
   (c) D_2O is cheaper
   (d) The neutron absorbing ability of D_2O is higher
9. Consider the following statements :
   1. Atomic hydrogen is obtained by passing hydrogen through an electric arc.
   2. Hydrogen gas will not reduce heated aluminium oxide.
   3. Finely divided palladium adsorbs large volume of hydrogen gas
   4. Pure nascent hydrogen is best obtained by reacting Na with C_2H_5OH

   Which of the above statements is/are correct ?
   (a) only 1 (b) only 2
   (c) 1, 2 and 3 (d) 2, 3 and 4
10. The low density of ice compared to water is due to
    (a) hydrogen bonding interactions
    (b) dipole – dipole interactions
    (c) dipole – induced dipole interactions
    (d) induced dipole – induced dipole interactions
11. What is formed when calcium carbide reacts with heavy water?
    (a) C_2D_2 (b) CaD_2 (c) Ca_2D_2O (d) CD_2
12. Which of the following is formed on reaction of carbon monoxide gas with dihydrogen in presence of cobalt as a catalyst?
    (a) Methanal (b) Methanol
    (c) Methane (d) Formic acid
13. Water possesses a high dielectric constant, therefore
    (a) it always contains ions
    (b) it is a universal solvent
    (c) can dissolve covalent compounds
    (d) can conduct electricity
14. The m.p. of most of the solid substances increase with an increase of pressure . However ice melts at a temperature lower than its usual melting point when pressure is increased. This is because
    (a) ice is less denser than H_2O
    (b) pressure generates heat
    (c) the chemical bonds break under pressure
    (d) ice is not a true solid
15. In context with the industrial preparation of hydrogen from water gas ($CO + H_2$), which of the following is the correct statement?
    (a) CO and H_2, are fractionally separated using differences in their densities
    (b) CO is removed by absorption in aqueous Cu_2Cl_2 solution
    (c) H_2 is removed through occlusion with Pd
    (d) CO is oxidised to CO_2 with steam in the presence of a catalyst followed by absorption of of CO_2 in alkali
16. Calculate the normality of 10 volume H_2O_2 ?
    (a) 1.7 N (b) 12 N (c) 30.3 N (d) 0.0303 N
17. The hydride ion H^- is stronger base than its hydroxide ion OH^-. Which of the following reactions will occur if sodium hydride (NaH) is dissolved in water ?
    (a) $H^-(aq) + H_2O \rightarrow H_3O^-$
    (b) $H^-(aq) + H_2O(l) \rightarrow OH^- + H_2$
    (c) $H^- + H_2O \rightarrow$ No reaction
    (d) None of these

RESPONSE GRID					
	6. ⓐⓑⓒⓓ	7. ⓐⓑⓒⓓ	8. ⓐⓑⓒⓓ	9. ⓐⓑⓒⓓ	10. ⓐⓑⓒⓓ
	11. ⓐⓑⓒⓓ	12. ⓐⓑⓒⓓ	13. ⓐⓑⓒⓓ	14. ⓐⓑⓒⓓ	15. ⓐⓑⓒⓓ
	16. ⓐⓑⓒⓓ	17. ⓐⓑⓒⓓ			

Space for Rough Work

18. Match list I with list II and select the correct answer using the codes given below the lists :

List I	List II
A. Heavy water	I. Bicarbonates of Mg and Ca in water
B. Temporary hard water	II. No foreign ions in water
C. Soft water	III. D_2O
D. Permanent hard water	IV. Sulphates & chlorides of Mg & Ca in water

(a) A–III; B–IV; C–II; D–I (b) A–II; B–I; C–III; D–IV
(c) A–II; B–IV; C–III; D–I (d) A–III; B–I; C–II; D–IV

19. When a substance A reacts with water it produces a combustible gas B and a solution of substance C in water. When another substance D reacts with this solution of C, it also produces the same gas B on warming but D can produce gas B on reaction with dilute sulphuric acid at room temperature. A imparts a deep golden yellow colour to a smokeless flame of Bunsen burner. A, B, C and D respectively are
(a) Na , H_2, NaOH, Zn (b) K, H_2, KOH, Al
(c) Ca, H_2, $Ca(OH)_2$, Sn (d) CaC_2, C_2H_2, $Ca(OH)_2$, Fe

20. At its melting point ice is lighter than water because
(a) H_2O molecules are more closely packed in solid state
(b) ice crystals have hollow hexagonal arrangement of H_2O molecules.
(c) on melting of ice the H_2O molecule shrinks in size
(d) ice froms mostly heavy water on first melting

21. H_2O_2 is commonly prepared in lab. by the reaction of
(a) $PbO_2 + H_2SO_4$ (b) $MnO_2 + H_2SO_4$
(c) $BaO_2 + H_2O + CO_2$ (d) $Na_2O_2 + H_2O$

22. Which of the following is formed by the action of water on sodium peroxide
(a) H_2 (b) N_2 (c) O_2 (d) CO_2

23. The reaction, $2H_2O_2 \rightarrow 2H_2O + O_2$
shows that H_2O_2 :
(a) acts as reducing agent (b) acts as oxidising agent
(c) is decomposed (d) None of these

24. True peroxide is
(a) BaO_2 (b) MnO_2 (c) PbO_2 (d) NO_2

25. The component present in greater proportion in water gas is
(a) CH_4 (b) CO_2 (c) CO (d) H_2

26. Which physical property of dihydrogen is wrong ?
(a) Odourless gas (b) Tasteless gas
(c) Colourless gas (d) Non–inflammable gas

27. In which of the following reactions, H_2O_2 acts as a reducing agent?
(a) $PbO_2(s) + H_2O_2(aq) \rightarrow PbO(s) + H_2O(l) + O_2(g)$
(b) $Na_2SO_3(aq) + H_2O_2(aq) \rightarrow Na_2SO_4(aq) + H_2O(l)$
(c) $2KI(aq) + H_2O_2(aq) \rightarrow 2KOH(aq) + I_2(s)$
(d) $KNO_2(aq) + H_2O_2(aq) \rightarrow KNO_3(aq) + H_2O(l)$

28. In which of the following reactions, H_2O_2 is acting as a reducing agent
(a) $H_2O_2 + SO_2 \rightarrow H_2SO_4$
(b) $2KI + H_2O_2 \rightarrow 2KOH + I_2$
(c) $PbS + 4H_2O_2 \rightarrow PbSO_4 + 4H_2O$
(d) $Ag_2O + H_2O_2 \rightarrow 2Ag + H_2O + O_2$

29. Commercial 10 volume H_2O_2 is a solution with a strength of approximately
(a) 15% (b) 3%
(c) 1% (d) 10%

30. Which of the following is not true?
(a) D_2O freezes at lower temperature than H_2O
(b) Reaction between H_2 and Cl_2 is much faster than D_2 and Cl_2
(c) Ordinary water gets electrolysed more rapidly than D_2O
(d) Bond dissociation energy of D_2 is greater than H_2

31. When zeolite (hydrated sodium aluminium silicate) is treated with hard water the sodium ions are exchanged with
(a) H^+ ions (b) Ca^{2+} ions
(c) SO_4^{2-} ions (d) OH^- ions

32. The oxide that gives H_2O_2 on treatment with a dil. acid is
(a) Na_2O_2 (b) PbO_2 (c) TiO_2 (d) MnO_2

RESPONSE GRID					
	18. ⓐⓑⓒⓓ	19. ⓐⓑⓒⓓ	20. ⓐⓑⓒⓓ	21. ⓐⓑⓒⓓ	22. ⓐⓑⓒⓓ
	23. ⓐⓑⓒⓓ	24. ⓐⓑⓒⓓ	25. ⓐⓑⓒⓓ	26. ⓐⓑⓒⓓ	27. ⓐⓑⓒⓓ
	28. ⓐⓑⓒⓓ	29. ⓐⓑⓒⓓ	30. ⓐⓑⓒⓓ	31. ⓐⓑⓒⓓ	32. ⓐⓑⓒⓓ

Space for Rough Work

33. Which statement is wrong?
(a) Ordinary hydrogen is an equilibrium mixture of ortho and para hydrogen
(b) In ortho hydrogen spin of two nuclei is in same direction
(c) Ortho and para forms do not resemble in their chemical properties
(d) In para hydrogen spin of two nuclei is in opposite direction.

34. Water contracts on heating
(a) to 100°C (b) from 0°C to 4°C
(c) to 273 K (d) from 10°C to 20°C

35. Water is :
(a) more polar than H_2S
(b) more or less identical in polarity with H_2S
(c) less polar than H_2S
(d) None of these

36. $LiAlH_4$ is used as :
(a) An oxidizing agent (b) A reducing agent
(c) A mordant (d) A water softener

37. Hydrogen is not obtained when Zn reacts with
(a) cold water (b) dil H_2SO_4
(c) dil. HCl (d) 20% NaOH

38. An inorganic compound gives off O_2 when heated, turns an acidic solution of KI violet and reduces acidified $KMnO_4$. The compound is
(a) SO_3 (b) KNO_3
(c) H_2O_2 (d) All of these

39. The species that does not contain peroxide ions
(a) PbO_2 (b) H_2O_2 (c) SrO_2 (d) BaO_2

40. Metal hydrides are ionic, covalent or molecular in nature. Among LiH, NaH, KH, RbH, CsH, the correct order of increasing ionic character is
(a) LiH > NaH > CsH > KH > RbH
(b) LiH < NaH < KH < RbH < CsH
(c) RbH > CsH > NaH > KH > LiH
(d) NaH > CsH > RbH > LiH > KH

41. Which of the following in incorrect statement?
(a) s-block elements, except Be and Mg, form ionic hydride
(b) BeH_4, MgH_2, CuH_2, ZnH_2, CaH_2 and HgH_2 are intermediate hydride
(c) p-block elements form covalent hydride
(d) d-and f-block elements form ionic hydride

42. The decomposition of H_2O_2 is accelerated by –
(a) glycerine (b) alcohol
(c) phosphoric acid (d) Pt powder

43. The molarity of a 100 ml solution containing 5.1 g of hydrogen peroxide is
(a) 0.15 M (b) 1.5 M (c) 3.0 M (d) 50.0 M

44. Permanent hardness of water can be removed by adding Calgon $(NaPO_3)_n$. This is an example of
(a) adsorption (b) exchange of ion
(c) precipitation (d) None of these.

45. The oxidation states of most electronegative element in the products of reaction BaO_2 with dil. H_2SO_4 are
(a) 0 and – 1 (b) –1 and – 2
(c) – 2 and 0 (d) – 2 and + 1

RESPONSE GRID					
	33. ⓐⓑⓒⓓ	34. ⓐⓑⓒⓓ	35. ⓐⓑⓒⓓ	36. ⓐⓑⓒⓓ	37. ⓐⓑⓒⓓ
	38. ⓐⓑⓒⓓ	39. ⓐⓑⓒⓓ	40. ⓐⓑⓒⓓ	41. ⓐⓑⓒⓓ	42. ⓐⓑⓒⓓ
	43. ⓐⓑⓒⓓ	44. ⓐⓑⓒⓓ	45. ⓐⓑⓒⓓ		

CHEMISTRY CHAPTERWISE SPEED TEST-37			
Total Questions	45	Total Marks	180
Attempted		Correct	
Incorrect		Net Score	
Cut-off Score	42	Qualifying Score	66
Success Gap = Net Score – Qualifying Score			
Net Score = (Correct × 4) – (Incorrect × 1)			

Space for Rough Work

CHEMISTRY

s-Block Elements

Speed TEST 38 Chapter-wise

No. of Questions	Maximum Marks	Time
45	180	1 Hour

GENERAL INSTRUCTIONS

- This test contains 45 MCQ's. For each question only one option is correct. Darken the correct circle/ bubble in the Response Grid provided on each page.
- You have to evaluate your Response Grids yourself with the help of solutions provided at the end of this book.
- Each correct answer will get you 4 marks and 1 mark shall be deduced for each incorrect answer. No mark will be given/ deducted if no bubble is filled. Keep a timer in front of you and stop immediately at the end of 60 min.
- The sheet follows a particular syllabus. Do not attempt the sheet before you have completed your preparation for that syllabus.
- After completing the sheet check your answers with the solution booklet and complete the Result Grid. Finally spend time to analyse your performance and revise the areas which emerge out as weak in your evaluation.

1. Which of the following has lowest melting point?
   (a) Li (b) Na (c) K (d) Cs
2. Lithium is strongest reducing agent among alkali metals due to which of the following factor?
   (a) Ionization energy (b) Electron affinity
   (c) Hydration energy (d) Lattice energy
3. KO_2 (potassium super oxide) is used in oxygen cylinders in space and submarines because it
   (a) absorbs CO_2 and increases O_2 content
   (b) eliminates moisture
   (c) absorbs CO_2
   (d) produces ozone.
4. The alkali metals form salt-like hydrides by the direct synthesis at elevated temperature. The thermal stability of these hydrides decreases in which of the following orders ?
   (a) CsH > RbH > KH > NaH > LiH
   (b) KH > NaH > LiH > CsH > RbH
   (c) NaH > LiH > KH > RbH > CsH
   (d) LiH > NaH > KH > RbH > CsH
5. Match the columns

	Column-I (Metal)		Column-II (Oxide formed on burning)
A.	Caesium	I.	Superoxide
B.	Lithium	II.	Peroxide
C.	Sodium	III.	Monoxide

   (a) A – II; B – I; C – III
   (b) A – III; B – II; C – I
   (c) A – I; B – III; C – II
   (d) A – II; B – III; C – I
6. Which of the following alkaline earth metal hydroxides is amphoteric in character
   (a) $Be(OH)_2$ (b) $Ca(OH)_2$
   (c) $Sr(OH)_2$ (d) $Ba(OH)_2$
7. Which of the following statements is **incorrect**?
   (a) Pure sodium metal dissolves in liquid ammonia to give blue solution.
   (b) NaOH reacts with glass to give sodium silicate
   (c) Aluminium reacts with excess NaOH to give $Al(OH)_3$
   (d) $NaHCO_3$ on heating gives Na_2CO_3

RESPONSE GRID					
	1. ⓐⓑⓒⓓ	2. ⓐⓑⓒⓓ	3. ⓐⓑⓒⓓ	4. ⓐⓑⓒⓓ	5. ⓐⓑⓒⓓ
	6. ⓐⓑⓒⓓ	7. ⓐⓑⓒⓓ			

Space for Rough Work

8. Which of the following statements about Na_2O_2 is not correct?
(a) It is diamagnetic in nature
(b) It is derivative of H_2O_2
(c) Na_2O_2 oxidises Cr^{3+} to CrO_4^{2-} in acid medium.
(d) It is the super oxide of sodium

9. Which of the following does not form an oxide on heating ?
(a) $ZnCO_3$ (b) $CaCO_3$
(c) Li_2CO_3 (d) Na_2CO_3

10. Sodium carbonate solution in water is alkaline due to
(a) hydrolysis of Na^+
(b) hydrolysis of CO_3^{2-}
(c) hydrolysis of both Na^+ and CO_3^{2-} ions
(d) None of these

11. A white solid reacts with dil.HCl to give colourless gas that decolourises aqueous bromine. The solid is most likely to be
(a) sodium carbonate (b) sodium chloride
(c) sodium acetate (d) sodium thiosulphate

12. Match the columns

Column-I (Alkali metal)		**Column-II (Colour imparted to an oxidizing flame)**	
A.	Cs	I.	Yellow
B.	Rb	II.	Blue
C.	K	III.	Violet
D.	Na	IV.	Red violet
E.	Li	V	Crimson red

(a) A – II; B – IV; C – III; D – I; E – V
(b) A – IV; B – II; C – III; D – I; E – V
(c) A – V; B – III; C – IV; D – I; E – II
(d) A – II; B – IV; C – III; D – I; E – V

13. Select the correct statements
(i) Cs^+ is more highly hydrated that the other alkali metal ions
(ii) Among the alkali metals Li, Na, K and Rb, lithium has the highest melting point
(iii) Among the alkali metals only lithium forms a stable nitride by direct combination with nitrogen
(a) (i), (ii) and (iii) (b) (i) and (ii)
(c) (i) and (iii) (d) (ii) and (iii)

14. When sulphur is heated with NaOH (aq). The compounds formed are
(a) $Na_2S + H_2O$
(b) $Na_2SO_3 + H_2O$
(c) $Na_2S + Na_2S_2O_3 + H_2O$
(d) $Na_2S_2O_3 + H_2O$

15. The raw materials in Solvay Process are :
(a) $Na_2CO_3, CaCO_3$ and NH_3
(b) $Na_2SO_4, CaCO_3$ and NH_3
(c) NaCl, NH_3 and $CaCO_3$.
(d) NaOH, CaO and NH_3.

16. A metal X on heating in nitrogen gas gives Y. Y on treatment with H_2O gives a colourless gas which when passed through $CuSO_4$ solution gives a blue colour. Y is
(a) $Mg(NO_3)_2$ (b) Mg_3N_2
(c) NH_3 (d) MgO

17. Acidified solution of sodium thiosulphate is unstable because in thiosulphate
(a) the sulphur atoms are at unstable oxidation state of +2
(b) the two sulphur atoms are at different oxidation states of + 6 and – 2
(c) the S – S bond are unstable bonds.
(d) sulphur is in zero oxidation state.

RESPONSE GRID					
	8. ⓐⓑⓒⓓ	9. ⓐⓑⓒⓓ	10. ⓐⓑⓒⓓ	11. ⓐⓑⓒⓓ	12. ⓐⓑⓒⓓ
	13. ⓐⓑⓒⓓ	14. ⓐⓑⓒⓓ	15. ⓐⓑⓒⓓ	16. ⓐⓑⓒⓓ	17. ⓐⓑⓒⓓ

Space for Rough Work

18. Which one of the following is least soluble in water?
(a) BaF_2 (b) MgF_2 (c) CaF_2 (d) SrF_2

19. Bleaching powder is obtained by the interaction of chlorine with
(a) dil. solution of $Ca(OH)_2$
(b) dry CaO
(c) conc. solution of $Ca(OH)_2$
(d) dry slaked lime

20. Which of the following statement is false ?
(a) Strontium decomposes water readily than beryllium
(b) Barium carbonate melts at a higher temperature than calcium carbonate
(c) Barium hydroxide is more soluble in water than magnesium hydroxide
(d) Beryllium hydroxide is more basic than barium hydroxide.

21. Melting point of calcium halides decreases in the order
(a) $CaF_2 > CaCl_2 > CaBr_2 > CaI_2$
(b) $CaI_2 > CaBr_2 > CaCl_2 > CaF_2$
(c) $CaBr_2 > CaI_2 > CaF_2 > CaCl_2$
(d) $CaCl_2 > CaBr_2 > CaI_2 > CaF_2$

22. Which of the following are found in biological fluids Na^+, Mg^{2+}, Ca^{2+}, K^+, Sr^{2+}, Li^+ and Ba^{2+}
(a) Mg^{2+}, Ca^{2+}, and Sr^{2+}
(b) Na^{2+} and K^+
(c) Na^+, K^+, Mg^{2+} and Ca^{2+}
(d) Sr^+, Li and Ba^{2+}

23. Chemical A is used for water softening to remove temporary hardness. A reacts with Na_2CO_3 to generate caustic soda. When CO_2 is bubbled through A, it turns cloudly. What is the chemical formula of A
(a) $CaCO_3$ (b) CaO (c) $Ca(OH)_2$ (d) $Ca(HCO_3)_2$

24. Which of the following statements is incorrect?
(a) Alkali metal hydroxide are hygroscopic
(b) Dissolution of alkali metal hydroxide is endothermic
(c) Aqueous solution of alkali metal hydroxides are strongly basic
(d) Alkali metal hydroxides form ionic crystals

25. Which of the following statement(s) is/are correct regarding Li_2CO_3 and Na_2CO_3 ?
(a) Sodium salt evolve CO_2 at higher temperature.
(b) Polarization of Na^+ is lesser than that of Li^+.
(c) Both are are highly stable to heat
(d) All of the above

26. Calcitonin and parathyroid hormone regulate concentration of which of the following element in plasma?
(a) Calcium (b) Magnesium
(c) Sodium (d) Potassium

27. Oxygen is obtained from bleaching powder by
(a) the action of dilute acid
(b) the action of alkali
(c) heating it with lime
(d) heating it with cobalt salt

28. Substance which absorbs CO_2 and violently reacts with H_2O with sound is :
(a) H_2SO_4 (b) $CaCO_3$ (c) ZnO (d) CaO.

29. The electric cookers have a coating that protects them against fire. The coating is made of
(a) Heavy lead (b) Zinc oxide
(c) Magnesium oxide (d) Sodium sulphate

30. Which among the following is most soluble in water?
(a) $CsClO_4$ (b) $NaClO_4$ (c) $LiClO_4$ (d) $KClO_4$

31. Which of the following is incorrect?
(a) Mg burns in air releasing dazzling light rich in UV rays.
(b) $CaCl_2.6H_2O$ when mixed with ice gives freezing mixture
(c) Mg cannot form complexes
(d) Be can form complexes due to its very small size

32. Electrolysis of fused KCl. $MgCl_2$. $6H_2O$ gives
(a) potassium only
(b) magnesium only
(c) magnesium and chlorine
(d) potassium, magnesium and chlorine

RESPONSE GRID					
	18. ⓐⓑⓒⓓ	19. ⓐⓑⓒⓓ	20. ⓐⓑⓒⓓ	21. ⓐⓑⓒⓓ	22. ⓐⓑⓒⓓ
	23. ⓐⓑⓒⓓ	24. ⓐⓑⓒⓓ	25. ⓐⓑⓒⓓ	26. ⓐⓑⓒⓓ	27. ⓐⓑⓒⓓ
	28. ⓐⓑⓒⓓ	29. ⓐⓑⓒⓓ	30. ⓐⓑⓒⓓ	31. ⓐⓑⓒⓓ	32. ⓐⓑⓒⓓ

Space for Rough Work

33. Beryllium shows diagonal relationship with aluminium. Which of the following similarity is incorrect ?
(a) Be forms beryllates and Al forms aluminates
(b) $Be(OH)_2$ like $Al(OH)_3$ is basic.
(c) Be like Al is rendered passive by HNO_3 .
(d) Be_2C like Al_4C_3 yields methane on hydrolysis.

34. Amongst the following hydroxides, the one which is insoluble is
(a) $Ca(OH)_2$ (b) $Mg(OH)_2$
(c) $Be(OH)_2$ (d) $Ba(OH)_2$

35. A and B are two salts. A with dil. HCl and A and B with conc. H_2SO_4 react to give reddish brown vapours, hence A and B respectively are :
(a) $NaNO_3$, NaBr (b) NaBr, $NaNO_3$
(c) NaBr, $NaNO_2$ (d) $NaNO_2$, NaBr

36. In crystals of which one of the following ionic compounds would you expect maximum distance between centres of cations and anions?
(a) LiF (b) CsF (c) CsI (d) LiI

37. Alkaline earth metal compounds are less soluble in water than corresponding alkali metal compounds because former have
(a) lower lattice energy
(b) higher I.P.
(c) higher covalent character
(d) lower covalent character.

38. The following compounds have been arranged in order of their increasing thermal stabilities. Identify the correct order.
(I) K_2CO_3 (II) $MgCO_3$
(III) $CaCO_3$ (IV) $BeCO_3$
(a) I<II<III<IV (b) IV<II<III<I
(c) IV<II<I<III (d) II<IV<III<I

39. Covalent radii of atoms varies in range of 72 pm to 133 pm from F to I while that of noble gases He to Xe varies from 120pm to 220pm. This is because in case of noble gases
(a) covalent radius is very large
(b) van der Waal radius is considered
(c) metallic radii is considered
(d) None of these

40. Among KO_2, AlO_2^-, BaO_2 and NO_2^+, unpaired electron is present in
(a) NO_2^+ and BaO_2 (b) KO_2 and AlO_2^-
(c) KO_2 only (d) BaO_2 only

41. A certain metal M is used to prepare an antacid, which is used as a medicine in acidity. This metal accidently catches fire which cannot be put out by using CO_2 based extinguishers. The metal M is
(a) Ca (b) Mg
(c) C (d) All of these

42. Choose the compound which does not possess a peroxide group
(a) Na_2O_2 (b) CrO_5 (c) Fe_2O_3 (d) BaO_2

43. Which of the following has correct increasing basic strength?
(a) MgO<BeO<CaO<BaO (b) BeO<MgO<CaO<BaO
(c) BaO<CaO<MgO<BeO (d) CaO<BaO<BeO<MgO

44. Which one of the following orders presents the correct sequence of the increasing basic nature of the given oxides?
(a) $Al_2O_3 < MgO < Na_2O < K_2O$
(b) $MgO < K_2O < Al_2O_3 < Na_2O$
(c) $Na_2O < K_2O < MgO < Al_2O_3$
(d) $K_2O < Na_2O < Al_2O_3 < MgO$

45. Which liberates ammonia when treated with water?
(a) Li_3N (b) Mg_3N_2 (c) $CaCN_2$ (d) All

RESPONSE GRID					
	33. ⓐⓑⓒⓓ	34. ⓐⓑⓒⓓ	35. ⓐⓑⓒⓓ	36. ⓐⓑⓒⓓ	37. ⓐⓑⓒⓓ
	38. ⓐⓑⓒⓓ	39. ⓐⓑⓒⓓ	40. ⓐⓑⓒⓓ	41. ⓐⓑⓒⓓ	42. ⓐⓑⓒⓓ
	43. ⓐⓑⓒⓓ	44. ⓐⓑⓒⓓ	45. ⓐⓑⓒⓓ		

CHEMISTRY CHAPTERWISE SPEED TEST-38

Total Questions	45	Total Marks	180
Attempted		Correct	
Incorrect		Net Score	
Cut-off Score	36	Qualifying Score	58
Success Gap = Net Score – Qualifying Score			
Net Score = (Correct × 4) – (Incorrect × 1)			

Space for Rough Work

CHEMISTRY

p-Block Elements

Speed TEST 39 Chapter-wise

No. of Questions	Maximum Marks	Time
45	180	1 Hour

GENERAL INSTRUCTIONS

- This test contains 45 MCQ's. For each question only one option is correct. Darken the correct circle/ bubble in the Response Grid provided on each page.
- You have to evaluate your Response Grids yourself with the help of solutions provided at the end of this book.
- Each correct answer will get you 4 marks and 1 mark shall be deduced for each incorrect answer. No mark will be given/ deducted if no bubble is filled. Keep a timer in front of you and stop immediately at the end of 60 min.
- The sheet follows a particular syllabus. Do not attempt the sheet before you have completed your preparation for that syllabus.
- After completing the sheet check your answers with the solution booklet and complete the Result Grid. Finally spend time to analyse your performance and revise the areas which emerge out as weak in your evaluation.

1. Which of the following hydroxide is acidic ?
   (a) $Al(OH)_3$ (b) $Ca(OH)_3$
   (c) $Tl(OH)_3$ (d) $B(OH)_3$
2. Boric acid is polymeric due to
   (a) its acidic nature
   (b) the presence of hydrogen bonds
   (c) its monobasic nature
   (d) its geometry
3. The $I.E_1$ among the group 13 member follows as
   (a) $B > Al < Ga < Tl$ (b) $B > Al > Ga > Tl$
   (c) $B > Ga > Al > Tl$ (d) $B > Ga < Al < Tl$
4. In aluminates, the coordination number of Al is
   (a) 4 (b) 6
   (c) 3 (d) 1
5. Match the columns

	Column-I		Column-II
A.	Carbon	I.	Metal
B.	Silicon	II.	Non-metal
C.	Germanium	III.	Metalloid
D.	Tin		
E.	Lead		

   (a) A – II; B – II; C – III; D – I; E – I
   (b) A – II; B – III; C – III; D – I; E – I
   (c) A – I; B – III; C – III; D – I; E – II
   (d) A – I; B – II; C – II; D – III; E – I
6. The melting pt. of group 13 follows the order
   (a) $B > Al > Ga > In > Tl$ (b) $B > Al < Ga > In > Tl$
   (c) $B > Al > Tl > In > Ga$ (d) $B > Al < Ga < In < Tl$
7. The stability of dihalides of Si, Ge, Sn and Pb increases steadily in the sequence
   (a) $PbX_2 << SnX_2 << GeX_2 << SiX_2$
   (b) $GeX_2 << SiX_2 << SnX_2 << PbX_2$
   (c) $SiX_2 << GeX_2 << PbX_2 << SnX_2$
   (d) $SiX_2 << GeX_2 << SnX_2 << PbX_2$.
8. The catenation tendency of C,Si and Ge is in the order Ge < Si < C. The bond energies (in kJ mol^{-1}) of C-C, Si-Si and Ge-Ge bonds, respectively are
   (a) 167, 180, 348 (b) 180, 167, 348
   (c) 348, 167, 180 (d) 348, 180, 167
9. Which is not the use of orthoboric acid?
   (a) As an antiseptic and eye wash.
   (b) In glass industry.
   (c) In glazes for pottery.
   (d) In borax - bead test.

RESPONSE GRID					
	1. ⓐⓑⓒⓓ	2. ⓐⓑⓒⓓ	3. ⓐⓑⓒⓓ	4. ⓐⓑⓒⓓ	5. ⓐⓑⓒⓓ
	6. ⓐⓑⓒⓓ	7. ⓐⓑⓒⓓ	8. ⓐⓑⓒⓓ	9. ⓐⓑⓒⓓ	

Space for Rough Work

10. On adding ammonium hydroxide solution to $Al_2(SO_4)_3(aq)$:
(a) A precipitate is formed which does not dissolve in excess of ammonium hydroxide
(b) A precipitate is formed which dissolves in excess of ammonia solution
(c) No precipitate is formed
(d) None of these

11. Heating an aqueous solution of aluminium chloride to dryness will give
(a) $Al(OH)Cl_2$ (b) Al_2O_3
(c) Al_2Cl_6 (d) $AlCl_3$

12. Which of the following statement(s) is/are incorrect ?
(i) Higher boranes are not flammable.
(ii) Boranes are hydrolysed by water to give orthoboric acid.
(iii) Boranes undergoes cleavage reactions with Lewis bases to give borane adducts.
(a) (i) only (b) (ii) and (iii)
(c) (iii) only (d) (i) and (ii)

13. Which among the following oxides react with alkali? B_2O_3, Al_2O_3 and Tl_2O
(a) B_2O_3 and Al_2O_3 (b) Al_2O_3 and Tl_2O
(c) Only B_2O_3 (d) B_2O_3 and Tl_2O

14. In the following sets of reactants which two sets best exhibit the amphoteric characters of $Al_2O_3.xH_2O$?
Set 1: $Al_2O_3.xH_2O$ (s) and OH^- (aq)
Set 2: $Al_2O_3.xH_2O$ (s) and H_2O (*l*)
Set 3: $Al_2O_3.xH_2O$ (s) and H^+ (aq)
Set 4: $Al_2O_3.xH_2O$ (s) and NH_3 (aq)
(a) 1 and 2 (b) 1 and 3
(c) 2 and 4 (d) 3 and 4

15. Aluminium is extracted from alumina (Al_2O_3) by electrolysis of a molten mixture of:
(a) $Al_2O_3 + HF + NaAlF_4$
(b) $Al_2O_3 + CaF_2 + NaAlF_4$
(c) $Al_2O_3 + Na_3AlF_6 + CaF_2$
(d) $Al_2O_3 + KF + Na_3AlF_6$

16. Which of the following has the minimum heat of dissociation:
(a) $(CH_3)_3N: \rightarrow BF_3$
(b) $(CH_3)_3N: \rightarrow B(CH_3)_2F$
(c) $(CH_3)_3N: \rightarrow B(CH_3)_3$
(d) $(CH_3)_3N: \rightarrow B(CH_3)F_2$

17. The hybridisation of boron atom in orthoboric acid is
(a) sp (b) sp^2
(c) sp^3 (d) sp^3d

18. Which among the following can act as reducing agent (A)$SnCl_2$, (B)CO and (C)$PbCl_2$?
(a) (A) and (B) (b) (B) and (C)
(c) (C) and (A) (d) Only (B)

19. What is the oxidation state and hybridisation of boron in compound formed when BCl_3 undergoes reaction with the water?
(a) 3, sp^2d (b) 3, sp^3
(c) 4, sp^3 (d) 3, sp^2d

20. Identify the statement that is not correct as far as structure of diborane is concerned
(a) There are two bridging hydrogen atoms and four terminal hydrogen atoms in diborane
(b) Each boron atom forms four bonds in diborane
(c) The hydrogen atoms are not in the same plane in diborane
(d) All, B – H bonds in diborane are similar

21. Specify the coordination geometry around and hybridization of N and B atoms in a 1 : 1 complex of BF_3 and NH_3
(a) N : tetrahedral, sp^3; B : tetrahedral, sp^3
(b) N : pyramidal, sp^3; B : pyramidal, sp^3
(c) N : pyramidal, sp^3; B : planar, sp^3
(d) N : pyramidal, sp^3; B : tetrahedral, sp^3

RESPONSE GRID					
	10. ⓐⓑⓒⓓ	11. ⓐⓑⓒⓓ	12. ⓐⓑⓒⓓ	13. ⓐⓑⓒⓓ	14. ⓐⓑⓒⓓ
	15. ⓐⓑⓒⓓ	16. ⓐⓑⓒⓓ	17. ⓐⓑⓒⓓ	18. ⓐⓑⓒⓓ	19. ⓐⓑⓒⓓ
	20. ⓐⓑⓒⓓ	21. ⓐⓑⓒⓓ			

Space for Rough Work

22. Which of the following shows bond in silicon :
(a) Si – Si – Si – Si (b) – Si – O – Si – O – Si
(c) Si – C – Si – C – Si (d) Si – C – Si – O – Si

23. CO_2 and N_2 are non-supporters of combustion. However for putting out fires CO_2 is preferred over N_2 because CO_2
(a) does not burn
(b) forms non-combustible products with burning substances
(c) is denser than nitrogen
(d) is a more reactive gas

24. Which of the following statement(s) is/are incorrect ?
(i) Trichlorides on hydrolysis in water form tetrahedral $[M(OH)_4]^-$ species.
(ii) Hybridisation state of metal in tetrahedral species is sp^3.
(iii) Aluminium chloride in acidified aqueous solution forms $[Al(OH)_4]^-$ ion.
(a) (i) and (ii) (b) (ii) only
(c) (iii) only (d) (i) and (iii)

25. _____ helps to maintain pH of blood between 7.26 to 7.42
(a) CO_2 (b) H_2CO_3
(c) CO_3^{2-} (d) H_2CO_3/HCO_3^-

26. The soldiers of Napolean army while at Alps during freezing winter suffered a serious problem as regards to the tin buttons of their uniforms. White metallic tin buttons got converted to grey powder. This transformation is related to
(a) a change in the partial pressure of oxygen in the air
(b) a change in the crystalline structure of tin
(c) an interaction with nitrogen of the air at very low temperature
(d) an interaction with water vapour contained in the humid air

27. On addition of excess of sodium hydroxide solution to stannous chloride solution, we obtain :
(a) $Sn(OH)_2$ (b) $SnO_2.H_2O$
(c) Na_2SnO_2 (d) None of these

28. The reducing power of divalent species decreases in the order
(a) Ge > Sn > Pb (b) Sn > Ge > Pb
(c) Pb > Sn > Ge (d) None of these

29. The gas evolved on heating CaF_2 and SiO_2 with concentrated H_2SO_4, on hydrolysis gives a white gelatinous precipitate. The precipitate is:
(a) hydrofluosilicic acid (b) silica gel
(c) silicic acid (d) calciumfluorosilicate

30. In view of the signs of $\Delta_r G^\circ$ for the following reactions :

$$PbO_2 + Pb \rightarrow 2PbO, \quad \Delta_r G^\circ < 0$$
$$SnO_2 + Sn \rightarrow 2SnO, \quad \Delta_r G^\circ > 0$$

Which oxidation states are more characteristics for lead and tin ?
(a) For lead + 2, for tin + 2 (b) For lead + 4, for tin + 4
(c) For lead + 2, for tin + 4 (d) For lead + 4, for tin + 2

31. A metal, M forms chlorides in its +2 and +4 oxidation states. Which of the following statements about these chlorides is correct?
(a) MCl_2 is more ionic than MCl_4
(b) MCl_2 is more easily hydrolysed than MCl_4
(c) MCl_2 is more volatile than MCl_4
(d) MCl_2 is more soluble in anhydrous ethanol than MCl_4

32. Which of the following statements about H_3BO_3 is not correct ?
(a) It is a strong tribasic acid.
(b) It is prepared by acidifying an aqueous solution of borax.
(c) It has a layer structure in which planar BO_3 units are joined by hydrogen bonds.
(d) It does not act as proton donor but acts as a Lewis acid by accepting a lone pair of electrons.

33. Pyrosilicate ion is
(a) SiO_2^{2-} (b) SiO_4^{2-} (c) $Si_2O_6^{7-}$ (d) $Si_2O_7^{6-}$

RESPONSE GRID					
	22. ⓐⓑⓒⓓ	23. ⓐⓑⓒⓓ	24. ⓐⓑⓒⓓ	25. ⓐⓑⓒⓓ	26. ⓐⓑⓒⓓ
	27. ⓐⓑⓒⓓ	28. ⓐⓑⓒⓓ	29. ⓐⓑⓒⓓ	30. ⓐⓑⓒⓓ	31. ⓐⓑⓒⓓ
	32. ⓐⓑⓒⓓ	33. ⓐⓑⓒⓓ			

Space for Rough Work

34. For making good quality mirrors, plates of float glass are used. These are obtained by floating molten glass over a liquid metal which does not solidify before glass. The metal used can be

(a) tin (b) sodium
(c) magnesium (d) mercury

35. PbF_4, $PbCl_4$ exist but $PbBr_4$ and PbI_4 do not exist because of

(a) large size of Br^- and I^-
(b) strong oxidising character of Pb^{4+}
(c) strong reducing character of Pb^{4+}
(d) low electronegativity of Br^- and I^-.

36. Ge(II) compounds are powerful reducing agents whereas Pb(IV) compounds are strong oxidants .It is because

(a) Pb is more electropositive than Ge
(b) ionization potential of lead is less than that of Ge
(c) ionic radii of Pb^{2+} and Pb^{4+} are larger than those of Ge^{2+} and Ge^{4+}
(d) of more pronounced inert pair effect in lead than in Ge

37. The structure and hybridization of $Si(CH_3)_4$ is

(a) Bent, sp (b) Trigonal, sp^2
(c) Octahedral, d^2sp^3 (d) Tetrahedral, sp^3

38. In reaction

$$8BF_3 + 6LiH \xrightarrow{\Delta} X + LiBF_4$$

(a) B_4H_{10} (b) B_2H_6 (c) BH_3 (d) B_3H_8

39. Which of the following gas is used in artificial respiration ?

(a) O_2 (b) CO_2
(c) Helium (d) All of these

40. Graphite conducts electricity because of

(a) weak van der Waal's forces between layers
(b) covalent bonding between carbon atoms of layers
(c) delocalized electrons in each layer
(d) sp^2 hybridisation of carbon atoms in a layer

41. A group 14 element is oxidised to form corresponding oxide which is gaseous in nature, when dissolved in water pH of the water decreases further addition of group 2 hydroxides leads to precipitation. This oxide can be

(a) GeO_2 (b) CO
(c) CO_2 (d) SnO_2

42. Carborundum is

(a) $Al_2(SO_4)_3$ (b) $Al_2O_3.2H_2O$
(c) $AlCl_3$ (d) SiC

43. R_3SiCl on hydrolysis forms

(a) R_3SiOH (b) $R_3Si-O-SiR_3$
(c) $R_2Si=O$ (d) None of these

44. Which of the following species exists (A) $[SiF_6]^{2-}$, (B) $[GeCl_6]^{2-}$ and (C) $[CCl_6]^{2-}$?

(a) (A) and (B) (b) (B) and (C)
(c) Only (C) (d) (A) and (C)

45. Which of the following attacks glass

(a) HCl (b) HF
(c) HI (d) HBr

RESPONSE GRID					
	34. ⓐⓑⓒⓓ	35. ⓐⓑⓒⓓ	36. ⓐⓑⓒⓓ	37. ⓐⓑⓒⓓ	38. ⓐⓑⓒⓓ
	39. ⓐⓑⓒⓓ	40. ⓐⓑⓒⓓ	41. ⓐⓑⓒⓓ	42. ⓐⓑⓒⓓ	43. ⓐⓑⓒⓓ
	44. ⓐⓑⓒⓓ	45. ⓐⓑⓒⓓ			

CHEMISTRY CHAPTERWISE SPEED TEST-39

Total Questions	45	Total Marks	180
Attempted		Correct	
Incorrect		Net Score	
Cut-off Score	38	Qualifying Score	65
Success Gap = Net Score – Qualifying Score			
Net Score = (Correct × 4) – (Incorrect × 1)			

Space for Rough Work

CHEMISTRY

Organic Chemistry - Some Basic Principles and Techniques

Speed TEST 40

Chapter-wise

No. of Questions	Maximum Marks	Time
45	180	1 Hour

GENERAL INSTRUCTIONS

- This test contains 45 MCQ's. For each question only one option is correct. Darken the correct circle/ bubble in the Response Grid provided on each page.
- You have to evaluate your Response Grids yourself with the help of solutions provided at the end of this book.
- Each correct answer will get you 4 marks and 1 mark shall be deduced for each incorrect answer. No mark will be given/ deducted if no bubble is filled. Keep a timer in front of you and stop immediately at the end of 60 min.
- The sheet follows a particular syllabus. Do not attempt the sheet before you have completed your preparation for that syllabus.
- After completing the sheet check your answers with the solution booklet and complete the Result Grid. Finally spend time to analyse your performance and revise the areas which emerge out as weak in your evaluation.

1. The correct decreasing order of priority for the functional groups of organic compounds in the IUPAC system of nomenclature is
   (a) $-COOH, -SO_3H, -CONH_2, -CHO$
   (b) $-SO_3H, -COOH, -CONH_2, -CHO$
   (c) $-CHO, -COOH, -SO_3H, -CONH_2$
   (d) $-CONH_2, -CHO, -SO_3H, -COOH$
2. The IUPAC name of the compound

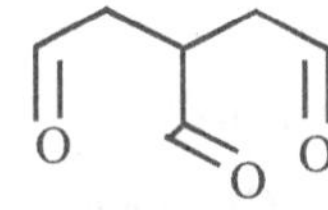

   (a) 1, 2, 3 – triformyl propane
   (b) Propane – 1, 2, 3 – tricarbaldehyde
   (c) 3 – formyl – 1, 5 – pentane dial
   (d) Propane – 1, 2, 3 – trial
3. Vinylcarbinol is
   (a) $HO-CH_2-CH=CH_2$
   (b) $CH_3C(OH)=CH_2$
   (c) $CH_3-CH=CH-OH$
   (d) $CH_3-C(CH_2OH)=CH_2$
4. The compound 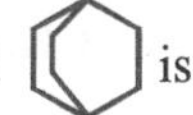 is known by which of the following names ?
   (a) Bicyclo [2.2.2] octane
   (b) Bicyclo [2.2.1] octane
   (c) Bicyclo [1.2.1] octane
   (d) Bicyclo [1.1.1] octane
5. The stability of the compounds

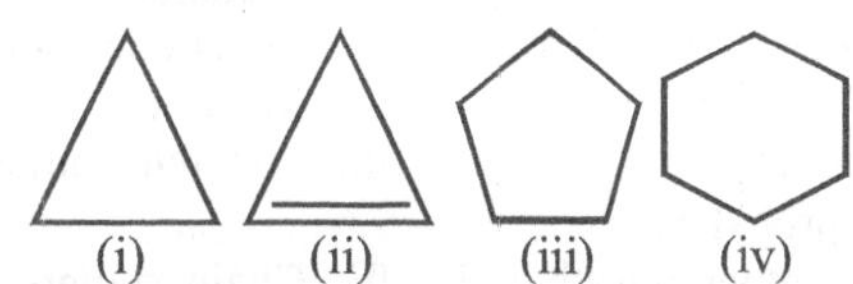

   (a) (iv) > (iii) > (i) > (ii) (b) (i) > (iii) > (ii) > (iv)
   (c) (ii) > (iii) > (i) > (iv) (d) (iv) > (i) > (iii) > (ii)
6. Fractional distillation is used when
   (a) there is a large difference in the boiling point of liquids
   (b) there is a small difference in the boiling points of liquids
   (c) boiling points of liquids are same
   (d) liquids form a constant boiling mixture
7. Rate of the reaction

$$R-\overset{\overset{O}{\|}}{C}-Z + Nu^{\ominus} \longrightarrow R-\overset{\overset{O}{\|}}{C}-Nu + Z^{\ominus}$$

   is fastest when Z is
   (a) OC_2H_5 (b) NH_2 (c) Cl^- (d) $OCOCH_3$
8. The order of activity of the various o- and p-director is
   (a) $-O^- > -OH > -OCOCH_3 > -COCH_3$
   (b) $-OH > -O^- > -OCOCH_3 > -COCH_3$
   (c) $-OH > -O^- > -COCH_3 > -OCOCH_3$
   (d) $-O^- > -COCH_3 > -OCOCH_3 > -OH$

RESPONSE GRID					
	1. ⓐⓑⓒⓓ	2. ⓐⓑⓒⓓ	3. ⓐⓑⓒⓓ	4. ⓐⓑⓒⓓ	5. ⓐⓑⓒⓓ
	6. ⓐⓑⓒⓓ	7. ⓐⓑⓒⓓ	8. ⓐⓑⓒⓓ		

Space for Rough Work

9. The general formula $C_nH_{2n}O_2$ could be for open chain
   (a) carboxylic acids (b) diols
   (c) dialdehydes (d) diketones

10. $C_6H_5CHO + HCN \longrightarrow C_6H_5 - \underset{OH}{\overset{H}{\overset{|}{\underset{|}{C}}}} - CN$
   The product would be
   (a) a racemate
   (b) optically active
   (c) a meso compound
   (d) a mixture of diastereomers

11. The number of possible open chain (acyclic) isomeric compounds for molecular formula C_5H_{10} would be
   (a) 8 (b) 7 (c) 6 (d) 5

12. Which one of the following is the stablest structure of cyclohexatriene ?
   (a) Chair form (b) Boat form
   (c) Halfchair form (d) Planar form

13. The compound formed in the positive test for nitrogen with the Lassaigne solution of an organic compound is
   (a) $Fe_4[Fe(CN)_6]_3$ (b) $Na_3[Fe(CN)_6]$
   (c) $Fe(CN)_3$ (d) $Na_4[Fe(CN)_5NOS]$

14. 2.79 g of an organic compound when heated in Carius tube with conc. HNO_3 and H_3PO_4 formed converted into $MgNH_4.PO_4$ ppt. The ppt. on heating gave 1.332 g of $Mg_2P_2O_7$. The percentage of P in the compound is
   (a) 23.33% (b) 13.33% (c) 33.33% (d) 26.66%

15. Match the columns

	Column-I		Column-II
A.	CH_3COOH & $HCOOCH_3$	I.	Functional isomers
B.	1-butene & 2-butene	II.	Metamers
C.	diethyl ether & methyl propyl ether	III.	Position isomers
D.	dimethyl ether and ethanol	IV.	Chain isomers

   (a) A – I; B – III; C – II; D – IV
   (b) A – II; B – III; C – IV; D – I
   (c) A – II; B – IV; C – I; D – III
   (d) A – II; B – I; C – IV; D – III

16. The accepted IUPAC name of the camphor is

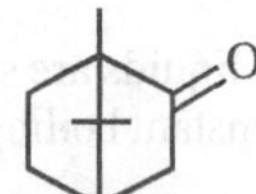

   (a) 1, 7, 7 – trimethyl bicyclo [2. 2. 1] heptan – 2 – one
   (b) 1, 7, 7, – trimethyl bicyclo [2. 1. 2] heptan – 2 – one
   (c) 1, 2, 2 – trimethyl bicyclo [2. 2. 1] heptan – 6 – one
   (d) None of these

17. The pair of structures given below represent

   (Newman projections — first: front H, CH$_3$ (top), Cl; back H, H, CH$_3$ (bottom). Second: front H, CH$_3$ (top), H; back H, H, CH$_2$Cl (bottom).)

   (a) enantiomers
   (b) diastereomers
   (c) structural isomers
   (d) two molecules of the same compound.

18. Which of the following compounds exhibits geometrical isomerism ?
   (a) C_2H_5Br (b) $(CH)_2(COOH)_2$
   (c) CH_3CHO (d) $(CH_2)_2(COOH)_2$

19. Chlorine in vinyl chloride is less reactive because
   (a) sp^2 - hybridised carbon has more acidic character than sp^3 - hybridised carbon
   (b) C - Cl bond develops partial double bond character
   (c) of resonance
   (d) All are correct

20. The best method for the separation of naphthalene and benzoic acid from their mixture is:
   (a) distillation (b) sublimation
   (c) chromatography (d) crystallisation

21. The percentage of sulphur in an organic compound whose 0.32 g produces 0.233 g of $BaSO_4$ [At. wt. Ba = 137, S = 32] is
   (a) 1.0 (b) 10.0 (c) 23.5 (d) 32.1

22. Indicate the wrongly named compound
   (a) $CH_3-\underset{CH_3}{\underset{|}{CH}}-CH_2-CH_2-CHO$
   (4-methyl -1- pentanal)
   (b) $CH_3-\underset{CH_3}{\underset{|}{CH}}-C\equiv C-COOH$
   (4- methyl -2- pentyne -1- oic acid)
   (c) $CH_3CH_2CH_2-\underset{CH_3}{\underset{|}{CH}}-COOH$
   (2- methyl -1- pentanoic acid)
   (d) $CH_3-CH_2-CH=CH-\overset{O}{\overset{||}{C}}-CH_3$
   (3- hexen -5- one)

RESPONSE GRID					
	9. ⓐⓑⓒⓓ	10. ⓐⓑⓒⓓ	11. ⓐⓑⓒⓓ	12. ⓐⓑⓒⓓ	13. ⓐⓑⓒⓓ
	14. ⓐⓑⓒⓓ	15. ⓐⓑⓒⓓ	16. ⓐⓑⓒⓓ	17. ⓐⓑⓒⓓ	18. ⓐⓑⓒⓓ
	19. ⓐⓑⓒⓓ	20. ⓐⓑⓒⓓ	21. ⓐⓑⓒⓓ	22. ⓐⓑⓒⓓ	

Space for Rough Work

23. The (R)- and (S)- enantiomers of an optically active compound differ in
(a) their reactivity with achiral reagents
(b) their optical rotation of plane polarized light
(c) their melting points
(d) None of these

24. But-2-ene exhibits cis-trans-isomerism due to
(a) rotation around $C_3 - C_4$ sigma bond
(b) restricted rotation around C = C bond
(c) rotation around $C_1 - C_2$ bond
(d) rotation around $C_2 - C_3$ double bond

25. Which of the following compounds undergoes nucleophilic substitution reaction most easily ?

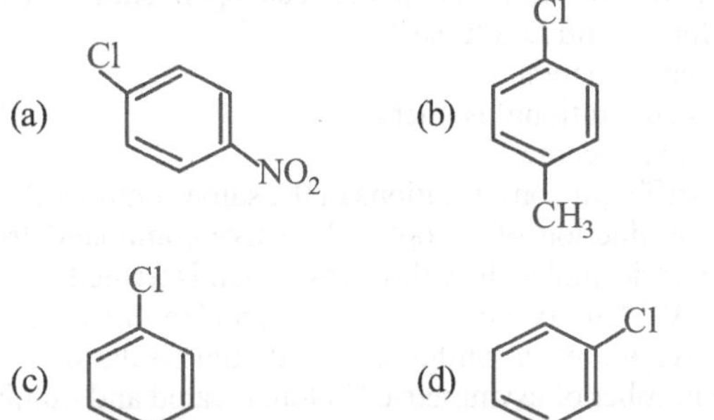

26. An organic compound contains C = 40%, H = 13.33% and N = 46.67%. Its empirical formula would be
(a) CHN (b) C_2H_2N (c) CH_4N (d) C_3H_7N

27. The IUPAC name of

$$CH_3-\overset{\overset{CH_3}{|}}{CH}-\overset{\overset{O}{||}}{C}-CH_2-CH_2OH$$ is

(a) 1- Hydroxy -4- methyl -3- pentanone
(b) 2- Methyl -5- hydroxy -3- pentanone
(c) 4- Methyl -3- oxo -1- pentanol
(d) Hexanol -1 - one -3

28. An important chemical method to resolve a racemic mixture makes use of the formation of
(a) a meso compound (b) enantiomers
(c) diastereomers (d) racemate

29. The Lassaigne's extract is boiled with dil. HNO_3 before testing for halogens because
(a) Silver halides are soluble in HNO_3
(b) Na_2S and NaCN are decomposed by HNO_3
(c) Ag_2S is soluble in HNO_3
(d) AgCN is soluble is HNO_3

30. What is the decreasing order of strength of the bases OH^-, NH_2^-, $HC \equiv C^-$ and $CH_3CH_2^-$?
(a) $CH_3CH_2^- > HC \equiv C^- > NH_2^- > OH^-$
(b) $HC \equiv C^- > CH_3CH_2^- > NH_2^- > OH^-$
(c) $OH^- > NH_2^- > HC \equiv C^- > CH_3CH_2^-$
(d) $NH_2^- > HC \equiv C^- > OH^- > CH_3CH_2^-$

31. Given

(I) 4,4-dimethylcyclohex-2-en-1-one (CH_3, CH_3 on ring carbon; C=O)
(II) cyclohexenone with two CH_3 groups
(III) cyclohexenone with two CH_3 groups

Which of the given compounds can exhibit tautomerism?
(a) I and III (b) II and III
(c) I, II and III (d) I and II

32. Cyclohexanol (I), acetic acid (II), 2, 4, 6-trinitrophenol (III) and phenol (IV) are given. In these the order of decreasing acidic character will be :
(a) III > II > IV > I (b) II > III > I > IV
(c) II > III > IV > I (d) III > IV > II > I

33. Some *meta*-directing substituents in aromatic substitution are given. Which one is most deactivating?
(a) $-SO_3H$ (b) –COOH (c) $-NO_2$ (d) $-C \equiv N$

34. Consider thiol anion (RS^-) and alkoxy anion (RO^-). Which of the following statements is correct ?
(a) RS^- is less basic but more nucleophilic than RO^-
(b) RS^- is more basic and more nucleophilic than RO^-
(c) RS^- is more basic but less nucleophilic than RO^-
(d) RS^- is less basic and less nucleophilic than RO^-

35. Consider the following compounds.

(i) C_6H_5COCl (ii) $O_2N-C_6H_4-COCl$
(iii) $H_3C-C_6H_4-COCl$ (iv) $OHC-C_6H_4-COCl$

The correct decreasing order of their reactivity towards hydrolysis is
(a) (i) > (ii) > (iii) > (iv) (b) (iv) > (ii) > (i) > (iii)
(c) (ii) > (iv) > (i) > (iii) (d) (ii) > (iv) > (iii) > (i)

36. The order of stability of the following tautomeric compounds is :

$$\underset{I}{CH_2=\overset{\overset{OH}{|}}{C}-CH_2-\overset{\overset{O}{||}}{C}-CH_3} \rightleftharpoons \underset{II}{CH_3-\overset{\overset{O}{||}}{C}-CH_2-\overset{\overset{O}{||}}{C}-CH_3} \rightleftharpoons \underset{III}{CH_3-\overset{\overset{OH}{|}}{C}=CH-\overset{\overset{O}{||}}{C}-CH_3}$$

(a) III > II > I (b) II > I > III
(c) II > III > I (d) I > II > III

RESPONSE GRID				
23. ⓐⓑⓒⓓ	24. ⓐⓑⓒⓓ	25. ⓐⓑⓒⓓ	26. ⓐⓑⓒⓓ	27. ⓐⓑⓒⓓ
28. ⓐⓑⓒⓓ	29. ⓐⓑⓒⓓ	30. ⓐⓑⓒⓓ	31. ⓐⓑⓒⓓ	32. ⓐⓑⓒⓓ
33. ⓐⓑⓒⓓ	34. ⓐⓑⓒⓓ	35. ⓐⓑⓒⓓ	36. ⓐⓑⓒⓓ	

Space for Rough Work

37. Match the columns

	Column - I		Column - II
A.	Duma's method	I.	$\frac{80 \times m_1 \times 100}{188 \times m}$
B.	Kjeldahl's method	II.	$\frac{31 \times m_1 \times 100}{1877 \times m}\%$
C.	Carius method for bromine	III.	$\frac{1.4 \times M \times 2\left(v - \frac{v_1}{2}\right)}{m}\%$
D.	Percentage of phosphorus	IV.	$\frac{28 \times V \times 100}{22400 \times m}\%$

(a) A – IV; B – III; C – I; D – II
(b) A – III; B – IV; C – II; D – I
(c) A – IV; B – I; C – II; D – III
(d) A – I; B – III; C – II; D – IV

38. Which of the following represents the correct order of stability of the given carbocations ?

(a) $F_3\overset{+}{C} > F_3C-\overset{+}{\underset{|}{\overset{|}{C}}} > \overset{+}{C}H_3$ (b) $H_3\overset{+}{C} > F_3C-\overset{+}{\underset{|}{\overset{|}{C}}} > F_3\overset{+}{C}$

(c) $F_3C-\overset{+}{\underset{|}{\overset{|}{C}}} > F_3\overset{+}{C} > H_3\overset{+}{C}$ (d) $F_3C-\overset{+}{\underset{|}{\overset{|}{C}}} > H_3\overset{+}{C} > F_3\overset{+}{C}$

39. $(CH_3)_4N^+$ is neither an electrophile, nor a nucleophile because it
(a) does not have electron pair for donation as well as can not attract electron pair
(b) neither has electron pair available for donation nor can accommodate electron since all shells of N are fully occupied
(c) can act as Lewis acid and base
(d) None of these

40. In Kjeldahl's method for the estimation of N_2, potassium sulphate and copper sulphate are used. On the basis of their functions which of the following statement(s) is/are correct?
(i) Potassium sulphate raises the b.pt. and ensures complete reaction.
(ii) Copper sulphate acts as catalyst.
(iii) Potassium sulphate acts as catalyst and copper sulphate raises the b.pt.
(a) Only (iii) is correct (b) (i) and (ii) are correct
(c) Only (ii) is correct (d) None is correct

41. What is the relationship between open chain forms of D-glucose and D-altrose ?
(a) enantiomers
(b) constitutional isomers
(c) diastereomers
(d) different conformations of the same compound

42. The production of an optically active compound from a symmetric molecule without resolution is termed
(a) Walden inversion (b) Partial racemisation
(c) Asymmetric synthesis (d) Partial resolution

43. The number of asymmetric C-atom created and number of possible stereoisomers when benzil (Ph CO CO Ph) is reduced with $LiAlH_4$.
(a) 2, 3 (b) 2, 2 (c) 2, 4 (d) 3, 2

44. Among the following, the true property about $(CH_3)_2\overset{+}{C}-CH_3$ is
(a) it is non-planar
(b) its C^+ is sp^2-hybridized
(c) an electrophile can attack on its C^+
(d) it does not undergo hydrolysis

45. The compound which contains all the four 1°, 2°, 3° and 4° carbon atoms is
(a) 2, 3-dimethylpentane
(b) 3-chloro-2, 3-dimethylpentane
(c) 2, 3, 4-trimethylpentane
(d) 3, 3- dimethylpentane

RESPONSE GRID					
	37. ⓐⓑⓒⓓ	38. ⓐⓑⓒⓓ	39. ⓐⓑⓒⓓ	40. ⓐⓑⓒⓓ	41. ⓐⓑⓒⓓ
	42. ⓐⓑⓒⓓ	43. ⓐⓑⓒⓓ	44. ⓐⓑⓒⓓ	45. ⓐⓑⓒⓓ	

CHEMISTRY CHAPTERWISE SPEED TEST-40

Total Questions	45	Total Marks	180
Attempted		Correct	
Incorrect		Net Score	
Cut-off Score	35	Qualifying Score	60
Success Gap = Net Score – Qualifying Score			
Net Score = (Correct × 4) – (Incorrect × 1)			

Space for Rough Work

CHEMISTRY

Hydrocarbons

Speed TEST 41 Chapter-wise

No. of Questions	Maximum Marks	Time
45	180	1 Hour

GENERAL INSTRUCTIONS

- This test contains 45 MCQ's. For each question only one option is correct. Darken the correct circle/ bubble in the Response Grid provided on each page.
- You have to evaluate your Response Grids yourself with the help of solutions provided at the end of this book.
- Each correct answer will get you 4 marks and 1 mark shall be deduced for each incorrect answer. No mark will be given/ deducted if no bubble is filled. Keep a timer in front of you and stop immediately at the end of 60 min.
- The sheet follows a particular syllabus. Do not attempt the sheet before you have completed your preparation for that syllabus.
- After completing the sheet check your answers with the solution booklet and complete the Result Grid. Finally spend time to analyse your performance and revise the areas which emerge out as weak in your evaluation.

1. When neo-pentyl bromide is subjected to Wurtz reaction, the product formed is
   (a) 2,2,4,4-tetramethylhexane
   (b) 2,2,4,4-tetramethylpentane
   (c) 2,2,5,5-tetramethylhexane
   (d) 2,2,3,3-tetramethylhexane
2. The conversion of 2, 3-dibromobutane to 2-butene with Zn and alcohol is
   (a) redox reaction (b) α-elimination
   (c) β-elimination (d) Both (a) and (b)
3. 1, 3-Butadiene when treated with Br_2 gives
   (a) 1, 4-dibromo-2-butene (b) 1, 3-dibromo-2-butene
   (c) 3, 4-dibromo-1-butene (d) 2, 3-dibromo-2-butene
4. An alkene having molecular formula C_7H_{14} was subjected to ozonolysis in the presence of zinc dust. An equimolar amount of the following two compounds was obtained CH_3COCH_3 and $CH_3COC_2H_5$
   The IUPAC name of the alkene is
   (a) 3,4-dimethyl-3-pentene (b) 3,4-dimethyl-2-pentene
   (c) 2,3-dimethyl-3-pentene (d) 2,3-dimethyl-2-pentene
5. Acid catalyzed hydration of alkenes except ethene leads to the formation of
   (a) mixture of secondary and tertiary alcohols
   (b) mixture of primary and secondary alcohols
   (c) secondary or tertiary alcohol
   (d) primary alcohol
6. In a reaction
   $$CH_2=CH_2 \xrightarrow[\text{acid}]{\text{Hypochlorous}} M \xrightarrow{R} \begin{array}{l} CH_2-OH \\ | \\ CH_2-OH \end{array}$$
   Where M = molecule; R = reagent; M and R are
   (a) CH_3CH_2Cl and NaOH
   (b) CH_2Cl-CH_2OH and aq. $NaHCO_3$
   (c) CH_3CH_2OH and HCl
   (d) $CH_2=CH_2$ and heat
7. The negative part of an addendum adds on to the carbon atom joined to the least number of hydrogen atoms. This statement is called
   (a) Thiele's theory (b) Peroxide effect
   (c) Markownikoff's rule (d) Baeyer's strain theory
8. Match the columns

	Column-I		Column-II
A.	$CH\equiv CH+H_2\rightarrow CH_2=CH_2$	I.	Zn
B.	$CH_3CH_2Br\rightarrow CH_2=CH_2$	II.	Conc. H_2SO_4
C.	$CH_2BrCH_2Br\rightarrow CH_2=CH_2$	III.	Pd/C
D.	$CH_3CH_2OH\rightarrow CH_2=CH_2$	IV.	Alc. KOH

   (a) A – III; B – IV; C – I; D – II
   (b) A – IV; B – III; C – II; D – I
   (c) A – II; B – I; C – IV; D – III
   (d) A – III; B – IV; C – II; D – I

RESPONSE GRID	
	1. ⓐⓑⓒⓓ 2. ⓐⓑⓒⓓ 3. ⓐⓑⓒⓓ 4. ⓐⓑⓒⓓ 5. ⓐⓑⓒⓓ
	6. ⓐⓑⓒⓓ 7. ⓐⓑⓒⓓ 8. ⓐⓑⓒⓓ

Space for Rough Work

9. Which of the following will yield a mixture of 2-chlorobutene and 3-chlorobutene on treatment with HCl ?
(a) $CH_2=C=CH-CH_3$ (b) $H_2C=C(CH_3)-CH=CH_2$
(c) $CH_2=CH-CH=CH_2$ (d) $HC\equiv C-CH=CH_2$

10. Lindlar's catalyst is
(a) Na in alcohol (b) Raney nickel
(c) $Pd/BaSO_4$ (d) Na/liq. NH_3

11. The treatment of CH_3MgX with $CH_3C\equiv C-H$ produces
(a) $CH_3-CH=CH_2$ (b) $CH_3C\equiv C-CH_3$
(c) $CH_3-HC=CH-CH_3$ (d) CH_4

12. A group which deactivates the benzene ring towards electrophilic substitution but which directs the incoming group principally to the o- and p-positions is
(a) $-NH_2$ (b) $-Cl$ (c) $-NO_2$ (d) $-C_2H_5$

13. Isopropyl alcohol is obtained by reacting which of the following alkenes with conc. H_2SO_4 and H_2O
(a) Ethylene (b) Propylene
(c) 2-methyl propene (d) Isoprene

14. In the preparation of alkanes from hydrogenation of alkenes and alkynes. Finely divided catalysts are used which of the following statement(s) is/are correct regarding these catalysts
(i) Platinum and palladium catalyse the reaction at room temperature.
(ii) Nickel catalyse the reaction at relatively higher temperature and pressure.
(iii) Platinum and palladium catalyse the reaction at higher temperature.
(a) (i) and (iii) (b) (i) and (ii)
(c) (ii) and (iii) (d) (i) only

15. Which one of the following reactions is expected to readily give a hydrocarbon product in good yields ?
(a) $RCOOK \xrightarrow[\text{oxidation}]{\text{Electrolytic}}$ (b) $RCOO^-Ag^+ \xrightarrow{Br_2}$
(c) $CH_3CH_3 \xrightarrow[h\upsilon]{Cl_2}$ (d) $(CH_3)_3CCl \xrightarrow{C_2H_5OH}$

16. Which of the following change is correct
(a) $>C=C< \xrightarrow[\text{wet } CH_3COOH]{I_2,\ CH_3COOAg} >C(OH)-C(OH)<$
(b) $>C=C< \xrightarrow[\text{dry } CH_3COOH]{I_2,\ CH_3COOAg} >C(OH)-C(OH)<$
(c) Both (a) and (b) one correct
(d) Neither (a) nor (b)

17. The products obtained via oxymercuration ($HgSO_4$ + H_2SO_4) of 1-butyne would be
(a) $CH_3-CH_2-CO-CH_3$
(b) $CH_3-CH_2-CH_2-CHO$
(c) $CH_3-CH_2-CHO+HCHO$
(d) $CH_3CH_2COOH+HCOOH$

18. The number of optically active products obtained from the **complete** ozonolysis of the given compound is :

$$CH_3-CH=CH-\underset{H}{\overset{CH_3}{C}}-CH=CH-\underset{CH_3}{\overset{H}{C}}-CH=CH-CH_3$$

(a) 0 (b) 1 (c) 2 (d) 4

19. Propyne on polymerisation gives
(a) Mesitylene (b) Benzene
(c) Ethyl benzene (d) Propyl benzene

20. The electrophilic substitutions reactions of benzene takes place via
(i) generation of electrophile
(ii) generation of nucleophile
(iii) formation of carbocation intermediate
(iv) removal of proton from the carbocation intermediate
(a) (i), (iii) and (iv) (b) (ii), (iii) and (iv)
(c) (i) and (iv) (d) (ii) and (iv)

21. Two organic compounds A and B both containing only carbon and hydrogen, on quantitative analysis gave the same percentage composition by weight :
$C=(12/13)\times 100\%$, $H=(1/13)\times 100\%$
A decolourises bromine water but B does not. A and B respectively are
(a) C_2H_2 and C_6H_6 (b) C_6H_6 and C_2H_2
(c) C_2H_4 and C_2H_6 (d) C_2H_2 and C_2H_6

22. The major product of the following reaction

$$H_3C-C\equiv CH \xrightarrow[\text{ether}]{CH_3CH_2MgCl} \xrightarrow[H_3O^+]{\text{cyclopentanone}}$$

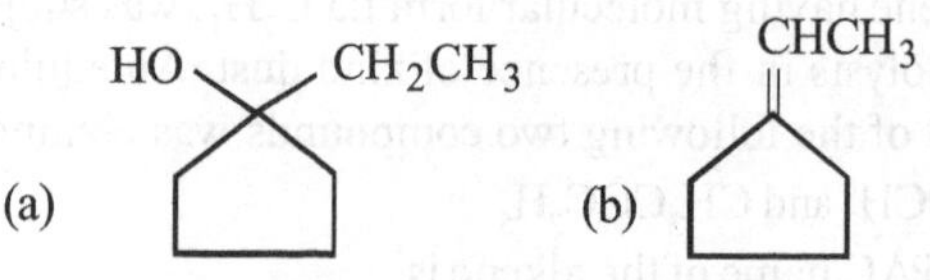

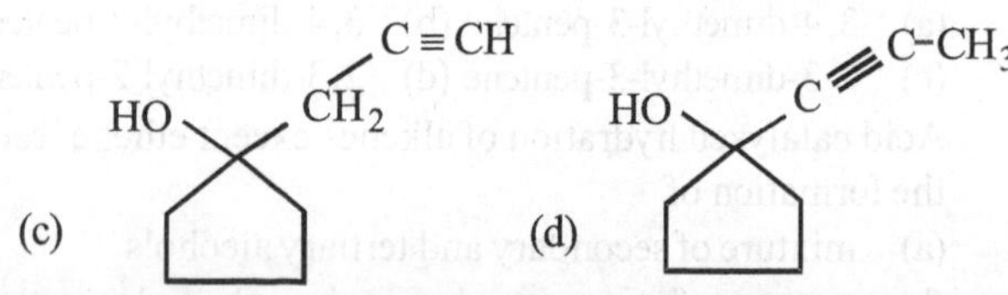

RESPONSE GRID

9. ⓐⓑⓒⓓ 10. ⓐⓑⓒⓓ 11. ⓐⓑⓒⓓ 12. ⓐⓑⓒⓓ 13. ⓐⓑⓒⓓ
14. ⓐⓑⓒⓓ 15. ⓐⓑⓒⓓ 16. ⓐⓑⓒⓓ 17. ⓐⓑⓒⓓ 18. ⓐⓑⓒⓓ
19. ⓐⓑⓒⓓ 20. ⓐⓑⓒⓓ 21. ⓐⓑⓒⓓ 22. ⓐⓑⓒⓓ

Space for Rough Work

23. 2,3-Dimethyl-2-butene can be prepared by heating which of the following compounds with a strong acid ?

(a) $(CH_3)_2CH-\underset{\substack{| \\ CH_3}}{CH}-CH=CH_2$

(b) $(CH_3)_3C-CH=CH_2$

(c) $(CH_3)_2C=CH-CH_2-CH_3$

(d) $(CH_3)_2CH-CH_2-CH=CH_2$

24. Which C-atom is the most electronegative in this structure?

$$\overset{III}{CH_3}-\overset{II}{CH_2}-\overset{I}{C}\equiv CH$$

(a) I

(b) II

(c) III

(d) all are equal electronegative

25. Which of the following will have least hindered rotation around carbon - carbon bond ?

(a) Ethane (b) Ethylene

(c) Acetylene (d) Hexachloroethane

26. Match the columns

	Column - I		Column - II
A.	Alkyl + Acid halide in presence of dry ether	I.	Sulphonation
B.	Arene + Acid halide in presence of $AlCl_3$	II.	Wurtz reaction
C.	Arene + Fuming sulphuric in presence of $AlCl_3$	III.	Catalytic hydrogenation
D.	Arene + Hydrogen in presence of Ni	IV.	Friedel-Crafts reaction

(a) A – I; B – III; C – II; D – IV

(b) A – IV; B – II; C – III; D – I

(c) A – III; B – I; C – IV; D – II

(d) A – II; B – IV; C – I; D – III

27. Of the three isomeric C_3H_4 hydrocarbons shown below how many can exist with all carbon and hydrogen nuclei located in a single plane

$$H_2C=C=CH_2\ ,\ \begin{matrix} CH \\ \| \\ CH \end{matrix}\!\!>CH_2\ ,\ H_3C-C\equiv CH$$

(a) 0 (b) 1 (c) 2 (d) 3

28. Excess of CH_3COOH is reacted with $CH\equiv CH$ in presence of Hg^{2+}, the product is

(a) $CH_3CH(OCOCH_3)_2$

(b) $CH_2=CH(OCOCH_3)$

(c) $(CH_3COO)CH_2-CH_2(OOCCH_3)$

(d) None of these

29. Which one of the following contain isopropyl group?

(a) 2, 2, 3, 3-tetramethylpentane

(b) 2, 4-dimethylhexone

(c) 2, 2, 3-trimethylpentane

(d) 3, 3-dimethylpentane

30. 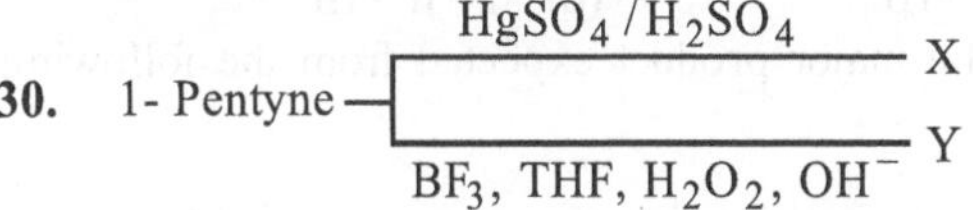

X and Y can be distinguished by

(a) Silver-mirror test (b) Iodoform test

(c) Both (d) None

31. The major product obtained in the photo catalysed bromination of 2-methylbutane is:

(a) 1-bromo-2-methylbutane

(b) 1-bromo-3-methylbutane

(c) 2-bromo-3-methylbutane

(d) 2-bromo-2-methylbutane

32. Acetylenic hydrogens are acidic because

(a) Sigma electron density of C – H bond in acetylene is nearer to carbon, which has 50% *s*-character

(b) Acetylene has only open hydrogen in each carbon

(c) Acetylene contains least number of hydrogens among the possible hydrocarbons having two carbons

(d) Acetylene belongs to the class of alkynes with molecular formula, C_nH_{2n-2}.

33. Which of the following will be most easily attacked by an electrophile?

(a) C_6H_6 (b) C_6H_5Cl (c) C_6H_5OH (d) $C_6H_5CH_3$

34. Name of the following reaction is

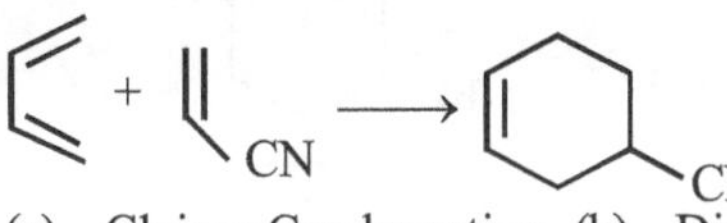

(a) Claisen Condensation (b) Diel's Alder reaction

(c) Dieckmann cyclisation (d) Michael addition reaction

35. The most suitable catalyst for the hydrogenation of 2-Hexyne ⟶ 2-cis-Hexene is

(a) Pd–$BaSO_4$ (b) $(Ph_3P)_3RhCl$

(c) 10% Pd—C (d) Raney Ni

36. NH_2 + Excess of Et. MgBr → ?

(a) 1 mole of Ethane

(b) 3 mole of ethane

(c) $EtC\equiv CCH_2CH_2NHEt$

(d) 4 mole of ethane

RESPONSE GRID					
	23. ⓐⓑⓒⓓ	24. ⓐⓑⓒⓓ	25. ⓐⓑⓒⓓ	26. ⓐⓑⓒⓓ	27. ⓐⓑⓒⓓ
	28. ⓐⓑⓒⓓ	29. ⓐⓑⓒⓓ	30. ⓐⓑⓒⓓ	31. ⓐⓑⓒⓓ	32. ⓐⓑⓒⓓ
	33. ⓐⓑⓒⓓ	34. ⓐⓑⓒⓓ	35. ⓐⓑⓒⓓ	36. ⓐⓑⓒⓓ	

Space for Rough Work

37. Among the following compounds (I – III), the correct order of reactivity with an electrophile is

$C_6H_5OCH_3$ (I) $\quad$ C_6H_6 (II) $\quad$ $C_6H_5NO_2$ (III)

(a) II > III > I (b) III < I < II
(c) I > II > III (d) I = II > III

38. What is the major product expected from the following reaction ?

CH_3 (1-methylcyclopentene) $\xrightarrow{D-Cl}$

Where D is an isotope of hydrogen

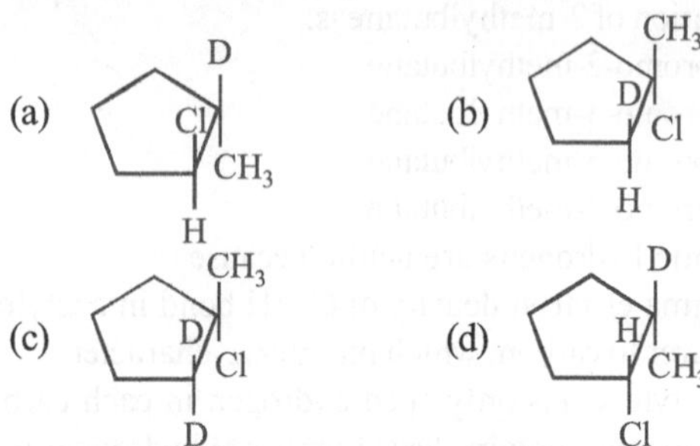

39. The product of the reaction given below is:

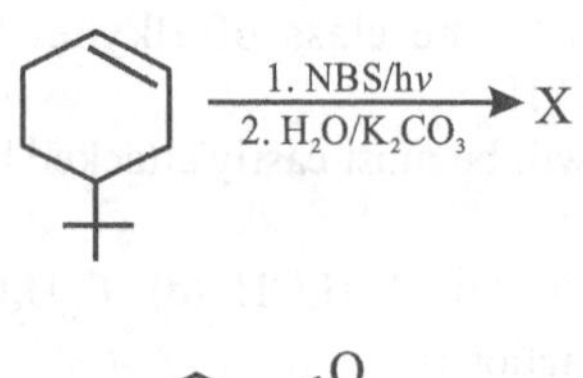

(a) 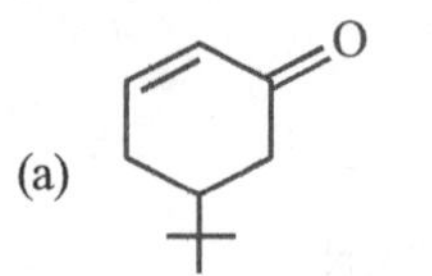
(b) 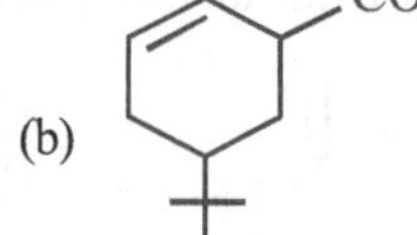
(c) 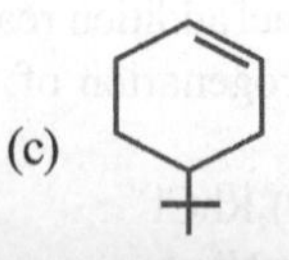
(d) 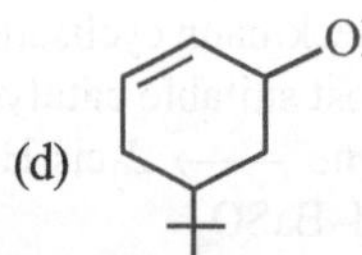

40. $CH_3C \equiv CCH_3 \xrightarrow[\text{(ii) } H_2O/Zn]{\text{(i) X}}$ $H_3C.\overset{\overset{O}{||}}{C}-\overset{\overset{O}{||}}{C}.CH_3$ In the above reaction X is

(a) HNO_3 (b) O_2 (c) O_3 (d) $KMnO_4$

41. Which of the following represent the correct order of acidic strength ?

(i) $HC \equiv CH > H_2C = CH_2 > CH_3 - CH_3$
(ii) $HC \equiv CH > CH_3 - CH_3 > H_2C = CH_2$
(iii) $CH_3C \equiv CH > HC \equiv CH > CH_3 - C \equiv C - CH_3$
(iv) $HC \equiv CH > CH_3 - C \equiv CH > CH_3 - C \equiv C - CH_3$

(a) (i) and (iii) (b) (ii) and (iv)
(c) (i) and (iv) (d) (i) and (iv)

42. Which one of the following compounds would have the highest heat of hydrogenation ?

(a) $CH_2 = CH_2$
(b) $CH_3 - CH_2 - CH = CH_2$
(c) $CH_3CH = CHCH_3$
(d) $(CH_3)_2C = C(CH_3)_2$

43. On mixing a certain alkane with chlorine and irradiating it with ultraviolet light, it forms only one monochloroalkane. This alkane could be

(a) pentane (b) isopentane
(c) neopentane (d) propane

44. Acetylene gives

(a) white ppt with $AgNO_3$ and red ppt with Cu_2Cl_2
(b) white ppt with Cu_2Cl_2 and red ppt with $AgNO_3$
(c) white ppt with both
(d) red ppt with both

45. Sodium ethoxide is a specific reagent for

(a) dehydration (b) dehydrogenation
(c) dehydrohalogenation (d) dehalogenation

RESPONSE GRID					
	37. ⓐⓑⓒⓓ	38. ⓐⓑⓒⓓ	39. ⓐⓑⓒⓓ	40. ⓐⓑⓒⓓ	41. ⓐⓑⓒⓓ
	42. ⓐⓑⓒⓓ	43. ⓐⓑⓒⓓ	44. ⓐⓑⓒⓓ	45. ⓐⓑⓒⓓ	

CHEMISTRY CHAPTERWISE SPEED TEST-41

Total Questions	45	Total Marks	180
Attempted		Correct	
Incorrect		Net Score	
Cut-off Score	37	Qualifying Score	62
Success Gap = Net Score – Qualifying Score			
Net Score = (Correct × 4) – (Incorrect × 1)			

Space for Rough Work

CHEMISTRY

Environmental Chemistry

Speed TEST 42

Chapter-wise

No. of Questions	Maximum Marks	Time
45	180	1 Hour

GENERAL INSTRUCTIONS

- This test contains 45 MCQ's. For each question only one option is correct. Darken the correct circle/ bubble in the Response Grid provided on each page.
- You have to evaluate your Response Grids yourself with the help of solutions provided at the end of this book.
- Each correct answer will get you 4 marks and 1 mark shall be deduced for each incorrect answer. No mark will be given/ deducted if no bubble is filled. Keep a timer in front of you and stop immediately at the end of 60 min.
- The sheet follows a particular syllabus. Do not attempt the sheet before you have completed your preparation for that syllabus.
- After completing the sheet check your answers with the solution booklet and complete the Result Grid. Finally spend time to analyse your performance and revise the areas which emerge out as weak in your evaluation.

1. The substance which is a primary pollutant?
   (a) H_2SO_4 (b) CO
   (c) PAN (d) Aldehydes
2. Ozone layer of stratosphere requires protection from indiscriminate use of
   (a) balloons
   (b) pesticides
   (c) atomic explosions
   (d) aerosols and high flying jets
3. Which of the following acts as a sink for CO?
   (a) Plants
   (b) Haemoglobin
   (c) Microorganisms present in the soil
   (d) Oceans
4. The viable particulate among the following is
   (a) fumes (b) algae
   (c) smoke (d) mist
5. Which of the following statements is not true about classical smog?
   (a) Its main components are produced by the action of sunlight on emissions of automobiles and factories.
   (b) Produced in cold and humid climate.
   (c) It contains compounds of reducing nature.
   (d) It contains smoke fog and sulphur dioxide.
6. Match the columns

	Column-I		Column-II
A.	Nitrous oxide from car exhausts	I.	Secondary pollutant
B.	Chlorofluorocarbon (CFCs)	II.	Combustion of fossil fuels, wood, etc
C.	Methane	III.	Denitrification
D.	Ozone (O_3)	IV.	Refrigerators, aerosol, sprays
E.	Carbon dioxide	V.	Cattle, rice fields, toilets.

   (a) A – III; B – IV; C – V; D – I; E – II
   (b) A – V; B – I; C – III; D – IV; E – II
   (c) A – IV; B – V; C – I; D – II; E – III
   (d) A – I; B – III; C – IV; D – V; E – II

RESPONSE GRID	1. ⓐⓑⓒⓓ 2. ⓐⓑⓒⓓ 3. ⓐⓑⓒⓓ 4. ⓐⓑⓒⓓ 5. ⓐⓑⓒⓓ 6. ⓐⓑⓒⓓ

Space for Rough Work

7. Which of the following sequence of T and F is correct for given statements. Here T stands for True statement and F stands for False statement.
   (i) Troposphere is the lowest region of atmosphere in which the human beings along with other organisms live.
   (ii) Troposphere extends up to the height of 10 km from sea level.
   (iii) Stratosphere lies above troposphere, between 10 and 20 km above sea level.
   (iv) Troposphere contains much little water vapour, dinitrogen, dioxygen and ozone
   (v) Stratosphere contains ozone, and cloud formation also takes place in this region.
   (a) TTTTT (b) TFTFF
   (c) TTFFF (d) TFTFT
8. Green chemistry means such reactions which :
   (a) produce colour during reactions
   (b) reduce the use and production of hazardous chemicals
   (c) are related to the depletion of ozone layer
   (d) study the reactions in plants
9. Photochemical smog consists of excessive amount of X, in addition to aldehydes, ketones, peroxyacetyl nitrate (PAN), and so forth, X is :
   (a) CO (b) CH_4 (c) O_3 (d) CO_2
10. Which of the following statements about polar stratosphere clouds (PSCs) is not correct?
   (a) PSCs do not react with chlorine nitrate and HCl
   (b) Type I clouds are formed at about –77°C and contain solid $HNO_3 . 3H_2O$
   (c) Type II clouds are formed at about –85°C and contain some ice
   (d) A tight whirlpool of wind called Polar Vortex is formed which surrounds Antarctica
11. Match the columns

	Column-I		Column-II
A.	Oxides of sulphur	I.	Global warming
B.	Nitrogen dioxide	II.	Damage to kidney
C.	Carbon dioxide	III.	'Blue baby' syndrome
D.	Nitrate in drinking water	IV.	Respiratory diseases
E.	Lead	V.	Red haze in traffic and congested areas

   (a) A–V.; B–I.; C–III.; D–IV.; E–II.
   (b) A–IV.; B–V.; C–I.; D–III.; E–II.
   (c) A–IV.; B–II.; C–I.; D–V.; E–III.
   (d) A–II.; B–IV.; C–V.; D–III.; E–I.
12. Which of the following statements are not correct?
   (i) F^- ion concentration above 2ppm causes brown mottling in teeth.
   (ii) Excessive F^- (over 10 ppm) causes harmful effect to bones and teeth.
   (iii) Excessive lead in drinking water causes disease methemoglobinemia
   (iv) Deficiency of sulphate in drinking water causes laxative effect.
   (a) (ii) and (iv) (b) (ii) and (iii)
   (c) (ii), (iii) and (iv) (d) (iii) and (iv)
13. The gas leaked from a storage tank of the Union Carbide plant in Bhopal gas tragedy was :
   (a) Methyl isocyanate (b) Methylamine
   (c) Ammonia (d) Phosgene
14. Minamata disease is due to pollution of
   (a) aresenic into the atmosphere
   (b) organic waste into drinking water
   (c) oil spill in water
   (d) industrial waste mercury into fishing water
15. Eutrophication causes reduction in
   (a) dissolved oxygen (b) nutrients
   (c) dissolved salts (d) All the above
16. Which of the following is/are formed when ozone reacts with the unburnt hydrocarbons in polluted air ?
   (i) Formaldehyde (ii) Acrolein
   (iii) Peroxyacetyl nitrate (iv) Formic acid
   (a) (i) and (iv) (b) (ii) only
   (c) (iii) only (d) (i), (ii) and (iii)
17. Use of which of the following solvent in dry cleaning will result in less harm to ground water ?
   (a) $Cl_2C=CCl_2$ (b) Liquid CO_2
   (c) H_2O_2 (d) None of these
18. Which among the following statements is *false*?
   (a) Oil slick in sea water increases D.O. value
   (b) The main reason for river water pollution is industrial and domestic sewage discharge
   (c) Surface water contains a lot of organic matter mineral nutrients and radioactive materials
   (d) Oil spill in sea water causes heavy damage to fishery
19. The false statement among the followings :
   (a) The average residence time of NO is one month
   (b) Limestone acts as a sink for SO_x
   (c) SO_x can be removed from flue gases by passing through a solution of citrate ions
   (d) Ammonia acts as a sink for NO_x

RESPONSE GRID				
7. ⓐⓑⓒⓓ	8. ⓐⓑⓒⓓ	9. ⓐⓑⓒⓓ	10. ⓐⓑⓒⓓ	11. ⓐⓑⓒⓓ
12. ⓐⓑⓒⓓ	13. ⓐⓑⓒⓓ	14. ⓐⓑⓒⓓ	15. ⓐⓑⓒⓓ	16. ⓐⓑⓒⓓ
17. ⓐⓑⓒⓓ	18. ⓐⓑⓒⓓ	19. ⓐⓑⓒⓓ		

Space for Rough Work

20. The aromatic compounds present as particulates are
(a) polycyclic aromatic hydrocarbons
(b) benzene
(c) toluene
(d) nitrobenzene

21. Which one of the following pairs is mismatched ?
(a) Fossil fuel burning - release of CO_2
(b) Nuclear power - radioactive wastes
(c) Solar energy - Greenhouse effect
(d) Biomass burning - release of CO_2

22. Which one of the following statement is **not** true ?
(a) pH of drinking water should be between 5.5 – 9.5.
(b) Concentration of DO below 6 ppm is good for the growth of fish.
(c) Clean water would have a BOD value of less than 5 ppm.
(d) Oxides of sulphur, nitrogen and carbon are the most widespread air pollutant.

23. Surface water contains
(a) suspended impurity (b) salt + organic matter
(c) only salt (d) organic matter

24. Formation of London smog takes place in
(a) winter during day time
(b) summer during day time
(c) summer during morning time
(d) winter during morning time

25. Dinitrogen and dioxygen are main constituents of air but these do not react with each other to form oxides of nitrogen because __________.
(a) the reaction is endothermic and requires very high temperature.
(b) the reaction can be initiated only in presence of a catalyst.
(c) oxides of nitrogen are unstable.
(d) N_2 and O_2 are unreactive

26. Which one of the following statements is correct ?
(a) Extensive use of chemical fertilizers may lead to eutrophication of nearby water bodies
(b) Both Azotobacter and Rhizobium fix atmospheric nitrogen in root nodules of plants
(c) Cyanobacteria such as Anabaena and Nostoc are important mobilizers of phosphates and potassium for plant nutrition in soil
(d) At present it is not possible to grow maize without chemical fertilizers

27. Lichens do not like to grow in cities
(a) because of absence of the right type of algae and fungi
(b) because of lack of moisture
(c) because of SO_2 pollution
(d) because natural habitat is missing

28. Which of the following statements about the depletion of ozone layer is correct?
(a) The problem of ozone depletion is less serious at poles because NO_2 solidifies and is not available for consuming $ClO^\bullet$ radicals.
(b) The problem of ozone depletion is more serious at poles because ice crystals in the clouds over poles act as catalyst for photochemical reactions involving the decomposition of ozone of $Cl^\bullet$ and $ClO^\bullet$ radicals.
(c) Freons and chlorofluorocarbons are inert. Chemically, they do not react with ozone in stratosphere.
(d) Oxides of nitrogen also do not react with ozone in stratosphere.

29. Acid rain is caused by or recent reports of acid rain in some industrial cities are due to the effect of atmospheric pollution by
(a) excessive release of CO_2 by burning of fuels like wood and charcoal, cutting of forests and increased animal population
(b) excessive release of NO_2 and SO_2 in atmosphere by burning of fossil fuel
(c) excessive release of NH_3 by industrial plants and coal gas
(d) excessive release of CO in atmosphere by incomplete combustion of coke, charcoal and other carbonaceous fuel in paucity of oxygen.

30. A water sample has ppm level concentration of following anions
$F^- = 10$; $SO_4^{2-} = 100$; $NO_3^- = 50$
the anion/anions that make/makes the water sample unsuitable for drinking is/are :
(a) only NO_3^- (b) both SO_4^{2-} and NO_3^-
(c) only F^- (d) only SO_4^{2-}

31. Which of the following is the major cause of global warming?
(a) re-radiation of U.V. rays by CO_2 and H_2O
(b) re-radiation of I.R. rays by CO_2 and H_2O
(c) re-radiation of I.R. rays by O_2 and N_2
(d) re-radiation of U.V. rays by O_2 and N_2

RESPONSE GRID					
	20. ⓐⓑⓒⓓ	21. ⓐⓑⓒⓓ	22. ⓐⓑⓒⓓ	23. ⓐⓑⓒⓓ	24. ⓐⓑⓒⓓ
	25. ⓐⓑⓒⓓ	26. ⓐⓑⓒⓓ	27. ⓐⓑⓒⓓ	28. ⓐⓑⓒⓓ	29. ⓐⓑⓒⓓ
	30. ⓐⓑⓒⓓ	31. ⓐⓑⓒⓓ			

Space for Rough Work

32. Identify the incorrect statement from the following :
(a) Ozone absorbs the intense ultraviolet radiation of the sun.
(b) Depletion of ozone layer is because of its chemical reactions with chlorofluoro alkanes.
(c) Ozone absorbs infrared radiation.
(d) Oxides of nitrogen in the atmosphere can cause the depletion of ozone layer.

33. BOD is connected with
(a) microbes and organic matter
(b) organic matter
(c) microbes
(d) None of the above

34. Which of the following is not a common component of Photochemical Smog?
(a) Ozone (b) Acrolein
(c) Peroxyacetyl nitrate (d) Chlorofluorocarbons

35. In which of the following regions hydrogen and helium are found?
(a) Stratosphere (b) Mesosphere
(c) Exosphere (d) Troposphere

36. Formation of ozone in the upper atmosphere from oxygen takes place by the action of
(a) nitrogen oxides (b) ultraviolet rays
(c) cosmic rays (d) free radicals

37. Which of the following is/are the hazardous pollutant(s) present in automobile exhaust gases?
(i) N_2 (ii) CO
(iii) CH_4 (iv) Oxides of nitrogen
(a) (ii) and (iii) (b) (i) and (ii)
(c) (ii) and (iv) (d) (i) and (iii)

38. The non-viable particulate among the following is
(a) dust (b) bacteria
(c) moulds (d) fungi

39. The region containing water vapour is
(a) thermosphere (b) stratosphere
(c) troposphere (d) mesosphere

40. The biggest particulate matter is
(a) HNO_3 droplets (b) soot
(c) H_2SO_4 droplets (d) fly ash

41. How many time oxyhaemoglobin is less stable than carboxyhaemoglobin?
(a) 50 (b) 200
(c) 500 (d) 300

42. When rain is accompanied by a thunderstorm, the collected rain water will have a pH value
(a) slightly lower than that of rain water without thunderstorm
(b) slightly higher than that when the thunderstorm is not there
(c) uninfluenced by occurrence of thunderstorm
(d) which depends upon the amount of dust in air

43. Which of the following can control the photochemical smog?
(A) Use of catalytic converters in automobiles.
(B) Plantation of trees like *pinus*, *pyrus* and *vitis* etc.
(C) Using less sulphur containing fossil fuels.
(a) A and C (b) B
(c) A and B (d) A, B and C

44. Which of the following statement is false?
(a) London smog is oxidising in nature
(b) Photochemical smog causes irritation in eyes
(c) London smog is a mixture of smoke and fog
(d) Photochemical smog results in the formation of PAN

45. Depletion of ozone layer causes
(a) Breast cancer (b) Blood cancer
(c) Lung cancer (d) Skin cancer

RESPONSE GRID					
	32. ⓐⓑⓒⓓ	33. ⓐⓑⓒⓓ	34. ⓐⓑⓒⓓ	35. ⓐⓑⓒⓓ	36. ⓐⓑⓒⓓ
	37. ⓐⓑⓒⓓ	38. ⓐⓑⓒⓓ	39. ⓐⓑⓒⓓ	40. ⓐⓑⓒⓓ	41. ⓐⓑⓒⓓ
	42. ⓐⓑⓒⓓ	43. ⓐⓑⓒⓓ	44. ⓐⓑⓒⓓ	45. ⓐⓑⓒⓓ	

CHEMISTRY CHAPTERWISE SPEED TEST-42

Total Questions	45	Total Marks	180
Attempted		Correct	
Incorrect		Net Score	
Cut-off Score	45	Qualifying Score	68
Success Gap = Net Score – Qualifying Score			
Net Score = (Correct × 4) – (Incorrect × 1)			

Space for Rough Work

CHEMISTRY

The Solid State

Speed TEST 43

Chapter-wise

No. of Questions	Maximum Marks	Time
45	180	1 Hour

GENERAL INSTRUCTIONS

- This test contains 45 MCQ's. For each question only one option is correct. Darken the correct circle/ bubble in the Response Grid provided on each page.
- You have to evaluate your Response Grids yourself with the help of solutions provided at the end of this book.
- Each correct answer will get you 4 marks and 1 mark shall be deduced for each incorrect answer. No mark will be given/ deducted if no bubble is filled. Keep a timer in front of you and stop immediately at the end of 60 min.
- The sheet follows a particular syllabus. Do not attempt the sheet before you have completed your preparation for that syllabus.
- After completing the sheet check your answers with the solution booklet and complete the Result Grid. Finally spend time to analyse your performance and revise the areas which emerge out as weak in your evaluation.

1. If Germanium crystallises in the same way as diamond, then which of the following statement is not correct?
   (a) Every atom in the structure is tetrahedrally bonded to 4 atoms.
   (b) Unit cell consists of 8 Ge atoms and co-ordination number is 4.
   (c) All the octahedral voids are occupied.
   (d) All the octahedral voids and 50% tetrahedral voids remain unoccupied.
2. If we mix a pentavalent impurity in a crystal lattice of germanium, what type of semiconductor formation will occur?
   (a) p-type (b) n-type
   (c) both (a) and (b) (d) None of the two.
3. Packing efficiency by arrangement of atoms in two dimensional hexagonal close packing is
   (a) 60.43 (b) 65.78
   (c) 59.78 (d) 68.76
4. The radius of a calcium ion is 94 pm and of the oxide ion is 146 pm. The possible crystal structure of calcium oxide will be
   (a) tetrahedral (b) trigonal
   (c) octahedral (d) pyramidal
5. The interionic distance for cesium chloride crystal will be
   (a) a (b) $\frac{a}{2}$
   (c) $\frac{\sqrt{3}a}{2}$ (d) $\frac{2a}{\sqrt{3}}$

RESPONSE GRID	1. ⓐⓑⓒⓓ	2. ⓐⓑⓒⓓ	3. ⓐⓑⓒⓓ	4. ⓐⓑⓒⓓ	5. ⓐⓑⓒⓓ

Space for Rough Work

6. The pure crystalline substance on being heated gradually first forms a turbid liquid at constant temperature and still at higher temperature turbidity completely disappears. The behaviour is a characteristic of substance forming.
   (a) Allotropic crystals (b) Liquid crystals
   (c) Isomeric crystals (d) Isomorphous crystals.
7. The radius of Li^+ ion is 60 pm and that of F^- is 136 pm. Structure of LiF and coordination number is
   (a) Like NaCl, C.No. = 6 (b) Like CsCl, C.No. = 8
   (c) Anti fluoride, C.No. = 8 (d) None of these
8. Among the following which is the best description of water in the solid phase?
   (a) Covalent solid (b) Molecular solid
   (c) Ionic solid (d) Network solid
9. Which one of the following statements about packing in solids is **incorrect**?
   (a) Coordination number in bcc mode of packing is 8.
   (b) Coordination number in hcp mode of packing is 12.
   (c) Void space in hcp mode of packing is 32%.
   (d) Void space is ccp mode of packing is 26%.
10. The packing fraction for a body-centred cubic is
   (a) 0.42 (b) 0.53
   (c) 0.68 (d) 0.82
11. What is the energy gap between valence band and conduction band in crystal of insulators ?
   (a) Both the bands are overlapped with each other
   (b) Very small
   (c) Infinite
   (d) Very large
12. Among solids, the highest melting point is exhibited by
   (a) Covalent solids (b) Ionic solids
   (c) Pseudo solids (d) Molecular solids
13. Which of the following solids is not an electrical conductor?
   (a) Mg (s) (b) TiO (s)
   (c) I_2 (s) (d) H_2O (s)
14. The range of radius ratio (cationic to anionic) for an octahedral arrangement of ions in an ionic solid is
   (a) 0 – 0.155 (b) 0.155 – 0.225
   (c) 0.225 – 0.414 (d) 0.414 – 0.732
15. Which of the following has Frenkel defects?
   (a) Sodium chloride (b) Graphite
   (c) Silver bromide (d) Diamond
16. The cubic unit cell of a metal (molar mass = 63.55 g mol^{-1}) has an edge length of 362 pm. Its density is 8.92 g cm^{-3}. The type of unit cell is
   (a) primitive (b) face centered
   (c) body centered (d) end centered
17. Which of the folliowing metal oxides is anti-ferromagnetic in nature?
   (a) MnO_2 (b) TiO_2
   (c) VO_2 (d) CrO_2
18. Which of the following amorphous solid is used as photovoltaic material for conversion of sunlight into electricity?
   (a) Quartz glass (b) Quartz
   (c) Silicon (d) Both (a) and (b)
19. The number of octahedral voids present in a lattice is _A_. The number of closed packed particles, the number of tetrahedral voids generated is _B_ the number of closed packed particles
   (a) A- equal, B- half (b) A- twice, B- equal
   (c) A- twice , B- half (d) A- equal, B- twice
20. A metal crystallizes in 2 cubic phases fcc and bcc whose unit cell lengths are 3.5 Å and 3.0Å respectively. The ratio of their densities is
   (a) 0.72 (b) 2.04
   (c) 1.26 (d) 3.12

RESPONSE GRID					
	6. ⓐⓑⓒⓓ	7. ⓐⓑⓒⓓ	8. ⓐⓑⓒⓓ	9. ⓐⓑⓒⓓ	10. ⓐⓑⓒⓓ
	11. ⓐⓑⓒⓓ	12. ⓐⓑⓒⓓ	13. ⓐⓑⓒⓓ	14. ⓐⓑⓒⓓ	15. ⓐⓑⓒⓓ
	16. ⓐⓑⓒⓓ	17. ⓐⓑⓒⓓ	18. ⓐⓑⓒⓓ	19. ⓐⓑⓒⓓ	20. ⓐⓑⓒⓓ

Space for Rough Work

21. Which of the following is not a crystalline solid?
(a) KCl (b) CsCl
(c) Glass (d) Rhombic S

22. The second order Bragg diffraction of X-rays with $\lambda = 1.0$Å from a set of parallel planes in a metal occurs at an angle of 60°. The distance between the scattering planes in the crystal is
(a) 0.575Å (b) 1.00Å
(c) 2.00Å (d) 1.15Å

23. The sharp melting point of crystalline solids is due to _____.
(a) a regular arrangement of constituent particles observed over a short distance in the crystal lattice.
(b) a regular arrangement of constituent particles observed over a long distance in the crystal lattice.
(c) same arrangement of constituent particles in different directions.
(d) different arrangement of constituent particles in different directions.

24. Solid CH_4 is
(a) ionic solid (b) covalent solid
(c) molecular solid (d) does not exist

25. When electrons are trapped into the crystal in anion vacancy, the defect is known as :
(a) Schottky defect (b) Frenkel defect
(c) Stoichiometric defect (d) F-centre

26. A metal has a fcc lattice. The edge length of the unit cell is 404 pm. The density of the metal is 2.72 g cm^{-3}. The molar mass of the metal is :
(N_A Avogadro's constant = 6.02×10^{23} mol^{-1})
(a) 30 g mol^{-1} (b) 27 g mol^{-1}
(c) 20 g mol^{-1} (d) 40 g mol^{-1}

27. If one end of a piece of a metal is heated the other end becomes hot after some time. This is due to
(a) Energised electrons moving to the other part of the metal
(b) resistance of the metal
(c) mobility of atoms, in the metal
(d) minor perturbation in the energy of atoms.

28. Among the following which one has the highest cation to anion size ratio?
(a) NaF (b) CsI
(c) CsF (d) LiF

29. Among the following the incorrect statement is
(a) Density of crystals remains unaffected due to Frenkel defect.
(b) In bcc unit cell the void space is 32%.
(c) Density of crystals decreases due to Schottky defect.
(d) Electrical conductivity of metals increases with increase in temperature.

30. Doping of AgCl crystals with $CdCl_2$ results in
(a) Frenkel defect
(b) Schottky defect
(c) Substitutional cation vacancy
(d) Formation of F - centres

31. How many unit cells are present in a cube-shaped ideal crystal of NaCl of mass 1.00 g ?
[Atomic masses : Na = 23, Cl = 35.5]
(a) 5.14×10^{21} unit cells (b) 1.28×10^{21} unit cells
(c) 1.71×10^{21} unit cells (d) 2.57×10^{21} unit cells

32. Which of the following expression is correct for CsCl unit cell with lattice parameter a
(a) $r_{Cs^+} + r_{Cl^-} = \frac{3a}{2}$ (b) $r_{Cs^+} + r_{Cl^-} = \frac{\sqrt{3}a}{2}$
(c) $r_{Cs^+} + r_{Cl^-} = \frac{a}{\sqrt{2}}$ (d) $r_{Cs^+} + r_{Cl^-} = 2a$

33. Which of the following compound is like metallic copper in its conductivity and appearance?
(a) VO_3 (b) TiO_3
(c) ReO_3 (d) CrO_2

RESPONSE GRID					
	21. ⓐⓑⓒⓓ	22. ⓐⓑⓒⓓ	23. ⓐⓑⓒⓓ	24. ⓐⓑⓒⓓ	25. ⓐⓑⓒⓓ
	26. ⓐⓑⓒⓓ	27. ⓐⓑⓒⓓ	28. ⓐⓑⓒⓓ	29. ⓐⓑⓒⓓ	30. ⓐⓑⓒⓓ
	31. ⓐⓑⓒⓓ	32. ⓐⓑⓒⓓ	33. ⓐⓑⓒⓓ		

Space for Rough Work

34. Which of the following oxides shows electrical properties like metals ?
(a) SiO_2 (b) MgO
(c) $SO_2(s)$ (d) CrO_2

35. Which of the following exists as covalent crystals in the solid state ?
(a) Iodine (b) Silicon
(c) Sulphur (d) Phosphorus

36. NaCl is doped with 2×10^{-3} mole % of $SrCl_2$. The concentration of cation vacancies is
(a) 12.04×10^{20} per mole
(b) 3.01×10^{18} per mole
(c) 6.02×10^{18} per mole
(d) 12.04×10^{18} per mole

37. Na and Mg crystallize in bcc and fcc type crystals respectively, then the number of atoms of Na and Mg present in the unit cell of their respective crystal is
(a) 4 and 2 (b) 9 and 14
(c) 14 and 9 (d) 2 and 4.

38. Copper crystallises in fcc with a unit length of 361pm. What is the radius of copper atom ?
(a) 157 pm (b) 128 pm
(c) 108 pm (d) 181 pm

39. Which of the following represents correct order of conductivity in solids ?
(a) $K_{metals} >> K_{insulators} < K_{semiconductors}$
(b) $K_{metals} << K_{insulators} < K_{semiconductors}$
(c) $K_{metals} > K_{insulators} > K_{semiconductors} = zero$
(d) $K_{metals} < K_{semiconductors} > K_{insulators} \neq zero$

40. The number of carbon atoms per unit cell of diamond unit cell is :
(a) 8 (b) 6
(c) 1 (d) 4

41. Percentages of free space in cubic close packed structure and in body centered packed structure are respectively
(a) 30% and 26% (b) 26% and 32%
(c) 32% and 48% (d) 48% and 26%

42. The edge length of a face centered cubic cell of an ionic substance is 508 pm. If the radius of the cation is 110 pm, the radius of the anion is
(a) 288 pm (b) 398 pm
(c) 618 pm (d) 144 pm

43. The correct statement for the molecule, CsI_3 is:
(a) It is a covalent molecule.
(b) It contains Cs^+ and I_3^- ions.
(c) It contains Cs^{3+} and I^- ions.
(d) It contains Cs^+, I^- and lattice I_2 molecule.

44. Which of the following type of substances can be permanently magnetised?
(a) Diamagnetic (b) Ferromagnetic
(c) Ferrimagnetic (d) Antiferromagnetic

45. AB crystallizes in a body centred cubic lattice with edge length 'a' equal to 387 pm. The distance between two oppositely charged ions in the lattice is :
(a) 335 pm (b) 250 pm
(c) 200 pm (d) 300 pm

RESPONSE GRID					
	34. ⓐⓑⓒⓓ	35. ⓐⓑⓒⓓ	36. ⓐⓑⓒⓓ	37. ⓐⓑⓒⓓ	38. ⓐⓑⓒⓓ
	39. ⓐⓑⓒⓓ	40. ⓐⓑⓒⓓ	41. ⓐⓑⓒⓓ	42. ⓐⓑⓒⓓ	43. ⓐⓑⓒⓓ
	44. ⓐⓑⓒⓓ	45. ⓐⓑⓒⓓ			

CHEMISTRY CHAPTERWISE SPEED TEST-43

Total Questions	45	Total Marks	180
Attempted		Correct	
Incorrect		Net Score	
Cut-off Score	40	Qualifying Score	58

Success Gap = Net Score – Qualifying Score

Net Score = (Correct × 4) – (Incorrect × 1)

Space for Rough Work

CHEMISTRY

Solutions

No. of Questions	Maximum Marks	Time
45	180	1 Hour

Speed TEST 44

Chapter-wise

GENERAL INSTRUCTIONS

- This test contains 45 MCQ's. For each question only one option is correct. Darken the correct circle/ bubble in the Response Grid provided on each page.
- You have to evaluate your Response Grids yourself with the help of solutions provided at the end of this book.
- Each correct answer will get you 4 marks and 1 mark shall be deduced for each incorrect answer. No mark will be given/ deducted if no bubble is filled. Keep a timer in front of you and stop immediately at the end of 60 min.
- The sheet follows a particular syllabus. Do not attempt the sheet before you have completed your preparation for that syllabus.
- After completing the sheet check your answers with the solution booklet and complete the Result Grid. Finally spend time to analyse your performance and revise the areas which emerge out as weak in your evaluation.

1. How many grams of concentrated nitric acid solution should be used to prepare 250 mL of 2.0M HNO_3 ? The concentrated acid is 70% HNO_3

(a) 90.0 g conc. HNO_3 (b) 70.0 g conc. HNO_3
(c) 54.0 g conc. HNO_3 (d) 45.0 g conc. HNO_3

2. For a solution of two liquids A and B it was proved that $P_S = x_A(p°_A - p°_B) + p°_B$. The resulting solution will be

(a) Non -ideal (b) ideal
(c) semi-ideal (d) None of these

3. If the elevation in boiling point of a solution of 10 gm of solute (mol. wt. = 100) in 100 gm of water is ΔT_b, the ebullioscopic constant of water is

(a) 10 (b) $10\,\Delta T_b$
(c) ΔT_b (d) $\frac{\Delta T_b}{10}$

4. Which of the following aqueous solution will have highest depression in freezing point?

(a) 0.1 M Urea (b) 0.1 M Sucrose
(c) 0.1 M $AlCl_3$ (d) 0.1 M $K_4[Fe(CN)_6]$

5. Two liquids *X* and *Y* form an ideal solution. At 300 K, vapour pressure of the solution containing 1 mol of *X* and 3 mol of *Y* is 550 *mm*Hg. At the same temperature, if 1 mol of *Y* is further added to this solution, vapour pressure of the solution increases by 10 *mm*Hg. Vapour pressure (in *mm*Hg) of *X* and *Y* in their pure states will be, respectively:

(a) 300 and 400 (b) 400 and 600
(c) 500 and 600 (d) 200 and 300

6. 6.02×10^{20} molecules of urea are present in 100 ml of its solution. The concentration of urea solution is

(a) 0.02 M (b) 0.01 M
(c) 0.001 M (d) 0.1 M

(Avogadro constant, $N_A = 6.02 \times 10^{23}$ mol^{-1})

7. To neutralise completely 20 mL of 0.1 M aqueous solution of phosphorous acid (H_3PO_3), the value of 0.1 M aqueous KOH solution required is

(a) 40mL (b) 20mL
(c) 10mL (d) 60mL

RESPONSE GRID	
	1. ⓐⓑⓒⓓ 2. ⓐⓑⓒⓓ 3. ⓐⓑⓒⓓ 4. ⓐⓑⓒⓓ 5. ⓐⓑⓒⓓ
	6. ⓐⓑⓒⓓ 7. ⓐⓑⓒⓓ

Space for Rough Work

8. Two 1-litre flask A and B are connected to each other by a valve which is closed. Flask A has benzene in equilibrium with its vapours at 30°C. The flask B, is evacuated, and the valve is opened. Which of the following is true. If temperature is kept constant.'
(a) Some of the benzene molecules would move to flask B from flask A.
(b) Vapour pressure will be half the initial value.
(c) The vapour pressure remains unchanged
(d) Some more of the liquid benzene in flask A would evaporate.

9. Two Aqueous solutions S_1 and S_2 are separated by a semipermeable membrane. Solution S_1 has got a greater vapour pressure than solution S_2. Water will be flowing
(a) from S_1 to S_2
(b) from S_2 to S_1
(c) in both the directions
(d) in either direction depending upon the nature of the solute

10. Henry's law constant of oxygen is 1.4×10^{-3} mol. lit^{-1}. atm^{-1} at 298 K. How much of oxygen is dissolved in 100 ml at 298 K when the partial pressure of oxygen is 0.5 atm?
(a) 1.4 g (b) 3.2 g
(c) 22.4 mg (d) 2.24 mg

11. Which of the following liquid pairs shows a positive deviation from Raoult's law?
(a) Water - nitric acid
(b) Benzene - methanol
(c) Water - hydrochloric acid
(d) Acetone - chloroform

12. Dissolving 120 g of urea (mol. wt. 60) in 1000 g of water gave a solution of density 1.15 g/mL. The molarity of the solution is
(a) 1.78 M (b) 2.00 M
(c) 2.05 M (d) 2.22 M

13. The vapour pressure of a solution of the liquids A ($p° = 80$ mm Hg and $x_A = 0.4$) and B ($p° = 120$ mm Hg and $x_B = 0.6$) is found to be 100 mm Hg. It shows that the solution exhibits
(a) positive deviation from ideal behaviour
(b) negative deviation from ideal behaviour
(c) ideal behaviour
(d) positive deviation for lower conc. and negative for higher conc.

14. The vapour pressure of two liquids X and Y are 80 and 60 torr respectively. The total vapour pressure of the ideal solution obtained by mixing 3 moles of X and 2 moles of Y would be
(a) 68 Torr (b) 140 Torr
(c) 48 Torr (d) 72 Torr

15. Iodine and sulphur dissolve in
(a) water (b) benzene
(c) carbon disulphide (d) ethanol

16. A 5% solution of cane sugar (molar mass 342) is isotonic with 1% of a solution of an unknown solute. The molar mass of unknown solute in g/mol is :
(a) 171.2 (b) 68.4 (c) 34.2 (d) 136.2

17. Coolent used in car radiator is aqueous solution of ethylene glycol. In order to prevent the solution from freezing at – 0.3 °C. How much ethylene glycol must be added to 5 kg of water ? ($K_f = 1.86$ K kg mol^{-1})
(a) 50 kg (b) 55 g
(c) 45 g (d) 40 g

18. A solution of urea (mol. mass 56 g mol^{-1}) boils at 100.18°C at the atmospheric pressure. If K_f and K_b for water are 1.86 and 0.512 K kg mol^{-1} respectively, the above solution will freeze at
(a) 0.654°C (b) –0.654°C
(c) 6.54°C (d) –6.54°C

19. A solution is prepared by mixing 8.5 g of CH_2Cl_2 and 11.95 g of $CHCl_3$. If vapour pressure of CH_2Cl_2 and $CHCl_3$ at 298 K are 415 and 200 mmHg respectively, the mole fraction of $CHCl_3$ in vapour form is :
(Molar mass of Cl = 35.5 g mol^{-1})
(a) 0.162 (b) 0.675 (c) 0.325 (d) 0.486

20. If α is the degree of dissociation of Na_2SO_4, the Vant Hoff's factor (i) used for calculating the molecular mass is
(a) $1+\alpha$ (b) $1-\alpha$ (c) $1+2\alpha$ (d) $1-2\alpha$

RESPONSE GRID					
	8. ⓐⓑⓒⓓ	9. ⓐⓑⓒⓓ	10. ⓐⓑⓒⓓ	11. ⓐⓑⓒⓓ	12. ⓐⓑⓒⓓ
	13. ⓐⓑⓒⓓ	14. ⓐⓑⓒⓓ	15. ⓐⓑⓒⓓ	16. ⓐⓑⓒⓓ	17. ⓐⓑⓒⓓ
	18. ⓐⓑⓒⓓ	19. ⓐⓑⓒⓓ	20. ⓐⓑⓒⓓ		

Space for Rough Work

21. The molecular mass of a solute cannot be calculated by which of the following?

(a) $M_B = \frac{W_B \times RT}{\pi V}$ (b) $M_B = \frac{p^o W_B M_A}{(p^o - p) W_A}$

(c) $M_B = \frac{\Delta T_b W_B \times 1000}{K_b W_A}$ (d) $M_B = \frac{K_b W_B \times 1000}{\Delta T_b \times W_A}$

22. We have three aqueous solutions of NaCl labelled as 'A', 'B' and 'C' with concentrations 0.1M, 0.01M and 0.001M, respectively. The value of van't Hoff factor for these solutions will be in the order ________.

(a) $i_A < i_B < i_C$ (b) $i_A > i_B > i_C$
(c) $i_A = i_B = i_C$ (d) $i_A < i_B > i_C$

23. The value of Henry's constant K_H is ________.
(a) greater for gases with higher solubility.
(b) greater for gases with lower solubility.
(c) constant for all gases.
(d) not related to the solubility of gases.

24. Which one of the following gases has the lowest value of Henry's law constant?
(a) N_2 (b) He (c) H_2 (d) CO_2

25. A binary liquid solution is prepared by mixing *n*-heptane and ethanol. Which one of the following statements is correct regarding the behaviour of the solution?
(a) The solution is non-ideal, showing – ve deviation from Raoult's Law.
(b) The solution is non-ideal, showing + ve deviation from Raoult's Law.
(c) *n*-heptane shows + ve deviation while ethanol shows – ve deviation from Raoult's Law.
(d) The solution formed is an ideal solution.

26. Which one of the following salts will have the same value of van't Hoff factor (*i*) as that of $K_4[Fe(CN)_6]$.
(a) $Al_2(SO_4)_3$ (b) NaCl
(c) $Al(NO_3)_3$ (d) Na_2SO_4.

27. Relation between partial pressure and mole fraction is stated by
(a) Graham's law (b) Raoult's law
(c) Le-Chatelier (d) Avogadro law

28. Which is an application of Henry's law?
(a) Spray paint (b) Bottled water
(c) Filling up atire (d) Soft drinks (soda)

29. For which of the following parameters the structural isomers C_2H_5OH and CH_3OCH_3 would be expected to have the same values?
(Assume ideal behaviour)
(a) Boiling points
(b) Vapour pressure at the same temperature
(c) Heat of vapourization
(d) Gaseous densities at the same temperature and pressure

30. 5 g of Na_2SO_4 was dissolved in x g of H_2O. The change in freezing point was found to be 3.82°C. If Na_2SO_4 is 81.5% ionised, the value of x
(K_f for water = 1.86°C kg mol^{-1}) is approximately :
(molar mass of S = 32 g mol^{-1} and that of Na = 23 g mol^{-1})
(a) 15 g (b) 25 g (c) 45 g (d) 65 g

31. The vapour pressure of acetone at 20°C is 185 torr. When 1.2 g of a non-volatile substance was dissolved in 100 g of acetone at 20°C, its vapour pressure was 183 torr. The molar mass (g mol^{-1}) of the substance is :
(a) 128 (b) 488 (c) 32 (d) 64

32. In mixture *A* and *B* components show -ve deviation as
(a) $\Delta V_{mix} > 0$
(b) $\Delta H_{mix} < 0$
(c) *A* – *B* interaction is weaker than *A* – *A* and *B* – *B* interaction
(d) *A* – *B* interaction is stronger than *A* – *A* and *B* – *B* interaction.

33. Which among the following will show maximum osmotic pressure?
(a) 1 M NaCl (b) 1 M $MgCl_2$
(c) 1 M $(NH_4)_3PO_4$ (d) 1 M Na_2SO_4

34. At 80° C, the vapour pressure of pure liquid 'A' is 520 mm Hg and that of pure liquid 'B' is 1000 mm Hg. If a mixture of solution of 'A' and 'B' boils at 80° C and 1 atm pressure, the amount of 'A' in the mixture is (1 atm = 760 mm Hg)
(a) 52 mol percent (b) 34 mol percent
(c) 48 mol percent (d) 50 mol percent

RESPONSE GRID					
	21. ⓐⓑⓒⓓ	22. ⓐⓑⓒⓓ	23. ⓐⓑⓒⓓ	24. ⓐⓑⓒⓓ	25. ⓐⓑⓒⓓ
	26. ⓐⓑⓒⓓ	27. ⓐⓑⓒⓓ	28. ⓐⓑⓒⓓ	29. ⓐⓑⓒⓓ	30. ⓐⓑⓒⓓ
	31. ⓐⓑⓒⓓ	32. ⓐⓑⓒⓓ	33. ⓐⓑⓒⓓ	34. ⓐⓑⓒⓓ	

Space for Rough Work

35. The observed osmotic pressure for a 0.10 M solution of $Fe(NH_4)_2(SO_4)_2$ at 25°C is 10.8 atm. The expected and experimental (observed) values of van't Hoff factor (i) will be respectively:
($R = 0.082 L atm k^{-1} mol^{-1}$)
(a) 5 and 4.42 (b) 4 and 4.00
(c) 5 and 3.42 (d) 3 and 5.42

36. The freezing point of equimolal aqueous solution will be highest for
(a) $C_6H_5NH_3^+Cl^-$ (b) $Ca(NO_3)_2$
(c) $La(NO_3)_2$ (d) $C_6H_{12}O_6$

37. If the solution boils at a temperature T_1 and the solvent at a temperature T_2 the elevation of boiling point is given by
(a) $T_1 + T_2$ (b) $T_1 - T_2$
(c) $T_2 - T_1$ (d) $T_1 + T_2$

38. The freezing point of a 1.00 m aqueous solution of HF is found to be –1.91°C. The freezing point constant of water, K_f is 1.86 K kg mol^{-1}. The percentage dissociation of HF at this concentration is
(a) 30% (b) 10% (c) 5.2% (d) 2.7%

39. A solution containing 0.85 g of $ZnCl_2$ in 125.0 g of water freezes at –0.23°C. The apparent degree of dissociation of the salt is (K_f for water = 1.86 K kg mol^{-1}, atomic mass: Zn = 65.3 and Cl = 35.5)
(a) 1.36% (b) 73.5% (c) 7.35% (d) 2.47%

40. During depression of freezing point in a solution the following are in equilibrium
(a) liquid solvent, solid solvent
(b) liquid solvent, solid solute
(c) liquid solute, solid solute
(d) liquid solute, solid solvent

41. The molecular weight of benzoic acid in benzene as determined by depression in freezing point method corresponds to
(a) ionization of benzoic acid
(b) dimerization of benzoic acid
(c) trimerization of benzoic acid
(d) solvation of benzoic acid

42. How many grams of methyl alcohol should be added to 10 litre tank of water to prevent its freezing at 268 K ? (K_f for water is 1.86 K kg mol^{-1})
(a) 880.07 g (b) 899.04 g
(c) 886.02 g (d) 868.06 g

43. The solubility of N_2 in water at 300 K and 500 torr partial pressure is 0.01 g L^{-1}. The solubility (in g L^{-1}) at 750 torr partial pressure is :
(a) 0.0075 (b) 0.005 (c) 0.02 (d) 0.015

44. When mercuric iodide is added to the aqueous solution of potassium iodide then
(a) freezing point is raised.
(b) freezing point is lowered.
(c) freezing point does not change.
(d) boiling point does not change.

45. Azeotropic mixture of HCl and H_2O has
(a) 48% HCl (b) 22.2% HCl
(c) 36% HCl (d) 20.2% HCl

RESPONSE GRID					
	35. ⓐⓑⓒⓓ	36. ⓐⓑⓒⓓ	37. ⓐⓑⓒⓓ	38. ⓐⓑⓒⓓ	39. ⓐⓑⓒⓓ
	40. ⓐⓑⓒⓓ	41. ⓐⓑⓒⓓ	42. ⓐⓑⓒⓓ	43. ⓐⓑⓒⓓ	44. ⓐⓑⓒⓓ
	45. ⓐⓑⓒⓓ				

CHEMISTRY CHAPTERWISE SPEED TEST-44			
Total Questions	45	Total Marks	180
Attempted		Correct	
Incorrect		Net Score	
Cut-off Score	42	Qualifying Score	63
Success Gap = Net Score – Qualifying Score			
Net Score = (Correct × 4) – (Incorrect × 1)			

Space for Rough Work

CHEMISTRY

Electrochemistry

Speed TEST 45

Chapter-wise

No. of Questions	Maximum Marks	Time
45	180	1 Hour

GENERAL INSTRUCTIONS

- This test contains 45 MCQ's. For each question only one option is correct. Darken the correct circle/ bubble in the Response Grid provided on each page.
- You have to evaluate your Response Grids yourself with the help of solutions provided at the end of this book.
- Each correct answer will get you 4 marks and 1 mark shall be deduced for each incorrect answer. No mark will be given/ deducted if no bubble is filled. Keep a timer in front of you and stop immediately at the end of 60 min.
- The sheet follows a particular syllabus. Do not attempt the sheet before you have completed your preparation for that syllabus.
- After completing the sheet check your answers with the solution booklet and complete the Result Grid. Finally spend time to analyse your performance and revise the areas which emerge out as weak in your evaluation.

1. A gas X at 1 atm is bubbled through a solution containing a mixture of 1 M Y^- and 1 M Z^- at 25°C. If the reduction potential of Z > Y > X, then,
   (a) Y will oxidize X and not Z
   (b) Y will oxidize Z and not X
   (c) Y will oxidize both X and Z
   (d) Y will reduce both X and Z
2. On the basis of the following E° values, the strongest oxidizing agent is :
   $[Fe(CN)_6]^{4-} \rightarrow [Fe(CN)_6]^{3-} + e^-$; E° = – 0.35 V
   $Fe^{2+} \rightarrow Fe^{3+} + e^-$; E° = – 0.77 V
   (a) $[Fe(CN)_6]^{4-}$ (b) Fe^{2+}
   (c) Fe^{3+} (d) $[Fe(CN)_6]^{3-}$
3. Resistance of a conductivity cell filled with a solution of an electrolyte of concentration 0.1 M is 100 Ω. The conductivity of this solution is 1.29 S m^{-1}. Resistance of the same cell when filled with 0.2 M of the same solution is 520 Ω. The molar conductivity of 0.2 M solution of electrolyte will be
   (a) 1.24×10^{-4} S m^2 mol^{-1} (b) 12.4×10^{-4} S m^2 mol^{-1}
   (c) 124×10^{-4} S m^2 mol^{-1} (d) 1240×10^{-4} S m^2 mol^{-1}
4. For the electrochemical cell, $M | M^+ || X^- | X$,
   $E^o_{M^+/M} = 0.44$ V and $E^o_{X/X^-} = 0.33$ V.
   From this data one can deduce that
   (a) $M + X \rightarrow M^+ + X^-$ is the spontaneous reaction
   (b) $M^+ + X^- \rightarrow M + X$ is the spontaneous reaction
   (c) $E_{cell} = 0.77$ V
   (d) $E_{cell} = -0.77$ V
5. What will be the emf for the given cell
   $Pt | H_2 (P_1) | H^+ (aq) || H_2 (P_2) | Pt$
   (a) $\frac{RT}{F}\log_e \frac{P_1}{P_2}$ (b) $\frac{RT}{2F}\log_e \frac{P_1}{P_2}$
   (c) $\frac{RT}{F}\log_e \frac{P_2}{P_1}$ (d) None of these
6. What is the standard cell potential E° for an electrochemical cell in which the following reaction takes place spontaneously ?
   $Cl_2(g) + 2Br^- \rightarrow Br_2(aq) + 2Cl^-$, $\Delta G° = -50.6$ kJ
   (a) 1.2V (b) 0.53 V
   (c) 0.26V (d) –0.53 V

RESPONSE GRID	1. ⓐⓑⓒⓓ 2. ⓐⓑⓒⓓ 3. ⓐⓑⓒⓓ 4. ⓐⓑⓒⓓ 5. ⓐⓑⓒⓓ 6. ⓐⓑⓒⓓ

Space for Rough Work

7. The unit of equivalent conductivity is
(a) ohm cm
(b) $ohm^{-1}\ cm^2\ (g\ equivalent)^{-1}$
(c) $ohm\ cm^2\ (g\ equivalent)$
(d) $S\ cm^{-2}$

8. The variation of equivalent conductance of strong electrolyte with $(concentration)^{1/2}$ is represented by

(a) 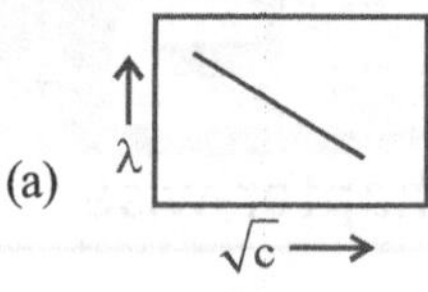
(b) 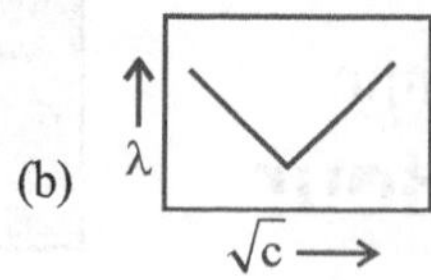

(c) 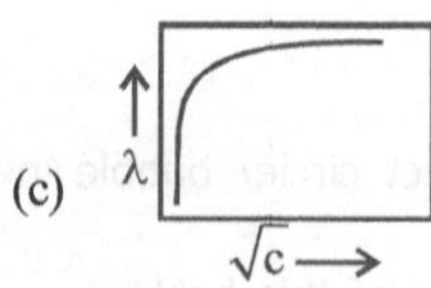
(d) 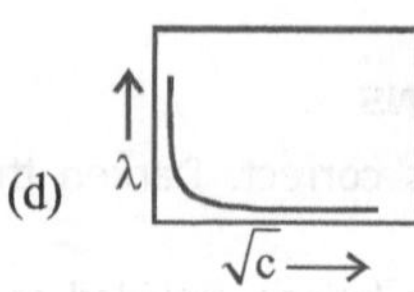

9. Consider the following cell reaction:

$$2Fe(s) + O_2(g) + 4H^+(aq) \rightarrow 2Fe^{2+}(aq) + 2H_2O(l); E^\circ = 1.67\ V$$

At $[Fe^{2+}] = 10^{-3}$ M, $p(O_2) = 0.1$ atm and pH = 3, the cell potential at 25°C is
(a) 1.47V (b) 1.77V (c) 1.87V (d) 1.57V

10. The electrical properties and their respective SI units are given below. Identify the wrongly matched pair.

	Electrical property	SI unit
(a)	Specific conductance	$S\ m^{-1}$
(b)	Conductance	S
(c)	Equivalent conductance	$S\ m^2\ g\ equiv^{-1}$
(d)	Cell constant	m

11. Limiting molar conductivity of NH_4OH $\left(i.e., \Lambda^\circ_{m(NH_4OH)}\right)$ is equal to :
(a) $\Lambda^\circ_{m(NH_4Cl)} + \Lambda^\circ_{m(NaCl)} - \Lambda^\circ_{m(NaOH)}$
(b) $\Lambda^\circ_{m(NaOH)} + \Lambda^\circ_{m(NaCl)} - \Lambda^\circ_{m(NH_4Cl)}$
(c) $\Lambda^\circ_{m(NH_4OH)} + \Lambda^\circ_{m(NH_4Cl)} - \Lambda^\circ_{m(HCl)}$
(d) $\Lambda^\circ_{m(NH_4Cl)} + \Lambda^\circ_{m(NaOH)} - \Lambda^\circ_{m(NaCl)}$

12. A lead storage battery containing 5.0 L of (1N) H_2SO_4 solution is operated for 9.65×10^5 s with a steady current of 100 mA. Assuming volume of the solution remaining constant, normality of H_2SO_4 will
(a) remain unchanged (b) increases by 0.20
(c) increase by unity (d) decrease by 0.40

13. The electrode potential $E_{(Zn^{2+}/Zn)}$ of a zinc electrode at 25°C with an aqueous solution of 0.1 M $ZnSO_4$ is $[E^\circ_{(Zn^{2+}/Zn)} = -0.76$ V. Assume $\frac{2.303RT}{F} = 0.06$ at 298 K].
(a) +0.73 (b) −0.79 (c) −0.82 (d) −0.70

14. A battery is constructed of Cr and $Na_2Cr_2O_7$. The unbalanced chemical equation when such a battery discharges is following:

$$Na_2Cr_2O_7 + Cr + H^+ \rightarrow Cr^{3+} + H_2O + Na^+$$

If one Faraday of electricity is passed through the battery during the charging, the number of moles of Cr^{3+} removed from the solution is
(a) $\frac{4}{3}$ (b) $\frac{1}{3}$ (c) $\frac{3}{3}$ (d) $\frac{2}{3}$

15. Which of the following reaction is possible at anode?
(a) $2Cr^{3+} + 7H_2O \rightarrow Cr_2O_7^{2-} + 14H^+$
(b) $F_2 \rightarrow 2F^-$
(c) $(1/2)O_2 + 2H^+ \rightarrow H_2O$
(d) none of these.

16. In a hydrogen-oxygen fuel cell, combustion of hydrogen occurs to
(a) produce high purity water
(b) create potential difference between two electrodes
(c) generte heat
(d) remove adsorbed oxygen from electron surfaces

17. E° for the cell,

$Zn \mid Zn^{2+}(aq) \mid\mid Cu^{2+}(aq) \mid Cu$ is 1.10 V at 25°C. The equilibrium constant for the cell reaction

$$Zn + Cu^{2+}(aq) \rightleftharpoons Cu + Zn^{2+}(aq)$$

is of the order of
(a) 10^{-37} (b) 10^{37} (c) 10^{-17} (d) 10^{17}

18. The correct order of $E^\circ_{M^{2+}/M}$ values with negative sign for the four successive elements Cr, Mn, Fe and Co is
(a) Mn > Cr > Fe > Co (b) Cr < Fe > Mn > Co
(c) Fe > Mn > Cr > Co (d) Cr > Mn > Fe > Co

RESPONSE GRID					
	7. ⓐⓑⓒⓓ	8. ⓐⓑⓒⓓ	9. ⓐⓑⓒⓓ	10. ⓐⓑⓒⓓ	11. ⓐⓑⓒⓓ
	12. ⓐⓑⓒⓓ	13. ⓐⓑⓒⓓ	14. ⓐⓑⓒⓓ	15. ⓐⓑⓒⓓ	16. ⓐⓑⓒⓓ
	17. ⓐⓑⓒⓓ	18. ⓐⓑⓒⓓ			

Space for Rough Work

19. For a spontaneous reaction the ΔG, equilibrium constant (K) and E°_{Cell} will be respectively
(a) –ve, >1, –ve (b) –ve, <1, –ve
(c) +ve, >1, –ve (d) –ve, >1, +ve

20. If the E°_{cell} for a given reaction has a negative value, then which of the following gives the correct relationships for the values of ΔG° and K_{eq} ?
(a) $\Delta G^\circ > 0; K_{eq} > 1$ (b) $\Delta G^\circ < 0; K_{eq} > 1$
(c) $\Delta G^\circ < 0; K_{eq} < 1$ (d) $\Delta G^\circ > 0; K_{eq} < 1$

21. Which of the following expressions correctly represents the equivalent conductance at infinite dilution of $Al_2(SO_4)_3$, Given that $\Lambda^\circ_{Al^{3+}}$ and $\Lambda^\circ_{SO_4^{2-}}$ are the equivalent conductances at infinite dilution of the respective ions?
(a) $\frac{1}{3}\Lambda^\circ_{Al^{3+}} + \frac{1}{2}\Lambda^\circ_{SO_4^{2-}}$ (b) $2\Lambda^\circ_{Al^{3+}} + 3\Lambda^\circ_{SO_4^{2-}}$
(c) $\Lambda^\circ_{Al^{3+}} + \Lambda^\circ_{SO_4^{2-}}$ (d) $\left(\Lambda^\circ_{Al^{3+}} + \Lambda^\circ_{SO_4^{2-}}\right) \times 6$

22. Given : $E^\circ_{Cr^{3+}/Cr} = -0.74$ V; $E^\circ_{MnO_4^-/Mn^{2+}} = 1.51$ V
$E^\circ_{Cr_2O_7^{2-}/Cr^{3+}} = 1.33$ V; $E^\circ_{Cl/Cl^-} = 1.36$ V
Based on the data given above, strongest oxidising agent will be :
(a) Cl (b) Cr^{3+}
(c) Mn^{2+} (d) MnO_4^-

23. The standard electrode potentials $\left(E^\circ_{M^+/M}\right)$ of four metals A, B, C and D are – 1.2 V, 0.6 V, 0.85 V and – 0.76 V, respectively. The sequence of deposition of metals on applying potential is:
(a) A, C, B, D (b) B, D, C, A
(c) C, B, D, A (d) D, A, B, C

24. Which of the following statements is correct?
(a) Oxidation number of oxygen in KO_2 is +1
(b) The specific conductance of an electrolyte solution decreases with increase in dilution
(c) Sn^{2+} oxidises Fe^{3+}
(d) $Zn/ZnSO_4$ is a reference electrode

25. Molar ionic conductivities of a two-bivalent electrolytes x^{2+} and y^{2-} are 57 and 73 respectively. The molar conductivity of the solution formed by them will be
(a) 130 S cm² mol⁻¹ (b) 65 S cm² mol⁻¹
(c) 260 S cm² mol⁻¹ (d) 187 S cm² mol⁻¹

26. The cell, $Zn \mid Zn^{2+} (1\ M) \parallel Cu^{2+} (1\ M) \mid Cu$ ($E^\circ_{cell} = 1.10$ V) was allowed to be completely discharged at 298 K. The relative concentration of Zn^{2+} to Cu^{2+} $\left(\frac{[Zn^{2+}]}{[Cu^{2+}]}\right)$ is
(a) 9.65×10^4 (b) antilog (24.08)
(c) 37.3 (d) $10^{37.3}$.

27. Which of the following statements is true for an electrochemical cell?
(a) Reduction occurs at H_2 electrode
(b) H_2 is cathode and Cu is anode
(c) H_2 is anode and Cu is cathode
(d) Oxidation occurs at Cu electrode

28. Given
$Fe^{3+} (aq) + e^- \rightarrow Fe^{2+} (aq); E^\circ = +0.77$ V
$Al^{3+} (aq) + 3e^- \rightarrow Al(s); E^\circ = -1.66$ V
$Br_2(aq) + 2e^- \rightarrow 2Br^-; E^\circ = +1.09$ V
Considering the electrode potentials, which of the following represents the correct order of reducing power?
(a) $Fe^{2+} < Al < Br^-$ (b) $Br^- < Fe^{2+} < Al$
(c) $Al < Br^- < Fe^{2+}$ (d) $Al < Fe^{2+} < Br^-$

29. Standard free energies of formation (in kJ/mol) at 298 K are – 237.2, – 394.4 and – 8.2 for $H_2O(l)$, $CO_2(g)$ and pentane (g), respectively. The value E°_{cell} for the pentane-oxygen fuel cell is :
(a) 1.968 V (b) 2.0968 V (c) 1.0968 V (d) 0.0968 V

30. Given $E^\circ_{Cr^{3+}/Cr} = -0.72$ V, $E^\circ_{Fe^{2+}/Fe} = -0.42$ V. The potential for the cell
$Cr|Cr^{3+} (0.1M)|| Fe^{2+} (0.01\ M)| Fe$ is
(a) 0.26 V (b) 0.336 V (c) –0.339 V (d) 0.26 V

31. Electrolysis of dilute aqueous NaCl solution was carried out by passing 10 milli ampere current. The time required to liberate 0.01 mole of H_2 gas at the cathode is
(1 Faraday = 96500 C mol⁻¹)
(a) 9.65×10^4 sec (b) 19.3×10^4 sec
(c) 28.95×10^4 sec (d) 38.6×10^4 sec

32. Which of the following reaction occurs at the cathode during the charging of lead storage battery?
(a) $Pb^{2+} + 2e^- \longrightarrow Pb$
(b) $Pb^{2+} + SO_4^{2-} \longrightarrow PbSO_4$
(c) $Pb \longrightarrow Pb^{2+} + 2e^-$
(d) $PbSO_4 + 2H_2O \longrightarrow 2PbO_2 + 4H^+ + SO_4^{2-} + 2e^-$

RESPONSE GRID					
	19. ⓐⓑⓒⓓ	20. ⓐⓑⓒⓓ	21. ⓐⓑⓒⓓ	22. ⓐⓑⓒⓓ	23. ⓐⓑⓒⓓ
	24. ⓐⓑⓒⓓ	25. ⓐⓑⓒⓓ	26. ⓐⓑⓒⓓ	27. ⓐⓑⓒⓓ	28. ⓐⓑⓒⓓ
	29. ⓐⓑⓒⓓ	30. ⓐⓑⓒⓓ	31. ⓐⓑⓒⓓ	32. ⓐⓑⓒⓓ	

Space for Rough Work

33. Conductance of 0.1 M KCl (conductivity = X $ohm^{-1}cm^{-1}$) filled in a conductivity cell is Y ohm^{-1}. If the conductance of 0.1 M NaOH filled in the same cell is Z ohm^{-1}, the molar conductance of NaOH will be
(a) $10^3\frac{XZ}{Y}$ (b) $10^4\frac{XZ}{Y}$ (d) $10\frac{XZ}{Y}$ (d) $0.1\frac{XZ}{Y}$

34. How much charge is required, when 1 mole of $Cr_2O_7^{2-}$ reduce to form 1 mole of Cr^{3+}?
(a) 6F (b) 3F (c) 1F (d) 2F

35. In electrolysis of dilute H_2SO_4 using platinum electrodes
(a) H_2 is evolved at cathode
(b) NH_3 is produced at anode
(c) Cl_2 is obtained at cathode
(d) O_2 is produced

36. The resistance of 0.1 N solution of a salt is found to be 2.5×10^3 ohm. The equivalent conductance of the solution is (cell constant = 1.15 cm^{-1})
(a) 4.6 (b) 5.6 (c) 6.6 (d) 7.6

37. The highest electrical conductivity of the following aqueous solutions is of
(a) 0.1 M difluoroacetic acid
(b) 0.1 M fluoroacetic acid
(c) 0.1 M chloroacetic acid
(d) 0.1 M acetic acid

38. When during electrolysis of a solution of $AgNO_3$ 9650 coulombs of charge pass through the electroplating bath, the mass of silver deposited on the cathode will be
(a) 10.8 g (b) 21.6 g (c) 108 g (d) 1.08 g

39. The reduction potential of hydrogen half-cell will be negative if:
(a) $p(H_2) = 1$ atm and $[H^+] = 2.0$ M
(b) $p(H_2) = 1$ atm and $[H^+] = 1.0$ M
(c) $p(H_2) = 2$ atm and $[H^+] = 1.0$ M
(d) $p(H_2) = 2$ atm and $[H^+] = 2.0$ M

40. When electric current is passed through acidified water, 112 mL of hydrogen gas at STP collected at the cathode in 965 seconds. The current passed in amperes is
(a) 1.0 (b) 0.5 (c) 0.1 (d) 2.0

41. An electrolytic cell contains a solution of Ag_2SO_4 and has platinum electrodes. A current is passed until 1.6 g of O_2 has been liberated at anode. The amount of silver deposited at cathode would be
(a) 107.88 g (b) 1.6 g
(c) 0.8 g (d) 21.60 g

42. Which of the following pair(s) is/are incorrectly matched?
(i) R (resistance) – ohm (Ω)
(ii) ρ (resistivity) – ohm metre (Ωm)
(iii) G (conductance) – seimens or ohm (S)
(iv) κ (conductivity) – seimens metre^{-1} (Sm^{-1})
(a) (i), (ii) and (iii) (b) (ii) and (iii)
(c) (i), (ii) and (iv) (d) (iii) only

43. One Faraday of electricity is passed through molten Al_2O_3, aqueous solution of $CuSO_4$ and molten NaCl taken in three different electrolytic cells connected in series. The mole ratio of Al, Cu and Na deposited at the respective cathode is
(a) 2 : 3 : 6 (b) 6 : 2 : 3 (c) 6 : 3 : 2 (d) 1 : 2 : 3

44. If ρ is the resistance in ohm of a centimeter cube, generally called the specific resistance of the substance constituting the conductor, the resistance r of the layer containing "a" cubes is given by
(a) $\frac{1}{r}=\frac{1}{\rho}+\frac{1}{\rho}+......$ (b) $\frac{1}{r}=\frac{1}{\rho a}+\frac{1}{\rho a}+...$
(c) $r = a/\rho$ (d) $r=\rho+\rho+......$

45. Which of the following statements is wrong ?
(a) Electrolysis of an aqueous sodium hydroxide solution liberates H_2 gas at the cathode and O_2 gas at the anode.
(b) Electrolysis of dil. H_2SO_4 liberates $H_2(g)$ at cathode and O_2 (g) at the anode
(c) ΔG° = nFE° for a spontaneous reaction
(d) $E=E^\circ-\frac{0.059}{n}\log Q$, Where Q = reaction quotient.

RESPONSE GRID					
	33. ⓐⓑⓒⓓ	34. ⓐⓑⓒⓓ	35. ⓐⓑⓒⓓ	36. ⓐⓑⓒⓓ	37. ⓐⓑⓒⓓ
	38. ⓐⓑⓒⓓ	39. ⓐⓑⓒⓓ	40. ⓐⓑⓒⓓ	41. ⓐⓑⓒⓓ	42. ⓐⓑⓒⓓ
	43. ⓐⓑⓒⓓ	44. ⓐⓑⓒⓓ	45. ⓐⓑⓒⓓ		

CHEMISTRY CHAPTERWISE SPEED TEST-45

Total Questions	45	Total Marks	180
Attempted		Correct	
Incorrect		Net Score	
Cut-off Score	36	Qualifying Score	65
Success Gap = Net Score – Qualifying Score			
Net Score = (Correct × 4) – (Incorrect × 1)			

Space for Rough Work

CHEMISTRY

Chemical Kinetics

Speed TEST 46

Chapter-wise

No. of Questions	Maximum Marks	Time
45	180	1 Hour

GENERAL INSTRUCTIONS

- This test contains 45 MCQ's. For each question only one option is correct. Darken the correct circle/ bubble in the Response Grid provided on each page.
- You have to evaluate your Response Grids yourself with the help of solutions provided at the end of this book.
- Each correct answer will get you 4 marks and 1 mark shall be deduced for each incorrect answer. No mark will be given/ deducted if no bubble is filled. Keep a timer in front of you and stop immediately at the end of 60 min.
- The sheet follows a particular syllabus. Do not attempt the sheet before you have completed your preparation for that syllabus.
- After completing the sheet check your answers with the solution booklet and complete the Result Grid. Finally spend time to analyse your performance and revise the areas which emerge out as weak in your evaluation.

1. The decomposition of a substance follows first order kinetics. Its concentration is reduced to 1/8th of its initial value in 24 minutes. The rate constant of the decomposition process is

   (a) $1/24\ min^{-1}$ (b) $\frac{0.692}{24}\ min^{-1}$

   (c) $\frac{2.303}{24}\log\left(\frac{1}{8}\right)\ min^{-1}$ (d) $\frac{2.303}{24}\log\left(\frac{8}{1}\right)\ min^{-1}$

2. Consider the reaction, $2A + B \rightarrow$ products. When concentration of B alone was doubled, the half-life did not change. When the concentration of A alone was doubled, the rate increased by two times. The unit of rate constant for this reaction is

   (a) s^{-1} (b) $L\ mol^{-1}\ s^{-1}$
   (c) no unit (d) $mol\ L^{-1}\ s^{-1}$.

3. A reaction involving two different reactants can never be

   (a) bimolecular reaction (b) second order reaction
   (c) first order reaction (d) unimolecular reaction

4. Select the rate law that corresponds to the data shown for the following reaction $A + B \longrightarrow C$

Expt. No.	*(A)*	*(B)*	*Initial Rate*
1	0.012	0.035	0.10
2	0.024	0.070	0.80
3	0.024	0.035	0.10
4	0.012	0.070	0.80

   (a) $Rate = k[B]^3$ (b) $Rate = k[B]^4$
   (c) $Rate = k[A][B]^3$ (d) $Rate = k[A]^2[B]^2$

5. Consider the reaction

   $N_2(g) + 3H_2(g) \rightarrow 2NH_3(g)$

   The equality relationship between $\frac{d[NH_3]}{dt}$ and $-\frac{d[H_2]}{dt}$ is

   (a) $+\frac{d[NH_3]}{dt} = -\frac{2}{3}\frac{d[H_2]}{dt}$ (b) $+\frac{d[NH_3]}{dt} = -\frac{3}{2}\frac{d[H_2]}{dt}$

   (c) $\frac{d[NH_3]}{dt} = -\frac{d[H_2]}{dt}$ (d) $\frac{d[NH_3]}{dt} = -\frac{1}{3}\frac{d[H_2]}{dt}$

6. Diazonium salt decomposes as

   $C_6H_5N_2^+Cl^- \rightarrow C_6H_5Cl + N_2$

   At 0°C, the evolution of N_2 becomes two times faster when the initial concentration of the salt is doubled. Therefore, it is

   (a) a first order reaction
   (b) a second order reaction
   (c) independent of the initial concentration of the salt
   (d) a zero order reaction

RESPONSE GRID	
	1. ⓐⓑⓒⓓ 2. ⓐⓑⓒⓓ 3. ⓐⓑⓒⓓ 4. ⓐⓑⓒⓓ 5. ⓐⓑⓒⓓ
	6. ⓐⓑⓒⓓ

Space for Rough Work

7. $CHCl_3 + Cl_2 \longrightarrow CCl_4 + HCl$
Rate law for above reaction will be
$$\text{Rate} = k[CHCl_3][Cl_2]^{\frac{1}{2}}$$
On the basis of information provided which of the following option will be correct ?
(a) Rate law for any chemical reaction can be predicted accurately by looking at balanced chemical equation.
(b) Rate law for a chemical reaction has to determine experimentally.
(c) Either determined experimentally or obtained from balanced chemical reaction, rate law will be same.
(d) None of the above is correct.

8. Which of the following statements is incorrect?
(a) Activation energy for the forward reaction equals to activation energy for the reverse reaction
(b) For a reversible reaction, an increase in temperature increases the reaction rate for both the forward and the backward reaction
(c) The larger the initial reactant concentration for a second order reaction, the shorter is its half-life.
(d) When Δt is infinitesimally small, the average rate equals the instantaneous rate

9. In a reaction $A \rightarrow$ Products, when start is made from 8.0×10^{-2} M of A, half-life is found to be 120 minute. For the initial concentration 4.0×10^{-2} M, the half-life of the reaction becomes 240 minute. The order of the reaction is :
(a) zero (b) one (c) two (d) 0.5

10. During decomposition of an activated complex.
(i) energy is always released
(ii) energy is always absorbed
(iii) energy does not change
(iv) reactants may be formed
(a) (i), (ii) and (iii) (b) (i) and (iv)
(c) (ii) and (iii) (d) (ii), (iii) and (iv)

11. Which of the following statements is incorrect ?
(a) Energy is always released when activated complex decomposes to form products.
(b) Peak of the energy distribution curve corresponds to the most probable potential energy.
(c) Peak of the energy distribution curve corresponds to the most probable kinectic energy.
(d) When the temperature is raised maximum of energy distribution curve moves to higher energy value and broadens out.

12. A catalyst increases rate of reaction by
(a) decreasing enthalpy
(b) decreasing internal energy
(c) decreasing activation energy
(d) increasing activation energy

13. Consider a reaction $aG + bH \rightarrow$ Products. When concentration of both the reactants G and H is doubled, the rate increases by eight times. However, when concentration of G is doubled keeping the concentration of H fixed, the rate is doubled. The overall order of the reaction is
(a) 0 (b) 1 (c) 2 (d) 3

14. For a first order reaction (A) $\rightarrow$ products the concentration of A changes from 0.1 M to 0.025 M in 40 minutes. The rate of reaction when the concentration of A is 0.01 M is :
(a) 1.73×10^{-5} M/min (b) 3.47×10^{-4} M/min
(c) 3.47×10^{-5} M/min (d) 1.73×10^{-4} M/min

15. The given reaction
$2FeCl_3 + SnCl_2 \longrightarrow 2FeCl_2 + SnCl_4$
is an example of
(a) first order reaction (b) second order reaction
(c) third order reaction (d) None of these

16. In a first-order reaction A $\rightarrow$ B, if k is rate constant and inital concentration of the reactant A is 0.5 M, then the half-life is
(a) $\frac{\log 2}{k}$ (b) $\frac{\log 2}{k\sqrt{0.5}}$ (c) $\frac{\ln 2}{k}$ (d) $\frac{0.693}{0.5k}$

17. The integrated rate equations can be determined for
(a) zero order reactions (b) first order reactions
(c) second order reactions (d) Both (a) and (b)

18. The rate constant, the activation energy and the arrhenius parameter of a chemical reaction at 25°C are $3.0 \times 10^{-4} s^{-1}$, 104.4 kJ mol^{-1} and $6.0 \times 10^{14} s^{-1}$ respectively. The value of the rate constant as $T \rightarrow \infty$ is
(a) $2.0 \times 10^{18} s^{-1}$ (b) $6.0 \times 10^{14} s^{-1}$
(c) Infinity (d) $3.6 \times 10^{30} s^{-1}$

19. According to the adsorption theory of catalysis, the speed of the reaction increases because
(a) in the process of adsorption, the activation energy of the molecules becomes large
(b) adsorption produces heat which increases the speed of the reaction
(c) adsorption lowers the activation energy of the reaction
(d) the concentration of product molecules at the active centres of the catalyst becomes high due to adsorption.

20. Consider a general chemical change 2A + 3B $\rightarrow$ products. The rate with respect to A is r_1 and that with respect to B is r_2. The rates r_1 and r_2 are related as
(a) $3r_1 = 2r_2$ (b) $r_1 = r_2$
(c) $2r_1 = 3r_2$ (d) $r_1^2 = 2r_2^2$

21. In a first order reaction, the concentration of the reactant, decreases from 0.8 M to 0.4 M in 15 minutes. The time taken for the concentration to change from 0.1 M to 0.025 M is
(a) 7.5 minutes (b) 15 minutes
(c) 30 minutes (d) 60 minutes

22. Activation energy (E_a) and rate constants (k_1 and k_2) of a chemical reaction at two different temperatures (T_1 and T_2) are related by :
(a) $\ln\frac{k_2}{k_1} = -\frac{E_a}{R}\left(\frac{1}{T_1} - \frac{1}{T_2}\right)$ (b) $\ln\frac{k_2}{k_1} = -\frac{E_a}{R}\left(\frac{1}{T_2} - \frac{1}{T_1}\right)$
(c) $\ln\frac{k_2}{k_1} = -\frac{E_a}{R}\left(\frac{1}{T_2} + \frac{1}{T_1}\right)$ (d) $\ln\frac{k_1}{k_2} = \frac{E_a}{R}\left(\frac{1}{T_1} - \frac{1}{T_2}\right)$

RESPONSE GRID

7. ⓐⓑⓒⓓ	8. ⓐⓑⓒⓓ	9. ⓐⓑⓒⓓ	10. ⓐⓑⓒⓓ	11. ⓐⓑⓒⓓ
12. ⓐⓑⓒⓓ	13. ⓐⓑⓒⓓ	14. ⓐⓑⓒⓓ	15. ⓐⓑⓒⓓ	16. ⓐⓑⓒⓓ
17. ⓐⓑⓒⓓ	18. ⓐⓑⓒⓓ	19. ⓐⓑⓒⓓ	20. ⓐⓑⓒⓓ	21. ⓐⓑⓒⓓ
22. ⓐⓑⓒⓓ				

Space for Rough Work

23. $t_{\frac{1}{4}}$ can be taken as the time taken for the concentration of a reactant to drop to $\frac{3}{4}$ of its initial value. If the rate constant for a first order reaction is k, the $t_{\frac{1}{4}}$ can be written as
(a) $0.75/k$ (b) $0.69/k$ (c) $0.29/k$ (d) $0.10/k$

24. The decomposition of ammonia on tungsten surface at 500 K follows zero order kinetics. The half-life period of this reaction is 45 minutes when the initial pressure is 4 bar. The half-life period (minutes) of the reaction when the initial pressure is 16 bar at the same temperature is
(a) 120 (b) 60 (c) 240 (d) 180

25. In a 1st order reaction, reactant concentration C varies with time t as :
(a) $\frac{1}{C}$ increases linearly with t
(b) $\log C$ decreases linearly with t
(c) C decreases with $\frac{1}{t}$
(d) $\log C$ decreases with $\frac{1}{t}$

26. For a reaction $A \rightarrow$ Product, a plot of $\log t_{1/2}$ versus $\log a_0$ is shown in the figure. If the initial concentration of A is represented by a_0, the order of the reaction is

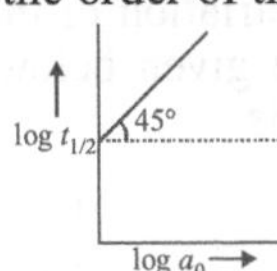

(a) one (b) zero (c) two (d) three

27. The rate of a chemical reaction doubles for every 10°C rise of temperature. If the temperature is raised by 50°C, the rate of the reaction increases by about :
(a) 10 times (b) 24 times (c) 32 times (d) 64 times

28. For a first order reaction $t_{0.75}$ is 1368 seconds, therefore, the specific rate constant in sec^{-1} is
(a) 10^{-3} (b) 10^{-2} (c) 10^{-9} (d) 10^{-5}

29. The integrated rate equation is
$Rt = \log C_0 - \log C_t$.
The straight line graph is obtained by plotting
(a) time Vs $\log C_t$ (b) $\frac{1}{\text{time}}$ Vs C_t
(c) time Vs C_t (d) $\frac{1}{\text{time}}$ Vs $\frac{1}{C_t}$

30. The energies of activation for forward and reverse reactions for $A_2 + B_2 \rightleftharpoons 2AB$ are 180 kJ mol^{-1} and 200 kJ mol^{-1} respectively. The presence of a catalyst lowers the activation energy of both (forward and reverse) reactions by 100 kJ mol^{-1}. The enthalpy change of the reaction ($A_2 + B_2 \rightarrow 2AB$) in the presence of a catalyst will be (in kJ mol^{-1})
(a) 20 (b) 300 (c) 120 (d) 280

31. The half-life period of a first order reaction is 15 minutes. The amount of substance left after one hour will be:
(a) $\frac{1}{4}$ of the original amount
(b) $\frac{1}{8}$ of the original amount
(c) $\frac{1}{16}$ of the original amount
(d) $\frac{1}{32}$ of the original amount

32. Reaction rate between two substance A and B is expressed as following:
rate $= k[A]^n[B]^m$
If the concentration of A is doubled and concentration of B is made half of initial concentration, the ratio of the new rate to the earlier rate will be:
(a) $m+n$ (b) $n-m$ (c) $\frac{1}{2^{(m+n)}}$ (d) $2^{(n-m)}$

33. The reaction of ozone with oxygen atoms in the presence of chlorine atoms can occur by a two step process shown below :
$O_3(g) + Cl^*(g) \rightarrow O_2(g) + ClO^*(g)$ ...(i)
$[K_i = 5.2 \times 10^9\ L\ mol^{-1}\ s^{-1}]$
$ClO^*(g) + O^*(g) \rightarrow O_2(g) + Cl^*(g)$ ...(ii)
$[K_{ii} = 2.6 \times 10^{10}\ L\ mol^{-1}\ s^{-1}]$
The closest rate constant for the overall reaction $O_3(g) + O^*(g) \rightarrow 2O_2(g)$ is :
(a) $1.4 \times 10^{20}\ L\ mol^{-1}\ s^{-1}$ (b) $3.1 \times 10^{10}\ L\ mol^{-1}\ s^{-1}$
(c) $5.2 \times 10^9\ L\ mol^{-1}\ s^{-1}$ (d) $2.6 \times 10^{10}\ L\ mol^{-1}\ s^{-1}$

34. The temperature dependence of rate constant (k) of a chemical reaction is written in terms of Arrhenius equation, $k = A.e^{-E_a}$ Activation energy (E_a) of the reaction can be calculated by plotting
(a) k vs. $\frac{1}{\log T}$ (b) log k vs $\frac{1}{T}$
(c) log k vs. $\frac{1}{\log T}$ (d) k vs. T

35. For the reaction system :
$2NO(g) + O_2(g) \rightarrow 2NO_2(g)$ volume is suddenly reduced to half its value by increasing the pressure on it. If the reaction is of first order with respect to O_2 and second order with respect to NO, the rate of reaction will
(a) diminish to one-eighth of its initial value
(b) increase to eight times of its initial value
(c) increase to four times of its initial value
(d) diminish to one-fourth of its initial value

36. In the reaction of formation of sulphur trioxide by contact process $2SO_2 + O_2 \rightleftharpoons 2SO_3$ the rate of reaction was measured as
$\frac{d[O_2]}{dt} = -2.5 \times 10^{-4}\ mol\ L^{-1} s^{-1}$. The rate of reaction is terms of $[SO_2]$ in mol $L^{-1}\ s^{-1}$ will be:
(a) -1.25×10^{-4} (b) -2.50×10^{-4}
(c) -3.75×10^{-4} (d) -5.00×10^{-4}

RESPONSE GRID					
	23. ⓐⓑⓒⓓ	24. ⓐⓑⓒⓓ	25. ⓐⓑⓒⓓ	26. ⓐⓑⓒⓓ	27. ⓐⓑⓒⓓ
	28. ⓐⓑⓒⓓ	29. ⓐⓑⓒⓓ	30. ⓐⓑⓒⓓ	31. ⓐⓑⓒⓓ	32. ⓐⓑⓒⓓ
	33. ⓐⓑⓒⓓ	34. ⓐⓑⓒⓓ	35. ⓐⓑⓒⓓ	36. ⓐⓑⓒⓓ	

Space for Rough Work

37. A reactant (A) froms two products :

$$A \xrightarrow{k_1} B, \text{ Activation Energy } Ea_1$$

$$A \xrightarrow{k_2} C, \text{ Activation Energy } Ea_2$$

If $Ea_2 = 2\ Ea_1$, then k_1 and k_2 are related as :

(a) $k_2 = k_1 e^{Ea_1/RT}$ (b) $k_2 = k_1 e^{Ea_2/RT}$

(c) $k_1 = Ak_2 e^{Ea_1/RT}$ (d) $k_1 = 2k_2 e^{Ea_2/RT}$

38. Consider an endothermic reaction $X \to Y$ with the activation energies E_b and E_f for the backward and forward reactions, respectively. In general

(a) there is no definite relation between E_b and E_f

(b) $E_b = E_f$

(c) $E_b > E_f$

(d) $E_b < E_f$

39. Which of the following influences the rate of a chemical reaction performed in solution?

(a) Temperature

(b) Activation energy

(c) Presence of a catalyst

(d) All of the above influence the rate

40. The rate of a reaction quadruples when the temperature changes from 300 to 310 K. The activation energy of this reaction is : (Assume activation energy and pre-exponential factor are independent of temperature; ln 2 = 0.693; $R = 8.314\ J\ mol^{-1}\ K^{-1}$)

(a) $107.2\ kJ\ mol^{-1}$ (b) $53.6\ kJ\ mol^{-1}$

(c) $26.8\ kJ\ mol^{-1}$ (d) $214.4\ kJ\ mol^{-1}$

41. Consider the reaction :

$$Cl_2(aq) + H_2S(aq) \to S(s) + 2H^+(aq) + 2Cl^-(aq)$$

The rate equation for this reaction is

rate = $k[Cl_2][H_2S]$

Which of these mechanisms is/are consistent with this rate equation?

A. $Cl_2 + H_2S \to H^+ + Cl^- + Cl^+ + HS^-$ (slow)

$Cl^+ + HS^- \to H^+ + Cl^- + S$ (fast)

B. $H_2S \rightleftharpoons H^+ + HS^-$ (fast equilibrium)

$Cl_2 + HS^- \to 2Cl^- + H^+ + S$ (Slow)

(a) B only (b) Both A and B

(c) Neither A nor B (d) A only

42. The slope in Arrhenius plot, is equal to:

(a) $-\dfrac{E_a}{2.303R}$ (b) $\dfrac{E_a}{R}$

(c) $-\dfrac{R}{2.303E_a}$ (d) None of these

43. A schematic plot of $\ln K_{eq}$ versus inverse of temperature for a reaction is shown below

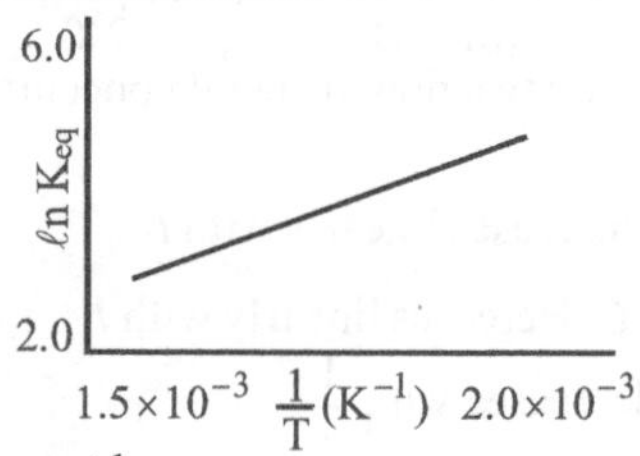

The reaction must be

(a) highly spontaneous at ordinary temperature

(b) one with negligible enthalpy change

(c) endothermic

(d) exothermic

44. Plots showing the variation of the rate constant (k) with temperature (T) are given below. The plot that follows Arrhenius equation is

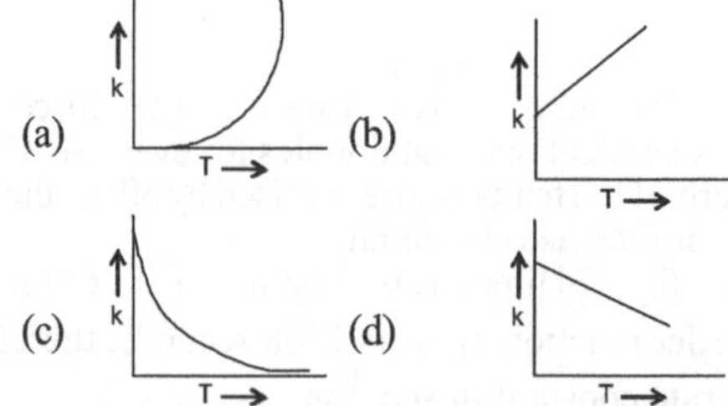

45. The reaction $2N_2O_5(g) \to 4NO_2(g) + O_2(g)$ follows first order kinetics. The pressure of a vessel containing only N_2O_5 was found to increase from 50 mm Hg to 87.5 mm Hg in 30 min. The pressure exerted by the gases after 60 min. will be (assume temperature remains constant) :

(a) 106.25 mm Hg (b) 150 mm Hg

(c) 125 mm Hg (d) 116.25 mm Hg

RESPONSE GRID					
	37. ⓐⓑⓒⓓ	38. ⓐⓑⓒⓓ	39. ⓐⓑⓒⓓ	40. ⓐⓑⓒⓓ	41. ⓐⓑⓒⓓ
	42. ⓐⓑⓒⓓ	43. ⓐⓑⓒⓓ	44. ⓐⓑⓒⓓ	45. ⓐⓑⓒⓓ	

CHEMISTRY CHAPTERWISE SPEED TEST-46			
Total Questions	45	Total Marks	180
Attempted		Correct	
Incorrect		Net Score	
Cut-off Score	38	Qualifying Score	64
Success Gap = Net Score – Qualifying Score			
Net Score = (Correct × 4) – (Incorrect × 1)			

Space for Rough Work

CHEMISTRY

Surface Chemistry

Speed TEST 47

Chapter-wise

No. of Questions	Maximum Marks	Time
45	180	1 Hour

GENERAL INSTRUCTIONS

- This test contains 45 MCQ's. For each question only one option is correct. Darken the correct circle/ bubble in the Response Grid provided on each page.
- You have to evaluate your Response Grids yourself with the help of solutions provided at the end of this book.
- Each correct answer will get you 4 marks and 1 mark shall be deduced for each incorrect answer. No mark will be given/ deducted if no bubble is filled. Keep a timer in front of you and stop immediately at the end of 60 min.
- The sheet follows a particular syllabus. Do not attempt the sheet before you have completed your preparation for that syllabus.
- After completing the sheet check your answers with the solution booklet and complete the Result Grid. Finally spend time to analyse your performance and revise the areas which emerge out as weak in your evaluation.

1. Which of the following statements is *not* true about the oil-in-water type emulsion?
 (a) On addition of small amount of water, no separate layer of water appears
 (b) On addition of oil, separate layer of oil is formed
 (c) Addition of an electrolyte causes the conductivity of the emulsion to increase
 (d) Addition of small amount of oil soluble dye renders the entire emulsion coloured.

2. Which of the following is **not** a favourable condition for physical adsorption ?
 (a) High pressure
 (b) Negative ΔH
 (c) Higher critical temperature of adsorbate
 (d) High temperature

3. The disperse phase in colloidal iron (III) hydroxide and colloidal gold is positively and negatively charged, respectively. Which of the following statements is NOT correct ?
 (a) Coagulation in both sols can be brought about by electrophoresis
 (b) Mixing the sols has no effect
 (c) Sodium sulphate solution causes coagulation in both sols
 (d) Magnesium chloride solution coagulates, the gold sol more readily than the iron (III) hydroxide sol

4. Among the following, correct statement is :
 (a) Brownian movement is more pronounced for smaller particles than for bigger–particles.
 (b) Sols of metal sulphides are lyophilic.
 (c) Hardy Schulze law states that bigger the size of the ons, the greater is its coagulating power.
 (d) One would expect charcoal to adsorb chlorine more than hydrogen sulphide.

5. One desires to prepare a positively charged sol of silver iodide. This can be achieved by
 (a) adding small amount of $AgNO_3$ solution to KI solution in slight excess
 (b) adding small amount of KI solution to $AgNO_3$ solution in slight excess
 (c) mixing equal volumes of equimolar solutions of $AgNO_3$ and KI
 (d) None of these

RESPONSE GRID	1. ⓐⓑⓒⓓ	2. ⓐⓑⓒⓓ	3. ⓐⓑⓒⓓ	4. ⓐⓑⓒⓓ	5. ⓐⓑⓒⓓ

Space for Rough Work

6. How many layers are adsorbed in chemical adsorption ?
(a) One (b) Two
(c) Many (d) Zero

7. Adsorption of gases on solid surface is exothermic reaction because
(a) free energy increases (b) enthalpy is positive
(c) entropy increases (d) enthalpy is negative

8. Cod Liver oil is
(a) fat dispersed in water (b) water dispersed in fat
(c) water dispersed in oil (d) fat dispersed in fat.

9. Physical adsorption of a gaseous species may change to chemical adsorption with ________.
(a) decrease in temperature
(b) increase in temperature
(c) increase in surface area of adsorbent
(d) decrease in surface area of adsorbent

10. Hydrolysis of urea is an example of
(a) homogenous catalysis (b) heterogenous catalysis
(c) biochemical catalysis (d) zeolite catalysis

11. Alum helps in purifying water by
(a) forming Si complex with clay particles
(b) sulphate part which combines with the dirt and removes it
(c) aluminium which coagulates the mud particiles
(d) making mud water soluble

12. The efficiency of an enzyme in catalysing a reaction is due to its capacity
(a) to form a strong enzyme-substrate complex
(b) to decrease the bond energies of substrate molecule
(c) to change the shape of the substrate molecule
(d) to lower the activation energy of the reaction

13. Tyndall effect is shown by
(a) sol (b) solution
(c) plasma (d) precipitate

14. The cause of Brownian movement is
(a) Heat changes in liquid state
(b) Convectional currents
(c) The impact of molecules of the dispersion medium on the colloidal particles.
(d) Attractive forces between the colloidal particles and molecules of dispersion medium.

15. Which of the following curves is in accordance with Freundlich adsorption isotherm ?

(a) [graph: log x/m → vs p →]
(b) [graph: log x/m → vs p →]
(c) [graph: log x/m → vs log p′ →]
(d) [graph: log x/m → vs log p →]

16. Which of the following kind of catalysis can be explained by the adsorption theory ?
(a) Homogeneous catalysis
(b) Acid - base catalysis
(c) Heterogeneous catalysis
(d) Enzyme catalysis

17. The electrolytic impurities of a sol can most easily be separated by
(a) dialysis (b) electrosmosis
(c) electrophoresis (d) electrodialysis

18. Which of the following constitutes irreversible colloidal system in water as dispersion medium?
(a) Clay (b) Platinum
(c) $Fe(OH)_3$ (d) All of these

19. If x is amount of adsorbate and m is amount of adsorbent, which of the following relations is not related to adsorption process ?
(a) $x/m = f(p)$ at constant T.
(b) $x/m = f(\mathrm{T})$ at constant p.
(c) $p = f(\mathrm{T})$ at constant (x/m).
(d) $\frac{x}{m} = p \times T$

20. Gold numbers of some colloids are : Gelatin : 0.005 – 0.01, Gum arabic : 0.15 – 0.25; Oleate : 0.04 – 1.0; Starch : 15 – 25. Which among these is a better protective colloid ?
(a) Gelatin (b) Starch
(c) Oleate (d) Gum arabic

RESPONSE GRID					
	6. ⓐⓑⓒⓓ	7. ⓐⓑⓒⓓ	8. ⓐⓑⓒⓓ	9. ⓐⓑⓒⓓ	10. ⓐⓑⓒⓓ
	11. ⓐⓑⓒⓓ	12. ⓐⓑⓒⓓ	13. ⓐⓑⓒⓓ	14. ⓐⓑⓒⓓ	15. ⓐⓑⓒⓓ
	16. ⓐⓑⓒⓓ	17. ⓐⓑⓒⓓ	18. ⓐⓑⓒⓓ	19. ⓐⓑⓒⓓ	20. ⓐⓑⓒⓓ

Space for Rough Work

21. Colloidal gold is prepared by
(a) Mechanical dispersion (b) Peptisation
(c) Bredig's Arc method (d) Hydrolysis

22. Freundlich equation for adsorption of gases (in amount of x g) on a solid (in amount of m g) at constant temperature can be expressed as
(a) $\log\frac{x}{m} = \log p + \frac{1}{n}\log K$ (b) $\log\frac{x}{m} = \log K + \frac{1}{n}\log p$
(c) $\frac{x}{m} \propto p^n$ (d) $\frac{x}{m} = \log p + \frac{1}{n}\log K$

23. Given below, catalyst and corresponding process/reaction are matched. The one with mismatch is
(a) $[RhCl(PPh_3)_2]$: Hydrogenation
(b) $TiCl_4 + Al(C_2H_5)_3$: Polymerization
(c) V_2O_5 : Haber-Bosch process
(d) Nickel : Hydrogenation

24. Which of the following does not contain a hydrophobic structure ?
(a) Linseed oil (b) Lanolin
(c) Glycogen (d) Rubber

25. The heats of adsorption in physisorption lie in the range (in kJ/mol)
(a) 40 - 400 (b) 40 - 100
(c) 10 - 40 (d) 1 - 10

26. Which one of the following characteristics is **not** correct for physical adsorption ?
(a) Adsorption increases with increase in temperature
(b) Adsorption is spontaneous
(c) Both enthalpy and entropy of adsorption are negative
(d) Adsorption on solids is reversible

27. Under ambient conditions, which among the following surfactants will form micelles in aqueous solution at lowest molar concentration?
(a) $CH_3-(CH_2)_8-COO^-Na^+$
(b) $CH_3(CH_2)_{11}\overset{\oplus}{N}(CH_3)_3Br^-$
(c) $CH_3-(CH_2)_{13}-OSO_3^- Na^+$
(d) $CH_3(CH_2)_{15}\overset{\oplus}{N}(CH_3)_3Br^-$

28. Flocculation value of $BaCl_2$ is much less than that of KCl for sol A and flocculation value of Na_2SO_4 is much less than that of NaBr for sol B. The correct statement among the following is :
(a) Both the sols A and B are negatively charged.
(b) Sol A is positively charged and Sol B is negatively charged.
(c) Both the sols A and B are positively charged.
(d) Sol A is negatively charged and sol B is positively charged.

29. The density of gold is 19 g/cm^3. If 1.9×10^{-4} g of gold is dispersed in one litre of water to give a sol having spherical gold particles of radius 10 nm, then the number of gold particles per mm^3 of the sol will be
(a) 1.9×10^{12} (b) 6.3×10^{14}
(c) 6.3×10^{10} (d) 2.4×10^{6}

30. The stablity of lyophillic colloids is due to which of the following?
(a) Charge on their particles
(b) Large size of their particles
(c) Small size of their particles
(d) A layer of dispersion medium

31. Colloid of which one of the following can be prepared by electrical dispersion method as well as reduction method ?
(a) Sulphur (b) Ferric hydroxide
(c) Arsenious sulphide (d) Gold

32. Example of intrinsic colloid is
(a) glue (b) sulphur
(c) Fe (d) As_2S_3

33. A particular adsorption process has the following characteristics : (i) It arises due to van der Waal's forces and (ii) it is reversile. Identify the correct statement that describes the above adsorption process :
(a) Adsorption is monolayer.
(b) Adsorption increases with increase in temperature.
(c) Enthalpy of adsorption is greater than 100 kJ mol^{-1}
(d) Energy of activation is low.

34. In petrochemical industry alcohols are directly converted to gasoline by passing over heated
(a) Platinum (b) ZSM-5
(c) Iron (d) Nickel

RESPONSE GRID					
	21. ⓐⓑⓒⓓ	22. ⓐⓑⓒⓓ	23. ⓐⓑⓒⓓ	24. ⓐⓑⓒⓓ	25. ⓐⓑⓒⓓ
	26. ⓐⓑⓒⓓ	27. ⓐⓑⓒⓓ	28. ⓐⓑⓒⓓ	29. ⓐⓑⓒⓓ	30. ⓐⓑⓒⓓ
	31. ⓐⓑⓒⓓ	32. ⓐⓑⓒⓓ	33. ⓐⓑⓒⓓ	34. ⓐⓑⓒⓓ	

Space for Rough Work

35. Match the columns

	Column-I		Column-II
A.	As_2S_3 sol	I.	Bredig's Arc method
B.	$Fe(OH)_3$ sol	II.	Double decomposition
C.	Colloidal sols of metals like Au, Ag, Pt, etc.	III.	Peptization
D.	Conversion of freshly prepared precipitate into a colloidal sol	IV.	Hydrolysis

(a) A – II; B – IV; C – III; D – I
(b) A – II; B – I; C – IV; D – III
(c) A – IV; B – II; C – I; D – III
(d) A – II; B – IV; C – I; D – III

36. In Langmuir's model of adsorption of a gas on a solid surface
(a) the mass of gas striking a given area of surface is proportional to the pressure of the gas
(b) the mass of gas striking a given area of surface is independent of the pressure of the gas
(c) the rate of dissociation of adsorbed molecules from the surface does not depend on the surface covered
(d) the adsorption at a single site on the surface may involve multiple molecules at the same time

37. Which of the following electrolytes is least effective in coagulating ferric hydroxide solution?
(a) KBr (b) K_2SO_4
(c) K_2CrO_4 (d) $K_4[Fe(CN)_6]$

38. .... is a silver sol used as an eye lotion.
(a) Amytol (b) Argyrol
(c) Ciprofloxacin (d) Cylol

39. Which of the following is not emulsifying agent for W/O emulsion?
(a) Lampblack
(b) Long chain alcohol
(c) Proteins
(d) Heavy metal salts of fatty acids

40. Among the following, the surfactant that will form micelles in aqueous solution at the lowest molar concentration at ambient condition is : -
(a) $CH_3(CH_2)_{15}N^+(CH_3)_3Br^-$
(b) $CH_3(CH_2)_{11}OSO_3^-Na^+$
(c) $CH_3(CH_2)_6COO^-Na^+$
(d) $CH_3(CH_2)_{11}N^+(CH_3)_3Br^-$

41. At low pressure, the fraction of the surface covered follows
(a) zero-order reaction (b) second-order reaction
(c) first-order reaction (d) fractional order

42. The following statements relate to the adsorption of gases on a solid surface. Identify the incorrect statement among them:
(a) Enthalpy of adsorption is negative
(b) Energy appears as heat
(c) On adsorption, the residual forces on the surface are increased
(d) Entropy of adsorption is negative

43. Peptization involves
(a) precipitation of colloidal particles
(b) disintegration of colloidal aggregates
(c) evaporation of dispersion medium
(d) impact of molecules of the dispersion medium on the colloidal particles

44. The isoelectric-point of a colloidally dispersed material is the pH value at which
(a) the dispersed phase migrate in an electric field
(b) the dispersed phase does not migrate in an electric field
(c) the dispersed phase has pH equal to 7
(d) the dispersed phase has pH equal to zero

45. When solution of 5g of iodine in CS_2 was shaken with the same volume of water. The amount of iodine in water is (Distribution coefficient $C_{CS_2}/C_{H_2O} = 420.0$)
(a) 1.19 (b) 0.0019 (c) 0.0119 (d) 0.119

RESPONSE GRID					
	35. ⓐⓑⓒⓓ	36. ⓐⓑⓒⓓ	37. ⓐⓑⓒⓓ	38. ⓐⓑⓒⓓ	39. ⓐⓑⓒⓓ
	40. ⓐⓑⓒⓓ	41. ⓐⓑⓒⓓ	42. ⓐⓑⓒⓓ	43. ⓐⓑⓒⓓ	44. ⓐⓑⓒⓓ
	45. ⓐⓑⓒⓓ				

CHEMISTRY CHAPTERWISE SPEED TEST-47

Total Questions	45	Total Marks	180
Attempted		Correct	
Incorrect		Net Score	
Cut-off Score	46	Qualifying Score	68
Success Gap = Net Score – Qualifying Score			
Net Score = (Correct × 4) – (Incorrect × 1)			

Space for Rough Work

CHEMISTRY

General Principles and Processes of Isolation of Elements

Speed TEST 48

Chapter-wise

No. of Questions	Maximum Marks	Time
45	180	1 Hour

GENERAL INSTRUCTIONS

- This test contains 45 MCQ's. For each question only one option is correct. Darken the correct circle/ bubble in the Response Grid provided on each page.
- You have to evaluate your Response Grids yourself with the help of solutions provided at the end of this book.
- Each correct answer will get you 4 marks and 1 mark shall be deduced for each incorrect answer. No mark will be given/ deducted if no bubble is filled. Keep a timer in front of you and stop immediately at the end of 60 min.
- The sheet follows a particular syllabus. Do not attempt the sheet before you have completed your preparation for that syllabus.
- After completing the sheet check your answers with the solution booklet and complete the Result Grid. Finally spend time to analyse your performance and revise the areas which emerge out as weak in your evaluation.

1. Bronze is a mixture of
   (a) Pb + Sn (b) Cu + Sn
   (c) Cu + Zn (d) Pb + Zn
2. Which of the following pair is incorrectly matched ?
   (a) Magnetite – Fe_3O_4 (b) Copper glance – Cu_2S
   (c) Calamine – $ZnCO_3$ (d) Zincite – ZnS
3. Which of the following factors is of ***no significance*** for roasting sulphide ores to the oxides and not subjecting the sulphide ores to carbon reduction directly?
   (a) Metal sulphides are thermodynamically more stable than CS_2
   (b) CO_2 is thermodynamically more stable than CS_2
   (c) Metal sulphides are less stable than the corresponding oxides
   (d) CO_2 is more volatile than CS_2
4. Aluminothermic process is used for the extraction of metals , whose oxides are
   (a) fusible
   (b) not easily reduced by carbon
   (c) not easily reduced by hydrogen
   (d) strongly basic.
5. Which reagent is used in Bayer's process?
   (a) Na_2CO_3 (b) Carbon
   (c) NaOH (d) Silica
6. Which of the following reaction takes place in blast furnace during extraction of copper ?
   (a) $2Cu_2S + 3O_2 \longrightarrow 2Cu_2O + 2SO_2$
   (b) $2FeS + 3O_2 \longrightarrow 2FeO + 2SO_2$
   (c) $2Cu_2O + Cu_2S \longrightarrow 6Cu + SO_2$
   (d) All of these
7. When an aqueous solution of sodium chloride is electrolysed using platinum electrodes, the ion discharged at the electrodes are
   (a) sodium and hydrogen (b) sodium and chloride
   (c) hydrogen and chloride (d) hydroxyl and chloride
8. Which of the following elements is present as the impurity to the maximum extent in the pig iron ?
   (a) Manganese (b) Carbon
   (c) Silicon (d) Phosphorus

RESPONSE GRID	
	1. ⓐⓑⓒⓓ 2. ⓐⓑⓒⓓ 3. ⓐⓑⓒⓓ 4. ⓐⓑⓒⓓ 5. ⓐⓑⓒⓓ
	6. ⓐⓑⓒⓓ 7. ⓐⓑⓒⓓ 8. ⓐⓑⓒⓓ

Space for Rough Work

9. Thomas slag is
(a) $Ca_3(PO_4)_2$
(b) $CaSiO_3$
(c) Mixture of (a) and (b)
(d) $FeSiO_3$

10. Brine is electrolysed by using inert electrodes. The reaction at anode is ________.
(a) $Cl^-(aq) \longrightarrow \frac{1}{2}Cl_2(g) + e^-;$ $E^\circ_{Cell} = 1.36V$
(b) $2H_2O(l) \longrightarrow O_2(g) + 4H^+ + 4e^-;$ $E^\circ_{Cell} = 1.23V$
(c) $Na^+(aq) + e^- \longrightarrow Na(s);$ $E^\circ_{Cell} = 2.71V$
(d) $H^+(aq) + e^- \longrightarrow \frac{1}{2}H_2(g);$ $E^\circ_{Cell} = 0.00V$

11. Pb and Sn are extracted from their chief ore by
(a) carbon reduction and self reduction.
(b) self reduction and carbon reduction.
(c) electrolysis and self reduction.
(d) self reduction and electrolysis.

12. In the commercial electrochemical process for aluminium extraction the electrolyte used is
(a) $Al(OH)_3$ in NaOH solution
(b) An aqueous solution of $Al_2(SO_4)_3$
(c) A molten mixture of Al_2O_3 and Na_3AlF_6
(d) A molten mixture of Al_2O_3 and $Al(OH)_3$

13. Aluminium is extracted from alumina (Al_2O_3) by electrolysis of a molten mixture of
(a) $Al_2O_3 + HF + NaAlF_4$
(b) $Al_2O_3 + CaF_2 + NaAlF_4$
(c) $Al_2O_3 + Na_3AlF_6 + CaF_2$
(d) $Al_2O_3 + KF + Na_3AlF_6$

14. A coupled reaction is takes place as follow–
$A + B \longrightarrow C + D,$ $\Delta G^\circ = +x\,kJ$
$D + E \longrightarrow F$ $\Delta G^\circ = -y\,kJ$
for the spontaneity of reaction $A + B + E \longrightarrow C + F$, which of the following is correct?
(a) $2x = y$
(b) $x < y$
(c) $x > y$
(d) $x = (y) \times T\Delta S$

15. The most electropositive metals are isolated from their ores by
(a) high temperature reduction with carbon
(b) self reduction
(c) thermal decomposition
(d) electrolysis of fused ionic salts

16. Which of the following pairs of metals is purified by van Arkel method ?
(a) Ga and In
(b) Zr and Ti
(c) Ag and Au
(d) Ni and Fe

17. Match list I with list II and select the correct answer using the codes given below the lists:

List I	List II
A. Cyanide process	I. Ultrapure Ge
B. Floatation process	II. Pine oil
C. Electrolytic reduction	III. Extraction of Al
D. Zone refining	IV. Extraction of Au

(a) A-III; B-I; C-IV; D-II
(b) A-IV; B-II; C-III; D-I
(c) A-III; B-II; C-IV; D-I
(d) A-IV; B-I; C-III; D-II

18. Blister copper is
(a) Impure Cu
(b) Cu alloy
(c) Pure Cu
(d) Cu having 1% impurity

19. Electrometallurgical process is used to extract
(a) Fe
(b) Pb
(c) Na
(d) Ag

20. Sulphide ores of metals are usually concentrated by froth flotation process. Which one of the following sulphide ores offer an exception and concentrated by chemical leaching?
(a) Galena
(b) Copper pyrite
(c) Sphalerite
(d) Argentite

21. Which of the following reactions is an example for calcination process ?
(a) $2Ag + 2HCl + (O) \rightarrow 2AgCl + H_2O$
(b) $2Zn + O_2 \rightarrow 2ZnO$
(c) $2ZnS + 3O_2 \rightarrow 2ZnO + 2SO_2$
(d) $MgCO_3 \rightarrow MgO + CO_2$

RESPONSE GRID					
	9. ⓐⓑⓒⓓ	10. ⓐⓑⓒⓓ	11. ⓐⓑⓒⓓ	12. ⓐⓑⓒⓓ	13. ⓐⓑⓒⓓ
	14. ⓐⓑⓒⓓ	15. ⓐⓑⓒⓓ	16. ⓐⓑⓒⓓ	17. ⓐⓑⓒⓓ	18. ⓐⓑⓒⓓ
	19. ⓐⓑⓒⓓ	20. ⓐⓑⓒⓓ	21. ⓐⓑⓒⓓ		

Space for Rough Work

22. In the metallurgy of Zn, Zn dust obtained from roasting and reduction of zinc sulphide contains some ZnO. It is removed by
(a) absorbance of ultraviolet light- and reemission of white light
(b) shock cooling by contact with a shower of molten lead.
(c) X-ray method
(d) smelting.

23. The electrolytic reduction technique is used in the extraction of
(a) highly electronegative elements
(b) highly electropositive elements
(c) metalloids
(d) transition metals.

24. Which of the following metal is leached by cyanide process
(a) Ag (b) Na (c) Al (d) Cu

25. $\Delta G°$ vs T plot in the Ellingham's diagram slopes downward for the reaction
(a) $Mg + \frac{1}{2}O_2 \rightarrow MgO$ (b) $2Ag + \frac{1}{2}O_2 \rightarrow Ag_2O$
(c) $C + \frac{1}{2}O_2 \rightarrow CO$ (d) $CO + \frac{1}{2}O_2 \rightarrow CO_2$

26. Process followed before reduction of carbonate ore is
(a) calcination (b) roasting
(c) liquation (d) polling

27. Which of the following metal is used in the manufacture of dye-stuffs and paints ?
(a) Copper (b) Zinc
(c) Aluminium (d) Magnesium

28. Silver containing lead as an impurity is removed by
(a) poling (b) cupellation
(c) lavigation (d) distillation

29. Among the following groups of oxides, the group containing oxides that cannot be reduced by carbon to give the respective metals is
(a) Cu_2O, SnO_2 (b) Fe_2O_3, ZnO
(c) CaO, K_2O (d) PbO, Fe_3O_4

30. Which of the following condition favours the reduction of a metal oxide to metal?
(a) $\Delta H = +ve, T\Delta S = +ve$ at low temperature
(b) $\Delta H = +ve, T\Delta S = -ve$ at any temperature
(c) $\Delta H = -ve, T\Delta S = -ve$ at high temperature
(d) $\Delta H = -ve, T\Delta S = +ve$ at any temperature

31. Match the columns.

Column-I	Column-II
(A) Blisterred Cu	I. Aluminium
(B) Blast furnace	II. $2Cu_2O + Cu_2S \rightarrow 6Cu + SO_2$
(C) Reverberatory furnace	III. Iron
(D) Hall-Heroult process	IV. $FeO + SiO_2 \rightarrow FeSiO_3$
	V. $2Cu_2S + 3O_2 \rightarrow 2Cu_2O + 2SO_2$

(a) A – II ; B – III ; C – IV ; D – I
(b) A – I ; B – II ; C – III ; D – V
(c) A – V ; B – IV ; C – III ; D – II
(d) A – IV ; B – V ; C – III ; D – II

32. In the extraction of copper from its sulphide ore, the metal is finally obtained by the reduction of cuprous oxide with :
(a) Copper (I) sulphide (Cu_2S)
(b) Sulphur dioxide (SO_2)
(c) Iron sulphide (FeS)
(d) Carbon monoxide (CO)

33. In electro-refining of metal the impure metal is made the anode and a strip of pure metal, the cathode, during the electrolysis of an aqueous solution of a complex metal salt. This method cannot be used for refining of
(a) silver (b) copper
(c) aluminium (d) sodium

34. According to Ellingham diagram, the oxidation reaction of carbon to carbon monoxide may be used to reduce which one of the following oxides at the lowest temperature ?
(a) Al_2O_3 (b) Cu_2O
(c) MgO (d) ZnO

35. Hematite is the ore of
(a) Pb (b) Cu
(c) Fe (d) Au

RESPONSE GRID					
	22. ⓐⓑⓒⓓ	23. ⓐⓑⓒⓓ	24. ⓐⓑⓒⓓ	25. ⓐⓑⓒⓓ	26. ⓐⓑⓒⓓ
	27. ⓐⓑⓒⓓ	28. ⓐⓑⓒⓓ	29. ⓐⓑⓒⓓ	30. ⓐⓑⓒⓓ	31. ⓐⓑⓒⓓ
	32. ⓐⓑⓒⓓ	33. ⓐⓑⓒⓓ	34. ⓐⓑⓒⓓ	35. ⓐⓑⓒⓓ	

Space for Rough Work

36. Which of the following is chalcopyrite?
(a) $CuFeS_2$ (b) FeS_2
(c) $KMgCl_3.6H_2O$ (d) $Al_2O_3.2H_2O$

37. Main function of roasting is
(a) to remove volatile substances
(b) oxidation
(c) reduction
(d) slag formation

38. Method used for obtaining highly pure silicon used as a semiconductor material, is
(a) Oxidation (b) Electrochemical
(c) Crystallization (d) Zone refining

39. After partial roasting the sulphide of copper is reduced by
(a) cyanide process (b) electrolysis
(c) reduction with carbon (d) self reduction

40. Cast iron is
(a) made by melting pig iron with scrap iron and coke using hot air blast
(b) having slightly lower carbon content (about 3%) as compared to pig iron
(c) extremely hard and brittle
(d) All of the above statements are true

41. The following reactions take place in the blast furnace in the preparation of impure iron. Identify the reaction pertaining to the formation of the slag.
(a) $Fe_2O_3(s) + 3\,CO(g) \rightarrow 2\,Fe\,(l) + 3\,CO_2\,(g)$
(b) $CaCO_3\,(s) \rightarrow CaO\,(s) + CO_2\,(g)$
(c) $CaO\,(s) + SiO_2(s) \rightarrow CaSiO_3(s)$
(d) $2C(s) + O_2\,(g) \rightarrow 2\,CO(g)$

42. Before introducing FeO in blast furnace, it is converted to Fe_2O_3 by roasting so that
(a) it may not be removed as slag with silica
(b) it may not evaporate in the furnace
(c) presence of it may increase the m.pt. of charge
(d) None of these.

43. When a metal is to be extracted from its ore and the gangue associated with the ore is silica, then
(a) an acidic flux is needed
(b) a basic flux is needed
(c) both acidic and basic fluxes are needed
(d) Neither of them is needed

44. $Cu_2S + 2Cu_2O \longrightarrow 6Cu + SO_2$
In which process of metallurgy of copper, above equation is involved?
(a) Roasting (b) Self reduction
(c) Refining (d) Purification

45. When the sample of copper with zinc impurity is to be purified by electrolysis, the appropriate electrodes are

	Cathode	Anode
(a)	pure zinc	pure copper
(b)	impure sample	pure copper
(c)	impure zinc	impure sample
(d)	pure copper	impure sample.

RESPONSE GRID					
	36. ⓐⓑⓒⓓ	37. ⓐⓑⓒⓓ	38. ⓐⓑⓒⓓ	39. ⓐⓑⓒⓓ	40. ⓐⓑⓒⓓ
	41. ⓐⓑⓒⓓ	42. ⓐⓑⓒⓓ	43. ⓐⓑⓒⓓ	44. ⓐⓑⓒⓓ	45. ⓐⓑⓒⓓ

CHEMISTRY CHAPTERWISE SPEED TEST-48

Total Questions	45	Total Marks	180
Attempted		Correct	
Incorrect		Net Score	
Cut-off Score	43	Qualifying Score	63
Success Gap = Net Score – Qualifying Score			
Net Score = (Correct × 4) – (Incorrect × 1)			

Space for Rough Work

CHEMISTRY

p-Block Elements (Group 15, 16, 17 and 18)

Speed TEST 49

Chapter-wise

No. of Questions	Maximum Marks	Time
45	180	1 Hour

GENERAL INSTRUCTIONS

- This test contains 45 MCQ's. For each question only one option is correct. Darken the correct circle/ bubble in the Response Grid provided on each page.
- You have to evaluate your Response Grids yourself with the help of solutions provided at the end of this book.
- Each correct answer will get you 4 marks and 1 mark shall be deduced for each incorrect answer. No mark will be given/ deducted if no bubble is filled. Keep a timer in front of you and stop immediately at the end of 60 min.
- The sheet follows a particular syllabus. Do not attempt the sheet before you have completed your preparation for that syllabus.
- After completing the sheet check your answers with the solution booklet and complete the Result Grid. Finally spend time to analyse your performance and revise the areas which emerge out as weak in your evaluation.

1. The brown ring test for NO_2^- and NO_3^- is due to the formation of complex ion with a formula

(a) $[Fe(H_2O)_6]^{2+}$ (b) $[Fe(NO)(CN)_5]^{2+}$

(c) $[Fe(H_2O)_5NO]^{2+}$ (d) $[Fe(H_2O)(NO)_5]^{2+}$

2. Which of the following shows nitrogen with its increasing order of oxidation number?

(a) $NO < N_2O < NO_2 < NO_3^- < NH_4^+$

(b) $NH_4^+ < N_2O < NO_2 < NO_3^- < NO$

(c) $NH_4^+ < N_2O < NO < NO_2 < NO_3^-$

(d) $NH_4^+ < NO < N_2O < NO_2 < NO_3^-$

3. Which one of the following is the correct decreasing order of boiling point?

(a) $H_2Te > H_2O > H_2Se > H_2S$

(b) $H_2O > H_2S > H_2Se > H_2Te$

(c) $H_2Te > H_2Se > H_2S > H_2O$

(d) $H_2O > H_2Te > H_2Se > H_2S$

4. The true statement for the acids of phosphorus. H_3PO_2, H_3PO_3, and H_3PO_4 is :

(a) the order of their acidity is $H_3PO_4 < H_3PO_3 <, H_3PO_2$

(b) all of them are reducing in nature

(c) all of them are tribasic acids

(d) the geometry of phosphorus is tetrahedral in all the three

5. The acid which forms two series of salts is

(a) H_3PO_4 (b) H_3PO_3 (c) H_3BO_3 (d) $H_3PO_2^-$

RESPONSE GRID	1. ⓐⓑⓒⓓ	2. ⓐⓑⓒⓓ	3. ⓐⓑⓒⓓ	4. ⓐⓑⓒⓓ	5. ⓐⓑⓒⓓ

Space for Rough Work

6. The nitrogen oxides that contain(s) N–N bond(s) is /are
(i) N_2O (ii) N_2O_3 (iii) N_2O_4 (iv) N_2O_5
(a) (i), (ii) (b) (ii), (iii), (iv)
(c) (iii), (iv) (d) (i), (ii) and (iii)

7. The geometry of ClO_3^- according to valence shell electron pair repulsion (VSEPR) theory will be
(a) planar triangle (b) pyramidal
(c) tetrahedral (d) square planar

8. It is possible to obtain oxygen from air by fractional distillation because
(a) oxygen is in a different group of the periodic table from nitrogen
(b) oxygen is more reactive than nitrogen
(c) oxygen has higher b.p. than nitrogen
(d) oxygen has a lower density than nitrogen

9. Which of the following is the most basic oxide?
(a) Sb_2O_3 (b) Bi_2O_3 (c) SeO_2 (d) Al_2O_3

10. Which compound is used in photography?
(a) Na_2SO_5 (b) $Na_2S_2O_8$
(c) $Na_2S_2O_6$ (d) $Na_2S_2O_3$

11. The oxyacid of phosphorous in which phosphorous has the lowest oxidation state is
(a) hypophosphorous acid
(b) orthophosphoric acid
(c) pyrophosphoric acid
(d) metaphosphoric acid

12. Which of the following statements is not valid for oxoacids of phosphorus?
(a) Orthophosphoric acid is used in the manufacture of triple superphosphate.
(b) Hypophosphorous acid is a diprotic acid.
(c) All oxoacids contain tetrahedral four coordinated phosphorus.
(d) All oxoacids contain atleast one P = O and one P — OH group.

13. Which one of the following reactions of xenon compounds is not feasible?
(a) $3XeF_4 + 6H_2O \longrightarrow 2Xe + XeO_3 + 12HF + 1.5O_2$
(b) $2XeF_2 + 2H_2O \longrightarrow 2Xe + 4HF + O_2$
(c) $XeF_6 + RbF \longrightarrow Rb[XeF_7]$
(d) $XeO_3 + 6HF \longrightarrow XeF_6 + 3H_2O$

14. The compound of sulphur that can be used as refrigerant is
(a) SO_2 (b) SO_3 (c) S_2Cl_2 (d) H_2SO_4

15. Which of the following on thermal decomposition gives oxygen gas ?
(a) Ag_2O (b) Pb_3O_4
(c) PbO_2 (d) All of these

16. Which of the following statements are correct?
(i) Arsenic and antimony are metalloids.
(ii) Phosphorus, arsenic and antimony are found mainly as sulphide minerals.
(iii) Covalent radii increases equally from N to Bi.
(iv) Elements of group 15 have extra stability and higher ionisation energy due to exactly half filled ns^2np^3 electronic configuration.
(v) In group 15 elements only nitrogen is gas whereas all others are solids.
(a) (i), (iv) and (v) (b) (ii), (iii) and (iv)
(c) (i), (ii) and (iii) (d) (ii), (iii) and (v)

17. The formation of $O_2^+[PtF_6]^-$ is the basis for the formation of xenon fluorides. This is because
(a) O_2 and Xe have comparable sizes
(b) both O_2 and Xe are gases
(c) O_2 and Xe have comparable ionisation energies
(d) Both (a) and (c)

18. Oxidation of thiosulphate by iodine gives
(a) tetrathionate ion (b) sulphide ion
(c) sulphate ion (d) sulphite ion

19. The hybridization in ICl_7 is
(a) sp^3d^3 (b) d^2sp^3 (c) sp^3d (d) sp^3

RESPONSE GRID					
	6. ⓐⓑⓒⓓ	7. ⓐⓑⓒⓓ	8. ⓐⓑⓒⓓ	9. ⓐⓑⓒⓓ	10. ⓐⓑⓒⓓ
	11. ⓐⓑⓒⓓ	12. ⓐⓑⓒⓓ	13. ⓐⓑⓒⓓ	14. ⓐⓑⓒⓓ	15. ⓐⓑⓒⓓ
	16. ⓐⓑⓒⓓ	17. ⓐⓑⓒⓓ	18. ⓐⓑⓒⓓ	19. ⓐⓑⓒⓓ	

Space for Rough Work

20. Match the columns.

	Column-I		Column-II
A.	Pb_3O_4	I.	Neutral oxide
B.	N_2O	II.	Acidic oxide
C.	Mn_2O_7	III.	Basic oxide
D.	Bi_2O_3	IV.	Mixed oxide

(a) A – I; B – II; C – III; D – IV
(b) A – IV; B – I; C – II; D – III
(c) A – III; B – II; C – IV; D – I
(d) A – IV; B – III; C – I; D – II

21. Which one of the following arrangements does not give the correct picture of the trends indicated against it ?
(i) $F_2 > Cl_2 > Br_2 > I_2$: Oxidizing power
(ii) $F_2 > Cl_2 > Br_2 > I_2$: Electron gain enthalpy
(iii) $F_2 > Cl_2 > Br_2 > I_2$: Bond dissociation energy
(iv) $F_2 > Cl_2 > Br_2 > I_2$: Electronegativity.
(a) (ii) and (iv) (b) (i) and (iii)
(c) (ii) and (iii) (d) (ii), (iii) and (iv)

22. Which of the following is a saline oxide ?
(a) Na_2O_2 (b) BaO_2 (c) Na_2O (d) Fe_2O_3

23. Shape of $XeOF_4$ is
(a) octahedral (b) square pyramidal
(c) pyramidal (d) T-shaped

24. Which among the following is paramagnetic ?
(a) Cl_2O (b) ClO_2 (c) Cl_2O_7 (d) Cl_2O_6

25. The molecule having smallest bond angle is :
(a) NCl_3 (b) $AsCl_3$ (c) $SbCl_3$ (d) PCl_3

26. Which one of the following orders correctly represents the increasing acid strengths of the given acids?
(a) $HOClO < HOCl < HOClO_3 < HOClO_2$
(b) $HOClO_2 < HOClO_3 < HOClO < HOCl$
(c) $HOClO_3 < HOClO_2 < HOClO < HOCl$
(d) $HOCl < HOClO < HOClO_2 < HOClO_3$

27. The ease of liquefaction of noble gases increases in the order
(a) He < Ne < Ar < Kr < Xe
(b) Xe < Kr < Ne < Ar < He
(c) Kr < Xe < He < Ne < Ar
(d) Ar < Kr < Xe < Ne < He

28. A certain compound (X) when treated with copper sulphate solution yields a brown precipitate. On adding hypo solution, the precipitate turns white. The compound is
(a) K_2CO_3 (b) KI (c) KBr (d) K_3PO_4

29. Which of the following species is not a pseudo halide
(a) CNO^- (b) $RCOO^-$ (c) OCN^- (d) NNN^-

30. Which of the following is used to produce and sustain powerful superconducting magnets to form an essential part of NMR spectrometer ?
(a) Ar (b) Ne (c) Rn (d) He

31. The product obtained as a result of a reaction of nitrogen with CaC_2 is
(a) $Ca(CN)_2$ (b) CaCN (c) $CaCN_3$ (d) Ca_2CN

32. Which of the following noble gases has the highest negative electron gain enthalpy value?
(a) Helium (b) Krypton
(c) Argon (d) Neon

33. Gaseous HCl is a poor conductor of electricity while its aqueous solution is a good conductor this is because
(a) H_2O is a good conductor of electricity
(b) a gas cannot conduct electricity but a liquid can
(c) HCl gas does not obey Ohm's law, whereas the solution does
(d) HCl ionises in aqueous solution

34. Density of nitrogen gas prepared from air is slightly greater than that of nitrogen prepared by chemical reaction from a compound of nitrogen due to the presence of
(a) argon
(b) carbon dioxide
(c) some N_3 molecules analogous to O_3
(d) greater amount of N_2 molecules derived from N-15 isotope

RESPONSE GRID					
	20. ⓐⓑⓒⓓ	21. ⓐⓑⓒⓓ	22. ⓐⓑⓒⓓ	23. ⓐⓑⓒⓓ	24. ⓐⓑⓒⓓ
	25. ⓐⓑⓒⓓ	26. ⓐⓑⓒⓓ	27. ⓐⓑⓒⓓ	28. ⓐⓑⓒⓓ	29. ⓐⓑⓒⓓ
	30. ⓐⓑⓒⓓ	31. ⓐⓑⓒⓓ	32. ⓐⓑⓒⓓ	33. ⓐⓑⓒⓓ	34. ⓐⓑⓒⓓ

Space for Rough Work

35. The correct order of acidic strength is
(a) $Cl_2O_7 > SO_2 > P_4O_{10}$
(b) $CO_2 > N_2O_5 > SO_3$
(c) $Na_2O > MgO > Al_2O_3$
(d) $K_2O > CaO > MgO$

36. Sulphur trioxide can be obtained by which of the following reaction :
(a) $CaSO_4 + C \xrightarrow{\Delta}$ (b) $Fe_2(SO_4)_3 \xrightarrow{\Delta}$
(c) $S + H_2SO_4 \xrightarrow{\Delta}$ (d) $H_2SO_4 + PCl_5 \xrightarrow{\Delta}$

37. The correct order of increasing bond angles in the following species are :
(a) $Cl_2O < ClO_2 < ClO_2^-$
(b) $ClO_2 < Cl_2O < ClO_2^-$
(c) $Cl_2O < ClO_2^- < ClO_2$
(d) $ClO_2^- < Cl_2O < ClO_2$

38. Which one of the following oxides of chlorine is obtained by passing dry chlorine over silver chlorate at 90°C ?
(a) Cl_2O (b) ClO_3 (c) ClO_2 (d) ClO_4

39. The shape of XeO_2F_2 molecule is
(a) trigonal bipyramidal (b) square planar
(c) tetrahedral (d) see-saw

40. Number of lone pairs of electrons on Xe atoms XeF_2, XeF_4 and XeF_6 molecules are respectively
(a) 3, 2 and 1 (b) 4, 3 and 2
(c) 2, 3 and 1 (d) 3, 2 and 0

41. Match the interhalogen compounds of column-I with the geometry in column II and assign the correct code.

	Column-I		Column-II
A.	XX'	I.	T-shape
B.	XX'_3	II.	Pentagonal bipyramidal
C.	XX'_5	III.	Linear
D.	XX'_7	IV.	Square-pyramidal
		V.	Tetrahedral

(a) A – III; B – I; C – IV; D – II
(b) A – V; B – IV; C – III; D – II
(c) A – IV; B – III; C – II; D – I
(d) A – III; B – IV; C – I; D – II

42. The crystals of ferrous sulphate on heating give :
(a) $FeO + SO_2 + H_2O$
(b) $FeO + SO_3 + H_2SO_4 + H_2O$
(c) $Fe_2O_3 + SO_2 + H_2SO_4 + H_2O$
(d) $Fe_2O_3 + H_2SO_4 + H_2O$

43. One mole of fluorine is reacted with two moles of hot and concentrated KOH. The products formed are KF, H_2O and O_2. The molar ratio of KF, H_2O and O_2 respectively is
(a) 1 : 1 : 2 (b) 2 : 1 : 0.5
(c) 1 : 2 : 1 (d) 2 : 1 : 2

44. A greenish yellow gas reacts with an alkali metal hydroxide to form a halate which can be used in fire works safety matches. The gas and halate respectively are
(a) $Br_2, KBrO_3$ (b) $Cl_2, KClO_3$
(c) $I_2, NaIO_3$ (d) $Cl_2, NaClO_3$

45. Yellow ammonium sulphide is
(a) $(NH_4)_2S_8$ (b) $(NH_4)_2S$
(c) $(NH_4)_2S_x$ (d) $(NH_4)_2S_4$

RESPONSE GRID				
35. ⓐⓑⓒⓓ	36. ⓐⓑⓒⓓ	37. ⓐⓑⓒⓓ	38. ⓐⓑⓒⓓ	39. ⓐⓑⓒⓓ
40. ⓐⓑⓒⓓ	41. ⓐⓑⓒⓓ	42. ⓐⓑⓒⓓ	43. ⓐⓑⓒⓓ	44. ⓐⓑⓒⓓ
45. ⓐⓑⓒⓓ				

CHEMISTRY CHAPTERWISE SPEED TEST-49			
Total Questions	45	Total Marks	180
Attempted		Correct	
Incorrect		Net Score	
Cut-off Score	37	Qualifying Score	58
Success Gap = Net Score – Qualifying Score			
Net Score = (Correct × 4) – (Incorrect × 1)			

Space for Rough Work

CHEMISTRY

The d- and f-Block Elements

Speed TEST 50

Chapter-wise

No. of Questions	Maximum Marks	Time
45	180	1 Hour

GENERAL INSTRUCTIONS

- This test contains 45 MCQ's. For each question only one option is correct. Darken the correct circle/ bubble in the Response Grid provided on each page.
- You have to evaluate your Response Grids yourself with the help of solutions provided at the end of this book.
- Each correct answer will get you 4 marks and 1 mark shall be deduced for each incorrect answer. No mark will be given/ deducted if no bubble is filled. Keep a timer in front of you and stop immediately at the end of 60 min.
- The sheet follows a particular syllabus. Do not attempt the sheet before you have completed your preparation for that syllabus.
- After completing the sheet check your answers with the solution booklet and complete the Result Grid. Finally spend time to analyse your performance and revise the areas which emerge out as weak in your evaluation.

1. Which one of the elements with the following outer orbital configurations may exhibit the largest number of oxidation states?

(a) $3d^5 4s^1$ (b) $3d^5 4s^2$ (c) $3d^2 4s^2$ (d) $3d^3 4s^2$

2. The addition of excess of aqueous HNO_3 to a solution containing $[Cu(NH_3)_4]^{2+}$ produces

(a) Cu^+ (b) $[Cu(H_2O)_4]^{2+}$

(c) $Cu(OH)_2$ (d) $Cu(NO_3)_2$

3. The "spin-only" magnetic moment [in units of Bohr magneton, (μ_B)] of Ni^{2+} in aqueous solution would be (At. No. Ni = 28)

(a) 6 (b) 1.73 (c) 2.84 (d) 4.90

4. In the form of dichromate, Cr (VI) is a strong oxidising agent in acidic medium but Mo (VI) in MoO_3 and W (VI) in WO_3 are not because ____________ .

(i) Cr (VI) is more stable than Mo(VI) and W (VI).

(ii) Mo (VI) and W(VI) are more stable than Cr(VI).

(iii) Higher oxidation states of heavier members of group-6 of transition series are more stable.

(iv) Lower oxidation states of heavier members of group-6 of transition series are more stable.

(a) (i) and (ii) (b) (ii) and (iii)

(c) (i) and (iv) (d) (ii) and (iv)

5. Of the following outer electronic configurations of atoms, the highest oxidation state is achieved by which one of them ?

(a) $(n-1)d^3 ns^2$ (b) $(n-1)d^5 ns^1$

(c) $(n-1)d^8 ns^2$ (d) $(n-1)d^5 ns^2$

6. $(n-1)d^{10}ns^2$ is the general electronic configuration of

(a) Fe, Co, Ni (b) Cu, Ag, Au

(c) Zn, Cd, Hg (d) Se, Y, La

RESPONSE GRID	
	1. ⓐⓑⓒⓓ 2. ⓐⓑⓒⓓ 3. ⓐⓑⓒⓓ 4. ⓐⓑⓒⓓ 5. ⓐⓑⓒⓓ
	6. ⓐⓑⓒⓓ

Space for Rough Work

7. In the following salts the highest value of magnetic moment is observed in
(a) $MnSO_4.4H_2O$ (b) $CuSO_4.5H_2O$
(c) $FeSO_4.6H_2O$ (d) $ZnSO_4.7H_2O$

8. Which one of the following transition metal ions shows magnetic moment of 5.92 BM?
(a) Mn^{2+} (b) Ti^{3+} (c) Cr^{3+} (d) Cu^{2+}

9. Which of the following statements is incorrect?
(a) Zn,Cd and Hg due to presence of completely filled *d*-orbitals $[(n-1)d^{10}ns^2]$ are not studied along with other transition metals.
(b) Zn, Cd and Hg have low m.p and are comparitively softer than other transition metals.
(c) Metallic bond made by elements with d^5 configuration is stronger as compared to metalic bond made by elements with d^3 configuration.
(d) Metals of 5*d* series forms strong metallic bonds as compared with metals of 3*d* series.

10. Super conductors are derived from compounds of
(a) p-Block elements (b) lanthanides
(c) actinides (d) transition elements

11. Which of the following compounds has colour but no unpaired electrons?
(a) $KMnO_4$ (b) K_2MnO_4
(c) $MnSO_4$ (d) $MnCl_2$

12. What is the percentage of lanthanoid metal in mischmetall?
(a) 90% (b) 20% (c) 5% (d) 95%

13. Which of the following in its oxidation state shows the paramagnetism ?
(a) Tb(IV) (b) Lu(III) (c) Ce(IV) (d) La(III)

14. In neutral or faintly alkaline medium, thiosulphate is quantitatively oxidized by $KMnO_4$ to
(a) SO_3^{2-} (b) SO_4^{2-} (c) SO_2 (d) SO_5^{2-}

15. Wrought iron, pig iron and steel differ in properties due to
(a) carbon content (b) malleability
(c) conductivity (d) softness

16. The lanthanide contraction is responsible for the fact that
(a) Zr and Zn have the same oxidation state
(b) Zr and Hf have about the same radius
(c) Zr and Nb have similar oxidation state
(d) Zr and Y have about the same radius

17. $KMnO_4$ can be prepared from K_2MnO_4 as per the reaction:
$$3MnO_4^{2-} + 2H_2O \rightleftharpoons 2MnO_4^{2-} + MnO_2 + 4OH^-$$
The reaction can go to completion by removing OH^- ions by adding.
(a) KOH (b) CO_2 (c) SO_2 (d) HCl

18. On the basis of data given below,
$$E^\circ_{Sc^{3+}/Sc^{2+}} = -0.37\text{ V},\ E^\circ_{Mn^{3+}/Mn^{2+}} = +1.57\text{ V}$$
$$E^\circ_{Cr^{2+}/Cr} = -0.90\text{ V},\ E^\circ_{Cu^{2+}/Cu} = 0.34\text{ V}$$
Which of the following statements is incorrect?
(a) Sc^{3+} has good stability due of $[Ar]3d^04s^0$ configuration.
(b) Mn^{3+} is more stable than Mn^{2+}.
(c) Cr^{2+} is reducing in nature.
(d) Copper does not give H_2 on reaction with dil. H_2SO_4

19. Green vitriol is
(a) $FeSO_4.7H_2O$ (b) $ZnSO_4.7H_2O$
(c) $CaSO_4.2H_2O$ (d) $CuSO_4.5H_2O$

20. Number of moles of $K_2Cr_2O_7$ reduced by one mole of Sn^{2+} ions is
(a) $\frac{1}{3}$ (b) 3 (c) $\frac{1}{6}$ (d) 6

21. Four successive members of the first series of the transition metals are listed below. For which one of them the standard potential $\left(E^\circ_{M^{2+}/M}\right)$ value has a positive sign?
(a) Co (Z = 27) (b) Ni (Z = 28)
(c) Cu (Z = 29) (d) Fe (Z = 26)

RESPONSE GRID					
	7. ⓐⓑⓒⓓ	8. ⓐⓑⓒⓓ	9. ⓐⓑⓒⓓ	10. ⓐⓑⓒⓓ	11. ⓐⓑⓒⓓ
	12. ⓐⓑⓒⓓ	13. ⓐⓑⓒⓓ	14. ⓐⓑⓒⓓ	15. ⓐⓑⓒⓓ	16. ⓐⓑⓒⓓ
	17. ⓐⓑⓒⓓ	18. ⓐⓑⓒⓓ	19. ⓐⓑⓒⓓ	20. ⓐⓑⓒⓓ	21. ⓐⓑⓒⓓ

Space for Rough Work

22. Which of the following factors may be regarded as the main cause of lanthanoide contraction?
(a) Greater shielding of 5*d* electrons by 4*f* electrons
(b) Poorer shielding of 5*d* electrons by 4*f* electrons.
(c) Effective shielding of one of 4*f* electrons by another in the subshell
(d) Poor shielding of one of 4*f* electron by another in the subshell

23. AgCl is soluble in NH_4OH solution. The solubility is due to the formation of
(a) AgOH (b) Ag_2O
(c) $\left[Ag(NH_3)_2\right]^+$ (d) NH_4Cl

24. Oxidation states of the metal in the minerals haematite and magnetite, respectively, are
(a) II, III in haematite and III in magnetite
(b) II, III in haematite and II in magnetite
(c) II in haematite and II, III in magnetite
(d) III in haematite and II, III in magnetite

25. In acidic medium $KMnO_4$ oxidises $FeSO_4$ solution. Which of the following statements is correct?
(a) 10 mL of 1N $KMnO_4$ solution oxidises 10 mL of 5 N $FeSO_4$ solution
(b) 10 mL of 1M $KMnO_4$ solution oxidises 10 mL of 5 N $FeSO_4$ solution
(c) 10 mL of 1M $KMnO_4$ solution oxidises 10 mL of 1M $FeSO_4$ solution
(d) 10 mL of 1N $KMnO_4$ solution oxidises 10 mL of 0.1M $FeSO_4$ solution

26. In which of the following lanthanides oxidation state +2 is most stable?
(a) Ce (b) Eu (c) Tb (d) Dy

27. Acidified solution of chromic acid on treatment with H_2O_2 gives blue colour which is due to
(a) $CrO_3 + H_2O + O_2$ (b) $CrO_5 + H_2O$
(c) $H_2Cr_2O_7 + H_2O + O_2$ (d) None of these

28. Which of the following is used in the preparation of chlorine?
(a) Only MnO_2
(b) Only $KMnO_4$
(c) Both MnO_2 and $KMnO_4$
(d) Either MnO_2 or $KMnO_4$

29. An explosion take place when conc. H_2SO_4 is added to $KMnO_4$. Which of the following is formed?
(a) Mn_2O_7 (b) MnO_2
(c) $MnSO_4$ (d) M_2O_3

30. Which of the following statements are correct ?
(i) Chromium has the highest melting point among the series 1 metals.
(ii) Number of unpaired electrons is greater in Cr than other elements of series 1.
(iii) In any row the melting point of transition metal increases as the atomic number increases.
(a) (i) and (iii) (b) (i) and (ii)
(c) (ii) and (iii) (d) (i), (ii) and (iii)

31. In the laboratory, manganese (II) salt is oxidised to permanganate ion in aqueous solution by
(a) hydrogen peroxide (b) conc. nitric acid
(c) peroxodisulphate (d) dichromate

32. Which of the following statements about the interstitial compounds is incorrect ?
(a) They are chemically reactive.
(b) They are much harder then the pure metal.
(c) They have higher melting points than the pure metal.
(d) They retain metallic conductivity.

33. Which of the following elements shows maximum number of different oxidation states in its compounds?
(a) Eu (b) Ld (c) Gd (d) Am

34. Identify the product and its colour when MnO_2 is fused with solid KOH in the presence of O_2.
(a) $KMnO_4$, purple (b) K_2MnO_4, dark green
(c) MnO, colourless (d) Mn_2O_3, brown

RESPONSE GRID					
	22. ⓐⓑⓒⓓ	23. ⓐⓑⓒⓓ	24. ⓐⓑⓒⓓ	25. ⓐⓑⓒⓓ	26. ⓐⓑⓒⓓ
	27. ⓐⓑⓒⓓ	28. ⓐⓑⓒⓓ	29. ⓐⓑⓒⓓ	30. ⓐⓑⓒⓓ	31. ⓐⓑⓒⓓ
	32. ⓐⓑⓒⓓ	33. ⓐⓑⓒⓓ	34. ⓐⓑⓒⓓ		

Space for Rough Work

35. In the extraction of silver from argentite ore. The ore is treated with dil. solution of NaCN in water in the presence of Y, whereby the following reaction takes place :
$Ag_2X + 4NaCN + 2Y \rightarrow 2Na[Ag(CN)_2] + Na_2XO_4 \cdot X$ and Y in this reaction are respectively :
(a) Sb and S (b) S and O_2
(c) O and O_2 (d) O and S

36. Which of the following compound is called Turnbull's blue?
(a) Ferricyanide (b) Ferrous ferricyanide
(c) Ferrous cyanide (d) Ferri-ferrocyanide

37. Which of the following element is responsible for oxidation of water to O_2 in biological process?
(a) Fe (b) Mn (c) Cu (d) Mo

38. Consider the following statements
(i) $La(OH)_3$ is the least basic among hydroxides of lanthanides.
(ii) Zr^{4+} and Hf^{4+} posses almost the same ionic radii.
(iii) Ce^{4+} can act as an oxidizing agent.
Which of the above is/are true ?
(a) (i) and (iii) (b) (ii) and (iii)
(c) (ii) only (d) (i) and (ii)

39. For making Ag from $AgNO_3$, which of the following is used
(a) PH_3 (b) phosphonium iodide
(c) Na_2CO_3 (d) NH_3

40. Which of the following conversions can be carried out by both acidified $K_2Cr_2O_4$ and acidified $KMnO_4$?
(i) $Fe^{2+} \rightarrow Fe^{3+} + e^-$
(ii) $I^- \rightarrow IO_3^-$
(iii) $I^- \rightarrow I_2$ (iv) $H_2S \rightarrow S$
(a) (i) and (iii) (b) (ii) and (iv)
(c) (i), (iii) and (iv) (d) (i), (ii) and (iii)

41. The catalytic activity of transition metals and their compounds is mainly due to :
(a) their magnetic behaviour
(b) their unfilled *d*-orbitals
(c) their ability to adopt variable oxidation state
(d) their chemical reactivity

42. Match the columns

	Column-I		Column-II
A.	Metal of the 3*d*-series which does not form MO type oxide.	I.	Manganese
B.	Metal of the 3*d*-series which forms most covalent oxide.	II.	Vanadium
C.	Metal of the 3*d*-series which forms the amphoteric oxide.	III.	Scandium

(a) A – I; B – III; C – II (b) A – III; B – I; C – II
(c) A – III; B – II; C – I (d) A – II; B – I; C – III

43. The basic character of the transition metal monoxides follows the order
(Atomic Nos., Ti = 22, V = 23, Cr = 24, Fe = 26)
(a) TiO > VO > CrO > FeO (b) VO > CrO > TiO > FeO
(c) CrO > VO > FeO > TiO (d) TiO > FeO > VO > CrO

44. Excited state configuration of Mn^{2+} is
(a) t_{2g}^4 (b) $t_{2g}^3e_g^2$ (d) $t_{2g}^4e_g^2$ (d) $t_{2g}^5e_g^0$

45. What would happen when a solution of potassium chromate is treated with an excess of dilute nitric acid?
(a) $Cr_2O_7^{2-}$ and H_2O are formed
(b) CrO_4^{2-} is reduced to +3 state of Cr
(c) CrO_4^{2-} is oxidized to +7 state of Cr
(d) Cr^{3+} and $Cr_2O_7^{2-}$ are formed

RESPONSE GRID					
	35. ⓐⓑⓒⓓ	36. ⓐⓑⓒⓓ	37. ⓐⓑⓒⓓ	38. ⓐⓑⓒⓓ	39. ⓐⓑⓒⓓ
	40. ⓐⓑⓒⓓ	41. ⓐⓑⓒⓓ	42. ⓐⓑⓒⓓ	43. ⓐⓑⓒⓓ	44. ⓐⓑⓒⓓ
	45. ⓐⓑⓒⓓ				

CHEMISTRY CHAPTERWISE SPEED TEST-50

Total Questions	45	Total Marks	180
Attempted		Correct	
Incorrect		Net Score	
Cut-off Score	42	Qualifying Score	65
Success Gap = Net Score – Qualifying Score			
Net Score = (Correct × 4) – (Incorrect × 1)			

Space for Rough Work

CHEMISTRY

Coordination Compounds

Speed TEST 51

Chapter-wise

No. of Questions	Maximum Marks	Time
45	180	1 Hour

GENERAL INSTRUCTIONS

- This test contains 45 MCQ's. For each question only one option is correct. Darken the correct circle/ bubble in the Response Grid provided on each page.
- You have to evaluate your Response Grids yourself with the help of solutions provided at the end of this book.
- Each correct answer will get you 4 marks and 1 mark shall be deduced for each incorrect answer. No mark will be given/ deducted if no bubble is filled. Keep a timer in front of you and stop immediately at the end of 60 min.
- The sheet follows a particular syllabus. Do not attempt the sheet before you have completed your preparation for that syllabus.
- After completing the sheet check your answers with the solution booklet and complete the Result Grid. Finally spend time to analyse your performance and revise the areas which emerge out as weak in your evaluation.

1. The compounds $[PtCl_2(NH_3)_4]Br_2$ and $[PtBr_2(NH_3)_4]Cl_2$ constitutes a pair of
   (a) coordination isomers (b) linkage isomers
   (c) ionization isomers (d) optical isomers
2. Which of the following species is not expected to be a ligand?
   (a) NO (b) NH_4^+
   (c) $NH_2CH_2CH_2NH_2$ (d) Both (a) and (b)
3. In which of the following complexes of the Co (At. no. 27), will the magnitude of Δ_o be the hightest?
   (a) $[Co(CN)_6]^{3-}$ (b) $[Co(C_2O_4)_3]^{3-}$
   (c) $[Co(H_2O)_6]^{3+}$ (d) $[Co(NH_3)_6]^{3+}$
4. Which of the following carbonyls will have the strongest C – O bond ?
   (a) $Mn(CO)_6^+$ (b) $Cr(CO)_6$
   (c) $V(CO)_6^-$ (d) $Fe(CO)_5$
5. A square planar complex is formed by hybridisation of which atomic orbitals?
   (a) s, p_x, p_y, d_{yz} (b) $s, p_x, p_y, d_{x^2-y^2}$
   (c) s, p_x, p_y, d_{z^2} (d) s, p_y, p_z, d_{xy}
6. The type of isomerism present in Pentamminenitrochromium (III) chloride is
   (a) optical (b) linkage
   (c) ionisation (d) polymerisation.
7. In the silver plating of copper, $K[Ag(CN)_2]$ is used instead of $AgNO_3$. The reason is
   (a) a thin layer of Ag is formed on Cu
   (b) more voltage is required
   (c) Ag^+ ions are completely removed from solution
   (d) less availability of Ag^+ ions, as Cu cannot displace Ag from $[Ag(CN)_2]^-$ ion.
8. The spin only magnetic moment value (in Bohr magneton units) of $Cr(CO)_6$ is
   (a) 0 (b) 2.84 (c) 4.90 (d) 5.92
9. Low spin complex of d^6-cation in an octahedral field will have the following energy :
   (a) $\frac{-12}{5}\Delta_0 + P$ (b) $\frac{-12}{5}\Delta_0 + 3P$
   (c) $\frac{-2}{5}\Delta_0 + 2P$ (d) $\frac{-2}{5}\Delta_0 + P$
   (Δ_0 = Crystal Field Splitting Energy in an octahedral field, P = Electron pairing energy)

RESPONSE GRID	
1. ⓐⓑⓒⓓ 2. ⓐⓑⓒⓓ 3. ⓐⓑⓒⓓ 4. ⓐⓑⓒⓓ 5. ⓐⓑⓒⓓ	
6. ⓐⓑⓒⓓ 7. ⓐⓑⓒⓓ 8. ⓐⓑⓒⓓ 9. ⓐⓑⓒⓓ	

Space for Rough Work

10. An example of double salt is
(a) Bleaching powder (b) $K_4[Fe(CN)_6]$
(c) Hypo (d) Potash alum

11. The ionisation isomer of $[Cr(H_2O)_4Cl(NO_2)]Cl$ is
(a) $[Cr(H_2O)_4(O_2N)]Cl_2$
(b) $[Cr(H_2O)_4Cl_2](NO_2)$
(c) $[Cr(H_2O)_4Cl(ONO)]Cl$
(d) $[Cr(H_2O)_4Cl_2(NO_2)].H_2O$

12. $[Co(NH_3)_4(NO_2)_2]Cl$ exhibits
(a) linkage isomerism, ionization isomerism and geometrical isomerism
(b) ionization isomerism, geometrical isomerism and optical isomerism
(c) linkage isomerism, geometrical isomerism and optical isomerism
(d) linkage isomerism, ionization isomerism and optical isomerism

13. The IUPAC name of $K_3[Ir(C_2O_4)_3]$ is
(a) potassium trioxalatoiridium (III)
(b) potassium trioxalatoiridate (III)
(c) potassium tris (oxalato) iridium (III)
(d) potassium tris (oxalato) iridate (III)

14. Consider the following complex $[Co(NH_3)_5CO_3]ClO_4$. The coordination number, oxidation number, number of *d*-electrons and number of unpaired *d*-electrons on the metal are respectively
(a) 6, 3, 6, 0 (b) 7, 2, 7, 1 (c) 7, 1, 6, 4 (d) 6, 2, 7, 3

15. Which of the following species represent the example of dsp^2 - hybridisation ?
(a) $[Fe(CN)_6]^{3-}$ (b) $[Ni(CN)_4]^{2-}$
(c) $[Ag(CN)_2]^-$ (d) $[Co(CN)_6]^{3-}$

16. When $AgNO_3$ is added to a solution of $Co(NH_3)_5Cl_3$, the precipitate of AgCl shows two ionisable chloride ions. This means :
(a) Two chlorine atoms satisfy primary valency and one secondary valency
(b) One chlorine atom satisfies primary as well as secondary valency
(c) Three chlorine atoms satisfy primary valency
(d) Three chlorine atoms satisfy secondary valency

17. The value of the 'spin only' magnetic moment for one of the following configurations is 2.82 B.M. The correct one is
(a) d^5 (in strong ligand field)
(b) d^3 (in weak as well as in strong fields)
(c) d^4 (in weak ligand fields)
(d) d^4 (in strong ligand fields)

18. Consider the following complex ions, P, Q and R.
$P = [FeF_6]^{3-}$, $Q = [V(H_2O)_6]^{2+}$ and $R = [Fe(H_2O)_6]^{2+}$
The correct order of the complex ions, according to their spin-only magnetic moment values (in B.M.) is
(a) $R < Q < P$ (b) $Q < R < P$
(c) $R < P < Q$ (d) $Q < P < R$

19. Which of the following is organo-metallic compound ?
(a) $Ti(C_2H_4)_4$ (b) $Ti(OC_2H_5)_4$
(c) $Ti(OCOCH_3)_4$ (d) $Ti(OC_6H_5)_4$

20. Which of the following statements is correct ? (Atomic number of Ni = 28)
(a) $Ni(CO)_4$ is diamagnetic and $[NiCl_4]^{2-}$ and $[Ni(CN)_4]^{2-}$ are paramagnetic
(b) $Ni(CO)_4$ and $[Ni(CN)_4]^{2-}$ are diamagnetic and $[NiCl_4]^{2-}$ is paramagnetic
(c) $Ni(CO)_4$ and $[NiCl_4]^{2-}$ are diamagnetic and $[Ni(CN)_4]^{2-}$ is paramagnetic
(d) $[NiCl_4]^{2-}$ and $[Ni(CN)_4]^{2-}$ are diamagnetic and $Ni(CO)_4$ is paramagnetic

21. The correct order for the wavelength of absorption in the visible region is :
(a) $[Ni(NO_2)_6]^{4-} < [Ni(NH_3)_6]^{2+} < [Ni(H_2O)_6]^{2+}$
(b) $[Ni(NO_2)_6]^{4-} < [Ni(H_2O)_6]^{2+} < [Ni(NH_3)_6]^{2+}$
(c) $[Ni(H_2O)_6]^{2+} < [Ni(NH_3)_6]^{2+} < [Ni(NO_2)_6]^{4-}$
(d) $[Ni(NH_3)_6]^{2+} < [Ni(H_2O)_6]^{2+} < [Ni(NO_2)_6]^{4-}$

22. The compound which is not coloured is
(a) $K_4Fe(CN)_6$ (b) $K_3Fe(CN)_6$
(c) Na_2CdCl_4 (d) Na_2CuCl_4

RESPONSE GRID					
	10. ⓐⓑⓒⓓ	11. ⓐⓑⓒⓓ	12. ⓐⓑⓒⓓ	13. ⓐⓑⓒⓓ	14. ⓐⓑⓒⓓ
	15. ⓐⓑⓒⓓ	16. ⓐⓑⓒⓓ	17. ⓐⓑⓒⓓ	18. ⓐⓑⓒⓓ	19. ⓐⓑⓒⓓ
	20. ⓐⓑⓒⓓ	21. ⓐⓑⓒⓓ	22. ⓐⓑⓒⓓ		

Space for Rough Work

23. Which is not π - bonded complex ?
(a) Zeise's salt (b) Ferrocene
(c) Dibenzene chromiun (d) Tetraethyl lead

24. Which of the following are inner orbital complex (i.e., involving d^2sp^3 hybridisation) and is paramagnetic in nature?
(a) $[Mn(CN)_6]^{3-}$, $[Fe(CN)_6]^{3-}$, $[Co(C_2O_4)_3]^{3-}$
(b) $[MnCl_6]^{3-}$, $[FeF_6]^{3-}$, $[CoF_6]^{3-}$
(c) $[Mn(CN)_6]^{3-}$, $[Fe(CN)_6]^{3-}$
(d) $[MnCl_6]^{3-}$, $[Fe(CN)_6]^{3-}$, $[Co(C_2O_4)_3]^{3-}$

25. Give name of the complex, name should specify the position of ligands.

H_3P .... CO
Ir
Cl .... PH_3

(a) bistransphosphinecarbonylchloroiridium (II)
(b) carbonylchlorobistransphosphineiridium (III)
(c) carbonylchlorobistransphosphineiridium (I)
(d) chlorocarbonylbistransphosphineiridium (I)

26. Which of the following coordination compounds would exhibit optical isomerism?
(a) pentamminenitrocobalt(III) iodide
(b) diamminedichloroplatinum(II)
(c) trans-dicyanobis (ethylenediamine) chromium (III) chloride
(d) tris-(ethylendiamine) cobalt (III) bromide

27. An excess of $AgNO_3$ is added to 100 mL of a 0.01 M solution of dichlorotetraaquachromium (iii) chloride. The number of moles of AgCl precipitated would be :
(a) 0.002 (b) 0.003 (c) 0.01 (d) 0.001

28. The most stable complex among the following is
(a) $K_3[Al(C_2O_4)_3]$ (b) $[Pt(en)_2]Cl$
(c) $[Ag(NH_3)_2]Cl$ (d) $K_2[Ni(EDTA)]$

29. Which one of the following has largest number of isomers ?
(a) $[Ir(PR_3)_2H(CO)]^{2+}$ (b) $[Co(NH_3)_5Cl]^{2+}$
(c) $[Ru(NH_3)_4Cl_2]^+$ (d) $[Co(en)_2Cl_2]^+$
(R = alkyl group, en = ethylenediamine)

30. Which of the following statements related to crystal field splitting in octahedral coordination entities is incorrect?
(a) The $d_{x^2-y^2}$ and d_{z^2} orbitals has more energy as compared to d_{xy}, d_{yz} and d_{xz} orbitals.
(b) Crystal field spitting energy (Δ_o) depends directly on the charge of the metal ion and on the field produced by the ligand.
(c) In the presence of Br^- as a ligand the distribution of electrons for d^4 configuration will be t_{2g}^3, e_g^1,
(d) In the presence of CN^- as a ligand $\Delta_o < P$.

31. Calculate the value of log K_3 when log values of K_2, K_1, K_4 and β_4 respectively are 2.0, 3.20, 4.0 and 11.9 ?
(a) 2.0 (b) 2.7 (c) 3.0 (d) 2.5

32. Which of the following does **not** have a metal- carbon bond?
(a) $Al(OC_2H_5)_3$ (b) C_2H_5MgBr
(c) $K[Pt(C_2H_4)Cl_3]$ (d) $Ni(CO)_4$

33. In $Fe(CO)_5$, the Fe – C bond possesses
(a) ionic character (b) σ-character only
(c) π-character (d) both σ and π characters

34. The geometry of $Ni(CO)_4$ and $Ni(PPh_3)_2Cl_2$ are
(a) both square planar
(b) tetrahedral and square planar
(c) both tetrahedral
(d) None of these

35. The crystal field splitting energy for octahedral (Δ_0) and tetrahedral (Δ_t) complexes is related as
(a) $\Delta_t = -\frac{1}{2}\Delta_0$ (b) $\Delta_t = -\frac{4}{9}\Delta_0$
(c) $\Delta_t = -\frac{3}{5}\Delta_0$ (d) $\Delta_t = -\frac{2}{5}\Delta_0$

RESPONSE GRID					
	23. ⓐⓑⓒⓓ	24. ⓐⓑⓒⓓ	25. ⓐⓑⓒⓓ	26. ⓐⓑⓒⓓ	27. ⓐⓑⓒⓓ
	28. ⓐⓑⓒⓓ	29. ⓐⓑⓒⓓ	30. ⓐⓑⓒⓓ	31. ⓐⓑⓒⓓ	32. ⓐⓑⓒⓓ
	33. ⓐⓑⓒⓓ	34. ⓐⓑⓒⓓ	35. ⓐⓑⓒⓓ		

Space for Rough Work

36. Match the columns.

	Column-I		Column-II
A.	$[Ni(CN)_4]^{2-}$	I.	Ti^{4+}
B.	Chlorophyll	II.	sp^3; paramagnetic
C.	Ziegler - Natta catalyst	III.	Non-planar
D.	$[NiCl_4]^{2-}$	IV.	Mg^{2+}
E.	Deoxyhaemoglobin	V.	Planar
		(VI)	dsp^2; diamagnetic

(a) A – VI; B – IV; C – I; D – II; E – III
(b) A – II; B – IV; C – I; D – VI; E – III
(c) A – II; B – IV; C – I; D – VI; E – V
(d) A – VI; B – IV; C – I; D – II; E – V

37. If magnetic moment of $[MnBr_4]^{2-}$ is 5.9 BM. Predict the number of electrons?
(a) 2 (b) 3 (c) 6 (d) 5

38. The correct structure of ethylenediaminetetraacetic acid (EDTA) is

(a) $(HOOC-H_2C)_2N-CH=CH-N(CH_2-COOH)_2$

(b) $(HOOC)_2N-CH_2-CH_2-N(COOH)_2$

(c) $(HOOC-H_2C)_2N-CH_2-CH_2-N(CH_2-COOH)_2$

(d) $HOOC-H_2C(H)N-CH(CH_2COOH)-CH(CH_2COOH)-N(H)CH_2-COOH$

39. The hypothetical complex chloro-diaquatriamminecobalt (III) chloride can be represented as
(a) $[CoCl(NH_3)_3(H_2O)_2]Cl_2$
(b) $[Co(NH_3)_3(H_2O)Cl_3]$
(c) $[Co(NH_3)_3(H_2O)_2Cl]$
(d) $[Co(NH_3)_3(H_2O)_3]Cl_3$

40. Which of the following is incorrect regarding spectrochemical series?
(a) $NH_3 > H_2O$ (b) $F^- > C_2O_4^{2-}$
(c) $NCS^- > SCN^-$ (d) $en > EDTA^{4-}$

41. Which of the following is the limitation of crystal field theory?
(i) Ligands are assumed as point charges.
(ii) It does not accounts for the covalent character of bonding between the ligand and the central atom.
(iii) It does not explain how colour of coordination compounds depends on ligand attached to central metal atom/ion.
(a) (i) and (ii) (b) (ii) and (iii)
(c) (ii) only (d) (i), (ii) and (iii)

42. For $[Co_2(CO)_8]$, what is the total number of metal – carbon bonds and number of metal–metal bonds.
(a) 10, 1 (b) 8, 2 (c) 8, 1 (d) 10, 0

43. Which will give a white precipitate with $AgNO_3$ in aqueous solution
(a) $[Co(NH_3)_5Cl](NO_2)_2$ (b) $[Pt(NH_3)_6]Cl_4$
(c) $[Pt(en)Cl_2]$ (d) $[Cu(NH_3)_4]SO_4$

44. $[NiCl_2\{P(C_2H_5)_2(C_6H_5)\}_2]$ exhibits temperature dependent magnetic behaviour (paramagnetic/diamagnetic). The coordination geometries of Ni^{2+} in the paramagnetic and diamagnetic states are respectively
(a) tetrahedral and tetrahedral
(b) square planar and square planar
(c) tetrahedral and square planar
(d) square planar and tetrahedral

45. Which one of the following coordination compounds is used to inhibit the growth of tumours?
(a) Trans-platin (b) EDTA complex of calcium
(c) $[(Ph_3P)_3RhCl]$ (d) Cis-platin

RESPONSE GRID					
	36. ⓐⓑⓒⓓ	37. ⓐⓑⓒⓓ	38. ⓐⓑⓒⓓ	39. ⓐⓑⓒⓓ	40. ⓐⓑⓒⓓ
	41. ⓐⓑⓒⓓ	42. ⓐⓑⓒⓓ	43. ⓐⓑⓒⓓ	44. ⓐⓑⓒⓓ	45. ⓐⓑⓒⓓ

CHEMISTRY CHAPTERWISE SPEED TEST-51

Total Questions	45	Total Marks	180
Attempted		Correct	
Incorrect		Net Score	
Cut-off Score	39	Qualifying Score	64
Success Gap = Net Score – Qualifying Score			
Net Score = (Correct × 4) – (Incorrect × 1)			

Space for Rough Work

CHEMISTRY

Haloalkanes and Haloarenes

Speed TEST 52

Chapter-wise

No. of Questions	Maximum Marks	Time
45	180	1 Hour

GENERAL INSTRUCTIONS

- This test contains 45 MCQ's. For each question only one option is correct. Darken the correct circle/ bubble in the Response Grid provided on each page.
- You have to evaluate your Response Grids yourself with the help of solutions provided at the end of this book.
- Each correct answer will get you 4 marks and 1 mark shall be deduced for each incorrect answer. No mark will be given/ deducted if no bubble is filled. Keep a timer in front of you and stop immediately at the end of 60 min.
- The sheet follows a particular syllabus. Do not attempt the sheet before you have completed your preparation for that syllabus.
- After completing the sheet check your answers with the solution booklet and complete the Result Grid. Finally spend time to analyse your performance and revise the areas which emerge out as weak in your evaluation.

1. *o*-Methoxybromobenzene is treated with sodamide and then with ammonia. The product formed is
   (a) *o*-Methoxyaniline (b) Aniline
   (c) Methoxybenzene (d) *m*-Methoxyaniline
2. Gem-dibromide is
   (a) $CH_3CH(Br)CH_2(Br)$ (b) $CH_3CBr_2CH_3$
   (c) $CH_2(Br)CH_2CH_2$ (d) CH_2BrCH_2Br
3. Arrange the following compounds in order of increasing dipole moment :
   Toluene (I)
   m-dichlorobenzene (II)
   o-dichlorobenzene (III)
   p-dichlorobenzene (IV)
   (a) I < IV < II < III (b) IV < I < II < III
   (c) IV < I < III < II (d) IV < II < I < III
4. The compound formed on heating chlorobenzene with chloral in the presence of concentrated sulphuric acid, is
   (a) freon (b) DDT
   (c) gammexene (d) hexachloroethane
5. Which among MeX, RCH_2X, R_2CHX and R_3CX is most reactive towards S_N2 reaction?
   (a) MeX (b) RCH_2X
   (c) R_2CHX (d) R_3CX
6. In the preparation of chlorobenzene from aniline, the most suitable reagent is
   (a) Chlorine in the presence of ultraviolet light
   (b) Chlorine in the presence of $AlCl_3$
   (c) Nitrous acid followed by heating with Cu_2Cl_2
   (d) HCl and Cu_2Cl_2
7. On sulphonation of C_6H_5Cl
   (a) *m*-Chlorobenzenesulphonic acid is formed
   (b) Benzenesulphonic acid is formed
   (c) *o*-Chlorobenzenesulphonic acid is formed
   (d) *o*- and *p*-Chlorobenzenesulphonic acid is formed
8. Compound (A), C_8H_9Br, gives a white precipitate when warmed with alcoholic $AgNO_3$. Oxidation of (A) gives an acid (B), $C_8H_6O_4$. (B) easily forms anhydride on heating. Identify the compound (A).
   (a) 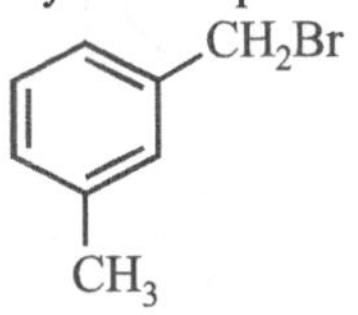 [benzene ring with CH_2Br and CH_3 meta] (b) 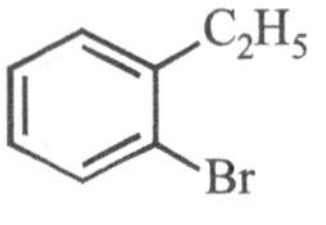 [benzene ring with C_2H_5 and Br ortho]
   (c) [benzene ring with CH_2Br and CH_3 para] (d) 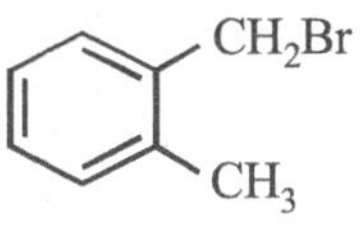 [benzene ring with CH_2Br and CH_3 ortho]

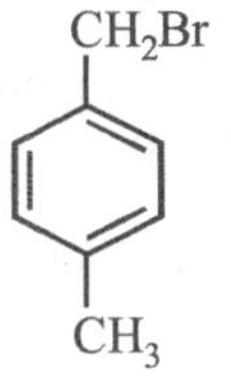

RESPONSE GRID	
1. ⓐⓑⓒⓓ 2. ⓐⓑⓒⓓ 3. ⓐⓑⓒⓓ 4. ⓐⓑⓒⓓ 5. ⓐⓑⓒⓓ	
6. ⓐⓑⓒⓓ 7. ⓐⓑⓒⓓ 8. ⓐⓑⓒⓓ	

Space for Rough Work

9. The reaction of $C_6H_5N_2^+Cl^-$ with CuCl gives
(a) C_6H_5Cl (b) C_6H_6
(c) $C_6H_5-C_6H_5$ (d) $C_6H_4Cl_2$

10. Conant Finkelstein reaction for the preparation of alkyl iodide is based upon the fact that
(a) Sodium iodide is soluble in methanol, while sodium chloride is insoluble in methanol
(b) Sodium iodide is soluble in methanol, while NaCl and NaBr are insoluble in methanol
(c) Sodium iodide is insoluble in methanol, while NaCl and NaBr are soluble
(d) The three halogens differ considerably in their electronegativity

11. Tertiary alkyl halides are practically inert to substitution by S_N2 mechanism because of
(a) steric hindrance (b) inductive effect
(c) instability (d) insolubility

12. Which one is most reactive towards S_N1 reaction ?
(a) $C_6H_5CH(C_6H_5)Br$ (b) $C_6H_5CH(CH_3)Br$
(c) $C_6H_5C(CH_3)(C_6H_5)Br$ (d) $C_6H_5CH_2Br$

13. The major product of the following reaction is :

$$CH_3\underset{\displaystyle Br}{\underset{|}{C}}HCH_2\underset{\displaystyle Br}{\underset{|}{C}}HCH_2CH_3 \xrightarrow[\text{heat}]{KOH, CH_3OH}$$

(a) $CH_2=CHCH_2CH=CHCH_3$
(b) $CH_2=CHCH=CHCH_2CH_3$
(c) $CH_3CH=C=CHCH_2CH_3$
(d) $CH_3CH=CH-CH=CHCH_3$

14. Which of the following is an example of S_N2 reaction?
(a) $CH_3Br + OH^- \longrightarrow CH_3OH + Br^-$
(b) $CH_3-\underset{\displaystyle Br}{\underset{|}{CH}}-CH_3 + OH^- \longrightarrow CH_3-\underset{\displaystyle OH}{\underset{|}{CH}}-CH_3$
(c) $CH_3CH_2OH \xrightarrow{-H_2O} CH_2=CH_2$
(d) $(CH_3)_3C-Br + OH^- \longrightarrow (CH_3)_3COH + Br^-$

15. What would be the product formed when 1–bromo–3–chlorocyclobutane reacts with two equivalents of metallic sodium in ether?

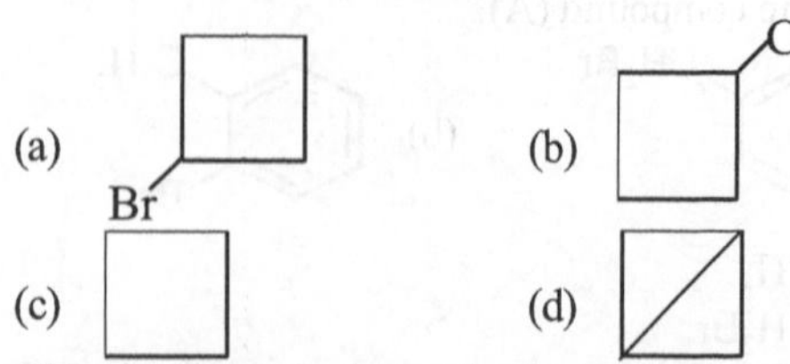

16. Chlorination of toluene in the presence of light and heat followed by treatment with aqueous NaOH gives
(a) *o*-Cresol (b) *p*-Cresol
(c) 2,4-Dihydroxytoluene (d) Benzoic acid

17. The starting substance for the preparation of iodoform is any one of the following, except
(a) $CH_3CH(OH)CH_3$ (b) CH_3CH_2OH
(c) HCH_2OH (d) CH_3COCH_3

18. The following reaction proceeds through the intermediate

$$RCOOAg + Br_2 \longrightarrow RBr + CO_2 + AgBr$$

(a) $RCOO^\bullet$ (b) $R^\bullet$ (c) $Br^\bullet$ (d) All

19. The major product of the following reaction is :

$$C_6H_5CH_2-\underset{\displaystyle Br}{\underset{|}{\overset{\displaystyle CH_3}{\overset{|}{C}}}}-CH_2-CH_3 \xrightarrow[C_2H_5OH]{C_2H_5ONa}$$

(a) $C_6H_5CH_2-\underset{\displaystyle OC_2H_5}{\underset{|}{\overset{\displaystyle CH_3}{\overset{|}{C}}}}-CH_2-CH_3$

(b) $C_6H_5CH=\underset{\displaystyle CH_3}{\underset{|}{C}}-CH_2-CH_3$

(c) $C_6H_5CH_2-\underset{\displaystyle CH_3}{\underset{|}{C}}=CHCH_3$

(d) $C_6H_5CH_2-\underset{\displaystyle CH_2CH_3}{\underset{|}{C}}=CH_2$

20. The reaction :

$$C_2H_5OH + SOCl_2 \xrightarrow{\text{Pyridine}} C_2H_5Cl + SO_2 + HCl$$

is known as
(a) Kharasch effect (b) Williamson's synthesis
(c) Darzen's procedure (d) Hunsdiecker reaction

21. If chloroform is left open in air in the presence of sunlight, it gives
(a) carbon tetrachloride (b) carbonyl chloride
(c) mustard gas (d) lewisite

22. In the following reaction sequence :

$$\underset{(C_3H_6Cl_2)}{I} \xrightarrow{KOH(aq)} II \xrightarrow[\text{(ii) } H_2O/H^+]{\text{(i) } CH_3MgBr} III \xrightarrow{\text{Anhy.}ZnCl_2 + \text{Conc.}HCl} \text{given turbidity immediately}$$

The compound I is :
(a) $\underset{\displaystyle Cl}{\underset{|}{CH_2}}-\underset{\displaystyle Cl}{\underset{|}{CH}}-CH_3$ (b) $CH_2-\underset{\displaystyle Cl}{\underset{|}{CH_2}}-\underset{\displaystyle Cl}{\underset{|}{CH_3}}$

(c) $CH-\underset{\displaystyle Cl}{\underset{|}{CH}}-CH_2-CH_3$ (d) $CH_3-\underset{\displaystyle Cl}{\underset{|}{\overset{\displaystyle Cl}{\overset{|}{C}}}}-CH_3$

RESPONSE GRID					
	9. ⓐⓑⓒⓓ	10. ⓐⓑⓒⓓ	11. ⓐⓑⓒⓓ	12. ⓐⓑⓒⓓ	13. ⓐⓑⓒⓓ
	14. ⓐⓑⓒⓓ	15. ⓐⓑⓒⓓ	16. ⓐⓑⓒⓓ	17. ⓐⓑⓒⓓ	18. ⓐⓑⓒⓓ
	19. ⓐⓑⓒⓓ	20. ⓐⓑⓒⓓ	21. ⓐⓑⓒⓓ	22. ⓐⓑⓒⓓ	

Space for Rough Work

23. Mg reacts with RBr best in
(a) $C_2H_5OC_2H_5$ (b) $C_6H_5OCH_3$
(c) $C_6H_5N(CH_3)_2$ (d) Equally in all the three

24. Which chloride is least reactive with the hydrolysis point of view?
(a) CH_3Cl (b) CH_3CH_2Cl
(c) $(CH_3)_3CCl$ (d) $CH_2=CH-Cl$

25. $CH_3-CH_2-\underset{\displaystyle Cl}{\underset{|}{CH}}-CH_3$ obtained by chlorination of n-butane, will be
(a) *l*-form (b) *d*-form
(c) Meso form (d) Racemic mixture

26. The reaction of toluene with Cl_2 in presence of $FeCl_3$ gives 'X' and reaction in presence of light gives 'Y'. Thus, 'X' and 'Y' are:
(a) X = Benzal chloride, Y = *o* – Chlorotoluene
(b) X = *m* – Chlorotoluene, Y = *p* –Chlorotoluene
(c) X = o –and *p* – Chlorotoluene, Y = Trichloromethylbenzene
(d) X = Benzyl chloride, Y = *m* – Chlorotoluene

27. Which reagent cannot be used to prepare an alkyl halide from an alcohol ?
(a) $HCl + ZnCl_2$ (b) NaCl (c) PCl_5 (d) $SOCl_2$

28. A is an optically inactive alkyl chloride which on reaction with aqueous KOH gives B. B on heating with Cu at 300°C gives on alkene C, what are A and C
(a) $CH_3CH_2Cl,\ CH_2=CH_2$
(b) Me_3CCl, MeCH=CH.Me
(c) $Me_3CCl,\ Me_2C=CH_2$
(d) $Me_2CH.CH_2Cl,\ Me_2C=CH_2$

29. $CH_3Br + Nu^- \longrightarrow CH_3-Nu + Br^-$ The decreasing order of the rate of the above reaction with nucleophiles (Nu^-) A to D is
[Nu^- = (A) PhO^-, (B) AcO^-, (C) HO^-, (D) CH_3O^-]
(a) A > B > C > D (b) B > D > C > A
(c) D > C > A > B (d) D > C > B > A

30. Which of the following will have a mesoisomer also?
(a) 2, 3- Dichloropentane (b) 2, 3-Dichlorobutane
(c) 2-Chlorobutane (d) 2-Hydroxypropanoic acid

31. The major product formed when 1, 1, 1-trichloro-propane is treated with aqueous potassium hydroxide is:
(a) Propyne (b) 1-Propanol
(c) 2-Propanol (d) Propionic acid

32. The major product obtained in the following reaction is :

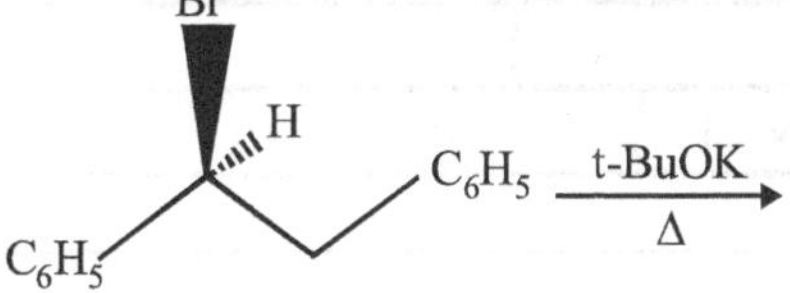

(a) $(\pm)C_6H_5CH(O^tBu)CH_2C_6H_5$
(b) $C_6H_5CH=CHC_6H_5$
(c) $(+)C_6H_5CH(O^tBu)CH_2C_6H_5$
(d) $(-)C_6H_5CH(O^tBu)CH_2C_6H_5$

33. A major component of Borsch reagent is obtained by reacting hydrazine hydrate with which of the following ?

(a) Cl, NO_2 (b) Cl, O_2N, NO_2

(c) Cl, NO_2, NO_2 (d) Cl, O_2N, NO_2, NO_2

34. Bottles containing C_6H_5I and $C_6H_5CH_2I$ lost their original labels. They were labelled A and B for testing. A and B were separately taken in test tubes and boiled with NaOH solution. The end solution in each tube was made acidic with dilute HNO_3 and then some $AgNO_3$ solution was added. Substance B gave a yellow precipitate. Which one of the following statements is true for this experiment ?
(a) A and $C_6H_5CH_2I$
(b) B and C_6H_5I
(c) Addition of HNO_3 was unnecessary
(d) A was C_6H_5I

35. Aryl fluoride may be prepared from arene diazonium chloride using :
(a) HBF_4/Δ (b) $HBF_4/NaNO_2, Cu, \Delta$
(c) CuF/HF (d) Cu/HF

36. The reagent(s) for the following conversion,
Br⌄⌃⌄Br $\xrightarrow{?}$ H—≡—H
is/are
(a) alcoholic KOH
(b) alcoholic KOH followed by $NaNH_2$
(c) aqueous KOH followed by $NaNH_2$
(d) Zn/CH_3OH

37. An organic compound A (C_4H_9Cl) on reaction with Na/diethyl ether gives a hydrocarbon which on monochlorination gives only one chloro derivative, then A is
(a) tert-butyl chloride (b) sec-butyl chloride
(c) isobutyl chloride (d) n-butyl chloride

RESPONSE GRID					
	23. ⓐⓑⓒⓓ	24. ⓐⓑⓒⓓ	25. ⓐⓑⓒⓓ	26. ⓐⓑⓒⓓ	27. ⓐⓑⓒⓓ
	28. ⓐⓑⓒⓓ	29. ⓐⓑⓒⓓ	30. ⓐⓑⓒⓓ	31. ⓐⓑⓒⓓ	32. ⓐⓑⓒⓓ
	33. ⓐⓑⓒⓓ	34. ⓐⓑⓒⓓ	35. ⓐⓑⓒⓓ	36. ⓐⓑⓒⓓ	37. ⓐⓑⓒⓓ

Space for Rough Work

38. Read the following statements and choose the correct answer
(i) The boiling points of isomeric haloalkanes decrease with increase in branching.
(ii) Among isomeric dihalobenzenes the para-isomers have higher melting point than their ortho and meta-isomers.
(iii) The isomeric dihalobenzene have large difference in their boiling and melting points
(iv) The isomeric dihalobenzene have nearly same boiling point.
(a) (i), (ii) and (iii) are correct
(b) (i) and (iii) are correct
(c) (ii) and (iv) are correct
(d) (i), (ii) and (iv) are correct

39. Chloroform cannot be prepared from which of the following?
(a) CH_3OH (b) C_2H_5OH
(c) CH_3CHO (d) $(CH_3)_2CO$

40. Silver benzoate reacts with bromine to form

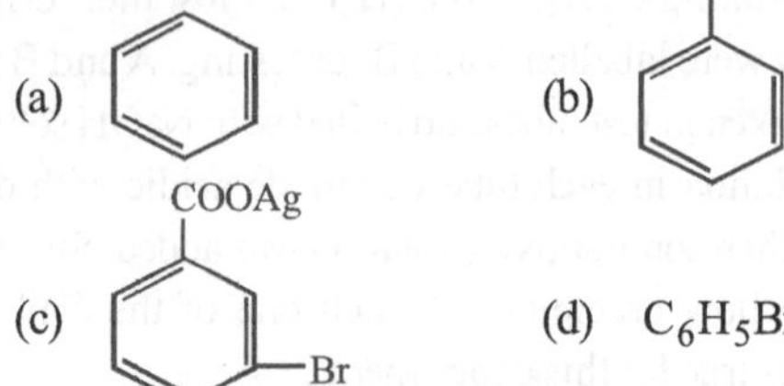

(d) C_6H_5Br

41. Benzene reacts with n-propyl chloride in the presence of anhydrous $AlCl_3$ to give
(a) 3 – Propyl – 1 – chlorobenzene
(b) n-Propylbenzene
(c) No reaction
(d) Isopropylbenzene

42. Match the columns

Column - I	Column - II
A. $C_2H_6 \xrightarrow{Cl_2/UV\ light} C_2H_5Cl$	I. Finkelstein reaction
B. $C_6H_5NH_2 \xrightarrow[273-278K]{NaNO_2+HCl/Cu_2Cl_2} C_6H_5Cl$	II. Free radical substitution
C. $CH_3Cl + NaI \longrightarrow CH_3I + NaCl$	III. Swarts reaction
D. $CH_3 - Br + AgF \longrightarrow CH_3F + AgBr$	IV. Sandmeyer's reaction

(a) A – II; B – IV; C – I; D – III
(b) A – II; B – III; C – I; D – IV
(c) A – III; B – I; C – IV; D – II
(d) A – IV; B – III; C – I; D – II

43. Which of the following statements is correct?
(a) S_N2 reactions of optically active halides are accompanied by inversion of configuration.
(b) S_N1 reactions of optically active halides are accompanied by racemisation.
(c) Carbocation formed in S_N1 reaction is sp^2 hybridized.
(d) All of the above.

44. The reaction is described as

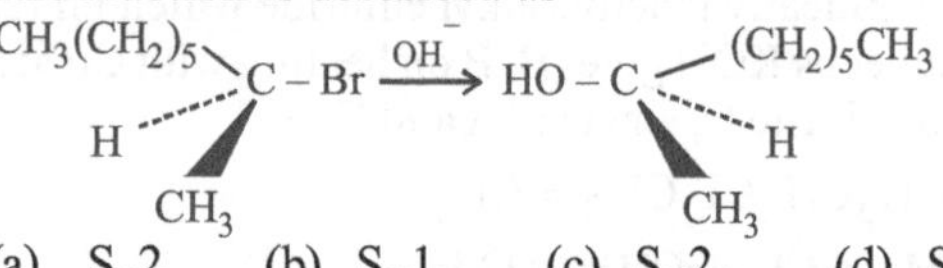

(a) S_E2 (b) S_N1 (c) S_N2 (d) S_N0

45. Which of the following is not used in Friedel-Crafts reaction?
(a) N–Phenyl acetanilide (b) Bromobenzene
(c) Benzene (d) Chlorobenzene

RESPONSE GRID					
	38. ⓐⓑⓒⓓ	39. ⓐⓑⓒⓓ	40. ⓐⓑⓒⓓ	41. ⓐⓑⓒⓓ	42. ⓐⓑⓒⓓ
	43. ⓐⓑⓒⓓ	44. ⓐⓑⓒⓓ	45. ⓐⓑⓒⓓ		

CHEMISTRY CHAPTERWISE SPEED TEST-52

Total Questions	45	Total Marks	180
Attempted		Correct	
Incorrect		Net Score	
Cut-off Score	37	Qualifying Score	59
Success Gap = Net Score – Qualifying Score			
Net Score = (Correct × 4) – (Incorrect × 1)			

Space for Rough Work

CHEMISTRY

Alcohols, Phenols and Ethers

Speed TEST 53

Chapter-wise

No. of Questions	Maximum Marks	Time
45	180	1 Hour

GENERAL INSTRUCTIONS

- This test contains 45 MCQ's. For each question only one option is correct. Darken the correct circle/ bubble in the Response Grid provided on each page.
- You have to evaluate your Response Grids yourself with the help of solutions provided at the end of this book.
- Each correct answer will get you 4 marks and 1 mark shall be deduced for each incorrect answer. No mark will be given/ deducted if no bubble is filled. Keep a timer in front of you and stop immediately at the end of 60 min.
- The sheet follows a particular syllabus. Do not attempt the sheet before you have completed your preparation for that syllabus.
- After completing the sheet check your answers with the solution booklet and complete the Result Grid. Finally spend time to analyse your performance and revise the areas which emerge out as weak in your evaluation.

1. Diethyl ether reacts, inspite of its usual inert nature, with :
   (a) Dilute suphuric acid
   (b) Dilute sodium hydroxide
   (c) Boron trifluoride
   (d) Metallic sodium
2. *n*-Propyl alcohol and isopropyl alcohol can be chemically distinguished by which reagent?
   (a) PCl_5
   (b) Reduction
   (c) Oxidation with potassium dichromate
   (d) Ozonolysis
3. Which of the following reactions will not result in the formation of anisole?
   (a) Phenol + dimethyl sulphate in presence of a base
   (b) Sodium phenoxide is treated with methyl iodide
   (c) Reaction of diazomethane with phenol
   (d) Reaction of methylmagnesium iodide with phenol
4. Intermolecular hydrogen bonding is strongest in :
   (a) Methylamine (b) Phenol
   (c) Formaldehyde (d) Methanol
5. Vinyl carbinol is
   (a) $HO-CH_2-CH=CH_2$
   (b) $CH_3C(OH)=CH_2$
   (c) $CH_3-CH=CH-OH$
   (d) $CH_3-C(CH_2OH)=CH_2$
6. Lucas reagent is
   (a) Conc. HCl and anhydrous $ZnCl_2$
   (b) Conc. HNO_3 and hydrous $ZnCl_2$
   (c) Conc. HCl and hydrous $ZnCl_2$
   (d) Conc. HNO_3 and anhydrous $ZnCl_2$
7. The order of reactivity of the following alcohols towards conc. HCl is

F, CH_3, OH

(I)

F, CH_3, OH

(II)

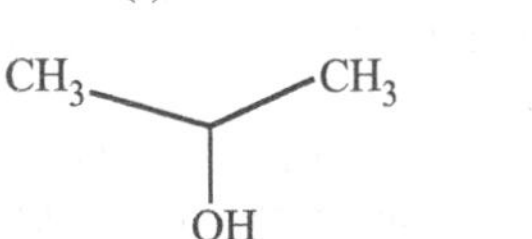

(III)

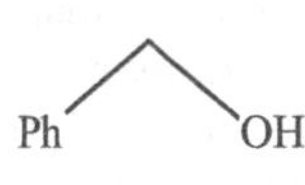

(IV)

(a) I > II > III > IV (b) I > III > II > IV
(c) IV > III > II > I (d) IV > III > I > II

RESPONSE GRID	
1. ⓐⓑⓒⓓ 2. ⓐⓑⓒⓓ 3. ⓐⓑⓒⓓ 4. ⓐⓑⓒⓓ 5. ⓐⓑⓒⓓ	
6. ⓐⓑⓒⓓ 7. ⓐⓑⓒⓓ	

Space for Rough Work

8. What is the major product M in the following reaction ?

$$CH_3\text{-}C_6H_4\text{-}Br \xrightarrow[CCl_4,\ heat]{NBS,\ benzoyl\ peroxide} X \xrightarrow[CH_3CH_2OH]{CH_3CH_2ONa} M$$

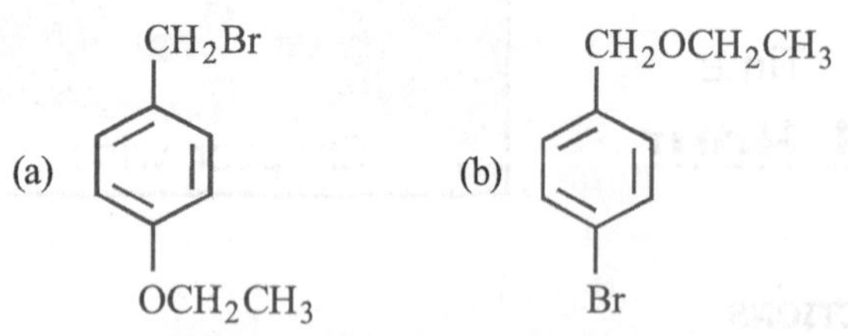

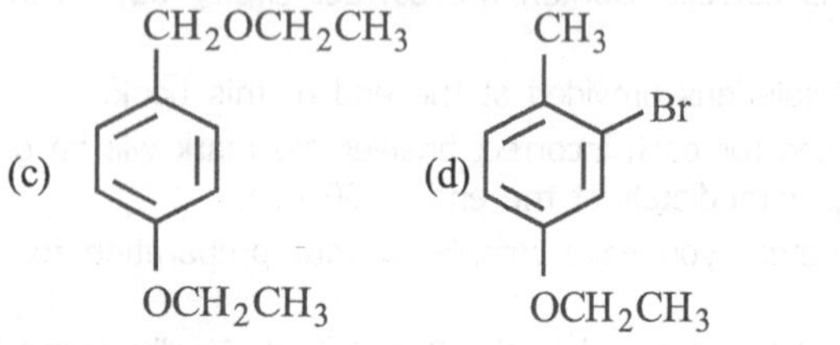

9. Epichlorohydrin is
   (a) 3-Chloropropane
   (b) 3-Chloropropan-1-ol
   (c) 3-Chloro-1, 2-epoxypropane
   (d) None of these

10. CH_3CH_2OH can be converted into CH_3CHO by________
    (a) catalytic hydrogenation
    (b) treatment with $LiAlH_4$
    (c) treatment with pyridinium chlorochromate
    (d) treatment with $KMnO_4$

11. In Williamson synthesis if tertiary alkyl halide is used than
    (a) ether is obtained in good yield
    (b) ether is obtained in poor yield
    (c) alkene is the only reaction product
    (d) a mixture of alkene as a major product and ether as a minor product forms.

12. Denaturation of alcohol is the
    (a) mixing of $CuSO_4$ (a foul smelling solid) and pyridine (to give the colour) to make the commercial alcohol unfit for drinking
    (b) mixing of $CuSO_4$ (to give the colour) and pyridine (a foul smelling solid) to make the commercial alcohol unfit for drinking
    (c) mixing of $Cu(OAc)_2$ and ammonia to make the commercial alcohol unfit for drinking
    (d) mixing of $Cu(OAc)_2$ and pyridine to make the commercial alcohol unfit for drinking

13. 2-Phenylethanol may be prepared by the reaction of phenylmagnesium bromide with
    (a) HCHO (b) CH_3CHO
    (c) CH_3COCH_3 (d) ethylene oxide (epoxide ring with O)

14. Arrange the following in increasing order of their acidity? *o*–cresol(a), salicyclic acid(b), phenol(c)
    (a) c < a < b (b) b < c < a
    (c) a < b < a (d) a < c < b

15. Which of the following is most reactive towards aqueous HBr ?
    (a) 1-Phenyl-1-propanol
    (b) 1-Phenyl-2-propanol
    (c) 3-Phenyl-1-propanol
    (d) All are equally reactive

16. The ionization constant of phenol is higher than that of ethanol because :
    (a) phenoxide ion is bulkier than ethoxide
    (b) phenoxide ion is stronger base than ethoxide
    (c) phenoxide ion is stabilized through delocalization
    (d) phenoxide ion is less stable than ethoxide

17. Rectified spirit is a mixture of
    (a) 95% ethyl alcohol + 5% water
    (b) 94% ethyl alcohol + 4.53 water
    (c) 94.4% ethyl alcohol + 5.43% water
    (d) 95.87% ethyl alcohol + 4.13% water

18. Ethanol is prepared industrially by
    (a) hydration of ethylene (b) fermentation of sugar
    (c) Both the above (d) None of these

19. Mechanism of acid catalysed hydration reaction involves
    (i) Protonation of alkene to form carbocation by electrophilic attack of H_3O^+
    (ii) Nucleophilic attack of water on carbocation.
    (iii) Deprotonation to form alcohol.
    (a) (i) and (ii) (b) (i) and (iii)
    (c) (i), (ii) and (iii) (d) (ii) and (iii)

RESPONSE GRID					
	8. ⓐⓑⓒⓓ	9. ⓐⓑⓒⓓ	10. ⓐⓑⓒⓓ	11. ⓐⓑⓒⓓ	12. ⓐⓑⓒⓓ
	13. ⓐⓑⓒⓓ	14. ⓐⓑⓒⓓ	15. ⓐⓑⓒⓓ	16. ⓐⓑⓒⓓ	17. ⓐⓑⓒⓓ
	18. ⓐⓑⓒⓓ	19. ⓐⓑⓒⓓ			

Space for Rough Work

20. Match the columns

	Column-I		Column-II
A.	Methanol	I.	Conversion of phenol to *o*-hydroxysalicylic acid
B.	Kolbe's reaction	II.	Wood spirit
C.	Williamson's synthesis	III.	Heated copper at 573 K
D.	Conversion of 2° alcohol to ketone	IV.	Reaction of alkyl halide with sodium alkoxide

(a) A – IV; B – III; C – II; D – I
(b) A – II; B – IV; C – I; D – III
(c) A – II; B – I; C – IV; D – III
(d) A – III; B – II; C – I; D – IV

21. Absolute alcohol (100% alcohol) is prepared by distilling rectified spirit over
(a) Na (b) $CaCl_2$
(c) Mg (d) $Mg(OC_2H_5)_2$

22. *p*-cresol reacts with chloroform in alkaline medium to give the compound A which adds hydrogen cyanide to form, the compound B. The latter on acidic hydrolysis gives chiral carboxylic acid. The structure of the carboxylic acid is

(a) CH_3, CH_2COOH, OH
(b) CH_3, CH_2COOH, OH
(c) CH_3, CH(OH)COOH, OH
(d) CH_3, CH(OH)COOH, OH

23. Which one of the following will show the highest pH value ?
(a) *m*–nitrophenol. (b) *p*–nitrophenol.
(c) *o*–nitrophenol. (d) Both (b) and (c).

24. Which of the following compounds is resistant to nucleophilic attack by hydroxyl ions?
(a) Methyl acetate (b) Acetonitrile
(c) Acetamide (d) Diethyl ether

25. Zerevitinov's determination of active hydrogen in a compound is based upon its reaction with
(a) Na (b) CH_3MgI
(c) Zn (d) Al

26. Williamson's synthesis is used to prepare
(a) acetone (b) diethyl ether
(c) P.V.C. (d) bakelite

27. Which of the following statements are correct ?
(i) Ethanol mixed with methanol is called denatured alcohol.
(ii) Excess of methanol in body may cause blindness.
(iii) In the body methanol is oxidised to methanoic acid.
(iv) A methanol poisoned patient is treated by giving intravenous injections of ethanoic acid.
(a) (i), (ii) and (iii) (b) (ii), (iii) and (iv)
(c) (i) and (v) (d) (i), (iii) and (iv)

28. In the following sequence of reactions,

$$CH_3CH_2OH \xrightarrow{P+I_2} A \xrightarrow[\text{ether}]{Mg} B \xrightarrow{HCHO} C \xrightarrow{H_2O} D$$

the compound D is
(a) propanal (b) butanal
(c) *n*-butyl alcohol (d) *n*-propyl alcohol

29. When wine is put in air, it becomes sour due to
(a) bacteria
(b) oxidation of C_2H_5OH to CH_3COOH
(c) virus
(d) formic acid formation

30. Which of the following diols would cleave into two fragments with HIO_4
(a) 1, 3-hexanediol (b) 2, 4-hexanediol
(c) 1, 6-hexanediol (d) 3, 4-hexanediol

31. The major product of the following reaction is

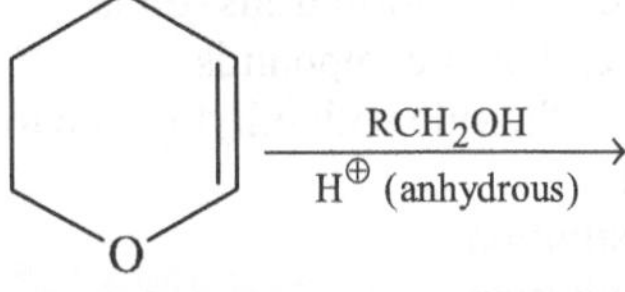

(a) a hemiacetal (b) an acetal
(c) an ether (d) an ester

32. $H_2COH \cdot CH_2OH$ on heating with periodic acid gives:
(a) 2 HCOOH (b) CHO–CHO
(c) 2 $H_2C=O$ (d) 2 CO_2

33. Victor Meyer's test is not given by
(a) $(CH_3)_3COH$ (b) C_2H_5OH
(c) $(CH_3)_2CHOH$ (d) $CH_3CH_2CH_2OH$

RESPONSE GRID					
	20. ⓐⓑⓒⓓ	21. ⓐⓑⓒⓓ	22. ⓐⓑⓒⓓ	23. ⓐⓑⓒⓓ	24. ⓐⓑⓒⓓ
	25. ⓐⓑⓒⓓ	26. ⓐⓑⓒⓓ	27. ⓐⓑⓒⓓ	28. ⓐⓑⓒⓓ	29. ⓐⓑⓒⓓ
	30. ⓐⓑⓒⓓ	31. ⓐⓑⓒⓓ	32. ⓐⓑⓒⓓ	33. ⓐⓑⓒⓓ	

Space for Rough Work

34. What is X in the following reaction ?

$$CH_2\overset{O}{\triangle}\underset{\underset{CH_3}{|}}{C}-CH_3 \xrightarrow{X} H_2C-\overset{\overset{OH}{|}}{}\underset{\underset{CH_3}{|}}{\overset{\overset{OCH_3}{|}}{C}}-CH_3$$

(a) CH_3OH, H_2SO_4
(b) $CH_3OH, CH_3O^-\overset{+}{Na}$
(c) H_2O/H_2SO_4 followed by CH_3OH
(d) CH_3MgBr / ether followed by H_3O^+

35. Which of the following pairs of reagents would give 4-methyl-2-pentanol ?
(a) $(CH_3)_2CHLi, CH_3COCH_3$
(b) $(CH_3)_2CHCH_2Li, CH_3CHO$
(c) $(CH_3)_2CHLi, CH_3CH_2CHO$
(d) $CH_3CH_2Li, (CH_3)_2CH.CHO$

36. Which of the following cannot be made by reduction of ketone or aldehyde with $NaBH_4$ in methanol ?
(a) 1 - butanol (b) 2 - butanol
(c) 2 - methyl - 1- propanol (d) 2 - methyl - 2- propanol

37. Osmium tetraoxide is a reagent used for
(a) hydroxylation of acetylenes
(b) hydroxylation of olefins to give *cis*-diols
(c) hydroxylation of olefins to form trans- diols
(d) hydroxylation of carbonyl compounds

38. The reaction of sodium ethoxide with ethyl iodide to form diethyl ether is termed
(a) electrophilic substitution
(b) nucleophilic substitution
(c) electrophilic addition
(d) radical substitution

39. The IUPAC name of $CH_3-\underset{\underset{OH}{|}}{CH}-CH_2-\underset{\underset{OH}{|}}{\overset{\overset{CH_3}{|}}{C}}-CH_3$ is
(a) 1, 1-dimethyl-1, 3-butanediol
(b) 2-methyl-2, 4-pentanediol
(c) 4-methyl-2, 4-pentanediol
(d) 1, 3, 3-trimethyl-1, 3-propanediol

40. Give IUPAC name of the compound given below

$$CH_3-\underset{\underset{Cl}{|}}{CH}-CH_2-CH_2-\underset{\underset{OH}{|}}{CH}-CH_3$$

(a) 2-Chloro-5-hydroxyhexane
(b) 2-Hydroxy-5-chlorohexane
(c) 5-Chlorohexane-2-ol
(d) 2-Chlorohexan-5-ol

41. Aspirin is an acetylation product of
(a) p-Dihydroxybenzene (b) o-Hydroxybenzoic acid
(c) o-Dihydroxybenzene (d) m-Hydroxybenzoic acid

42. Acetic anhydride reacts with diethyl ether in the presence of anhydrous $AlCl_3$ to give
(a) CH_3COOCH_3 (b) $CH_3CH_2COOCH_3$
(c) $CH_3COOCH_2CH_3$ (d) CH_3CH_2OH

43. Formation of which compound given below from 1 - butanol needs an oxidising agent?
(a) $CH_3CH_2CH_2CH_2Br$ (b) $CH_3CH_2CH_2CH=O$
(c) $(CH_3CH_2CH_2CH_2)_2O$ (d) $CH_3-CH_2CH=CH_2$

44. $o-\text{Xylene} \xrightarrow{HNO_3} X \xrightarrow[H_2SO_4]{\text{Phenol}} Y$. The product Y is
(a) Phthalic acid (b) Isophthalic acid
(c) Phenolphthalein (d) o-Hydroxysulphonic acid

45. Which of the following , upon treatment with tert-BuONa followed by addition of bromine water, fails to decolourize the colour of bromine?

(a) O, Br

(b) 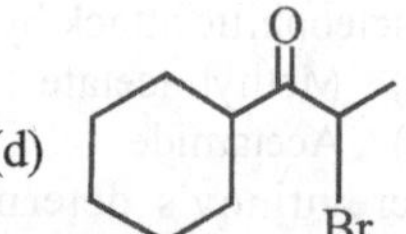

(c) O, Br

(d) O, Br

RESPONSE GRID	34. ⓐⓑⓒⓓ	35. ⓐⓑⓒⓓ	36. ⓐⓑⓒⓓ	37. ⓐⓑⓒⓓ	38. ⓐⓑⓒⓓ
	39. ⓐⓑⓒⓓ	40. ⓐⓑⓒⓓ	41. ⓐⓑⓒⓓ	42. ⓐⓑⓒⓓ	43. ⓐⓑⓒⓓ
	44. ⓐⓑⓒⓓ	45. ⓐⓑⓒⓓ			

CHEMISTRY CHAPTERWISE SPEED TEST-53

Total Questions	45	Total Marks	180
Attempted		Correct	
Incorrect		Net Score	
Cut-off Score	38	Qualifying Score	62
Success Gap = Net Score – Qualifying Score			
Net Score = (Correct × 4) – (Incorrect × 1)			

Space for Rough Work

CHEMISTRY

Aldehydes, Ketones and Carboxylic Acids

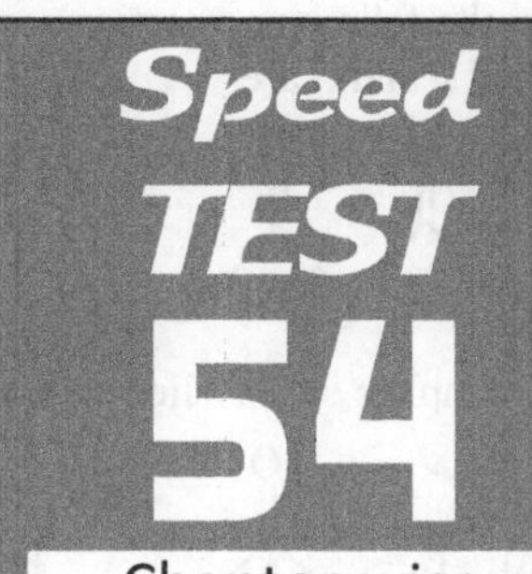

No. of Questions	Maximum Marks	Time
45	180	1 Hour

GENERAL INSTRUCTIONS

- This test contains 45 MCQ's. For each question only one option is correct. Darken the correct circle/ bubble in the Response Grid provided on each page.
- You have to evaluate your Response Grids yourself with the help of solutions provided at the end of this book.
- Each correct answer will get you 4 marks and 1 mark shall be deduced for each incorrect answer. No mark will be given/ deducted if no bubble is filled. Keep a timer in front of you and stop immediately at the end of 60 min.
- The sheet follows a particular syllabus. Do not attempt the sheet before you have completed your preparation for that syllabus.
- After completing the sheet check your answers with the solution booklet and complete the Result Grid. Finally spend time to analyse your performance and revise the areas which emerge out as weak in your evaluation.

1. Which of the following compounds is most reactive towards nucleophilic addition reactions?

(a) $CH_3-\overset{O}{\overset{\|}{C}}-H$ (b) $CH_3-\overset{O}{\overset{\|}{C}}-CH_3$

(c) $C_6H_5-\overset{O}{\overset{\|}{C}}-H$ (d) $C_6H_5-\overset{O}{\overset{\|}{C}}-CH_3$

2. Arrange the following in order of decreasing acidity

(A) cyclopentanone (B) cyclopentane-1,3-dione (C) methylenecyclopentane ($=CH_2$)

(a) B>A>C (b) C>B>A

(c) A>C>B (d) A>B>C

3. A and B in the following reactions are

$$R-\underset{\underset{O}{\|}}{C}-R' \xrightarrow[KCN]{HCN} A \xrightarrow{B} R-\underset{R'}{\overset{}{C}}\begin{smallmatrix}OH\\CH_2NH_2\end{smallmatrix}$$

(a) $A = RR'C\begin{smallmatrix}CN\\OH\end{smallmatrix}$, $B = LiAlH_4$

(b) $A = RR'C\begin{smallmatrix}OH\\COOH\end{smallmatrix}$, $B = NH_3$

(c) $A = RR'C\begin{smallmatrix}CN\\OH\end{smallmatrix}$, $B = H_3O^{\oplus}$

(d) $A = RR'CH_2CN, B = NaOH$

4. Acetaldehyde reacts with
   (a) Electrophiles only
   (b) Nucleophiles only
   (c) Free radicals only
   (d) Both electrophiles and nucleophiles

5. $C_6H_5CH{=}CHCHO \xrightarrow{X} C_6H_5CH{=}CHCH_2OH$
   In the above sequence X can be :
   (a) H_2/Ni (b) $NaBH_4$
   (c) $K_2Cr_2O_7/H^+$ (d) Both (a) and (b)

6. Which one of the following can be oxidised to the corresponding carbonyl compound?
   (a) 2-hydroxy-propane
   (b) Ortho-nitro-phenol
   (c) Phenol
   (d) 2-methyl-2 hydroxy-propane

RESPONSE GRID	1. ⓐⓑⓒⓓ	2. ⓐⓑⓒⓓ	3. ⓐⓑⓒⓓ	4. ⓐⓑⓒⓓ	5. ⓐⓑⓒⓓ
	6. ⓐⓑⓒⓓ				

Space for Rough Work

7. In the following reaction sequence, the correct structures of E, F and G are

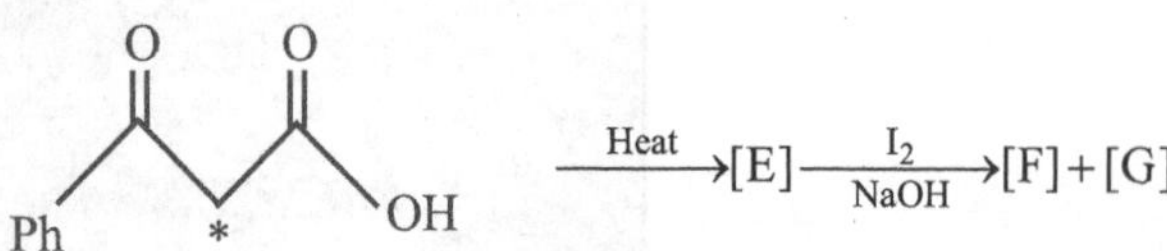

[* implies ^{13}C labelled carbon)

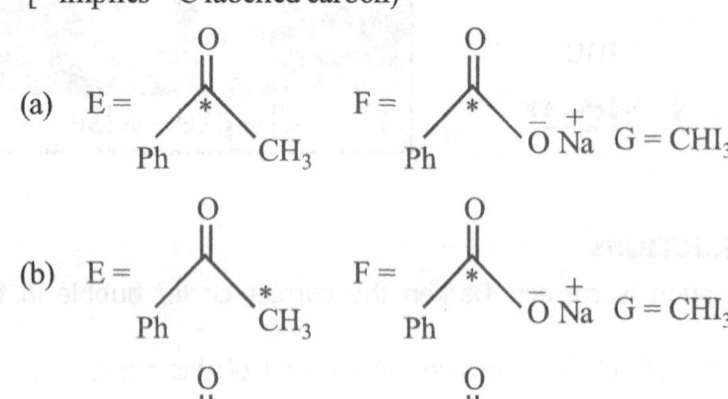

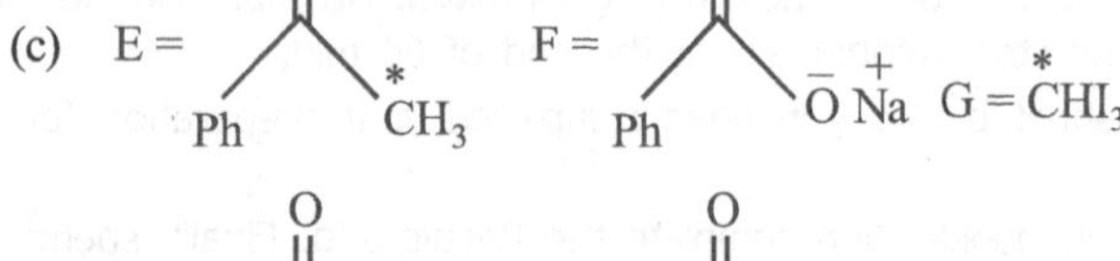

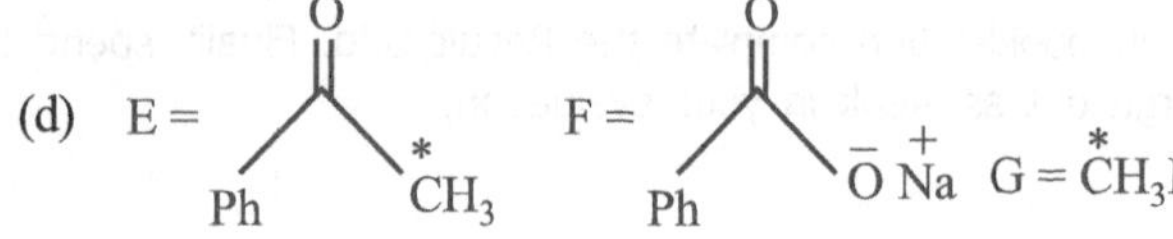

8. Ketones
$[R-\underset{\underset{O}{\|}}{C}-R_1$, where $R = R_1$ = alkyl groups]
can be obtained in one step by
(a) oxidation of primary alcohols
(b) hydrolysis of esters
(c) oxidation of tertiary alcohols
(d) reaction of acid halides with alcohols

9. The compound that neither forms semicarbazone nor oxime is
(a) HCHO (b) CH_3COCH_2Cl
(c) CH_3CHO (d) $CH_3CONHCH_3$

10. Ethyl ester $\xrightarrow[\text{excess}]{CH_3MgBr}$ P. The product P will be

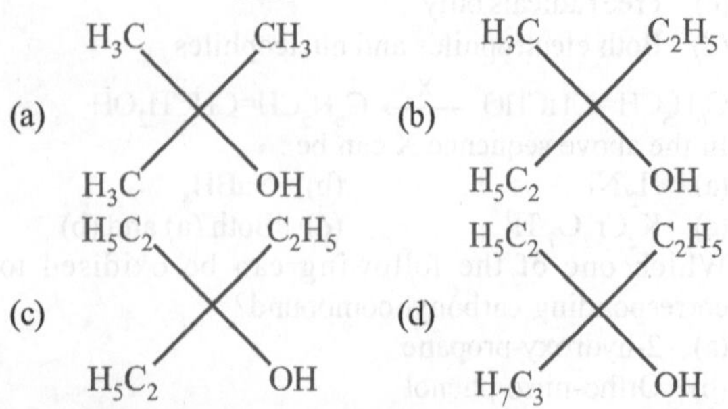

11. Which of the following compounds when heated with CO at 150°C and 500 atm pressure in presence of BF_3 forms ethyl propionate ?
(a) C_2H_5OH (b) CH_3OCH_3
(c) $C_2H_5OC_2H_5$ (d) $CH_3OC_2H_5$

12. Benzaldehyde is obtained from Rosenmund's reduction of

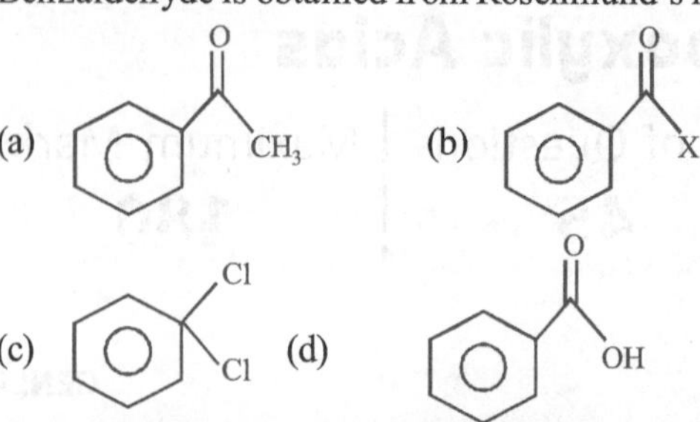

13. Acetone oxime is obtained by reacting acetone with
(a) NH_3 (b) NH_2OH (c) NH_2Na (d) $NH_2.NH_2$

14. $2C_6H_5CHO \xrightarrow[H_2O]{OH^-} C_6H_5CH_2OH + C_6H_5COO^-$
Which of the following statements are correct regarding the above reduction of benzaldehyde to benzyl alcohol?
(i) One hydrogen is coming from H_2O as H^+ and another from C_6H_5CHO as H^-
(ii) One hydrogen is coming from H_2O as H^- and another from C_6H_5CHO as H^+
(iii) One hydrogen from H_2O and another from C_6H_5CHO, both in the form of H^-
(iv) The reduction is an example of disproportionation reaction
(a) (i), (ii) and (iii) (b) (i) and (iv)
(c) (ii), (iii) and (iv) (d) (iii) and (iv)

15. A carboxylic acid can best be converted into acid chloride by using
(a) PCl_5 (b) $SOCl_2$
(c) HCl (d) ClCOCOCl

16. Among the given compounds, the most susceptible to nucleophilic attack at the carbonyl group is
(a) MeCOCl (b) MeCHO
(c) MeCOOMe (d) MeCOOCOMe

17. Find out B in the given reactions

$C_6H_6 + CH_3-X \xrightarrow{AlCl_3} A \xrightarrow[H_3O^{\oplus}]{CrO_3 \text{ in } (CH_3CO)_2O} B$

(a) acetophenone
(b) benzaldehyde
(c) cyclohexyl carbaldehyde
(d) benzoic acid

18. Pinacolone is
(a) 2, 3-Dimethyl-2, 3-butanediol
(b) 3,3-Dimethyl-2-butanone
(c) 1-Phenyl-2-propanone
(d) 1, 1-Diphenyl-1, 2-ethandiol

RESPONSE GRID					
	7. ⓐⓑⓒⓓ	8. ⓐⓑⓒⓓ	9. ⓐⓑⓒⓓ	10. ⓐⓑⓒⓓ	11. ⓐⓑⓒⓓ
	12. ⓐⓑⓒⓓ	13. ⓐⓑⓒⓓ	14. ⓐⓑⓒⓓ	15. ⓐⓑⓒⓓ	16. ⓐⓑⓒⓓ
	17. ⓐⓑⓒⓓ	18. ⓐⓑⓒⓓ			

Space for Rough Work

19. The correct sequence of reagents for the following conversion will be :

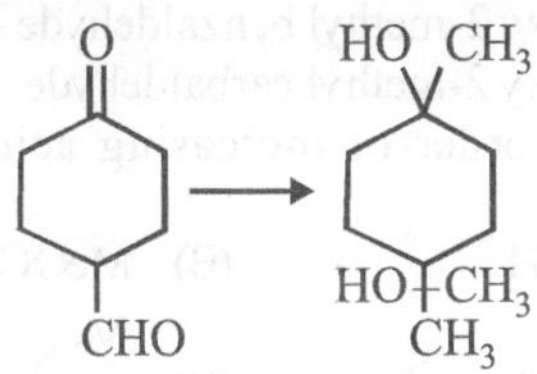

(a) $[Ag(NH_3)_2]^+ OH^-$, H^+/CH_3OH, CH_3MgBr
(b) CH_3MgBr, H^+/CH_3OH, $[Ag(NH_3)_2]^+ OH^-$
(c) CH_3MgBr, $[Ag(NH_3)_2]^+ OH^-$, H^+/CH_3OH
(d) $[Ag(NH_3)_2]^+ OH^-$, CH_3MgBr, H^+/CH_3OH

20. Benzaldehyde reacts with ethanoic KCN to give
(a) $C_6H_5CHOHCN$ (b) $C_6H_5CHOHCOC_6H_5$
(c) $C_6H_5CHOHCOOH$ (d) $C_6H_5CHOHCHOHC_6H_5$

21. Which gives lactic acid on hydrolysis after reacting with HCN?
(a) HCHO (b) CH_3CHO
(c) C_6H_5CHO (d) CH_3COCH_3

22. Reduction of $>C=O$ to $>CH_2$ can be carried out with
(a) catalytic reduction
(b) Na/C_2H_5OH
(c) Wolff-Kishner reduction
(d) $LiAlH_4$

23. The end product B in the sequence of reactions

$$R-X \xrightarrow{CN^-} A \xrightarrow{NaOH} B \text{ is}$$

(a) an alkane
(b) a carboxylic acid
(c) sodium salt of carboxylic acid
(d) a ketone

24. Phenylmethyl ketone can be converted into ethylbenzene in one step by which of the following reagents?
(a) $LiAlH_4$ (b) Zn-Hg/HCl
(c) $NaBH_4$ (d) CH_3MgI

25. Conversion of acetaldehyde into ethyl acetate in presence of aluminium ethoxide is called
(a) Aldol condensation (b) Cope reaction
(c) Tischenko reaction (d) Benzoin condensation

26. Match the columns

	Column-I		Column-II
A.	Etard reaction	I.	Alcoholic KOH
B.	Hydroxylation	II.	Anhydrous $AlCl_3$
C.	Dehydrohalogenation	III.	Chromyl chloride
D.	Friedel-Crafts reaction	IV.	Dilute alkaline $KMnO_4$

(a) A – I; B – II; C – III; D – II
(b) A – IV; B – III; C – I; D – II
(c) A – III; B – IV; C – I; D – II
(d) A – II; B – I; C – IV; D – III

27. An organic compound A upon reacting with NH_3 gives B. On heating B gives C. C in presence of KOH reacts with Br_2 to given $CH_3CH_2NH_2$. A is :
(a) CH_3COOH (b) $CH_3CH_2CH_2COOH$
(c) $CH_3-\underset{\underset{CH_3}{|}}{CH}-COOH$ (d) CH_3CH_2COOH

28. Which one of the following can be oxidised to the corresponding carbonyl compound?
(a) 2-hydroxypropane
(b) Ortho-nitrophenol
(c) Phenol
(d) 2-methyl-2 hydroxypropane

29. The reagent which can be used to distinguish acetophenone from benzophenone is
(a) 2,4- dinitrophenylhydrazine
(b) aqueous solution of $NaHSO_3$
(c) benedict reagent
(d) $I_2$and Na_2CO_3

30. $R-CH_2-CH_2OH$ can be converted into RCH_2CH_2COOH. The correct sequence of reagents is
(a) PBr_3,KCN,H^+ (b) PBr_3, KCN, H_2
(c) KCN,H^+ (d) HCN,PBr_3,H^+

31. Sodium salt of an organic acid 'X' produces effervescence with conc. H_2SO_4. 'X' reacts with the acidified aqueous $CaCl_2$ solution to give a white precipitate which decolourises acidic solution of $KMnO_4$. 'X' is :
(a) C_6H_5COONa (b) HCOONa
(c) CH_3COONa (d) $Na_2C_2O_4$

32. In a set of the given reactions, acetic acid yielded a product C.

$$CH_3COOH + PCl_5 \longrightarrow A \xrightarrow[\text{Anh. }AlCl_3]{C_6H_6} B \xrightarrow[\text{Ether}]{C_2H_5MgBr} C$$

Product C would be
(a) $CH_3-\overset{\overset{C_2H_5}{|}}{C}(OH)C_6H_5$ (b) $CH_3CH(OH)C_2H_5$
(c) $CH_3COC_6H_5$ (d) $CH_3CH(OH)C_6H_5$

33. Which one of the following will most readily be dehydrated in acidic condition ?

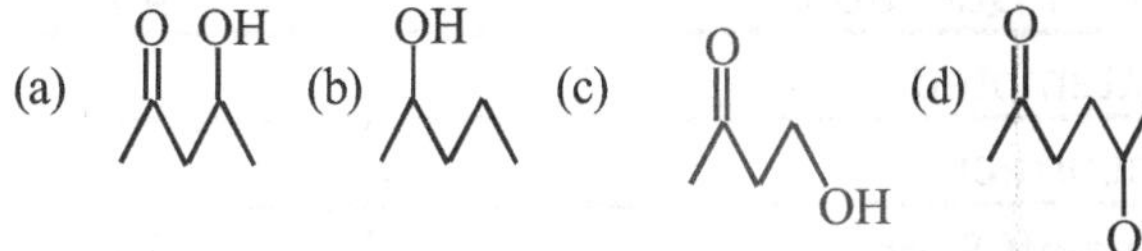

RESPONSE GRID					
	19. ⓐⓑⓒⓓ	20. ⓐⓑⓒⓓ	21. ⓐⓑⓒⓓ	22. ⓐⓑⓒⓓ	23. ⓐⓑⓒⓓ
	24. ⓐⓑⓒⓓ	25. ⓐⓑⓒⓓ	26. ⓐⓑⓒⓓ	27. ⓐⓑⓒⓓ	28. ⓐⓑⓒⓓ
	29. ⓐⓑⓒⓓ	30. ⓐⓑⓒⓓ	31. ⓐⓑⓒⓓ	32. ⓐⓑⓒⓓ	33. ⓐⓑⓒⓓ

Space for Rough Work

34. Which of the following contain an aldehyde?
(a) Vanilla beans (b) Meadow sweet
(c) Cinnamon (d) All of these

35. Heating mixture of sodium benzoate and soda-lime gives
(a) benzene (b) methane
(c) sodium phenoxide (d) calcium benzoate

36. Observe the following structures and pick up the correct statement.

$>C=O$ (I) $>C=\overset{+}{O}H$ (II)

(a) Carbonyl carbon of I is more electrophilic than that of II
(b) Carbonyl carbon of I is less electrophilic than that of II
(c) Carbonyl carbon of both structures have equal electrophilic character
(d) It depends upon the complete structure of the compound

37. An enantiomerically pure acid is treated with a racemic mixture of an alcohol having one chiral carbon. The ester formed will be
(a) Optically active mixture (b) Pure enantiomer
(c) Meso compound (d) Racemic mixture

38. *m*-Chlorobenzaldehyde on reaction with conc. KOH at room temperature gives
(a) potassium *m*-chlorobenzoate and *m*-hydroxybenzaldehyde
(b) *m*-hydroxybenzaldehyde and *m*-chlorobenzyl alcohol
(c) *m*-chlorobenzyl alcohol and *m*-hydroxybenzyl alcohol
(d) potassium *m*-chlorobenzoate and *m*-chlorobenzyl alcohol.

39. IUPAC name of following will be

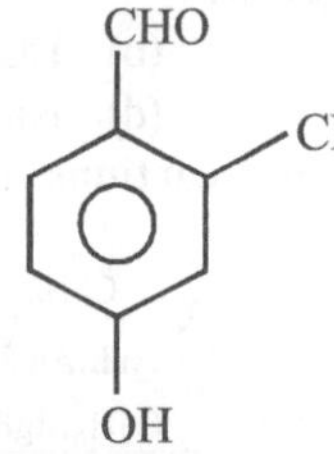

(Benzene ring with CHO at top, CH_3 at adjacent position, OH at para position)

(a) 4-formyl 3-methyl 1-hydroxy benzene
(b) 4-formyl 3-methyl phenol
(c) 4-hydroxy 2-methyl benzaldehyde
(d) 4-hydroxy 2-methyl carbaldehyde

40. The correct order of increasing acid strength of the compounds
(A) CH_3CO_2H (B) $MeOCH_2CO_2H$
(C) CF_3CO_2H (D) $(Me)_2CH{-}CO_2H$ is
(a) D<A<B<C (b) A<D<B<C
(c) B<D<A<C (d) D<A<C<B

41. The increasing order of the rate of HCN addition to compound A – D is
(A) HCHO (B) CH_3COCH_3
(C) $PhCOCH_3$ (D) PhCOPh
(a) D<C<B<A (b) C<D<B<A
(c) A<B<C<D (d) D<B<C<A

42. The carboxyl functional group (– COOH) is present in
(a) picric acid (b) barbituric acid
(c) ascorbic acid (d) aspirin

43. Which alkene on ozonolysis gives CH_3CH_2CHO and $CH_3\underset{\underset{O}{\|}}{C}CH_3$
(a) $CH_3CH_2CH=C(CH_3)_2$ (b) $CH_3CH_2CH=CHCH_2CH_3$
(c) $CH_3CH_2CH=CHCH_3$ (d) $CH_3-\underset{\underset{CH_3}{|}}{C}=CHCH_3$

44. Which one of the following is reduced with zinc and hydrochloric acid to give the corresponding hydrocarbon?
(a) Acetamide (b) Acetic acid
(c) Ethyl acetate (d) Butan-2-one

45. Acetal is produced by reacting an alcohol in the presence of dry HCl with
(a) acetaldehyde (b) ketone
(c) ether (d) carboxylic acid

RESPONSE GRID					
	34. ⓐⓑⓒⓓ	35. ⓐⓑⓒⓓ	36. ⓐⓑⓒⓓ	37. ⓐⓑⓒⓓ	38. ⓐⓑⓒⓓ
	39. ⓐⓑⓒⓓ	40. ⓐⓑⓒⓓ	41. ⓐⓑⓒⓓ	42. ⓐⓑⓒⓓ	43. ⓐⓑⓒⓓ
	44. ⓐⓑⓒⓓ	45. ⓐⓑⓒⓓ			

CHEMISTRY CHAPTERWISE SPEED TEST-54

Total Questions	45	Total Marks	180
Attempted		Correct	
Incorrect		Net Score	
Cut-off Score	35	Qualifying Score	57
Success Gap = Net Score – Qualifying Score			
Net Score = (Correct × 4) – (Incorrect × 1)			

Space for Rough Work

CHEMISTRY

Amines

Speed TEST 55

Chapter-wise

No. of Questions	Maximum Marks	Time
45	**180**	**1 Hour**

GENERAL INSTRUCTIONS

- This test contains 45 MCQ's. For each question only one option is correct. Darken the correct circle/ bubble in the Response Grid provided on each page.
- You have to evaluate your Response Grids yourself with the help of solutions provided at the end of this book.
- Each correct answer will get you 4 marks and 1 mark shall be deduced for each incorrect answer. No mark will be given/ deducted if no bubble is filled. Keep a timer in front of you and stop immediately at the end of 60 min.
- The sheet follows a particular syllabus. Do not attempt the sheet before you have completed your preparation for that syllabus.
- After completing the sheet check your answers with the solution booklet and complete the Result Grid. Finally spend time to analyse your performance and revise the areas which emerge out as weak in your evaluation.

1. The reduction of nitro compounds is most preferred in the presence of
   (a) Pd/H_2 in ethanol (b) Sn + HCl
   (c) finely divided Ni (d) iron scrap and HCl.
2. Ortho-Nitrophenol is less soluble in water than *p*- and *m*- Nitrophenols because :
   (a) *o*-Nitrophenol is more volatile than those of *m*- and *p*-isomers.
   (b) *o*-Nitrophenol shows intramolecular H-bonding
   (c) *o*-Nitrophenol shows intermolecular H-bonding
   (d) Melting point of *o*-Nitrophenol is lower than those of *m*- and *p*-isomers.
3. In a reaction of aniline a coloured product C was obtained.

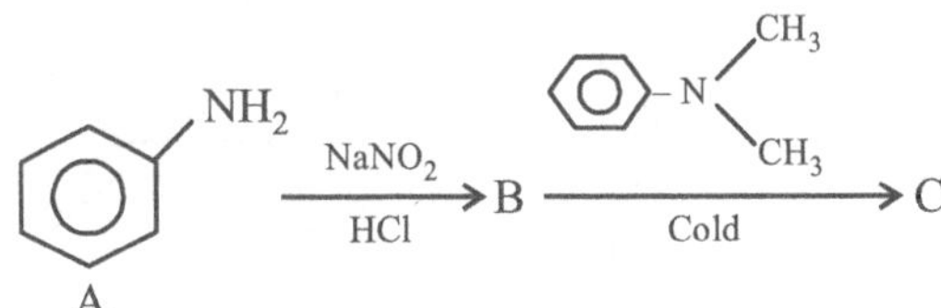

The structure of C would be :

(a) $C_6H_5-N=N-CH_2-N(CH_3)-C_6H_5$

(b) CH_3-substituted benzene $-N=N-$ CH_3-substituted benzene (both CH_3 ortho to the azo group)

(c) $C_6H_5-NH-NH-C_6H_4-N(CH_3)_2$

(d) $C_6H_5-N=N-C_6H_4-N(CH_3)_2$

4. The number of primary amines of formula $C_4H_{11}N$ is :
   (a) 1 (b) 3 (c) 4 (d) 2
5. Which of the following reactions will not give a primary amine?
   (a) $CH_3CONH_2 \xrightarrow{Br_2/KOH}$
   (b) $CH_3CN \xrightarrow{LiAlH_4}$
   (c) $CH_3NC \xrightarrow{LiAlH_4}$
   (d) $CH_3CONH_2 \xrightarrow{LiAlH_4}$
6. Which one of the following methods is neither meant for the synthesis nor for separation of amines?
   (a) Curtius reaction (b) Wurtz reaction
   (c) Hofmann method (d) Hinsberg method
7. Amongst the following the most basic compound is
   (a) p -nitroaniline (b) acetanilide
   (c) aniline (d) benzylamine
8. Which of the following is not correct ?
   (a) Ethyl amine and aniline both have $-NH_2$ group
   (b) Ethyl amine and aniline dissolve in HCl
   (c) Ethyl amine and aniline both react with $CHCl_3$ and KOH to form unpleasant smelling compound
   (d) Ethyl amine and aniline both react with HNO_2 in cold to give hydroxy compounds

RESPONSE GRID					
	1. ⓐⓑⓒⓓ	2. ⓐⓑⓒⓓ	3. ⓐⓑⓒⓓ	4. ⓐⓑⓒⓓ	5. ⓐⓑⓒⓓ
	6. ⓐⓑⓒⓓ	7. ⓐⓑⓒⓓ	8. ⓐⓑⓒⓓ		

Space for Rough Work

9. Arrange the following amines in the order of increasing basicity.

(a) $CH_3NH_2 < C_6H_5NH_2 < p\text{-}CH_3OC_6H_4NH_2 < p\text{-}O_2NC_6H_4NH_2$

(b) $p\text{-}CH_3OC_6H_4NH_2 < p\text{-}O_2NC_6H_4NH_2 < C_6H_5NH_2 < CH_3NH_2$

(c) $p\text{-}O_2NC_6H_4NH_2 < C_6H_5NH_2 < p\text{-}CH_3OC_6H_4NH_2 < CH_3NH_2$

(d) $C_6H_5NH_2 < p\text{-}CH_3OC_6H_4NH_2 < p\text{-}O_2NC_6H_4NH_2 < CH_3NH_2$

10. When bromination of aniline is carried out by protecting $-NH_2$. The product is
(a) o-bromoaniline
(b) 2, 4, 6-tribromoaniline
(c) p-bromoaniline
(d) mixture of o-and p-bromoaniline

11. Ethyl isocyanide on hydrolysis in acidic medium generates
(a) propanoic acid and ammonium salt
(b) ethanoic acid and ammonium salt
(c) methylamine salt and ethanoic acid
(d) ethylamine salt and methanoic acid

12. Which one of the following is the strongest base in aqueous solution ?
(a) Methylamine (b) Trimethylamine
(c) Aniline (d) Dimethylamine

13. Tautomerism will be exhibited by
(a) $(CH_3)_3CNO$ (b) $(CH_3)_2NH$
(c) R_3CNO_2 (d) RCH_2NO_2

14. Amongst the compounds given, the one that would form a brilliant colored dye on treatment with $NaNO_2$ in dil. HCl followed by addition to an alkaline solution of β-naphthol is

(a) 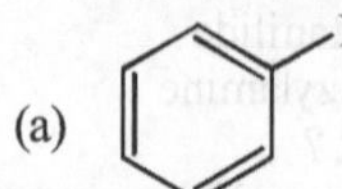

(b) 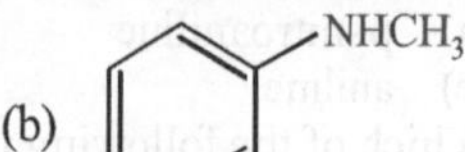

(c) $H_3C-C_6H_4-NH_2$ (d) $C_6H_5CH_2NH_2$

15. Amongst the given set of reactants, the most appropriate for preparing 2° amine is ________.
(a) 2°R–Br + NH_3
(b) 2°R–Br + NaCN followed by H_2/Pt
(c) 1°R–NH_2 + RCHO followed by H_2/Pt
(d) 1°R–Br (2 mol) + Potassium phthalimide followed by H_3O^+/heat

16. In the chemical reaction,
$CH_3CH_2NH_2 + CHCl_3 + 3KOH \rightarrow$
(A) + (B) + $3H_2O$, the compounds (A) and (B) are respectively
(a) C_2H_5NC and 3KCl
(b) C_2H_5CN and 3KCl
(c) $CH_3CH_2CONH_2$ and 3KCl
(d) C_2H_5NC and K_2CO_3

17. Which of the following is not an explosive?
(a) Nitroglycerine (b) o-Aminotoluene
(c) Dynamite (d) Trinitrotoluene

18. Which of the following reagents will be useful to distinguish between
$H_3C-C_6H_4-NH_2$ and $-C_6H_4-CH_2NH_2$?
(a) Dilute HCl
(b) $C_6H_5SO_2Cl$ and OH^-/H_2O
(c) HONO then β -naphthol
(d) $AgNO_3$ in H_2O

19. High basicity of Me_2NH relative to Me_3N is attributed to:
(a) effect of solvent (b) inductive effect of Me
(c) shape of Me_2NH (d) shape of Me_3N

20. The major product of the reaction

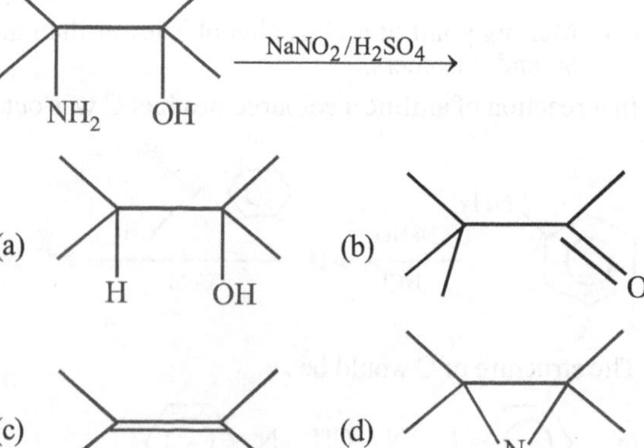

RESPONSE GRID					
	9. ⓐⓑⓒⓓ	10. ⓐⓑⓒⓓ	11. ⓐⓑⓒⓓ	12. ⓐⓑⓒⓓ	13. ⓐⓑⓒⓓ
	14. ⓐⓑⓒⓓ	15. ⓐⓑⓒⓓ	16. ⓐⓑⓒⓓ	17. ⓐⓑⓒⓓ	18. ⓐⓑⓒⓓ
	19. ⓐⓑⓒⓓ	20. ⓐⓑⓒⓓ			

Space for Rough Work

21. Which reaction sequence would be best to prepare 3-chloroanilne from benzene ?
(a) Chlorination, nitration, reduction
(b) Nitration, chlorination, reduction
(c) Nitration, reduction, chlorination
(d) Nitration, reduction, acetylation, chlorination, hydrolysis

22. In the following reaction, X is

$$X \xrightarrow{\text{Bromination}} Y \xrightarrow{NaO_2/HCl} Z \xrightarrow[C_2H_5OH]{\text{Boiling}} \text{Tribromobenzene}$$

(a) Benzoic acid (b) Salicyclic acid
(c) Phenol (d) Aniline

23. $R-NH_2 + \underset{(excess)}{CH_3COCl} \longrightarrow A$
The product (A) will be –
(a) $RNHCOCH_3$ (b) $RN(COCH_3)_2$
(c) $R\overset{+}{N}(COCH_3)_3Cl^-$ (d) $R-CONH_2$

24. 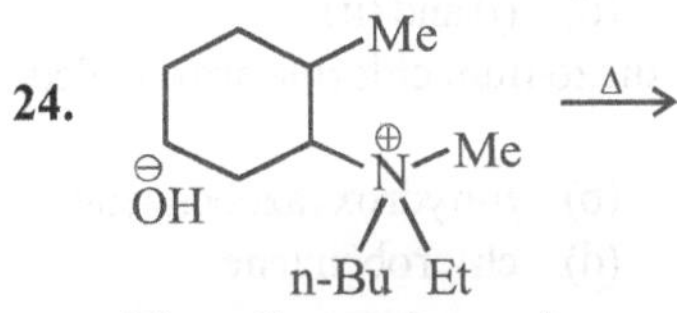

The alkene formed as a major product in the above elimination reaction is
(a) 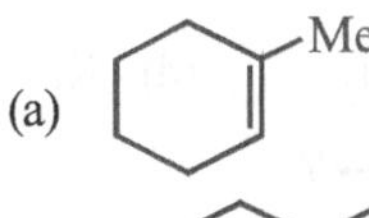

(b) 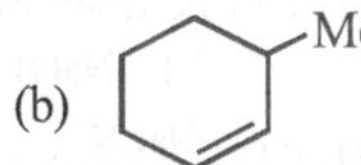

(c) Me (allyl structure) (d) $CH_2=CH_2$

25. N– ethyl benzene sulphonyl amide is strongly acidic and soluble in alkali due to presence of
(a) strong electron donating sulphonyl group.
(b) strong electron withdrawing sulphonyl group.
(c) weak electron donating sulphonyl group.
(d) weak electron withdrawing sulphonyl group.

26. Match the columns

	Column-I		Column-II
A.	Benzene sulphonyl chloride	I.	Zwitter ion
B.	Sulphanilic acid	II.	Hinsberg reagent
C.	Alkyl diazonium salts	III.	Dyes
D.	Aryl diazonium salts	IV.	Conversion to alcohols

(a) A – IV; B – II; C – III; D – I
(b) A – II; B – I; C – IV; D – III
(c) A – III; B – IV; C – I; D – II
(d) A – IV; B – I; C – III; D – II

27. Primary amines can be distinguished from secondary and tertiary amines by reacting with
(a) Chloroform and alcoholic KOH
(b) Methyl iodide
(c) Chloroform alone
(d) Zinc dust

28. The indicator that is obtained by coupling the diazonium salt of sulphanilic acid with N, N-dimethylaniline is
(a) phenanthroline (b) methyl orange
(c) methyl red (d) phenolphthalein

29. Among the following compounds, the increasing order of their basic strength is :

(I) 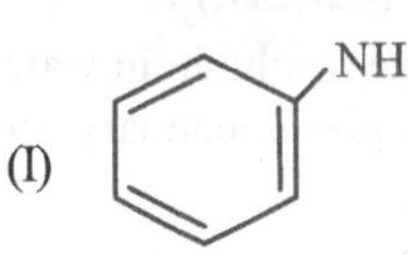

(II) 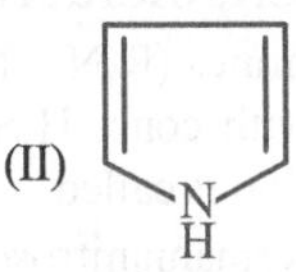

(III) 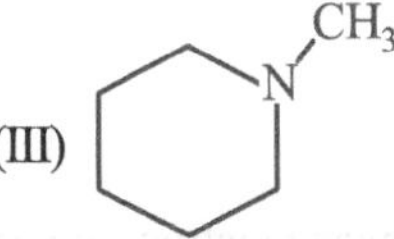

(IV) 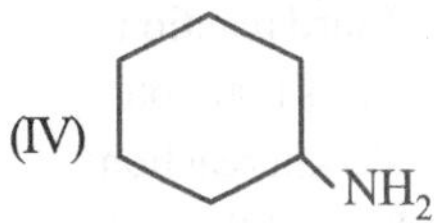

(a) (I) < (II) < (IV) < (III)
(b) (I) < (II) < (III) < (IV)
(c) (II) < (I) < (IV) < (III)
(d) (II) < (I) < (III) < (IV)

30. The correct order of basicity of the following compounds

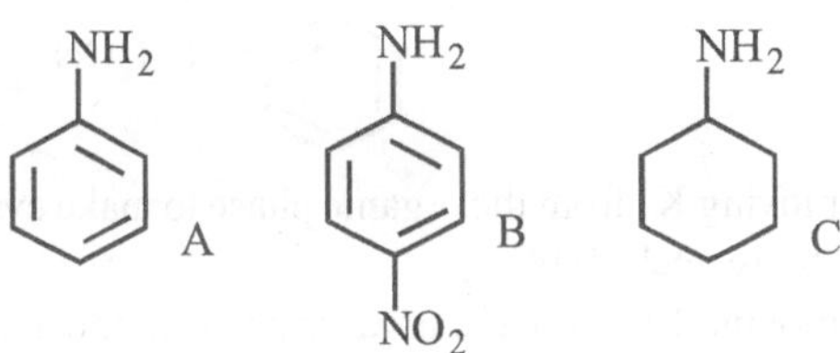

(a) B > A > C (b) A > B > C
(c) C > A > B (d) C > B > A

31. Which of the following compounds cannot be identified by carbylamine test?
(a) $CH_3CH_2NH_2$ (b) $CHCl_3$
(c) $C_6H_5NH_2$ (d) $C_6H_5–NH–C_6H_5$

32. A compound with molecular mass 180 is acylated with CH_3COCl to get a compound with molecular mass 390. The number of amino groups present per molecule of the former compound is :
(a) 2 (b) 5 (c) 4 (d) 6

33. Reaction of cyclohexanone with dimethylamine in the presence of catalytic amount of an acid forms a compound if water during the reaction is continuously removed. The compound formed is generally known as
(a) an amine (b) an imine
(c) an anemine (d) a Schiff's base

34. Match the compounds in List I with their nature from List II, as seen in aqueous medium

	List I		List II
A.	Acetamide	I.	Acidic
B.	Benzonitrile	II.	Basic
C.	Triethylamine	III.	Neutral
D.	Phenol		

(a) A–III; B–III; C–II; D–I
(b) A–II; B–III; C–III; D–I
(c) A–III; B–II; C–II; D–III
(d) A–I; B–I; C–III; D–II

RESPONSE GRID				
21. ⓐⓑⓒⓓ	22. ⓐⓑⓒⓓ	23. ⓐⓑⓒⓓ	24. ⓐⓑⓒⓓ	25. ⓐⓑⓒⓓ
26. ⓐⓑⓒⓓ	27. ⓐⓑⓒⓓ	28. ⓐⓑⓒⓓ	29. ⓐⓑⓒⓓ	30. ⓐⓑⓒⓓ
31. ⓐⓑⓒⓓ	32. ⓐⓑⓒⓓ	33. ⓐⓑⓒⓓ	34. ⓐⓑⓒⓓ	

Space for Rough Work

35. An organic amino compound reacts with aqueous nitrous acid at low temperature to produce an oily nitrosoamine. The compound is
(a) CH_3NH_2 (b) $CH_3CH_2NH_2$
(c) $CH_3CH_2NHCH_2CH_3$ (d) $(CH_3CH_2)_3N$

36. Nitrosoamines ($R_2N-N=O$) are insoluble in water. On heating with conc. H_2SO_4, they give secondary amines. The reaction is called
(a) Liebermann nitroso reaction
(b) Etard reaction
(c) Fries reaction
(d) Perkin reaction

37. In which of the following two phase reaction, the catalyst works by ?

$$C_6H_5CH_2Br + KCN \xrightarrow[H_2O/heptane]{C_6H_5CH_2\overset{+}{N}(CH_3)_3\overline{Cl}} C_6H_5CH_2CN + KBr$$

(a) Removing K^+ from the organic phase to make cyanide ion more nucleophilic.
(b) Removing Br^- from the organic phase to the aqueous phase.
(c) Transferring CN^- from the aqueous phase to organic phase containing $C_6H_5CH_2Br$.
(d) Transferring $C_6H_5CH_2Br$ from the organic phase to the aqueous phase containing CN^-

38. Match the compounds in List I with the appropriate test that will be answered by each one of them in List II

	List I		List II
A.	Propyne Fehling's	I.	Reduces solutions
B.	Ethyl benzoate	II.	Forms a precipitate with $AgNO_3$ in ethanol
C.	Acetaldehyde	III.	Insoluble in water but dissolves in aqueous NaOH solution upon heating
D.	Aniline	IV.	Dissolves in dilute HCl in the cold and is reprecipitated by the addition of alkali

(a) A–I; B–IV; C–II; D–I (b) A–I; B–IV; C–III; D–II
(c) A–IV; B–II; C–III; D–I (d) A–II; B–III; C–I; D–IV

39. All three amines 1°, 2°, 3° react with
1. H_2O 2. R–X 3. HCl 4. $(CH_3CO)_2O$
(a) 1,2 (b) 4 only (c) 1, 2, 4 (d) 1, 2, 3

40. Hinsberg reagent is
(a) $C_6H_5SO_3H$ (b) C_6H_5NO
(c) $C_6H_5SO_2Cl$ (d) $C_6H_5N_2Cl$

41. Which of the following amines can be prepared by Gabriel method ?
(i) $CH_3CH_2NH_2$ (ii) $(CH_3)_2CHNH_2$
(iii) $(CH_3)_3CNH_2$ (iv) $C_6H_5NH_2$
(a) (i) and (iii) (b) (ii) and (iv)
(c) (i), (ii) and (iii) (d) (i) and (ii)

42. When phenol and benzene diazonium chloride are coupled, the main product is :
(a) aniline (b) *p*-hydroxyazobenzene
(c) azobenzene (d) chlorobenzene

43. Replacement of $-N_2^+Cl^-$ from benzene diazonium chloride by iodine can be done by using
(a) HI (b) NaOI (c) PI_3 (d) KI

44. $CH_3CH_2Cl \xrightarrow{NaCN} X \xrightarrow{Ni/H_2} Y \xrightarrow{\text{acetic anhydride}} Z$

Z in the above reacting sequence is
(a) $CH_3CH_2CH_2NHCOCH_3$
(b) $CH_3CH_2CH_2NH_2$
(c) $CH_3CH_2CH_2CONHCH_3$
(d) $CH_3CH_2CH_2CONHCOCH_3$

45. Towards electrophilic substitution, the most reactive will be
(a) Nitrobenzene
(b) Aniline
(c) Aniline hydrochloride
(d) N-Acetylaniline

RESPONSE GRID					
	35. ⓐⓑⓒⓓ	36. ⓐⓑⓒⓓ	37. ⓐⓑⓒⓓ	38. ⓐⓑⓒⓓ	39. ⓐⓑⓒⓓ
	40. ⓐⓑⓒⓓ	41. ⓐⓑⓒⓓ	42. ⓐⓑⓒⓓ	43. ⓐⓑⓒⓓ	44. ⓐⓑⓒⓓ
	45. ⓐⓑⓒⓓ				

CHEMISTRY CHAPTERWISE SPEED TEST-55

Total Questions	45	Total Marks	180
Attempted		Correct	
Incorrect		Net Score	
Cut-off Score	34	Qualifying Score	55

Success Gap = Net Score – Qualifying Score

Net Score = (Correct × 4) – (Incorrect × 1)

Space for Rough Work

CHEMISTRY

Biomolecules

Speed TEST 56 Chapter-wise

No. of Questions	Maximum Marks	Time
45	180	1 Hour

GENERAL INSTRUCTIONS

- This test contains 45 MCQ's. For each question only one option is correct. Darken the correct circle/ bubble in the Response Grid provided on each page.
- You have to evaluate your Response Grids yourself with the help of solutions provided at the end of this book.
- Each correct answer will get you 4 marks and 1 mark shall be deduced for each incorrect answer. No mark will be given/ deducted if no bubble is filled. Keep a timer in front of you and stop immediately at the end of 60 min.
- The sheet follows a particular syllabus. Do not attempt the sheet before you have completed your preparation for that syllabus.
- After completing the sheet check your answers with the solution booklet and complete the Result Grid. Finally spend time to analyse your performance and revise the areas which emerge out as weak in your evaluation.

1. Chemically amylose is a _________ with 200–1000 α-D-(+)-glucose units held by ______ glycosidic linkage
   (a) long unbranched chain, C1– C6.
   (b) branched chain, C1 – C4.
   (c) long unbranched chain, C1– C4.
   (d) branched chain, C1– C6.
2. Which is wrongly matched?
   (a) Insulin - steroid hormone
   (b) Estrone - control the uterine cycle in women
   (c) Oxytocin - contraction of uterus
   (d) Pot. metabisulphite - food preservative
3. In nucleic acids, the sequence is
   (a) phosphate - base - sugar
   (b) sugar- base-phosphate
   (c) base- sugar - phosphate
   (d) base- phosphate - sugar
4. Read the following statements and choose the correct– option?
   (i) Starch is a polymer of α – glucose.
   (ii) Starch consists of amylose and amylopectin.
   (iii) Amylose is insoluble in water.
   (iv) Amylopectin is soluble in water.
   (a) (i) (iii) and (iv) (b) (i), (ii) and (iii)
   (c) (i) and (ii) (d) (iii) and (iv)
5. An acidic amino acid among the following is
   (a) glycine (b) valine
   (c) proline (d) histidine
6. If one strand of DNA has the sequence ATGCTTGA, the sequence in the complimentary strand would be
   (a) TACGAACT (b) TCCGAACT
   (c) TACGTACT (d) TACGTAGT
7. The hormone produced by pancreas
   (a) Adrenaline (b) Glucogen
   (c) Thyroxene (d) Cortisone

RESPONSE GRID	
1. ⓐⓑⓒⓓ 2. ⓐⓑⓒⓓ 3. ⓐⓑⓒⓓ 4. ⓐⓑⓒⓓ 5. ⓐⓑⓒⓓ	
6. ⓐⓑⓒⓓ 7. ⓐⓑⓒⓓ	

Space for Rough Work

8. Match the columns

	Column - I (Enzymes)		Column - II (Reactions)
(A)	Invertase	I.	Decomposition of urea into NH_3 and CO_2
(B)	Maltase	II.	Conversion of glucose into ethyl alcohol
(C)	Pepsin	III.	Hydrolysis of maltose into glucose
(D)	Urease	IV.	Hydrolysis of cane sugar
(E)	Zymase	V.	Hydrolysis of proteins into peptides

(a) A – IV; B – III; C – V; D – I; E – II
(b) A – III; B – II; C – IV; D – I; E – V
(c) A – II; B – I; C – III; D – IV; E – V
(d) A – IV; B – I; C – V; D – II; E – III

9. Which of the following structures represents thymine ?

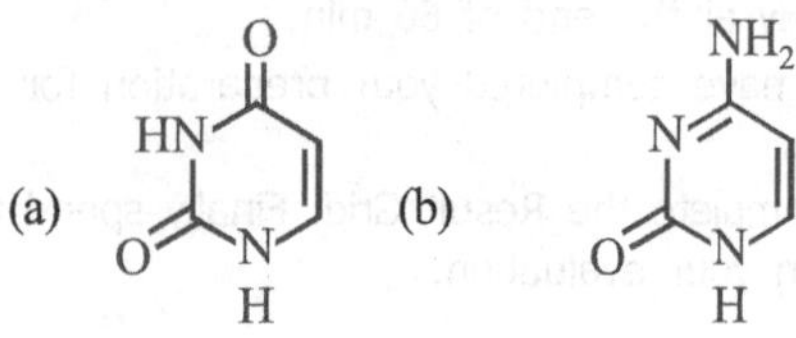

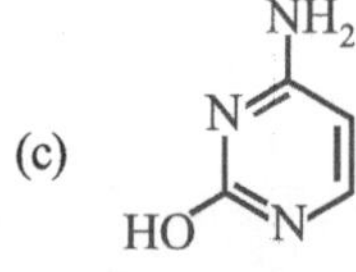

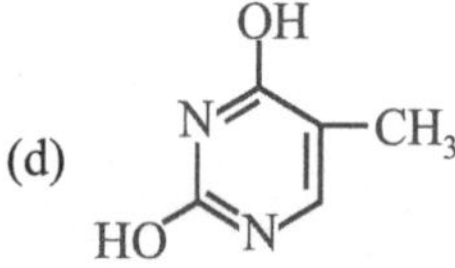

10. Which statement is incorrect about peptide bond?
(a) C–N bond length in proteins is longer than usual C–N bond length
(b) Spectroscopic analysis shows planar structure of $-\underset{\underset{O}{\|}}{C}-NH-$ bond
(c) C–N bond length in proteins is smaller than usual C–N bond length
(d) None of these

11. The presence or absence of hydroxyl group on which carbon atom of sugar differentiates RNA and DNA?
(a) 1st (b) 2nd
(c) 3rd (d) 4th

12. Which of the following compounds can be detected by Molisch's Test ?
(a) Nitro compounds (b) Sugars
(c) Amines (d) Primary alcohols

13. Night blindness is caused by deficiency of vitamin :
(a) Vit – B_{12} (b) Vit – A
(c) Vit – C (d) Vit – E

14. Which of the following is correct about H-bonding in nucleotide?
(a) A --- A and T --- T (b) G --- T and A --- C
(c) A --- G and T --- C (d) A --- T and G --- C

15. In an amino acid, the carboxyl group ionises at $pK_{a_1} = 2.34$ and ammonium ion at $pK_{a_2} = 9.60$. The isoelectric point of the amino acid is at pH
(a) 5.97 (b) 2.34
(c) 9.60 (d) 6.97

16. The secondary structure of a protein refers to
(a) fixed configuration of the polypeptide backbone
(b) α – helical backbone
(c) hydrophobic interactions
(d) sequence of α – amino acids.

17. Which of the following statements regarding DNA fingerprinting is incorrect?
(a) It is used in forensic laboratories for identification of criminals.
(b) It cannot be altered by surgery.
(c) It is different for every cell and cannot be altered by any known treatment.
(d) It is used to determine paternity of an individual.

18. The artificial sweetener that has the highest sweetness value in comparison to cane sugar is :
(a) Sucralose (b) Aspartane
(c) Saccharin (d) Alitame

19. The term invert sugar refers to an equimolar mixture of
(a) D-glucose and D-galactose
(b) D-glucose and D-fructose
(c) D-glucose and D-mannose
(d) D-glucose and D-ribose

RESPONSE GRID				
8. ⓐⓑⓒⓓ	9. ⓐⓑⓒⓓ	10. ⓐⓑⓒⓓ	11. ⓐⓑⓒⓓ	12. ⓐⓑⓒⓓ
13. ⓐⓑⓒⓓ	14. ⓐⓑⓒⓓ	15. ⓐⓑⓒⓓ	16. ⓐⓑⓒⓓ	17. ⓐⓑⓒⓓ
18. ⓐⓑⓒⓓ	19. ⓐⓑⓒⓓ			

Space for Rough Work

20. Which of the following compounds will behave as a reducing sugar in an aqueous KOH solution?

(a) 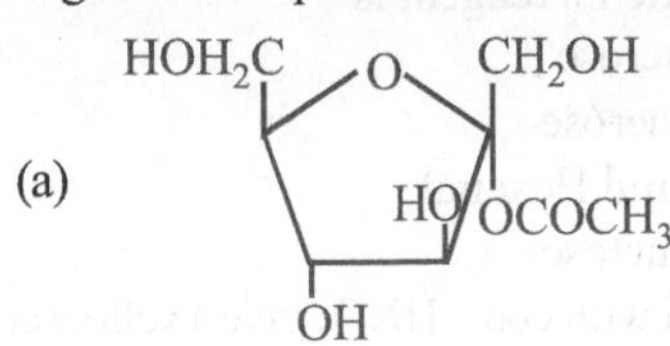

(b) 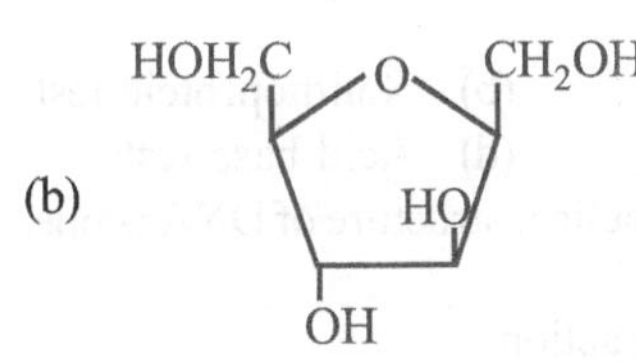

(c) HOH_2C O CH_2OH HO OCH_3 OH

(d) HOH_2C O CH_2OCH_3 OH OH OH

21. For osazone formation, the effective structural unit necessary is

(a) CH_2OCH_3 | CO |
(b) CH_2OH | CO |
(c) CH_2OH | $CHOCH_3$ |
(d) CHO | $CHOCH_3$ |

22. Which of the following statements about vitamin B_{12} is incorrect ?

(a) It has a cobalt atom
(b) It also occurs in plants
(c) It is also present in rain water
(d) It is needed for human body in very small amounts

23. The following carbohydrate is

H, OH, H, O, HO, HO, OH, H, OH, H, H

(a) a ketohexose (b) an aldohexose
(c) an α-furanose (d) an α-pyranose

24. The two functional groups present in a typical carbohydrate are:

(a) – CHO and – COOH (b) >C = O and – OH
(c) – OH and – CHO (d) – OH and – COOH

25. Deficiency of vitamin E causes :

(a) Beriberi (b) Scurvy
(c) Sterility (d) None

26. Which of the following terms indicates to the arrangement of different protein subunits in a multiprotein complex ?

(a) primary structure (b) secondary structure
(c) tertiary structure (d) quaternary structure

27. The term anomers of glucose refers to

(a) enantiomers of glucose
(b) isomers of glucose that differ in configuration at carbon one (C-1)
(c) isomers of glucose that differ in configurations at carbons one and four (C-1 and C-4)
(d) a mixture of (D)-glucose and (L)-glucose

28. In both DNA and RNA, heterocyclic base and phosphate ester linkages are at –

(a) C_5' and C_1' respectively of the sugar molecule
(b) C_1' and C_5' respectively of the sugar molecule
(c) C_2' and C_5' respectively of the sugar molecule
(d) C_5' and C_2' respectively of the sugar molecule

29. An amine hormone is

(a) Cortisone (b) Adrenaline
(c) Insulin (d) Estrone

30. Amino acids generally exist in the form of Zwitter ions. This means they contain

(a) basic—NH_2 group and acidic —COOH group
(b) the basic— $\overset{+}{N}H_3$ group and acidic —COO^- group
(c) basic—NH_2 and acidic —H^+ group
(d) basic–COO^- group and acidic — $\overset{+}{N}H_3$ group

31. The change in the optical rotation (with time) of freshly prepared solution of sugar is known as

(a) Specific rotation (b) Inversion
(c) Rotatory motion (d) Mutarotation

32. Phospholipids are esters of glycerol with

(a) two carboxylic acid residues and one phosphate group
(b) one carboxylic acid residue and two phosphate groups
(c) three phosphate groups
(d) three carboxylic acid residues

RESPONSE GRID					
	20. ⓐⓑⓒⓓ	21. ⓐⓑⓒⓓ	22. ⓐⓑⓒⓓ	23. ⓐⓑⓒⓓ	24. ⓐⓑⓒⓓ
	25. ⓐⓑⓒⓓ	26. ⓐⓑⓒⓓ	27. ⓐⓑⓒⓓ	28. ⓐⓑⓒⓓ	29. ⓐⓑⓒⓓ
	30. ⓐⓑⓒⓓ	31. ⓐⓑⓒⓓ	32. ⓐⓑⓒⓓ		

Space for Rough Work

33. When glucose reacts with bromine water, the main product is
(a) gluconic acid (b) glyceraldehyde
(c) saccharic acid (d) acetic acid

34. Among the following vitamins the one whose deficiency causes rickets (bone deficiency) is
(a) Vitamin A (b) Vitamin B
(c) Vitamin D (d) Vitamin C

35. Three cyclic structures of monosaccharides are given below which of these are anomers

(I)	(II)	(III)
H—C—OH	HO—C—H	HO—C—H
H—C—OH	H—C—OH	HO—C—H
HO—C—H	HO—C—H	HO—C—H
H—C—OH	H—C—OH	H—C—OH
H—C (ring O)	H—C (ring O)	HO—C—H
CH_2OH	CH_2OH	H—C (ring O)
		CH_2OH

(a) I and II (b) II and III
(c) I and III (d) III is anomer of I and II

36. Glucose molecule reacts with X number of molecules of phenylhydrazine to yield osazone. The value of X is
(a) three (b) two
(c) one (d) four

37. Which of the following indicates to 'regions of ordered structure within a protein'.
(a) Primary structure (b) Secondary structure
(c) Tertiary structure (d) Quaternary structure

38. Denaturation of proteins leads to loss of its biological activity by
(a) Formation of amino acids
(b) Loss of primary structure
(c) Loss of both primary and secondary structures
(d) Loss of both secondary and tertiary structures

39. The pair of compounds in which both the compounds give positive test with Tollen's reagent is
(a) Glucose and Sucrose
(b) Fructose and Sucrose
(c) Acetophenone and Hexanal
(d) Glucose and Fructose

40. Proteins when heated with conc. HNO_3 give a yellow colour. This is
(a) Oxidizing test (b) Xanthoproteic test
(c) Hoppe's test (d) Acid base test

41. The reason for double helical structure of DNA is operation of
(a) dipole-dipole interaction
(b) hydrogen bonding
(c) electrostatic attractions
(d) van der Waals' forces

42. Which of the statements about "Denaturation" given below are correct ?
(i) Denaturation of proteins causes loss of secondary and tertiary structures of the protein.
(ii) Denaturation leads to the conversion of double strand of DNA into single strand
(iii) Denaturation affects primary strucrture which gets distorted
(a) (ii) and (iii) (b) (i) and (iii)
(c) (i) and (ii) (d) (i), (ii) and (iii)

43. Which of the following protein destroy the antigen when it enters in body cell?
(a) Antibodies (b) Insulin
(c) Chromoprotein (d) Phosphoprotein

44. Glucose can't be classified as
(a) hexose (b) carbohydrate
(c) aldose (d) oligosaccharide

45. Hydrolysis of sucrose is called
(a) hydration (b) saponification
(c) esterification (d) inversion

RESPONSE GRID					
	33. (a)(b)(c)(d)	34. (a)(b)(c)(d)	35. (a)(b)(c)(d)	36. (a)(b)(c)(d)	37. (a)(b)(c)(d)
	38. (a)(b)(c)(d)	39. (a)(b)(c)(d)	40. (a)(b)(c)(d)	41. (a)(b)(c)(d)	42. (a)(b)(c)(d)
	43. (a)(b)(c)(d)	44. (a)(b)(c)(d)	45. (a)(b)(c)(d)		

CHEMISTRY CHAPTERWISE SPEED TEST-56

Total Questions	45	Total Marks	180
Attempted		Correct	
Incorrect		Net Score	
Cut-off Score	38	Qualifying Score	58

Success Gap = Net Score – Qualifying Score

Net Score = (Correct × 4) – (Incorrect × 1)

Space for Rough Work

CHEMISTRY

Polymers

Speed TEST 57

Chapter-wise

No. of Questions	Maximum Marks	Time
45	180	1 Hour

GENERAL INSTRUCTIONS

- This test contains 45 MCQ's. For each question only one option is correct. Darken the correct circle/ bubble in the Response Grid provided on each page.
- You have to evaluate your Response Grids yourself with the help of solutions provided at the end of this book.
- Each correct answer will get you 4 marks and 1 mark shall be deduced for each incorrect answer. No mark will be given/ deducted if no bubble is filled. Keep a timer in front of you and stop immediately at the end of 60 min.
- The sheet follows a particular syllabus. Do not attempt the sheet before you have completed your preparation for that syllabus.
- After completing the sheet check your answers with the solution booklet and complete the Result Grid. Finally spend time to analyse your performance and revise the areas which emerge out as weak in your evaluation.

1. Which of the following catalyst is used in preparation of high density polythene ?
   (a) Peroxide catalyst
   (b) Ziegler - Natta catalyst
   (c) Wilkinson's catalyst
   (d) Pd - catalyst
2. Among cellulose, polyvinyl chloride, nylon and natural rubber, the polymer in which the intermolecular force of attraction is weakest is
   (a) nylon (b) polyvinyl chloride
   (c) cellulose (d) natural Rubber
3. Polyvinylalcohol can be prepared by
   (a) polymerization of vinyl alcohol
   (b) alkaline hydrolysis of polyvinyl acetate
   (c) polymerization of acetylene
   (d) reaction of acetylene with H_2SO_4 in presence of $HgSO_4$
4. Which of the following polymer is an example of fibre ?
   (a) Silk (b) Dacron
   (c) Nylon-6, 6 (d) All of these
5. Which compound/set of compounds is used in the manufacture of nylon 6?
   (a) $C_6H_5-CH=CH_2$
   (b) $HOOC(CH_2)_4COOH + NH_2(CH_2)_6NH_2$
   (c) $CH_2=CH-\underset{|}{\overset{CH_3}{C}}=CH_2$
   (d) cyclohexanone (cyclohexane ring with C=O)
6. The polymer containing strong intermolecular forces e.g. hydrogen bonding, is
   (a) teflon (b) nylon 6, 6
   (c) polystyrene (d) natural rubber
7. Which one of the following polymers is prepared by condensation polymerisation?
   (a) Teflon (b) Natural rubber
   (c) Styrene (d) Nylon-6, 6
8. Three dimensional molecules with cross links are formed in the case of a
   (a) thermoplastic (b) thermosetting plastic
   (c) both (a) and (b) (d) none of the above
9. In elastomer, intermolecular forces are
   (a) strong (b) weak
   (c) nil (d) none of these
10. Nylon 6, 6 is a polyamide obtained by the reaction of
    (a) $COOH(CH_2)_4COOH + NH_2C_6H_4NH_2$
    (b) $COOH(CH_2)_4COOH + NH_2(CH_2)_6NH_2$
    (c) $COOH(CH_2)_6COOH + NH_2(CH_2)_4NH_2$
    (d) $COOHC_6H_4COOH\text{-}(p) + NH_2(CH_2)_6NH_2$

RESPONSE GRID					
	1. ⓐⓑⓒⓓ	2. ⓐⓑⓒⓓ	3. ⓐⓑⓒⓓ	4. ⓐⓑⓒⓓ	5. ⓐⓑⓒⓓ
	6. ⓐⓑⓒⓓ	7. ⓐⓑⓒⓓ	8. ⓐⓑⓒⓓ	9. ⓐⓑⓒⓓ	10. ⓐⓑⓒⓓ

Space for Rough Work

11. Buna-N synthetic rubber is a copolymer of :
(a) $H_2C=CH-CH=CH_2$ and $H_5C_6-CH=CH_2$
(b) $H_2C=CH-CN$ and $H_2C=CH-CH=CH_2$
(c) $H_2C=CH-CN$ and $H_2C=CH-C(CH_3)=CH_2$
(d) $H_2C=CH-C(Cl)=CH_2$ and $H_2C=CH-CH=CH_2$

12. Interparticle forces present in nylon-6, 6 are
(a) van der Waal's
(b) hydrogen bonding
(c) dipole-dipole interactions
(d) None of the above

13. Monomer of $\left[-\underset{CH_3}{\overset{CH_3}{C}}-CH_2-\right]_n$ is
(a) 2-Methylpropene (b) Styrene
(c) Propylene (d) Ethene

14. Which of the following is not correctly matched?
(a) Neoprene; $\left[-CH_2-\underset{Cl}{C}=CH-CH_2-\right]_n$
(b) Nylon-6, 6: $\left[-NH-(CH_2)_6-NH-CO-(CH_2)_4-\overset{O}{\overset{||}{C}}-O-\right]_n$
(c) Terylene; $\left[-OCH_2-CH_2-O-\overset{O}{\overset{||}{C}}-C_6H_4-\overset{O}{\overset{||}{C}}-\right]_n$
(d) PMMA : $\left[-CH_2-\underset{COOCH_3}{\overset{CH_3}{C}}-\right]_n$

15. Which of the following compound is used for preparation of melamine formaldehyde polymer ?
(a) $C_6H_5NH_2$ (aniline)
(b) triazine ring (N–N=N) with three NH_2 groups
(c) 2,4,6-triamino-1,3,5-triazine (ring of three N with three NH_2 groups)
(d) pyridine ring with two NH_2 groups

16. Acrilan is a hard, horny and a high melting material. Which of the following represents its structure?
(a) $\left(-CH_2-\underset{COOCH_3}{\overset{CH_3}{C}}-\right)_n$ (b) $\left(-CH_2-\underset{COOC_2H_5}{CH}-\right)_n$
(c) $\left(-CH_2-\underset{Cl}{CH}-\right)_n$ (d) $\left(-CH_2-\underset{CN}{CH}-\right)_n$

17. Bakelite is obtained from phenol by reacting with
(a) $(CH_2OH)_2$ (b) CH_3CHO
(c) CH_3COCH_3 (d) HCHO

18. Polymer formation from monomers starts by
(a) condensation reaction between monomers
(b) coordinate reaction between monomers
(c) conversion of monomer to monomer ions by protons
(d) hydrolysis of monomers.

19. Melamine plastic crockery is a codensation polymer of
(a) HCHO and melamine
(b) HCHO and ethylene
(c) melamine and ethylene
(d) None of these

RESPONSE GRID				
11. ⓐⓑⓒⓓ	12. ⓐⓑⓒⓓ	13. ⓐⓑⓒⓓ	14. ⓐⓑⓒⓓ	15. ⓐⓑⓒⓓ
16. ⓐⓑⓒⓓ	17. ⓐⓑⓒⓓ	18. ⓐⓑⓒⓓ	19. ⓐⓑⓒⓓ	

Space for Rough Work

20. Which of the following is a polyamide?
(a) Bakelite (b) Terylene
(c) Nylon-6, 6 (d) Teflon

21. Terylene is a condensation polymer of ethylene glycol and
(a) benzoic acid (b) phthalic acid
(c) salicyclic acid (d) terephthalic acid

22. The monomer of the polymer;

$$\sim\sim CH_2-\underset{CH_3}{\overset{CH_3}{|}{C}}-CH_2-\overset{\oplus}{C}(CH_3)_2 \text{ is}$$

(a) $H_2C=C(CH_3)_2$ (b) $CH_3CH{=}CHCH_3$
(c) $CH_3CH=CH_2$ (d) $(CH_3)_2C=C(CH_3)_2$

23. Generally, molecular mass of a polymer is over
(a) 100 (b) 500
(c) 1,000 (d) 10,000

24. Plexiglas (PMMA) is a polymer of
(a) acrylic acid (b) methyl acrylate
(c) methyl methacrylate (d) None of these

25. Which one of the following is not a condensation polymer ?
(a) Melamine (b) Glyptal
(c) Dacron (d) Neoprene

26. Dacron is obtained by the condensation polymerisation of:
(a) Dimethyl terephthalate and ethylene glycol
(b) Terephthalic acid and formaldehyde
(c) Phenol and phthalic acid
(d) Phenol and formaldehyde

27. Which of the following is not a copolymer?
(a) Buna–S (b) Baketite
(c) Neoprene (d) Dacron

28. Ziegler-Natta catalyst is
(a) $K[PtCl_3(C_2H_4)]$ (b) $(Ph_3P)_3RhCl$
(c) $Al_2(C_2H_5)_6+TiCl_4$ (d) $Fe(C_5H_5)_2$

29. Dacron is a –
(a) crease resistant
(b) polyamide
(c) addition polymer
(d) polymer of ethylene glycol and phthalic acid

30. The turbidity of a polymer solution measures
(a) the light scattered by solution
(b) the light absorbed by a solution
(c) the light transmitted by a solution
(d) None of these

31. Which of the following polymers do not involve cross linkages?
(a) Melmac (b) Bakelite
(c) Polythene (d) Vulcanised rubber

32. Which of the following statements are correct?
(i) Buna–N being resistant to the action of petrol, lubricating oil and organic solvents is used in making oil seals.
(ii) Biodegradable polymers are manufactured because of low chemical resistance, strength and durability of conventional polymers.
(iii) PHBV is a copolymer used in the manufacture of orthopaedic devices.
(iv) Nylon 2–nylon 6 is a biodegradable polymer.
(a) (i), (ii) and (iii) (b) (ii), (iii) and (iv)
(c) (i), (iii) and (iv) (d) (i) and (iv)

33. Arrange the following in increasing order of their melting point.
(1) Nylon 2,2; (2) Nylon 2,4; (3) Nylon 2,6; (4) Nylon 2,10
(a) 1, 2, 3, 4 (b) 3, 4, 2, 1
(c) 2, 1, 3, 4 (d) 4, 3, 2, 1

34. A copolymer of isobutylene and isoprene is called:
(a) butyl rubber (b) buna-S
(c) buna-N (d) thiokol

35. Ebonite is
(a) natural rubber
(b) synthetic rubber
(c) highly vulcanized rubber
(d) polypropene

36. Orlon is a polymer of
(a) styrene (b) tetrafluoroethylene
(c) vinyl chloride (d) acrylonitrile

37. Among the following polymers the strongest molecular forces are present in
(a) elastomers (b) fibres
(c) thermoplastics (d) thermosetting polymers

RESPONSE GRID					
	20. ⓐⓑⓒⓓ	21. ⓐⓑⓒⓓ	22. ⓐⓑⓒⓓ	23. ⓐⓑⓒⓓ	24. ⓐⓑⓒⓓ
	25. ⓐⓑⓒⓓ	26. ⓐⓑⓒⓓ	27. ⓐⓑⓒⓓ	28. ⓐⓑⓒⓓ	29. ⓐⓑⓒⓓ
	30. ⓐⓑⓒⓓ	31. ⓐⓑⓒⓓ	32. ⓐⓑⓒⓓ	33. ⓐⓑⓒⓓ	34. ⓐⓑⓒⓓ
	35. ⓐⓑⓒⓓ	36. ⓐⓑⓒⓓ	37. ⓐⓑⓒⓓ		

Space for Rough Work

38. Caprolactam polymerises to give
(a) terylene (b) teflon
(c) glyptal (d) Nylon-6

39. Match Column-I (Monomer) with Colum-II (Polymer) and select the correct answer using the codes given below the lists:

	Column-I		Column-II
A.	Hexamethylenediamine	I.	Bakelite
B.	Phenol	II.	Dacron
C.	Phthalic acid	III.	Glyptal
D.	Terephthalic acid	IV.	Melamine
		V.	Nylon

(a) A – V; B – I; C – II; D – III
(b) A – V; B – I; C – III; D – II
(c) A – IV; B – III; C – I; D – II
(d) A – IV; B – III; C – II; D – I

40. Which of the following is novolac ?

(a) [Structure: two benzene rings joined by CH_2, each bearing CH_3 and –O– substituents]

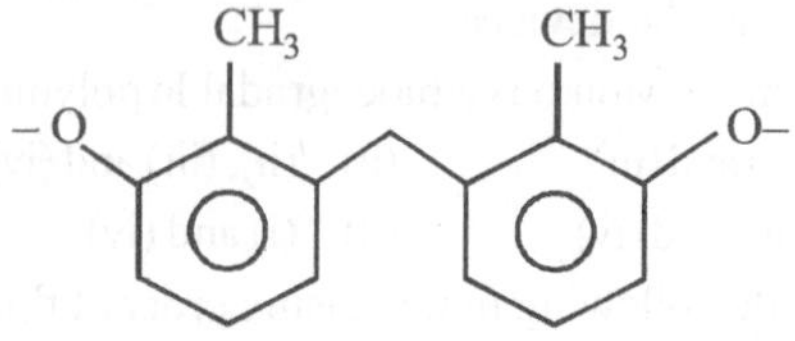

(b) [Structure: benzene ring with OH, $-H_2C$ and CH_3 substituents]

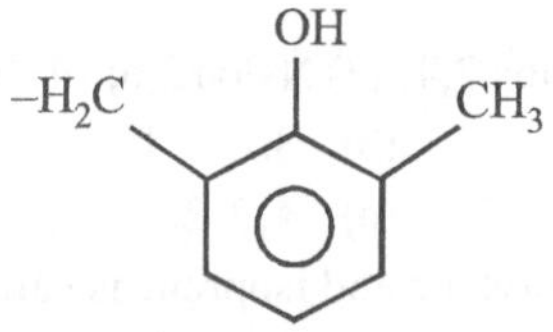

(c) [Structure: benzene ring with OH, CH_2- (ortho) and CH_2- (para) substituents]

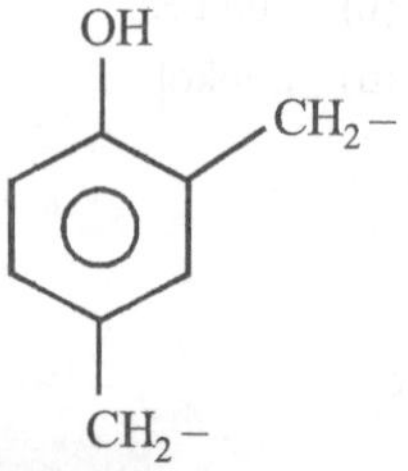

(d) [Structure: $-H_2C$–(phenol ring with OH)–CH_2–(phenol ring with OH)–CH_2-]

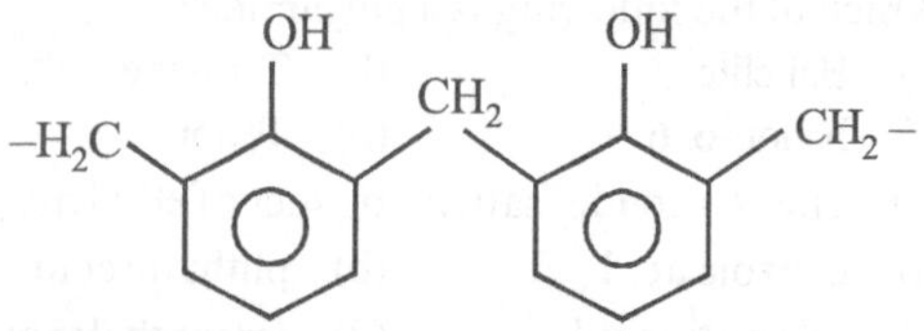

41. Match the polymers given in Column-I with their chemical names given in Column-II

	Column-I		Column-II
A.	Nylon 6	I.	Polyvinyl chloride
B.	PVC	II.	Polyacrylonitrile
C.	Acrolein	III.	Polycaprolactum
D.	Natural rubber	IV.	Low density polythene
E.	LDP	V.	cis-polyisoprene

(a) A – III; B – I; C – II; D – V; E – IV
(b) A – IV; B – II; C – V; D – III; E – I
(c) A – V; B – IV; C – I; D – II; E – III
(d) A – IV; B – V; C – III; D – II; E – I

42. Two condensation polymers are made
(1) ethylene diamine + ethane–1, 2– dicarboxylic acid
(2) trimethylenediamine + ethane–1, 2– dicarboxylic acid
if both polymers of same molecular weight are obtained then which of the following statements is/are correct ?
(i) Polymer (1) is found to melt at lower temperature.
(ii) Polymer (2) is found to melt at lower temperature.
(iii) H-bonding is major factor.
(a) (i), (ii) and (iii) (b) Only (ii)
(c) (i) and (iii) (d) (ii) and (iii)

43. Which of the following polymer is used for making phonograph records ?
(a) Bakelite (b) Dacron
(c) Teflon (d) PVC

44. Which of the following statements is not true about low density polythene?
(a) Tough
(b) Hard
(c) Poor conductor of electricity
(d) Highly branched structure

45. Polymer used in bullet proof glass is
(a) PMMA (b) Lexan
(c) Nomex (d) Kevlar

RESPONSE GRID					
	38. ⓐⓑⓒⓓ	39. ⓐⓑⓒⓓ	40. ⓐⓑⓒⓓ	41. ⓐⓑⓒⓓ	42. ⓐⓑⓒⓓ
	43. ⓐⓑⓒⓓ	44. ⓐⓑⓒⓓ	45. ⓐⓑⓒⓓ		

CHEMISTRY CHAPTERWISE SPEED TEST-57

Total Questions	45	Total Marks	180
Attempted		Correct	
Incorrect		Net Score	
Cut-off Score	46	Qualifying Score	65
Success Gap = Net Score – Qualifying Score			
Net Score = (Correct × 4) – (Incorrect × 1)			

Space for Rough Work

CHEMISTRY

Chemistry in Everyday Life

Speed TEST 58 Chapter-wise

No. of Questions	Maximum Marks	Time
45	180	1 Hour

GENERAL INSTRUCTIONS

- This test contains 45 MCQ's. For each question only one option is correct. Darken the correct circle/ bubble in the Response Grid provided on each page.
- You have to evaluate your Response Grids yourself with the help of solutions provided at the end of this book.
- Each correct answer will get you 4 marks and 1 mark shall be deduced for each incorrect answer. No mark will be given/ deducted if no bubble is filled. Keep a timer in front of you and stop immediately at the end of 60 min.
- The sheet follows a particular syllabus. Do not attempt the sheet before you have completed your preparation for that syllabus.
- After completing the sheet check your answers with the solution booklet and complete the Result Grid. Finally spend time to analyse your performance and revise the areas which emerge out as weak in your evaluation.

1. Which of the following is a hypnotic drug?
   (a) luminal (b) salol
   (c) catechol (d) chemisol
2. Phenolic antibacterial used in body deodrants is
   (a) 2, 4-Dichlorophenol
   (b) p-Chloro-m-xylenol
   (c) p-Chlorophenol
   (d) p-Nitro-m-xylenol
3. Most of the deodorants contain aluminium salts because they
   (a) act as antiperspirants
   (b) act as anti-bacterial agents
   (c) mask body odour
   (d) All the these
4. An example of a psychedelic agent is
   (a) DNA (b) LSD
   (c) DDT (d) TN
5. Which of the following is a bactericidal antibiotic ?
   (a) Ofloxacin
   (b) Tetracycline
   (c) Chloramphenicol
   (d) Erythromycin

RESPONSE GRID	1. ⓐⓑⓒⓓ	2. ⓐⓑⓒⓓ	3. ⓐⓑⓒⓓ	4. ⓐⓑⓒⓓ	5. ⓐⓑⓒⓓ

Space for Rough Work

6. The following compound is used as

(a) an anti-inflammatory compound
(b) analgesic
(c) hypnotic
(d) antiseptic

7. The substance which is not an artificial sweetener
(a) sucralose (b) alitame
(c) saccharin (d) sucrose

8. Alum is used by dyers for cloth
(a) for fire- proofing fabrics
(b) as first aid for cuts
(c) for softening hard water
(d) as mordant

9. Which of the following compounds is not an antacid ?
(a) Phenelzine (b) Ranitidine
(c) Aluminium hydroxide (d) Cimetidine

10. Washing soap can be prepared by saponification with alkali of which of the following oil
(a) Rose oil (b) Paraffin oil
(c) Groundnut oil (d) Kerosene oil

11. The cationic detergent that is used in hair conditioners is
(a) sodium dodecylbenzene sulphonate
(b) sodium lauryl sulphate
(c) tetramethyl ammonium chloride
(d) cetyltrimethyl ammonium bromide

12. Which of the following is not true ?
(a) Some disinfectants can be used as antiseptics
(b) Sulphadiazine is a synthetic antibacterial
(c) Aspirin is analgesic as well as antipyretic
(d) Polystyrene is used to make non-stick cookware

13. Which artificial sweetener contains chlorine ?
(a) Sucralose (b) Alitame
(c) Aspartame (d) Saccharin

14. Which one of the following is used as Antihistamine?
(a) Omeprazole (b) Chloranphenicol
(c) Diphenhydramine (d) Norethindrone

15. Commonly used antiseptic 'Dettol' is a mixture of
(a) *o*-chlorophenozylenol + terpeneol
(b) *o*-cresol + terpeneol
(c) phenol + terpeneol
(d) chloroxylenol + terpeneol

16. Which of the following ceramics possesses good strength, translucency and very low porosity
(a) whiteware (b) earthenware
(c) stoneware (d) bricks and tiles

17. Various phenol derivatives, tincture of iodine (2 – 3%) I_2 in (water / alcohol) and some dyes like methylene blue are
(a) antiseptics (b) disinfectants
(c) analgesics (d) antipyretics

18. Bithional is an example of
(a) disinfectant (b) antiseptic
(c) antibiotic (d) analgesic

19. The structure given below is known as

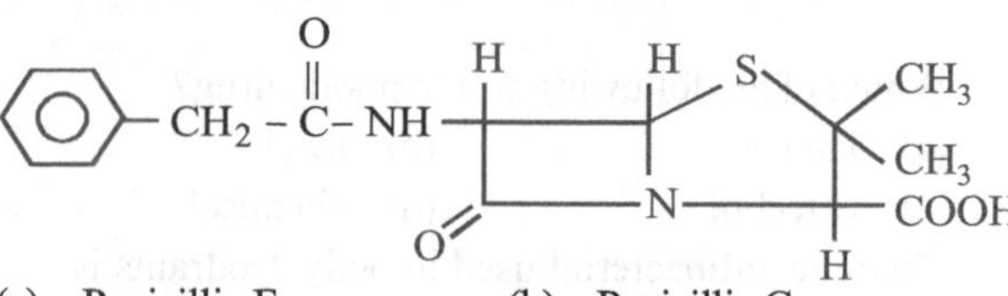

(a) Penicillin F (b) Penicillin G
(c) Penicillin K (d) Ampicillin

20. Chemical substances used by insects for communication are called
(a) pheromones (b) hormones
(c) enzymes (d) nucleoproteins

RESPONSE GRID					
	6. ⓐⓑⓒⓓ	7. ⓐⓑⓒⓓ	8. ⓐⓑⓒⓓ	9. ⓐⓑⓒⓓ	10. ⓐⓑⓒⓓ
	11. ⓐⓑⓒⓓ	12. ⓐⓑⓒⓓ	13. ⓐⓑⓒⓓ	14. ⓐⓑⓒⓓ	15. ⓐⓑⓒⓓ
	16. ⓐⓑⓒⓓ	17. ⓐⓑⓒⓓ	18. ⓐⓑⓒⓓ	19. ⓐⓑⓒⓓ	20. ⓐⓑⓒⓓ

Space for Rough Work

21. Aminoglycosides are usually used as:
(a) antibiotic (b) analgesic
(c) hypnotic (d) antifertility

22. Which type of detergent is formed when stearic acid reacts with polyethylene glycol?
(a) Cationic detergent (b) Anionic detergent
(c) Non– ionic detergent (d) None of these

23. Which of the following statements are correct?
(i) Before 1970 for treatment of stomach acidity $Al(OH)_3$ is a better antacid in comparison to $NaHCO_3$.
(ii) Discovery of cimetidine was a major break through in the treatment of hyperacidity.
(iii) Terfenadine is a drug which competes with histamine for binding sites of receptor.
(iv) Antidepressant drugs like equanil inhibit the enzymes which catalyze the degradation of noradernaline.
(v) Veronal and luminal belongs to the class of tranquilizers called barbiturates.
(a) (i), (ii) and (iii) (b) (i), (iii) and (v)
(c) (ii), (iii) and (iv) (d) (ii), (iv) and (v)

24. Detergents are prepared by the action of H_2SO_4 on which of the following?
(a) Cholesterol (b) Lauryl alcohol
(c) Cyclohexanol (d) *p*-Nitrophenol

25. Which of the following statements about aspirin is **not** true?
(a) It is effective in relieving pain.
(b) It is a neurologically active drug.
(c) It has antiblood clotting action.
(d) It belongs to narcotic analgesics.

26. Parathion is
(a) an orgnic phosphorus compound
(b) chlorinated aromatic compound
(c) chlorinated aliphatic compound
(d) benzene derivative

27. Which of the following add nutritive value to food?
(a) Sweeteners (b) Antioxidants
(c) Fat emulsifiers (d) None of these

28. Which one of the following compounds is an anti-fertility drug?
(a) Aspirin (b) Chloromycetin
(c) Saheli (d) Penicillin

29. Which of the following represents a synthetic detergent?
(a) $C_{15}H_{31}COOK$
(b) $CH_3[CH_2]_{16}COONa$
(c) $C_{12}H_{25}-C_6H_4-SO_3Na$
(d) None of these

30. Sulphonamides act as
(a) Antiseptic (b) Analgesic
(c) Antimicrobials (d) Antipyretic

31. Which of the following compound is an antioxidant?
(a) BHA (b) DDB
(c) ABS (d) CFRP

32. Which of the following statements are correct?
(i) Antiseptics are not ingested like antibiotics.
(ii) 1% solution of iodine in alcohol–water mixture is known as tincture of iodine.
(iii) SO_2 in low concentrations are used as antiseptics whereas in higher concentration are used as disinfectants.
(iv) Birth control pills essentially contain a mixture of synthetic estrogen and progesterone derivates.
Which of the following is the correct code for the statements above ?
(a) (i) & (iii) (b) (ii) & (iv)
(c) (i) & (iv) (d) (iii) & (iv)

RESPONSE GRID				
21. (a)(b)(c)(d)	22. (a)(b)(c)(d)	23. (a)(b)(c)(d)	24. (a)(b)(c)(d)	25. (a)(b)(c)(d)
26. (a)(b)(c)(d)	27. (a)(b)(c)(d)	28. (a)(b)(c)(d)	29. (a)(b)(c)(d)	30. (a)(b)(c)(d)
31. (a)(b)(c)(d)	32. (a)(b)(c)(d)			

Space for Rough Work

33. Arsenic containing medicine used for the treatment of syphilis, is
(a) erythromycin (b) ofloxacin
(c) tetracycline (d) salvarsan

34. Artificial sweetner which is stable under cold conditions only is :
(a) Saccharine (b) Sucralose
(c) Aspartame (d) Alitame

35. Zinc salts used in deodorants act as
(a) antiperspirants and astringents
(b) astringents as well as antiseptics
(c) antibacterials as well as antiperspirants
(d) antiperspirants and antiseptics

36. Synthetic detergents are more effective in hard water than soaps because
(a) they are non-ionic
(b) their Ca^{++} and Mg^{++} salts are insoluble in water
(c) their Ca^{++} and Mg^{++} salts are water soluble
(d) they are highly soluble in water

37. An antibiotic with a broad spectrum
(a) Kills the antibodies
(b) Acts on a specific antigen
(c) Acts on different antigens
(d) Acts on both the antigens and antibodies

38. Which of the following is an analgesic?
(a) Novalgin (b) Penicillin
(c) Streptomycin (d) Chloromycetin

39. Which one of the following types of drugs reduces fever ?
(a) Tranquiliser (b) Antibiotic
(c) Antipyretic (d) Analgesic

40. Antiseptics and disinfectants either kill or prevent growth of microorganisms. Identify which of the following statements **is not true:**
(a) Chlorine and iodine are used as strong disinfectants.
(b) Dilute solutions of Boric acid and Hydrogen Peroxide are strong antiseptics.
(c) Disinfectants harm the living tissues.
(d) A 0.2% solution of phenol is an antiseptic while 1% solution acts as a disinfectant.

41. A medicine which promotes the secretion of urine is called
(a) Uretic (b) Monouretic
(c) Diuretic (d) Triuretic

42. Saccharine contains
(a) C and H (b) C, H, N and O
(c) C, H, N, O & S (d) C, O and H

43. Which one of the following can possibly be used as analgesic without causing addiction and mood modification ?
(a) Diazepam
(b) Morphine
(c) N-Acetyl-para-aminophenol
(d) Tetrahydrocannabinol

44. Which one of the following is employed as a tranquilizer drug?
(a) Promethazine (b) Valium
(c) Naproxen (d) Mifepristone

45. Match List I with List II and select the correct answer using the codes gives below the lists :

	List I		List II
I.	Iodoform	A.	Anaesthetic
II.	Methyl salicylate	B.	Antiseptic
III.	Diethyl ether	C.	Insecticide
IV.	Hexachlorocyclohexane	D.	Detergent
		E.	Pain balm

Codes :
(a) I-B, II-E, III-C, IV-D (b) I-D, II-B, III-A, IV-C
(c) I-B, II-E, III-A, IV-C (d) I-C, II-A, III-D, IV-B

RESPONSE GRID				
33. ⓐⓑⓒⓓ	34. ⓐⓑⓒⓓ	35. ⓐⓑⓒⓓ	36. ⓐⓑⓒⓓ	37. ⓐⓑⓒⓓ
38. ⓐⓑⓒⓓ	39. ⓐⓑⓒⓓ	40. ⓐⓑⓒⓓ	41. ⓐⓑⓒⓓ	42. ⓐⓑⓒⓓ
43. ⓐⓑⓒⓓ	44. ⓐⓑⓒⓓ	45. ⓐⓑⓒⓓ		

CHEMISTRY CHAPTERWISE SPEED TEST-58

Total Questions	45	Total Marks	180
Attempted		Correct	
Incorrect		Net Score	
Cut-off Score	46	Qualifying Score	68
Success Gap = Net Score – Qualifying Score			
Net Score = (Correct × 4) – (Incorrect × 1)			

Space for Rough Work

BIOLOGY

The Living World

Speed TEST 59

Chapter-wise

No. of Questions	Maximum Marks	Time
45	180	1 Hour

GENERAL INSTRUCTIONS

- This test contains 45 MCQ's. For each question only one option is correct. Darken the correct circle/ bubble in the Response Grid provided on each page.
- You have to evaluate your Response Grids yourself with the help of solutions provided at the end of this book.
- Each correct answer will get you 4 marks and 1 mark shall be deduced for each incorrect answer. No mark will be given/ deducted if no bubble is filled. Keep a timer in front of you and stop immediately at the end of 60 min.
- The sheet follows a particular syllabus. Do not attempt the sheet before you have completed your preparation for that syllabus.
- After completing the sheet check your answers with the solution booklet and complete the Result Grid. Finally spend time to analyse your performance and revise the areas which emerge out as weak in your evaluation.

1. The living organisms can be unexceptionally distinguished from the non-living things on the basis of their ability for
   (a) interaction with the environment and progressive evolution
   (b) reproduction
   (c) growth and movement
   (d) responsiveness to touch.
2. Which one of the following animals is correctly matched with its particular named taxonomic category ?
   (a) Tiger - *tigris*, the species
   (b) Cuttle fish - mollusca, a class
   (c) Humans - primata, the family
   (d) Housefly - musca, an order
3. Taxonomic hierarchy refers to
   (a) Step-wise arrangement of all categories for classification of plants and animals
   (b) A group of senior taxonomists who decide the nomenclature of plants and animals
   (c) A list of botanists or zoologists who have worked on taxonomy of a species or group
   (d) Classification of a species based on fossil record
4. Choose correct scientific name of mango.
   (a) *Mangifera Indica*
   (b) *Mangifera indica* Linn
   (c) *Mangifera indica* Hook.
   (d) *Mangifera indica* L

RESPONSE GRID	1. ⓐⓑⓒⓓ	2. ⓐⓑⓒⓓ	3. ⓐⓑⓒⓓ	4. ⓐⓑⓒⓓ

Space for Rough Work

5. Arrange the following taxonomic categories in increasing number of common characteristics w.r.t. plant mango
A. Dicotyledonae
B. Polymoniales
C. *Mangifera*
D. Angiospermae
E. Anacardiaceae
(a) A→D→B→E→C
(b) A→D→C→B→E
(c) D→A→B→E→C
(d) D→A→C→E→B

6. The common characteristics between brinjal and wheat can be observed maximum at the level of their.
(a) Division (b) Phylum
(c) Kingdom (d) Both (b) and (c)

7. Study of number of chromosomes for resolving difficulties in classification is used in
(a) Chemotaxonomy
(b) Morphotaxonomy
(c) Cytotaxonomy
(d) Biochemical taxonomy

8. Most names in biological nomenclature of living organisms are taken from which language?
(a) Hindi (b) Latin
(c) German (d) French

9. The main objective of plant taxonomy is
(a) to study the world's flora
(b) to provide a method for identification and nomenclature
(c) to provide Latin 'scientific' names for every group of plants in the world
(d) all of these

10. Which one of the following has least similar characters?
(a) Family (b) Class
(c) Genus (d) Species

11. The ascending or descending arrangement of taxonomic categories is called as
(a) classification (b) taxonomy
(c) hierarchy (d) key

12. Select the false statement
(a) Carolus Linnaeus described plants and classified them on the basis of their sexual parts
(b) Some facts established by accurate and repeated observations do not require further verification
(c) Study of the vestigeal organs is called teleology
(d) 'White Revolution' resulted in enhanced production of milk

13. Animal taxonomists have named the animals according to:
(a) International class for Zoology Nomenclature
(b) Indian code for Zoology Nomenclature
(c) International classification for Zoological Nomenclature
(d) International code for Zoological Nomenclature

14. Which of the following statement is not true?
(a) Homeostasis is a fundamental property of life
(b) When the external temperature is warm, the superficial blood vessels constrict to prevent loss of body heat
(c) Human beings are endothermic
(d) Human beings are homeothermic

15. Species is :
(a) population of individuals having same genotypes and phenotypes
(b) a group of individuals inhabiting a geographical area
(c) a group of interbreeding populations
(d) population of one type

16. The usage of binomial names, for plant species was accepted by all after the publication of the work by :
(a) Hooker (b) Linnaeus
(c) Bentham (d) Darwin

17. Which of the following is less general in characters as compared to genus ?
(a) Species (b) Division
(c) Class (d) Family

RESPONSE GRID					
	5. ⓐⓑⓒⓓ	6. ⓐⓑⓒⓓ	7. ⓐⓑⓒⓓ	8. ⓐⓑⓒⓓ	9. ⓐⓑⓒⓓ
	10. ⓐⓑⓒⓓ	11. ⓐⓑⓒⓓ	12. ⓐⓑⓒⓓ	13. ⓐⓑⓒⓓ	14. ⓐⓑⓒⓓ
	15. ⓐⓑⓒⓓ	16. ⓐⓑⓒⓓ	17. ⓐⓑⓒⓓ		

Space for Rough Work

18. A taxon with reference to classification of living organisms can be defined as
(a) a group of similar genera
(b) a group of similar species
(c) a group of organisms based on chromosome numbers
(d) a group of any one rank of organisms

19. Species are considered as
(a) Real units of classification devised by taxonomists
(b) Real basic units of classification
(c) The lowest units of classification
(d) Artificial concept of human mind which cannot be defined in absolute terms

20. Linneaus system of classification is :
(a) Natural (b) Artificial
(c) Phylogenetic (d) Progressive

21. The book systema naturae was written by
(a) Carolus Von Linnaeus
(b) Hutchinson
(c) Engler and Prantl
(d) Bentham & Hooker

22. "Ordines Anomali" of Bentham and Hooker includes :
(a) Seed plants showing abnormal forms of growth and development
(b) Plants represented only in fossil state
(c) Plants described in the literature but which Bentham and Hooker did not see in original
(d) A few orders which could not be placed satisfactory in the classification.

23. What is true for individuals of same species?
(a) Live in same niche
(b) Live in same habitat
(c) Interbreeding
(d) Live in different habitat

24. Biosystematics aims at
(a) Identification and arrangement of organisms on the basis of their cytological characteristics
(b) The classification of organisms based on broad morphological characters
(c) Delimiting various taxa of organisms and establishing their relationships
(d) The classification of organisms based on their evolutionary history and establishing their phylogeny on the totality of various parameters from all fields of studies

25. An animal with same generic, specific and subspecific names is
(a) man (b) gorilla
(c) rabbit (d) elephant

26. Two similar holotypes are called
(a) Isotypes (b) Neotypes
(c) Syntypes (d) Mesotypes

27. Which of the following is not a taxon?
(a) Carnivora (b) Insectivora
(c) Herbivora (d) Mastigophora

28. The category which includes related families is
(a) Class (b) Phylum
(c) Order (d) Kingdom

29. NBRI is situated at
(a) Calcutta (b) Bombay
(c) Madras (d) Lucknow

30. A duplicate of nomenclature type is termed by a taxonomist as
(a) Syntype (b) Neotype
(c) Paratype (d) Isotype

31. Classification based on sequencing of DNA and chemical nature of protein is
(a) Chemotaxonomy
(b) Cytotaxonomy
(c) Adansonian taxonomy
(d) Karyotaxonomy

RESPONSE GRID					
	18. ⓐⓑⓒⓓ	19. ⓐⓑⓒⓓ	20. ⓐⓑⓒⓓ	21. ⓐⓑⓒⓓ	22. ⓐⓑⓒⓓ
	23. ⓐⓑⓒⓓ	24. ⓐⓑⓒⓓ	25. ⓐⓑⓒⓓ	26. ⓐⓑⓒⓓ	27. ⓐⓑⓒⓓ
	28. ⓐⓑⓒⓓ	29. ⓐⓑⓒⓓ	30. ⓐⓑⓒⓓ	31. ⓐⓑⓒⓓ	

Space for Rough Work

32. *Rattus rattus* scientific name is an example of
(a) Autonyms (b) Tautonyms
(c) Synonyms (d) Homonyms

33. Species belonging to different time period are called
(a) Syntype (b) Paratype
(c) Lectotype (d) Isotype

34. A new nomenclatural type submitted when the original material is missing is known as
(a) Holotype (b) Isotype
(c) Paratype (d) Neotype

35. Choose the incorrect statement regarding herbarium
(a) Dried specimens are poisoned by using DDT
(b) The collections are kept inside metallic vasculum
(c) Herbarium sheet is 41 × 29 cm
(d) It is used for alpha taxonomic research

36. No non-living object is capable of reproduction or replication by itself. Although reproduction can not be an all-inclusive defining characteristics of living organisms because
(a) Organisms like mules do not reproduce
(b) It brings about variation in offsprings
(c) Clones are blueprints of their parents
(d) Drones (male honey bees) are produced parthenogenetically

37. Which of the following have more characters in common ?
(a) Order (b) Class
(c) Phylum (d) Family

38. Mark the odd one in the following:
(a) Family (b) Class
(c) Taxon (d) Phylum

39. Which of the following is a name for a taxon that is identical to other such name?
(a) Autonym (b) Synonym
(c) Homonym (d) Tautonym

40. Which of the following is an automatically created name?
(a) Autonym
(b) Synonym
(c) Homonym
(d) Tautonym

41. When the specific epithet exactly repeats generic name, it is called
(a) Basionym (b) Synonym
(c) Homonym (d) Tautonym

42. Which of the following is most important for speciation ?
(a) Seasonal isolation
(b) Reproductive isolation
(c) Behavioural isolation
(d) Temporal isolation

43. Species occurring in different geographical areas are called as
(a) Sibling (b) Sympatric
(c) Allopatric (d) Neopatric

44. All members of different species of plants and animals present in particular area make up
(a) Population (b) Community
(c) Ecosystem (d) Biosphere

45. The study of the kind of life in outer space is known as :
(a) ecology (b) evolution
(c) anthropology (d) exobiology

RESPONSE GRID					
	32. ⓐⓑⓒⓓ	33. ⓐⓑⓒⓓ	34. ⓐⓑⓒⓓ	35. ⓐⓑⓒⓓ	36. ⓐⓑⓒⓓ
	37. ⓐⓑⓒⓓ	38. ⓐⓑⓒⓓ	39. ⓐⓑⓒⓓ	40. ⓐⓑⓒⓓ	41. ⓐⓑⓒⓓ
	42. ⓐⓑⓒⓓ	43. ⓐⓑⓒⓓ	44. ⓐⓑⓒⓓ	45. ⓐⓑⓒⓓ	

BIOLOGY CHAPTERWISE SPEED TEST-59

Total Questions	45	Total Marks	180
Attempted		Correct	
Incorrect		Net Score	
Cut-off Score	45	Qualifying Score	60
Success Gap = Net Score – Qualifying Score			
Net Score = (Correct × 4) – (Incorrect × 1)			

Space for Rough Work

BIOLOGY

Biological Classification

Speed TEST 60

Chapter-wise

No. of Questions	Maximum Marks	Time
45	180	1 Hour

GENERAL INSTRUCTIONS

- This test contains 45 MCQ's. For each question only one option is correct. Darken the correct circle/ bubble in the Response Grid provided on each page.
- You have to evaluate your Response Grids yourself with the help of solutions provided at the end of this book.
- Each correct answer will get you 4 marks and 1 mark shall be deduced for each incorrect answer. No mark will be given/ deducted if no bubble is filled. Keep a timer in front of you and stop immediately at the end of 60 min.
- The sheet follows a particular syllabus. Do not attempt the sheet before you have completed your preparation for that syllabus.
- After completing the sheet check your answers with the solution booklet and complete the Result Grid. Finally spend time to analyse your performance and revise the areas which emerge out as weak in your evaluation.

1. Which of the following processes are involved in the reproduction of protista?
   (a) Binary fission and fragmentation
   (b) Cell fusion and zygote formation
   (c) Spore formation and fragmentation
   (d) Budding and spore formation
2. In prokaryotes, the genetic material is
   (a) linear DNA with histones
   (b) circular DNA with histones
   (c) linear DNA without histones
   (d) circular DNA without histones
3. Which of the following bacteria carry out oxygenic photosynthesis by means of a photosynthetic apparatus similar to the eukaryotes?
   (a) Purple sulphur bacteria
   (b) Green sulphur bacteria
   (c) Cyanobacteria
   (d) More than one option is correct
4. Bacteria is a group of prokaryotic organisms which is characterised by
   (a) 70 S ribosomes
   (b) Peptidoglycan cell wall
   (c) Simple structure and complex behaviour
   (d) All of the above.
5. What may be a 'photosynthetic protistian' to one biologist may be 'a plant' to another? Which of the given below features of slime moulds shows linkage with plant?
   (a) Presence of holozoic nutrition
   (b) Presence of diverse sexual reproduction
   (c) Slime moulds have cellulosic spore wall
   (d) Formation of fruiting bodies

RESPONSE GRID	1. ⓐⓑⓒⓓ	2. ⓐⓑⓒⓓ	3. ⓐⓑⓒⓓ	4. ⓐⓑⓒⓓ	5. ⓐⓑⓒⓓ

Space for Rough Work

6. Choose the correct match
   (a) *Gonyaulax* – Red sea
   (b) *Euglena* – Chlorophyll a & c
   (c) Desmids – Chrysophytes
   (d) *Gymnodinium* – Hemicellulosic plates in wall
7. Nuclear dimorphism is shown by
   (a) *Paramecium* (b) *Amoeba*
   (c) *Plasmodium* (d) *Trypanosoma*
8. Most common type of genetic material present in bacteriophages is
   (a) ds RNA (b) ss RNA
   (c) ds DNA (d) ss DNA
9. Which of the following statement about Mycoplasma is true:
   (a) They are smallest, disease causing thin walled organisms
   (b) They differ from viruses in being cellular in organisation
   (c) Insensitive to several antibiotics as they have 70S ribosomes
   (d) They can survive without photosynthetic pigments and genetic material
10. Consider the following characters:
    Non-motile spores, saprophytic unicellular eukaryotes, transfer of gametes by wind currents, Differentiation of plasmodium under suitable conditions.
    How many of the characters given in box belong to slime moulds?
    (a) Four (b) One
    (c) Three (d) Two
11. Eubacteria can be differentiated from archaebacteria on the basis of
    (a) Ribosomes (b) Gene of tRNA
    (c) Cell wall (d) Nutrition
12. Select the pair that consists of plant or animal bacterial diseases.
    (a) Cholera and typhoid
    (b) Citrus canker and crown gall
    (c) Malaria and dengue
    (d) Both (a) and (b)
13. Cyanobacteria are classified under which of the following kingdoms?
    (a) Monera (b) Protista
    (c) Algae (d) Plantae
14. _______ are important decomposers that cause decay and decomposition of dead bodies of plants and animals.
    (a) Saprotrophic bacteria
    (b) Saprotrophic fungi
    (c) Plants, like *Sarracenia*
    (d) Both (a) and (b)
15. Chrysophytes are
    (a) planktons (b) nektons
    (c) benthic organisms (d) rooted submerged.
16. Eukaryotic, achlorophyllous and heterotrophic organisms are grouped under which of the following kingdoms?
    (a) Monera (b) Protista
    (c) Fungi (d) Plantae
17. Virion is
    (a) nulceic acid of virus
    (b) antiviral agent
    (c) protein of virus
    (d) completely assembled virus outside host.
18. In the five-kingdom system of classification, which single kingdom out of the following can include blue, green algae, nitrogen-fixing bacteria and methanogenic archaebacteria?
    (a) Fungi (b) Plantae
    (c) Protista (d) Monera
19. Viruses that infect bacteria, multiply and cause their lysis, are called
    (a) Lysozymes (b) Lipolytic
    (c) Lytic (d) Lysogenic
20. Phenetic classification of organisms is based on
    (a) Observable characteristics of existing organisms
    (b) The ancestral lineage of existing organisms
    (c) Dendogram based on DNA characteristics
    (d) Sexual characteristics
21. The practical purpose of classification of living organisms is to
    (a) explain the origin of living organisms
    (b) trace the evolution of living organisms
    (c) name the living organisms
    (d) facilitate identification of unknown organisms

RESPONSE GRID					
	6. ⓐⓑⓒⓓ	7. ⓐⓑⓒⓓ	8. ⓐⓑⓒⓓ	9. ⓐⓑⓒⓓ	10. ⓐⓑⓒⓓ
	11. ⓐⓑⓒⓓ	12. ⓐⓑⓒⓓ	13. ⓐⓑⓒⓓ	14. ⓐⓑⓒⓓ	15. ⓐⓑⓒⓓ
	16. ⓐⓑⓒⓓ	17. ⓐⓑⓒⓓ	18. ⓐⓑⓒⓓ	19. ⓐⓑⓒⓓ	20. ⓐⓑⓒⓓ
	21. ⓐⓑⓒⓓ				

Space for Rough Work

22. A system of classification in which a large number of traits are considered, is
(a) artificial system (b) synthetic system
(c) natural system (d) phylogenetic system
23. In five kingdom system, the main basis of classification is
(a) structure of nucleus (b) mode of nutrition
(c) structure of cell wall (d) asexual reproduction
24. Phenetic classification is based on
(a) Sexual characteristics
(b) The ancestral lineage of existing organisms
(c) Observable characteristics of existing organisms
(d) Dendograms based on DNA characteristics
25. In which kingdom would you classify the archaebecteria and nitrogen-fixing organisms. If the five-kingdom system of classification is used ?
(a) Monera (b) Plantae
(c) Fungi (d) Protista
26. Which of the following statements is not true for retroviruses?
(a) DNA is not present at any stage in the life cycle of retroviruses
(b) Retroviruses carry gene for RNA-dependent DNA polymerase
(c) The genetic material in mature retroviruses is RNA
(d) Retroviruses are causative agents for certain kinds of cancer in man
27. On how many criteria living organisms have been classified into five kingdoms ?
(a) Two (b) Four
(c) Five (d) Three
28. First true phylogenetic system of classification was given by
(a) Eichler (b) Engler and Prantl
(c) de Jussiaeu (d) de Candolle
29. Which of the following is not a protist ?
(a) *Taenia* (b) *Amoeba*
(c) *Paramecium* (d) *Euglena*
30. Which of the following is not correctly matched?
(a) Root knot disease - *Meloidogyne javanica*
(b) Smut of bajra - *Tolysporium penicillariae*
(c) Covered smut of barley - *Ustilago nuda*
(d) Late blight of potato - *Phytophthora infestans*
31. Which one of the following character was not used by R.H. Whittaker for biological classification ?
(a) Cell structure
(b) Physiological characters
(c) Thallus organisation
(d) Phylogenetic relationships
32. The first organisms to appear on earth were
(a) photoautotrophs (b) chemoautotrophs
(c) chemoheterotrophs (d) heterotrophs
33. 'Comma' shaped bacteria are known as
(a) coccus (b) spiral
(c) spirillum (d) vibrio
34. Slime moulds in the division myxomycota (true slime moulds) have
(a) pseudoplasmodia.
(b) spores that develop into free living amoeboid cells.
(c) spores that develop into flagellated gametes.
(d) feeding stages consisting of solitary individual cells.
35. Which one of the following statements about Mycoplasma is wrong ?
(a) They are pleomorphic.
(b) They are sensitive to penicillin.
(c) They cause diseases in plants.
(d) They are also called (Pleuro pneumonia like organisms) PPLO.
36. African sleeping sickness is due to
(a) *Plasmodium vivax* transmitted by Tse-tse fly
(b) *Trypanosoma lewsii* transmitted by Bed Bug
(c) *Trypanosoma gambiense* transmitted by *Glossina palpalis*
(d) *Entamoeba gingivalis* spread by Housefly

RESPONSE GRID					
	22. ⓐⓑⓒⓓ	23. ⓐⓑⓒⓓ	24. ⓐⓑⓒⓓ	25. ⓐⓑⓒⓓ	26. ⓐⓑⓒⓓ
	27. ⓐⓑⓒⓓ	28. ⓐⓑⓒⓓ	29. ⓐⓑⓒⓓ	30. ⓐⓑⓒⓓ	31. ⓐⓑⓒⓓ
	32. ⓐⓑⓒⓓ	33. ⓐⓑⓒⓓ	34. ⓐⓑⓒⓓ	35. ⓐⓑⓒⓓ	36. ⓐⓑⓒⓓ

Space for Rough Work

37. Which one single organism or the pair of organisms is **correctly** assigned to its taxonomic group?
(a) *Paramecium* and *Plasmodium* belong to the same kingdom as that of *Penicillium*
(b) Lichen is a composite organism formed from the symbiotic association of an algae and a protozoan
(c) Yeast used in making bread and beer is a fungus
(d) *Nostoc* and *Anabaena* are examples of protista

38. Two animals which are the members of the same order must also be the members of the same :
(a) Class (b) Family
(c) Genus (d) Species

39. Bacteria lack alternation of generation because there is
(a) neither syngamy nor reduction division.
(b) distinct chromosomes are absent.
(c) no conjugation.
(d) no exchange of genetic material.

40. Capsid is
(a) genetic material of virus
(b) protein cover of virus
(c) extra genetic material of bacterium
(d) house keeping genome of bacterium

41. A group of fungi with septate mycelium in which sexual reproduction is either unknown or lacking are classified under
(a) phycomycetes (b) deuteromycetes
(c) ascomycetes (d) basidiomycetes

42. A few organisms are known to grow and multiply at temperatures of 100–105°C. They belong to
(a) marine archaebacteria
(b) thermophilic sulphur bacteria
(c) blue-green algae (cyanobacteria)
(d) thermophilic, subaerial fungi

43. Mycoplasma is pleuromorphic due to
(a) absence of cell wall
(b) presence of three layered cell membrane
(c) the presence of sterol
(d) None of these

44. Refer to the given figures of bacteria cell and *Nostoc* and choose the option which shows correct label for the structures marked as A, B, C, D and E ?

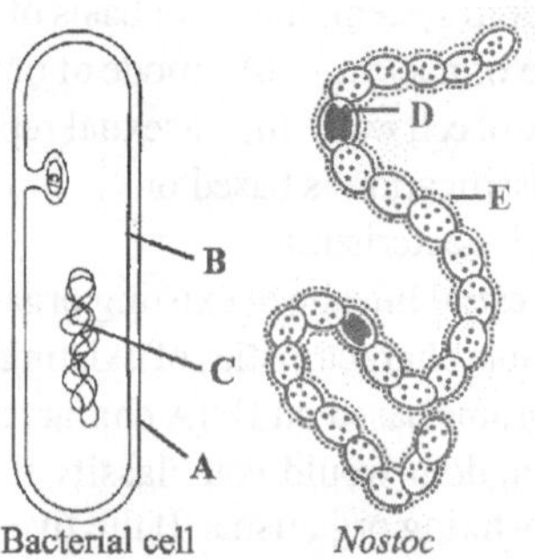

(a) A – Cell wall, B – Cell membrane, C – Heterocyst, D – DNA, E – Mucilagenous sheath
(b) A – Cell wall, B – Cell membrane, C – DNA, D – Heterocyst, E – Mucilagenous sheath
(c) A – Mucilagenous sheath, B – Cell membrane, C – DNA, D – Heterocyst, E – Cell wall
(d) A – Cell membrane, B – Cell wall, C – DNA, D – Heterocyst, E – Mucilagenous sheath

45. Choose the correct names of the different bacteria given below according to their shapes.

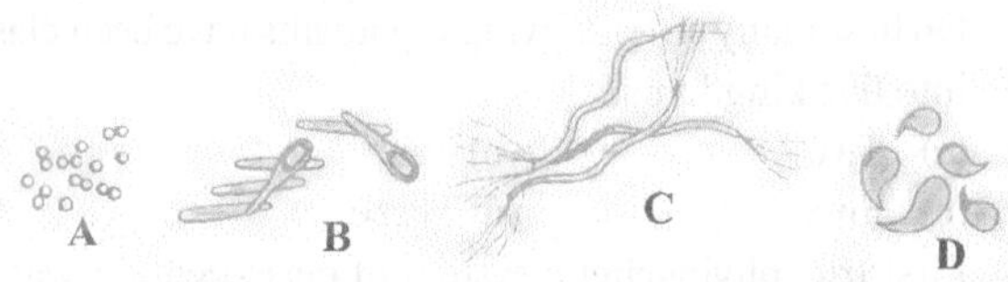

(a) A – Cocci, B – Bacilli, C – Spirilla, D – Vibrio
(b) A – Bacilli, B – Cocci, C – Spirilla, D – Vibrio
(c) A – Spirilla, B – Bacilli, C – Cocci, D – Vibrio
(d) A – Spirilla, B – Vibrio, C – Cocci, D – Bacilli

RESPONSE GRID					
	37. ⓐⓑⓒⓓ	38. ⓐⓑⓒⓓ	39. ⓐⓑⓒⓓ	40. ⓐⓑⓒⓓ	41. ⓐⓑⓒⓓ
	42. ⓐⓑⓒⓓ	43. ⓐⓑⓒⓓ	44. ⓐⓑⓒⓓ	45. ⓐⓑⓒⓓ	

BIOLOGY CHAPTERWISE SPEED TEST-60			
Total Questions	45	Total Marks	180
Attempted		Correct	
Incorrect		Net Score	
Cut-off Score	45	Qualifying Score	60
Success Gap = Net Score – Qualifying Score			
Net Score = (Correct × 4) – (Incorrect × 1)			

Space for Rough Work

BIOLOGY

Plant Kingdom

No. of Questions	Maximum Marks	Time
45	180	1 Hour

Speed TEST 61

Chapter-wise

GENERAL INSTRUCTIONS

- This test contains 45 MCQ's. For each question only one option is correct. Darken the correct circle/ bubble in the Response Grid provided on each page.
- You have to evaluate your Response Grids yourself with the help of solutions provided at the end of this book.
- Each correct answer will get you 4 marks and 1 mark shall be deduced for each incorrect answer. No mark will be given/ deducted if no bubble is filled. Keep a timer in front of you and stop immediately at the end of 60 min.
- The sheet follows a particular syllabus. Do not attempt the sheet before you have completed your preparation for that syllabus.
- After completing the sheet check your answers with the solution booklet and complete the Result Grid. Finally spend time to analyse your performance and revise the areas which emerge out as weak in your evaluation.

1. Floridean starch is found in
   (a) Chlorophyceae
   (b) Rhodophyceae
   (c) Phaeophyceae
   (d) Cyanophyceae
2. Peat moss is another name of
   (a) *Sphagnum* (b) *Marchantia*
   (c) *Riccia* (d) *Dryopteris*
3. Pteridophytes differ from mosses/bryophytes in possessing
   (a) independent gametophyte
   (b) well developed vascular system
   (c) archegonia structure
   (d) flagellate spermatozoids
4. Most plants are green in colour because
   (a) the atmosphere filters out all the colours of the visible light spectrum except green.
   (b) green light is the most effective wavelength region of the visible spectrum in sunlight for photosynthesis.
   (c) chlorophyll is least effective in absorbing green light.
   (d) green light allows maximum photosynthesis.
5. In Chlorophyceae, sexual reproduction occurs by
   (a) isogamy and anisogamy
   (b) isogamy, anisogamy and oogamy
   (c) oogamy only
   (d) anisogamy and oogamy

RESPONSE GRID	1. ⓐⓑⓒⓓ	2. ⓐⓑⓒⓓ	3. ⓐⓑⓒⓓ	4. ⓐⓑⓒⓓ	5. ⓐⓑⓒⓓ

Space for Rough Work

6. A water fern which is used as a green manure in rice fields is
   (a) *Salvinia* (b) *Mucor*
   (c) *Aspergillus* (d) *Azolla*
7. The largest flower found is known as
   (a) *Rafflesia* (b) *Tecoma*
   (c) *Musa* (d) Cauliflower
8. In fern, spores are formed in
   (a) sporangium (b) oogonium
   (c) archegonium (d) stomium
9. *Laminaria* (kelp) and *Fucus* (rock weed) are the examples of
   (a) red algae
   (b) brown algae
   (c) green algae
   (d) golden brown algae
10. People recovering from long illness are often advised to include the alga *Spirulina* in their diet because it
    (a) makes the food easy to digest.
    (b) is rich in proteins.
    (c) has antibiotic properties.
    (d) restores the intestinal microflora.
11. Which of the following cell organelle remains enveloped by a single unit membrane?
    (a) Mitochondria (b) Lysosomes
    (c) Nucleus (d) Chloroplast
12. Consider the following statements regarding the major pigments and stored food in the different groups of algae and choose the correct option.
    (i) In Chlorophyceae, the stored food material is starch and the major pigments are chlorophyll-*a* and *d.*
    (ii) In Phaeophyceae, laminarin is the stored food and major pigments are chlorophyll-*a* and *b.*
    (iii) In Rhodophyceae, floridean starch is the stored food and the major pigments are chlorophyll-*a*, *d* and phycoerythrin.
    (a) (i) is correct, but (ii) and (iii) are wrong.
    (b) (i) and (ii) are correct, but (iii) is wrong.
    (c) (i) and (iii) are correct, but (ii) is wrong.
    (d) (iii) is correct, but (i) and (ii) are wrong.
13. Algae have cell wall made up of
    (a) cellulose, galactans and mannans
    (b) hemicellulose, pectins and proteins
    (c) pectins, cellulose and proteins
    (d) cellulose, hemicellulose and pectins.
14. Which plays an important role in the dispersal of spores in *Funaria*?
    (a) Operculum
    (b) Capsule
    (c) Peristome and annulus
    (d) Sporogonium
15. Read the following five statements (i – v) and answer the question.
    (i) In *Equisetum* the female gametophyte is retained on the parent sporophyte.
    (ii) In *Ginkgo* male gametophyte is not independent.
    (iii) The sporophyte in *Riccia* is more developed than that in *Polytrichum.*
    (iv) Sexual reproduction in *Volvox* is isogamous.
    (v) The spores of slime molds lack cell walls.
    How many of the above statements are correct?
    (a) Two (b) Three
    (c) Four (d) One
16. Which one of the following is common to multicellular fungi, filamentous algae and protonema of mosses?
    (a) Diplontic life cycle
    (b) Members of kingdom plantae
    (c) Mode of Nutrition
    (d) Multiplication by fragmentation
17. Which one of the following is a correct statement ?
    (a) Pteridophyte gametophyte has a protonemal and leafy stage
    (b) In gymnosperms female gametophyte is free-living
    (c) Antheridiophores and archegoniophores are present in pteridophytes
    (d) Origin of seed habit can be traced in pteridophytes

RESPONSE GRID					
	6. ⓐⓑⓒⓓ	7. ⓐⓑⓒⓓ	8. ⓐⓑⓒⓓ	9. ⓐⓑⓒⓓ	10. ⓐⓑⓒⓓ
	11. ⓐⓑⓒⓓ	12. ⓐⓑⓒⓓ	13. ⓐⓑⓒⓓ	14. ⓐⓑⓒⓓ	15. ⓐⓑⓒⓓ
	16. ⓐⓑⓒⓓ	17. ⓐⓑⓒⓓ			

Space for Rough Work

18. What is the similarity between gymnosperms and angiosperms ?
(a) Phloem of both have companian cells.
(b) Endosperm is formed before fertilization in both.
(c) Origin of ovule and seed is similar in both.
(d) Both have leaves, stem and roots.

19. In Chlorophyceae, sexual reproduction occurs by
(a) isogamy and anisogamy
(b) isogamy, anisogamy and oogamy
(c) oogamy only
(d) anisogamy and oogamy

20. In gymnosperms, the ovule is naked because
(a) ovary wall is absent (b) integuments are absent
(c) perianth is absent (d) nucellus is absent

21. How many meiotic division would be required to produce 101 female gametophytes in an angiosperm?
(a) 101 (b) 26
(c) 127 (d) None of these

22. Which one of the following is the major difference between mosses and ferns ?
(a) Ferns lack alternation of generation while mosses show the same.
(b) Mosses are facultative aerobes while ferns are obligate aerobes.
(c) Vascular bundles of ferns show xylem vessels while those of mosses lack it.
(d) Sporophytes of ferns live much longer as compared to the sporophytes of mosses.

23. Red snow causing alga is
(a) *Chlamydomonas nivalis*
(b) *Chlamydomonas reinhardtii*
(c) *Chlamydomonas debaryanum*
(d) *Chalmydomonas media*

24. Alginates (alginin), used as highly efficient gauze in internal operations are obtained from cell walls of
(a) Cyanophyceae (b) Phaeophyceae
(c) Rhodophyceae (d) All of these

25. Bryophytes resemble algae in the following aspects
(a) Filamentous body, presence of vascular tissues and autotrophic nutrition
(b) Differentiation of plant body into root, stem and leaves and autotrophic nutrition
(c) Thallus like plant body, presence of root and autotrophic nutrition
(d) Thallus like plant body, lack of vascular tissues and autotrophic nutrition

26. In sexual life cycle of *Agaricus*, dikaryotization (n + n) is brought about by
(a) Fusion of male and female sex organs
(b) Fusion of vegetative cells of different genotypes
(c) Somatogamy between basidiospores
(d) Fusion of motile gametes

27. Read the following features properly
A. Free living
B. Mostly photosynthetic
C. Mostly parasitic
D. Inconspicuous
E. Unicellular
How many of the given features are correct for prothallus of pteridophytes?
(a) Three (b) Five
(c) Four (d) Two

28. Identify the correctly matched pair:

	Class	Example	Feature
(a)	Psilopsida	*Lycopodium*	Seed habit
(b)	Sphenopsida	*Selaginella*	Strobilus
(c)	Lycopsida	*Psilotum*	Homosporous
(d)	Pteropsida	*Dryopteris*	Macrophylls

29. Angiosperms have dominated the land flora primarily because of their
(a) power of adaptability in diverse habitat
(b) property of producing large number of seeds
(c) nature of self pollination
(d) domestication by man

RESPONSE GRID					
	18. ⓐⓑⓒⓓ	19. ⓐⓑⓒⓓ	20. ⓐⓑⓒⓓ	21. ⓐⓑⓒⓓ	22. ⓐⓑⓒⓓ
	23. ⓐⓑⓒⓓ	24. ⓐⓑⓒⓓ	25. ⓐⓑⓒⓓ	26. ⓐⓑⓒⓓ	27. ⓐⓑⓒⓓ
	28. ⓐⓑⓒⓓ	29. ⓐⓑⓒⓓ			

Space for Rough Work

30. Which out of the following are included under tracheophyta i.e., vascular plants?
(a) Pteridophytes (b) Gymnosperms
(c) Angiosperms (d) All of these

31. At least a half of the total CO_2 fixation on earth is carried out through photosynthesis by
(a) angiosperms (b) gymnosperms
(c) algae (d) bryophytes

32. The embryonic development in bryophytes takes place in the
(a) protonema (b) sporangium
(c) antheridium (d) archegonium.

33. The spread of living pteridophytes is limited and is restricted to narrow geographical region because of
(a) gametophytic growth needs cool, damp and shady places
(b) requirement of water for fertilization
(c) absence of stomata in leaf and absence of vascular tissue
(d) both (a) and (b)

34. Gymnosperm called as a living fossil is
(a) *Cycas* (b) *Ginkgo*
(c) *Juniperus* (d) Both (a) and (b).

35. The sporophyte is the dominant phase in
(a) pteridophytes (b) gymnosperms
(c) angiosperms (d) all of these.

36. Which kind of life-cycle pattern is exhibited by seed-bearing plants?
(a) Haplontic (b) Diplontic
(c) Haplo-diplontic (d) All of these

37. Plants reproducing by spores such as mosses and ferns are grouped under the general term
(a) Thallophytes (b) Cryptogams
(c) Bryophytes (d) Sporophytes

38. Angiosperms have dominated the land flora primarily because of their
(a) Power of adaptability in diverse habitat
(b) Property of producing large number of seeds
(c) Nature of self pollination
(d) Domestication by man

39. Many blue-green algae occur in thermal springs (hot water springs). The temperature tolerance of these algae have been attributed to their
(a) cell wall structure
(b) mitochondrial structure
(c) modern cell organization
(d) importance of homopolar bonds in their proteins

40. Which of the following occurs both in fresh as well as in marine water ?
(a) Spirogyra (b) *Cladophora*
(c) Oedogonium (d) *Cephaleuros*

41. The pyrenoids are made up of
(a) proteinaceous centre and starchy sheath
(b) core of protein surrounded by fatty sheath
(c) core of starch surrounded by sheath of protein
(d) core of nucleic acid surrounded by protein sheath

42. Blue green algae have
(a) chlorophyll (b) xanthyophyll
(c) phycocyanin (d) fucoxanthin

43. Parasitic alga is
(a) *Volvox* (b) Ulothrix
(c) *Porphyra* (d) *Cephaleuros*

44. Which one of the following pairs of plants are not seed producers?
(a) *Funaria* and *Pinus* (b) Fern and *Funaria*
(c) *Funaria* and *Ficus* (d) *Ficus* and *Chlamydomonas*

45. Neck canal cells are absent in archegonia of–
(a) Bryophytes (b) Gymnosperms
(c) Pteridophytes (d) All of these

RESPONSE GRID	30. ⓐⓑⓒⓓ	31. ⓐⓑⓒⓓ	32. ⓐⓑⓒⓓ	33. ⓐⓑⓒⓓ	34. ⓐⓑⓒⓓ
	35. ⓐⓑⓒⓓ	36. ⓐⓑⓒⓓ	37. ⓐⓑⓒⓓ	38. ⓐⓑⓒⓓ	39. ⓐⓑⓒⓓ
	40. ⓐⓑⓒⓓ	41. ⓐⓑⓒⓓ	42. ⓐⓑⓒⓓ	43. ⓐⓑⓒⓓ	44. ⓐⓑⓒⓓ
	45. ⓐⓑⓒⓓ				

BIOLOGY CHAPTERWISE SPEED TEST-61			
Total Questions	45	Total Marks	180
Attempted		Correct	
Incorrect		Net Score	
Cut-off Score	35	Qualifying Score	50
Success Gap = Net Score – Qualifying Score			
Net Score = (Correct × 4) – (Incorrect × 1)			

Space for Rough Work

BIOLOGY

Animal Kingdom

Speed TEST 62 Chapter-wise

No. of Questions	Maximum Marks	Time
45	180	1 Hour

GENERAL INSTRUCTIONS

- This test contains 45 MCQ's. For each question only one option is correct. Darken the correct circle/ bubble in the Response Grid provided on each page.
- You have to evaluate your Response Grids yourself with the help of solutions provided at the end of this book.
- Each correct answer will get you 4 marks and 1 mark shall be deduced for each incorrect answer. No mark will be given/ deducted if no bubble is filled. Keep a timer in front of you and stop immediately at the end of 60 min.
- The sheet follows a particular syllabus. Do not attempt the sheet before you have completed your preparation for that syllabus.
- After completing the sheet check your answers with the solution booklet and complete the Result Grid. Finally spend time to analyse your performance and revise the areas which emerge out as weak in your evaluation.

1. Classification of Porifera is based on
   (a) branching (b) spicules
   (c) reproduction (d) symmetry
2. A chordate character is
   (a) gills (b) spiracles
   (c) postanal tail (d) chitinous exoskeleton
3. Which one of the following pairs of animals comprises 'jawless fishes'?
   (a) Mackerals and Rohu (b) Lampreys and hag fishes
   (c) Guppies and hag fishes (d) Lampreys and eels
4. Leech is
   (a) carnivorous (b) sanguivorous
   (c) ectoparasite (d) Both (b) and (c)
5. Which one of the following groups of animals is bilaterally symmetrical and triploblastic?
   (a) Aschelminthes (round worms)
   (b) Ctenophores
   (c) Sponges
   (d) Coelenterates (Cnidarians)
6. Which of the following animal is cold blooded and has 4 - chambered heart?
   (a) Salamander (b) *Ornithorhynchus*
   (c) Crocodile (d) *Calotes*
7. Which one of the following is NOT a characteristic of phylum Annelida?
   (a) Closed circulatory system
   (b) Segmentation
   (c) Pseudocoelom
   (d) Ventral nerve cord

RESPONSE GRID					
	1. ⓐⓑⓒⓓ	2. ⓐⓑⓒⓓ	3. ⓐⓑⓒⓓ	4. ⓐⓑⓒⓓ	5. ⓐⓑⓒⓓ
	6. ⓐⓑⓒⓓ	7. ⓐⓑⓒⓓ			

Space for Rough Work

8. Which one of the following characters is not typical of the class mammalia?
(a) Thecodont dentition
(b) Alveolar lungs
(c) Ten pairs of cranial nerves
(d) Seven cervical vertebrae

9. Which one of following feature is possessed by Crustaceans and not by insects?
(a) Paired limbs
(b) Two pairs of antenna
(c) Chitinous exoskeleton
(d) Bilateral symmetry

10. Poison glands of snake are modified
(a) Linguals (b) Sublinguals
(c) Maxillaries (d) Parotids

11. The adults are radially symmetrical but larvae exhibit bilateral symmetry in
(a) Mollusca (b) Hemichordata
(c) Echinodermata (d) Cephalochordata

12. Which one of the following categories of animals, is correctly described with no single exception in it?
(a) All sponges are marine and have collared cells.
(b) All mammals are viviparous and possess diaphragm for breathing.
(c) All bony fishes have four pairs of gills and an operculum on each side.
(d) All reptiles possess scales, have a three chambered heart and are cold blooded (poikilothermal).

13. Solenocytes and metanephridia are excretory organs of
(a) Annelida and Arthropoda
(b) Platyhelminthes and Annelida
(c) Coelenterata and Mollusca
(d) Aschelminthes and Annelida

14. Radial symmetry occurs in
(a) Porifera and Coelenterata
(b) Coelenterata and Echinodermata
(c) Coelenterata and Platyhelminthes
(d) Arthropoda and Mollusca

15. Which of the following statements is/are not true?
(i) In Urochordata, notochord is present in larval tail.
(ii) In Cephalochordata, notochord extends from head to tail region.
(iii) *Branchiostoma* belongs to hemichordata.
(iv) Only one class of living members, class Cyclostomata represents the super class agnatha
(a) (ii) and (iv) (b) (i), (iii) and (iv)
(c) (iii) only (d) (i) and (iv)

16. In *Amoeba* and *Paramecium* osmoregulation occurs through
(a) pseudopodia (b) nucleus
(c) contractile vacuole (d) general surface

17. Animals with metameric segmentation, bilateral symmetry and closed circulatory system belong to phylum
(a) Annelida (b) Echinodermata
(c) Arthropoda (d) Mollusca

18. Which one of the following characters is **not** typical of the class Mammalia?
(a) Thecodont dentition
(b) Alveolar lungs
(c) Ten pairs of cranial nerves
(d) Seven cervical vertebrae

19. The segments of earthworms are
(a) Apparent in the embryo but not in the adult
(b) Specialised for different functions and are present in endoderm only
(c) Present in mesoderm but not in the ectoderm
(d) Repetitive, with serial repetition of at least some organs

20. The evolution of an internal body cavity/coelom offered an advantage in animal body design in all areas, except
(a) Evolution of effecient organ systems
(b) Provides space within which the gonads can expand and large number of gametes stored
(c) Circulation
(d) Greater freedom of movement

RESPONSE GRID					
	8. ⓐⓑⓒⓓ	9. ⓐⓑⓒⓓ	10. ⓐⓑⓒⓓ	11. ⓐⓑⓒⓓ	12. ⓐⓑⓒⓓ
	13. ⓐⓑⓒⓓ	14. ⓐⓑⓒⓓ	15. ⓐⓑⓒⓓ	16. ⓐⓑⓒⓓ	17. ⓐⓑⓒⓓ
	18. ⓐⓑⓒⓓ	19. ⓐⓑⓒⓓ	20. ⓐⓑⓒⓓ		

Space for Rough Work

21. Animals like bats have/are
(a) Hollow skeleton
(b) Feathers which are modified reptilian scales
(c) Endothermic
(d) Efficient respiration. Non-vascular air sacs are connected to lungs to supplement respiration

22. Which of the following is incorrect match of animal group/life style/structure/function?

	Animal	Lifestyle	Structure/functions group
(a)	Sponges	Sessile filter feeders	Amoebocytes/carry food and wastes Spicules/support and protection spongin / support
(b)	Cnidarians	Free floating or attached	Gastrovascular cavity/digestion Cnidocytes/ protection and food getting
(c)	Flatworms	Free living or parasite	Flame cells/ excretion Tegument/ protection
(d)	Molluscs	Terrestrial, marine, fresh water inhabitants	Radula/feeding mantle/motility

23. Complete the following analogy : Pigeon's milk : Crop :: Song :
(a) Syrinx (b) Trachea
(c) Proventriculus (d) Anterior air sacs

24. Which of the following is not correct matching of phylum and its three examples?
(a) Annelida : *Aphrodite, Chaetopterus, Bonnelia*
(b) Mollusca : *Teredo, Aplysia, Chaetopleura*
(c) Aschelminthes : *Ancylostoma, Enterobius, Tubifex*
(d) Arthropoda : *Buthus, Lepisma, Leptocorisa*

25. Hemichordates differ from chordates, in that hemichordates
(a) Are gill breathers
(b) Fertilisation is external and development is indirect
(c) Do not possess notochord
(d) Are bilaterally symmetrical, triploblastic and coelomate animals

26. All birds have
(a) Oil gland at the base of tail
(b) Feather on their body and can fly
(c) Nests to care their babies
(d) Internal fertilization, are oviparous and eggs are covered with calcareous shell

27. Which one of the following is a coelenterate?
(a) Sea mouse (b) Sea anemone
(c) Sea urchin (d) Sea cucumber

28. Presence of external ear pinna, body hairs, four chambered heart are the characters of
(a) *Macropus* (b) *Balaenoptera*
(c) *Psittacula* (d) *Aptenodytes*

29. Which one of the following statements about certain given animals is correct?
(a) Round worms are pseudo-coelomates
(b) Molluscs are acoelomates
(c) Insects are pseudo-coelomates
(d) Flatworms are coelomates

30. Which one of the following phyla is correctly matched with its two general characteristics?
(a) Echinodermata – pentamerous radial symmetry and mostly internal fertilization
(b) Mollusca – normally oviparous and development through a trochophore or veliger larva
(c) Arthropoda – body divided into head, thorax and abdomen and respiration by mouth
(d) Chordata – notochord persists throughout and separate anal and urinary openings to the outside

31. Amphibians share with reptiles all of the following characters expect
(a) ventral heart
(b) external fertilization and indirect development
(c) dioecious, oviparous
(d) cold blooded or poikilotherms.

RESPONSE GRID					
	21. ⓐⓑⓒⓓ	22. ⓐⓑⓒⓓ	23. ⓐⓑⓒⓓ	24. ⓐⓑⓒⓓ	25. ⓐⓑⓒⓓ
	26. ⓐⓑⓒⓓ	27. ⓐⓑⓒⓓ	28. ⓐⓑⓒⓓ	29. ⓐⓑⓒⓓ	30. ⓐⓑⓒⓓ
	31. ⓐⓑⓒⓓ				

Space for Rough Work

32. Which of the following statements about the body cavity of animals is true ?
(a) The body cavity of coelomates develops from the embryonic ectoderm.
(b) The acoelomates' body cavity is filled with liquid.
(c) The pseudocoel of the pseudocoelomates have a peritoneum.
(d) The acoelomates do not have an enclosed body cavity.

33. Sponges have a very simple body plan. Which of the following statements about sponge structure or function is false ?
(a) Choanocytes are flagellated cells that play a role in feeding.
(b) Large species are found in areas of heavy wave action, where food is most abundant.
(c) Individual sponges are both male and female.
(d) Water enters a sponge through pores and exits via one or more oscula.

34. Which of the following traits is not shared by the Ctenophora and the Cnidaria ?
(a) Both are diploblastic
(b) Both have radial symmetry
(c) Both have complete guts.
(d) Both have feeding tentacles.

35. Earthworm has
(a) Two eyes (b) Many eyes
(c) No eyes (d) One eye.

36. Which of the following statements is not true of the Rotifera ?
(a) They have a complete gut with an anterior mouth and posterior anus.
(b) They are coelomates
(c) The corona is a ciliated organ used in acquiring food.
(d) They use a hydrostatic skeleton.

37. The combination of a true coelom and repeating body segmentation allows the annelids (unlike the anatomically "simpler" worms) to do which of the following ?
(a) Attain complex body shapes and thus locomote more precisely
(b) Move through loose marine sediments
(c) Be hermaphroditic
(d) Inject paralytic poisons into their prey

38. An animal is divided along its main body axis to produce similar halves. Which of the following types of symmetry could apply ?
(a) Spherical (b) Radial
(c) Radial or biradial (d) Bilateral

39. Cephalization is a characteristic mainly associated with which of the following types of body symmetry in animals ?
(a) Asymmetric (b) Radial
(c) Biradial (d) Bilateral

40. Amphids present on ventrolateral lips of *Ascaris* are
(a) Chemoreceptors (b) Olfactoreceptors
(c) Tactoreceptors (d) Gustatoreceptors

41. Corals are common representatives of the cnidarian class______.
(a) Scyphozoa (b) Anthozoa
(c) Porifera (d) Placozoa

42. Which of the following characteristics is unique to the phylum Cnidaria ?
(a) Sexual reproduction
(b) Symbiotic associations with other organisms
(c) Sedentary body forms
(d) Nematocysts

43. Which of the following statements is true of all flatworms ?
(a) Flatworms are biradially symmetric
(b) Flatworms have a complete digestive system
(c) Flatworms tend to have large, thickened bodies
(d) Flatworms are triploblastic

44. Which of the following structures is absent from a typical gastropod mollusk (e.g., a garden snail) ?
(a) Protective shell (b) Head
(c) Radula (d) None of these

45. Which two of the following are found in the mesophyl or protein matrix and serve as structural support for a sponge ?
(a) spicule, spongin (b) osculum, spicule
(c) medusa, polyp (d) polyp, osculum

RESPONSE GRID					
	32. ⓐⓑⓒⓓ	33. ⓐⓑⓒⓓ	34. ⓐⓑⓒⓓ	35. ⓐⓑⓒⓓ	36. ⓐⓑⓒⓓ
	37. ⓐⓑⓒⓓ	38. ⓐⓑⓒⓓ	39. ⓐⓑⓒⓓ	40. ⓐⓑⓒⓓ	41. ⓐⓑⓒⓓ
	42. ⓐⓑⓒⓓ	43. ⓐⓑⓒⓓ	44. ⓐⓑⓒⓓ	45. ⓐⓑⓒⓓ	

BIOLOGY CHAPTERWISE SPEED TEST-62			
Total Questions	45	Total Marks	180
Attempted		Correct	
Incorrect		Net Score	
Cut-off Score	40	Qualifying Score	65
Success Gap = Net Score – Qualifying Score			
Net Score = (Correct × 4) – (Incorrect × 1)			

Space for Rough Work

BIOLOGY

Morphology of Flowering Plants

Speed TEST 63

Chapter-wise

No. of Questions	Maximum Marks	Time
45	180	1 Hour

GENERAL INSTRUCTIONS

- This test contains 45 MCQ's. For each question only one option is correct. Darken the correct circle/ bubble in the Response Grid provided on each page.
- You have to evaluate your Response Grids yourself with the help of solutions provided at the end of this book.
- Each correct answer will get you 4 marks and 1 mark shall be deduced for each incorrect answer. No mark will be given/ deducted if no bubble is filled. Keep a timer in front of you and stop immediately at the end of 60 min.
- The sheet follows a particular syllabus. Do not attempt the sheet before you have completed your preparation for that syllabus.
- After completing the sheet check your answers with the solution booklet and complete the Result Grid. Finally spend time to analyse your performance and revise the areas which emerge out as weak in your evaluation.

1. Which one of the following is a true fruit?
   (a) Apple (b) Pear
   (c) Cashew nut (d) Coconut
2. Pulses are belong to the family
   (a) fabaceae (b) asteraceae
   (c) poaceae (d) solanaceae
3. In a cereal grain the single cotyledon of embryo is represented by
   (a) scutellum (b) prophyll
   (c) coleoptile (d) coleorrhiza
4. Perisperm is
   (a) remnant of endosperm
   (b) persistant nucellus
   (c) remnant of embryo
   (d) part of endosperm
5. The mode of catching insects in *Drosera* plants is by means of
   (a) sensitive glandular hairs which secrete a sweet, viscous, shining substance.
   (b) specially sensitive trigger hairs.
   (c) leaves which are modified into pitcher.
   (d) leaf segments modified into bladder.
6. Insectivorous plants grow in
   (a) calcium deficient soil
   (b) carbon deficient soil
   (c) magnesium deficient soil
   (d) nitrogen deficient soil
7. Which part of the coconut produces coir?
   (a) Seed coat (b) Mesocarp
   (c) Epicarp (d) Pericarp

RESPONSE GRID	
	1. ⓐⓑⓒⓓ 2. ⓐⓑⓒⓓ 3. ⓐⓑⓒⓓ 4. ⓐⓑⓒⓓ 5. ⓐⓑⓒⓓ
	6. ⓐⓑⓒⓓ 7. ⓐⓑⓒⓓ

Space for Rough Work

8. Pineapple (ananas) fruit develops from
   (a) a multipistillate syncarpous flower
   (b) a cluster of compactly borne flowers on a common axis
   (c) a multilocular monocarpellary flower
   (d) a unilocular polycarpellary flower
9. Scutellum is a/an
   (a) protective covering of radicle
   (b) protective covering of plumule
   (c) endosperm of gymnosperms
   (d) shield-shaped cotyledon
10. Fibrous root system is better adopted than tap root system for
   (a) transport of organic matter
   (b) absorption of water and minerals
   (c) storage of food
   (d) anchorage of plant to soil
11. Velamen is found in
   (a) roots of screwpine
   (b) aerial and terrestrial roots of orchids
   (c) leaves of *Ficus elastica*
   (d) only aerial roots of orchids
12. Hypanthodium is
   (a) thalamus (b) fruit
   (c) inflorescence (d) ovary
13. Which of the following statement (s) is/are incorrect?
   (i) Calyx and corolla are reproductive organs of a flower.
   (ii) Zygomorphic flower can be divided into two equal radial halves in any radial plane.
   (iii) Flowers without bracts are termed as bracteate.
   (iv) Parthenocarpic fruit is formed after fertilization of the ovary.
   (v) In legumes, seed is non-endospermic.
   (vi) Radical buds develop on roots.
   (a) (i), (ii), (iii) and (iv) (b) (i), (ii) and (v)
   (c) (iii), (iv) and (vi) (d) (i), (iv) and (v)
14. Milky water of green coconut is
   (a) liquid nucellus
   (b) liquid of female gametophyte
   (c) liquid endosperm
   (d) liquid embryo
15. Clove is
   (a) flower bud (b) axillary bud
   (c) thalamus (d) ovule
16. When gynoecium is present in the top most position of thalamus, the flower is known as
   (a) inferior (b) epigynous
   (c) perigynous (d) hypogynous
17. Which is not a stem modification ?
   (a) Rhizome of ginger (b) Corm of *Colocasia*
   (c) Pitcher of *Nepenthes* (d) Tuber of potato
18. Which option is correctly matched with the diagrams?

   A B C D

   (a) A-Valvate B-Twisted, C-Imbricate, D-Vexillary
   (b) A-Vexillary, B-Valvate, C-Twisted, D-Imbricate
   (c) A-Imbricate, B-Vexillary, C-Valvate, D-Twisted
   (d) A-Twisted, B-Imbricate, C-Vexillary, D-Valvate

RESPONSE GRID					
	8. ⓐⓑⓒⓓ	9. ⓐⓑⓒⓓ	10. ⓐⓑⓒⓓ	11. ⓐⓑⓒⓓ	12. ⓐⓑⓒⓓ
	13. ⓐⓑⓒⓓ	14. ⓐⓑⓒⓓ	15. ⓐⓑⓒⓓ	16. ⓐⓑⓒⓓ	17. ⓐⓑⓒⓓ
	18. ⓐⓑⓒⓓ				

Space for Rough Work

19. Given below are the diagrammatic representation of position of floral parts on thalamus, condition of ovary and example. Find the correctly matched combination?

	Position of floral parts on thalamus	Condition of ovary	Example
(a)	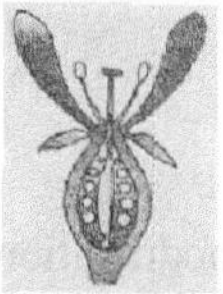	$\overline{G}$	Cucumber
(b)	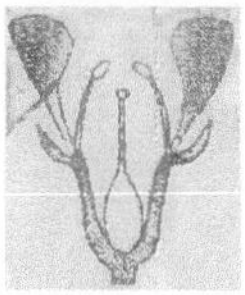	G–	Brinjal
(c)	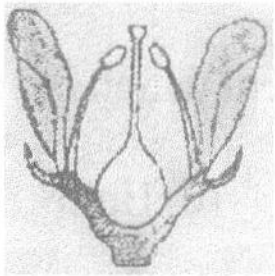	$\underline{G}$	Plum
(d)	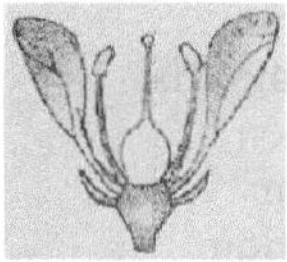	$\overline{G}$	Rose

20. Match Column-I with Column-II and select the correct option from the codes given below.

	Column-I		Column-II
A.	Thorns	I.	Vegetative propagation
B.	Phylloclades	II.	Defensive mechanism
C.	Runners	III.	Mechanical support
D.	Stilt roots	IV.	Absorption of nutrition
E.	Haustoria	V.	Photosynthesis

(a) A-I; B-IV; C-III; D-II; E-I
(b) A-II; B-V; C-III; D-I; E-IV
(c) A-II; B-V; C-I; D-III; E-IV
(d) A-III; B-V; C-IV; D-I; E-II

21. Maize grain is a fruit known as
(a) cypsela (b) caryopsis
(c) legume (d) achene

22. Monocotyledonous root differs from dicot root in which of the following internal features (a to d)?
(a) Presence of parenchymatous pericycle.
(b) Absence of fewre xylem bundle.
(c) Presence of large and well-developed pith.
(d) Presence of parenchymatous cortex without intercellular spaces.

23. Select correct match w.r.t column I & II.

	Column I		Column II
A.	Modified tap root for respiration	I.	Zea mays
B.	Storage tap root	II.	ipomoea
C.	Modified aventitious root for mechanical support	III.	Rhizophora
D.	Modified adventitious root for food storge	IV.	Turnip

(a) A-III; B-IV; C-I; D-II
(b) A-III; B-IV; C-II; D-I
(c) A-IV; B-II; C-I; D-III
(d) A-III; B-II; C-I; D-IV

24. The modified stem in some plants of arid region is
(a) Tendril for climbring as in *Passiflora*
(b) Spines for defence mechanism
(c) Phylloclade for food synthesis
(d) Phyllode for food synthesis

25. The modified stem in grasses, strawberry and *Crysanthemum* is concerned with special functions i.e.,
i. Food storage
ii. Vegetative propagation
iii. Assimilation
iv. Spread to new niches
v. Perennation
(a) ii, iv (b) i, ii, v
(c) ii, iv, v (d) iii, iv, v

RESPONSE GRID	19. ⓐⓑⓒⓓ	20. ⓐⓑⓒⓓ	21. ⓐⓑⓒⓓ	22. ⓐⓑⓒⓓ	23. ⓐⓑⓒⓓ
	24. ⓐⓑⓒⓓ	25. ⓐⓑⓒⓓ			

Space for Rough Work

26. In which of the following type of flowers stamens are superior in position?
(a) Hypogynous (b) Perigynous
(c) Epigynous (d) Protogynous

27. Inner layer of pericarp is hard and stony in
(a) Dateplam, Almond (b) Wood, apple, Pea
(c) Mango, Coconut (d) Pear, Litchi

28. Find out the incorrect match.
(a) Sterile stamen – Staminode
(b) Stamens attached to petals – Epipetalous
(c) Stamens attached to perianth – Episepalous
(d) Free stamens – Polyandrous

29. Ovary is said to be half inferior in which of the following conditions?
(a) Hypogynous (b) Perigynous
(c) Epigynous (d) Both (b) and (c)

30. Identify the family which shows the following diagnostic features.
Flowers pentamerous, gynoecium-bicarpellary, syncarpous, ovary placed obliquely, placentation axile, placenta swollen.
(a) Solanaceae (b) Le guminosae
(c) Papilionaceae (d) Liliaceae

31. Select the pair which contains monocotyledonous families.
(a) Solanaceae and Brassicaceae
(b) Fabaceae and Asteraceae
(c) Liliaceae and Poaceae
(d) None of these

32. In Nepenthes (pitcher plant), the pitcher is formed due to modification of
(a) leaf petiole (b) leaf lamina
(c) tendril (d) leaflet

33. Example for tuberous adventitious roots
(a) Dahlia (b) Carrot
(c) Radish (d) Beet

34. A root-cap is usually absent in the roots of
(a) Hydrophytes (b) Epiphytes
(c) Parasites (d) All of the above

35. An example of negatively geotropic root
(a) Coralloid root of *Cycas*
(b) Pneumatophore of mangroves
(c) Assimilatory roots *of Trapa*
(d) More than one of the above.

36. *Santalum album* is normally considered as a
(a) Complete root parasite
(b) Partial root parasite
(c) Complete stem parasite
(d) Partial stem parasite

37. An example of tuberous root that is a modification of tap foot
(a) Radish (b) *Mirabilis*
(c) Sweet Potato (d) *Ipomoea*

38. Ginger is a stem and not a root because
(a) It stores food
(b) It is bitter in taste
(c) It has nodes and internodes
(d) It is non-green in colour.

39. In *Allium*, the leafless part of the stem which bears flower is called
(a) Culm (b) Scape (c) Caudex (d) Bulb

40. Sweet Potato is a modification of
(a) Root (b) Stem
(c) Bud (d) Flowering axis

41. Epiphyllous buds serve the function of
(a) Respiration (b) Nutrition
(c) Reproduction (d) Absorption

42. In a potato plant the tubers develop on
(a) Primary root (b) Secondary root
(c) Tertiary root (d) Stolon

43. Root is the prolongation of
(a) Plumule (b) Radicle
(c) Stem (d) Branches

44. Food stored in a bulb is within
(a) A swollen stem (b) Swollen leaf-bases
(c) Enlarged roots (d) In the inflorescence

45. Cladode is the modification of
(a) Whole stem (b) Axillary bud
(c) Leaf (d) Leaflets.

RESPONSE GRID					
	26. ⓐⓑⓒⓓ	27. ⓐⓑⓒⓓ	28. ⓐⓑⓒⓓ	29. ⓐⓑⓒⓓ	30. ⓐⓑⓒⓓ
	31. ⓐⓑⓒⓓ	32. ⓐⓑⓒⓓ	33. ⓐⓑⓒⓓ	34. ⓐⓑⓒⓓ	35. ⓐⓑⓒⓓ
	36. ⓐⓑⓒⓓ	37. ⓐⓑⓒⓓ	38. ⓐⓑⓒⓓ	39. ⓐⓑⓒⓓ	40. ⓐⓑⓒⓓ
	41. ⓐⓑⓒⓓ	42. ⓐⓑⓒⓓ	43. ⓐⓑⓒⓓ	44. ⓐⓑⓒⓓ	45. ⓐⓑⓒⓓ

BIOLOGY CHAPTERWISE SPEED TEST-63			
Total Questions	45	Total Marks	180
Attempted		Correct	
Incorrect		Net Score	
Cut-off Score	45	Qualifying Score	60
Success Gap = Net Score – Qualifying Score			
Net Score = (Correct × 4) – (Incorrect × 1)			

Space for Rough Work

BIOLOGY

Anatomy of Flowering Plants

Speed TEST 64

Chapter-wise

No. of Questions	Maximum Marks	Time
45	**180**	**1 Hour**

GENERAL INSTRUCTIONS

- This test contains 45 MCQ's. For each question only one option is correct. Darken the correct circle/ bubble in the Response Grid provided on each page.
- You have to evaluate your Response Grids yourself with the help of solutions provided at the end of this book.
- Each correct answer will get you 4 marks and 1 mark shall be deduced for each incorrect answer. No mark will be given/ deducted if no bubble is filled. Keep a timer in front of you and stop immediately at the end of 60 min.
- The sheet follows a particular syllabus. Do not attempt the sheet before you have completed your preparation for that syllabus.
- After completing the sheet check your answers with the solution booklet and complete the Result Grid. Finally spend time to analyse your performance and revise the areas which emerge out as weak in your evaluation.

1. During formation of leaves and elongation of stem, some cells ' left behind' from the shoot apical meristem, constitute ____
   (a) Lateral meristem (b) Axillary bud
   (c) Cork cambium (d) Fascicular cambium
2. Function of companion cells is
   (a) providing energy to sieve elements for active transport.
   (b) providing water to phloem.
   (c) loading of sucrose into sieve elements by passive transport.
   (d) loading of sucrose into sieve elements.
3. The cork cambium, cork and secondary cortex are collectively called
   (a) phelloderm (b) phellogen
   (c) periderm (d) phellem
4. Which of the following does not have stomata ?
   (a) Hydrophytes (b) Mesophytes
   (c) Xerophytes (d) Submerged hydrophytes
5. The chief water conducting elements of xylem in gymnosperms are :
   (a) vessels (b) fibres
   (c) transfusion tissue (d) tracheids
6. Which is correct about transport or conduction of substances?
   (a) Organic food moves up through phloem.
   (b) Organic food moves up through phloem
   (c) Inorganic food moves upwardly and downwardly through xylem
   (d) Organic food moves upwardly and downwardly through phloem

RESPONSE GRID	
	1. ⓐⓑⓒⓓ 2. ⓐⓑⓒⓓ 3. ⓐⓑⓒⓓ 4. ⓐⓑⓒⓓ 5. ⓐⓑⓒⓓ
	6. ⓐⓑⓒⓓ

Space for Rough Work

7. A narrow layer of thin walled cells found between phloem/ bark and wood of a dicot is
(a) cork cambium (b) vascular cambium
(c) endodermis (d) pericycle

8. Which of the following statements is true?
(a) Vessels are multicellular with narrow lumen.
(b) Tracheids are multicellular with narrow lumen.
(c) Vessels are unicellular with wide lumen.
(d) Tracheids are unicellular with wide lumen.

9. The quiescent centre in root meristem serves as a
(a) site for storage of food which is utilized during maturation.
(b) reservoir of growth hormones.
(c) reserve for replenishment of damaged cells of the meristem.
(d) region for absorption of water.

10. Root hair arises from
(a) pericycle (b) endodermis
(c) cortex (d) epiblema

11. Phellogen and phellem respectively denote
(a) cork and cork cambium
(b) cork cambium and cork
(c) secondary cortex and cork
(d) cork and secondary cortex

12. The common bottle cork is a product of :
(a) Dermatogen (b) Phellogen
(c) Xylem (d) Vascular cambium

13. A vascular bundle in which the protoxylem is pointing to the periphery is called
(a) endarch (b) exarch
(c) radial (d) closed

14. Which of the following does not have stomata?
(a) Hydrophytes
(b) Mesophytes
(c) Xerophytes
(d) Submerged hydrophytes

15. Collenchyma differs from parenchyma in having
(a) living protoplasm
(b) cellulose walls
(c) vacuoles
(d) pectin deposits at corners

16. Which of the following plant shows multiple epidermis?
(a) *Croton* (b) *Allium*
(c) *Nerium* (d) *Cucurbita*

17. Epidermis is absent in
(a) root tip and shoot tip (b) shoot bud and floral bud
(c) ovule and seed (d) petiole and pedicel

18. Which of the following layer is present nearest of plasma membrane in plant cell?
(a) Secondary wall (b) Middle lamella
(c) Primary wall (d) Tonoplast

19. Which one of the following statement is false?
(i) Epidermal cell has small amount of cytoplasm and a large vacuole.
(ii) Waxy cuticle layer is absent in roots.
(iii) Root hairs are unicellular, while stem hairs / trichomes are multicellular.
(iv) Trichomes may be branched or unbranched, soft or stiff and prevent transpiration.
(v) Guard cells are dumbell shaped in dicots and bean-shaped in monocots.
(a) (i) only (b) (iv) only
(c) (iii) only (d) (v) only

20. Which option is true about heart wood/duramen?
(i) It does not help in water and mineral conduction.
(ii) It is dark coloured but soft.
(iii) It has tracheary elements filled with tannins, resins, gums, oil, etc.
(iv) It is a peripheral part.
(v) Sensitive to microbes and insects, hence least durable.
(a) (i) and (iii) (b) (ii) and (iii)
(c) (iv) and (v) (d) (iii) and (iv)

RESPONSE GRID					
	7. ⓐⓑⓒⓓ	8. ⓐⓑⓒⓓ	9. ⓐⓑⓒⓓ	10. ⓐⓑⓒⓓ	11. ⓐⓑⓒⓓ
	12. ⓐⓑⓒⓓ	13. ⓐⓑⓒⓓ	14. ⓐⓑⓒⓓ	15. ⓐⓑⓒⓓ	16. ⓐⓑⓒⓓ
	17. ⓐⓑⓒⓓ	18. ⓐⓑⓒⓓ	19. ⓐⓑⓒⓓ	20. ⓐⓑⓒⓓ	

21. In land plants, the guard cells differ from other epidermal cells in having
(a) cytoskeleton (b) mitochondria
(c) endoplasmic reticulum (d) chloroplasts

22. Which of the following statement(s) is/are true?
(i) Uneven thickening of cell wall is characteristic of sclerenchyma.
(ii) Periblem forms cortex of the stem and the root.
(iii) Tracheids are the chief water transporting elements in gymnosperms.
(iv) Companion cell is devoid of nucleus at maturity.
(v) The Commercial cork is obtained from *Quercus suber.*
(a) (i) and (iv) only (b) (ii) and (v) only
(c) (iii) and (iv) only (d) (ii), (iii) and (v) only

23. In endarch condition of xylem, protoxylem lies ______ of metaxylem.
(a) on inner side
(b) on outer side
(c) both on inner and outer side
(d) in centre

24. Y-shaped arrangement of xylem vessels is found in
(a) monocot stem (b) dicotstem
(c) monocot root (d) dicot root

25. Study carefully the following statements and select the incorrect one(s).
(i) Lateral roots develop from pericycle.
(ii) Endodermis is the innermost layer of cortex.
(iii) Sap wood is the central, dark coloured, non-conducting part of secondary xylem
(a) (i) and (ii) (b) (ii) and (iii)
(c) (i) only (d) (iii) only

26. Removed parts of grasses by the grazing herbivores are regenerated fast by
(a) Both apical and intercalary meristems
(b) Lateral meristems only
(c) Secondary meristems
(d) Intercallary meristems

27. Which of the following statement for early wood is correct?
(a) Xylary elements having narrow vessels
(b) Darker with higher density
(c) Lighter in colour and has high density
(d) Having vessels with wider cavities

28. Choose correct option w.r.t origin and position of meristem reponsible for the regeneration of parts removed by the grazing herbivores.

	Origin	Position
(a)	Secondary	Lateral
(b)	Primary	Apical
(c)	Secondary	Apical
(d)	Primary	Intercalated

29. Companion cells are
(a) Thin, parrenchymatous, enucleated cells
(b) Thick, sclerenchymatous, nucleated cells
(c) Thin, parenchymatous, nucleated cells
(d) Thick, collenchymatous, enucleated cells

30. Conjoint type of vascular bundle are present in
(a) Root, stem (b) Root, leaves
(c) Stem, leaves (d) Root only

31. Activity of cambium is controlled by
(a) Physiological and environmental factors
(b) Hormonal and external factors
(c) Internal and external factors
(d) Move than one option is correct

32. Epidermal and ground tissue system are made of
(a) Meristem and simple permanet tissue
(b) Primary and secondary meristem
(c) Simple and complex permanent tissue
(d) Simple permanent tissues

RESPONSE GRID					
	21. ⓐⓑⓒⓓ	22. ⓐⓑⓒⓓ	23. ⓐⓑⓒⓓ	24. ⓐⓑⓒⓓ	25. ⓐⓑⓒⓓ
	26. ⓐⓑⓒⓓ	27. ⓐⓑⓒⓓ	28. ⓐⓑⓒⓓ	29. ⓐⓑⓒⓓ	30. ⓐⓑⓒⓓ
	31. ⓐⓑⓒⓓ	32. ⓐⓑⓒⓓ			

33. Root region with thin-walled, small cells having dense cytoplasm is
(a) Region of cell elongation
(b) Maturation region
(c) Proximal to cell elongation zone
(d) Distal to cell elongation zone

34. Periderm includes
(a) Cork and secondary cortex
(b) Only cork cambium
(c) Cork cambium and cork only
(d) Cork, phellogen and secondary cortex

35. Choose incorrect statement from the given below
I. In dicot stem, the innemost layer of cortex is endodermis.
II. Endodermis with casparian strips is found in dicot stem.
III. In dicot stem, the cells of endodermis are rich in starch grain.
(a) I & II (b) II & III
(c) I & III (d) Only II

36. The cells which lie between xylem and phloem in dicot root are
(a) Pith rays
(b) Conjuctive tissue
(c) Interfascicular cambium
(d) Intrafascicular cambium

37. Which tissue of the dicot root is involved in the formation of vascular cambium?
(a) Pericyle part above primary phloem
(b) Whole pericycle
(c) Thich walled parenchymatous cells of pith
(d) Portion of pericycle above the protoxylem

38. Vascular bundles in dicot leaves are
(a) Conjoint, bicollateral, closed
(b) Radia, open
(c) Conjoint, collateral, closed
(d) Conjoint, collaterl, open

39. Which of the following represents the functions of veins in the leaves?
(a) Transport of water and minerals
(b) Mechanical support
(c) Transport of organic food material
(d) All of these

40. In *Cuscuta* the nodes give rise to special roots which penetrate the host tissue upto
(a) Cortex (b) Phloem
(c) Epidermis (d) Pericycle

41. A tylose is formed form :
(a) ray parenchyma
(b) inner parenchyma
(c) paratracheal parenchyma
(d) metatracheal parenchyma

42. Which of the following plant shows multiple epidermis?
(a) *Croton* (b) *Allium*
(c) *Nerium* (d) *Cucurbita*

43. In the monocot root, we obseve
(a) suberized exodermis, polyarch xylem , pith
(b) exodermis, endarch, tetarch closed bundles
(c) conjoint, collateral, open, polyarch vascular bundle
(d) suberized exodermis, casparian strip, passage cells, cambium

44. In a dicotyledonous stem, the sequence of tissues from the outside to the inside is :
(a) phellem-pericycle-endodermis-phloem
(b) phellem-phloem-endodermis-pericycle
(c) phellem-endodermis-pericycle-phloem
(d) pericycle-phellem-endodermis-phloem

45. The tunica corpus theory was proposed by :
(a) Nageli
(b) Hanstein
(c) Schmidt
(d) Haberlandt

RESPONSE GRID					
	33. ⓐⓑⓒⓓ	34. ⓐⓑⓒⓓ	35. ⓐⓑⓒⓓ	36. ⓐⓑⓒⓓ	37. ⓐⓑⓒⓓ
	38. ⓐⓑⓒⓓ	39. ⓐⓑⓒⓓ	40. ⓐⓑⓒⓓ	41. ⓐⓑⓒⓓ	42. ⓐⓑⓒⓓ
	43. ⓐⓑⓒⓓ	44. ⓐⓑⓒⓓ	45. ⓐⓑⓒⓓ		

BIOLOGY CHAPTERWISE SPEED TEST-64			
Total Questions	45	Total Marks	180
Attempted		Correct	
Incorrect		Net Score	
Cut-off Score	45	Qualifying Score	60
Success Gap = Net Score – Qualifying Score			
Net Score = (Correct × 4) – (Incorrect × 1)			

Space for Rough Work

BIOLOGY

Structural Organisation in Animals

Speed TEST 65 Chapter-wise

No. of Questions	Maximum Marks	Time
45	180	1 Hour

GENERAL INSTRUCTIONS

- This test contains 45 MCQ's. For each question only one option is correct. Darken the correct circle/ bubble in the Response Grid provided on each page.
- You have to evaluate your Response Grids yourself with the help of solutions provided at the end of this book.
- Each correct answer will get you 4 marks and 1 mark shall be deduced for each incorrect answer. No mark will be given/ deducted if no bubble is filled. Keep a timer in front of you and stop immediately at the end of 60 min.
- The sheet follows a particular syllabus. Do not attempt the sheet before you have completed your preparation for that syllabus.
- After completing the sheet check your answers with the solution booklet and complete the Result Grid. Finally spend time to analyse your performance and revise the areas which emerge out as weak in your evaluation.

1. The kind of epithelium which forms the inner walls of blood vessels is
   (a) cuboidal epithelium
   (b) columnar epithelium
   (c) ciliated columnar epithelium
   (d) squamous epithelium
2. The cell junctions called tight, adhering and gap junctions are found in
   (a) connective tissue (b) epithelial tissue
   (c) neural tissue (d) muscular tissue
3. Housefly possesses
   (a) two pairs of wings (b) one pair of wings
   (c) three pairs of wings (d) four pair of wings
4. Excretory organs of Cockroach are
   (a) flame cells
   (b) nephridia
   (c) hreen glands
   (d) malpighian tubules
5. Myoglobin is present in
   (a) all muscle fibres
   (b) white muscle fibres only
   (c) red muscle fibres only
   (d) both white and red muscle fibres
6. Intercalated discs are the communication junctions between the cells of
   (a) cardiac muscles
   (b) striped muscles
   (c) adipose tissue
   (d) nerve and striated muscles

RESPONSE GRID	1. ⓐⓑⓒⓓ 2. ⓐⓑⓒⓓ 3. ⓐⓑⓒⓓ 4. ⓐⓑⓒⓓ 5. ⓐⓑⓒⓓ 6. ⓐⓑⓒⓓ

Space for Rough Work

7. What is common among silverfish, scorpion, crab and honey bee?
   (a) Compound eyes (b) Poison glands
   (c) Jointed legs (d) Metamorphosis
8. Mast cells are associated with
   (a) exocrine glands
   (b) endocrine glands
   (c) areolar connective tissue
   (d) neural tissue
9. Lymph differs from blood in possessing
   (a) only WBCs.
   (b) more RBCs and WBCs.
   (c) more RBCs and few WBCs.
   (d) more WBCs and few RBCs.
10. Pseudostratified epithelium is found in
   (a) oesophagus (b) respiratory tract
   (c) urinary tract (d) kidney
11. Given below are four matchings of an animal and its kind of respiratory organ :
   (i) Silver fish – trachea
   (ii) Scorpion – book lung
   (iii) Sea squirt – pharyngeal gills
   (iv) Dolphin – skin
   The correct matchings are
   (a) (iii) and (iv) (b) (i) and (iv)
   (c) (i), (ii) and (iii) (d) (ii) and (iv)
12. Tendons and ligaments are the examples of
   (a) areolar connective tissue
   (b) adipose tissue
   (c) dense regular connective tissue
   (d) loose connective tissue
13. Major inorganic component of vertebrate bone is
   (a) calcium carbonate
   (b) calcium phosphate
   (c) sodium hydroxide
   (d) potassium hydroxide
14. Histamine is secreted by
   (a) mast cells (b) fibroblast
   (c) histocytes (d) melanocytes
15. Which of the following is not a granulocyte?
   (a) Lymphocyte (b) Neutrophil
   (c) Basophil (d) Eosinophil
16. The type of epithelial cells which line inner surface of fallopian tubes, bronchioles and small bronchi are known as
   (a) squamous epithelium (b) columnar epithelium
   (c) ciliated epithelium (d) cubical epithelium
17. Male and female cockroaches can be distinguished externally through
   (a) anal styles in male
   (b) anal cerci in female
   (c) anal style and antennae in females
   (d) both (b) and (c)
18. The long bones are hollow and connected by air passage. They are characteristic of
   (a) aves (b) mammalia
   (c) reptilia (d) sponges
19. The most active phagocytic white blood cells are
   (a) neutrophils and monocytes
   (b) neutrophils and eosinophils
   (c) lymphocytes and macrophages
   (d) eosinophils and lymphocytes
20. In the mouthparts of the cockroach, the organ of mastication is
   (a) labium (b) maxillae
   (c) mandibles (d) labrum
21. Which one of the following groups of structures/organs have similar function?
   (a) Typhlosole in earthworm, intestinal villi in rat and contractile vacuole in *Amoeba.*
   (b) Nephridia in earthworm, malpighian tubules in cockroach and urinary tubules in rat.
   (c) Antennae of cockroach, tympanum of frog and clitellum of earthworm.
   (d) Incisors of rat, gizzard (proventriculus) of cockroach and tube feet of starfish.

RESPONSE GRID					
	7. ⓐⓑⓒⓓ	8. ⓐⓑⓒⓓ	9. ⓐⓑⓒⓓ	10. ⓐⓑⓒⓓ	11. ⓐⓑⓒⓓ
	12. ⓐⓑⓒⓓ	13. ⓐⓑⓒⓓ	14. ⓐⓑⓒⓓ	15. ⓐⓑⓒⓓ	16. ⓐⓑⓒⓓ
	17. ⓐⓑⓒⓓ	18. ⓐⓑⓒⓓ	19. ⓐⓑⓒⓓ	20. ⓐⓑⓒⓓ	21. ⓐⓑⓒⓓ

Space for Rough Work

22. Which of the following statements are wrong?
(i) Leucocytes disintegrate in the spleen and liver.
(ii) RBC, WBC and blood platelets are produced by bone marrow.
(iii) Neutrophils bring about destruction and detoxification of toxins of protein origin.
(iv) The important function of lymphocytes is to produce antibodies.
(a) (i) and (ii) only (b) (i) and (iv) only
(c) (i) and (iii) only (d) (ii) and (iii) only

23. Malpighian tubules are the excretory organs in
(a) Cockroach (b) Platyhelminthes
(c) *Ascaris* (d) *Pila*

24. Young one of the cockroach is called
(a) Naid (b) Grub
(c) Nymph (d) Maggot

25. Cilia, Flagella and microvilli are associated with the
(a) Connective tissue (b) Epithelial tissue
(c) Nervous tissue (d) Muscular tissue

26. In which of the following animals, respiration occurs without any respiratory organ?
(a) Frog (b) Fish
(c) Cockroach (d) Earthworm

27. Which of the following type of cell junction is not found in animal tissues ?
(a) Desmosome (b) Tight junction
(c) Gap junction (d) Plasmodesmata

28. Which one of the following cellular components of the blood is responsible for the production of antibodies?
(a) Thrombocyte (b) Lymphocyte
(c) Monocyte (d) Erythrocyte

29. Sprain is caused due to the excessive pulling of
(a) Muscles (b) Tendons
(c) Ligaments (d) All of the above

30. In cockroach, the corpora allata is
(a) A sense organ (b) A tactile organ
(c) An endocrine organ (d) A digestive gland

31. Which of the following is incorrect w.r.t stucture/gland of cockroach and its total number in body?
(a) Collateral glands in female cockroach - 2
(b) Malpighian tubules - 100- 150
(c) Spiracles - 10
(d) Ommatidia in each compound eye - 2000

32. The function of basement membrane in epithelial tissue is to
(a) Facilitate communication of cells with each other
(b) Allow rapid ion transfer among cells
(c) Separate the epithellal tissue from underlying connective tissue
(d) Produce multiple layers of cells in a compound epithelium

33. All among the following are function of connective tissue except
(a) Binding support
(b) Fat storage
(c) Body defense and transport
(d) Propelling mucus towards the pharynx

34. Mark the statement that is incorrect for smooth muscles.
(a) Smooth muscles from the muscular component of the visceral organs such as blood vessels, urinary bladder, ciliary body etc.
(b) Smooth muscles cells do not have the troponin-tropomyosin mechanism of controlling contraction
(c) Irritability is shown by all smooth muscles except ciliary muscles
(d) Hair root muscles and muscles on the large blood vessels are in example of multi-unit smooth muscles

35. The avascular nature of cartilage is responsible for its
(a) Flexibility
(b) Slow repair
(c) Suitability for embryonic endoskeleton
(d) Transparent consistency

RESPONSE GRID					
	22. ⓐⓑⓒⓓ	23. ⓐⓑⓒⓓ	24. ⓐⓑⓒⓓ	25. ⓐⓑⓒⓓ	26. ⓐⓑⓒⓓ
	27. ⓐⓑⓒⓓ	28. ⓐⓑⓒⓓ	29. ⓐⓑⓒⓓ	30. ⓐⓑⓒⓓ	31. ⓐⓑⓒⓓ
	32. ⓐⓑⓒⓓ	33. ⓐⓑⓒⓓ	34. ⓐⓑⓒⓓ	35. ⓐⓑⓒⓓ	

Space for Rough Work

36. Match Column-I with Column-II and select the correct option from the codes given below.

	Column-I		Column-II
A.	Hyaline cartilage	I.	Pectoral girdle of frog
B.	Fibrous cartilage	II.	Long bones; sternum; ribs
C.	Elastic cartilage	III.	Pubic symphysis
D.	Calcified cartilage	IV.	Eustachain tube; epiglottis

(a) A-I; B-II; C-III; D-IV
(b) A-II; B-III; C-IV; D-I
(c) A-II; B-IV; C-III; D-I
(d) A-IV; B-III; C-II; D-I

37. The type of epithelial cells which line the inner surface of Fallopian tubes, bronchioles and small bronchi are known as
(a) squamous epithelium
(b) columnar epithelium
(c) ciliated epithelium
(d) cubical epithelium

38. The wall of heart is thick due to
(a) Pericardium (b) Epicardium
(c) Myocardium (d) Endocardium

39. The strongest cartilage is
(a) Hyaline cartilage
(b) Elastic cartilage
(c) Fibrous cartilage
(d) None of the above

40. Nissl's granules are found in cyton of nerve cells. These have affinity for basic dyes. The granules are made up of
(a) Protein (b) DNA
(c) Amino acids (d) RNA

41. The inability to absorb digested nutrients may be due to damage of which type of epithelium?
(a) Ciliated columnar
(b) Simple columnar
(c) Simple squamous
(d) Simple cuboidal

42. The presence of a basement membrane is typical of most
(a) Epithelial tissues
(b) Connective tissues
(c) Nervous tissues
(d) Muscle tissues

43. The most appropriate definition of Neuroglial cells are that they are
(a) Nonsensory supporting cells
(b) Secretory cells
(c) Sensory cells
(d) Sensory and supporting cells

44. Covering around bone is called
(a) Perichondrion
(b) Periosteum
(c) Epiosteum
(d) Endosteum

45. The figure given below shows the head region of cockroach. Identify A to F.

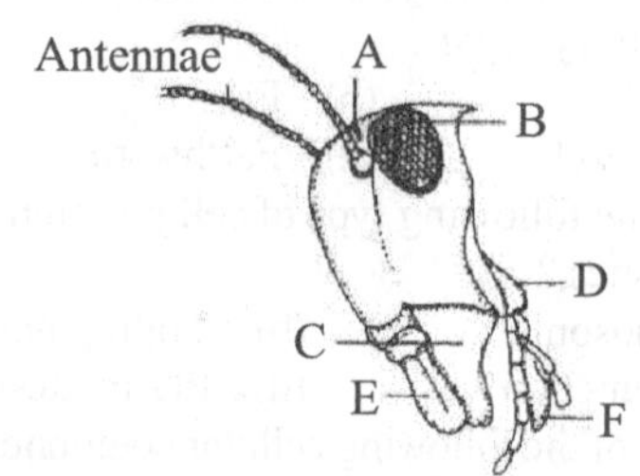

(a) A- Compound eye, B-Ocellus, C-Maxilla, D-Mandible, E-Labrum, F-Labium
(b) A- Ocellus, B-Compound eye, C-Mandible, D-Maxilla, E-Labrum, F-Labium
(c) A- Ocellus, B-Compound eye, C-Mandible, D-Maxilla, E-Labium, F-Labrum
(d) A- Ocellus, B-Compound eye, C-Maxilla, D-Mandible, E-Labrum, F-Labium

RESPONSE GRID					
	36. ⓐⓑⓒⓓ	37. ⓐⓑⓒⓓ	38. ⓐⓑⓒⓓ	39. ⓐⓑⓒⓓ	40. ⓐⓑⓒⓓ
	41. ⓐⓑⓒⓓ	42. ⓐⓑⓒⓓ	43. ⓐⓑⓒⓓ	44. ⓐⓑⓒⓓ	45. ⓐⓑⓒⓓ

BIOLOGY CHAPTERWISE SPEED TEST-65			
Total Questions	45	Total Marks	180
Attempted		Correct	
Incorrect		Net Score	
Cut-off Score	40	Qualifying Score	55
Success Gap = Net Score – Qualifying Score			
Net Score = (Correct × 4) – (Incorrect × 1)			

Space for Rough Work

BIOLOGY

CELL: The Unit of Life

Speed TEST 66

Chapter-wise

No. of Questions	Maximum Marks	Time
45	180	1 Hour

GENERAL INSTRUCTIONS

- This test contains 45 MCQ's. For each question only one option is correct. Darken the correct circle/ bubble in the Response Grid provided on each page.
- You have to evaluate your Response Grids yourself with the help of solutions provided at the end of this book.
- Each correct answer will get you 4 marks and 1 mark shall be deduced for each incorrect answer. No mark will be given/ deducted if no bubble is filled. Keep a timer in front of you and stop immediately at the end of 60 min.
- The sheet follows a particular syllabus. Do not attempt the sheet before you have completed your preparation for that syllabus.
- After completing the sheet check your answers with the solution booklet and complete the Result Grid. Finally spend time to analyse your performance and revise the areas which emerge out as weak in your evaluation.

1. The cell organelle involved in glycosylation of protein is
(a) ribosome
(b) peroxisome
(c) endoplasmic reticulum
(d) mitochondria

2. The outer layer of vacuole is called
(a) cell wall (b) tonoplast
(c) plasmalayer (d) leucoplast

3. Which of the following cell organelle remains enveloped by a single unit membrane?
(a) Mitochondria (b) Lysosomes
(c) Nucleus (d) Chloroplast

4. Choose the correct option.
(i) Lysosomes are double membranous vesicles budded off from Golgi apparatus and contain digestive enzymes.
(ii) Endoplasmic reticulum consists of a network of membranous tubule and helps in transport, synthesis and secretion.
(iii) Leucoplasts are bound by two membranes, lack pigment but contain their own DNA and protein synthesising machinery.
(iv) Sphaerosomes are single membrane bound organelle which are associated with synthesis and storage of lipids.
(a) (i) only (b) (i) and (ii)
(c) (ii), (iii) and (iv) (d) All of these

5. The nucleolus is the site of formation of
(a) spindle fibres (b) chromosomes
(c) ribosomes (d) peroxisomes

RESPONSE GRID	1. ⓐⓑⓒⓓ	2. ⓐⓑⓒⓓ	3. ⓐⓑⓒⓓ	4. ⓐⓑⓒⓓ	5. ⓐⓑⓒⓓ

Space for Rough Work

6. Which one of the following combination is mismatched?
   (a) Glycocalyx - may be capsule or slime layer
   (b) Pili - Reproduction
   (c) Cell wall - Protective, determines shape, prevents from bursting
   (d) Flagella, Pili and Fimbriae - Surface structures of bacterial cell
7. The fluidity of membranes in a plant in cold weather may be maintained by
   (a) increasing the number of phospholipids with unsaturated hydrocarbon tails
   (b) increasing the proportion of integral proteins
   (c) increasing concentration of cholesterol in membrane
   (d) increasing the number of phospholipids with saturated hydrocarbon tail
8. The cell as a basic unit of structure of living beings was discovered by
   (a) Aristotle
   (b) Robert Hooke
   (c) Schleiden and Schwann
   (d) Gregore Mendel
9. Which pair of structures are usually found in both plant and animal cells?
   (a) Cell membrane and nucleolus
   (b) Cell membrane and cell wall
   (c) Nucleolus and chloroplast
   (d) Nucleus and cell wall
10. Most abundant lipid in the cell membrane is
   (a) cholesterol (b) phospholipids
   (b) glycolipids (d) cerebrosides
11. If you remove the fimbriae from the bacterial cell, which of the following would you expect to happen?
   (a) The bacteria could no longer swim
   (b) The bacteria would not adhere to the host tissue
   (c) Transportation of molecules across the membrane would stop
   (d) The shape of bacteria would change
12. Cell recognition and adhesion are facilitated by components of plasma membrane. These components are generally
   (a) protein molecules alone
   (b) lipids alone
   (c) both lipids and proteins
   (d) glycolipids and glycoproteins
13. Smooth endoplasmic reticulum is well developed in the cells which synthesize
   (a) sterolds (b) proteins
   (c) carbohydrates (d) all of these.
14. Select the option with correct labelling of given structure of Golgi apparatus.

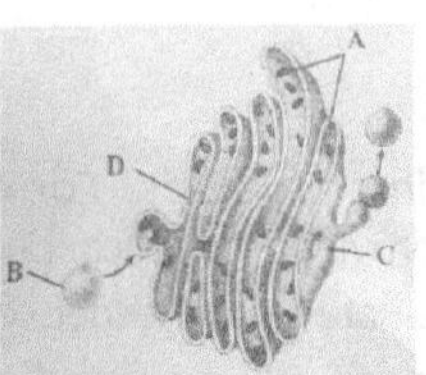

	A	B	C	D
(a)	Cisternae	Vesicle	*trans* face	*cis* face
(b)	Cisternae	Vesicle	*cis* face	*trans* face
(c)	Vesicle	Cisternae	*cis* face	*trans* face
(d)	Tubules	Vesicle	*trans* face	*cis* face

15. The molecules in the membrane that limit its permeability are the
   (a) carbohydrates (b) phospholipids
   (c) proteins (d) water
16. pH of vacuolar cell sap is
   (a) neutral and isotonic.
   (b) alkaline and isotonic.
   (c) acidic and hypertonic.
   (d) equal to cytoplasm and isotonic.
17. All plastids have essentially the same structure because
   (a) they have to perform the same function
   (b) they are localised in the aerial parts of plants
   (c) one type of plastids can differentiate into another type of plastids depending upon the cell requirements
   (d) all plastids have to store starch, lipids and proteins

RESPONSE GRID					
	6. ⓐⓑⓒⓓ	7. ⓐⓑⓒⓓ	8. ⓐⓑⓒⓓ	9. ⓐⓑⓒⓓ	10. ⓐⓑⓒⓓ
	11. ⓐⓑⓒⓓ	12. ⓐⓑⓒⓓ	13. ⓐⓑⓒⓓ	14. ⓐⓑⓒⓓ	15. ⓐⓑⓒⓓ
	16. ⓐⓑⓒⓓ	17. ⓐⓑⓒⓓ			

Space for Rough Work

18. A Semi-autonomous organelle.
B Have linear DNA as well as RNA
C Carry out ATP synthesis.
D Have quantasomes embedded in thylakoid membrane
E Occurs in all photosynthetic organisms.
Find the correct number of statements w.r.t. plastids.
(a) One (b) Two
(c) Three (d) Four

19. Select incorrect matching
(a) Elaioplasts - Oils
(b) Chromoplasts - Fat soluble anthocyanin pigments
(c) Mitochondria - Fission in G_2 phase
(d) Contractile vacuole - Excretion

20. Quasi-fluid nature of membrane is due to
(a) Phospholipid (b) Integral protein
(c) Peripheral protein (d) Sugar moiety

21. Gas vacuole is present in
(a) Blue green algae
(b) Purple photosynthetic bacteria
(c) Green photosynthetic bacteria
(d) All of the above

22. Which of the following feature is not associated with centrosome?
(a) Pericentriolar material
(b) Two cylindrical structures
(c) Two centriole
(d) Lipid bilayer covering

23. What is the site of DNA and centriole duplication respectively?
(a) Nucleus, nucleus
(b) Nucleus, cytoplasm
(c) Cytoplasm, nucleus
(d) Nucleus, nucleolous

24. Cell wall
(a) Helps in cell to cell interaction
(b) Protects the cell from infection
(c) Contains minerals like calcium carbonate in certain algae
(d) All are correct

25. Read the following statements carefully and choose the correct options w.r.t. eukaryotic cell.
I. All eukaryotic cells are identical in structure
II. Mitochondria and plastids are semi-autonomous organelles
III. Ribosomes are associated with plasma membrane
IV. There is an extensive compartmentalization of cytoplasm through the presence of membrane bound organelles
(a) I & IV (b) II & IV
(c) I & III (d) II & III

26. Golgi bodies are involved in
(a) Recycling of broken plasma membrane during endocytosis
(b) Synthesis of glycolipids
(c) Modification of proteins
(d) All of the above

27. Which of the following organelles lack membrane in eukaryotic cell?
A. Cilia B. Lysosome
C. RER D. Ribosomes
E. Flagella F. Centrioles
(a) D & F (b) C & D
(c) A & D (d) A & E

28. Aleuroplasts, amyloplasts and elaioplasts
(a) Divide by multiple fission
(b) Store protein, starch and fat respectively
(c) Help in photolysis of water
(d) Store reserve food and pigments

29. Reformation of nucleolus, golgi complex and ER occurs in
(a) Telophase (b) Metaphase
(c) Prophase (d) Anaphase

30. Ribosomes of the cytoplasm, chloroplast and mitochondrion are respectively
(a) 80S, 80S and 70S (b) 80S, 70S and 70S
(c) 70S in all (d) 80S in all

31. Integral cell membrane proteins
(a) are partially embedded in lipid layers
(b) are completely embedded in lipid layers
(c) show lateral but not vertical movements within bilayer of lipid
(d) All of these

RESPONSE GRID					
	18. ⓐⓑⓒⓓ	19. ⓐⓑⓒⓓ	20. ⓐⓑⓒⓓ	21. ⓐⓑⓒⓓ	22. ⓐⓑⓒⓓ
	23. ⓐⓑⓒⓓ	24. ⓐⓑⓒⓓ	25. ⓐⓑⓒⓓ	26. ⓐⓑⓒⓓ	27. ⓐⓑⓒⓓ
	28. ⓐⓑⓒⓓ	29. ⓐⓑⓒⓓ	30. ⓐⓑⓒⓓ	31. ⓐⓑⓒⓓ	

Space for Rough Work

32. Which group of organelles is involved in synthesis of substances needed by cell?
(a) Lysosome, vacuole, ribosome
(b) Vacuole, RER, SER
(c) Ribosome, RER, SER
(d) RER, lysosome, vacuole

33. Who gave the lamellar or sandwich model of cell membrane?
(a) Singer and Nicolson
(b) Danielle and Davson
(c) J. Robertson
(d) None of these

34. Microtubules are absent in
(a) mitochondria (b) flagella
(c) spindle fibres (d) centriole

35. Which of the following contributes to differences in the two sides of the cell membrane?
(a) Differences in peripheral proteins
(b) Different domains expressed on the ends of integral proteins
(c) Differences in phospholipid types
(d) All of the above

36. Which of the following cell membrane components serve as recognition signals for interactions between cells?
(a) Recognition proteins
(b) Glycolipids or glycoproteins
(c) Phospholipids
(d) Integral proteins

37. Channel proteins allow ions that would not normally pass through the cell membrane to go through the channel. What properties of the proteins are responsible for this?
(a) The channels are often composed of charged or polar R groups.
(b) The channels are often composed of hydrophobic R groups.
(c) a and b
(d) None of the above

38. Which of the following is present in both prokaryotes and eukaryotes?
(a) Lysosome (b) Vesicles
(c) Chloroplast (d) Plasma membrane

39. Both chloroplasts and mitochondria
(a) have multiple membranes.
(b) have highly structured innermost membranes.
(c) are found only in eukaryotic cells.
(d) All of the above

40. Microtubules, motor proteins, and actin filaments are all part of the
(a) mechanism of photosynthesis that occurs in chloroplasts.
(b) rough ER in prokaryotic cells.
(c) cytoskeleton of eukaryotic cells.
(d) process that moves small molecules across cell membranes.

41. The cell wall of both bacteria and cyanobacteria contains
(a) Lipid (b) Pectin
(c) Protein (d) Muramic acid

42. Mesosomes were taken as
(a) Golgi bodies (b) Plastids
(c) Mitochondria (d) Endoplasmic reticulum

43. Pit membrane of simple pit is formed by :
(a) Secondary cell wall (b) Middle lamella
(c) Primary cell wall (d) Plasma

44. Which one of the following cell organelles found only in plants?
(a) Golgi complex (b) Mitochondria
(c) Plastids (d) Ribosomes

45. Peroxisomes are rich in
(a) DNA (b) RNA
(c) Catalytic enzymes (d) Oxidative enzymes

RESPONSE GRID					
	32. ⓐⓑⓒⓓ	33. ⓐⓑⓒⓓ	34. ⓐⓑⓒⓓ	35. ⓐⓑⓒⓓ	36. ⓐⓑⓒⓓ
	37. ⓐⓑⓒⓓ	38. ⓐⓑⓒⓓ	39. ⓐⓑⓒⓓ	40. ⓐⓑⓒⓓ	41. ⓐⓑⓒⓓ
	42. ⓐⓑⓒⓓ	43. ⓐⓑⓒⓓ	44. ⓐⓑⓒⓓ	45. ⓐⓑⓒⓓ	

BIOLOGY CHAPTERWISE SPEED TEST-66

Total Questions	45	Total Marks	180
Attempted		Correct	
Incorrect		Net Score	
Cut-off Score	45	Qualifying Score	60
Success Gap = Net Score – Qualifying Score			
Net Score = (Correct × 4) – (Incorrect × 1)			

Space for Rough Work

BIOLOGY

Biomolecules

Speed TEST 67

Chapter-wise

No. of Questions	Maximum Marks	Time
45	180	1 Hour

GENERAL INSTRUCTIONS

- This test contains 45 MCQ's. For each question only one option is correct. Darken the correct circle/ bubble in the Response Grid provided on each page.
- You have to evaluate your Response Grids yourself with the help of solutions provided at the end of this book.
- Each correct answer will get you 4 marks and 1 mark shall be deduced for each incorrect answer. No mark will be given/ deducted if no bubble is filled. Keep a timer in front of you and stop immediately at the end of 60 min.
- The sheet follows a particular syllabus. Do not attempt the sheet before you have completed your preparation for that syllabus.
- After completing the sheet check your answers with the solution booklet and complete the Result Grid. Finally spend time to analyse your performance and revise the areas which emerge out as weak in your evaluation.

1. A nucleotide is formed of
   (a) Purine, pyrimidine and phosphate
   (b) Purine, sugar and phosphate
   (c) Nitrogen base, sugar and phosphate
   (d) Pyrimidine, sugar and phosphate
2. Glycogen is a polymer of
   (a) galactose (b) glucose
   (c) fructose (d) sucrose
3. Most abundant organic compound on earth is
   (a) Protein (b) Cellulose
   (c) Lipids (d) Steroids
4. Protein synthesis in a cell takes place
   (a) only in the cytoplasm
   (b) in the nucleolus as well as in cytoplasm
   (c) in cytoplasm as well as in mitochondria
   (d) only on ribosomes attached to the nuclear envelope
5. In RNA, thymine is replaced by
   (a) Adenine (b) Guanine
   (c) Cytosine (d) Uracil
6. Which of the following is a reducing sugar?
   (a) Galactose (b) Gluconic acid
   (c) β-methyl galactoside (d) Sucrose
7. An enzyme that can stimulate germination of barley seeds is
   (a) lipase (b) protease
   (c) invertase (d) α-amylase
8. Carrier ions like Na^+ facilitate the absorption of substances like:
   (a) amino acids and glucose
   (b) glucose and fatty acids
   (c) fatty acids and glycerol
   (d) fructose and some amino acids

RESPONSE GRID					
	1. ⓐⓑⓒⓓ	2. ⓐⓑⓒⓓ	3. ⓐⓑⓒⓓ	4. ⓐⓑⓒⓓ	5. ⓐⓑⓒⓓ
	6. ⓐⓑⓒⓓ	7. ⓐⓑⓒⓓ	8. ⓐⓑⓒⓓ		

Space for Rough Work

9. An enzyme brings about
   (a) decrease in reaction time
   (b) increase in reaction time
   (c) increase in activation energy
   (d) reduction in activation energy
10. The enzymes hexokinase which catalyses glucose to glucose-6-phosphate in glycolysis is inhibited by glucose-6-phosphate. This is an example of
   (a) competitive inhibition
   (b) non-competitive inhibition
   (c) feedback allosteric inhibition
   (d) positive feedback
11. The enormous diversity of protein molecules is due mainly to the diversity of
   (a) amino groups on the amino acids
   (b) R groups on the amino acids
   (c) amino acid sequences within the protein molecule
   (d) peptide bonds
12. Length of one turn of the helix in a B-form DNA is approximately
   (a) 3.4 nm (b) 2 nm
   (c) 0.34 nm (d) 20 nm
13. The catalytic efficiency of two different enzymes can be compared by the
   (a) formation of the product
   (b) pH optimum value
   (c) K_m value
   (d) molecular size of the enzyme
14. Which of the following sets contains polysaccharides?
   (a) Glucose, fructose, lactose
   (b) Starch, glycogen, cellulose
   (c) Sucrose, maltose, cellulose
   (d) Galactose, starch, sucrose
15. Sigmoid growth curve is represented by
   (a) dN/dt = rN
   (b) dN/dt = rN (1 – N/K)
   (c) $Nt = N_o + B + I - D - E$
   (d) dN/dt = 1 – N/K
16. A coenzyme is
   (a) Same enzyme that occurs in different tissues such as heart and muscle
   (b) One that shares the function of other enzyme
   (c) Organic or inorganic in nature and helps activate metabolic enzymes
   (d) Organic non-protein in nature and helps to activate metabolic enzymes
17. The most basic amino acid is
   (a) Arginine (b) Histidine
   (c) Glycine (d) Glutamine
18. Which of the following is not an aromatic amino acid?
   (a) Valine (b) Tyrosine
   (c) Phenylalanine (d) Tryptophan
19. The class of enzymes that catalyze the removal of a group from a substrate without addition of water, leaving double bonds, is
   (a) Transferases (b) Dehydrogenases
   (c) Hydrolases (d) Lyases
20. Which of the following is a component of vitamin (thiamine, biotin), Acetyl CoA, cysteine, methionine and ferredoxin?
   (a) Fe (b) S
   (c) Co (d) K
21. The helical structure of protein is stabilized by
   (a) Ester (b) Peptide bonds
   (c) Disulphide bonds (d) Hydrogen bonds
22. Cellulose is a polymer of
   (a) α-glucose (b) α-D-glucose
   (c) β-D-glucose (d) β-L-glucose

RESPONSE GRID					
	9. ⓐⓑⓒⓓ	10. ⓐⓑⓒⓓ	11. ⓐⓑⓒⓓ	12. ⓐⓑⓒⓓ	13. ⓐⓑⓒⓓ
	14. ⓐⓑⓒⓓ	15. ⓐⓑⓒⓓ	16. ⓐⓑⓒⓓ	17. ⓐⓑⓒⓓ	18. ⓐⓑⓒⓓ
	19. ⓐⓑⓒⓓ	20. ⓐⓑⓒⓓ	21. ⓐⓑⓒⓓ	22. ⓐⓑⓒⓓ	

Space for Rough Work

23. The given graph shows the effect of substrate concentration on the rate of reaction of the enzyme green -gram - phosphatase. What does the graph indicate ?

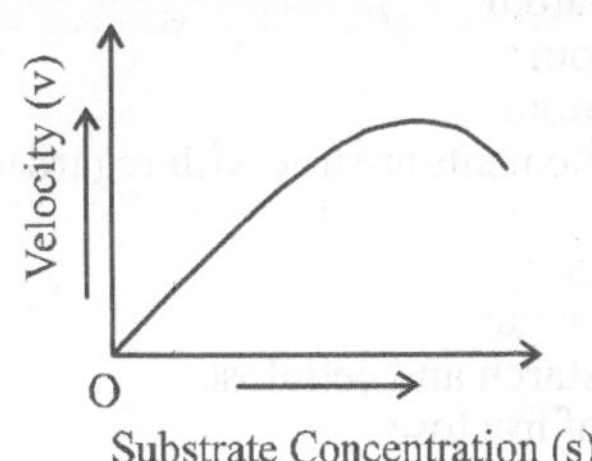

(a) The rate of enzyme reaction is directly proportional to the substrate concentration
(b) Presence of an enzyme inhibitor in the reaction mixture
(c) Formation of an enzyme-substrate complex
(d) At higher substrate-concentration the pH increases.

24. The Km value of the enzyme is the value of the substrate concentration at which the reaction reaches to
(a) Zero (b) 2 Vmax
(c) ½ Vmax (d) ¼ Vmax

25. Which group contains biocatalysts?
(a) Myosin, oxytocin, adrenalin
(b) Peptidase, amylase, rennin
(c) Glucose, amino acids, fatty acids
(d) Rhodopsin, pepsin, steapsin

26.

```
                              O
                              ||
        O        CH2—O—C—R1
        ||         |
R2— C—O— CH       O
                   |       ||
                 CH2—O—P—O—CH2—CH2
                           |              |
                          OH             N+
                                       /  |  \
                                   CH3 CH3 CH3
```

Given structural formula is correctly identified alongwith its related function by which of the following options?
(a) Cholesterol – A component of animal cell membrane
(b) Lecithin – A component of cell membrane
(c) Triglyceride – An energy source
(d) Adenosine – A component of nucleic acids

27. Select the option that correctly identifies the chemical bonds present in the given biomolecules.
Polysaccharides – A, Proteins – B, Fats – C, Water – D

	A	B	C	D
(a)	Ester	Peptide	Glycosidic	Hydrogen
(b)	Glycosidic	Peptide	Ester	Hydrogen
(c)	Glycosidic	Peptide	Hydrogen	Ester
(d)	Hydrogen	Ester	Peptide	Glycosidic

28. Which of the following statements is not correct regarding chitin?
(a) It is a storage polysaccharide
(b) It is a homopolysccharide
(c) It is a constituent of arthropod exoskeleton and fungal cell wall
(d) It is the second most abundant carbohydrate on earth

29. Which of the following secondary metabolites are used as drugs?
(a) Abrin and ricin
(b) Vinblastin and curcumin
(c) Anthocyanins
(d) Gums and cellulose

30. Enzymes that catalyse removal of groups from substrates by mechanisms other than hydrolysis, and addition of groups to double bonds, are called
(a) ligases (b) lyases
(c) hydrolases (d) dehydrogenases

31. Which of the following statement is incorrect w.r.t. starch?
(a) Starch consists of unbranched amylose and branched amylopectin
(b) It is a polymer of α-D-glucose
(c) Successive glucose units are linked together by α 1 → 6 linkage and at branching α 1 → 4 linkage is found
(d) Starch turns black with iodine

RESPONSE GRID					
	23. ⓐⓑⓒⓓ	24. ⓐⓑⓒⓓ	25. ⓐⓑⓒⓓ	26. ⓐⓑⓒⓓ	27. ⓐⓑⓒⓓ
	28. ⓐⓑⓒⓓ	29. ⓐⓑⓒⓓ	30. ⓐⓑⓒⓓ	31. ⓐⓑⓒⓓ	

Space for Rough Work

32. Cellulose differs from chitin in
(a) Branching
(b) Type of glycosidic bond
(c) Type of monomer unit
(d) Abundancy in biosphere

33. Oils are rich in
(a) Glycerol that possesses three hydroxyl groups
(b) Saturated fatty acids
(c) Fats that are generally liquid at room temperature
(d) Esters of fatty acids

34. Bonds that do not exist in tertiary structure of proteins
(a) Covalent bonds
(b) Phosphodiester bonds
(c) Hydrophobic etnractions
(d) Ionic bonds

35. Cleavage of specific covalent bonds and removal of groups without hydrolysis is the property of
(a) Isomerases (b) Lyases
(c) Hydrolases (d) Transferases

36. The catalytic efficiency of two different enzymes can be compared by the
(a) K_m value
(b) pH value
(c) Formation of the product
(d) Molecular size of the enzyme

37. Which of the following is an example of isozyme?
(a) α-Amylase
(b) Glucokinase
(c) Lactate dehydrogenase
(d) All of these

38. Essential amino acids include
(a) leucine (b) valine
(c) tryptophan (d) all of these

39. Acidic amino acids have two –COOH groups and one –NH_2 group per molecule. Select the pair that consists of acidic amino acids.
(a) Aspartic acid, glutamic acid
(b) Lysine, arginine
(c) Glycine, alanine
(d) Both (a) and (b)

40. The structure of glucose and galactose are same except with regard to
(a) First carbon atom
(b) Second carbon atom
(c) Third carbon atom
(d) Fourth carbon atom

41. All the following statements are true with regard to glucose, except :
(a) It is an aldohexose
(b) It is a reducing sugar
(c) It is present in starch and cellulose
(d) It is an epimer of fructose

42. Guanylic acid is a
(a) Nucleoside of purine
(b) Nucleoside of pyrimidine
(c) Nucleotide of purine
(d) Nucleotide of pyrimidine

43. Long chain molecules of fatty acids are formed by
(a) Polymerisation of 2 carbon compounds
(b) Decomposition of fats
(c) Polymerisation of glycogen
(d) Conversion of glycogen

44. Read the following four statements (A to D) and mark the option that has both correct statements
A. Blood conc. of glucose in a normal healthy man is 4.5 to 5.0 mM
B. In proteins only left handed helices are observed
C. The pitch of B- DNA is 3.4 Angstrom
D. At each step of ascent the strand of DNA turns 36 degree
(a) A, B (b) B, C (c) C, D (d) A, D

45. Which one of the following biomolecules is correctly characterized?
(a) Lecithin - A phosphorylated glyceride found in cell membrane.
(b) Palmitic acid - An unsaturated fatty acid with 18 carbon atoms.
(c) Adenylic acid - Adenosine with a glucose phosphate molecule.
(d) Alanine amino acid - Contains an amino group and an acidic group anywhere in the molecule.

RESPONSE GRID					
	32. ⓐⓑⓒⓓ	33. ⓐⓑⓒⓓ	34. ⓐⓑⓒⓓ	35. ⓐⓑⓒⓓ	36. ⓐⓑⓒⓓ
	37. ⓐⓑⓒⓓ	38. ⓐⓑⓒⓓ	39. ⓐⓑⓒⓓ	40. ⓐⓑⓒⓓ	41. ⓐⓑⓒⓓ
	42. ⓐⓑⓒⓓ	43. ⓐⓑⓒⓓ	44. ⓐⓑⓒⓓ	45. ⓐⓑⓒⓓ	

BIOLOGY CHAPTERWISE SPEED TEST-67			
Total Questions	45	Total Marks	180
Attempted		Correct	
Incorrect		Net Score	
Cut-off Score	45	Qualifying Score	55
Success Gap = Net Score – Qualifying Score			
Net Score = (Correct × 4) – (Incorrect × 1)			

Space for Rough Work

BIOLOGY

Cell Cycle and Cell Division

Speed TEST 68

Chapter-wise

No. of Questions	Maximum Marks	Time
45	180	1 Hour

GENERAL INSTRUCTIONS

- This test contains 45 MCQ's. For each question only one option is correct. Darken the correct circle/ bubble in the Response Grid provided on each page.
- You have to evaluate your Response Grids yourself with the help of solutions provided at the end of this book.
- Each correct answer will get you 4 marks and 1 mark shall be deduced for each incorrect answer. No mark will be given/ deducted if no bubble is filled. Keep a timer in front of you and stop immediately at the end of 60 min.
- The sheet follows a particular syllabus. Do not attempt the sheet before you have completed your preparation for that syllabus.
- After completing the sheet check your answers with the solution booklet and complete the Result Grid. Finally spend time to analyse your performance and revise the areas which emerge out as weak in your evaluation.

1. In cell cycle, DNA replication takes place in
   (a) G_1 phase (b) G_2 phase
   (c) mitotic metaphase (d) S phase
2. During cell division, the spindle fibres attach to the chromosome at a region called
   (a) chromocentre (b) kinetochore
   (c) centriole (d) chromomere
3. Chromosome duplication without nuclear division refers to
   (a) meiosis (b) mitosis
   (c) androgenesis (d) endomitosis
4. During which stages (or prophase I substages) of meiosis do you expect to find the bivalents and DNA replication respectively?
   (a) Pachytene and interphase (between two meiotic divisions)
   (b) Pachytene and interphase (just prior to prophase I)
   (c) Pachytene and S phase (of interphase just prior to prophase I)
   (d) Zygotene and S phase (of interphase prior to prophase I)
5. The two chromatids of a metaphase chromosome represent
   (a) replicated chromosomes to be separated at anaphase
   (b) homologous chromosomes of a diploid set
   (c) non-homologous chromosomes joined at the centromere
   (d) maternal and paternal chromosomes joined at the centromere
6. Recombination of genes occur at
   (a) prophase in mitosis
   (b) prophase I in meiosis
   (c) prophase II in meiosis
   (d) metaphase II in meiosis

RESPONSE GRID	1. ⓐⓑⓒⓓ 2. ⓐⓑⓒⓓ 3. ⓐⓑⓒⓓ 4. ⓐⓑⓒⓓ 5. ⓐⓑⓒⓓ 6. ⓐⓑⓒⓓ

Space for Rough Work

7. Four daughter cells formed after meiosis are
(a) genetically similar (b) genetically different
(c) anucleate (d) multinucleate

8. In animal cells, cytokinesis involves
(a) the separation of sister chromatids
(b) the contraction of the contractile ring of microfilament
(c) depolymerisation of kinetochore microtubules
(d) a protein kinase that phosphorylates other enzymes

9. The number of chromatids in a chromosome at anaphase is
(a) 2 in mitosis and 1 in meiosis
(b) 1 in mitosis and 2 in meiosis
(c) 2 each in mitosis and meiosis
(d) 2 in mitosis and 4 in meiosis

10. During cell division, sometimes there will be failure of separation of sister chromatids. This event is called
(a) interference (b) complementation
(c) non-disjunction (d) coincidence

11. In which stage of the cell cycle histone proteins synthesized in a eukaryotic cell?
(a) During G_2 stage of prophase
(b) During S-phase
(c) During entire prophase
(d) During telophase

12. What is true about telophase stage?
(a) Chromosomes lose their identity as discrete elements
(b) Chromosomes cluster at opposite spindle poles
(c) Nuclear envelope, nucleolus, Golgi complex and ER reform
(d) All of these

13. Match Column-I with Column-II and select the correct option from the codes given below.

	Column-I		Column-II
A.	Disintegration of nuclear membrane	I.	Anaphase
B.	Appearance of nucleolus	II.	Prophase
C.	Division of centromere	III.	Telophase
D.	Replication of DNA	IV.	S-phase

(a) A-II; B-III; C-I; D-IV
(b) A-II; B-III; C-IV; D-I
(c) A-III; B-II; C-I; D-IV
(d) A-III; B-II; C-IV; D-I

14. The centromere is situated close to its ends and forming one extremely short and one very long arm in
(a) Metacentric chromosome
(b) Sub-metacentric chromosome
(c) Acrocentric chromosome
(d) Telocentric chromosome

15. Select the events that do not occur in interphase stage of cell-cycle
A. RNA and protein synthesis.
B. Cytoplasmic growth.
C. Polymerisation of spindle fibres protein.
D. Disappearance of Golgi bodies and ER.
E. DNA molecules in highly supercoiled stage.
(a) C, D & E (b) D & E only
(c) B, C & D (d) C & D only

16. The stage between two meiotic divisions is called interkinesis and
(a) Is long lived
(b) Is followed by prophase I
(c) Is generally short lived and followed by prophase II
(d) Involves duplication of genes and centrioles

17. Which is correct w.r.t. anaphase?
(a) Centromeres split and chromatids separate
(b) Spindle fibres attach to kinetochores
(c) Chromosomes are moved to spindle equator
(d) Chromatid splits by recombinase activity

18. Maximum cytoplasmic growth occurs in
(a) G_1-phase (b) S-phase
(c) G_2-phase (d) M-phase

19. Diagrammatic representation of chromosomes of a species, is called
(a) Karyotype (b) Crytogram
(c) Cladogram (d) Idiogram

20. Which one of the following events is incorrect for cell cycle?
(a) All events are under genetic control
(b) Maximum cell growth occurs in M-phase
(c) DNA synthesis occurs only during one specific
(d) Centriole duplication occurs in S-phase

RESPONSE GRID				
7. ⓐⓑⓒⓓ	8. ⓐⓑⓒⓓ	9. ⓐⓑⓒⓓ	10. ⓐⓑⓒⓓ	11. ⓐⓑⓒⓓ
12. ⓐⓑⓒⓓ	13. ⓐⓑⓒⓓ	14. ⓐⓑⓒⓓ	15. ⓐⓑⓒⓓ	16. ⓐⓑⓒⓓ
17. ⓐⓑⓒⓓ	18. ⓐⓑⓒⓓ	19. ⓐⓑⓒⓓ	20. ⓐⓑⓒⓓ	

Space for Rough Work

21. The sequence of events by which a cell duplicates its genome, synthesises other constituents of the cell and eventually divide into two daughter cell is termed as
(a) Karyochorists (b) I-phase
(c) Cell cycle (d) M-phase

22. Lampbrush chromosomes are seen in which typical stage?
(a) Mitotic anaphase (b) Mitotic prophase
(c) Mitotic metaphase (d) Meiotic prophase

23. In telophase of mitosis, the mitotic spindle breaks down and nuclear membranes form. This is essentially the opposite of what happens in
(a) prophase. (b) interphase.
(c) metaphase. (d) S phase.

24. Most cells divide if they receive the proper signal at a checkpoint in the _____ phase of the cell cycle.
(a) M (b) G_1 (c) S (d) G_2

25. Which of the following carry the same genetic information?
(a) sister chromatids
(b) X and Y chromosomes
(c) all autosomes
(d) homologous chromosomes

26. A zoologist examined an intestine cell from a crayfish and counted 200 chromosomes, each consisting of 2 chromatids, at prophase I of mitosis. What would he expect to see in each of the four cells at telophase II of meiosis if he looked in the crayfish ovary?
(a) 50 chromosomes, each consisting of 2 chromatids
(b) 50 chromosomes, each consisting of 1 chromatid
(c) 100 chromosomes, each consisting of 2 chromatids
(d) 100 chromosomes, each consisting of 1 chromatid

27. Which of the following is true of kineto-chores?
(a) They are localized at the centromere of each chromosome.
(b) They are the sites where microtubules attach to separate the chromosomes.
(c) They are organized so that there is one per sister chromatid in meiosis.
(d) All of the above

28. Chromosome movement during anaphase is the result of:
(a) the molecular motors at the kinetochores that move the chromosomes toward the poles.
(b) molecular motors at the centrosome that pull the microtubules toward the poles.
(c) shortening of the microtubules at the centrosome that pull the chromosomes toward the poles.
(d) a and c

29. Programmed cell death (apoptosis):
(a) occurs in cells that have been deprived of essential nutrients.
(b) occurs only in cells that have damaged DNA
(c) is a natural process during development.
(d) is signaled by the initiated of mitosis.

30. The following graph represents the changes in the quantity of DNA present in the cell cycle at different stages.

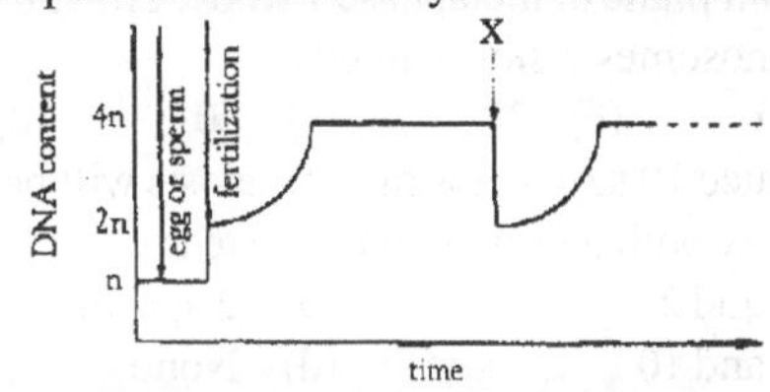

What stage takes place at X?
(a) anaphase (b) cytokinesis
(c) interphase (d) metaphase

31. The absence of centrioles from higher plant cells means that during somatic cell nuclear division there is:
(a) no apparent organiser of mitotic spindles
(b) no equatorial arrangement of chromo-somes at metaphase.
(c) no new cell wall laid down at telophase.
(d) no spindle formed.

32. The amount of DNA in a mammalian cell in early prophase I is x.
What is the amount of DNA in the same cell in anaphase I of meiosis?
(a) $\frac{x}{4}$ (b) $\frac{x}{2}$ (c) x (d) 2x

RESPONSE GRID					
	21. ⓐⓑⓒⓓ	22. ⓐⓑⓒⓓ	23. ⓐⓑⓒⓓ	24. ⓐⓑⓒⓓ	25. ⓐⓑⓒⓓ
	26. ⓐⓑⓒⓓ	27. ⓐⓑⓒⓓ	28. ⓐⓑⓒⓓ	29. ⓐⓑⓒⓓ	30. ⓐⓑⓒⓓ
	31. ⓐⓑⓒⓓ	32. ⓐⓑⓒⓓ			

Space for Rough Work

33. Fully differentiated cells which do not divide are supposed to be in :
(a) G_1 - phase (b) G_2 - phase
(c) S - phase (d) G_0 - phase

34. A cell can not divide if it does not cross :
(a) Hayflick limit (b) cytokinesis
(c) restriction point (d) G_0 - phase

35. Synapsis is of______ kind(s) :
(a) one (b) two (c) three (d) four

36. If a stock has 2n = 48 and scion microspore mother cell has 2n = 24; then root cell and the microspores will have_____ chromosomes respectively.
(a) 12, 48 (b) 48, 12 (c) 24, 12 (d) 24, 96

37. A plant has number of chromosome groups arranged at equatorial plane of metaphase-I whose 2n = 50; the number of chromosomes visible will be :
(a) 100 (b) 25 (c) 50 (d) 75

38. To produce 10 seeds how many meiosis will be needed and how many pollen grain will be wasted?
(a) 13 and 2 (b) 2 and 14
(c) 10 and 10 (d) None

39. Which one of the following list contain the correct order of meiotic events ?
(a) Separation of sister chromatids, recombination, formation of the synaptonemal complex, separation of homologous chromosomes
(b) Separation of homologous chromosomes, formation of the synaptonemal complex, recombination, separation of sister chromatids
(c) Formation of synaptonemal complex, recombination, separation of sister chromatids, separation of homologous chromosomes
(d) Formation of the synaptonemal complex, recombination, separation of homologous chromosomes, separation of sister chromatids.

40. In meiosis, actual haploidy in terms of DNA comes in
(a) Metaphase-I (b) Anaphase-II
(c) Anaphase-I (d) Interkinesis

41. Which of the following can not be considered as mitogen ?
(a) Cytokinin (b) Insulin
(c) Cholchicine (d) Auxin

42. G_2 phase is not assiciated with
(a) Synthesis of some non-histone proteins
(b) Synthesis of tubulin proteins for spindle fibres
(c) DNA synthesis
(d) Duplication of centrioles

43. Replication of centriole occurs during
(a) Early anaphase (b) Mid metaphase
(c) Late metaphase (d) Interphase

44. A cell in mitotic prophase can be distinguished from a cell in meiotic prophase by
(a) Formation of tetrad in a meiotic cell
(b) The terminalization of chiasmata in late prophase of mitosis
(c) Zipping in early prophase of mitosis
(d) Presence of only half as many chromosomes in the meiotic cell

45. The diagram shows a cell whose diploid chromosome number is four. Which one of the following option shows correct stage of cell ?

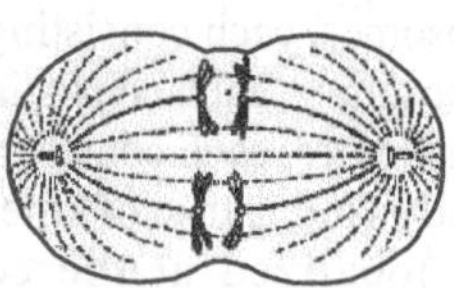

(a) Metaphase
(b) Anaphase of mitosis
(c) Anaphase I of meiosis
(d) Anaphase II of meiosis

RESPONSE GRID					
	33. ⓐⓑⓒⓓ	34. ⓐⓑⓒⓓ	35. ⓐⓑⓒⓓ	36. ⓐⓑⓒⓓ	37. ⓐⓑⓒⓓ
	38. ⓐⓑⓒⓓ	39. ⓐⓑⓒⓓ	40. ⓐⓑⓒⓓ	41. ⓐⓑⓒⓓ	42. ⓐⓑⓒⓓ
	43. ⓐⓑⓒⓓ	44. ⓐⓑⓒⓓ	45. ⓐⓑⓒⓓ		

BIOLOGY CHAPTERWISE SPEED TEST-68			
Total Questions	45	Total Marks	180
Attempted		Correct	
Incorrect		Net Score	
Cut-off Score	40	Qualifying Score	50
Success Gap = Net Score – Qualifying Score			
Net Score = (Correct × 4) – (Incorrect × 1)			

Space for Rough Work

BIOLOGY

Transport in Plants

Speed TEST 69

Chapter-wise

No. of Questions	Maximum Marks	Time
45	180	1 Hour

GENERAL INSTRUCTIONS

- This test contains 45 MCQ's. For each question only one option is correct. Darken the correct circle/ bubble in the Response Grid provided on each page.
- You have to evaluate your Response Grids yourself with the help of solutions provided at the end of this book.
- Each correct answer will get you 4 marks and 1 mark shall be deduced for each incorrect answer. No mark will be given/ deducted if no bubble is filled. Keep a timer in front of you and stop immediately at the end of 60 min.
- The sheet follows a particular syllabus. Do not attempt the sheet before you have completed your preparation for that syllabus.
- After completing the sheet check your answers with the solution booklet and complete the Result Grid. Finally spend time to analyse your performance and revise the areas which emerge out as weak in your evaluation.

1. Water potential is equal to
   (a) $\Psi_s + \text{O.P.}$ (b) $\Psi_s + \text{T.P.}$
   (c) $\Psi_p + \Psi_w$ (d) $\Psi_s + \Psi_p$
2. The movement of mineral ions into plant root cells as a result of diffusion is called
   (a) osmosis
   (b) active absorption
   (c) passive absorption
   (d) endocytosis
3. In soil, the water available for root absorption is
   (a) gravitational water (b) capillary water
   (c) hygroscopic water (d) combined water
4. Plasmolysis occurs when the cell is placed in
   (a) isotonic solution (b) hypotonic solution
   (c) hypertonic solution (d) None of the above
5. The rate of transpiration in plants is dependent upon
   (a) temperature and soil
   (b) light and temperature
   (c) wind, temperature and light
   (d) light, temperature, atmospheric humidity and wind
6. The water potential and osmotic potential of pure water are
   (a) zero and zero (b) 100 and 100
   (c) zero and 100 (d) 100 and zero
7. Stomata open and close due to
   (a) circadian rhythm
   (b) genetic clock
   (c) pressure of gases inside the leaves
   (d) turgor pressure of guard cells
8. Movement of ions or molecules in a direction opposite to that of prevailing electrochemical gradient is known as
   (a) diffusion (b) active transport
   (c) pinocytosis (d) brownian movement
9. Osmosis means movement of
   (a) solute from lower concentration to higher concentration.
   (b) solute from higher concentration to lower concentration.
   (c) solvent from low concentration of solution to higher concentration of solution.
   (d) solvent from higher concentration of solution to low concentration of solution.

RESPONSE GRID					
	1. ⓐⓑⓒⓓ	2. ⓐⓑⓒⓓ	3. ⓐⓑⓒⓓ	4. ⓐⓑⓒⓓ	5. ⓐⓑⓒⓓ
	6. ⓐⓑⓒⓓ	7. ⓐⓑⓒⓓ	8. ⓐⓑⓒⓓ	9. ⓐⓑⓒⓓ	

Space for Rough Work

10. Solution outside a cell has higher concentration than cytoplasm, then the solution is
(a) isotonic (b) acidic
(c) hypotonic (d) hypertonic

11. Which of the following is used as antitranspirant?
(a) Calcium carbonate
(b) Phenyl mercuric acetate
(c) Cobalt chloride
(d) Naphthol acetic acid

12. During $Na^+ - K^+$ pump
(a) $3Na^+$ and $2K^+$ are transported
(b) $1Na^+$ and $2K^+$ are transported
(c) $3Na^+$ and $3K^+$ are transported
(d) Depends on requirement of cell

13. In rainy season, door gets swelled due to
(a) imbibition (b) diffusion
(c) transpiration (d) respiration

14. Turgor pressure become equal to the wall pressure when
(a) water leaves the cell
(b) water enter the cell
(c) no exchange of water takes place
(d) solute goes from cell into water

15. Addition of a solute to pure water causes
(a) negative water potential.
(b) more negative water potential.
(c) positive water potential.
(d) more positive water potential.

16. Which one of the following process help the water- soluble inorganic nutrients go down into the soil horizon and get precipitated as unavailable salts?
(a) Fragmentation (b) Leaching
(c) Catabolism (d) Humification

17. Water logging of soil makes it physiologically dry because:
(a) this condition does not allow the capillary force to work
(b) this condition does not allow oxygen to enter the soil
(c) Both (a) and (b)
(d) None of the above

18. The productivity of a crop declines when leaves begin to wilt mainly because
(a) the chlorophyll of wilting leaves decomposes.
(b) flaccid mesophyll cells are incapable of photosynthesis.
(c) stomata close, preventing CO_2 from entering the leaf.
(d) photolysis, the water-splitting step of photosynthesis, cannot occur when there is a water deficiency.

19. The phenomenon of plasmolysis is evident when cells are kept in
(a) hypotonic solution
(b) hypertonic solution
(c) isotonic solution
(d) None of the above

20. What mechanism explains the movement of sucrose from source to sink ?
(a) Evaporation of water and active transport of sucrose from sink.
(b) Osmotic movement of water into the sucrose loaded sieve tube cells creating a higher hydrostatic pressure into the source than in the sink.
(c) Tension created by differences in hydrostatic pressure in the source and sink.
(d) Active transport of sucrose through the sieve tube membranes driven by proton pump.

21. Water will be absorbed by root hairs when
(a) concentration of salt in the soil is high.
(b) concentration of solutes in the cell sap is high.
(c) plant is rapidly respiring.
(d) they are separated from soil by a permeable membrane.

22. Proton pumps in the plasma membranes of plant cells may
(a) generate a membrane potential that helps drive cations into the cell through their specific carriers.
(b) be coupled to the movement of K^+ into guard cells.
(c) drive the accumulation of sucrose in sieve-tube members.
(d) be involved in all of the above

23. Which one of the following graphs most closely represents the relationship between the rate of transpiration of a mesophytic leaf and the atmospheric humidity ?

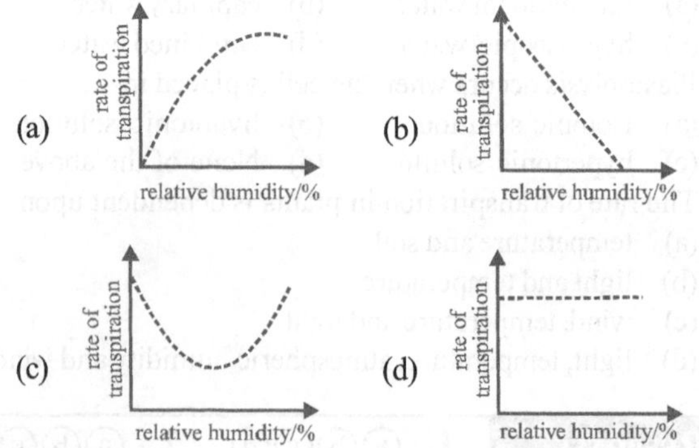

RESPONSE GRID					
	10. ⓐⓑⓒⓓ	11. ⓐⓑⓒⓓ	12. ⓐⓑⓒⓓ	13. ⓐⓑⓒⓓ	14. ⓐⓑⓒⓓ
	15. ⓐⓑⓒⓓ	16. ⓐⓑⓒⓓ	17. ⓐⓑⓒⓓ	18. ⓐⓑⓒⓓ	19. ⓐⓑⓒⓓ
	20. ⓐⓑⓒⓓ	21. ⓐⓑⓒⓓ	22. ⓐⓑⓒⓓ	23. ⓐⓑⓒⓓ	

Space for Rough Work

24. A plant cell placed in pure water will
(a) expand until the osmotic potential or solute potential reaches that of water.
(b) becomes more turgid until the pressure potential of cell reaches its osmotic potential.
(c) become more turgid until the osmotic potential reaches that of pure water.
(d) becomes less turgid until the osmotic potential reaches that of pure water.

25. The casparian strip prevents water and minerals from entering the stele through the
(a) plasmodesmata (b) apoplast
(c) symplast (d) xylem vessel

26. If a soft stemmed plant, is cut horizontally near the base of its stem with a sharp blade on early morning of a humid day, drops of solution ooze through cut stem. This is due to
(a) guttation (b) bleeding
(c) transpiration pull (d) root pressure

27. Which of the following statements is incorrect?
(a) Endodermis is impervious to water due to the presence of suberized Casparian stips.
(b) Xylem vessels and tracheids, being non-living, are parts of the apoplast
(c) Ascent of sap is best explained by root pressure theory.
(d) None of these

28. In part A of a plant, sugars are actively transported into the phloem tissue. In part B, sugars are actively transported out of the phloem. Which way will the phloem sap move under these conditions?
(a) From A to B
(b) From B to A
(c) First from A to B; then, once the pressure builds up, from B to A
(d) First from B to A; then, once the pressure builds up, from A to B

29. If the pressure potential is +0.16 megapascals (mPa) and the osmotic potential is –0.24 megapascals, then the water potential would be
(a) +0.4 mPa (b) +0.08 mPa
(c) –0.08 mPa (d) + 0.16 mPa.

30. The movement of water up the stems of tall plants is least dependent on which of the following factors ?
(a) Guttation
(b) Transpiration
(c) Cohesiveness of water molecules
(d) Tension within column of water molecules

31. As a leaf loses water, a series of events typically occurs leading to the closing of stomata. Which of the following shows the correct sequence of these events ?
(a) Potassium ions enter guard cells, water passively enters guard cells, abscisic acid is released by leaf cells, pressure potential in guard cells decreases
(b) Potassium ions enter guard cells, water passively leaves guard cells, pressure potential in guard cells decreases
(c) Water passively leaves guard cells, pressure potential in guard cells decreases, abscisic acid is released by leaf cells, potassium ions leave guard cells
(d) Abscisic acid is released by leaf cells, potassium ions leave guard cells, water passively leaves guard cells, pressure potential in guard cells decreases

32. Which of the following explains why the leaf cells of plants within the family Crassulaceae have a lower pH at night than during the day ?
(a) These plants keep their stomata open at night but clossed during the day.
(b) Carbon dioxide in these plants is chemically fixed in orgnanic acids during the night, but these acids are metabolized during the day.
(c) These plants have a buildup of abscisic acid at night.
(d) Because their stomata are closed during the day, excess carbon dioxide within the leaf forms carbonic acid.

33. Which of the following characteristics applies to both xylem and phloem transport ?
(a) Follows a water potential gradient
(b) Involves only living cells
(c) Can occur in both directions
(d) Involves active transport of solute with passive movement of water

34. Which of the following cell types would be the third cell type a sugar molecule is likely to encounter on its route from its site of production in a chloroplast to its site of storage in the root ?
(a) Mesophyll cell
(b) Companion cell
(c) Sieve tube element
(d) Parenchyma

35. The primary difference between the apoplast and the symplast is that the
(a) apoplast is nonliving spaces and cell walls.
(b) apoplast relies on active transport.
(c) symplast is nonliving spaces and cell walls.
(d) apoplast prevents passive diffusion.

RESPONSE GRID					
	24. ⓐⓑⓒⓓ	25. ⓐⓑⓒⓓ	26. ⓐⓑⓒⓓ	27. ⓐⓑⓒⓓ	28. ⓐⓑⓒⓓ
	29. ⓐⓑⓒⓓ	30. ⓐⓑⓒⓓ	31. ⓐⓑⓒⓓ	32. ⓐⓑⓒⓓ	33. ⓐⓑⓒⓓ
	34. ⓐⓑⓒⓓ	35. ⓐⓑⓒⓓ			

Space for Rough Work

36. Tension is a result of which of the following?
(a) Transpiration at the leaf surface
(b) The cohesive nature of water
(c) The narrowness of the xylem tube
(d) All of the above

37. Which of the following regulates stomatal opening and closing ?
(a) Abscisic acid levels
(b) Light levels
(c) Carbon dioxide concentrations
(d) All of the above

38. Regulators of stomatal opening and closing work by activating the
(a) proton pump in guard cells.
(b) proton pump in stomata
(c) sodium-potassium pump
(d) all of the above

39. Which of the following would not contribute to water uptake by a plant cell ?
(a) an increase in the water potential (ψ) of the surrounding solution
(b) a decrease in pressure on the cell exerted by the wall
(c) the uptake of solutes by the cell
(d) an increase in tension on the surrounding solution.

40. Which of the following does not appear to involve active transport across membranes?
(a) the movement of mineral nutrients from the apoplast to the symplast
(b) the movement of sugar from mesophyll cells into sieve-tube members in corn
(c) the movement of sugar from one sieve-tube member to the next
(d) K^+ uptake by guard cells during stomatal opening.

41. The productivity of a crop declines when leaves begin to wilt mainly because
(a) the chlorophyll of wilting leaves decomposes.
(b) flaccid mesophyll cells are incapable of photosynthesis
(c) stomata close, preventing CO_2 from entering the leaf.
(d) photolysis, the water-splitting step of photosynthesis, cannot occur when there is a water deficiency

42. Imagine cutting a live twig from a tree and examining the cut surface of the twig with a magnifying glass. You locate the vascular tissue and observe a growing droplet of fluid exuding from the cut surface. This fluid is probably
(a) phloem sap
(b) xylem sap
(c) guttation fluid
(d) fluid of the transpiration stream

43. Xylem moves its materials
(a) from the leaves to the roots.
(b) from the roots to the leaves.
(c) when the plant is actively photosynthesizing.
(d) if the proper pressure is maintained.

44. Primary and secondary active transport both
(a) Generate ATP
(b) Use ATP directly
(c) Can move solutes against their concentration gradient
(d) Include the passive movement of glucose molecule

45. Aquaporins are
(a) cytoplasmic connections between cortex cells.
(b) openings in the lower epidermis of leaves through which water vapour escapes.
(c) openings into root hairs through which water enters.
(d) water specific channels in membranes that may regulate the rate of osmosis.

RESPONSE GRID					
	36. ⓐⓑⓒⓓ	37. ⓐⓑⓒⓓ	38. ⓐⓑⓒⓓ	39. ⓐⓑⓒⓓ	40. ⓐⓑⓒⓓ
	41. ⓐⓑⓒⓓ	42. ⓐⓑⓒⓓ	43. ⓐⓑⓒⓓ	44. ⓐⓑⓒⓓ	45. ⓐⓑⓒⓓ

BIOLOGY CHAPTERWISE SPEED TEST-69

Total Questions	45	Total Marks	180
Attempted		Correct	
Incorrect		Net Score	
Cut-off Score	40	Qualifying Score	55
Success Gap = Net Score – Qualifying Score			
Net Score = (Correct × 4) – (Incorrect × 1)			

Space for Rough Work

BIOLOGY

Mineral Nutrition

Speed TEST 70

Chapter-wise

No. of Questions	Maximum Marks	Time
45	180	1 Hour

GENERAL INSTRUCTIONS

- This test contains 45 MCQ's. For each question only one option is correct. Darken the correct circle/ bubble in the Response Grid provided on each page.
- You have to evaluate your Response Grids yourself with the help of solutions provided at the end of this book.
- Each correct answer will get you 4 marks and 1 mark shall be deduced for each incorrect answer. No mark will be given/ deducted if no bubble is filled. Keep a timer in front of you and stop immediately at the end of 60 min.
- The sheet follows a particular syllabus. Do not attempt the sheet before you have completed your preparation for that syllabus.
- After completing the sheet check your answers with the solution booklet and complete the Result Grid. Finally spend time to analyse your performance and revise the areas which emerge out as weak in your evaluation.

1. Which of the following is a free living aerobic non-photosynthetic nitrogen-fixer?
   (a) *Rhizobium* (b) *Azotobacter*
   (c) *Azospirillum* (d) *Nostoc*
2. Which element is located at the centre of the porphyrin ring in chlorophyll ?
   (a) Manganese (b) Calcium
   (c) Magnesium (d) Potassium
3. Which one of the following mineral elements plays an important role in biological nitrogen fixation ?
   (a) Molybdenum (b) Copper
   (c) Manganese (d) Zinc
4. Leghaemoglobin helps in
   (a) nitrogen fixation
   (b) protecting nitrogenase from O_2
   (c) destroys bacteria
   (d) transport of food in plants
5. 'Whip-tail' disease in cauliflower is noted due to deficiency of
   (a) manganese (b) magnesium
   (c) molybdenum (d) nitrogen
6. Which of the following is correct set of micronutrient for plants?
   (a) Mg, Si, Fe, Cu, Ca (b) Cu, Fe, Zn, B, Mn
   (c) Mg, Fe, Zn, B, Mn (d) Mo, Zn, Cl, Mg, Ca

RESPONSE GRID	
	1. ⓐⓑⓒⓓ 2. ⓐⓑⓒⓓ 3. ⓐⓑⓒⓓ 4. ⓐⓑⓒⓓ 5. ⓐⓑⓒⓓ
	6. ⓐⓑⓒⓓ

Space for Rough Work

7. Which of the following statements about nitrification is not true ?
   (a) *Nitrobacter* oxidizes nitrite to nitrate.
   (b) *Nitrosomonas* and *Nitrosococcus* convert ammonium ions to nitrite.
   (c) Nitrification reactions are energy-producing (exergonic) reactions.
   (d) Heterotrophic plants are more directly dependent on the nitrifying bacteria for usable nitrogen than autotrophic plants.
8. A free living nitrogen-fixing cyanobacterium which can also form symbiotic association with the water fern *Azolla* is
   (a) *Tolypothrix* (b) *Chlorella*
   (c) *Nostoc* (d) *Anabaena*
9. *Azotobacter* and *Beijerinckia* are the examples of
   (a) symbiotic nitrogen-fixers
   (b) non-symbiotic nitrogen-fixers
   (c) ammonifying bacteria
   (d) disease causing bacteria
10. Which of the following is not performed by root hairs ?
   (a) Water uptake (b) Oxygen uptake
   (c) Mineral uptake (d) CO_2 uptake
11. The plant ash is an indication of.
   (a) organic matter of plant.
   (b) waste product.
   (c) mineral salts absorbed by plants.
   (d) None of the above
12. Plant obtains nitrogen from soil in the form of
   (a) nitrite (b) nitrate
   (c) ammonia (d) hydroxylamine
13. Hydroponics is
   (a) nutrient less culture (b) water less culture
   (c) soilless culture (d) none of these
14. Which element is required in the germination of pollen grain?
   (a) Chlorine (b) Potassium
   (c) Boron (d) Calcium
15. $N_2 + 8e^- + 8H^+ + 16\,ATP \rightarrow 2NH_4 + H_2 + 16ADP + 16Pi$
   The above equation refers to
   (a) ammonification (b) nitrification
   (c) nitrogen fixation (d) denitrification
16. A trace element essential for plant growth and radio-isotope, which is used in cancer therapy is
   (a) cobalt (b) calcium
   (c) sodium (d) iron
17. Which one of the following elements in plants is not remobilised?
   (a) Phosphorus (b) Calcium
   (c) Potassium (d) Sulphur
18. Element necessary for middle lamella is
   (a) Ca (b) Zn
   (c) K (d) Cu
19. Which of the following element is necessary for translocation of sugars in plants ?
   (a) Boron (b) Molybdenum
   (c) Manganese (d) Iron
20. Plants die from prolonged water-logging because
   (a) soil nutrients become very dilute.
   (b) root respiration stops.
   (c) cell sap in the plants becomes too dilute.
   (d) nutrients leach down due to excess water.
21. Conversion of ammonia into nitrates through *Nitrosomonas* is called
   (a) nitrogen fixation (b) nitrification
   (c) denitrification (d) ammonification

RESPONSE GRID					
	7. ⓐⓑⓒⓓ	8. ⓐⓑⓒⓓ	9. ⓐⓑⓒⓓ	10. ⓐⓑⓒⓓ	11. ⓐⓑⓒⓓ
	12. ⓐⓑⓒⓓ	13. ⓐⓑⓒⓓ	14. ⓐⓑⓒⓓ	15. ⓐⓑⓒⓓ	16. ⓐⓑⓒⓓ
	17. ⓐⓑⓒⓓ	18. ⓐⓑⓒⓓ	19. ⓐⓑⓒⓓ	20. ⓐⓑⓒⓓ	21. ⓐⓑⓒⓓ

Space for Rough Work

22. Which of the following is not a correct pairing of a macronutrient and the major functions it performs in the life of a plant ?
(a) Potassium-enzyme activation, water balance, ion balance.
(b) Calcium-activity of membranes and cytoskeleton, second messenger.
(c) Sulphur-in proteins and coenzymes.
(d) Iron-in active sites of many redox enzymes and electron carriers.

23. Which of the following minerals activate the enzymes involved in respiration?
(a) nitrogen and phosphorus
(b) magnesium and manganese
(c) potassium and calcium
(d) sulpur and iron

24. Soil can easily become deficient in_____________ because these ions are negatively charged and do not stick to negatively charged clay particles.
(a) Nitrate (b) Calcium
(c) Ammonium (d) Magnesium

25. Legumes' roots have swellings called nodules that
(a) produce antibiotics that protect the plant from soil bacteria
(b) provide a steady supply of sugar to the host plant
(c) increases the surface area for water uptake
(d) contain nitrogen-fixing bacteria

26. Macronutrients are_____ than micronutrients.
(a) Larger molecules
(b) Needed in greater quantities
(c) More essential
(d) More important for growth

27. 'Hunger signs' in plants are :
(a) Symptoms due to lesser water absorption in plants
(b) Sympotms due to poor photosynthesis in plants
(c) Deficiency symptoms of particular mineral nutrients
(d) None of the above

28. Death of stem and root tips occur due to deficiency of :
(a) Calcium (b) Nitrogen
(c) Carbon (d) Phosphorus

29. Which of the following is not involved in the phenomenon called ion exchange ?
(a) Negatively charged clay particles
(b) pH
(c) Cations like K^+, Mg^{2+}, and Ca^{2+}
(d) H_2S

30. Tea yellow is a disease of tea plants produced due to the deficiency of-
(a) Nitrogen (b) Sulphur
(c) Potassium (d) Phosphorus

31. Nitrogenase
(a) is insensitive to oxygen.
(b) contains magnesium
(c) releases two NH_3 molecules as products.
(d) requires an aerobic environment.

32. Deficiency of iron causes :
(a) interveinal chlorosis first on young leaves
(b) decrease in protein synthesis
(c) reduced leaves and stunted growth
(d) bending of stem tip

33. You notice that the young leaves of your tomato plants are very yellow. What type of deficiency does this suggest ?
(a) Nitrogen (b) Carbon
(c) Water (d) Iron

RESPONSE GRID				
22. (a)(b)(c)(d)	23. (a)(b)(c)(d)	24. (a)(b)(c)(d)	25. (a)(b)(c)(d)	26. (a)(b)(c)(d)
27. (a)(b)(c)(d)	28. (a)(b)(c)(d)	29. (a)(b)(c)(d)	30. (a)(b)(c)(d)	31. (a)(b)(c)(d)
32. (a)(b)(c)(d)	33. (a)(b)(c)(d)			

Space for Rough Work

34. Where does most nutrient uptake occur in roots ?
(a) At the root tip, where root tissue first encounters soil away from the zone of nutrient depletion.
(b) At the casparian strip, where ions must enter the symplast prior to entering xylem cells.
(c) In the symplastic and apoplastic pathways.
(d) In root hairs and in the zone of maturation.

35. It is possible to determine whether an element is essential by observing growth of plants
(a) On soil in which the particular element is removed
(b) On soil in which only the particular element is present
(c) On an inert medium to which solution of only the particular element is added
(d) On an inert medium to which a nutrient solution excluding that particular element, is added.

36. Terrestrial plants obtain all of the following nutrients from the soil except
(a) potassium (b) nitrogen
(c) phosphorus (d) carbon

37. For chlorophyll formation a plant needs :
(a) Fe, Ca & light (b) Fe, Mg & Light
(c) Ca, K & light (d) Mn & Cu

38. Which element essential for the stability of chromosome structure?
(a) Zn (b) Ca
(c) Mo (d) Fe

39. Which mineral nutrients are called critical element for crops?
(a) N, P, K (b) C, H, O
(c) N, S, Mg (d) K, Ca, Fe

40. Nitrogenase enzymes are extremely sensitive to ________ molecules -
(a) Hydrogen (b) Oxygen
(c) Water (d) CO_2

41. Gray spots of Oat are caused by deficiency of :
(a) Cu (b) Zn
(c) Mn (d) Fe

42. Which element participates in photolysis of water, ionic balance maintenance and solute concentration?
(a) Cl^- (b) B
(c) Na^+ (d) Mg^{2+}

43. "Reclamation" and "Little leaf" disease, caused by deficiency of
(a) Zn and Mo (b) Cu and Zn
(c) Cu and B (d) Mn and Cu

44. Brown heart rot of beets is due to deficiency of
(a) B (b) P
(c) Mg (d) Mo

45. Which element is related with Khaira disease of paddy & auxin synthesis?
(a) Fe (b) Zn
(c) B (d) Cu

RESPONSE GRID					
	34. ⓐⓑⓒⓓ	35. ⓐⓑⓒⓓ	36. ⓐⓑⓒⓓ	37. ⓐⓑⓒⓓ	38. ⓐⓑⓒⓓ
	39. ⓐⓑⓒⓓ	40. ⓐⓑⓒⓓ	41. ⓐⓑⓒⓓ	42. ⓐⓑⓒⓓ	43. ⓐⓑⓒⓓ
	44. ⓐⓑⓒⓓ	45. ⓐⓑⓒⓓ			

BIOLOGY CHAPTERWISE SPEED TEST-70			
Total Questions	45	Total Marks	180
Attempted		Correct	
Incorrect		Net Score	
Cut-off Score	40	Qualifying Score	55
Success Gap = Net Score – Qualifying Score			
Net Score = (Correct × 4) – (Incorrect × 1)			

Space for Rough Work

BIOLOGY

Photosynthesis in Higher Plants

Speed TEST 71 Chapter-wise

No. of Questions	Maximum Marks	Time
45	180	1 Hour

GENERAL INSTRUCTIONS

- This test contains 45 MCQ's. For each question only one option is correct. Darken the correct circle/ bubble in the Response Grid provided on each page.
- You have to evaluate your Response Grids yourself with the help of solutions provided at the end of this book.
- Each correct answer will get you 4 marks and 1 mark shall be deduced for each incorrect answer. No mark will be given/ deducted if no bubble is filled. Keep a timer in front of you and stop immediately at the end of 60 min.
- The sheet follows a particular syllabus. Do not attempt the sheet before you have completed your preparation for that syllabus.
- After completing the sheet check your answers with the solution booklet and complete the Result Grid. Finally spend time to analyse your performance and revise the areas which emerge out as weak in your evaluation.

1. Quantasomes are present in
(a) chloroplast (b) mitochondria
(c) golgi body (d) lysosome

2. The C_4 plants are photosynthetically more efficient than C_3 plants because:
(a) the CO_2 compensation point is more
(b) CO_2 generated during photorespiration is trapped and recycled through PEP carboxylase
(c) the CO_2 efflux is not prevented
(d) they have more chloroplasts

3. Photorespiration is favoured by
(a) high O_2 and low CO_2
(b) low light and high O_2
(c) low temperature and high O_2
(d) low O_2 and high CO_2

4. Which one is the correct summary equation of photosynthesis?
(a) $C_6H_{12}O_6 + 6O_2 \longrightarrow 6CO_2 + 6H_2O + \text{energy}$
(b) $C_6H_{12}O_6 + 6O_2 + 6H_2O \longrightarrow 6CO_2 + 12H_2O + \text{energy}$
(c) $6CO_2 + 6H_2O \longrightarrow 6H_2O + C_6H_{12}O_6$
(d) $6CO_2 + 12H_2O \xrightarrow[\text{Chlorophyll}]{\text{Light}} 6O_2 + C_6H_{12}O_6 + 6H_2O$

5. C_4 acid, formed in the mesophyll of C_4 plants leaf during photosynthesis is
(a) OAA or malic acid or aspartic acid
(b) pyruvic acid
(c) succinic acid
(d) fumaric acid

6. The organelles which take part in photo-respiration are
(a) chloroplast, mitochondria, nucleus
(b) chloroplast, mitochondria, lysosome
(c) mitochondria, chloroplast, peroxisome
(d) mitochondria, lysosomes, peroxisome

RESPONSE GRID	1. ⓐⓑⓒⓓ	2. ⓐⓑⓒⓓ	3. ⓐⓑⓒⓓ	4. ⓐⓑⓒⓓ	5. ⓐⓑⓒⓓ
	6. ⓐⓑⓒⓓ				

Space for Rough Work

7. Grana are present inside the :
(a) mitochondria (b) chloroplast
(c) endoplasmic reticulum (d) ribosome

8. Photosynthetically active radiation is represented by the range of wavelength of
(a) 340 - 450 nm (b) 400 - 700 nm
(c) 500 - 600 nm (d) 400 - 950 nm

9. Which of the following statement is incorrect ?
(a) C_3 plants respond to higher temperature, show higher photosynthetic rate while C_4 plants have lower optimum temperature.
(b) Tropical plants have higher temperature optimum than the plants adapted to temperate climate.
(c) Light reaction is less temperature sensitive than dark reaction.
(d) The effect of water as a factor is more through its effect on plant, rather than directly on photosynthesis.

10. Chemiosmotic hypothesis given by Peter Mitchell proposes the mechanism of
(a) synthesis of ATP (b) synthesis of $FADH_2$
(c) synthesis of NADH (d) synthesis of NADPH

11. RuBisCO stands for
(a) Ribulose Biphosphate Carboxylase Oxygenase
(b) Ribulose Phosphate Carboxylase Oxygenase
(c) Ribulose Phosphate Carboxylic Oxygenase
(d) None of the above

12. Which enzyme is most abundantly found on earth?
(a) Catalase (b) RuBisCo
(c) Nitrogenase (d) Invertase

13. The first carbon dioxide acceptor in C_4-plants is
(a) Phosphoenol-pyruvate
(b) Ribulose 1, 5-diphosphate
(c) Oxalo-acetic acid
(d) Phosphoglyceric acid

14. Which one of the following is essential for photolysis of water ?
(a) Manganese (b) Zinc
(c) Copper (d) Boron

15. Which element is required in the germination of pollen grain?
(a) Chlorine (b) Potassium
(c) Boron (d) Calcium

16. In a CAM plant, the concentration of organic acid
(a) increases during the day.
(b) decreases during the day.
(c) increases during night.
(d) decreases or increases during day.

17. Which of the following statements regarding photorespiration are **true**?
(a) Photorespiration is a metabolically expensive pathway.
(b) Photorespiration is avoided when CO_2 is abundant.
(c) Photorespiration results in a loss of usable carbon dioxide.
(d) All of the above

18. The Z-scheme refers to
(a) the type of photosynthesis occurs in plants found in areas with minimal precipitation.
(b) the pattern of grana within the chloroplasts of photosynthetic plants.
(c) the carbon-fixation process which is also known as the Calvin cycle.
(d) an energy diagram for the transfer of electrons in the light reactions of photosynthesis in plants.

19. Which one is a C_4-plant?
(a) Papaya (b) Pea
(c) Potato (d) Maize/Corn

20. In an experiment, mature leaves on the plant were enclosed for a fixed amount of time in a transparent bag that had radioactive CO_2. In which part of the plant will maximum radioactivity be found after some time?
(a) Actively growing leaves.
(b) Guard cells of all the leaves.
(c) In mature leaves.
(d) Senescing leaves and roots.

21. When a photosynthetic plant is transferred to an atmosphere of enriched O_2, its rate of
(a) photosynthesis would increase.
(b) photosynthesis would decrease.
(c) respiration would decrease.
(d) osmosis would increase.

RESPONSE GRID					
	7. ⓐⓑⓒⓓ	8. ⓐⓑⓒⓓ	9. ⓐⓑⓒⓓ	10. ⓐⓑⓒⓓ	11. ⓐⓑⓒⓓ
	12. ⓐⓑⓒⓓ	13. ⓐⓑⓒⓓ	14. ⓐⓑⓒⓓ	15. ⓐⓑⓒⓓ	16. ⓐⓑⓒⓓ
	17. ⓐⓑⓒⓓ	18. ⓐⓑⓒⓓ	19. ⓐⓑⓒⓓ	20. ⓐⓑⓒⓓ	21. ⓐⓑⓒⓓ

Space for Rough Work

22. In C_4 plants, agranal chloroplasts are found in
(a) mesophyll cells
(b) epidermal cell chloroplasts of green stem
(c) bundle sheath cells
(d) chloroplasts of guard cells

23. Oxysomes or $F_0 - F_1$ particles occur on
(a) thylakoids
(b) mitochondrial surface
(c) inner mitochondrial membrane
(d) chloroplast surface

24. Photorespiration is favoured by
(a) high O_2 and low CO_2
(b) low light and high O_2
(c) low temperature and high O_2
(d) low O_2 and high CO_2

25. In the leaves of C_4 plants, malic acid formation during CO_2 fixation occurs in the cells of
(a) bundle sheath (b) phloem
(c) epidermis (d) mesophyll

26. The graph shows the relation between light intensity and the giving off and taking up of carbon dioxide by the leaves of a plant. Why is most carbon dioxide given off when the light intensity is zero units ?

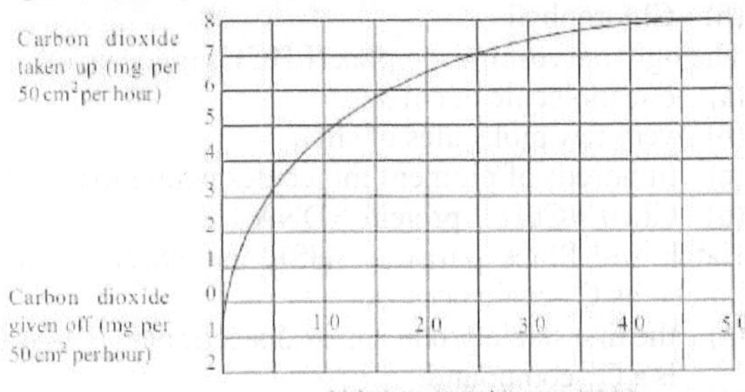

(a) Because it is just the start of the experiment.
(b) Only respiration is taking place at this intensity of light.
(c) Only photosynthesis is taking place at this intensity of light.
(d) The rate of photosynthesis is equivalent to the rate of respiration.

27. In photosystem-I the first electron acceptor is
(a) cytochrome (b) plastocyanin
(c) an iron-sulphur protein (d) ferredoxin

28. Which of the following statement is false?
(a) H_2S, not H_2O, is involved in photosynthesis of purple sulphur bacteria.
(b) Light and dark reactions are stopped in the absence of light.
(c) Calvin cycle occurs in the grana of chloroplast.
(d) ATP is produced during light reaction *via* chemiosmosis.

29. Given below is the pathway of light reaction. Identify the given blanks indicated by A, B, C, D and E.

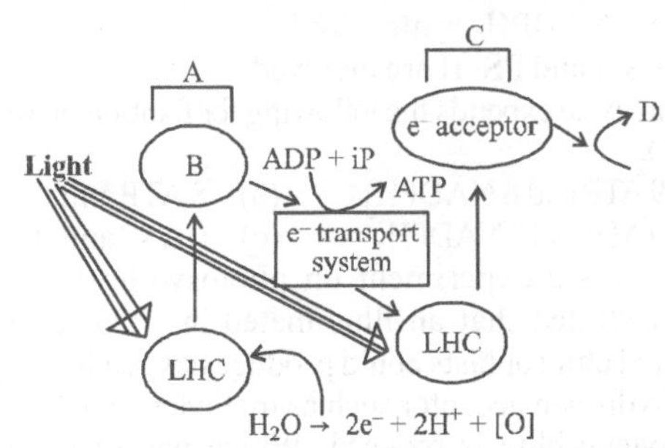

	A	B	C	D
(a)	P 700	H^+ acceptor	P680	$NADP^+$
(b)	Photosystem I	e^- acceptor	Photosystem II	$NADPH_2^+$ ATP
(c)	Photosystem II	H^+ acceptor	P700	NADPH
(d)	Photosystem II	e^- acceptor	Photosystem I	NADPH + H^+

30. Warburg effect refers to
(a) decreased photosynthetic rate at very high O_2 concentration
(b) increased photosynthetic rate at very high O_2 concentration
(c) decreased photosynthetic rate at very low O_2 concentration
(d) increased photosynthetic rate at very low O_2 concentration

RESPONSE GRID					
	22. ⓐⓑⓒⓓ	23. ⓐⓑⓒⓓ	24. ⓐⓑⓒⓓ	25. ⓐⓑⓒⓓ	26. ⓐⓑⓒⓓ
	27. ⓐⓑⓒⓓ	28. ⓐⓑⓒⓓ	29. ⓐⓑⓒⓓ	30. ⓐⓑⓒⓓ	

Space for Rough Work

31. Read the following statements and select the correct ones.
(i) PS I is involved in non-cyclic photophosphorylation only.
(ii) PS II is involved in both cyclic and non-cyclic photophosphorylation
(iii) Stroma lamellae membranes possess PS I only, whereas grana lamellae membranes possess both PS I and PS II.
(a) (i) only (b) (ii) only
(c) (iii) only (d) (i), (ii) and (iii)

32. Which is not correct for cyclic photophosporylation ?
(a) No O_2 given off
(b) No water consumed
(c) No $NADPH_2$ synthesized
(d) PS–I and PS–II are involved

33. Calvin cycle expends the following for fixation of 3-molecules of CO_2
(a) 9 ATP and 6 $NADPH_2$ (b) 8 ATP and 6 $NADPH_2$
(c) 9 ATP and 3 $NADPH_2$ (d) 6 ATP and 9 $NADPH_2$

34. In a classic experiment on photosynthesis, R. L. Hill demonstrated that an illuminated in *vitro* suspension of isolated chloroplasts could produce oxygen in the presence of a hydrogen acceptor such as methylene blue. In this case methylene blue is reduced. Which one of the following compounds replaces methylene blue in the intact photosynthesising plant ?
(a) adenosine triphosphate (ATP)
(b) carbon dioxide
(c) nicotinamide adenine dinucleotide phosphate (NADP)
(d) phosphoglyceric acid (PGA)

35. The key compound of Calvin cycle is
(a) PGA (b) PGAL
(c) DHAP (d) DPGA

36. Which one of the following is a correct outline of the main events in photosynthesis?
(a) Oxygen reacts with a carbohydrate to produce water and carbon dioxide in the presence of light.
(b) Light joins carbon dioxide to an acceptor compound which is then reduced by hydrogen obtained from water.
(c) Light splits water and the resulting hydroxyl group combines with a compound which has incorporated carbon dioxide
(d) Carbon dioxide combines with an acceptor compound and this is reduced by hydrogen split from water by light.

37. Who used prism, white light, green alga, *Cladophora* and aerobic bacteria and plotted the action spectra for photosynthesis?
(a) Sachs (b) Arnon
(c) Arnold (d) Englemann

38. Which one of the following pigment does not occur in the chloroplast?
(a) Carotene (b) Xanthophyll
(c) Chlorophyll '*b*' (d) Anthocyanin

39. Which pigment is water soluble?
(a) Chlorophyll (b) Carotene
(c) Anthocyanin (d) Xanthophyll

40. Generally CO_2 is not limiting for hydrophytes –
(a) Mesophytes plants fix H_2S in their photosynthesis.
(b) These plants also CO_2 have from water in the form of HCO_3.
(c) Glucose is not required for their respiration
(d) All of the above

41. Suspension of isolated thylakoids in culture medium containing CO_2 and H_2O does not produce hexose due to absence of
(a) ATP (b) Enzyme
(c) Proteins (d) Hill reagent

42. Stroma in the chloroplasts of higher plant contains
(a) Light-independent reaction enzymes
(b) Light-dependent reaction enzymes
(c) Ribosomes
(d) Chlorophyll

43. The light harvesting complex (LHC) is made up of
(a) one molecule of chl *a*.
(b) very few molecules of chl *a*.
(c) hundreds of pigment molecules bound to proteins.
(d) Chl *a* + Chl *c* + protein + DNA.

44. Hatch and Slack pathway (HSK pathway) is otherwise known as C_4-cycle because
(a) the first stable product is oxaloacetic acid / OAA which is a C_4-compound.
(b) the primary CO_2 acceptor is OAA, a C_4-compounds.
(c) all intermediate metabolites are C_4-compound.
(d) at one time $4CO_2$ molecules take part in carboxylation pathway.

45. The first acceptor of electrons from an excited chlorophyll molecule of photosystem II is –
(a) Quinone (b) Cytochrome
(c) Iron-sulphur protein (d) Ferredoxin

RESPONSE GRID					
	31. ⓐⓑⓒⓓ	32. ⓐⓑⓒⓓ	33. ⓐⓑⓒⓓ	34. ⓐⓑⓒⓓ	35. ⓐⓑⓒⓓ
	36. ⓐⓑⓒⓓ	37. ⓐⓑⓒⓓ	38. ⓐⓑⓒⓓ	39. ⓐⓑⓒⓓ	40. ⓐⓑⓒⓓ
	41. ⓐⓑⓒⓓ	42. ⓐⓑⓒⓓ	43. ⓐⓑⓒⓓ	44. ⓐⓑⓒⓓ	45. ⓐⓑⓒⓓ

BIOLOGY CHAPTERWISE SPEED TEST-71			
Total Questions	45	Total Marks	180
Attempted		Correct	
Incorrect		Net Score	
Cut-off Score	45	Qualifying Score	60
Success Gap = Net Score – Qualifying Score			
Net Score = (Correct × 4) – (Incorrect × 1)			

Space for Rough Work

BIOLOGY

Respiration in Plants

Speed TEST 72

Chapter-wise

No. of Questions	Maximum Marks	Time
45	180	1 Hour

GENERAL INSTRUCTIONS

- This test contains 45 MCQ's. For each question only one option is correct. Darken the correct circle/ bubble in the Response Grid provided on each page.
- You have to evaluate your Response Grids yourself with the help of solutions provided at the end of this book.
- Each correct answer will get you 4 marks and 1 mark shall be deduced for each incorrect answer. No mark will be given/ deducted if no bubble is filled. Keep a timer in front of you and stop immediately at the end of 60 min.
- The sheet follows a particular syllabus. Do not attempt the sheet before you have completed your preparation for that syllabus.
- After completing the sheet check your answers with the solution booklet and complete the Result Grid. Finally spend time to analyse your performance and revise the areas which emerge out as weak in your evaluation.

1. Respiratory Quotient (R.Q.) is defined as:
   (a) vol. of O_2/vol. of CO_2
   (b) vol. of CO_2 /vol. of O_2
   (c) vol. of O_2/vol. of N_2
   (d) vol. of N_2/vol. of CO_2
2. What is the end product of glycolysis of a glucose molecule?
   (a) Fructose 1, 6- diphosphate
   (b) Pyruvate and ATP
   (c) Phosphoglyceraldehyde
   (d) Lactic acid and ATP
3. Connecting link between glycolysis and Krebs cycle is/ before entering Krebs cycle pyruvate is changed to
   (a) oxaloacetate (b) phosphoenol pyruvate
   (c) pyruvate (d) acetyl CoA
4. Site of respiration in bacteria is
   (a) episome (b) ribosome
   (c) mesosome (d) microsome
5. Terminal cytochrome of respiratory chain which donates electrons to oxygen is
   (a) Cyt. b (b) Cyt. c
   (c) Cyt. a_1 (d) Cyt. a_3
6. Which of the following processes make direct use of oxygen ?
   (a) Glycolysis (b) Fermentation
   (c) Electron transport (d) citric acid cycle
7. Glycolysis is a
   (a) redox process (b) aerobic process
   (c) oxidative process (d) reductive process
8. In Kreb's cycle, the FAD participates as electron acceptor during the conversion of
   (a) succinyl CoA to succinic acid
   (b) α - ketoglutarate to succinyl CoA
   (c) fumaric acid to malic acid
   (d) succinic acid to fumaric acid
9. The major reason that glycolysis is not as energy productive as respiration is that
   (a) NAD^+ is regenerated by alcohol or lactate production, without the high-energy electrons passing through the electron transport chain.
   (b) it is the pathway common to fermentation and respiration.
   (c) it does not take place in a specialized membrane-bound organelle.
   (d) pyruvate is more reduced than CO_2; it still contains much of the energy from glucose.

RESPONSE GRID					
	1. ⓐⓑⓒⓓ	2. ⓐⓑⓒⓓ	3. ⓐⓑⓒⓓ	4. ⓐⓑⓒⓓ	5. ⓐⓑⓒⓓ
	6. ⓐⓑⓒⓓ	7. ⓐⓑⓒⓓ	8. ⓐⓑⓒⓓ	9. ⓐⓑⓒⓓ	

Space for Rough Work

10. Which of the following is a 4-carbon compound?
(a) Oxaloacetic acid (b) Citric acid
(c) Phosphoglyceric acid (d) Phosphoenol pyruvate

11. Which of the following is a biological uncoupler of oxidative phosphorylation ?
(a) Thermogenin
(b) 2, 4 – Dichlorophenoxy acetic acid
(c) 2, 4 – Dinitrophenol
(d) Ethylene diaminotetra acetic acid

12. Which of the following is not true for oxidative phosphorylation?
(a) It uses oxygen as the initial electron donor.
(b) It involves the redox reactions of electron transport chain.
(c) It involves an ATP synthase located in the inner mitochondrial membrane.
(d) It depends on chemiosmosis.

13. In which of the following reaction of glycolysis, a molecule of water is removed from the substrate ?
(a) Frucoste-6-phosphate → Fructose 1, 6-biphosphate
(b) 3-phosphate glyceraldehyde → 1, 3 biphosphoglyceric acid
(c) Phosphoenol-pyruvate → Pyruvic acid
(d) 2-phosphoglycerate → PEP

14. The first dicarboxylic acid in Krebs' cycle is
(a) isocitric acid (b) pyruvic acid
(c) oxalo acetic acid (d) α-ketoglutaric acid

15. Final electron acceptor in oxidative phosphorylation is
(a) hydrogen (b) dehydrogenase
(c) cytochrome (d) oxygen

16. Quantasomes are found in
(a) mitochondria (b) chloroplast
(c) lysosome (d) endoplasmic reticulum

17. Which of the following statement(s) is/are incorrect ?
(i) Proton channel of oxysome / complex V / ATP synthase is located in F_1.
(ii) Metabolic water is produced in terminal oxidation / produced in respiration.
(iii) CoQ accepts electron from NADH dehydrogenase (complex I) and also can accept electron from $FADH_2$/ succinate Q-reductase / complex II.
(iv) Cytochrome *c* is a small protein attached to outer surface of the inner mitochondrial membrane and acts as mobile carrier for transfer of electrons between complex I (Cyt *bc*, complex) and III.
(v) Complex IV refers to cytochrome *c* oxidase (cyt *a*, a_3 and 2 Cu per centre).
(vi) If a cell is treated with a drug that inhibits ATP synthase, the pH of mitochondrial matrix will increase.
(a) (i), (ii) and (iii) (b) (iii), (v) and (vi)
(c) (i) and (iv) (d) Only (iii)

18. Which of the following is an important intermediate found in all the types of respiration ?
(a) Acetyl CoA (b) Pyruvic acid
(c) Oxaloacetate (d) Tricarboxylic acid

19. Incomplete oxidation of glucose into pyruvic acid with several intermediate steps is known as
(a) TCA-pathway (b) Glycolysis
(c) HMS-pathway (d) Krebs cycle

20. Common enzyme in glycolysis and pentose phosphate pathways is
(a) hexokinase (b) aconitase
(c) fumarase (d) dehydrogenase

21. Out of 36 ATP molecules produced per glucose molecule during respiration
(a) 2 are produced outside glycolysis and 34 during respiratory chain.
(b) 2 are produced outside mitochondria and 34 inside mitochondria.
(c) 2 during glycolysis and 34 during Krebs cycle.
(d) all are formed inside mitochondria.

22. R.Q. is highest when respiratory substance is
(a) fat (b) malic acid
(c) glucose (d) protein

23. Electron transport chain is inhibited by
(a) rotenone and amytal
(b) antimycin-A
(c) cyanide (CN^-), azide (N^{3-}) and carbon monoxide (CO)
(d) All of the above

24. Though vertebrates are aerobes, but their __(i)__ show anaerobic respiration during __(ii)__. During this, __(iii)__ of skeletal muscle fibres is broken down to release lactic acid and energy. Lactic acid, if accumulates causes muscle fatigue.
Fill up the blanks in the above paragraph and select the correct option.

	(i)	(ii)	(iii)
(a)	skeletal muscles	heavy exercise	glucose
(b)	skeletal muscles	mild exercise	glycogen
(c)	skeletal muscles	heavy exercise	glycogen
(d)	cardiac muscles	heavy exercise	glycogen

RESPONSE GRID				
10. ⓐⓑⓒⓓ	11. ⓐⓑⓒⓓ	12. ⓐⓑⓒⓓ	13. ⓐⓑⓒⓓ	14. ⓐⓑⓒⓓ
15. ⓐⓑⓒⓓ	16. ⓐⓑⓒⓓ	17. ⓐⓑⓒⓓ	18. ⓐⓑⓒⓓ	19. ⓐⓑⓒⓓ
20. ⓐⓑⓒⓓ	21. ⓐⓑⓒⓓ	22. ⓐⓑⓒⓓ	23. ⓐⓑⓒⓓ	24. ⓐⓑⓒⓓ

Space for Rough Work

25. Identify A and B in the given diagram showing ATP synthesis in oxysomes

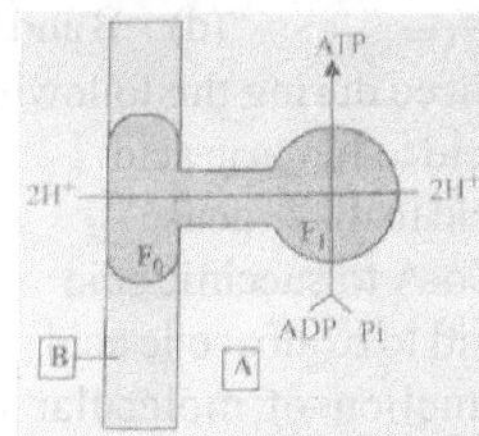

(a) A = Mitochondrial matrix
B = Outer mitochondrial membrane
(b) A = Mitochondrial matrix
B = Inner mitochondrial membrane
(c) A = Cell cytoplasm
B = Inner mitochondrial membrane
(d) A = Cell cytoplasm
B = Outer mitochondrial membrane

26. Potassium cyanide is known to interfere with the formation and use of ATP in cell metabolism.
If the use of potassium cyanide resulted in an accelerated entry of a solute into a cell, it may be reasonably assumed that, under normal circumstances, the solute enters by
(a) active transport (b) osmosis
(c) passive diffusion (d) pinocytosis

27. When yeast growing anaerobically in glucose-rich-environment is exposed to oxygen in sufficient quantity, its rate of glucose utilization decreases. This pheno-menon is known as the Pasteur effect. Adding an uncoupler of oxidative phosphorylation would have what effect on Pasteur effect?
(a) Pasteur effect will be enhanced
(b) Pasteur effect will remain unchanged
(c) Pasteur effect will not take place
(d) Variable effect

28. An inhibitor is added to a cell culture so that succinate accumulates. The enzyme catalysing the formation of which substance has been blocked?
(a) Citrate (b) Oxaloacetate
(c) α-ketoglutarate (d) Fumarate

29. One of the following is common to glycolysis as well as Krebs cycle in eukaryotes :
(a) Substrate level phosphorylation
(b) Photophosphorylation
(c) Localization in mitochondria
(d) Production of $FADH_2$

30. A mutant cell lacking mitochondria will show:
(a) Inability to oxidize carbohydrates
(b) Inability to oxidize fats
(c) Inability to oxidize carbohydrates and fats
(d) Inability to synthesize glucose

31. During the early stages of alcoholic fermentation there is a high rate of growth of yeast. After some time the rate decreases. Which of the following conditions in the culture medium is least likely to have caused this?
(a) Depletion of glucose
(b) Depletion of oxygen
(c) Depletion of mineral salts
(d) Accumulation of waste products

32. Hexose monophosphate shunt does not take place when :
(a) Oxygen is not enough
(b) Glucose is the substrate
(c) NAD is available
(d) NAD is not available due to shortage of oxygen

33. Chemiosmotic theory of ATP synthesis in the chloroplasts and mitochondria is based on
(a) membrane potential (b) accumulation of Na ions
(c) accumulation of K ions (d) proton gradient

34. During the stage in the complete oxidation of glucose are the greatest number of ATP molecules formed from ADP
(a) glycolysis
(b) krebs cycle
(c) conversion of pyruvic acid to acetyl Co-A
(d) electron transport chain

35. How many ATP molecules could maximally be generated from one molecule of glucose, if the complete oxidation of one mole of glucose to CO_2 and H_2O yields 686 kcal and the useful chemical energy available in the high energy phosphate bond of one mole of ATP is 12 kcal ?
(a) Thirty (b) Fifty-seven
(c) One (d) Two

36. All enzymes of TCA cycle are located in the mitochondrial matrix except one which is located in inner mitochondrial membranes in eukaryotes and in cytosol in prokaryotes. This enzyme is
(a) isocitrate dehydrogenase
(b) malate dehydrogenase
(c) succinate dehydrogenase
(d) lactate dehydrogenase.

37. The energy-releasing process in which the substrate is oxidised without an external electron acceptor is called
(a) fermentation (b) photorespiration
(c) aerobic respiration (d) glycolysis

RESPONSE GRID					
	25. ⓐⓑⓒⓓ	26. ⓐⓑⓒⓓ	27. ⓐⓑⓒⓓ	28. ⓐⓑⓒⓓ	29. ⓐⓑⓒⓓ
	30. ⓐⓑⓒⓓ	31. ⓐⓑⓒⓓ	32. ⓐⓑⓒⓓ	33. ⓐⓑⓒⓓ	34. ⓐⓑⓒⓓ
	35. ⓐⓑⓒⓓ	36. ⓐⓑⓒⓓ	37. ⓐⓑⓒⓓ		

Space for Rough Work

38. In TCA cycle the conversion of succinyl Co-A to succinic acid requires
(a) Acetyl Co-A + GTP + iP
(b) Acetyl Co-A + GDP + iP
(c) Co-A + GTP + iP
(d) GDP + iP

39. The diagram shows the reversible conversion of pyruvate to lactate by the enzyme lactate dehydrogenase.

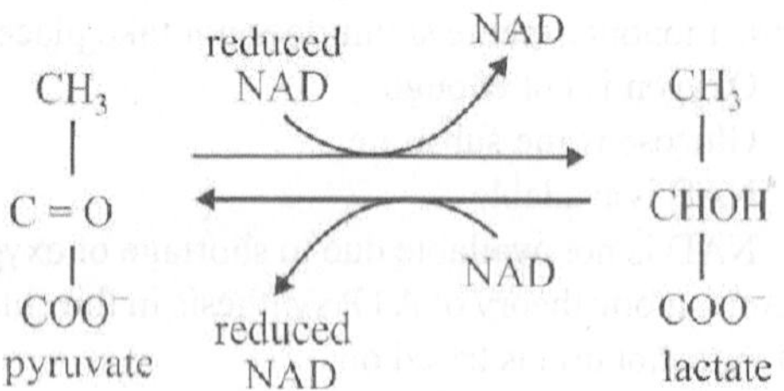

What would be the effect of inhibition of lactate dehydrogenase in a mammalian cell under anaerobic conditions?
(a) A decrease in cell pH, due to the accumulation of lactic acid.
(b) A decrease in glycolysis, due to the lack of NAD.
(c) An increase in ATP production, due to increased amounts of reduced NAD.
(d) An increase in the activity of the Krebs cycle, due to increased amounts of pyruvate.

40. The diagram summarises the pathway of glucose breakdown.

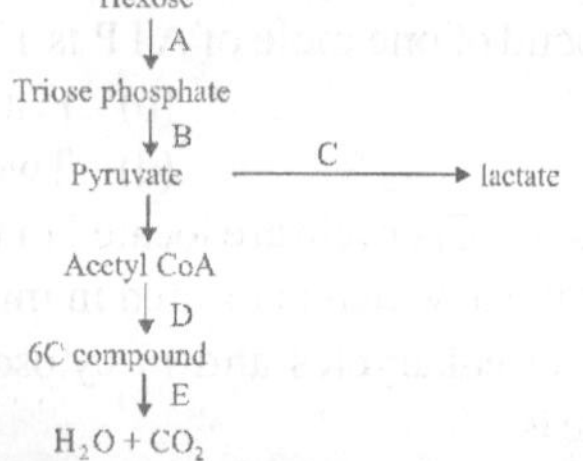

When two steps result in a net increase of ATP?
(a) A and C (b) A and D
(c) B and D (d) B and E

41. $FADH_2$ is produced during the following reaction
(a) Succinic acid to fumaric acid
(b) Fumaric acid to malic acid
(c) Succinyl Co-A to succinic acid
(d) Isocitric acid to oxaloacetic acid

42. What is the function of molecular oxygen in cellular respiration?
(a) It causes the breakdown of citric acid.
(b) To combine with glucose to produce carbon dioxide.
(c) To combine with carbon from organic molecules to produce carbon dioxide.
(d) To combine with hydrogen from organic molecules to produce water.

43. Sugars are not as good as fats as a source of energy for cellular respiration, because sugars
(a) produce toxic amino groups when broken down.
(b) contain more hydrogen.
(c) usually bypass glycolysis and the Krebs cycle.
(d) contain fewer hydrogen atoms and electrons.

44. For bacteria to continue growing rapidly when they are shifted from an environment containing O_2 to an anaerobic environment, they must
(a) produce more ATP per mole of glucose during glycolysis.
(b) produce ATP during oxidation of glucose.
(c) increase the rate of glycolysis.
(d) increase the rate of TCA cycle.

45. Protein is used as respiratory substrate only when
(a) Carbohydrates are absent
(b) Fats are absent
(c) Both carbohydrates and fats are exhausted
(d) Fats and carbohydrates are abundant

RESPONSE GRID	38. ⓐⓑⓒⓓ	39. ⓐⓑⓒⓓ	40. ⓐⓑⓒⓓ	41. ⓐⓑⓒⓓ	42. ⓐⓑⓒⓓ
	43. ⓐⓑⓒⓓ	44. ⓐⓑⓒⓓ	45. ⓐⓑⓒⓓ		

BIOLOGY CHAPTERWISE SPEED TEST-72			
Total Questions	45	Total Marks	180
Attempted		Correct	
Incorrect		Net Score	
Cut-off Score	45	Qualifying Score	60
Success Gap = Net Score – Qualifying Score			
Net Score = (Correct × 4) – (Incorrect × 1)			

BIOLOGY

Plant Growth and Development

Speed TEST 73

Chapter-wise

No. of Questions	Maximum Marks	Time
45	180	1 Hour

GENERAL INSTRUCTIONS

- This test contains 45 MCQ's. For each question only one option is correct. Darken the correct circle/ bubble in the Response Grid provided on each page.
- You have to evaluate your Response Grids yourself with the help of solutions provided at the end of this book.
- Each correct answer will get you 4 marks and 1 mark shall be deduced for each incorrect answer. No mark will be given/ deducted if no bubble is filled. Keep a timer in front of you and stop immediately at the end of 60 min.
- The sheet follows a particular syllabus. Do not attempt the sheet before you have completed your preparation for that syllabus.
- After completing the sheet check your answers with the solution booklet and complete the Result Grid. Finally spend time to analyse your performance and revise the areas which emerge out as weak in your evaluation.

1. Which one is a long day plant?
   (a) Tobacco (b) *Glycine max*
   (c) *Mirabilis jalapa* (d) Spinach
2. The hormone which controls cell division and cell differentiation is
   (a) ABA (b) auxin
   (c) gibberellin (d) cytokinin
3. Which one of the following is a long day plant?
   (a) Bajra (b) Soyabean
   (c) Tobacco (d) Wheat
4. A chemical believed to be involved in flowering is
   (a) gibberellin (b) kinetin
   (c) florigen (d) IBA
5. Which one of the following acids is a derivative of carotenoids ?
   (a) Indole-3 -acetic acid (b) Gibberellic acid
   (c) Abscisic acid (d) Indole butyric acid
6. Differentiation of shoot is controlled by
   (a) high gibberellin : cytokinin ratio
   (b) high auxin : cytokinin ratio
   (c) high cytokinin : auxin ratio
   (d) high gibberellin : auxin ratio
7. Which one of the following generally acts as an antagonist to gibberellins?
   (a) Zeatin (b) Ethylene
   (c) ABA (d) IAA
8. To avoid excessive water loss during severe drought stress, the closure of stomata is signalled by the production of
   (a) IAA (b) NAA
   (c) ABA (d) IBA

RESPONSE GRID					
	1. ⓐⓑⓒⓓ	2. ⓐⓑⓒⓓ	3. ⓐⓑⓒⓓ	4. ⓐⓑⓒⓓ	5. ⓐⓑⓒⓓ
	6. ⓐⓑⓒⓓ	7. ⓐⓑⓒⓓ	8. ⓐⓑⓒⓓ		

Space for Rough Work

9. In short day plants, flowering is induced by
(a) photoperiod less than 12 hours.
(b) photoperiod below a critical length and uninterrupted long night.
(c) long night.
(d) short photoperiod and interrupted long night.

10. Apical dominance in plants is caused by
(a) high concentration of auxins in the terminal bud.
(b) high concentration of gibberellins in the apical bud.
(c) high concentration of auxins in the lateral bud.
(d) absence of auxins and gibberellins in apical bud.

11. Primary precursor of IAA is
(a) phenylalanine (b) tyrosine
(c) tryptophan (d) leucine

12. In a plant growing under dark condition, the leaves turn light coloured, internodes become much elongated and it is termed as
(a) vernalization (b) etiolation
(c) phyllotaxy (d) chlorosis

13. Parthenocarpic fruit can be produced by the application of which of the following auxin?
(a) IBA (Indole butyric acid)
(b) IAA (Indole acetic acid)
(c) 2, 4-D (2-4 dichlorophenoxy acetic acid)
(d) All of the above.

14. The conditions necessary for vernalization are
(a) high temperature and water
(b) low temperature and oxygen
(c) water and carbon dioxide
(d) oxygen and water.

15. Which of the following hormones does not naturally occur in plants?
(a) 2,4–D (2, 4–dichloropheoxy acetic acid)
(b) IAA
(c) ABA
(d) GA

16. Which of the following types of phytohormones resemble the nucleic acids in some structural aspects ?
(a) Auxin (b) Cytokinin
(c) Gibberellin (d) ABA

17. Which one of the following statement regarding auxin is/are correct?
(a) IAA and IBA are natural but NAA, 2, 4-D and 2, 4, 5-T are synthetic auxins.
(b) IAA and NAA are natural but IBA, 2, 4, 5-T and 2, 4-D are synthetic auxins.
(c) NAA and 2, 4, 5-T are natural but IAA, IBA and 2, 4-D are synthetic auxins.
(d) IAA, NAA, IBA, 2, 4-D and 2, 4, 5-T are synthetic auxins.

18. Which one among the following chemicals is used for causing defoliation of forest trees?
(a) Phosphon-D
(b) Malic hydrazide
(c) 2, 4-dichlorophenoxy acetic acid
(d) Amo-1618

19. Which of the following hormone prevents ripening of fruit?
(a) Gibberellin (b) Ethylene
(c) Cytokinin (d) ABA

20. Gibberellin was first extracted from
(a) *Gibberella fujikuroi* (b) *Gelidium*
(c) *Gracelaria* (d) *Aspergillus*

21. A plant completing its life cycle before the onset of dry condition is said to be
(a) short day plant (b) long day plant
(c) drought escaping (d) All of these

22. Phytohormones are
(a) chemicals regulating flowering.
(b) chemicals regulating secondary growth.
(c) hormones regulating growth from seed to adulthood.
(d) regulators synthesized by plants and influencing physiological processes.

RESPONSE GRID					
	9. ⓐⓑⓒⓓ	10. ⓐⓑⓒⓓ	11. ⓐⓑⓒⓓ	12. ⓐⓑⓒⓓ	13. ⓐⓑⓒⓓ
	14. ⓐⓑⓒⓓ	15. ⓐⓑⓒⓓ	16. ⓐⓑⓒⓓ	17. ⓐⓑⓒⓓ	18. ⓐⓑⓒⓓ
	19. ⓐⓑⓒⓓ	20. ⓐⓑⓒⓓ	21. ⓐⓑⓒⓓ	22. ⓐⓑⓒⓓ	

Space for Rough Work

23. Which one of the following is a natural growth inhibitor?
(a) NAA (b) ABA
(c) IAA (d) GA

24. Select the incorrect statement among the following.
(a) Increase in growth per unit time is growth rate.
(b) A sigmoid growth curve is a characteristic of most living organisms in their natural environment.
(c) Rate of growth is constant during geometrical growth.
(d) Exponential phase is also called as log phase.

25. Cabbage is a biennial plant which produces flowers in second year of growth. In an attempt to make it flower in a single year, four potted plants (I, II, III and IV) of cabbage were subjected to different temperatures for several days as given in the table.

Potted plant	Temperature
I	5°C
II	20°C
III	30°C
IV	25°C

Which potted plant will show flowering?
(a) I (b) II
(c) III (d) IV

26. Etiolated seedlings are produced by germinating seeds and keeping them in total darkness. Under which of the following conditions will plants kept in the dark-begin to synthesize chlorophyll ?
(a) After being given a pulse of blue light
(b) After being given a pulse of red light
(c) After being given a pulse of red light followed by a pulse of far-red light
(d) After being given a pulse of far-red light followed by a pulse of red light

27. Which of the following may function to break dormancy in seeds ?
(a) Penetration of the seed coat
(b) Leaching of inhibitory compounds by water
(c) Exposure to fire
(d) All of the above

28. You have installed an outdoor gas burning grill on your back ratio next to your favorite camellia bush. After the first few chilly nights of using your grill you notice that your camellia, which does not normally lose its leaves, is beginning to do so. Which of the following is the best explanation for what is happening ?
(a) The bush is getting too warm next to your grill.
(b) Ethylene is a by-product of the gas you are burning and is causing senescence in your plant.
(c) Abscisic acid is a by-product of the gas you are burning and is causing senescence in your plant.
(d) The plant is a biennial and is bolting.

29. Cytokinins are known to :
(a) Inhibit cytoplasmic movement
(b) Help in retention of chlorophyll
(c) Influence water movement
(d) Promote abscission layer formation.

30. Which of the following schemes best represents how environmental cues are transduced to changes in a plant ?
(a) Receptors receive environmental cues, a signal transduction pathway is initiated, there is an alteration in the particular genes that are transcribed and translated and a cellular response is generated.
(b) Receptors are triggered, hormones are released, signal transduction pathways are initiated, there is an alteration in expression of genes and a cellular response is generated.
(c) Neither a nor b
(d) Both a and b

31. When a plant is not reproducing most of the cytokinins are produced in its :
(a) Lateral buds (b) Shoot apex
(c) Roots (d) Leaves

RESPONSE GRID					
	23. ⓐⓑⓒⓓ	24. ⓐⓑⓒⓓ	25. ⓐⓑⓒⓓ	26. ⓐⓑⓒⓓ	27. ⓐⓑⓒⓓ
	28. ⓐⓑⓒⓓ	29. ⓐⓑⓒⓓ	30. ⓐⓑⓒⓓ	31. ⓐⓑⓒⓓ	

Space for Rough Work

32. Which of the following light receptors is responsible for absorbing blue and ultraviolet light ?
(a) Phytochrome P_r (b) Photochrome P_{fr}
(c) Cryptochrome (c) Phototropin
33. Phototropic and geotropic movements in plants have been traced to be linked with:
(a) Enzymes (b) Starch
(c) Gibberellins (d) Auxins
34. The natural plant hormones were first isolated from :
(a) Corn germoil and human urine
(b) Cotton fruits, spinach leaves and rice plants
(c) Human urine and rice seedlings
(d) Spinach leaves and fungus Gibberella
35. Auxin regulates cell growth by which of the following mechanisms ?
(a) Altering the elasticity of cell walls
(b) Altering the plasticity of cell walls
(c) Synthesizing new cell walls
(d) Breaking down cell walls in growing cells
36. Which of the following were not observed in studies done on certain dwarf strains of plants ?
(a) Applications of extracts of normal strains promoted growth of dwarf strains.
(b) Dwarf strains grew normally if additional fertilizer was applied
(c) Application of gibberellin A1 promoted growth of dwarf strains
(d) Gibberellin caused little additional growth of normal strains.
37. The closure of lid of pitcher in pitcher plant is :
(a) A paratonic movement
(b) A tropic movement
(c) A turgor movement
(d) An autonomous movement
38. Which of the following instrument can be used to record plant growth by seconds?
(a) Arc auxanometer (b) Arc indicator
(c) Space marker disc (d) Crescograph
39. *Avena* coleoptile test to find out the quantity of growth promoting hormones was discovered by –
(a) F.W. Went (b) L.J. Oudus
(c) K.V. Thimann (d) F. Skoog
40. "Foolish seedling" disease of rice led to the discovery of
(a) ABA (b) 2,4-D
(c) IAA (d) GA
41. Which of the growth substance act as a stimulant during nodule formation in Leguminous plant ?
(a) Ethylene (b) ABA
(c) IAA (d) Morphactin
42. Indole-3 acetic acid called as auxin was first isolated from
(a) Human urine (b) Corn germ oil
(c) *Fusarium* (d) *Rhizopus*
43. Prunning of plants promotes branching, because the axillary buds get sensitized to –
(a) Ethylene (b) Gibberellin
(c) Cytokinin (d) IAA
44. Pineapple can be made to flower in off season by :
(a) Ethylene
(b) Zeatin
(c) Napthalene Acetic Acid (NAA)
(d) Temperature
45. Choose the wrongly matched pair from the following
(a) Auxins – "to grow"
(b) Gibberellins – "*Gibberella fujikuroi*"
(c) Cytokinins – Herring sperm DNA
(d) Abscisic acid – Flowering hormone

RESPONSE GRID					
	32. ⓐⓑⓒⓓ	33. ⓐⓑⓒⓓ	34. ⓐⓑⓒⓓ	35. ⓐⓑⓒⓓ	36. ⓐⓑⓒⓓ
	37. ⓐⓑⓒⓓ	38. ⓐⓑⓒⓓ	39. ⓐⓑⓒⓓ	40. ⓐⓑⓒⓓ	41. ⓐⓑⓒⓓ
	42. ⓐⓑⓒⓓ	43. ⓐⓑⓒⓓ	44. ⓐⓑⓒⓓ	45. ⓐⓑⓒⓓ	

BIOLOGY CHAPTERWISE SPEED TEST-73			
Total Questions	45	Total Marks	180
Attempted		Correct	
Incorrect		Net Score	
Cut-off Score	45	Qualifying Score	60
Success Gap = Net Score – Qualifying Score			
Net Score = (Correct × 4) – (Incorrect × 1)			

Space for Rough Work

BIOLOGY

Digestion and Absorption

Speed TEST 74

Chapter-wise

No. of Questions	Maximum Marks	Time
45	180	1 Hour

GENERAL INSTRUCTIONS

- This test contains 45 MCQ's. For each question only one option is correct. Darken the correct circle/ bubble in the Response Grid provided on each page.
- You have to evaluate your Response Grids yourself with the help of solutions provided at the end of this book.
- Each correct answer will get you 4 marks and 1 mark shall be deduced for each incorrect answer. No mark will be given/ deducted if no bubble is filled. Keep a timer in front of you and stop immediately at the end of 60 min.
- The sheet follows a particular syllabus. Do not attempt the sheet before you have completed your preparation for that syllabus.
- After completing the sheet check your answers with the solution booklet and complete the Result Grid. Finally spend time to analyse your performance and revise the areas which emerge out as weak in your evaluation.

1. Dark purplish gland lying on the left side of abdomen is called :
   (a) liver (b) spleen
   (c) gall bladder (d) appendix
2. Which of the following are water soluble vitamins?
   (a) B, C (b) A, D, K
   (c) A, D, E, K (d) K, B, A, E
3. Jaundice is a disorder of
   (a) Excretory system (b) Skin and eyes
   (c) Digestive system (d) Circulatory system
4. Which one of the following pairs of food components in humans reaches the stomach totally undigested ?
   (a) Starch and cellulose (b) Protein and starch
   (c) Starch and fat (d) Fat and cellulose
5. Which of following teeth are lophodont?
   (a) Incisor and canine (b) Premolar and molar
   (c) Canine and premolar (d) Premolar and incisor
6. Oxyntic cells are located in
   (a) Islets of Langerhans
   (b) Gastric epithelium and secrete pepsin
   (c) Kidneys and secrete renin
   (d) Gastric epithelium and secrete HCl
7. Continued consumption of a diet rich in butter, red meat and eggs for a long period may lead to
   (a) vitamin A toxicity
   (b) kidney stones
   (c) hypercholesterolemia
   (d) urine laden with ketone bodies
8. Which one of the following is a matching pair of a substrate and its particular digestive enzyme?
   (a) Starch — maltase (b) Lactose — rennin
   (c) Maltose — steapsin (d) Casein — chymotrypsin

RESPONSE GRID					
	1. ⓐⓑⓒⓓ	2. ⓐⓑⓒⓓ	3. ⓐⓑⓒⓓ	4. ⓐⓑⓒⓓ	5. ⓐⓑⓒⓓ
	6. ⓐⓑⓒⓓ	7. ⓐⓑⓒⓓ	8. ⓐⓑⓒⓓ		

Space for Rough Work

9. Which one of the following is a matching pair of a vitamin and the deficiency disease related with it ?
(a) Riboflavin — beri beri
(b) Thiamine — xerophthalmia
(c) Niacin — pellagra
(d) Calciferol — scurvy

10. Which one of the following pairs of the cells with their secretion is **correctly** matched?
(a) Oxyntic cells - A secretion with pH between 2.0 and 3.0.
(b) Alpha cells of Islets of Langerhans -Secretion that decreases blood sugar level.
(c) Kupffer cells - A digestive enzyme that hydrolysis nucleic acids.
(d) Sebaceous glands - A digestive enzyme that hydrolysis nucleic acids

11. "Kwashiorkar' and 'Beri-Beri' are
(a) communicable diseases
(b) infectious diseases
(c) deficiency diseases
(d) None of the above

12. First milk produced after child birth is called
(a) sebum (b) cerumen
(c) true milk (d) colostrum

13. Cirrhosis of liver is caused by the chronic intake of
(a) Opium
(b) Alcohol
(c) Tobacco (Chewing)
(d) Cocaine

14. The sphincter of Oddi is present between
(a) Oesophagus and cardiac stomach
(b) Pyloric stomach and duodenum
(c) Hepatic duct and cystic duct
(d) Hepatopancreatic duct and duodenum

15. The structure which prevents the entry of food into the windpipe is
(a) Gullet (b) Glottis
(c) Tonsil (d) Epiglottis

16. Layer of cells that secrete enamel of tooth is
(a) Osteoblast (b) Ameloblast
(c) Odontoblast (d) Dentoblast

17. Cow's milk is slightly yellowish in colour due to the presence of
(a) Carotene
(b) Riboflavin
(c) Xanthophyll
(d) Xanthophyll and Carotene

18. Accessory excretory organs of man are
(a) only skin
(b) only skin and liver
(c) only skin and lungs
(d) skin, lungs, liver and intestine

19. Cholecystokinin is secretion of
(a) Duodenum that causes contraction of gall bladder
(b) Globlet cells of ileum, stimulates secretion of succus entericus
(c) Liver and controls secondary sex characters
(d) Stomach that stimulates pancreas to release juice

20. Which of the following sets represents vestigial organs?
(a) Vermiform appendix, body hair and patella
(b) Wisdom teeth, body hair and atlas vertebra
(c) Ear muscles, cochlea and coccyx
(d) Vermiform appendix, ear muscles and coccyx.

21. Which part of the alimentary canal does not secrete any enzyme?
(a) Mouth (b) Oesophagus
(c) Stomach (d) Duodenum

22. The protein coated, water soluble fat globules are called
(a) Chylomicrons (b) Micelles
(c) Chyle (d) Monoglycerides

23. Where do certain symbiotic micro-organisms normally occur in human body?
(a) Caecum
(b) Oral lining and tongue surface
(c) Vermiform appendix and rectum
(d) Duodenum

RESPONSE GRID					
	9. ⓐⓑⓒⓓ	10. ⓐⓑⓒⓓ	11. ⓐⓑⓒⓓ	12. ⓐⓑⓒⓓ	13. ⓐⓑⓒⓓ
	14. ⓐⓑⓒⓓ	15. ⓐⓑⓒⓓ	16. ⓐⓑⓒⓓ	17. ⓐⓑⓒⓓ	18. ⓐⓑⓒⓓ
	19. ⓐⓑⓒⓓ	20. ⓐⓑⓒⓓ	21. ⓐⓑⓒⓓ	22. ⓐⓑⓒⓓ	23. ⓐⓑⓒⓓ

Space for Rough Work

24. Both the crown and root of a tooth is covered by a layer of bony hard substance. It is called
(a) enamel (b) dentine
(c) bony socket (d) cementum

25. Which one of the following pairs of the kind of cells and their secretion is correctly matched?
(a) Oxyntic cells—a secretion with pH between 2.0 and 3.0
(b) Alpha cells of islets of Langerhans—secretion that decreases blood sugar level
(c) Kupffer cell—a digestive enzyme that hydrolyses nucleic acids
(d) Sebaceous glands—a secretion that evaporates for cooling

26. Which one of the following is the correct matching of the site of action on the given substate, the enzyme acting upon it and the end product?
(a) Small intestine : Proteins $\xrightarrow{\text{Pepsin}}$ Amino acids
(b) Stomach : Fats $\xrightarrow{\text{Lipase}}$ Micelles
(c) Duodenum : Triglycerides $\xrightarrow{\text{Trypsin}}$ Monoglycerides
(d) Small intestine : Starch $\xrightarrow{\alpha\text{-Amylase}}$ Disaccharide (maltose)

27. Read the following four statements (i) - (iv) with certain mistakes in two of them.
(i) Fructose is generally absorbed by simple diffusion.
(ii) The digestive wastes, solidified into coherent faeces in the rectum initiate and endocrinal action causing an urge or desire for its removal
(iii) The food mixes thoroughly with the acidic gastric juice of the stomach by the churning movements of its muscular wall and is called the chyme.
(iv) The secretions of the brush border cells of the mucosa alongwith the secretions of the goblet cells constitute the succus entericus.

28. Which of the following dietary deficiencies will affect the functioning of enzymes in the human body most quickly?
(a) Too few carbohydrates
(b) Shortage of fat-soluble vitamins
(c) Shortage of water-soluble vitamins
(d) Insufficient variety of fats

29. Pancreatic cancer is an especially dangerous disease in people because the pancreas is
(a) the organ that produces and stores bile.
(b) the site of synthesis for all of the essential amino acids.
(c) one of the organs through which food must pass on its way to the colon.
(d) an organ in which many different kinds of digestive enzymes are manufacture

30. How does a gastrovascular cavity differ from an alimentary canal? The gastrovascular cavity
(a) stores food but does not digest it.
(b) is usually much larger.
(c) has only one opening.
(d) functions in digestion but not absorption.

31. The largest variety of digestive enzymes function in the
(a) large intestine. (b) oral cavity.
(c) stomach. (d) small intestine.

32. Certain amino acids are essential to the diet of animals because
(a) they prevent overnourishment
(b) they are cofactors and coenzymes that are required for normal physiological function.
(c) an animal cannot directly synthesize them through the transfer of an amino group to an appropriate carbon skeleton.
(d) animals need these substances in order to make the stored fats that are used during hibernation and migration

RESPONSE GRID					
	24. ⓐⓑⓒⓓ	25. ⓐⓑⓒⓓ	26. ⓐⓑⓒⓓ	27. ⓐⓑⓒⓓ	28. ⓐⓑⓒⓓ
	29. ⓐⓑⓒⓓ	30. ⓐⓑⓒⓓ	31. ⓐⓑⓒⓓ	32. ⓐⓑⓒⓓ	

Space for Rough Work

33. Protection of the walls of the stomach against the action of its own digestive juices
(a) results from the presence of an anti-enzyme chemical formed by the gastric glands
(b) results from the nervous reactions of the lining of the stomach.
(c) is controlled by a centre in the medulla of the brain.
(d) results from the neutralizing, buffering, and a coating mucus covering its inner surface

34. Most of the chemical digestion of food in humans is completed in the
(a) small intestine. (b) appendix.
(c) ascending colon (d) stomach

35. Which of the following is characteristic of the large intestine?
(a) It has almost no bacterial populations.
(b) It contains chyme.
(c) It absorbs much of the water remaining in waste materials.
(d) It is the site of most of digestion.

36. The innermost layer of the digestive tract is the
(a) serosa membrane.
(b) mucosa membrane.
(c) submucosa membrane.
(d) lumen.

37. The ______ is primarily a storage chamber within the digestive system, while the ______ reabsorbs water, ions, and generates the faeces.
(a) buccal cavity; midgut
(b) crop; midgut
(c) stomach; hindgut
(d) buccal cavity; hindgut

38. What does an increase in the secretion of insulin produce?
(a) a decrease in glucose metabolism
(b) a decrease in glucose permeability of cells
(c) an increase in blood sugar level
(d) an increase in glucose permeability of cells

39. Which function of the liver results in the production of bile pigments?
(a) breakdown of haemoglobin
(b) deamination of amino acids
(c) detoxification of metabolic poisons
(d) release of stored vitamin A

40. The centre of hunger or centre which regulates the amount of food we eat or out appetite is located in –
(a) Medulla (b) Cerebrum
(c) Hypothalamus (d) Alimentary canal

41. Fatty acid and glycerol are first taken up from alimentary canal by
(a) Villi (b) Blood capillaries
(c) Hepatic portal vein (d) Lymph vessels

42. Mammals may drink water and also get it from
(a) Breakdown of glycogen into glucose
(b) Secretion of saliva
(c) Oxidation of glucose
(d) Conversion of oxyhaemoglobin into haemoglobin

43. When a piece of bread in chewed it tastes sweet because
(a) The sugar contents are drawn out
(b) Saliva converts starch into maltose
(c) It does not taste sweet
(d) The taste buds are stimulated by chewing

44. Anxiety and eating spicy food together in an otherwise normal human, may lead to
(a) Indigestion (b) Jaundice
(c) Diarrhoea (d) Vomiting

45. A young infant may be feeding entirely on mothers milk which is white in colour but the stools which the infant passes out is quite yellowish. What is this yellow colour due to ?
(a) bile pigments passed through bile juice
(b) undigested milk protein casein
(c) pancreatic juice poured into duodenum
(d) intestinal juice

RESPONSE GRID					
	33. ⓐⓑⓒⓓ	34. ⓐⓑⓒⓓ	35. ⓐⓑⓒⓓ	36. ⓐⓑⓒⓓ	37. ⓐⓑⓒⓓ
	38. ⓐⓑⓒⓓ	39. ⓐⓑⓒⓓ	40. ⓐⓑⓒⓓ	41. ⓐⓑⓒⓓ	42. ⓐⓑⓒⓓ
	43. ⓐⓑⓒⓓ	44. ⓐⓑⓒⓓ	45. ⓐⓑⓒⓓ		

BIOLOGY CHAPTERWISE SPEED TEST-74			
Total Questions	45	Total Marks	180
Attempted		Correct	
Incorrect		Net Score	
Cut-off Score	45	Qualifying Score	60
Success Gap = Net Score – Qualifying Score			
Net Score = (Correct × 4) – (Incorrect × 1)			

Space for Rough Work

BIOLOGY

Breathing and Exchange of Gases

Speed TEST 75

Chapter-wise

No. of Questions	Maximum Marks	Time
45	180	1 Hour

GENERAL INSTRUCTIONS

- This test contains 45 MCQ's. For each question only one option is correct. Darken the correct circle/ bubble in the Response Grid provided on each page.
- You have to evaluate your Response Grids yourself with the help of solutions provided at the end of this book.
- Each correct answer will get you 4 marks and 1 mark shall be deduced for each incorrect answer. No mark will be given/ deducted if no bubble is filled. Keep a timer in front of you and stop immediately at the end of 60 min.
- The sheet follows a particular syllabus. Do not attempt the sheet before you have completed your preparation for that syllabus.
- After completing the sheet check your answers with the solution booklet and complete the Result Grid. Finally spend time to analyse your performance and revise the areas which emerge out as weak in your evaluation.

1. Bulk of carbon dioxide (CO_2) released from body tissues into the blood is present as
   (a) bicarbonate in blood plasma and RBCs
   (b) free CO_2 in blood plasma
   (c) 70% carbamino- haemoglobin and 30% as bicarbonate
   (d) carbamino-haemoglobin in RBCs
2. A large proportion of oxygen is left unused in the human blood even after its uptake by the body tissues. This O_2
   (a) acts as a reserve during muscular exercise
   (b) raise the pCO_2 of blood to 75 mm of Hg.
   (c) is enough to keep oxyhaemoglobin saturation at 96%
   (d) helps in releasing more O_2 to the epithelial tissues.
3. Oxygen dissociation curve of haemoglobin is
   (a) Sigmoid (b) Hyperbolic
   (c) Linear (d) Hypobolic
4. Which one of the following organs in the human body is most affected due to shortage of oxygen?
   (a) Intestine (b) Skin (c) Kidney (d) Brain
5. When CO_2 concentration in blood increases, breathing becomes
   (a) shallower and slow
   (b) there is no effect on breathing
   (c) slow and deep
   (d) faster and deeper
6. Although much CO_2 is carried in blood, yet blood does not become acidic, because
   (a) it is absorbed by the leucocytes
   (b) blood buffers play an important role in CO_2 transport.
   (c) it combines with water to form carbonic acid (H_2CO_3) which is neutralized by Na_2CO_3.
   (d) it is continuously diffused through tissues and is not allowed to accumulate.
7. Which one of the following is the correct statement for respiration in humans?
   (a) Workers in grinding and stone-breaking industries may suffer from lung fibrosis.
   (b) About 90% of carbon dioxide (CO_2) is carried by haemoglobin as carbaminohaemoglobin.
   (c) Cigarette smoking may lead to inflammation of bronchi.
   (d) Neural signals from pneumotoxic centre in pons region of brain can increase the duration of inspiration.
8. The largest quantity of air that can be expired after a maximal inspiratory effort is called
   (a) residual volume (b) tidal volume
   (c) vital capacity (d) total lung volume

RESPONSE GRID					
	1. ⓐⓑⓒⓓ	2. ⓐⓑⓒⓓ	3. ⓐⓑⓒⓓ	4. ⓐⓑⓒⓓ	5. ⓐⓑⓒⓓ
	6. ⓐⓑⓒⓓ	7. ⓐⓑⓒⓓ	8. ⓐⓑⓒⓓ		

Space for Rough Work

9. Which one of the following statements is incorrect ?
(a) The presence of non-respiratory air sacs, increases the efficiency of respiration in birds.
(b) In insects, circulating body fluids serve to distribute oxygen to tissues.
(c) The principle of countercurrent flow facilitates efficient respiration in gills of fishes.
(d) The residual air in lungs slightly decreases the efficiency of respriration in mammals.

10. During oxygen transport the oxyhaemoglobin at the tissue level liberates oxygen to the cells because in tissue
(a) O_2 concentration is high and CO_2 is low
(b) O_2 concentration is low and CO_2 is high
(c) O_2 tension is high and CO_2 tension is low
(d) O_2 tension is low and CO_2 tension is high

11. Emphysema developes mainly because of
(a) Allergy or hypersensitisation
(b) Spasm of the smooth muscles of bronchioles
(c) Cigarette smoking
(d) Inflammation of the alveoli

12. During inspiration the diaphragm
(a) relaxes to become dome-shaped
(b) contracts and flattens
(c) expands
(d) shows no change

13. The volume of air breathed in and out during normal breathing is called
(a) Vital capacity
(b) Inspiratory reserve volume
(c) Explratory reserve volume
(d) Tidal volume

14. What would happen if human blood becomes acidic (low pH)
(a) Oxygen carying capacity of haemoglobin increases
(b) Oxygen carrying capacity of haemoglobin decreases
(c) RBCs count increases
(d) RBCs count decreases

15. The respiratory centre, which regulates respiration, is located in
(a) Cerebral peduncle (b) Vagus nerve
(c) Pons (d) Medulla oblongata

16. Even when there is no air in it, human trachea does not collapse due to presence of
(a) Bony rings (b) Turgid pressure
(c) Chitinous rings (d) Cartilaginous rings

17. The structure which does not contribute to the breathing movements in mammals is
(a) Larynx (b) Ribs
(c) Diaphragm (d) Intercostal muscles

18. In emphysema –
(a) Gas exchange area of lungs is reduced
(b) Gas exchange area of lungs is increased
(c) Trachea gets narrowed
(d) Larynx is permanently closed

19. Which of the following changes occur in diaphragm and intercostal muscles when expiration of air takes place?
(a) External intercostal muscles relax and diaphargm contracts
(b) External intercostal muscles contract and diaphargm relaxes
(c) External intercostal muscles and diaphargm relax
(d) External intercostal muscles and diaphargm contract

20. The graph below shows how gaseous exchange in an amphibian varies with temperature.

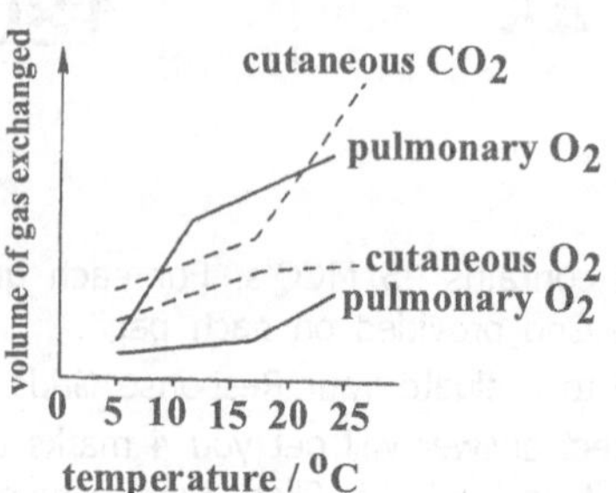

The graph shows that at all temperatures the lungs :
(a) absorb more oxygen than the skin
(b) absorb less oxygen than the skin
(c) release more carbon dioxide than the skin
(d) release less carbon dioxide than the skin

21. Which statement explains the significance of myoglobin in muscle tissue?
(a) Myoglobin can associate with oxygen in conditions of high carbon dioxide tension
(b) Myoglobin can dissociate from oxygen most readily under aerobic conditions
(c) Myoglobin acts as an oxygen store delaying the onset of anaerobic respiration
(d) Myoglobin acts as a buffer to hydrogen ions produced during anaerobic respiration

22. When you exhale, the diaphragm
(a) relaxes and arches.
(b) relaxes and flattens.
(c) contracts and arches.
(d) contracts and flattens.

23. Smoking destroys the cilia in the respiratory passageways. This
(a) makes it harder to move air in and out of the lungs.
(b) decreases the surface area for respiration.
(c) slows blood flow through lung blood vessels.
(d) makes it harder to keep the lungs clean.

RESPONSE GRID					
	9. ⓐⓑⓒⓓ	10. ⓐⓑⓒⓓ	11. ⓐⓑⓒⓓ	12. ⓐⓑⓒⓓ	13. ⓐⓑⓒⓓ
	14. ⓐⓑⓒⓓ	15. ⓐⓑⓒⓓ	16. ⓐⓑⓒⓓ	17. ⓐⓑⓒⓓ	18. ⓐⓑⓒⓓ
	19. ⓐⓑⓒⓓ	20. ⓐⓑⓒⓓ	21. ⓐⓑⓒⓓ	22. ⓐⓑⓒⓓ	23. ⓐⓑⓒⓓ

Space for Rough Work

24. The graph shows dissociation curves for four respiratory pigments.

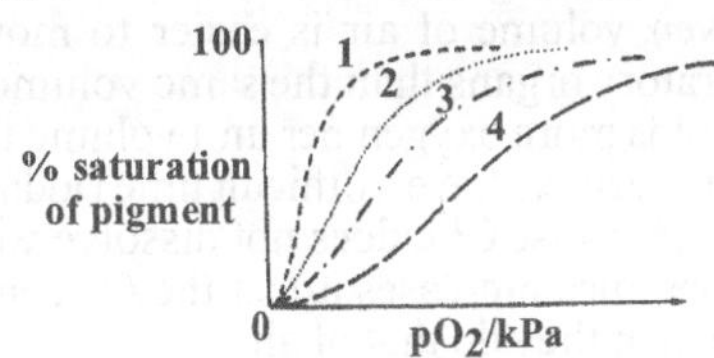

Which combination identifies the four curve?

adult haemoglobin with high CO_2	adult haemoglobin	myo-globin	foetal haemoglobin
(a) 1	2	3	4
(b) 2	1	4	3
(c) 3	2	1	4
(d) 3	4	2	1

25. Gas flows into the lungs of mammals during inspiration because
(a) The pressure in the lungs falls below atmospheric pressure.
(b) The volume of the lungs decreases.
(c) The pressure in the lungs rises above atmospheric pressure.
(d) The diaphragm moves upward toward the lungs.

26. The Bohr shift describes
(a) The outward movement of Cl^- from the blood cell in exchange for HCO_3^- moving into the cell.
(b) The leftward shift of the entire oxygen equilibrium curve when temperature rises.
(c) The rightward shift of the entire oxygen equilibrium curve when pH rises.
(d) The rightward shift of the entire oxygen equilibrium curve when pH falls.

27. The movement of O_2 and CO_2 between the blood in the tissue capillaries and the cells in tissues depends most directly upon
(a) active transport of O_2 and CO_2.
(b) total atmospheric (barometric) pressure differences across the cell membranes.
(c) diffusion of O_2 and CO_2 down a concentration gradient.
(d) diffusion of O_2 and CO_2 down a partial pressure gradient.

28. The function of the mucus elevator in the mammalian respiratory system is to
(a) move surfactant from the bronchi to the alveoli.
(b) produce negative pressure during inhalation.
(c) stimulate contraction of rib musculature during forcible exhalation.
(d) trap and remove particulate matter that has entered the respiratory system.

29. The oxygen-binding curve for myoglobin is steep and shifted to the left of the same curve for hemoglobin. This indicates that
(a) people with myoglobin are acclimated for life at high altitudes.
(b) myoglobin occurs in high concentration in the human foetus.
(c) myoglobin does not function well at high percent saturation of oxygen.
(d) myoglobin picks up and releases O_2 at lower Po_2 values than does haemoglobin.

30. The graph shows haemoglobin-oxygen dissociation curves at two different partial pressures of carbon dioxide

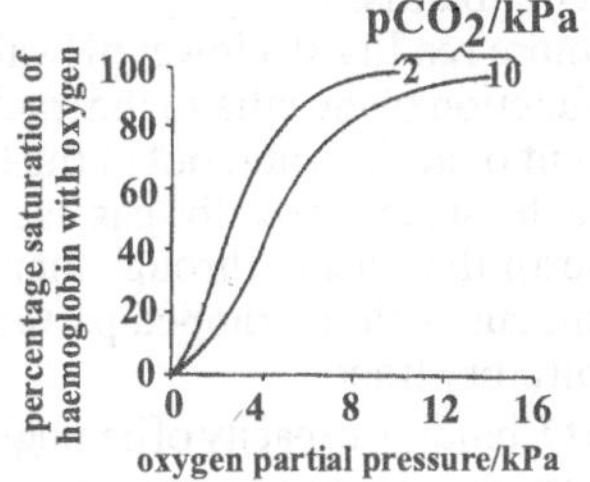

What is the advantage to the organism of the difference between the curve?
(a) CO_2 is readily released into the alveoli
(b) Haemoglobin removes more CO_2 from active tissues
(c) Haemoglobin can release oxygen to myoglobin
(d) Oxygen is readily released into active tissues

31. A person can hold his breath longer if he gradually exhales than if he keeps his lungs fully expanded. This phenomenon is due to the fact that :
(a) concentration of CO_2 in the blood decreases, lessening the excitatory input to the carotid bodies
(b) he is then using less O_2 as his thoracic muscles are not working as hard
(c) stretch receptors in his lungs are then not firing as much thus lessening the excitatory input to the expiratory centres
(d) he is preventing the pressure in his lungs from increasing too much

32. The alveoli contain specialized cells that secrete a phospholipoprotein complex known as pulmonary surfactant. The function of pulmonary surfactant is :
(a) to provide some rigidity to the alveoli to prevent lung collapse
(b) to decrease the surface tension of the alveoli, making it easier to expand them
(c) to facilitate the diffusion of O_2 and CO_2 by providing protein channels through which these gases flow
(d) to provide a sticky surface upon which dust and microbes are trapped and disposed of.

RESPONSE GRID					
	24. ⓐⓑⓒⓓ	25. ⓐⓑⓒⓓ	26. ⓐⓑⓒⓓ	27. ⓐⓑⓒⓓ	28. ⓐⓑⓒⓓ
	29. ⓐⓑⓒⓓ	30. ⓐⓑⓒⓓ	31. ⓐⓑⓒⓓ	32. ⓐⓑⓒⓓ	

Space for Rough Work

33. During inspiration, the air is brought into the lungs by the working of the thoracoabdominal pump whereby the :
(a) diaphragm contracts to lengthen the thoracic cavity
(b) chest muscles pull the ribs up and out to widen the thoracic cavity
(c) abdominal muscles relax
(d) all of the above

34. The binding of an O_2 atom to the first iron atom of a haemoglobin molecule
(a) occurs at a very low partial pressure of oxygen
(b) produces a conformational change that lowers the other subunits' affinity for oxygen
(c) is an example of cooperativity as O_2 readily binds to the other subunits.
(d) occurs more readily at a lower pH value.

35. What is the function of the cilia in the trachea and bronchi?
(a) movement of air into and out of the lungs
(b) increase the surface area for gas exchange
(c) filter the air that rushes through them
(d) sweep mucus with its trapped particles up and out of the respiratory tract

36. A shift in the O_2 binding capacity of hemoglobin as a function of pH is known as
(a) oxygen binding
(b) the Hering-Breuer reflex
(c) the Bohr effect.
(d) respiratory ventilation

37. The most important function of diaphragm is
(a) To divide body cavity into compartments
(b) To protect lungs
(c) To aid in digestion
(d) To aid in ventilation

38. Which is not a structure of the respiratory system ?
(a) the pharynx (b) the bronchus
(c) the larynx (d) the hyoid

39. The alveoli of the lungs do not contain "air" because
(a) we normally do not ventilate our lungs at a high enough rate.
(b) the lungs have too many alveoli to ventilate.
(c) there is "dead space" in the trachea and bronchi.
(d) the trachea and bronchi are too small in volume.

40. Which of the following is not a reason that breathing air is easier than breathing water?
(a) A given volume of air is easier to move across the respiratory organs than the same volume of water.
(b) Air holds more oxygen per unit volume than water.
(c) Water breathers have a difficult time ridding themselves of CO_2 because CO_2 does not dissolve well in water.
(d) Temperature increases affect the O_2 content of water more than they do that of air.

41. Which of the following represents a larger volume of air than is normally found in the resting tidal volume of a human lung ?
(a) Residual volume
(b) Inspiratory reserve volume
(c) Expiratory reserve volume
(d) All of the above

42. The graph shows four dissociation curves.

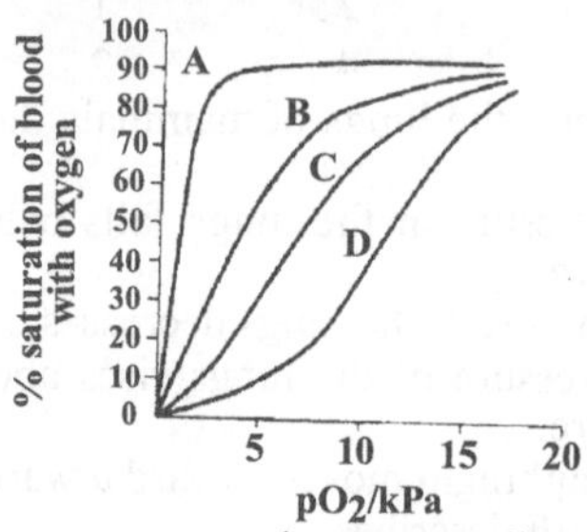

Which curve represents the oxygen dissociation curve for myoglobin?
(a) At A (b) At B (c) At C (d) At D

43. Functional residual capacity can be represented as
(a) TV+ERV (b) ERV+RV
(c) RV+IRV (d) ERV+TV+IRV

44. The process of migration of chloride ions from plasma to RBC and carbonate ions from RBC to plasma is
(a) chloride shift (b) ionic shift
(c) atomic shift (d) Na^+ pump

45. The quantity 1500 ml in the respiratory volumes of a normal human adult refers to
(a) maximum air that can be breathed in and breathed out
(b) residual volume
(c) expiratory reserve volume
(d) total lung capacity

RESPONSE GRID					
	33. ⓐⓑⓒⓓ	34. ⓐⓑⓒⓓ	35. ⓐⓑⓒⓓ	36. ⓐⓑⓒⓓ	37. ⓐⓑⓒⓓ
	38. ⓐⓑⓒⓓ	39. ⓐⓑⓒⓓ	40. ⓐⓑⓒⓓ	41. ⓐⓑⓒⓓ	42. ⓐⓑⓒⓓ
	43. ⓐⓑⓒⓓ	44. ⓐⓑⓒⓓ	45. ⓐⓑⓒⓓ		

BIOLOGY CHAPTERWISE SPEED TEST-75

Total Questions	45	Total Marks	180
Attempted		Correct	
Incorrect		Net Score	
Cut-off Score	50	Qualifying Score	65
Success Gap = Net Score – Qualifying Score			
Net Score = (Correct × 4) – (Incorrect × 1)			

Space for Rough Work

BIOLOGY

Body Fluids and Circulation

Speed TEST 76

Chapter-wise

No. of Questions	Maximum Marks	Time
45	180	1 Hour

GENERAL INSTRUCTIONS

- This test contains 45 MCQ's. For each question only one option is correct. Darken the correct circle/ bubble in the Response Grid provided on each page.
- You have to evaluate your Response Grids yourself with the help of solutions provided at the end of this book.
- Each correct answer will get you 4 marks and 1 mark shall be deduced for each incorrect answer. No mark will be given/ deducted if no bubble is filled. Keep a timer in front of you and stop immediately at the end of 60 min.
- The sheet follows a particular syllabus. Do not attempt the sheet before you have completed your preparation for that syllabus.
- After completing the sheet check your answers with the solution booklet and complete the Result Grid. Finally spend time to analyse your performance and revise the areas which emerge out as weak in your evaluation.

1. Blood pressure is measured by
   (a) sphygmomanometer (b) stethoscope
   (c) electrocardiogram (d) phonocardiogram
2. Coronary artery disease (CAD) is often referred to as
   (a) Heart failure (b) Cardiac arrest
   (c) Atherosclerosis (d) Thrombosis
3. Which one of the following is a **correct** matching pair?
   (a) Lubb - Sharp closure of AV valves at the beginning of ventricular systole.
   (b) Dup - Sudden opening of semilunar valves at the beginning of ventricular diastole.
   (c) Pulsation of the radial artery valves in the blood vessels.
   (d) Purkinje fibers - Initiation of the heart beat.
4. Child death may occur in the marriage between
   (a) Rh^+ man and Rh^+ woman
   (b) Rh^+ man and Rh^- woman
   (c) Rh^- man and Rh^- woman
   (d) Rh^- man and Rh^+ woman
5. Heart is covered by
   (a) Peritoneum (b) Pleural membrane
   (c) Pericardium (d) Visceral membrane
6. Which one of the components of ECG in human is correctly interpreted below ?
   (a) Complex QRS-One complete Pulse
   (b) Peak T - Initiation of total cardiac contraction
   (c) Peak P and Peak R together-Systolic and diastolic blood pressures
   (d) Peak P- Initiation of left atrial contraction only
7. Pacemaker of heart is
   (a) AV node (b) Bundle of His
   (c) SA node (d) Purkinje fibres
8. Uricotelism is found in
   (a) Frogs and toads
   (b) Mammals and birds
   (c) Birds, reptiles and insects
   (d) Fishes and fresh water protozoans

RESPONSE GRID					
	1. ⓐⓑⓒⓓ	2. ⓐⓑⓒⓓ	3. ⓐⓑⓒⓓ	4. ⓐⓑⓒⓓ	5. ⓐⓑⓒⓓ
	6. ⓐⓑⓒⓓ	7. ⓐⓑⓒⓓ	8. ⓐⓑⓒⓓ		

Space for Rough Work

9. Haemoglobin is having maximum affinity with:
(a) NH_3 (b) O_2
(c) CO_2 (d) CO

10. An adult human with average health has systolic and diastolic pressures as
(a) 80mm Hg and 80 mm Hg
(b) 70 mm Hg and 120 mm Hg
(c) 120 mm Hg and 80 mm Hg
(d) 50 mm Hg and 80 mm Hg

11. Blood group AB has
(a) no antigen
(b) no antibody
(c) neither antigen nor antibody
(d) both antigen and antibody

12. With reference to the blood in a normal person, which one of the following statements is correct?
(a) Compared to arteries, veins are less numerous and hold less of the body's blood at any given time.
(b) Blood cells constitute about 70 percent of the total volume of the blood.
(c) White blood cells (WBC) are made by lymph nodes only.
(d) The blood has more platelets than WBC.

13. Thickening of arteries due to cholesterol deposition is
(a) arteriosclerosis (b) rheumatic heart
(c) blood pressure (d) cardiac arrest

14. Hepatic portal system carries
(a) Oxygenated blood from liver to intestine
(b) Deoxygenated blood from liver to intestine
(c) Oxygenated blood from intestine to liver
(d) Deoxygenated blood from intestine to liver

15. 'Bundle of His' is a part of which one of the following organs in humans?
(a) Brain (b) Heart
(c) Kidney (d) Pancreas

16. Chordae tendinae are found in
(a) joints of legs (b) atria of heart
(c) ventricles of brain (d) ventricles of heart

17. The pattern of contraction and relaxation of the heart is referred to as
(a) blood pressure (b) arterial flow
(c) blood flow (d) cardiac cycle

18. Which of the following statements are true ?
(i) The blood transports CO_2 comparatively easily because of its higher solubility.
(ii) Approximately 8-9% of CO_2 is transported being dissolved in the plasma of blood.
(iii) The carbon dioxide produced by the tissues, diffuses passively into the blood stream and passes into red blood corpuscles and react with water to form H_2CO_3.
(iv) The oxyhaemoglobin (HbO_2) of the erythrocytes is basic.
(v) The chloride ions diffuse from plasma into the erythrocytes to maintain ionic balance.
(a) (i), (iii) and (v) are true, (ii) and (iv) are false
(b) (i), (iii) and (v) are false, (ii) and (iv) are true
(c) (i), (ii) and (iv) are true, (iii) and (v) are false
(d) (i), (ii) and (iv) are false, (iii) and (v) are true

19. About 70% of CO_2 is transported as
(a) Carbonic acid (b) Carboxyhaemoglobin
(c) Bicarbonates (d) Carbamino compounds

20. In human heart, which of the following valve remains in contact of the oxygenated blood only?
(a) Tricuspid valve (b) Semi lunar valve
(c) Eustachian valve (d) Mitral valve

21. Myocardial Infarction is caused by
(a) hardening of arteries
(b) lumpy thickness develop in the inner walls of arteries
(c) clot may occur in the lumen of a coronary artery
(d) sudden interruption in blood flow towards a portion of heart

22. The affinity of CO with Hb is more than oxygen by
(a) 2 times (b) 20 times
(c) 200 times (d) 2000 times

23. Life span of human RBCs is
(a) 120 days (b) 20 days
(c) 9 days (d) 90 days

RESPONSE GRID					
	9. ⓐⓑⓒⓓ	10. ⓐⓑⓒⓓ	11. ⓐⓑⓒⓓ	12. ⓐⓑⓒⓓ	13. ⓐⓑⓒⓓ
	14. ⓐⓑⓒⓓ	15. ⓐⓑⓒⓓ	16. ⓐⓑⓒⓓ	17. ⓐⓑⓒⓓ	18. ⓐⓑⓒⓓ
	19. ⓐⓑⓒⓓ	20. ⓐⓑⓒⓓ	21. ⓐⓑⓒⓓ	22. ⓐⓑⓒⓓ	23. ⓐⓑⓒⓓ

Space for Rough Work

24. Which one of the following is a incorrect matching pair?
 (a) Lubb-Sharp closure of AV valves at the beginning of atrial systole
 (b) Dub-Sudden opening of semilunar valves at the end of ventricular systole
 (c) Cardiac Output-Stroke volume and heart beat
 (d) Initiation of the heart beat -sino atrial node

25. Erythroblastosis foetalis occurs when
 (a) Mother is Rh negative and father is Rh positive
 (b) Father is Rh negative and mother is Rh positive
 (c) Both are Rh positive
 (d) Both are Rh negative

26. Which of the following set of animals has an incomplete double circulation system?
 (a) Frog and crocodile (b) Shark and whale
 (c) Lizard and pigeon (d) Toad and lizard

27. Find out the incorrect answer from the following?
 (a) Veins are typically larger in diameter than arteries
 (b) Because of their small size, capillaries contain blood that is moving more quickly than in other parts of the circulatory system
 (c) The walls of arteries are elastic, enabling them to stretch and shrink during changes in blood pressure
 (d) Veins contain more blood than any other part of the circulatory system

28. Given below are four statements (i-iv) regarding human blood circulatory system
 (i) Arteries are thick-walled and have narrow lumen as compared to veins
 (ii) Angina is acute chest pain when the blood circulation to the brain is reduced
 (iii) Persons with blood group AB can donate blood to any person with any blood group under ABO system
 (iv) Calcium ions play a very important role in blood clotting
 Which two of the above statements are correct?
 (a) (i) and (iv) (b) (i) and (iv)
 (c) (ii) and (iii) (d) (iii) and (iv)

29. Haldane effect plays more important role in promoting carbon dioxide transport than that of the Bohr's effect in promoting oxygen transport because
 (a) oxyhaemoglobin is a stronger acid which donates hydrogen ion (H^+) which in turn displace carbon dioxide from blood
 (b) carbaminohaemoglobin is a stronger acid which splits into hydrogen ion (H^+) and bicarbonate (HCO_3^-)
 (c) carbon dioxide reacts with water to form carbonic acid that lowers the pH in tissue
 (d) carbon dioxide is less soluble in venous blood than in arterial blood

30. Which of the following factors is known as Christmas factor?
 (a) Factor VIII (b) Factor XII
 (c) Factor IV (d) Factor IX

31. In veins, values are present to check backward flow to blood flowing at
 (a) high pressure (b) atmospheric pressure
 (c) low pressure (d) all of these

32. In a cardiac output of 5250 ml per minute, with 75 heartbeats per minute, the stroke volume is
 (a) 60 ml (b) 80 ml
 (c) 55 ml (d) 70 ml

33. Heart valves function to
 (a) keep blood moving forward through the heart.
 (b) mix blood thoroughly as it passes through the heart.
 (c) control the amount of blood pumped by the heart.
 (d) slow blood down as it passes through the heart.

34. The accompanying diagram shows a small part of a normal electrocardiogram. Which region represents a wave of excitation passing through the ventricles?

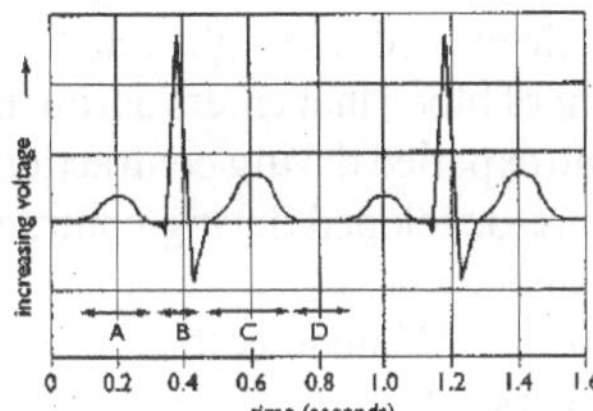

 (a) A (b) B
 (c) C (d) D

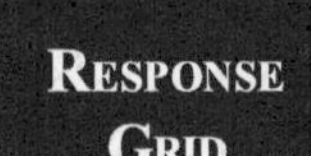

RESPONSE GRID

24. ⓐⓑⓒⓓ 25. ⓐⓑⓒⓓ 26. ⓐⓑⓒⓓ 27. ⓐⓑⓒⓓ 28. ⓐⓑⓒⓓ
29. ⓐⓑⓒⓓ 30. ⓐⓑⓒⓓ 31. ⓐⓑⓒⓓ 32. ⓐⓑⓒⓓ 33. ⓐⓑⓒⓓ
34. ⓐⓑⓒⓓ

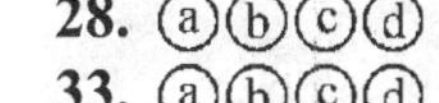

Space for Rough Work

35. Just after blood leaves the left ventricle of the human heart, it passes through the
(a) pulmonary artery (b) left atrium
(c) aorta (d) superior vena cava

36. In the human body, the highest blood pressure can be recorded in
(a) arteries near the heart
(b) veins returning to the heart
(c) capillaries of the body tissue
(d) the lungs

37. Blood flows rather rapidly as it leaves the human heart. Upon arriving at the capillaries, it slows dramatically. This reduction in speed is due largely to
(a) the loss of pressure as the blood gets farther away from the heart.
(b) changes in pressure that result from water evaporation on the skin.
(c) the resistance offered by the small diameter of the capillaries.
(d) differences in pressure caused by the sugar content of the blood.

38. The atrial walls are ___ than the ventricular wall, and pressure generated in the atrial chambers is ___ than in the ventricles.
(a) thinner, higher (b) thinner, lower
(c) thicker, higher (d) thicker, lower

39. Atheroma consist mainly of
(a) cholesterol and lipid hardened by calcium
(b) cholesterol and lipid hardened by iron
(c) glycogen and protein hardened by calcium
(d) glycogen and protein hardened by iron

40. The left ventricle exceeds the right ventricle in
(a) the amount of blood that enters during heart contraction.
(b) the volume expelled during contraction
(c) the pressure developed during contraction
(d) all of the above

41. The purpose of the AV node is to ____ and the purpose of the Purkinje fibers is to___.
(a) create simultaneous atrial and ventricular depolarization; speed up transmission of the cardiac impulse into the ventricle
(b) delay ventricular depolarization relative to atrial depolarization; insulate the cardiac impulse from the general ventricular fibers
(c) delay ventricular depolarization relative to atrial depolarization; transmit the cardiac impulse to very small localized groups of ventricular fibers
(d) delay atrial depolarization relative to ventricular depolarization; transmit the cardiac impulse to very small localized groups of ventricular fibers

42. Persons suffering from high blood pressure should take the following precaution to avoid excessive rise in their blood pressure
(a) sleep as much as possible
(b) avoid standing
(c) increase their weight
(d) avoid emotional disturbances and excitement

43. You are required to draw blood from a patient and to keep the blood in a test tube for analysis of corpuscles and plasma. You are also provided with the following four types of test tubes. Which of them will you not use for the purpose?
(a) Test tube containing calcium bicarbonate
(b) Chilled test-tube
(c) Test-tube containing heparin
(d) Test-tube containing sodium oxalate

44. A drop of each of the following, is placed separately on four slides. Which of them will not coagulate?
(a) Blood serum
(b) Sample from the thoracic duct of lymphatic system
(c) Whole blood from pulmonary vein
(d) Blood plasma

45. Examination of blood of a person suspected of having anemia, shows large, immature, nucleated erythrocytes without haemoglobin. Supplementing his diet with which of the following, is likely to alleviate his symptoms?
(a) Folic acid and cobalamine (b) Riboflavin
(c) Iron compounds (d) Thiamine

RESPONSE GRID					
	35. ⓐⓑⓒⓓ	36. ⓐⓑⓒⓓ	37. ⓐⓑⓒⓓ	38. ⓐⓑⓒⓓ	39. ⓐⓑⓒⓓ
	40. ⓐⓑⓒⓓ	41. ⓐⓑⓒⓓ	42. ⓐⓑⓒⓓ	43. ⓐⓑⓒⓓ	44. ⓐⓑⓒⓓ
	45. ⓐⓑⓒⓓ				

BIOLOGY CHAPTERWISE SPEED TEST-76			
Total Questions	45	Total Marks	180
Attempted		Correct	
Incorrect		Net Score	
Cut-off Score	50	Qualifying Score	60
Success Gap = Net Score – Qualifying Score			
Net Score = (Correct × 4) – (Incorrect × 1)			

Space for Rough Work

BIOLOGY

Excretory Products and Their Elimination

Speed TEST 77 Chapter-wise

No. of Questions	Maximum Marks	Time
45	180	1 Hour

GENERAL INSTRUCTIONS

- This test contains 45 MCQ's. For each question only one option is correct. Darken the correct circle/ bubble in the Response Grid provided on each page.
- You have to evaluate your Response Grids yourself with the help of solutions provided at the end of this book.
- Each correct answer will get you 4 marks and 1 mark shall be deduced for each incorrect answer. No mark will be given/ deducted if no bubble is filled. Keep a timer in front of you and stop immediately at the end of 60 min.
- The sheet follows a particular syllabus. Do not attempt the sheet before you have completed your preparation for that syllabus.
- After completing the sheet check your answers with the solution booklet and complete the Result Grid. Finally spend time to analyse your performance and revise the areas which emerge out as weak in your evaluation.

1. Toxic substances are detoxified in human body in
   (a) kidney (b) lungs (c) liver (d) stomach
2. The function of rennin is
   (a) vasodilation
   (b) reduce blood pressure
   (c) degradation of angiotensinogen
   (d) None of the above
3. Proximal and distal convoluted tubules are parts of
   (a) Seminiferous tubules (b) Nephron
   (c) Oviduct (d) Vas deferens
4. Antidiuretic hormone
   (a) Secretion is determined by plasma osmolarity
   (b) Increases permeability of renal collecting duct cells to water
   (c) Is secreted by nerve cells with their cell bodies in hypothalamus
   (d) All the above
5. Which one of the following is correctly matched pair of the given secretion and its primary role in human physiology?
   (a) Sebum — Sexual attraction
   (b) Sweat — Thermoregulation
   (c) Saliva — Tasting food
   (d) Tears — Excretion of salts
6. A person who is one along hunger strike and is surviving only on water, will have
   (a) less amino acids in his urine
   (b) more glucose in his blood
   (c) less urea in his urine
   (d) more sodium in his urine
7. Uricotelism is found in
   (a) Frogs and toads
   (b) Mammals and birds
   (c) Birds, reptiles and insects
   (d) Fishes and fresh water protozoans
8. If Henle's loop were absent from mammalian nephron which of the following is to be expected?
   (a) The urine will be more concentrated
   (b) The urine will be more dilute
   (c) There will be no urine formation
   (d) There will be hardly any change in the quality and quantity of urine formed
9. The basic functional unit of the human kidney is
   (a) nephron (b) nephridia
   (c) pyramid (d) Henle's loop

RESPONSE GRID					
	1. ⓐⓑⓒⓓ	2. ⓐⓑⓒⓓ	3. ⓐⓑⓒⓓ	4. ⓐⓑⓒⓓ	5. ⓐⓑⓒⓓ
	6. ⓐⓑⓒⓓ	7. ⓐⓑⓒⓓ	8. ⓐⓑⓒⓓ	9. ⓐⓑⓒⓓ	

Space for Rough Work

10. Reabsorption of water in distal parts of kidney tubules/urine formation is controlled by
(a) relaxin (b) calcitonin
(c) oxytocin (d) vasopressin

11. Urea from the blood can be removed by
(a) Uremia (b) Diuresis
(c) Dialysis (d) Micturition

12. In mammals, the urinary bladder opens into
(a) Uterus (b) Urethra
(c) Vestibule (d) Ureter

13. Which of the following components of blood does not enter into the nephron?
(a) urea (b) water
(c) glucose (d) plasma protein

14. Which one of the following correctly explains the function of a specific part of a human nephron ?
(a) Podocytes : create minute spaces (slite pores) for the filtration of blood into the Bowman's capsule.
(b) Henle's loop : most reabsorption of the major substances from the glomerular filtrate.
(c) Distal convoluted tubule : reabsorption of K^+ ions into the surrounding blood capillaries.
(d) Afferent arteriole : carries the blood away from the glomerular towards renal vein.

15. The condition of excess urea in blood is known as
(a) Polyuria (b) Haematuria
(c) Uraemia (d) Diuresis

16. Urine under normal conditions does not contain glucose because
(a) The normal blood sugar is fructose
(b) Glucose of blood is not filtered in the glomerulus
(c) Glucose in glomerular filtrate is reabsorbed in the uriniferous tubules
(d) Glucose in glomerular filtrate is converted into glycogen.

17. Which is not correct with respect to human kidney?
(a) The peripheral region is called cortex and central medulla
(b) Malpighian capsules are present in the cortex region
(c) Blood enters glomerulus through efferent arterioles
(d) The concave part of kidney is called hilus

18. Atrial natriuretic factor (ANF) is released in response to the increase in blood volume and blood pressure. Which of the following is not the function of ANF?
(a) Stimulates aldosterone secretion
(b) Inhibits the release of renin from JGA
(c) Stimulates salt loss in urine
(d) Inhibits sodium reabsorption from collecting duct

19. Reabsorption of chloride ions from glomerular filtrate in kidney tubule occurs by
(a) Active transport (b) Diffusion
(c) Osmosis (d) Brownian movement

20. Metanephric kidneys are found in
(a) Reptiles only (b) Birds only
(c) mammals only (d) All of these

21. In Prawn, excretion is carried out by
(a) Nephrons (b) Malpighian tubules
(c) Flame cells (d) Green glands

22. Consider the following four statements (i - iv) about certain desert animals such as kangaroo rat
(i) They have dark colour and high rate of reproduction and excrete solid urine
(ii) They do not drink water, breathe at a slow rate to conserve water and have their body covered with thick hairs
(iii) They feed on dry seeds and do not require drinking water
(iv) They excrete very concentrated urine and do not use water to regulate body temperature.

Which two of the above statements for such animals are true?
(a) (i) and (ii) (b) (iii) and (iv)
(c) (ii) and (iii) (d) (iii) and (i)

23. The longest loop of Henle is found in
(a) kangaroo rat (b) opposum
(c) rhesus monkey (d) porcupine

24. In peritoneal dialysis
(a) the blood is removed from the body and a natural filter is used
(b) the blood is not removed from the body and a natural filter is used
(c) the blood is not removed from the body and an artificial filter is used
(d) the blood is removed from the body and an artificial filter is used

25. Diabetes insipidus is a condition in which a person is unable to produce sufficient levels of the hormone ADH. The hormone increases the permeability to water of the second (distal) convoluted tubule and collecting duct in the kidney nephrons.
What is produced as a result?
(a) large volumes of concentrated urine
(b) large volumes of dilute urine
(c) small volumes of concentrated urine
(d) small volumes of dilute urine

RESPONSE GRID					
	10. ⓐⓑⓒⓓ	11. ⓐⓑⓒⓓ	12. ⓐⓑⓒⓓ	13. ⓐⓑⓒⓓ	14. ⓐⓑⓒⓓ
	15. ⓐⓑⓒⓓ	16. ⓐⓑⓒⓓ	17. ⓐⓑⓒⓓ	18. ⓐⓑⓒⓓ	19. ⓐⓑⓒⓓ
	20. ⓐⓑⓒⓓ	21. ⓐⓑⓒⓓ	22. ⓐⓑⓒⓓ	23. ⓐⓑⓒⓓ	24. ⓐⓑⓒⓓ
	25. ⓐⓑⓒⓓ				

Space for Rough Work

26. By definition, an ectotherm
    (a) is cold-blooded.
    (b) is warm-blooded.
    (c) obtains most of its heat from its environment.
    (d) derives most of its heat from its own metabolism.
27. Which region of the kidney nephron is the main site of amino acid reabsorption?
    (a) glomerulus
    (b) Bowman's capsule
    (c) proximal convoluted tubule
    (d) distal convoluted tubule
28. Long term kidney failure can be treated by introducing sterile dialysis fluid into the abdominal cavity. The fluid is drained and replaced regularly using a tube inserted surgically through the abdominal wall.
    Why does this method work well?
    (a) because osmoregulation and excretion are achieved by diffusion between the blood in the abdominal capillaries and the dialysis fluid.
    (b) because osmoregulation and excretion are achieved by the active transport of ions, water and urea between the abdominal capillaries and the dialysis fluid.
    (c) because the fluid is in direct contact with the kidneys, the urea and excess ions can pass into it without being filtered by the glomeruli.
    (d) because the fluid is in direct contact with the liver and the large intestine, and wastes and excess ions can pass into it from these organs.
29. Which of the following describes the route of urine out of the body after it leaves the kidney?
    (a) renal vein-urinary bladder-urethra-ureter
    (b) urethra-urinary bladder-ureter
    (c) renal vein-ureter-urinary bladder-urethra
    (d) ureter-urinary bladder-urethra
30. If the human kidneys filter 150 litres of plasma in a 24 hour period, what is the typical amount of urine produced and eliminated in that time period?
    (a) 0.15 litres (b) 1.5 litres
    (c) 15 litres (d) 30 litres
31. A number of hormones help to regulate water and solute uptake and release in the nephron. Antidiuretic hormone (ADH) promotes _____ in response to ______.
    (a) active transport of Cl^-, increased solute concetration
    (b) active transport of Na^+, increased blood pressure
    (c) increased permeability of the collecting duct to water, increased blood pressure
    (d) decreased permeability of the collecting duct to water, increased solute concetration
32. The filtrate formed by the nephrons in the kidney is not the same as urine. The filtrate is first refined and concentrated by the processes of ______, forming the urine that leaves the body.
    (a) filtration and secretion
    (b) reabsorption and secretion
    (c) reabsorption and excretion
    (d) filtration and reabsorption
33. What pathway is taken by water and solutes as they travel through a nephron?
    (a) Glomerulus, to Bowman's capsule, to proximal tubule, to loop of Henle, to distal tubule, to collecting ducts
    (b) Bowman's capsule, to glomerulus, to distal tubule, to loop of Henle, to proximal tubule, to collecting ducts
    (c) Glomerulus, to Bowman's capsule, to distal tubule, to loop of Henle, to proximal tubule, to collecting ducts
    (d) Glomerulus, to Bowman's capsule, to proximal tubule, to collecting ducts, to distal tubule, to loop of Henle
34. The kidney's filtration process is nonselective, so
    (a) many valuable substances are lost in the urine.
    (b) the proportions of substances in urine are the same as in blood.
    (c) urine is much less concentrated than blood.
    (d) useful substances must be selectively reabsorbed.
35. Na^+ and Cl^- are actively transported out of the tubules to help set up the countercurrent multiplier. Which the following are sites of active Na^+ and Cl^- transport in the nephron?
    (a) Proximal tubule, ascending limb of the loop of Henle
    (b) Descending limb of the loop of Henle, ascending limb of the loop of Henle
    (c) Ascending limb of the loop of Henle, proximal tubule
    (d) Collecting duct, descending limb of the loop of Henle
36. Which of the following is not a normal constituent of the glomerular filtrate?
    (a) Red blood cells (b) Urea
    (c) Sodium ion (d) Glucose
37. Kidneys help in the conservation of useful materials and excretion of wastes and therefore they receive 20% of the hearts output of blood (as much as the heart and brain combined). On a percentage basis which substance is most completely reabsorbed by the kidneys ?
    (a) Water (b) Glucose
    (c) Urea (d) Sodium
38. The sole mechanism for water reabsorption by the renal tubules is :
    (a) active tansport
    (b) osmosis.
    (c) cotransport with sodium ions
    (d) cotransport with bicarbonate ions

RESPONSE GRID					
	26. ⓐⓑⓒⓓ	27. ⓐⓑⓒⓓ	28. ⓐⓑⓒⓓ	29. ⓐⓑⓒⓓ	30. ⓐⓑⓒⓓ
	31. ⓐⓑⓒⓓ	32. ⓐⓑⓒⓓ	33. ⓐⓑⓒⓓ	34. ⓐⓑⓒⓓ	35. ⓐⓑⓒⓓ
	36. ⓐⓑⓒⓓ	37. ⓐⓑⓒⓓ	38. ⓐⓑⓒⓓ		

Space for Rough Work

39. Figure shown human urinary system with structures labelled A to D. Select option which correctly identifies them and gives their characteristics and /or functions.

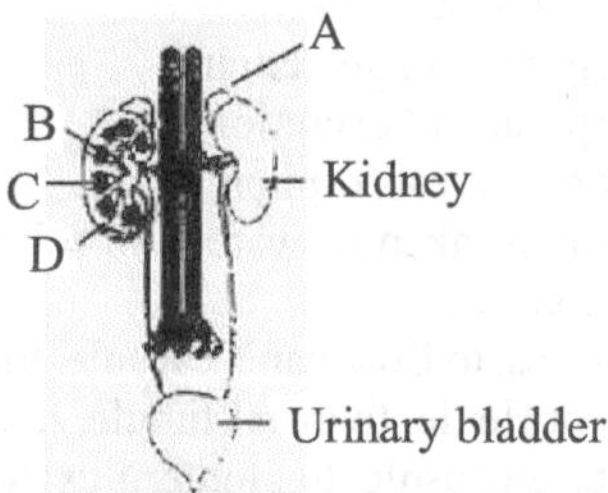

(a) B-pelvis-broad funnel shaped space inner to hilum, directly connected to loops of Henle.
(b) C-Medulla-inner zone of kidney and contains complex nephrons.
(c) D - Cortex - outer part of kidney and do not contain any part of nephrons
(d) A-Adrenal gland - located at the anterior part of kidney. Secrete Catecholamines which stimulate glycogen breakdown.

40. Refer the following diagram and identify the parts of a kidney indicated

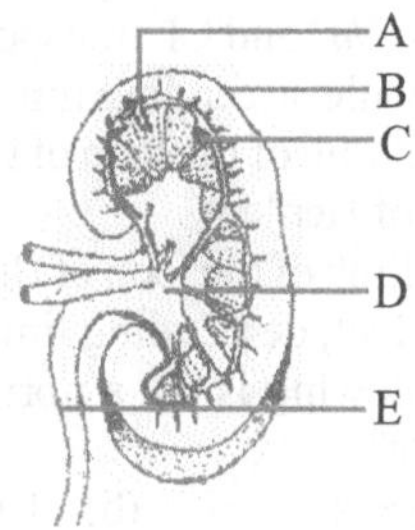

(a) A = cortex, B = nephron, C = pelvis, D= medulla, E = ureter
(b) A = cortex, B = medulla, C = nephron, D = pelvis, E = ureter
(c) A = nephron, B = cortex, C = medulla, D = ureter, E = pelvis
(d) A = nephron, B = cortex, C = medulla, D = pelvis, E = ureter

41. Select the option which shows correct matching of animal with excretory organs and excretory product

	Animal	Excretory organs	Excretory product
(a)	Housefly	Renal tubules	Uric acid
(b)	*Labeo* (Rohu)	Nephridial tubes	Ammonia
(c)	Salamander	Kidney	Urea
(d)	Peacock	Kidney	Urea

42. The appearance of albumin in the urine is most likely due to
(a) Increase in the blood pressure
(b) Decrease in the blood osmotic corpuscles
(c) Damage to the Malpighian corpuscles
(d) Damage to the proximal convoluted tubules

43. Kidney crystals are solid clusters of
(a) Calcium nitrate and uric acid
(b) Phosphate and uric acid
(c) Calcium carbonate and uric acid
(d) Calcium metabisulphite and uric acid

44. The liquid which is collected in the cavity of Bowman's capsule is
(a) Concentrated urine
(b) Blood plasma minus blood proteins
(c) Glycogen and water
(d) Sulphates and water

45. A person who is on a long hunger strike and is surviving only on water, will have –
(a) less amino acids in his urine
(b) more glucose in his blood
(c) less urea in his urine
(d) more sodium in his urine

RESPONSE GRID					
	39. ⓐⓑⓒⓓ	40. ⓐⓑⓒⓓ	41. ⓐⓑⓒⓓ	42. ⓐⓑⓒⓓ	43. ⓐⓑⓒⓓ
	44. ⓐⓑⓒⓓ	45. ⓐⓑⓒⓓ			

BIOLOGY CHAPTERWISE SPEED TEST-77

Total Questions	45	Total Marks	180
Attempted		Correct	
Incorrect		Net Score	
Cut-off Score	45	Qualifying Score	60
Success Gap = Net Score – Qualifying Score			
Net Score = (Correct × 4) – (Incorrect × 1)			

Space for Rough Work

BIOLOGY

Locomotion and Movement

Speed TEST 78
Chapter-wise

No. of Questions	Maximum Marks	Time
45	180	1 Hour

GENERAL INSTRUCTIONS

- This test contains 45 MCQ's. For each question only one option is correct. Darken the correct circle/ bubble in the Response Grid provided on each page.
- You have to evaluate your Response Grids yourself with the help of solutions provided at the end of this book.
- Each correct answer will get you 4 marks and 1 mark shall be deduced for each incorrect answer. No mark will be given/ deducted if no bubble is filled. Keep a timer in front of you and stop immediately at the end of 60 min.
- The sheet follows a particular syllabus. Do not attempt the sheet before you have completed your preparation for that syllabus.
- After completing the sheet check your answers with the solution booklet and complete the Result Grid. Finally spend time to analyse your performance and revise the areas which emerge out as weak in your evaluation.

1. Which ion is essential for muscle contraction?
   (a) Na^+ (b) K^+
   (c) Ca^{2+} (d) Cl^-
2. Elbow joint is an example of:
   (a) hinge joint (b) gliding joint
   (c) ball and socket joint (d) pivot joint
3. Two of the body parts which do not appear in MRI may be
   (a) molar teeth and eye lens
   (b) scapula and canines
   (c) ligaments and ribs
   (d) tendons and premolars
4. Which of the following is made up of a single bone in mammal?
   (a) Dentary (b) Hyoid
   (c) Upper jaw (d) All of these
5. Intercoastal muscles are found attached with
   (a) diaphragm (b) ribs
   (c) pleura (d) lungs
6. Ball and socket joint is found between
   (a) ribs and vertebral
   (b) femur and tibio-fibula
   (c) humerus and olecranon fossa
   (d) humerus and pectoral girdle
7. Which of the following is the contractile protein of a muscle?
   (a) Myosin (b) Tropomyosin
   (c) Actin (d) Tubulin

RESPONSE GRID					
	1. ⓐⓑⓒⓓ	2. ⓐⓑⓒⓓ	3. ⓐⓑⓒⓓ	4. ⓐⓑⓒⓓ	5. ⓐⓑⓒⓓ
	6. ⓐⓑⓒⓓ	7. ⓐⓑⓒⓓ			

Space for Rough Work

8. Myofibrils are made up of
   (a) Myosin and actin
   (b) Myosin and troponin
   (c) Actin and tropomyosin
   (d) All the above components

9. Which one of the following is the correct matching of three items and their grouping category?

	Items		Group
(a)	Ilium, ischium, pubis	-	coxal bones of pelvic girdle
(b)	Actin, myosin, rhodopsin.	-	muscle proteins
(c)	Cytosine, uracil, thiamine	-	pyrimidines
(d)	Malleus, incus, cochlea	-	ear ossicles

10. The number of floating ribs, in the human body, is
    (a) 6 pairs (b) 5 pairs
    (c) 3 pairs (d) 2 pairs

11. Select the **correct** statement regarding the specific disorder of muscular or skeletal system :
    (a) *Myasthenia gravis* - Autoimmune disorder which inhibits sliding of myosin filaments.
    (b) *Gout* - inflammation of joints due to extra deposition of calcium.
    (c) *Muscular dystrophy* - age related shortening of muscles.
    (d) *Osteoporosis* - decrease in bone mass and higher chances of fractures with advancing age.

12. The sensation of fatigue in the muscles after prolonged strenuous physical work, is caused by
    (a) a decrease in the supply of oxygen
    (b) minor wear and tear of muscle fibres
    (c) the depletion of glucose
    (d) the accumulation of lactic acid

13. Synovial fluid is found in
    (a) cranial cavity (b) spinal cavity
    (c) immovable joints (d) freely movable joints

14. Humerus differs from the femur in having:
    (a) Sigmoid notch (b) Trochanter
    (c) Deltoid ridge (d) None of these

15. The most abundant mineral in human body is
    (a) Magnesium (b) Sodium
    (c) Calcium (d) Potassium

16. Ankle joint is
    (a) Pivot Joint (b) Ball and socket joint
    (c) Hinge joint (d) Gliding joint

17. The major function of the intervertebral disc is to
    (a) Absorb shock
    (b) String the vertebrae together
    (c) Prevent injuries
    (d) Prevent hyperextension

18. Which one of the following pairs of chemical substances is correctly categorized?
    (a) Calcitonin and thymosin - Thyroid hormones
    (b) Pepsin and prolactin - Two digestive enzymes secreted in stomach
    (c) Troponin and myosin - Complex proteins in striated muscles
    (d) Secretin and rhodopsin - Polypeptide hormones

19. The functional unit of contractile system of a striated muscle is
    (a) Sarcomere (b) Z-band
    (c) Sarcosome (d) Myofibril

20. Joint between bones of human skull is
    (a) Hinge joint (b) Synovial joint
    (c) Cartilaginous joint (d) Fibrous joint

RESPONSE GRID					
	8. ⓐⓑⓒⓓ	9. ⓐⓑⓒⓓ	10. ⓐⓑⓒⓓ	11. ⓐⓑⓒⓓ	12. ⓐⓑⓒⓓ
	13. ⓐⓑⓒⓓ	14. ⓐⓑⓒⓓ	15. ⓐⓑⓒⓓ	16. ⓐⓑⓒⓓ	17. ⓐⓑⓒⓓ
	18. ⓐⓑⓒⓓ	19. ⓐⓑⓒⓓ	20. ⓐⓑⓒⓓ		

Space for Rough Work

21. Which one of the following is the *correct description* of a certain part of the normal human skeleton ?
(a) Parietal bone and the temporal bone of the skull are joined by fibrous joint
(b) First vertebra is axis which articulates with the occipital condyles
(c) The 9th and 10th pairs of ribs are called the floating ribs
(d) Glenoid cavity is a depression to which the thigh bone articulates.

22. Which of the following is an autoimmune disorder ?
(a) Myasthenia gravis (b) Osteoporosis
(c) Muscular dystrophy (d) Gout

23. The joint in our neck which allows us to rotate our head left to right is
(a) pivot joint (b) hinge joint
(c) saddle joint (d) ellipsoid joint

24. Read the following statements carefully and select the correct ones.
(i) Cardiac fibres are branched with one or more nuclei
(ii) Smooth muscles are unbranched and cylindrical
(iii) Skeletal muscles can be branched or unbranched
(iv) Smooth muscles are non-striated
(a) only (iv) (b) (ii) and (iii)
(c) (iii) and (iv) (d) only (iii)

25. A cricket player is fast chasing a ball in the field. Which one of the following groups of bones is directly contributing in this movement?
(a) Femur, malleus, tibia, metatarsals
(b) Pelvis, ulna, patella, tarsals
(c) Sternum, femur, tibia, fibula
(d) Tarsals, femur, metatarsals, tibia

26. Which of the following statement is incorrect w.r.t. bone?
(a) If born is kept in HCl it becomes soft
(b) Bone is made up of 60&70% organic matter and 30&40% inorganic matter
(c) If bone is heated then the organic part disappears and inorganic part is retained
(d) Hydroxyapatite salts and fluorapatite salts are found in matrix

27. One of the following is a location of most abundant cartilage in the human body.
(a) Tracheal rings and costal cartilages
(b) Intevertebral disc and public symphysis
(c) Pinna and tip of nose
(d) Pectoral girdle and pelvic girdle

28. Upon preventing acetylcholine from diffusing across a neuromuscular junction, which of the following will *not* result?
(a) No action potential will be produced in the affected muscle fibre's plasma membrane.
(b) The endoplasmic reticulum releases calcium ions (Ca^{2+}) into the cytoplasm.
(c) Myosin will not bind to actin in the affected muscle fibre.
(d) The affected muscle fiber will fail to contract.

29. Muscle A and muscle B are the same size, but muscle A is capable of much finer control than muscle B. Which one of the following is likely to be true of muscle A?
(a) It contains fewer motor units than muscle B.
(b) It has larger sarcomeres than muscle B.
(c) It is controlled by more neurons than muscle B.
(d) It is controlled by fewer neurons than muscle B.

30. Much discussion of muscle is related to 'striated' muscle, but 'smooth' muscles are also important for ________
(a) protecting and nourishing striated muscle cells.
(b) conveying action potentials from nerve endings to the deepest parts of striated muscle.
(c) involuntary activities, such as movement of food in the gut and controlling blood pressure.
(d) sheathing the striated muscles so that they do not damage each other as they slide past one another.

RESPONSE GRID					
	21. ⓐⓑⓒⓓ	22. ⓐⓑⓒⓓ	23. ⓐⓑⓒⓓ	24. ⓐⓑⓒⓓ	25. ⓐⓑⓒⓓ
	26. ⓐⓑⓒⓓ	27. ⓐⓑⓒⓓ	28. ⓐⓑⓒⓓ	29. ⓐⓑⓒⓓ	30. ⓐⓑⓒⓓ

Space for Rough Work

31. What is a hydrostatic skeleton largely composed of?
(a) Bone (b) Fluid
(c) Cartilage (d) Connective tissue

32 The only movable bone in the skull is:
(a) Mandible (b) Maxilla
(c) Ethmoid (d) None

33. The smallest irregular bone in man is:
(a) Patella (b) Stapes
(c) Nasal (d) Palatine

34. ATP provides the energy for muscle contraction by allowing for
(a) an action potential formation in the muscle cell.
(b) cross-bridge detachment of myosin from action.
(c) cross-bridge attachment of myosin to actin
(d) release of calcium by sarcoplasmic reticulum.

35. The primary difference between an endoskeleton and an exoskeleton has to do with
(a) the presence of both circular and longitudinal muscles.
(b) whether or not the skeleton is on the inside of the body.
(c) the presence or absence of joints.
(d) the amount of fluid in the body.

36. Deposition of uric acid crystals within the synovial joint causes:
(a) osteoarthritis (b) rheumatoid arthritis
(c) gout (d) paralysis

37. Total no. of muscles in our body is
(a) 256 muscles (b) 639 muscles
(c) 400 muscles (d) 421 muscles

38. The muscle band that remains unchanged during contraction and relaxation of the skeletal muscle is
(a) I (b) H
(c) A (d) Z line

39. What is not true about human skull ?
(a) It is dicondylic
(b) It includes 6 ear ossicles
(c) It includes 14 facial bones
(d) Hyoid is not included in skull bones

40. Which is part of pectoral girdle?
(a) Glenoid cavity (b) Sternum
(c) Ilium (d) Acetabulum

41. Number of bones in hind limb of human is-
(a) 21 (b) 24
(c) 30 (d) 14

42. Haversian system is diagnostic feature of-
(a) Avian bones (b) Reptilian bones
(c) Mammalian bones (d) Bones of all animal

43. In children the bones are more flexible and brittle because their bones have
(a) large quantity of salts and little organic substances
(b) large quantity of organic substances and little salts
(c) well developed haversian system
(d) large number of osteoblasts

44. Pneumatic bones are found in
(a) House lizard (b) Pigeon
(c) Flying fish (d) Frog's tadpole

45. Actin protein occurs in two forms
(a) Polymeric F- actin and monomeric G- actin
(b) Monomeric F- actin and polymeric G-actin
(c) The tail and a head
(d) F-actin and G- actin, but both globular

RESPONSE GRID					
	31. ⓐⓑⓒⓓ	32. ⓐⓑⓒⓓ	33. ⓐⓑⓒⓓ	34. ⓐⓑⓒⓓ	35. ⓐⓑⓒⓓ
	36. ⓐⓑⓒⓓ	37. ⓐⓑⓒⓓ	38. ⓐⓑⓒⓓ	39. ⓐⓑⓒⓓ	40. ⓐⓑⓒⓓ
	41. ⓐⓑⓒⓓ	42. ⓐⓑⓒⓓ	43. ⓐⓑⓒⓓ	44. ⓐⓑⓒⓓ	45. ⓐⓑⓒⓓ

BIOLOGY CHAPTERWISE SPEED TEST-78			
Total Questions	45	Total Marks	180
Attempted		Correct	
Incorrect		Net Score	
Cut-off Score	45	Qualifying Score	60
Success Gap = Net Score – Qualifying Score			
Net Score = (Correct × 4) – (Incorrect × 1)			

Space for Rough Work

BIOLOGY

Neural Control and Co-ordination

Speed TEST 79

Chapter-wise

No. of Questions	Maximum Marks	Time
45	180	1 Hour

GENERAL INSTRUCTIONS

- This test contains 45 MCQ's. For each question only one option is correct. Darken the correct circle/ bubble in the Response Grid provided on each page.
- You have to evaluate your Response Grids yourself with the help of solutions provided at the end of this book.
- Each correct answer will get you 4 marks and 1 mark shall be deduced for each incorrect answer. No mark will be given/ deducted if no bubble is filled. Keep a timer in front of you and stop immediately at the end of 60 min.
- The sheet follows a particular syllabus. Do not attempt the sheet before you have completed your preparation for that syllabus.
- After completing the sheet check your answers with the solution booklet and complete the Result Grid. Finally spend time to analyse your performance and revise the areas which emerge out as weak in your evaluation.

1. Afferent nerve fibres carry impulses from
   (a) effector organs to CNS (b) receptors to CNS
   (c) CNS to receptors (d) CNS to muscles
2. The nerve centres which control the body temperature and the urge for eating are contained in:
   (a) hypothalamus (b) pons
   (c) cerebellum (d) thalamus
3. Rods and cones of eyes are modified
   (a) multipolar neuron (b) unipolar neuron
   (c) bipolar neuron (d) None of these
4. The nerve transmitter, produced at the synapse and neuromuscular junction, is
   (a) GTP (b) ATP
   (c) acetylcholine (d) phosphokinase
5. Alzheimer disease in humans is associated with the deficiency of:
   (a) glutamic acid
   (b) acetylcholine
   (c) gamma aminobutyric acid (GABA)
   (d) dopamine
6. Which is the example of conditioned reflex ?
   (a) Eyes closed when anything enter into it.
   (b) Hand took up when piercing with needle.
   (c) Salivation in a hungry dog in response to ringing of a bell.
   (d) Digestion food goes forward in alimentary canal.
7. The black pigment in the eye which reduces the internal reflection is located in
   (a) retina (b) iris
   (c) cornea (d) sclerotic
8. Which one of the following does not act as a neurotransmitter ?
   (a) Epinephrine (b) Norepinephrine
   (c) Cortisone (d) Acetylcholine

RESPONSE GRID					
	1. ⓐⓑⓒⓓ	2. ⓐⓑⓒⓓ	3. ⓐⓑⓒⓓ	4. ⓐⓑⓒⓓ	5. ⓐⓑⓒⓓ
	6. ⓐⓑⓒⓓ	7. ⓐⓑⓒⓓ	8. ⓐⓑⓒⓓ		

Space for Rough Work

9. During the propagation of a nerve impulse, the action potential results from the movement of :
(a) K^+ ions from extracellular fluid to intracellular fluid.
(b) Na^+ ions from intracellular fluid to extracellular fluid.
(c) K^+ ions from intracellular fluid to extracellular fluid.
(d) Na^+ ions from extracellular fluid to intracellular fluid.

10. The cochlea of ear contains
(a) perilymph
(b) aqueous humour
(c) perilymph and endolymph
(d) only endolymph

11. Eustachian tube connects
(a) External ear with middle ear
(b) External ear with internal ear
(c) Middle ear with pharynx
(d) Internal pharyax

12. Mark the incorrect statement
(a) The ear ossicle attached to tympanic membrane is malleus
(b) Opsin (of Rhodopsin) develops from vitamin A
(c) The pressure on ear drum is equalized by eustachian tube
(d) Otolith organ consists of saccule and utricle

13. Frequency of sound is discriminated by
(a) The intensity of movement of basilar fibres of cochlea
(b) The type of fluid - perilymph or endolymph
(c) The site at the cochlear coil
(d) All of these

14. Which one of the following is the correct difference between rod cells and cone cells of our retina?

		Rod Cells	Cone Cells
(a)	Distribution	More concentrated in centre of retina	Evenly distributed all over retina
(b)	Visual activity	High	Low
(c)	Visual pigment contained	Iodopsin	Rhodopsin
(d)	Over all function	Vision in poor light	Colour vision and detailed vision in bright light

15. Saltatory conduction of nerve impulse takes place through :
(a) Myelinated fibre
(b) Non-myelinated fibre
(c) Grey fibres
(d) None of these

16. In which part of the brain corpora quadrigemina is located?
(a) Diencephalon (b) Mesencephalon
(c) Prosencephalon (d) Rhombencephalon

17. A person entering an empty room suddenly finds a snake right in front on opening the door. Which one of the following is likely to happen in his neuro-hormonal control system ?
(a) Sympathetic nervous system is activated releasing epinephrine and norepinephrine from adrenal medulla.
(b) Neurotransmitters diffuse rapidly across the cleft and transmit a nerve impulse.
(c) Hypothalamus activates the parasympathetic division of brain.
(d) Sympathetic nervous system is activated releasing epinephrine and norepinephrine from adrenal cortex.

18. The blind spot is the region where
(a) Image is formed
(b) Cones are numerous
(c) The optic nerve leaves out
(d) Image is formed during the dark

19. In myopia or short sightedness
(a) Image is formed slightly in front of retina because eye ball is longer
(b) Eye ball is normal but image is formed over blind spot
(c) Eye ball is normal but images is formed slightly behind the retina due to faulty lens
(d) Curvature of cornea becomes irregular

20. Sequence of meninges from inner to outside is
(a) Duramater – Archnoid – Piamater
(b) Duramater – Piamater – Arachnoid
(c) Arachnoid – Duramater - Piamater
(d) Piamater- Arachnoid - Duramater

21. Among which one of the following groups of chemicals, all are neurotransmitters?
(a) Glycine, dopamine, melatonin
(b) Somatostatin, serotonin, acetylcholine
(c) Noradrenaline, somatostatin, threonine
(d) Acetylcholine, noradrenaline, dopamine

RESPONSE GRID					
	9. ⓐⓑⓒⓓ	10. ⓐⓑⓒⓓ	11. ⓐⓑⓒⓓ	12. ⓐⓑⓒⓓ	13. ⓐⓑⓒⓓ
	14. ⓐⓑⓒⓓ	15. ⓐⓑⓒⓓ	16. ⓐⓑⓒⓓ	17. ⓐⓑⓒⓓ	18. ⓐⓑⓒⓓ
	19. ⓐⓑⓒⓓ	20. ⓐⓑⓒⓓ	21. ⓐⓑⓒⓓ		

Space for Rough Work

22. The enzyme required for the conduction of nerve impulse across synapse is:
(a) peroxidase (b) choline acetylase
(c) ascorbic acid oxidase (d) succinic dehydrogenase

23. The purplish red pigment rhodopsin contained in the rods type of photoreceptor cells of the human eye, is a derivative of
(a) Vitamin A (b) Vitamin B_1
(c) Vitamin C (d) Vitamin D

24. During stress condition which of the following nerves start working?
(a) Sympathetic nerves
(b) Parasympathetic nerves
(c) Autonomic nerves
(d) Cranial nerves

25. The gelatinous membrane covering the sensorys hair cells of the ear is known as
(a) Reissner's membrane
(b) tectorial membrane
(c) basilar membrane
(d) neuro-sensory membrane

26. Nerve cells do not divide because they do not have
(a) nucleus (b) centrosome
(c) Golgi body (d) mitochondria

27. Reflex arcs, which involve no processing in the brain, are beneficial because they permit
(a) instantaneous signaling to motor neurons.
(b) avoidance of dangerous stimuli, even without a previously "learned" response.
(c) immediate response to dangerous stimuli.
(d) All of the above

28. Drugs that alter the permeability of the plasma membrane of a neuron have which of the following effects on nerve impulse conduction?
(a) They prevent movement of sodium and potassium ions into and out of the cell, thereby stopping the transmission of the impulse.
(b) They primarily affect conduction along the axon.
(c) They prevent the release of neurotransmitters at synapses.
(d) All of the above

29. The local depolarization of a receptor-cell membrane is called as
(a) inhibitory postsynaptic potential (or IPSP).
(b) action potential.
(c) resting potential.
(d) threshold potential.

30. Action potentials travel along a neuron because ____________.
(a) the neuron cytoskeleton conducts electricity as long as an ion gradient is maintained by the sodium-potassium pump
(b) of cytoplasmic streaming within the neuron
(c) they are pulled along by positive-negative attraction
(d) depolarization of the membrane at one point causes an increase of permeability to sodium at the next point

31. Which one of the following structures constitutes the mammalian forebrain?
(a) Cerebrum and cerebellum
(b) Olfactory bulb
(c) Cerebellum and medulla
(d) Thalamus, hypothalamus, and cerebrum

32. If you electrically stimulate a resting neuron in the middle of its axon and cause it to fire an action potential, which of the following will happen ?
(a) The action potential will propagate toward the axon terminal.
(b) The action potential will propagate toward the cell body.
(c) The action potential will propagate toward both the axon terminal and the cell body.
(d) The action potential will not propagate at all.

33. The resting membrane potential for neuron A is –70mV, while the resting potential for neuron B is –50mV. The threshold voltage for the production of an action potential is –35mV for both neurons. Which of the following statements is *false* ?
(a) Neuron A must depolarize by 35mV to reach the threshold voltage.
(b) Neuron B must hyperpolarize by 15mV to reach the threshold voltage.
(c) The inside of both neurons is negatively charged with respect to the outside.
(d) A single EPSP received by neuron A would cause it to depolarize slightly.

RESPONSE GRID					
	22. ⓐⓑⓒⓓ	23. ⓐⓑⓒⓓ	24. ⓐⓑⓒⓓ	25. ⓐⓑⓒⓓ	26. ⓐⓑⓒⓓ
	27. ⓐⓑⓒⓓ	28. ⓐⓑⓒⓓ	29. ⓐⓑⓒⓓ	30. ⓐⓑⓒⓓ	31. ⓐⓑⓒⓓ
	32. ⓐⓑⓒⓓ	33. ⓐⓑⓒⓓ			

Space for Rough Work

34. You are sitting in biology class daydreaming. Your intrinsic heartbeat is controlled by.....
(a) the spinal cord.
(b) the cerebrum.
(c) the medulla.
(d) levels of adrenaline in the blood.

35. The threshold of a neuron is
(a) The amount of inhibitory neurotransmitter required to inhibit an action potential.
(b) The membrane voltage at which an axon potential will be suppressed.
(c) the amount of excitatory neurotransmitter required to elicit an action potential.
(d) The membrane voltage at which the membrane potential develops into an action potential.

36. Which of the following statements about gap juctions or electrical synapses is *false*?
(a) Connexons form molecular tunnels between two cells.
(b) Electrical synapses cannot be inhibitory
(c) Electrical synapses do not allow for temporal summation.
(d) Electrical transmission is very slow and is bidirectional.

37. All but one of the following chemicals are neurotransmitters that function in the human brain. Select the *exception*.
(a) Dopamine (b) Glycine
(c) Atropine (d) Glutamic acid

38. Which of the following cell stop dividing after birth ?
(a) Epithelium (b) Neuron
(c) Glial cells (d) Liver

39. Arbor vitae is composed of
(a) Neuroglea cells (b) Grey matter
(c) White matter (d) All of these

40. Twilight vision is also called
(a) Scotopic vision and is the function of rods
(b) Scotopic vision and is the function of cones
(c) Photopic vision and is the function of rods
(d) Photopic vision and is the function of cones

41. The white matter of the CNS is always
(a) deep to the grey matter
(b) unmyelinated
(c) arranged into tracts
(d) composed of sensory fibers only

42. The pneumotaxic centre in the body is
(a) Heart (b) Lung
(c) Medulla (d) Liver

43. Identify the organ/innervation mismatch
(a) Glossopharyngeal nerve-tongue
(b) Optic nerve-Eye
(c) Facial nerve-Olfactory epithelium
(d) Cochlear nerve-Spiral organ

44. Our ear can hear the frequency of sound waves
(a) 20 to 20,000 cycles/sec
(b) 1000 to 2000 cycles/sec
(c) 5000 to 7000 cycles/sec
(d) 5000 to 10,000 cycles/sec

45. Fenestra ovalis is the opening of –
(a) Cranium (b) Tympanum
(c) Tympanic cavity (d) Brain

RESPONSE GRID					
	34. ⓐⓑⓒⓓ	35. ⓐⓑⓒⓓ	36. ⓐⓑⓒⓓ	37. ⓐⓑⓒⓓ	38. ⓐⓑⓒⓓ
	39. ⓐⓑⓒⓓ	40. ⓐⓑⓒⓓ	41. ⓐⓑⓒⓓ	42. ⓐⓑⓒⓓ	43. ⓐⓑⓒⓓ
	44. ⓐⓑⓒⓓ	45. ⓐⓑⓒⓓ			

BIOLOGY CHAPTERWISE SPEED TEST-79			
Total Questions	45	Total Marks	180
Attempted		Correct	
Incorrect		Net Score	
Cut-off Score	45	Qualifying Score	60
Success Gap = Net Score – Qualifying Score			
Net Score = (Correct × 4) – (Incorrect × 1)			

Space for Rough Work

BIOLOGY

Chemical Co-ordination and Integration

Speed TEST 80

Chapter-wise

No. of Questions	Maximum Marks	Time
45	180	1 Hour

GENERAL INSTRUCTIONS

- This test contains 45 MCQ's. For each question only one option is correct. Darken the correct circle/ bubble in the Response Grid provided on each page.
- You have to evaluate your Response Grids yourself with the help of solutions provided at the end of this book.
- Each correct answer will get you 4 marks and 1 mark shall be deduced for each incorrect answer. No mark will be given/ deducted if no bubble is filled. Keep a timer in front of you and stop immediately at the end of 60 min.
- The sheet follows a particular syllabus. Do not attempt the sheet before you have completed your preparation for that syllabus.
- After completing the sheet check your answers with the solution booklet and complete the Result Grid. Finally spend time to analyse your performance and revise the areas which emerge out as weak in your evaluation.

1. Which hormone possesses anti-insulin effect?
   (a) Cortisol (b) Calcitonin
   (c) Oxytocin (d) Aldosterone
2. Which of the following is both exocrine and endocrine gland ?
   (a) Liver (b) Pancreas
   (c) Thyroid (d) Adrenal
3. Chemically hormones are
   (a) biogenic amines only
   (b) proteins, steroids and biogenic amines
   (c) proteins only
   (d) steroids only
4. The blood calcium level is lowered by the deficiency of
   (a) parathormone
   (b) thyroxine
   (c) both calcitonin and parathormone
   (d) calcitonin
5. The technique used for estimation of minute amounts of hormones and drugs is called
   (a) electrophoresis
   (b) electroencephalogram
   (c) fractionation
   (d) radioimmunoassay
6. Testosterone is produced by
   (a) sertoli cells (b) leydig's cells
   (c) oxyntic cells (d) pituitary gland
7. Which one of the following pairs correctly matches a hormone with a disease resulting from its deficiency?
   (a) Luteinizing - Failure of ovulation
   (b) Insulin - Diabetes insipidus
   (c) Thyroxine - Tetany
   (d) Parathyroid - Diabetes mellitus
8. Which one of the following is not a second messenger in hormone action ?
   (a) Calcium (b) Sodium
   (c) cAMP (d) cGMP

RESPONSE GRID	
	1. ⓐⓑⓒⓓ 2. ⓐⓑⓒⓓ 3. ⓐⓑⓒⓓ 4. ⓐⓑⓒⓓ 5. ⓐⓑⓒⓓ
	6. ⓐⓑⓒⓓ 7. ⓐⓑⓒⓓ 8. ⓐⓑⓒⓓ

Space for Rough Work

9. Which of the following statements regarding glucagon is false?
(a) It is secreted by α-cells islets of Langerhans.
(b) It acts antagonistically to insulin.
(c) It decreases blood sugar level.
(d) The gland responsible for its secretion is heterocrine gland.

10. Which one of the following statements is correct?
(a) Neurons regulate endocrine activity, but not *vice versa.*
(b) Endocrine glands regulate neural activity and nervous system regulates endocrine glands.
(c) Neither hormones control neural activity nor the neurons control endocrine activity.
(d) Endocrine glands regulate neural activity but not *vice versa.*

11. Match the source gland with respective hormone as well as the function correctly.

	Source gland	Hormone	Function
(a)	Anterior pituitary	Oxytocin	Contraction of uterus muscles during child birth
(b)	Posterior pituitary	Vasopressin	Stimulates reabsorption of water in the distal tubules in the nephron
(c)	Corpus luteum	Estrogen	Supports pregnancy
(d)	Thyroid	Thyroxine	Regulates blood calcium level

12. Which of the following is incorrect?
(a) Iodine is needed for thyroxine formation.
(b) Calcium regulates the excitibility of nerve fibres.
(c) Potassium plays an important role in the regulation of acid base balance in cell.
(d) Phosphorus helps to maintain the osmotic pressure of the body fluids.

13. Sertoli cells are found in
(a) ovaries and secrete progesterone
(b) adrenal cortex and secrete adrenaline
(c) seminiferous tubules and provide nutrition to germ cells
(d) pancreas and secrete cholecystokinin

14. The phase of menstrual cycle in humans that lasts for 7-8 days, is
(a) follicular phase (b) ovulatory phase
(c) luteal phase (d) menstruation

15. Blood glucose level in man is regulated by:
(a) insulin
(b) adrenaline
(c) glucagon and insulin
(d) All of the above

16. Which of the following glands grows to the maximum size at puberty and then diminishes gradually?
(a) Thymus (b) Pituitary
(c) Thyroid (d) Adrenal

17. Hypoglycemic hormone is
(a) Insulin (b) Glucagon
(c) Thyroxine (d) Calcitonin

18. Which of the following diseases is caused by the under secretion of cortisol?
(a) Anaemia
(b) Addison's disease
(c) Hyperglycemia
(d) Mental illness or retardation

19. Glycogen is converted to glucose by
(a) Insulin
(b) Glucagon
(c) Galactose
(d) Both glucagons and insulin

20. A decrease in the level of oestrogen and progesterone causes
(a) Growth and dilation of myometrium
(b) Growth of endometrium
(c) Constriction of uterine blood vessels leading to sloughing of endometrium or uterine epithelium
(d) Release of ovum from the ovary.

21. Which of the following is a minerelocorticoid?
(a) Calciferol (b) Progesterone
(c) Adrenalin (d) Aldosterone

22. Which hormone interacts with membrane bound receptor and does not normally enter the target cell ?
(a) Follicle stimulating hormone
(b) Estrogen
(c) Thyroxin
(d) Cortisol

RESPONSE GRID					
	9. ⓐⓑⓒⓓ	10. ⓐⓑⓒⓓ	11. ⓐⓑⓒⓓ	12. ⓐⓑⓒⓓ	13. ⓐⓑⓒⓓ
	14. ⓐⓑⓒⓓ	15. ⓐⓑⓒⓓ	16. ⓐⓑⓒⓓ	17. ⓐⓑⓒⓓ	18. ⓐⓑⓒⓓ
	19. ⓐⓑⓒⓓ	20. ⓐⓑⓒⓓ	21. ⓐⓑⓒⓓ	22. ⓐⓑⓒⓓ	

Space for Rough Work

23. The 24 hour (diurnal) rhythm of our body such as the sleep-wake cycle is regulated by the hormone
(a) Adrenaline (b) Melatonin
(c) Calcitonin (d) Prolactin

24. Steroid hormones transmit their information by
(a) stimulating the receptors present on cell membrance
(b) entering into the cell and modifying cellular contents
(c) entering into the cell and modifying nuclear organization
(d) the help of an intracellular second messenger

25. Increase in bleeding time and delay in blood coagulation is due to the deficiency of which hormone?
(a) Adrenaline (b) Noradrenaline
(c) Parathormone (d) Thyroxine

26. Estrogen and testosterone are steroid hormones, and most likely bind to
(a) membrane ion channels
(b) enzyme-linked membrane reseptors
(c) G-protein coupled membrane receptors
(d) cytoplasmic receptors

27. The only unicellular exocrine glands in our body are
(a) Sweat glands
(b) Mucus secreting goblet cells
(c) Mammary glands
(d) Sebaceous glands

28. Steroid-based hormones are able to act inside the cell. This is possible because
(a) there are no receptors for hormones on the cell surface.
(b) hormones must interact with the nucleus to have an effect.
(c) proteins carry them into the cell.
(d) steroid-based hormones are hydrophobic molecules that can pass through the cell membrane.

29. Every time you eat a cookie or candy bar, your blood sugar increases. This triggers an increase in the hormone
(a) thyroxine. (b) epinephrine.
(c) glucagon. (d) insulin.

30. Target cells
(a) react specifically to a chemical messenger.
(b) have receptors for chemical messengers
(c) secrete hormones
(d) Both a and b

31. Researchers have found increased levels of hormones from the _____ in the blood of students preparing for final exams. These hormones are produced in response to stress.
(a) thyroid gland (b) pineal gland
(c) posterior pituitary (d) adrenal glands

32. Hormones generally cause a response in a cell by
(a) interacting directly with the cell's DNA.
(b) binding with a receptor and stimulating protein production.
(c) changing the polarity of the cell membrane and causing a cascade of events within the cell.
(d) halting all other cellular activity except the required response

33. Hormones are produced at a particular centralized site and transported throughout the organism by means of
(a) a series of synapses
(b) an integrated neural pathway system.
(c) cellular communication
(d) an internal transport system

34. Injections of a hormone are sometimes given to strengthen contractions of the uterus during childbirth. What hormone might this be?
(a) adrenocorticotropic hormone (ACTH)
(b) thyroxine
(c) oxytocin (d) insulin

35. The graph below illustrates the changes in blood sugar concentration after a healthy man has drunk a glucose solution.

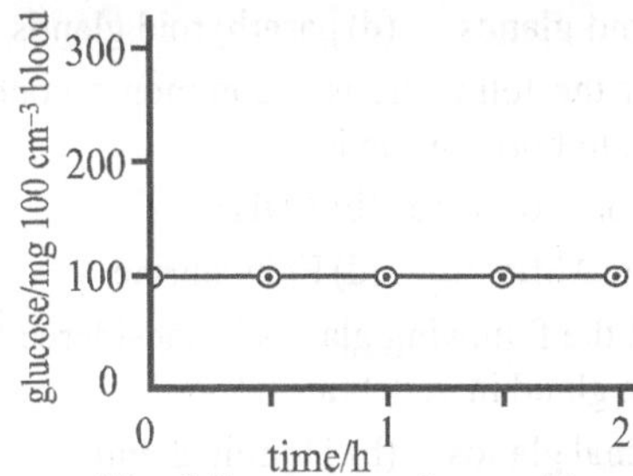

Which one of the following graphs would apply to a diabetic man in similar circumstances?

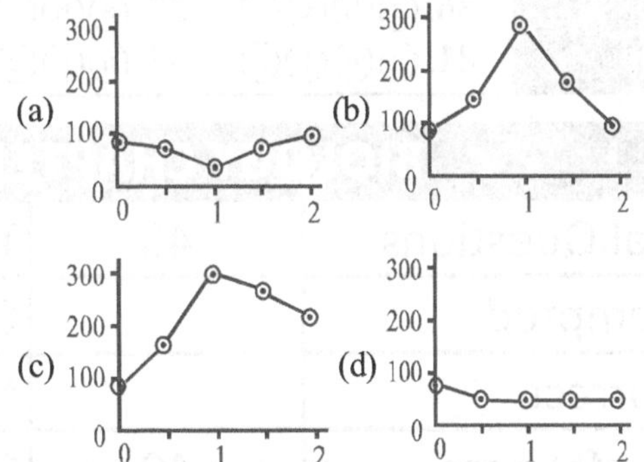

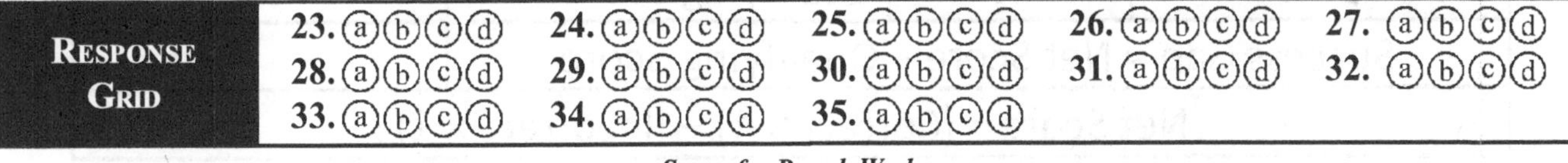
RESPONSE GRID
23. (a)(b)(c)(d) 24. (a)(b)(c)(d) 25. (a)(b)(c)(d) 26. (a)(b)(c)(d) 27. (a)(b)(c)(d)
28. (a)(b)(c)(d) 29. (a)(b)(c)(d) 30. (a)(b)(c)(d) 31. (a)(b)(c)(d) 32. (a)(b)(c)(d)
33. (a)(b)(c)(d) 34. (a)(b)(c)(d) 35. (a)(b)(c)(d)

Space for Rough Work

36. A paracrine hormone is
(a) a local hormone that acts on the cell that releases it.
(b) always acting on a wide variety of target tissues.
(c) a local hormone produced at one site but active at a different site in the body.
(d) none of the above

37. "Upregulation" of hormone receptors refers to
(a) increase in hormone receptor numbers with low hormone levels.
(b) increase in hormone receptor numbers with high neurotransmitter levels
(c) increase in hormone levels produced by increase in hormone receptor numbers
(d) decrease in hormone levels produced by decrease in hormone receptor numbers

38. In an experiment, researchers removed the ____ of young mice, and as a result, these mice were able to accept organ transplants without rejection.
(a) pineal glands (b) thymus glands
(c) thyroid glands (d) parathyroid glands

39. Which of the following is a common second messenger substance in hormone action ?
(a) Thyroid hormone (b) ADH
(c) Cyclic AMP (d) Epinephrine

40. Which of the following glands is considered the "master" endocrine gland in vertebrates ?
(a) Adrenal glands (b) Thyroid gland
(c) Hypothalamus (d) Pituitary gland

41. Through negative feedback, a hormone may shut off the secretion of an anterior pituitary hormone by :
(a) stimulating the release of a (hypothalamic) releasing hormone
(b) inhibiting the release of a (hypothalamic) inhibiting hormone
(c) inhibiting the release of a (hypothalamic) releasing hormone
(d) all of the preceding.

42. ANF is a peptide hormone and is secrected from
(a) Gastrointestinal tract (b) Kidney
(c) Post. Pituitary (d) None of these

43. Steroid hormones –
(a) have only cell surface receptors
(b) are lipophobic
(c) act through altering the activity of proteins in the target cell
(d) are produced by only adrenal cortex.

44. The hormones that initiate ejection of milk, stimulates milk production and growth of ovarian follicles are respectively known as
(a) PRL, OT and LH (b) OT, PRL and FSH
(c) LH, PRL and FSH (d) PRH, OT and LH

45. A pregnant female deliver a baby who suffers from stunted growth, mental retardation/low intelligence quotient and abnormal skin. This is the result of :
(a) Low secretion of growth hormone
(b) Cancer of the thyroid gland
(c) Over secretion of pars distalis
(d) Deficiency of iodine in diet

RESPONSE GRID					
	36. ⓐⓑⓒⓓ	37. ⓐⓑⓒⓓ	38. ⓐⓑⓒⓓ	39. ⓐⓑⓒⓓ	40. ⓐⓑⓒⓓ
	41. ⓐⓑⓒⓓ	42. ⓐⓑⓒⓓ	43. ⓐⓑⓒⓓ	44. ⓐⓑⓒⓓ	45. ⓐⓑⓒⓓ

BIOLOGY CHAPTERWISE SPEED TEST-80			
Total Questions	45	Total Marks	180
Attempted		Correct	
Incorrect		Net Score	
Cut-off Score	40	Qualifying Score	50
Success Gap = Net Score – Qualifying Score			
Net Score = (Correct × 4) – (Incorrect × 1)			

Space for Rough Work

BIOLOGY

Reproduction in Organism

Speed TEST 81

Chapter-wise

No. of Questions	Maximum Marks	Time
45	180	1 Hour

GENERAL INSTRUCTIONS

- This test contains 45 MCQ's. For each question only one option is correct. Darken the correct circle/ bubble in the Response Grid provided on each page.
- You have to evaluate your Response Grids yourself with the help of solutions provided at the end of this book.
- Each correct answer will get you 4 marks and 1 mark shall be deduced for each incorrect answer. No mark will be given/ deducted if no bubble is filled. Keep a timer in front of you and stop immediately at the end of 60 min.
- The sheet follows a particular syllabus. Do not attempt the sheet before you have completed your preparation for that syllabus.
- After completing the sheet check your answers with the solution booklet and complete the Result Grid. Finally spend time to analyse your performance and revise the areas which emerge out as weak in your evaluation.

1. Which one of the following is not a method of vegetative propagation?
(a) Budding (b) Layering
(c) Sowing (d) Tissue culture
2. A population of genetically identical individuals, obtained from asexual reproduction is
(a) Callus (b) Clone
(c) Deme (d) Aggregate
3. Natural parthenogenesis occurs in:
(a) Protozoans (b) Earthworm
(c) All insects (d) Honeybee
4. Retention of larval characters even after sexual maturity is called
(a) Parthenogenesis (b) Ontogenesis
(c) Paedogenesis (d) Neoteny
5. Asexual reproduction is an effective strategy in stable environments because
(a) gametogenesis is most efficient under these conditions.
(b) the offspring, genetically identical to their parents, are preadapted to the environment.
(c) asexual parthenogenesis produces a large amount of genetic diversity.
(d) animal cells tend to be more totipotent under stable conditions.
6. If you compared the genetic makeup of an animal produced by parthenogenesis with that of its mother, which of the following would you expect?
(a) About 100 percent genetic similarity
(b) About 50 percent genetic similarity
(c) No genetic similarity
(d) Parthenogenetic animals have no mother

RESPONSE GRID	1. ⓐⓑⓒⓓ 2. ⓐⓑⓒⓓ 3. ⓐⓑⓒⓓ 4. ⓐⓑⓒⓓ 5. ⓐⓑⓒⓓ 6. ⓐⓑⓒⓓ

Space for Rough Work

7. Which of the following statements about animals that utilize external fertilization is *false*?
   (a) They are divided equally between terrestrial and aquatic species.
   (b) Many produce large numbers of gametes to ensure successful reproduction.
   (c) The behaviours associated with mating are often highly synchronized.
   (d) The probability of any one egg being fertilized and developing into an adult can be low.
8. Which of the following statements about animal reproduction is *false* ?
   (a) Species that reproduce sexually cannot also reproduce asexually.
   (b) Viviparity, but not ovoviviparity, is common in mammals.
   (c) Male insects can remove spermatophores deposited in a female by other males.
   (d) Oogenesis and spermatogenesis both occur in simultaneous hermaphrodites.
9. Which of the following animals qualifies as a sexually reproducing, oviparous species ?
   (a) Human (b) Chicken
   (c) Kangaroo (d) Sea star
10. Benefits of asexual reproduction include all of the following except
   (a) it often allows for the production of many more offspring at the same time
   (b) it is advantageous in changing environments in which population variety is the key to successful propagation of a species
   (c) it is easier in certain environments to have offspring without searching for a mate
   (d) allowing the conservation of resources otherwise allocated to finding mates and performing ritualized courtship.
11. All the 'eyes' of a potato tuber are taken out and it is sown in the ground normally. New plants will
   (a) Not emerge (b) Emerge normally
   (c) Be weaker (d) Be healthier
12. Basal half of an onion bulb is removed and upper half is sown in the ground. New plant will
   (a) Emerge normally (b) Not emerge
   (c) Be without leaves (d) Be without flowers
13. A small portion of cane-sugar stem between the two successive nodes is cut off and sown in the soil normally. New plants will
   (a) Be formed normally (b) Not be formed
   (c) Be without juice (d) Without nodes
14. A cutting of rose plant is thoroughly waxed and planted in the soil normally, It will form
   (a) New rose plant
   (b) A dead piece of rose stem after some time
   (c) A rose plant of improved variety
   (d) None of these
15. When an ovary develops into a fruit, without fertilization, it is called
   (a) apospory (b) apogamy
   (c) parthenocarpy (d) porogamy
16. Asexual reproduction is the best strategy for plants
   (a) that are well adapted to their stable environment.
   (b) as winter approaches
   (c) when new genes must be introduced
   (d) that have underground stems.
17. Bamboo reproduces by
   (a) rhizomes (b) tubers
   (c) corms (d) stolons
18. Grafting is an example of asexual reproduction. Which of the following choices is an example of asexual reproduction involving nonvegetative parts of a plant ?
   (a) Apomixis (b) Production of corms
   (c) Production of bulbs (d) Production of rhizomes
19. What is necessary for successful grafting to occur ?
   (a) Each section must be able to form roots.
   (b) The grafted section must be able to form seeds.
   (c) Fusion of the two vascular tissues must occur.
   (d) Fusion of the two cambial tissues must occur.
20. Banana fruits are seedless, because
   (a) auxins are sprayed for rapid development of fruit.
   (b) vegetative propagation of plant.
   (c) they are triploid plants.
   (d) fruits are artificially ripened.

RESPONSE GRID					
	7. ⓐⓑⓒⓓ	8. ⓐⓑⓒⓓ	9. ⓐⓑⓒⓓ	10. ⓐⓑⓒⓓ	11. ⓐⓑⓒⓓ
	12. ⓐⓑⓒⓓ	13. ⓐⓑⓒⓓ	14. ⓐⓑⓒⓓ	15. ⓐⓑⓒⓓ	16. ⓐⓑⓒⓓ
	17. ⓐⓑⓒⓓ	18. ⓐⓑⓒⓓ	19. ⓐⓑⓒⓓ	20. ⓐⓑⓒⓓ	

Space for Rough Work

21. Consider the following statements and choose the correct option.
(i) The genetic constitution of a plant is unaffected in vegetative propagation.
(ii) Rhizome in ginger serves as an organ of vegetative reproduction.
(iii) Totipotency of cells enables us to micropropagate plants.
(a) Statements (i) and (ii) alone are true
(a) Statements (ii) and (iii) alone are true
(c) Statement (ii) alone is true
(d) All the three statements (i), (ii) and (iii) are true

22. Plants identical to mother plants can be obtained from
(a) seeds (b) stem cutting
(c) Both (a) and (b) (d) None of these

23. Ploidy of ovary, anther, egg, pollen, male gamete and zygote are respectively-
(a) 2n, 2n, n, 2n, n, 2n (b) 2n, 2n, n, n, n, 2n
(c) 2n, n, n, n, n, n (d) 2n, 2n, n, 2n, 2n, 2n

24. Offsprings of oviparous animals are at greater risk as compared to offsprings of viviparous animals because-
(a) Proper embryonic care and protection is lesser
(b) Embryo is not developed
(c) Progenies are with more variation
(d) Progenies are larger

25. The parameter(s) of senescence or old age is/are-
(a) End of the reproductive phase
(b) Concomitant change in body (like slowing metabolism)
(c) Failure of metabolism decreases
(d) Both (a) and (b)

26. The terms homothallic and monoecious are used to denote
(a) bisexual condition (b) unisexual condition
(c) staminate flowers (d) pistillate flowers

27. During regeneration, modification of an organ to other organ is known as
(a) Morphogenesis (b) Epimorphosis
(c) Morphallaxis (d) Accretionary growth

28. Cells become variable in morphology and function in different regions of the embryo. The process is
(a) differentiation (b) metamorphosis
(c) organisation (d) rearrangement

29. Earthworms, sponges, tapeworms are
(a) bisexual animals (b) unisexual animals
(c) hermaphrodites (d) Both (a) and (c)

30. The site of origin of the new plantlets in potato, dahlia, ginger and banana is-
(a) Floral buds present on stem
(b) Internodes of modified stem
(c) Nodes of modified stem
(d) Adventitious buds present on root

31. Among the following which one is not a method of vegetative propagation?
(a) Budding (b) Layering
(c) Sowing (d) Tissue culture

32. Vegetative propagation in mint occurs by:
(a) offset (b) rhizome
(c) sucker (d) runner

33. What is common between vegetative reproduction and apomixis?
(a) Both are applicable to only dicot plants
(b) Both bypass the flowering phase
(c) Both occur round the year
(d) Both produces progeny identical to the parent

34. Individuals of a clone-
(a) Are genetically similar but morphologically different
(b) Are morphologically similar but genetically different
(c) Are morphologically and genetically similar
(d) Are genetically and phenotypically different

35. Some organisms are capable of asexual or sexual reproduction. Under favourable conditions, reproduction proceeds asexually. When conditions become more stressful reproduction switchess to a sexual mode. Why?
(a) Sexual reproduction is simple and more rapid allowing larger numbers of offspring to be produced
(b) Sexual reproduction requires two separate individuals, who can mutually provide nutrient support during stress
(c) Sexual reproduction produces individuals with new combinations of recombined chromosomes increasing diversity
(d) Asexual reproduction requires more energy

RESPONSE GRID					
	21. ⓐⓑⓒⓓ	22. ⓐⓑⓒⓓ	23. ⓐⓑⓒⓓ	24. ⓐⓑⓒⓓ	25. ⓐⓑⓒⓓ
	26. ⓐⓑⓒⓓ	27. ⓐⓑⓒⓓ	28. ⓐⓑⓒⓓ	29. ⓐⓑⓒⓓ	30. ⓐⓑⓒⓓ
	31. ⓐⓑⓒⓓ	32. ⓐⓑⓒⓓ	33. ⓐⓑⓒⓓ	34. ⓐⓑⓒⓓ	35. ⓐⓑⓒⓓ

Space for Rough Work

36. Apomixis in plant means development of a plant
(a) from root cuttings
(b) without fusion of gametes
(c) from fusion of gametes
(d) from cuttings of stem

37. Which of the following is not vegetative propagule ?
(a) Rhizome and sucker
(b) Tuber and offset
(c) Bulbil (*e.g.* in *Agave*), leaf buds and bulb
(d) Antherozoid

38. Which of the following is false about external fertilization?
(a) Organisms showing external fertilization exhibit great synchrony between the sexes and release gametes.
(b) Gametes are produced in large number in water to enhance the chances of fertilization.
(c) A large number of gametes are wasted.
(d) A major advantage is that the offspring are protected from predators and there is a great chance of their survival upto adulthood.

39. Modified stem present in *Gladiolus* is:
(a) bulb (b) rhizome
(c) corm (d) bulbil

40. Which of the following are seasonal breeders?
(a) Frogs (b) Birds
(c) Lizards (d) All of these

41. Select the wrong statement:
(a) Anisogametes differ either in structure, function or behaviour.
(b) In oomycetes female gamete is smaller and motile, while male gamete is larger and non-motile.
(c) *Chalmydomonas* exhibits both isogamy and anisogamy and *Fucus* shows oogamy.
(d) Isogametes are similar in structure, function and behaviour.

42. Monoecious plant of *Chara* shows occurrence of :
(a) stamen and carpel of the same plant
(b) upper antheridium and lower oogonium on the same plant
(c) upper oogonium and lower antheridium on the same plant
(d) antheridiophore and archegoniophore on the same plant

43. Which of the following statement(s) is/are false about internal fertilization?
(i) Male gametes are motile.
(ii) Male gametes are non-motile.
(iii) Male gametes are produced in large number.
(iv) Male gametes are produced in small number.
(v) There is a significant reduction in the number of eggs produced.
(a) (i), (iii) and (v) (b) (iii) and (iv)
(c) (ii) and (iv) (d) Only (v)

44. Syngamy can occur outside the body of the organism in
(a) Fungi (b) Mosses
(c) Algae (d) Ferns

45. Select the correct sequence from the following.
(i) Juvenile phase → Senescent phase → Reproductive phase
(ii) Juvenile phase → Reproductive phase → Senescent phase
(iii) Reproductive phase → Juvenile phase → Senescent phase
(iv) Vegetative phase → Reproductive phase → Senescent phase
(a) (i) and (ii) (b) (i) and (iv)
(c) (iii) and (iv) (d) (ii) and (iv)

RESPONSE GRID					
	36. ⓐⓑⓒⓓ	37. ⓐⓑⓒⓓ	38. ⓐⓑⓒⓓ	39. ⓐⓑⓒⓓ	40. ⓐⓑⓒⓓ
	41. ⓐⓑⓒⓓ	42. ⓐⓑⓒⓓ	43. ⓐⓑⓒⓓ	44. ⓐⓑⓒⓓ	45. ⓐⓑⓒⓓ

BIOLOGY CHAPTERWISE SPEED TEST-81			
Total Questions	45	Total Marks	180
Attempted		Correct	
Incorrect		Net Score	
Cut-off Score	55	Qualifying Score	65
Success Gap = Net Score – Qualifying Score			
Net Score = (Correct × 4) – (Incorrect × 1)			

Space for Rough Work

BIOLOGY

Sexual Reproduction in Flowering Plants

Speed TEST 82

Chapter-wise

No. of Questions	Maximum Marks	Time
45	180	1 Hour

GENERAL INSTRUCTIONS

- This test contains 45 MCQ's. For each question only one option is correct. Darken the correct circle/ bubble in the Response Grid provided on each page.
- You have to evaluate your Response Grids yourself with the help of solutions provided at the end of this book.
- Each correct answer will get you 4 marks and 1 mark shall be deduced for each incorrect answer. No mark will be given/ deducted if no bubble is filled. Keep a timer in front of you and stop immediately at the end of 60 min.
- The sheet follows a particular syllabus. Do not attempt the sheet before you have completed your preparation for that syllabus.
- After completing the sheet check your answers with the solution booklet and complete the Result Grid. Finally spend time to analyse your performance and revise the areas which emerge out as weak in your evaluation.

1. Entry of pollen tube through micropyle is
   (a) Chalazogamy (b) Mesogamy
   (c) Porogamy (d) Pseudogamy
2. Dry indehiscent single-seeded fruit formed from bicarpellary syncarpous inferior ovary is
   (a) Caryopsis (b) Cypsela
   (c) Berry (d) Cremocarp
3. One of the most resistant biological material is
   (a) lignin (b) hemicellulose
   (c) lignocellulose (d) sporopollenin
4. When funiculum, chalaza, and micropyle lie in one straight line, then ovule is called –
   (a) Amphitropous (b) Orthotropous
   (c) Campylotropous (d) Anatropous
5. Which one of the following is a fruit ?
   (a) Ginger (b) Sweet potato
   (c) Radish (d) Lady's finger
6. Female gametophyte of angiosperms is represented by
   (a) Ovule
   (b) Megaspore mother cell
   (c) Embryo sac
   (d) Nucellus
7. Which of the following pair has haploid structures?
   (a) Nucellus and antipodal cells
   (b) Antipodal cells and egg cell
   (c) Antipodal cells and megaspore mother cell
   (d) Nucellus and primary endosperm nucleus
8. Polyembryony commonly occurs in
   (a) citrus (b) turmeric
   (c) tomato (d) potato

RESPONSE GRID					
	1. ⓐⓑⓒⓓ	2. ⓐⓑⓒⓓ	3. ⓐⓑⓒⓓ	4. ⓐⓑⓒⓓ	5. ⓐⓑⓒⓓ
	6. ⓐⓑⓒⓓ	7. ⓐⓑⓒⓓ	8. ⓐⓑⓒⓓ		

Space for Rough Work

9. Chasmogamy refers to the condition where –
   (a) Flowers remains closed
   (b) Flowers are absent
   (c) Flowers open
   (d) Flowers gamopetalous
10. In oogamy, fertilization involves
   (a) a small non-motile female gamete and a large motile male gamete
   (b) a large non-motile female gamete and a small motile male gamete
   (c) a large non-motile female gamete and a small nonmotile male gamete
   (d) a large motile female gamete and a small non-motile male gamete
11. Cotyledons and testa respectively are edible parts in
   (a) walnut and tamarind
   (b) french bean and coconut
   (c) cashew nut and litchi
   (d) groundnut and pomegranate
12. A *Polygonum* type of embryo sac is
   (a) 7-celled and 8-nucleate
   (b) 8-celled and 7-nucleate
   (c) 7-celled and 7-nucleate
   (d) 8-celled and 8-nucleate
13. In dicot embryo the radicle is formed by
   (a) epibasal tier of embryo
   (b) hypobasal tier of embryo
   (c) hypophysis of suspensor
   (d) terminal cell of suspensor
14. A drupe develops in
   (a) mango (b) wheat
   (c) pea (d) tomato
15. When pollen grains are not transferred from anthers to stigma in a flower, due to the barrier, it is called
   (a) herkogamy (b) heterogamy
   (c) cleistogamy (d) dichogamy
16. The parenchyma tissue which forms the bulk of ovule where the sporogenous tissue is produced is –
   (a) Megaspore mother cell
   (b) Nucellus
   (c) Ovule
   (d) Embryo sac
17. Unisexuality of flowers prevents
   (a) autogamy, but not geitonogamy
   (b) both geitonogamy and xenogamy
   (c) geitonogamy, but not xenogamy
   (d) autogamy and geitonogamy
18. Which one of the following represents an ovule, where the embryo sac becomes horse-shoe shaped and the funiculus and micropyle are close to each other?
   (a) Amphitropous (b) Circinotropous
   (c) Atropous (d) Anotropous
19. If an angiospermic male plant is diploid and female plant tetraploid, the ploidy level of endosperm will be
   (a) haploid (b) triploid
   (c) tetraploid (d) pentaploid
20. These plants flower and fruit only once in their life time and die after fruiting. These are
   (a) monocarpic plants
   (b) polycarpic plants
   (c) vegetative plants
   (d) reproductive plants
21. Select the mismatched pair.
   (a) Microsporangium — Pollen sac
   (b) Megasporangium — Nucellus
   (c) Pollen grain — Male gamete
   (d) Embryo sac — Female gametophyte

RESPONSE GRID					
	9. ⓐⓑⓒⓓ	10. ⓐⓑⓒⓓ	11. ⓐⓑⓒⓓ	12. ⓐⓑⓒⓓ	13. ⓐⓑⓒⓓ
	14. ⓐⓑⓒⓓ	15. ⓐⓑⓒⓓ	16. ⓐⓑⓒⓓ	17. ⓐⓑⓒⓓ	18. ⓐⓑⓒⓓ
	19. ⓐⓑⓒⓓ	20. ⓐⓑⓒⓓ	21. ⓐⓑⓒⓓ		

Space for Rough Work

22. A typical angiospermous ovule is attached to the placenta by means of a stalk called X. Body of the ovule fuses with X in the region called Y. Identify X and Y.

	X	Y
(a)	Funicle	Hilum
(b)	Hilum	Funicle
(c)	Funicle	Micropyle
(d)	Hilum	Chalaza

23. Which of the following options is correct?
    (a) Transfer of pollen grains from the anther to the stigma of the same flower – Autogamy.
    (b) Transfer of pollen grains from the anther of one flower to the stigma of another flower of same plant – Geitonogamy.
    (c) Transfer of pollen grains from the anther to the stigma of a genetically different plant – Xenogamy.
    (d) All of these
24. Which of the following is not a water pollinated plant?
    (a) *Zostera* (b) *Vallisneria*
    (c) *Hydrilla* (d) *Cannabis*
25. Identify the parts labelled A, B, C and D in the given figure and select the correct option.

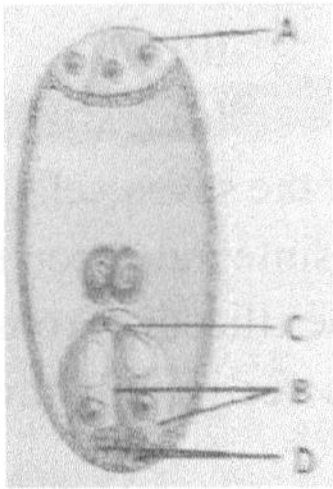

	A	B	C	D
(a)	Synergids	Antipodals	Egg	Filiform apparatus
(b)	Antipodals	Synergids	Egg	Filiform apparatus
(c)	Antipodals	Synergids	Filiform appartus	Egg
(d)	Polar nuclei	Antipodals	Filiform appartus	Egg

26. Growth of pollen tube towards embryo sac is
    (a) chemotropic (b) thigmotaxis
    (c) geotropic (d) none of these
27. The part of gynoecium that determines the complatible nature of pollen is
    (a) stigma (b) style
    (c) ovary (d) synergids
28. The innermost layer of anther is tapetum whose function is
    (a) dehiscence (b) mechanical
    (c) nutrition (d) protection
29. The female gametophyte of a typical dicot at the time of fertilization is
    (a) 8-celled (b) 7-celled
    (d) 6-celled (d) 5-celled
30. One of the most resistant biological material present in the exine of pollen grain is
    (a) pectocellulose (b) sporopollenin
    (c) suberin (d) cellulose
31. What is the function of germ pore?
    (a) Emergence of radicle
    (b) Absorption of water for seed germination
    (c) Initiation of pollen tube
    (d) All of these
32. How many meiotic divisions are required for the formation of 100 functional megaspores?
    (a) 100 (b) 50
    (c) 25 (d) 26
33. Study of pollen grains is called
    (a) micrology (b) anthology
    (c) palynology (d) pomology

RESPONSE GRID					
	22. ⓐⓑⓒⓓ	23. ⓐⓑⓒⓓ	24. ⓐⓑⓒⓓ	25. ⓐⓑⓒⓓ	26. ⓐⓑⓒⓓ
	27. ⓐⓑⓒⓓ	28. ⓐⓑⓒⓓ	29. ⓐⓑⓒⓓ	30. ⓐⓑⓒⓓ	31. ⓐⓑⓒⓓ
	32. ⓐⓑⓒⓓ	33. ⓐⓑⓒⓓ			

Space for Rough Work

34. Which of these is a condition that makes flowers invariably autogamous?
(a) Dioecy
(b) Self incompatibilty
(c) Cleistogamy
(d) Xenogamy

35. An embryo may sometimes develop from any cell of embryo sac other than egg. It is termed as
(a) apospory (b) apogamy
(c) parthenogenesis (d) parthenocarpy

36. Endosperm is completely consumed by the developing embryo in
(a) pea and groundnut
(b) maize and castor
(c) castor and groundnut
(d) maize and pea

37. The portion of embryonal axis between plumule (future shoot) and cotyledons is called
(a) hypocotyl (b) epicotyl
(c) coleohize (d) coleoptile

38. Stigma of a flower is removed before pollination. The flower will
(a) Form fruit normally
(b) Not form fruit
(c) Form deformed fruit
(d) Form fruit smaller than normal size

39. In a pea flower, all petals are removed before pollination. The flower will
(a) Form fruit normally
(b) Not form fruit
(c) Form smaller pod
(d) Form deformed pod

40. A drop of glue is placed on the stigma of a flower before pollination. The flower will
(a) Not form fruit
(b) Form normal fruit
(c) Form sticky fruit
(d) Form fruit filled with glue

41. An apomictic seed contains an embryo that is
(a) produced when two sperm fertilize one egg.
(b) developed from one egg alone.
(c) the result of parental self-fertilization
(d) genetically identical to its parent.

42. The embryo is carefully taken out of pea seed and sown in the soil and watered normally. New plant will
(a) Be healthier
(b) Be weaker
(c) Not be formed
(d) Be formed normally

43. Angiospermic plant has chromosome number of 24. The number of chromosomes in pollens will be
(a) 6 (b) 12
(c) 24 (d) 48

44. What is the fate of the seven cells of the embryo sac ?
(a) All but one disintegrate upon fertilization.
(b) Two become fertilized; the others disintegrate.
(c) Two become fertilized; the others fuse to form endosperm.
(d) All are involved in nuclear fusion events.

45. A close relation between flower and pollinating agent is best exhibited by :
(a) *Cocos* (b) *Salvia*
(c) *Yucca* (d) *Avena*

RESPONSE GRID					
	34. ⓐⓑⓒⓓ	35. ⓐⓑⓒⓓ	36. ⓐⓑⓒⓓ	37. ⓐⓑⓒⓓ	38. ⓐⓑⓒⓓ
	39. ⓐⓑⓒⓓ	40. ⓐⓑⓒⓓ	41. ⓐⓑⓒⓓ	42. ⓐⓑⓒⓓ	43. ⓐⓑⓒⓓ
	44. ⓐⓑⓒⓓ	45. ⓐⓑⓒⓓ			

BIOLOGY CHAPTERWISE SPEED TEST-82			
Total Questions	45	Total Marks	180
Attempted		Correct	
Incorrect		Net Score	
Cut-off Score	40	Qualifying Score	55
Success Gap = Net Score – Qualifying Score			
Net Score = (Correct × 4) – (Incorrect × 1)			

Space for Rough Work

BIOLOGY

Human Reproduction

Speed TEST 83

Chapter-wise

No. of Questions	Maximum Marks	Time
45	180	1 Hour

GENERAL INSTRUCTIONS

- This test contains 45 MCQ's. For each question only one option is correct. Darken the correct circle/ bubble in the Response Grid provided on each page.
- You have to evaluate your Response Grids yourself with the help of solutions provided at the end of this book.
- Each correct answer will get you 4 marks and 1 mark shall be deduced for each incorrect answer. No mark will be given/ deducted if no bubble is filled. Keep a timer in front of you and stop immediately at the end of 60 min.
- The sheet follows a particular syllabus. Do not attempt the sheet before you have completed your preparation for that syllabus.
- After completing the sheet check your answers with the solution booklet and complete the Result Grid. Finally spend time to analyse your performance and revise the areas which emerge out as weak in your evaluation.

1. Breast feeding suspends pregnancy due to
   (a) post pregnancy lower levels of FSH and LH
   (b) post pregnancy higher levels of FSH and LH which put negative check on ovulation
   (c) inhibiting the release of LH by prolactin and thus countering the effects of LH on the ovarian follicles
   (d) increasing the release of inhibin by prolactin and thus countering the effects of FSH on the ovarian follicles
2. The human embryo, with 8 to 16 blastomere is called
   (a) Morula (b) Blastula
   (c) Gastrula (d) Foetus
3. A person which shows the secondary sexual characters of both male and female is called –
   (a) Intersex (b) Hermaphrodite
   (c) Bisexual (d) Gynandromorph
4. Which one of the following is the correct matching of the events occurring during menstrual cycle?
   (a) Proliferative phase: Rapid regeneration of myometrium and maturation of Graffian follicle.
   (b) Development of corpus luteum : Secretory phase and increased secretion of progesterone.
   (c) Menstruation: Breakdown of myometrium and ovum not fertilised.
   (d) Ovulation: LH and FSH attain peak level and sharp fall in the secretion of progesterone.
5. The second maturation division of the mammalian ovum occurs:
   (a) in the graafian follicle following the first maturation division
   (b) shortly after ovulation before the ovum makes entry into the Fallopian tube
   (c) until after the ovum has been penetrated by a sperm
   (d) until the nucleus of the sperm has fused with that of the ovum

RESPONSE GRID	1. ⓐⓑⓒⓓ	2. ⓐⓑⓒⓓ	3. ⓐⓑⓒⓓ	4. ⓐⓑⓒⓓ	5. ⓐⓑⓒⓓ

Space for Rough Work

6. Foetal ejection reflex in human female is induced by
(a) release oxytocin from pituitary
(b) fully developed foetus and placenta
(c) differentiation of mammary glands
(d) pressure exerted by amniotic fluid

7. Which one of the following statements about human sperm is correct?
(a) Acrosome has a conical pointed structure used for piercing and penetrating the egg, resulting in fertilisation
(b) The sperm lysine in the acrosome dissolve the egg envelope facilitating fertilisation
(c) Acrosome serves as a sensory structure leading the sperm towards the ovum
(d) Acrosome serves no particular function

8. Sertoli cells are found in
(a) ovaries and secrete progesterone
(b) adrenal cortex and secrete adrenaline
(c) seminiferous tubules and provide nutrition to germ cells
(d) pancreas and secrete cholecystokinin

9. The phase of menstrual cycle in humans that lasts for 7-8 days, is
(a) follicular phase (b) ovulatory phase
(c) luteal phase (d) menstruation

10. Cessation of menstrual cycle in women is called
(a) menopause (b) lactation
(c) ovulation (d) parturition

11. In human female the blastocyst
(a) Forms placenta even before implantation
(b) Gets implanted into uterus 3 days after ovulation
(c) Gets nutrition from uterine endometrial secretion only after implantation
(d) Gets implanted in endometrium by the trophoblast cells

12. Bulbourethral gland is present in
(a) Males and is another name for Uterus masculina
(b) Females and is another name for Bertholin's gland
(c) Males and is another name for Cowper's gland
(d) None of these

13. Which one of the following are rich in fructose, calcium and some enzymes?
(a) Male accessory glands
(b) Liver
(c) Pancreas
(d) Salivary glands

14. Umbilical cord has
(a) Two arteries carrying blood to placenta and one vein returning blood to foetus
(b) One artery carrying blood to placenta and two veins returning blood to foetus
(c) Two arteries bringing blood to foetus and one vein carrying blood to placenta
(d) One artery bringing blood to foetus and two veins carrying blood to placenta

15. Which of the following induces parturition ?
(a) Vasopressin
(b) Oxytocin
(c) Growth hormone
(d) Thyroid stimulating hormone

16. What happens during fertilisation in humans after many sperms reach close to the ovum?
(a) Cells of corona radiata trap all the sperms except one
(b) Only two sperms nearest the ovum penetrate zona pellucida
(c) Secretions of acrosome helps one sperm enter cytoplasm of ovum through zona pellucida
(d) All sperms except the one nearest to the ovum lose their tails

17. The part of fallopian tube closest to the ovary is
(a) isthmus (b) infundibulum
(c) cervix (d) ampulla

18. The chemical substance found in the surface layer of cytoplasm of spermatozoa is:
(a) fertilizin (b) agglutinin
(c) antifertilizin (d) hyaluronidase

RESPONSE GRID					
	6. ⓐⓑⓒⓓ	7. ⓐⓑⓒⓓ	8. ⓐⓑⓒⓓ	9. ⓐⓑⓒⓓ	10. ⓐⓑⓒⓓ
	11. ⓐⓑⓒⓓ	12. ⓐⓑⓒⓓ	13. ⓐⓑⓒⓓ	14. ⓐⓑⓒⓓ	15. ⓐⓑⓒⓓ
	16. ⓐⓑⓒⓓ	17. ⓐⓑⓒⓓ	18. ⓐⓑⓒⓓ		

Space for Rough Work

19. Which of the following diseases is caused by the under secretion of cortisol?
(a) Anaemia
(b) Addison's disease
(c) Hyperglycemia
(d) Mental illness or retardation

20. Reabsorption of chloride ions from glomerular filtrate in kidney tubule occurs by
(a) Active transport (b) Diffusion
(c) Osmosis (d) Brownian movement

21. If for some reason, the vasa efferentia in the human reproductive system get blocked, the gametes will not be transported from
(a) testes to epididymis
(b) epididymis to vas deferens
(c) ovary to uterus
(d) vagina to uterus

22. The nutritive cells found in seminiferous tubules are
(a) Leydig's cells (b) atretic follicular cells
(c) Sertoli cells (d) chromaffin cells.

23. Seminal plasma in humans is rich in
(a) fructose and calcium but has no enzymes
(b) glucose and certain enzymes but has no calcium
(c) fructose and certain enzymes but poor in calcium
(d) fructose, calcium and certain enzymes

24. The function of the secretion of prostate gland is to
(a) inhibit sperm activity
(b) attract sperms
(c) stimulate sperm activity
(d) none of these

25. The head of the epididymis at the head of the testis is called
(d) cauda epididymis
(b) vas deferens
(c) caput epididymis
(d) gubernaculum

26. Which part of ovary in mammals acts as an endocrine gland after ovulation?
(a) Stroma
(b) Germinal epithelium
(c) Vitelline membrane
(d) Graafian follicle

27. The female external genitalia include
(i) Ovary (ii) Mammary gland
(iii) Mons pubis (iv) Clitoris
(a) (i) and (ii) (b) (ii) and (iii)
(c) (iii), (iv) and (v) (d) (ii), (iii) and (v)

28. 2n = 16 is in a primary spermatocyte which is in metaphase of first meiotic division. What shall be the total number of chromatids in each of the secondary spermatocyte?
(a) 16 (b) 24
(c) 32 (d) 8

29. In humans, at the end of the first meiotic division, the male germ cells differentiate into the
(a) spermatids
(b) spermatogonia
(c) primary spermatocytes
(d) secondary spermatocytes

30. The sperms undergo physiological maturation, acquiring increased motility and fertilizing capacity in
(a) seminiferous tubules
(b) vasa efferentia
(c) epididymis
(d) vagina

31. At what stage of life is oogenesis initiated in a human female?
(a) At puberty
(b) During menarch
(c) During menopause
(d) During embryonic development

32. The middle piece of the sperm contains
(a) proteins (b) mitochondria
(c) centriole (d) nucleus

RESPONSE GRID					
	19. ⓐⓑⓒⓓ	20. ⓐⓑⓒⓓ	21. ⓐⓑⓒⓓ	22. ⓐⓑⓒⓓ	23. ⓐⓑⓒⓓ
	24. ⓐⓑⓒⓓ	25. ⓐⓑⓒⓓ	26. ⓐⓑⓒⓓ	27. ⓐⓑⓒⓓ	28. ⓐⓑⓒⓓ
	29. ⓐⓑⓒⓓ	30. ⓐⓑⓒⓓ	31. ⓐⓑⓒⓓ	32. ⓐⓑⓒⓓ	

Space for Rough Work

33. Corpus luteum is developed from
(a) Graafian follicle (b) nephrostome
(c) oocyte (d) none of these

34. Spermatogenesis is induced by
(a) FSH (b) ICSH
(C) STH (d) ATH

35. Layers of an ovum from outside to inside is
(a) corona radiata, zona pellucida and vitelline membrane
(b) zona pellucida, corona radiata and vitelline membrane
(c) vitelline membrane, zona pellucida and corona radiata
(d) zona pellucida, vitelline membrane and corona radiata

36. Name the hormone that has no role in menstruation.
(a) LH (b) FSH
(c) Estradiol (d) TSH

37. The time for optimum chances of conception in a woman is ________ starting from the day of menstruation.
(a) 1st day (b) 4th day
(c) 14th day (d) 26th day

38. Repair of endometrium is undertaken by
(a) LH (b) FSH
(c) estrogen (d) prolactin

39. The sex of the foetus will be decided at
(a) fertilization by male gamete
(b) implantation
(c) fertilization by female gamete
(d) the start of cleavage

40. Match Column-I with Column-II and select the correct option from the codes given below.

Column-I	Column-II
A. Cleavage	(i) Fertilization
B. Morula	(ii) Mitotic divisions
C. Polyspermy	(iii) Endometric
D. Implantation	(iv) Little mulberry

(a) A-(ii), B-(iv), C-(i), D-(iii)
(b) A-(i), B-(iv), C-(ii), D-(iii)
(c) A-(iv), B-(ii), C-(i), D-(iii)
(d) A-(ii), B-(iv), C-(iii), D-(i)

41. Which part of the sperm plays an important role in penetrating the egg membrane?
(a) Allosome (b) Tail
(c) Autosome (d) Acrosome

42. Which of the following hormones is not a secretory product of human placenta?
(a) Human chorionic gonadotropin
(b) Prolactin
(c) Estrogen
(d) Progesterone

43. After birth, colostrum is released from mammary glands which is rich in
(a) fat and low in proteins
(b) proteins and low in fat
(c) proteins, antibodies and low in fat
(d) proteins, fat and low in antibodies

44. The correct sequence in the process of development of human embryo is
(a) fertilization—zygote—cleavage—morula—blastula—gastrula
(b) fertilization—cleavage—morula—zygote—blastula—gastrula
(c) fertilization—zygote—blastula—morula—cleavage—gastrula
(d) cleavage—zygote—fertilization—morula—blastula—gastrula

45. The given figure refers to which type of reproduction in yeast?

(a) Binary fission (b) Budding
(c) Layering (d) Fusion

RESPONSE GRID

33. ⓐⓑⓒⓓ 34. ⓐⓑⓒⓓ 35. ⓐⓑⓒⓓ 36. ⓐⓑⓒⓓ 37. ⓐⓑⓒⓓ
38. ⓐⓑⓒⓓ 39. ⓐⓑⓒⓓ 40. ⓐⓑⓒⓓ 41. ⓐⓑⓒⓓ 42. ⓐⓑⓒⓓ
43. ⓐⓑⓒⓓ 44. ⓐⓑⓒⓓ 45. ⓐⓑⓒⓓ

BIOLOGY CHAPTERWISE SPEED TEST-83

Total Questions	45	Total Marks	180
Attempted		Correct	
Incorrect		Net Score	
Cut-off Score	55	Qualifying Score	60
Success Gap = Net Score – Qualifying Score			
Net Score = (Correct × 4) – (Incorrect × 1)			

Space for Rough Work

BIOLOGY

Reproductive Health

Speed TEST 84

Chapter-wise

No. of Questions	Maximum Marks	Time
45	180	1 Hour

GENERAL INSTRUCTIONS

- This test contains 45 MCQ's. For each question only one option is correct. Darken the correct circle/ bubble in the Response Grid provided on each page.
- You have to evaluate your Response Grids yourself with the help of solutions provided at the end of this book.
- Each correct answer will get you 4 marks and 1 mark shall be deduced for each incorrect answer. No mark will be given/ deducted if no bubble is filled. Keep a timer in front of you and stop immediately at the end of 60 min.
- The sheet follows a particular syllabus. Do not attempt the sheet before you have completed your preparation for that syllabus.
- After completing the sheet check your answers with the solution booklet and complete the Result Grid. Finally spend time to analyse your performance and revise the areas which emerge out as weak in your evaluation.

1. Consider the statements given below regarding contraception and answer as directed thereafter:
   (i) Medical Termination of Pregnancy (MTP) during first trimester is generally safe
   (ii) Generally chances of conception are nil until mother breast-feeds the infant upto two years
   (iii) Intrauterine devices like copper-T are effective contraceptives
   (iv) Contraception pills may be taken upto one week after coitus to prevent conception
   Which two of the above statements are correct?
   (a) ii and iii (b) iii and iv
   (c) i and iii (d) i and ii
2. Amniocentesis is a technique
   (a) by which the essential amino acids in the body can be estimated
   (b) by which any chromosomal anomalies in the foetus can be detected
   (c) in which the sex of the foetus can be reversed
   (d) that can be used for correcting genetic disorders of the foetus
3. Tying up or removing a small part of fallopian duct is called
   (a) Vasectomy (b) Ductus arteriosus
   (c) Archidectomy (d) Tubectomy
4. Copper-T is a device that prevents
   (a) implantation of blastocyst
   (b) ovulation
   (c) fertilization
   (d) egg maturation
5. The diaphragm, cervical cap and vaults are
   (a) Disposable contraceptive devices
   (b) Reusable contraceptives
   (c) IUDs
   (d) Implants
6. The transfer of zygote or early embryo (up to 8 blastomere) into fallopian tube is
   (a) IVF and ET (b) ZIFT
   (c) GIFT (d) IUT

RESPONSE GRID	1. ⓐⓑⓒⓓ	2. ⓐⓑⓒⓓ	3. ⓐⓑⓒⓓ	4. ⓐⓑⓒⓓ	5. ⓐⓑⓒⓓ
	6. ⓐⓑⓒⓓ				

Space for Rough Work

7. The technique called gamete intrafallopian transfer (GIFT) is recommended for those females:
(a) who cannot produce an ovum
(b) who cannot retain the foetus inside uterus.
(c) whose cervical canal is too narrow to allow passage for the sperms
(d) who cannot provide suitable environment for fertilisation

8. The copper ions of IUDs
(a) Suppress the motility and fertilization capacity of sperms
(b) Make the uterus unsuitable for implantation
(c) Increase phagocytosis of sperms
(d) Make cervix hostile to sperms

9. Condoms are barriers that cover–
(a) Penis in male and ovary in female.
(b) Penis in male and cervix and vagina in female.
(c) Scrotum in male and cervix and vagina in female.
(d) Cervix in male and vagina in female.

10. Birth control pills check ovulation in female by inhibiting the secretion of –
(a) follicle stimulating hormone
(b) luteinizing hormone
(c) Both (a) and (b)
(d) None of the above

11. Identical twins are produced when
(a) One fertilized egg divides and two blastomeres separate
(b) One sperm fertilizes two eggs
(c) One egg is fertilized with two sperms
(d) Two eggs are fertilized

12. Progestasert and LNG-20 are
(a) Implants (b) Copper releasing IUDs
(c) Non-medicated IUDs (d) Hormone releasing IUDs

13. Read the following 4-statements and mark the option that has both correct statements
(i) MTP was legalized in 1971
(ii) Inability to conceive or produce children even after 2 years of unprotected sexual cohabitation is called infertility
(iii) Surgical method of contraception prevents gamete formation
(iv) MTPs are relatively safe up to 12 weeks of pregnancy
(a) (i) and (ii) (b) (ii) and (iii)
(c) (iii) and (iv) (d) (i) and (iii)

14. Medical Termination of Pregnancy (MTP) is considered safe up to how many weeks of pregnancy?
(a) Eight weeks (b) Twelve weeks
(c) Eighteen weeks (d) Six weeks

15. Ultrasound of how much frequency is beamed into human body for sonography ?
(a) 15 – 30 MHZ (b) 1 – 15 MHZ
(b) 45 – 70 MHZ (d) 30 – 45 MHZ.

16. What is the figure given below showing in particular ?

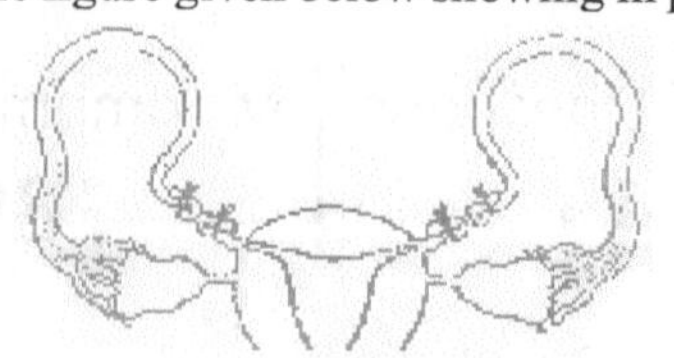

(a) Ovarian cancer (b) Uterine cancer
(c) Tubectomy (d) Vasectomy

17. *In vitro* fertilisation is a technique that involves transfer of which one of the following into the fallopian tube ?
(a) Zygote only
(b) Embryo only, upto 8 cell stage
(c) Either zygote or early embryo upto 8 cell stage
(d) Embryo of 32 cell stage

18. MTP is practised mainly to –
(a) get rid of unwanted female child legally.
(b) get rid of unwanted pregnancies due to failure of contraception.
(c) both (a) and (b).
(d) decrease population size.

19. In amniocentesis, the fluid is taken from –
(a) foetal blood
(b) mother's blood
(c) body fluid of mother
(d) fluid surrounding foetus

20. Which of the following is not *true* about the birth control pill ?
(a) The pill works by preventing ovulation.
(b) The pill works by preventing implantation.
(c) The ovarian cycle is suspended by the birth control pill.
(d) The birth control pill contains low doses of estrogen and progesterone.

21. Which of the following birth control measures can be considered as the safest?
(a) The rhythm method
(b) The use of physical barriers
(c) Temination of unwanted pregnancy
(d) Sterilization techniques

RESPONSE GRID					
	7. ⓐⓑⓒⓓ	8. ⓐⓑⓒⓓ	9. ⓐⓑⓒⓓ	10. ⓐⓑⓒⓓ	11. ⓐⓑⓒⓓ
	12. ⓐⓑⓒⓓ	13. ⓐⓑⓒⓓ	14. ⓐⓑⓒⓓ	15. ⓐⓑⓒⓓ	16. ⓐⓑⓒⓓ
	17. ⓐⓑⓒⓓ	18. ⓐⓑⓒⓓ	19. ⓐⓑⓒⓓ	20. ⓐⓑⓒⓓ	21. ⓐⓑⓒⓓ

Space for Rough Work

22. Using which contraceptive also provides protection from contracting STDs and AIDS ?
(a) Diaphragms (b) Spermicidal foams
(c) Condoms (d) Lactational amenorrhoea

23. Copper-T is a device that prevents
(a) implantation of blastocyst
(b) ovulation
(c) fertilization
(d) egg maturation

24. Cu ions released from copper - releasing Intra Uterine Devices (IUDs):
(a) make uterus unsuitable for implantation
(b) increase phagocytosis of sperms
(c) suppress sperm motility
(d) prevent ovulation

25. Which one of the following is the most widely accepted method of contraception in India, as at present ?
(a) Cervical caps
(b) Tubectomy
(c) Diaphragms
(d) IUDs. (Intra uterine devices)

26. The test-tube Baby Programme employs which one of the following techniques?
(a) Intra cytoplasmic sperm injection (ICSI)
(b) Intra uterine insemination (IUI)
(c) Gamete intra fallopian transfer (GIET)
(d) Zygote intra fallopian transfer (ZIFT)

27. Oral contraceptive pills are composed of
(a) progestrogens only
(b) progestrogen and estrogen combination
(c) progestrogen-testosterone combination
(d) both (a) or (b)

28. Which of the following cannot be detected in a developing foetus by amniocentesis?
(a) Sex of the foetus
(b) Down syndrome
(c) Jaundice
(d) Klinefelter syndrome

29. One of the legal methods of birth control is :
(a) by abstaining from coitus from day 10 to 17 of the menstrual cycle
(b) by having coitus at the time of day break
(c) by a premature ejaculation during coitus
(d) abortion by taking an appropriate medicine

30. One of the following is **not** a method of contraception – which one?
(a) Tubectomy
(b) Condoms
(c) Pills of a combination of oxytocin and vasopressin
(d) Lippes loop

31. Which one of the following statements is correct regarding Sexually Transmitted Diseases (STD)?
(a) The chances of a 5 year boy contacting a STD are very little
(b) A person may contact syphilis by sharing milk with one already suffering from the disease
(c) Haemophilia is one of the STD
(d) Genital herpes and sickle-cell anaemia are both STD

32. The stage transferred into the uterus after induced fertilization of ova in the laboratory is:
(a) Zygote
(b) Embryo at 4 blastomere stage
(c) Embryo at 2 blastomere stage
(d) Morula

33. Reproductive health in society can be improved by –
(i) Introduction of sex education in schools.
(ii) Increased medical assistance.
(iii) Awareness about contraception and STDs.
(iv) Equal opportunities to male and female child.
(v) Ban on aminocentesis.
(vi) Encouraging myths and misconceptions.
(a) All of these (b) (i), (ii), (iv) and (vi)
(c) (i), (ii), (iii), (iv) and (v) (d) (ii) and (v)

34. What is true for " Lactational amenorrhoea"?
(i) It means absence of menstruation.
(ii) Ovulation does not occur during the lactational period.
(iii) Chances of failure of contraception are almost nil upto six months following parturition.
(iv) Side effects are almost nil.
(v) Contraceptive efficiency reduces after the period of intense lactation.
(vi) It is natural method of contraception.
(vii) It increases phagocytosis of sperms
(a) (ii), (iii), (iv), (v) and (vi)
(b) All except (vii)
(c) (ii), (iii), (iv) and (v)
(d) All of these

35. IUDs-
(i) Increase phagocytosis of sperms.
(ii) Release Cu ions that suppress sperm motility and fertilising capacity of sperms.
(iii) Make the uterus unsuitable for implantation.
(iv) Make the cervix hostile to sperms.
(v) Prevent semen from entering the female reproductive tract.
(a) (i), (ii), (iii), (iv) and (v) (b) (i), (ii), (iii) and (iv)
(c) (i) and (ii) (d) (ii), (iii) and (iv)

RESPONSE GRID					
	22. ⓐⓑⓒⓓ	23. ⓐⓑⓒⓓ	24. ⓐⓑⓒⓓ	25. ⓐⓑⓒⓓ	26. ⓐⓑⓒⓓ
	27. ⓐⓑⓒⓓ	28. ⓐⓑⓒⓓ	29. ⓐⓑⓒⓓ	30. ⓐⓑⓒⓓ	31. ⓐⓑⓒⓓ
	32. ⓐⓑⓒⓓ	33. ⓐⓑⓒⓓ	34. ⓐⓑⓒⓓ	35. ⓐⓑⓒⓓ	

Space for Rough Work

36. Match Column -I with Column - II.

	Column I		Column II
A.	Non-medicated IUDs	(i)	Lippes loop
B.	Hormone releasing IUDs	(ii)	Multiload (iii)7
C.	Copper releasing IUDs	(iii)	CuT
		(iv)	Cu7
		(v)	LNG-(ii)0
		(vi)	Progestasert

(a) A-(i); B-(ii, vi); C-(iii, iv, v)
(b) A-(i); B-(v, vi); C-(ii, iii, iv)
(c) A-(ii); B-(v, vi); C-(i, iii, iv)
(d) A-(ii); B-(i, vi); C-(iii, iv, v)

37. Progesterone pill helps in preventing pregnancy by not allowing –
(a) ova formation (b) fertilization
(c) implantation (d) None of these

38. The permissible use of the technique amniocentesis is for
(a) detecting sex of the unborn foetus
(b) artificial insemination
(c) transfer of embryo into the uterus of the surrogate mother
(d) detecting any genetic abnormality

39. The family planning programmes in India were initiated in
(a) 1951 (b) 1961
(c) 1971 (d) 1981

40. RCH stands for
(a) Routine Check-up of Health
(b) Reproduction Cum Hygiene
(c) Reversible Contraceptive Hazards
(d) Reproductive and Child Health Care

41. 'Saheli' a new oral contraceptive developed by
(a) All Indian Institute of Medical Science
(b) Central Drug Research Institute
(c) Health Care Pvt. Ltd.
(d) Bharat Immunologicals & Biologicals corp. Ltd.

42. Artificial insemination mean
(a) transfer of sperms of husband to a test tube containing ova.
(b) artificial introduction of sperms of a healthy donor into the vagina.
(c) introduction of sperms of a healthy donor directly into the ovary.
(d) transfer of sperms of a healthy donor to a test tube containing ova.

43. What is true for an ideal contraceptive ?
(i) It should be user-friendly.
(ii) It should be easily available.
(iii) It should be ineffective and reversible with least side effects.
(iv) It should be effective and reversible with least side effects.
(v) It should interfere with the sexual act of the user.
(a) All of these (b) (i), (ii) and (iii)
(c) (i), (ii) and (iv) (d) (i),(ii), (iv) and (v)

44. Choose the correct statements –
(i) According to the WHO, reproductive health is total well-being in the physical, social, emotional, behavioural aspects of reproduction.
(ii) According to the WHO, reproductive health is total well being in the physical, social and emotional aspects of reproduction.
(iii) A reproductively healthy society has people with physically and functionally normal reproductive organs.
(iv) Reproductively healthy societies have abnormal sex-related emotional and behavioural interactions.
(a) (i), (ii) and (iii) (b) (ii) and (iv)
(c) (i) and (iii) (d) (i) only

45. Study the given reasons on the basis of which pregnancy can be terminated. Identify the correct reasons.
(i) To get rid of unwanted pregnancies.
(ii) To prevent the fatality or harmfulness to the mother or to foetus or both due to the continuation of pregnancy.
(iii) Termination of pregnancy is safe in each and every case.
(iv) If the foetus is male.
(v) It plays an important role in decreasing the population.
(a) (i), (ii), only (b) (ii), (iii) only
(c) (iii), (iv), (v) only (d) All of these

RESPONSE GRID					
	36. ⓐⓑⓒⓓ	37. ⓐⓑⓒⓓ	38. ⓐⓑⓒⓓ	39. ⓐⓑⓒⓓ	40. ⓐⓑⓒⓓ
	41. ⓐⓑⓒⓓ	42. ⓐⓑⓒⓓ	43. ⓐⓑⓒⓓ	44. ⓐⓑⓒⓓ	45. ⓐⓑⓒⓓ

BIOLOGY CHAPTERWISE SPEED TEST-84

Total Questions	45	Total Marks	180
Attempted		Correct	
Incorrect		Net Score	
Cut-off Score	48	Qualifying Score	55
Success Gap = Net Score – Qualifying Score			
Net Score = (Correct × 4) – (Incorrect × 1)			

Space for Rough Work

BIOLOGY

Speed TEST 85

Chapter-wise

Principles of Inheritance and Variation

No. of Questions	Maximum Marks	Time
45	180	1 Hour

GENERAL INSTRUCTIONS

- This test contains 45 MCQ's. For each question only one option is correct. Darken the correct circle/ bubble in the Response Grid provided on each page.
- You have to evaluate your Response Grids yourself with the help of solutions provided at the end of this book.
- Each correct answer will get you 4 marks and 1 mark shall be deduced for each incorrect answer. No mark will be given/ deducted if no bubble is filled. Keep a timer in front of you and stop immediately at the end of 60 min.
- The sheet follows a particular syllabus. Do not attempt the sheet before you have completed your preparation for that syllabus.
- After completing the sheet check your answers with the solution booklet and complete the Result Grid. Finally spend time to analyse your performance and revise the areas which emerge out as weak in your evaluation.

1. Cross between AaBB and aaBB will form
   (a) 1 AaBB : 1aaBB (b) All AaBB
   (c) 3 AaBB : 1 aaBB (d) 1 AaBB : 3 aaBB
2. Red (RR) *Antirrhinum* is crossed with white (WW) one. Offspring RW are pink. This is an example of
   (a) dominant -recessive
   (b) incomplete dominance
   (c) hybrid
   (d) supplementary genes
3. The dihybrid ratio in F_2 - generation is
   (a) 1 : 1 : 1 : 1 (b) 2 : 1 : 2 : 1
   (c) 3:1 (d) 9 : 3 : 3 : 1
4. Genetic map is one that
   (a) shows the distribution of various species in a region
   (b) establishes sites of the genes on a chromosome
   (c) establishes the various stages in gene evolution
   (d) show the stages during the cell division
5. A gene pair hides the effect of another gene. The phenomenon is
   (a) epistasis (b) dominance
   (c) mutation (d) None of the above
6. Independent assortment of genes does not take place when
   (a) genes are located on homologous chromosomes
   (b) genes are linked and located on same chromosomes
   (c) genes are located on non-homologous chromosomes
   (d) All the above
7. Extranuclear inheritance occurs in
   (a) peroxisome and ribosome
   (b) chloroplast and mitochondria
   (c) mitochondria and ribosome
   (d) chloroplast and lysosome
8. Test cross involves
   (a) crossing between two F_1 hybrids
   (b) crossing the F_1 hybrid with a double recessive genotype
   (c) crossing between two genotypes with dominant trait
   (d) crossing between two genotypes with recessive trait
9. When one gene controls two or more different characters simultaneously, the phenomenon is called
   (a) apomixis (b) pleiotropy
   (c) polyploidy (d) polyteny

RESPONSE GRID					
	1. ⓐⓑⓒⓓ	2. ⓐⓑⓒⓓ	3. ⓐⓑⓒⓓ	4. ⓐⓑⓒⓓ	5. ⓐⓑⓒⓓ
	6. ⓐⓑⓒⓓ	7. ⓐⓑⓒⓓ	8. ⓐⓑⓒⓓ	9. ⓐⓑⓒⓓ	

Space for Rough Work

10. ABO blood group system is due to
(a) multifactor inheritance
(b) incomplete dominance
(c) multiple allelism
(d) epistasis

11. In humans, male XXY and female XXXX occur due to
(a) aneuploidy
(b) euploidy
(c) Nutosomal syndrome
(d) none of these

12. Haemophilia is more common in males because it is a
(a) Recessive character carried by Y-chromosome
(b) Dominant character carried by Y-chromosome
(c) Dominant trait carried by X-chromosome
(d) Recessive trait carried by X-chromosome

13. The most striking example of point mutation is found in a disease called
(a) thalassemia (b) night blindness
(c) down's syndrome (d) sickle cell anaemia

14. In Down's syndrome of a male child, the sex complement is
(a) XO (b) 45 + XY
(c) 45 + XX (d) XXY

15. Barr body in mammals represents
(a) all the heterochromatin in female cells
(b) Y-chromosomes in somatic cells of male
(c) all heterochromatin in male and female cells
(d) one of the two X-chromosomes in somatic cells of females

16. A person with the sex chromosomes XXY suffers from
(a) Down's syndrome
(b) Klinefelter's syndrome
(c) Turner's syndrome
(d) Gynandromorphism

17. *Drosophila* flies with XXY genotype are females, but human beings with such genotype are abnormal males. It shows that
(a) Y-chromosome is essential for sex determination in *Drosophila.*
(b) Y-chromosome is female determinant in *Drosophila.*
(c) Y-chromosome is male determination in human beings.
(d) Y-chromosome has no role in sex determination either in *Drosophila* or in human beings.

18. Lack of independent assortment of two genes A and B in fruit fly *Drosophila* is due to
(a) repulsion (b) recombination
(c) linkage (d) crossing over

19. Select the **incorrect** statement from the following:
(a) Galactosemia is an inborn error of metabolism
(b) Small population size results in random genetic drift in a population
(c) Baldness is a sex -limited trait
(d) Linkage is an exception to the principle of independent assortment in heredity

20. The "Cri-du-Chat" syndrome is caused by change in chromosome structure involving
(a) deletion (b) duplication
(c) inversion (d) translocation

21. Biometric genetics deals with :
(a) the biochemical explanations of various genetical phenomena
(b) the effect of environment on genetic set up organisms
(c) the genetical radiations on the living organisms
(d) the inheritance of quantitative traits

22. Which one of the following conditions correctly describes the manner of determining the sex in the given example?
(a) Homozygous sex chromosomes (ZZ) determines female sex in birds.
(b) XO type of sex chromosomes determines male sex in grasshopper.
(c) XO condition in human as found in Turner syndrome, determines female sex.
(d) Homozygous sex chromosomes (XX) produces male in *Drosophila.*

23. Select the correct statement from the ones given below with respect to dihybrid cross.
(a) Tightly linked genes on the same chromosome show higher recombinations
(b) Genes far apart on the same chromosome show very few recombinations
(c) Genes loosely linked on the same chromosome show similar recombinations as the tightly linked ones
(d) Tightly linked genes on the same chromosome show very few recombinations

24. Chromosome complement with 2n – 1 is called
(a) Monosomy (b) Trisomy
(c) Nullisomy (d) Tetrasomy

RESPONSE GRID				
10. ⓐⓑⓒⓓ	11. ⓐⓑⓒⓓ	12. ⓐⓑⓒⓓ	13. ⓐⓑⓒⓓ	14. ⓐⓑⓒⓓ
15. ⓐⓑⓒⓓ	16. ⓐⓑⓒⓓ	17. ⓐⓑⓒⓓ	18. ⓐⓑⓒⓓ	19. ⓐⓑⓒⓓ
20. ⓐⓑⓒⓓ	21. ⓐⓑⓒⓓ	22. ⓐⓑⓒⓓ	23. ⓐⓑⓒⓓ	24. ⓐⓑⓒⓓ

Space for Rough Work

25. In a cross between AABB × aabb, the ratio of F_2 genotypes between AABB, AaBB, Aabb and aabb would be
(a) 9 : 3 : 3 : 1 (b) 2 : 1 : 1 : 2
(c) 1 : 2 : 2 : 1 (d) 7 : 5 : 3 : 1

26. The basis of karyotaxonomy is
(a) Number of nucleoli
(b) Sedimentation rate of ribosomes
(c) Chromosome banding
(d) Chromosome number

27. Study the pedigree chart given below:

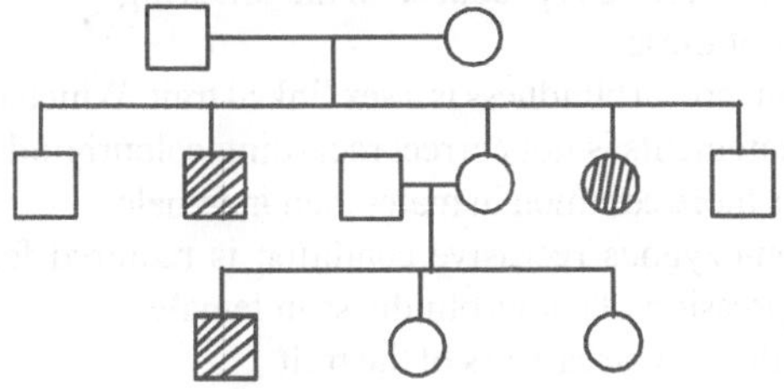

What does it show?
(a) Inheritance of a recessive sex-linked disease like haemophilia
(b) Inheritance of a sex-linked inborn error of metabolism like phenylketonuria
(c) Inheritance of a condition like phenylketonuria as an autosomal recessive trait
(d) The pedigree chart is wrong as this is not possible

28. Which one is a hereditary disease ?
(a) Cataract (b) Leprosy
(c) Blindness (d) Phenylketonuria

29. Diploid chromosome number in humans is
(a) 46 (b) 44
(c) 48 (d) 42

30. Given below is a pedigree chart showing the inheritance of a certain sex-linked trait in humans

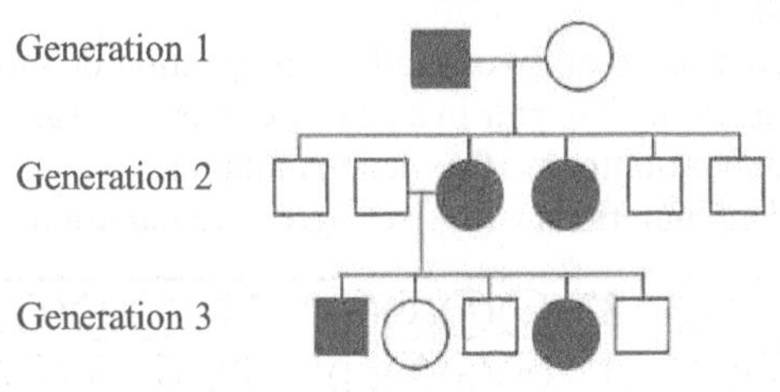

Key :

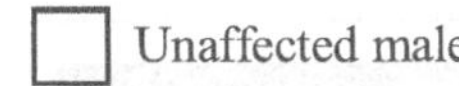

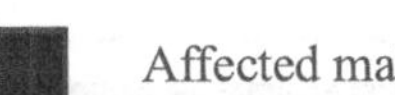

Unaffected female

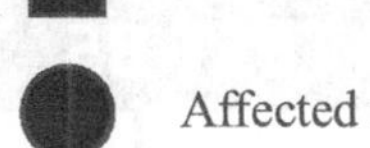

The trait traced in the above pedigree chart is
(a) dominant X - linked
(b) recessive X-linked
(c) dominant Y - linked
(d) recessive Y-linked

31. In maize, coloured endosperm (C) is dominant over coloureless (c); and full endosoperm (R) is dominant over shrunken (r). When a dihybrid of F_1 generation was test crossed, it produced your phenotypes in the following percentage:
Coloured full - 48% Coloured shrunken - 5%
Colourless full - 7% Colourless shrunken - 40%
From this data, what will be the distance between two non-allelic genes?
(a) 48 units (b) 5 units
(c) 7 units (d) 12 units

32. Inheritance of which of the following traits is shown in the given cross?

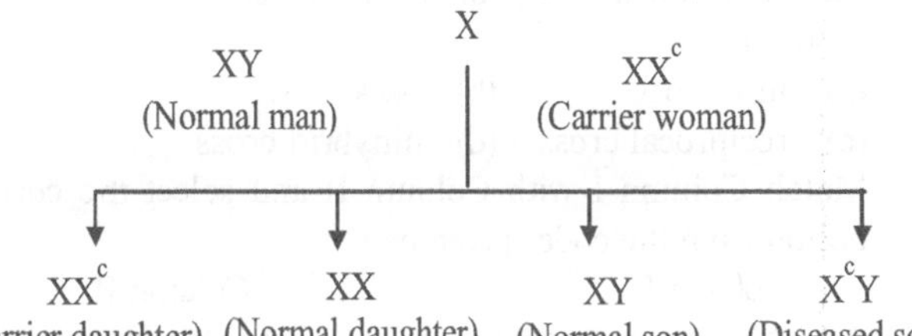

(a) X-linked dominant trait
(b) X-linked recessive trait
(c) Autosomal dominant trait
(d) Autosomal recessive trait

33. More than two alternate forms of a gene present on the same locus are called (i). They are produced due to repeated (ii) of the same gene but in different directions. Their well known example is (iii).

	(i)	(ii)	(iii)
(a)	Epistatic genes	Crossing over	polydactyly
(b)	Multiple alleles	mutations	human blood groups
(c)	Supplementary	mutations	hypertrichosis
(d)	Linked genes	Crossing over	aljaptonuria

RESPONSE GRID					
	25. ⓐⓑⓒⓓ	26. ⓐⓑⓒⓓ	27. ⓐⓑⓒⓓ	28. ⓐⓑⓒⓓ	29. ⓐⓑⓒⓓ
	30. ⓐⓑⓒⓓ	31. ⓐⓑⓒⓓ	32. ⓐⓑⓒⓓ	33. ⓐⓑⓒⓓ	

Space for Rough Work

34. In fruit files, long wing is dominant to vestigial wing. When heterozygous long-winged files were crossed with vestigial-winged files, 192 offsprings were produced. Of these, 101 had long wings and 91 had vestigial wings.
If an exact Mendelian ratio had been obtained, then the number of each phenotype would have been

	Long-winged	Vestigial-winged
(a)	64	128
(b)	96	96
(c)	128	64
(d)	192	0

35. Phenotypic and genotypic ratio is similar in case of
(a) complete dominance
(b) incomplete dominance
(c) over dominance
(d) epistasis

36. To determine the genotype of a tall plant of F_2 generation, Mendel crossed this plant with a dwarf plant. This coss represents a
(a) test cross (b) back cross
(c) reciprocal cross (d) dihybrid cross

37. Match Column-I with Column-II and select the correct option from the codes given below.

	Column-I		Column-II
A.	A single trait controlled by three or more than three alleles	(i)	Pleiotropy
B.	A single trait controlled by three or more than three genes	(ii)	Multiple alleles
C.	A single gene exhibits multiple phenotypic expression	(iii)	Polygenic inheritance

38. Chromosomal theory of inheritanc was given by
(a) Morgan et al (b) Sutton and Boveri
(c) Hugo de Vries (d) Gregor J. Mendel

39. What is true about the crossing over between linked genes?
(a) No crossing over at all
(b) High percentage of crossing over
(c) Hardly any crossing over
(d) None of these

40. Which of the following is incorrect regarding ZW-ZZ type of sex determination?
(a) It occurs in birds and some reptiles
(b) Females are homogametic and males are heterogametic
(c) 1 : 1 sex ratio is produced in the offsprings
(d) All of these

41. Red green colourblindness is a sex linked trait. Which of the given statements is not correct regarding colourblindness?
(a) It is more common in males than in females
(b) Homozygous recessive condition is required for the expression of colourblindness in females
(c) Males can be carriers of the trait
(d) Colourblind women always have colourblind father and always produce colourblind son.

42. At a particular locus, frequency of allele A is 0.6 and that of allele a is 0.4. What would be the frequency of heterozygotes in a random mating population at equilibrium?
(a) 0.36 (b) 0.16
(c) 0.24 (d) 0.48

43. The distance between the genes is measured by
(a) Angstrom (b) map unit
(c) Dobson unit (d) millimetre

44. Which of the following trait is controlled by dominant autosomal genes?
(a) Polydactyly
(b) Huntigton's chorea
(c) PTC (phenylthiocarbomide) tasting
(d) All of these

45. The mutations that involve addition, deletion or substitution of a single base pair in a gene are referred to as
(a) point mutations (b) lethal mutations
(c) silent mutations (d) retrogressive mutations

RESPONSE GRID					
	34. ⓐⓑⓒⓓ	35. ⓐⓑⓒⓓ	36. ⓐⓑⓒⓓ	37. ⓐⓑⓒⓓ	38. ⓐⓑⓒⓓ
	39. ⓐⓑⓒⓓ	40. ⓐⓑⓒⓓ	41. ⓐⓑⓒⓓ	42. ⓐⓑⓒⓓ	43. ⓐⓑⓒⓓ
	44. ⓐⓑⓒⓓ	45. ⓐⓑⓒⓓ			

BIOLOGY CHAPTERWISE SPEED TEST-85			
Total Questions	45	Total Marks	180
Attempted		Correct	
Incorrect		Net Score	
Cut-off Score	45	Qualifying Score	60
Success Gap = Net Score – Qualifying Score			
Net Score = (Correct × 4) – (Incorrect × 1)			

Space for Rough Work

BIOLOGY

Molecular Basis of Inheritance

Speed TEST 86 Chapter-wise

No. of Questions	Maximum Marks	Time
45	180	1 Hour

GENERAL INSTRUCTIONS

- This test contains 45 MCQ's. For each question only one option is correct. Darken the correct circle/ bubble in the Response Grid provided on each page.
- You have to evaluate your Response Grids yourself with the help of solutions provided at the end of this book.
- Each correct answer will get you 4 marks and 1 mark shall be deduced for each incorrect answer. No mark will be given/ deducted if no bubble is filled. Keep a timer in front of you and stop immediately at the end of 60 min.
- The sheet follows a particular syllabus. Do not attempt the sheet before you have completed your preparation for that syllabus.
- After completing the sheet check your answers with the solution booklet and complete the Result Grid. Finally spend time to analyse your performance and revise the areas which emerge out as weak in your evaluation.

1. Which form of RNA has a structure resembling clover leaf?
(a) rRNA (b) hn RNA
(c) m RNA (d) t RNA
2. Other than DNA polymerase, which is/ are the enzyme(s) involved in DNA synthesis?
(a) Topoisomerase (b) Helicase
(c) RNA primase (d) All of these
3. The enzyme used for joining two DNA fragments is called:
(a) ligase (b) restriction endonuclease
(c) DNA polymerase (d) gyrase
4. Nucleotide arrangement in DNA can be seen by
(a) X-ray crystallography
(b) electron microscope
(c) ultracentrifuge
(d) light microscope
5. The okazaki fragments in DNA chain growth
(a) polymerize in the 3' - to - 5' direction and forms replication fork
(b) prove semi-conservative nature of DNA replication
(c) polymerize in the 5' - to - 3' direction and explain 3' - to - 5' DNA replication
(d) result in transcription
6. Reverse transcriptase is
(a) RNA dependent RNA polymerase
(b) DNA dependent RNA polymerase
(c) DNA dependent DNA polymerase
(d) RNA dependent DNA polymerase
7. Telomerase is an enzyme which is a
(a) simple protein
(b) RNA
(c) ribonucleoprotein
(d) repetitive DNA
8. DNA template sequence of CTGATAGC is transcribed over mRNA as
(a) GUCTUTCG (b) GACUAUCG
(c) GAUTATUG (d) UACTATCU

RESPONSE GRID	
	1. ⓐⓑⓒⓓ 2. ⓐⓑⓒⓓ 3. ⓐⓑⓒⓓ 4. ⓐⓑⓒⓓ 5. ⓐⓑⓒⓓ
	6. ⓐⓑⓒⓓ 7. ⓐⓑⓒⓓ 8. ⓐⓑⓒⓓ

Space for Rough Work

9. During replication of a bacterial chromosome DNA synthesis starts from a replication origin site and
   (a) RNA primers are involved
   (b) is facilitated by telomerase
   (c) moves in one direction of the site
   (d) moves in bi-directional way
10. The enzyme, which helps to cut one strand of DNA duplex to release tension of coiling of two strands is
   (a) DNA ligase
   (b) DNA polymerase I
   (c) topoisomerase
   (d) helicase or unwindases
11. Histones are
   (a) glycoproteins (b) mucoproteins
   (c) basic proteins (d) acid proteins
12. One gene-one enzyme relationship was established for the first time in
   (a) *Salmonella typhimurium*
   (b) *Escherichia coli*
   (c) *Diplocococcus pneumoniae*
   (d) *Neurospora crassa.*
13. The transforming principle of *Pneumococcus* as found out by Avery, MacLeod and McCarty was
   (a) mRNA (b) DNA
   (c) protein (d) polysaccharide
14. How many pair of nucleotides are present in one helix of B- DNA?
   (a) 10 (b) 12
   (c) 5 (d) 6
15. Read the following four statements (i - iv).
   (i) In transcription, adenosine pairs with uracil.
   (ii) Regulation of *lac* operon by repressor is referred to as positive regulation.
   (iii) The human genome has approximately 50,000 genes.
   (iv) Haemophilia is a sex-linked recessive disease.
   How many of the above statements are correct?
   (a) Two (b) Three
   (c) Four (d) One
16. In negative operon
   (a) co-repressor binds with repressor
   (b) co-repressor does not bind with repressor
   (c) co-repressor binds with inducer
   (d) cAMP have negative effect on *lac* operon
17. Transfer of genetic material from one bacterium to another in the transduction process is through
   (a) conjugation
   (b) bacteriophages
   (c) another bacterium
   (d) physical contact between donor and recipient strain
18. Telomere and eukaryotic chromosome possesses short segments of
   (a) guanine rich repeats.
   (b) thymine rich repeats.
   (c) cytosine rich repeats.
   (d) adenine rich repeats.
19. Refer the given figure of nucleosome and select the option that correctly identifies the parts A, B and C.

	A	B	C
(a)	DNA	Histone octamer	H_1 histone
(b)	Histone octamer	H_1 histone	DNA
(c)	Histone	DNA	H_1 histone
(d)	DNA	H_1 histone octamer	Histone octamer

20. The process of transformation is not affected by which of the following enzymes?
   A. DNase B. RNase
   C. Peptidase D. Lipase
   (a) A, B (b) A, B, C, D
   (c) B, C, D (d) A, B, C
21. Select the incorrect statement regarding DNA replication
   (a) Leading strand is formed is 5' $\rightarrow$ 3' direction
   (b) Okazaki fragments are formed in 5' $\rightarrow$ 3' direction
   (c) DNA polymerase catalyses polymerisation in 5' $\rightarrow$ 3' direction
   (d) DNA polymerase catalyses polymerisation in 3' $\rightarrow$ 5' direction

RESPONSE GRID					
	9. ⓐⓑⓒⓓ	10. ⓐⓑⓒⓓ	11. ⓐⓑⓒⓓ	12. ⓐⓑⓒⓓ	13. ⓐⓑⓒⓓ
	14. ⓐⓑⓒⓓ	15. ⓐⓑⓒⓓ	16. ⓐⓑⓒⓓ	17. ⓐⓑⓒⓓ	18. ⓐⓑⓒⓓ
	19. ⓐⓑⓒⓓ	20. ⓐⓑⓒⓓ	21. ⓐⓑⓒⓓ		

Space for Rough Work

22. Identify the labels A, B, C and D in the given structure of tRNA and select the correct option.

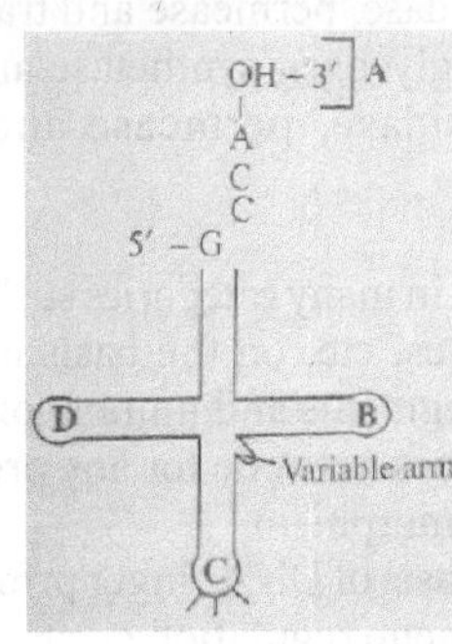

	A	B	C	D
(a)	Anticodon loop	TΨC loop	AA binding stie	DHU loop
(b)	AA binding site	TΨC loop	Anticodon loop	DHU loop
(c)	AA binding site	DHU loop	Anticodon loop	TΨC loop
(d)	AA binding site	DHU loop	TΨC loop	Anticodon loop

23. In one polynucleotide strand of a DNA molecule the ratio of A + T/G + C is 0.3. What is the A + G/T + C ratio of the entire DNA molecule?
(a) 0.3 (b) 0.6
(c) 1.2 (d) 1

24. Chemically, RNA is (i) reactive and (ii) stable as compared to DNA.
(a) (i) equally, (ii) equally
(b) (i) less, (ii) more
(c) (i) more, (ii) less
(d) (i) more, (ii) equally

25. Given diagram represents the components of a transcription unit. Select the correct answer regarding it.

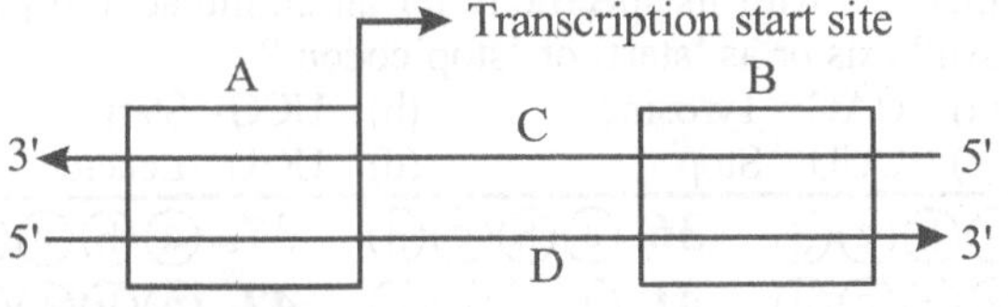

	A	B	C	D
(a)	Teminator	Promoter	Template strand	Coding strand
(b)	Promoter	Terminator	Coding strand	Template strand
(c)	Promoter	Terminator	Template strand	Coding strand
(d)	Terminator	Promoter	Coding strand	Template strand

26. In transcription in eukaryotes, heterogenous nuclear RNA (hnRNA) is transcribed by
(a) RNA polymerase I
(b) RNA polymerase II
(c) RNA polymerase III
(d) all of these

27. What would happen if in a gene encoding a polypeptide of 50 amino acids, 25th codon (UAU) is mutated to UAA?
(a) A polypeptide of 24 amino acids will be formed.
(b) Two polypeptides of 24 and 25 amino acids will be formed
(c) A polypeptide of 49 amino acids will be formed
(d) A polypeptide of 25 amino acids will be formed

28. Regulation of gene expression occurs at the level of
(a) transcription (b) processing/splicing
(c) translation (d) all of these

29. Find out the wrong sentence about heterochromatin.
(a) It is densely packed
(b) It stains dark
(c) It is transcriptionally active
(d) It is late replicating

30. Other than DNA polymerase, which are the enzymes involved in DNA synthesis?
(a) topoisomerase (b) helicase
(c) RNA primase (d) all of these

31. What does "*lac*" refer to in what we call the *lac* operon?
(a) The number 1,00,000 (b) Lactose
(c) Lactase (d) *Lac* insect

32. The error rate of changing an incorrect base with another incorrect base during proofreading is
(a) 1 in 10 bases (b) 1 in 100 bases
(c) 1 in 1,000 bases (d) 1 in 10,000 bases

RESPONSE GRID				
22. ⓐⓑⓒⓓ	23. ⓐⓑⓒⓓ	24. ⓐⓑⓒⓓ	25. ⓐⓑⓒⓓ	26. ⓐⓑⓒⓓ
27. ⓐⓑⓒⓓ	28. ⓐⓑⓒⓓ	29. ⓐⓑⓒⓓ	30. ⓐⓑⓒⓓ	31. ⓐⓑⓒⓓ
32. ⓐⓑⓒⓓ				

Space for Rough Work

33. DNA fingerprinting refers to
(a) molecular analysis of profiles of DNA samples
(b) analysis of DNA samples using imprinting devices
(c) techniques used for molecular analysis of different specimens of DNA
(d) techniques used for identification of fingerprints of individuals

34. In negative operon
(a) co-repressor binds with repressor
(b) co-repressor does not bind with repressor
(c) co-repressor binds with inducer
(d) cAMP have negative effect on *lac* operon

35. Genes that are involved in turning on or off the transcription of a set of structural genes are called
(a) Operator genes (b) Redundant genes
(c) Regulator genes (d) Polymorphic genes

36. If the gene encoding the *lac* repressor is mutated so that it can no longer bind the operator, will transcription of that operon occur?
(a) Yes, but only when lactose is present.
(b) No, because RNA polymerase is need to transcribe the genes.
(c) Yes, because the operator will not be bound by repressor and RNA polymerase can transcribe the *lac* operon.
(d) No, because cAMP levels are low when the repressor is nonfunctional.

37. Transcriptional regulation in prokaryotes can occur by
(a) a repressor binding an operator and preventing transcription.
(b) an activator binding upstream from a promoter and positively affecting transcription.
(c) different promoter sequences binding RNA polymerase more tightly, resulting in more effective transcriptional initiation.
(d) All of the above

38. Process used for amplication or multiplication of DNA for finger printing is
(a) polymerse chain reaction
(b) nesslerisation
(c) southern blotting
(d) northern blotting

39. Lactose operon produces enzymes
(a) β-galactosidase, permease and glycogen synthetase.
(b) β-galactosidase, permease and transacetylase.
(c) Permease, glycogen synthetase and transacetylase.
(d) β-galactosidase, permease and phosphoglucose isomerase.

40. Satellite DNA
(a) is classified in many categories such as micro-satellites, minisatellites, etc. on the basis of base composition length of segments and number of repetitive units.
(b) normally does not code for any protein.
(c) shows polymorphism.
(d) forms the basis of DNA finger printing.

41. In prokaryotes, gene regulation occurs at the level of
(a) transcription (b) translation
(c) post-transcription (d) post-translation

42. The regulation of tryptophan synthesis in *E. coli* is an example of affecting gene expression through
(a) translational control.
(b) transcriptional control.
(c) homeotic gene control.
(d) breaking down mRNA molecules.

43. Transcription in prokaryotic cell is :
(a) initiated at a promoter using one of three RNA polymerases (RNA polymerase II).
(b) initiated at a start codon with the help of initiation factors and the small subunit of the ribosome.
(c) initiated at a promoter and uses only one strand of DNA, the template strand, to synthesize a complementary RNA strand.
(d) is terminated at stop codons.

44. DNA replication is an ______ process and ______ energy.
(a) exergonic; does not require
(b) endothermic; does require
(c) endergonic; does require
(d) endothermic; does not require

45. Which one of the following triplet codes, is correctly matched with its specificity for an amino acid in protein synthesis or as 'start' or 'stop' codon ?
(a) UAC – Tyrosine (b) UCG – Start
(c) UUU – Stop (d) UGU – Leucine

RESPONSE GRID					
	33. ⓐⓑⓒⓓ	34. ⓐⓑⓒⓓ	35. ⓐⓑⓒⓓ	36. ⓐⓑⓒⓓ	37. ⓐⓑⓒⓓ
	38. ⓐⓑⓒⓓ	39. ⓐⓑⓒⓓ	40. ⓐⓑⓒⓓ	41. ⓐⓑⓒⓓ	42. ⓐⓑⓒⓓ
	43. ⓐⓑⓒⓓ	44. ⓐⓑⓒⓓ	45. ⓐⓑⓒⓓ		

BIOLOGY CHAPTERWISE SPEED TEST-86			
Total Questions	45	Total Marks	180
Attempted		Correct	
Incorrect		Net Score	
Cut-off Score	55	Qualifying Score	65
Success Gap = Net Score – Qualifying Score			
Net Score = (Correct × 4) – (Incorrect × 1)			

Space for Rough Work

BIOLOGY

Evolution

Speed TEST 87

Chapter-wise

No. of Questions	Maximum Marks	Time
45	180	1 Hour

GENERAL INSTRUCTIONS

- This test contains 45 MCQ's. For each question only one option is correct. Darken the correct circle/ bubble in the Response Grid provided on each page.
- You have to evaluate your Response Grids yourself with the help of solutions provided at the end of this book.
- Each correct answer will get you 4 marks and 1 mark shall be deduced for each incorrect answer. No mark will be given/ deducted if no bubble is filled. Keep a timer in front of you and stop immediately at the end of 60 min.
- The sheet follows a particular syllabus. Do not attempt the sheet before you have completed your preparation for that syllabus.
- After completing the sheet check your answers with the solution booklet and complete the Result Grid. Finally spend time to analyse your performance and revise the areas which emerge out as weak in your evaluation.

1. Genetic drift operates only in
   (a) smaller populations
   (b) larger populations
   (c) mendelian populations
   (d) island populations
2. *Archaeopteryx* is connecting link between
   (a) Reptiles and birds
   (b) Reptiles and mammals
   (c) Fishes and reptiles
   (d) Chordates and nonchordates
3. Which of the following is true?
   (a) Wings of birds and insects are homologous organs.
   (b) Human hands and bird's wings are analogous organs.
   (c) Human hands and bat's wings are analogous organs.
   (d) Flipper of seal and wing of birds are homologous organs.
4. Which one of the following phenomena supports Darwin's concept of natural selection in organic evolution?
   (a) Development of transgenic animals.
   (b) Production of 'Dolly', the sheep by cloning.
   (c) Prevalence of pesticide resistance insects.
   (d) Development of organs from 'stem cells' for organ transplantation.
5. What is the correct arrangement of periods of palaeozoic era in ascending order in geological time scale?
   (a) Cambrian → Devonian → Ordovician → Silurian → Carboniferous → Permian
   (b) Cambrian → Ordovician → Silurian → Devonian → Carboniferous → Permian
   (c) Cambrian → Ordovician → Devonian → Silurian → Carboniferous → Permian
   (d) Silurian → Devonian → Cambrian → Ordovician → Permian → Carboniferous
6. The brain capacity of *Homo erectus* was about
   (a) 650 cc (b) 900 cc
   (c) 1500 cc (d) 1400 cc

RESPONSE GRID	1. ⓐⓑⓒⓓ 2. ⓐⓑⓒⓓ 3. ⓐⓑⓒⓓ 4. ⓐⓑⓒⓓ 5. ⓐⓑⓒⓓ 6. ⓐⓑⓒⓓ

Space for Rough Work

7. Following is the digrammatic representation of the operation of natural selection on different traits. Which of the following options correctly identifies all the three graphs A, B and C.

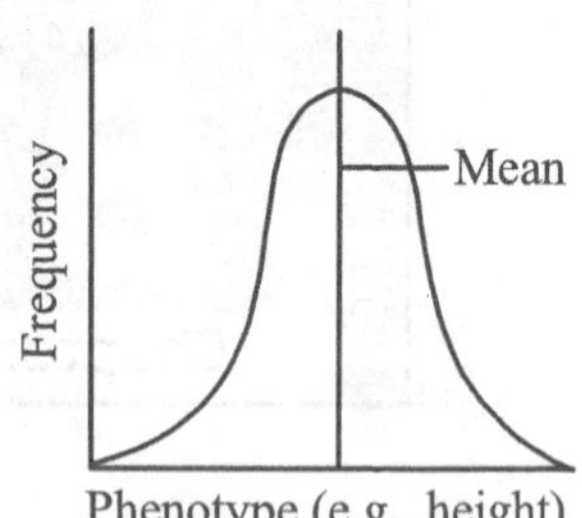

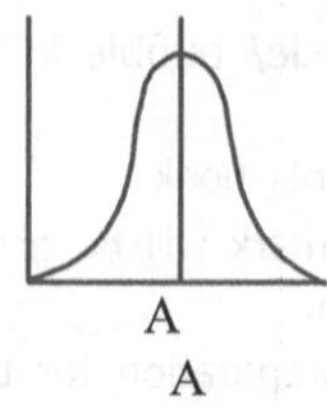

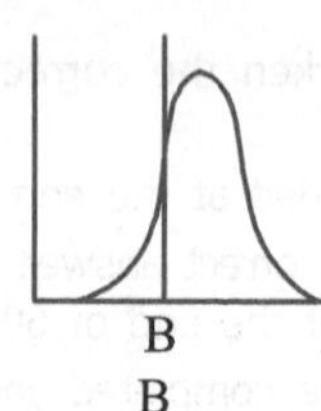

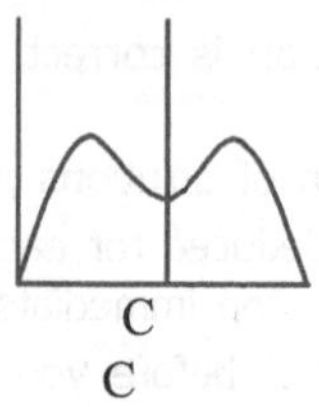

	A	B	C
(a)	Directional	Stabilizing	Disruptive
(b)	Stabilizing	Directional	Disruptive
(c)	Disruptive	Stabilizing	Directional
(d)	Directional	Disruptive	Stabilizing

8. First life form on earth was a
(a) cyanobacterium (b) chemoheterotroph
(c) autotroph (d) photoautotroph

9. The cranial capacity was largest among the
(a) Peking man (b) Java ape man
(c) African man (d) Neanderthal man

10. The Hardy-Weinberg principle cannot operate if
(a) the population is very large
(b) frequent mutations occur in the population
(c) the population has no chance of interaction with other populations
(d) free interbreeding occurs among all members of the population

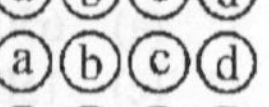

11. The different forms of interbreeding species that live in different geographical regions are called
(a) sibling species (b) sympatric species
(c) allopatric species (d) polytypic species

12. At a particular locus, frequency of allele A is 0.6 and that of allele a is 0.4. What would be the frequency of heterozygotes in a random mating population at equilibrium?
(a) 0.36 (b) 0.16
(c) 0.24 (d) 0.48

13. On the primitive earth, polymers such as proteins and nucleic acids in aqueous suspension formed the spherical aggregates. These are called
(a) primitosomes (b) liposomes
(c) primitogens (d) coacervates

14. Which of the following evidences does not favour the Lamarckian concept of inheritance of acquired characters?
(a) Lack of pigment in cave-dwelling animals
(b) Melanization in peppered moth
(c) Absence of limbs in snakes
(d) Presence of webbed toes in aquatic birds.

15. Genetic drift is change of
(a) gene frequency in same generation
(b) appearance of recessive genes
(c) gene frequency from one generation to next
(d) None of these

16. The Miller-Urey abiotic synthesis experiment (and other subsequent, similar experiments) showed that...
(a) simple organic molecules can form spontaneously under conditions like those thought to prevail early in the earth's history.
(b) the earliest life forms introduced large amounts of oxygen to the atmosphere.
(c) life can be created in a test tube.
(d) long chains of DNA can form under abiotic conditions.

17. In evolutionary terms, an organism's fitness is measured by its
(a) health
(b) contribution to the gene pool of the next generation
(c) mutation rate
(d) genetic variability

18. Frequency of a character or a mutant gene in a population is expected to increase if the phenotype or its gene is.
(a) dominant (b) favourably selected
(c) recessive (d) sex linked

RESPONSE GRID					
	7. ⓐⓑⓒⓓ	8. ⓐⓑⓒⓓ	9. ⓐⓑⓒⓓ	10. ⓐⓑⓒⓓ	11. ⓐⓑⓒⓓ
	12. ⓐⓑⓒⓓ	13. ⓐⓑⓒⓓ	14. ⓐⓑⓒⓓ	15. ⓐⓑⓒⓓ	16. ⓐⓑⓒⓓ
	17. ⓐⓑⓒⓓ	18. ⓐⓑⓒⓓ			

Space for Rough Work

19. In a population of bears, which would be considered the fittest?
(a) The biggest bear
(b) The bear having the largest number of mutations
(c) The bear that blends in with its environment the best
(d) The bear that leaves the most descendants

20. Presence of temporary gill pouches in embryos of snakes. birds and mammals indicates that
(a) these embryos need the pouches for breathing
(b) common ancestor of these animals had gill pouches
(c) lungs evolved from gills
(d) fluid medium in which these embryos develop has abundant

21. Which of the following statements is correct?
(a) Present apes are ancestors of man anatomically
(b) Proconsul was perhaps the common ancestor of apes and man
(c) Proconsul was the ancestor of man and not of apes
(d) None of these

22. What is common to whale, seal and shark?
(a) Thick subcutaneous fat
(b) Convergent evolution
(c) Homoiothermy
(d) Seasonal migration

23. One of the important consequences of geographical isolation is:
(a) preventing speciation
(b) speciation through reproductive isolation
(c) random creation of new species
(d) no change in the isolated fauna

24. Which one of the following in birds, indicates their reptilian ancestry?
(a) Scales on their hind limbs
(b) Eggs with a calcareous shell
(c) Four-chambered heart
(d) Both (a) and (b)

25. Jurassic period of the mesozoic era was characterised by:
(a) Radiation of reptiles and origin of mammal-like reptiles
(b) Dinosaurs become extinct and angiosperms appeared
(c) Flowering plants and first dinosaurs appeared
(d) Gymnosperms were dominant plants and first birds appeared

26. Which one of the following scientists name is correctly matched with the theory put forth by him?
(a) Weismann - Theory of continuity of Germplasm
(b) Pasteur - Inheritance of acquired characters
(c) De Vries - Natural selection
(d) Mendel - Theory of Pangenesis

27. The eye of octopus and eye of cat show different patterns of structure, yet they perform similar function. This is an example of:
(a) Homologous organs that have evolved due to divergent evolution.
(b) Analogous organs that have evolved due to convergent evolution.
(c) Analogous organs that have evolved due to divergent evolution.
(d) Homologous organs that have evolved due to convergent evolution.

28. Variation in gene frequencies within populations can occur by chance rather than by natural section. The is referred to as:
(a) genetic drift
(b) random mating
(c) genetic load
(d) genetic flow

29. The finch species of Galapagos Islands are grouped according to their food sources. Which of the following is not a finch food?
(a) Seeds (b) Carrion
(c) Insects (d) Tree buds

30. Evolution is
(a) progressive development of a race
(b) history and development of a race alongwith variations
(c) history of a race
(d) development of a race

31. Homologous organs are
(a) Wings of Insects and Bat
(b) Gills of Fish and lungs of Rabbit
(c) Pectoral fins of Fish and fore limbs of Horse
(d) Wings of Grasshopper and Crow

RESPONSE GRID					
	19. ⓐⓑⓒⓓ	20. ⓐⓑⓒⓓ	21. ⓐⓑⓒⓓ	22. ⓐⓑⓒⓓ	23. ⓐⓑⓒⓓ
	24. ⓐⓑⓒⓓ	25. ⓐⓑⓒⓓ	26. ⓐⓑⓒⓓ	27. ⓐⓑⓒⓓ	28. ⓐⓑⓒⓓ
	29. ⓐⓑⓒⓓ	30. ⓐⓑⓒⓓ	31. ⓐⓑⓒⓓ		

Space for Rough Work

32. Theory of inheritance of acquired characters was given by
(a) Wallace (b) Lamarck
(c) Darwin (d) De Vries

33. The kind of evolution in which two species of different geneology come to resemble one another closely, is termed as
(a) progressive evolution
(b) convergent evolution
(c) parallel evolution
(d) retrogressive evolution

34. The presence of gill slits in the embryos of all vertebrates, supports the theory of
(a) biogenesis
(b) recapitulation
(c) metamorphosis
(d) organic evolution

35. The change of the light-coloured variety of peppered moth *(Biston betularia)* to its darker variety *(Biston carbonaria)* is due to
(a) mutation (b) regeneration
(c) genetic isolation (d) temporal isolation

36. Which of the following primate is the closest relative of humans?
(a) Rhesus monkey (b) Orangutan
(c) Gorilla (d) Gibbon

37. Which of the following is the relatively most accurate method for dating of fossils?
(a) Radio-carbon method
(b) Potassium-argon method
(c) Electron-spin resonance method
(d) Uranium-lead method

38. Adaptive radiation refers to
(a) evolution of different species from a common ancestor
(b) migration of members of a species to different geographical areas
(c) power of adaptation in an individual to a variety of environments
(d) adaptations due to geographical isolation.

39. What was the most significant trend in evolution of modern man (*Homo sapiens*) from his ancestors ?
(a) Upright posture
(b) Shortening of jaws
(c) Binocular vision
(d) Increasing brain capacity

40. According to Oparin, which one of the following was ***not*** present in the primitive atmosphere of the earth?
(a) Methane (b) Oxygen
(c) Hydrogen (d) Water vapour

41. There is no life on moon due to the absence of
(a) O_2 (b) water
(c) light (d) temperature

42. Which one of the following statements is correct?
(a) Cro-Magnon man's fossil has been found in Ethiopia
(b) *Homo erectus* is the ancestor of man
(c) Neanderthal man is the direct ancestor of *Homo sapiens*
(d) *Australopithecus* is the real ancestor of modern man

43. Atmosphere of earth just before the origin of life consisted of
(a) water vapours, CH_4, NH_3 and oxygen.
(b) CO_2, NH_3, and CH_2
(c) CH_4, NH_3, H_2 and water vapours.
(d) CH_4, O_3, O_2 and water vapours.

44. The extinct human ancestor who ate only fruits and hunted with stone weapons was
(a) *Ramapithecus* (b) *Australopithecus*
(c) *Dryopithecus* (d) *Homo habilis*

45. Tasmanian Wolf is a marsupial while Wolf is a placental mammal. This shows
(a) convergent evolution
(b) divergent evolution
(c) inheritance of acquired characters
(d) None of these

RESPONSE GRID					
	32. ⓐⓑⓒⓓ	33. ⓐⓑⓒⓓ	34. ⓐⓑⓒⓓ	35. ⓐⓑⓒⓓ	36. ⓐⓑⓒⓓ
	37. ⓐⓑⓒⓓ	38. ⓐⓑⓒⓓ	39. ⓐⓑⓒⓓ	40. ⓐⓑⓒⓓ	41. ⓐⓑⓒⓓ
	42. ⓐⓑⓒⓓ	43. ⓐⓑⓒⓓ	44. ⓐⓑⓒⓓ	45. ⓐⓑⓒⓓ	

BIOLOGY CHAPTERWISE SPEED TEST-87			
Total Questions	45	Total Marks	180
Attempted		Correct	
Incorrect		Net Score	
Cut-off Score	45	Qualifying Score	60
Success Gap = Net Score – Qualifying Score			
Net Score = (Correct × 4) – (Incorrect × 1)			

Space for Rough Work

BIOLOGY

Human Health and Disease

Speed TEST 88

Chapter-wise

No. of Questions	Maximum Marks	Time
45	180	1 Hour

GENERAL INSTRUCTIONS

- This test contains 45 MCQ's. For each question only one option is correct. Darken the correct circle/ bubble in the Response Grid provided on each page.
- You have to evaluate your Response Grids yourself with the help of solutions provided at the end of this book.
- Each correct answer will get you 4 marks and 1 mark shall be deduced for each incorrect answer. No mark will be given/ deducted if no bubble is filled. Keep a timer in front of you and stop immediately at the end of 60 min.
- The sheet follows a particular syllabus. Do not attempt the sheet before you have completed your preparation for that syllabus.
- After completing the sheet check your answers with the solution booklet and complete the Result Grid. Finally spend time to analyse your performance and revise the areas which emerge out as weak in your evaluation.

1. A cell coded protein formed in response to infection with most animal viruses is
   (a) Antigen (b) Antibody
   (c) Interferon (d) Histone
2. A sexually transmitted disease caused by bacteria is
   (a) Leprosy (b) AIDS
   (c) Syphilis (d) Pertussis
3. What is true about T-lymphocytes in mammals?
   (a) These are produced in thyroid
   (b) There are of three main types — cytotoxic T-cells, helper T-cells and suppressor T-cells
   (c) These originate in lymphoid tissues
   (d) They scavenge damaged cells and cellular debris
4. Obstacle to large scale transplantation of organs is
   (a) insufficiency of organ donors
   (b) immunological rejection of foreign bodies
   (c) religious or ethnic considerations
   (d) lack of effective surgical techniques
5. The use of *Cannabis* products (bhang, ganja, charas, marijuana or hashish) causes
   (a) depression of brain activity and feeling of calmness
   (b) alters thoughts, perceptions and feelings
   (c) suppresses brain function and relieves pain
   (d) stimulates the nervous system and increases alertness and activity.
6. Which one of the following is an Indian medicinal plant ?
   (a) *Saccharum officinarum* (b) *Rauwolfia serpentina*
   (c) *Oryza sativa* (d) *Solanum melongena*
7. In which one of the following pairs of diseases both are caused by viruses ?
   (a) Tetanus and typhoid
   (b) Whooping cough and sleeping sickness
   (c) Syphilis and AIDS
   (d) Measles and Rabies
8. Hypersensitivity to an allergen is associated with
   (a) aberrant functioning of the immune mechanism
   (b) increase in ambient temperature
   (c) age of the individual
   (d) food habits

RESPONSE GRID					
	1. ⓐⓑⓒⓓ	2. ⓐⓑⓒⓓ	3. ⓐⓑⓒⓓ	4. ⓐⓑⓒⓓ	5. ⓐⓑⓒⓓ
	6. ⓐⓑⓒⓓ	7. ⓐⓑⓒⓓ	8. ⓐⓑⓒⓓ		

Space for Rough Work

9. Carcinoma refers to
(a) benign tumours of the connective tissue
(b) malignant tumours of the connective tissue
(c) malignant tumours of the skin or mucous membrane
(d) malignant tumours of the colon

10. Human immuno deficiency virus (HIV) has a protein coat and a genetic material which is
(a) single stranded DNA
(b) double stranded DNA
(c) single stranded RNA
(d) double stranded RNA

11. Short-lived immunity acquired from mother to foetus across placenta or through mother's milk to the infant is categorised as
(a) innate non-specific immunity
(b) active immunity
(c) passive immunity
(d) cellular immunity

12. Which one is a correctly match sexually transmitted disease with its pathogen?
(a) Syphilis – *Leishmania donovani*
(b) AIDS – *Bacillus anthracis*
(c) Urethritis – *Entamoeba gingivalis*
(d) Gonorrhoea – *Neisseria gonorrhoeae*

13. To which type of barriers under innate immunity, do the saliva in the mouth and the tears from the eyes, belong?
(a) Cytokine barriers
(b) Cellular barriers
(c) Physiological barriers
(d) Physical barriers

14. Widal test is used for the diagnosis of
(a) Malaria (b) Pneumonia
(c) Tuberculosis (d) Typhoid

15. Which one of the following depresses brain activity and produced feelings of calmness, relaxation and drowsiness?
(a) Morphine (b) Valium
(c) Amphetamines (d) Hashish

16. Antibodies in our body are complex
(a) steroids (b) prostaglandins
(c) glycoproteins (d) lipoproteins

17. Select the correct statement with respect to diseases and immunisation?
(a) If due to some reason B-and T-lymphocytes áre damaged, the body will not produce antibodies against a pathogen
(b) Injection of dead / inactivated pathogens causes passive immunity
(c) Certain protozoans have been used to mass produce hepatitis B vaccine.
(d) Injection of snake antivenom against snake bite is an example of active immunisation

18. Increased asthmatic attacks in certain seasons are related to
(a) eating fruits preserved in tin containers
(b) inhalation of seasonal pollen
(c) low temperature
(d) hot and humid environment.

19. A person likely to develop tetanus is immunised by administering
(a) preformed antibodies
(b) wide spectrum antibiotics
(c) weakened germs
(d) dead germs

20. Which one of the following statements is correct with respect to AIDS?
(a) The HIV can be transmitted through eating food together with an infected person
(b) Drug addicts are least susceptible to HIV infection .
(c) AIDS patients are being fully cured with proper care and nutrition
(d) The causative HIV retrovirus enters helper T-lymphocytes thus reducing their numbers

21. Damage to thymus in a child may lead to –
(a) a reduction in haemoglobin content of blood
(b) a reduction in stem cell production
(c) loss of antibody mediated immunity
(d) loss of cell mediated immunity

RESPONSE GRID					
	9. ⓐⓑⓒⓓ	10. ⓐⓑⓒⓓ	11. ⓐⓑⓒⓓ	12. ⓐⓑⓒⓓ	13. ⓐⓑⓒⓓ
	14. ⓐⓑⓒⓓ	15. ⓐⓑⓒⓓ	16. ⓐⓑⓒⓓ	17. ⓐⓑⓒⓓ	18. ⓐⓑⓒⓓ
	19. ⓐⓑⓒⓓ	20. ⓐⓑⓒⓓ	21. ⓐⓑⓒⓓ		

Space for Rough Work

22. Thromboplastin is secreted by
(a) platelets (b) lymphocytes
(c) helper T-cells (d) mast cells

23. Which one of the following techniques is safest for the detection of cancers?
(a) Magnetic resonance imaging (MRI)
(b) Radiography (X-ray)
(c) Computed tomography (CT)
(d) Histopathological studies

24. Common cold differs from pneumonia in, that
(a) Pneumonia is caused by a virus while the common cold is caused by the bacterium *Haemophilus influenzae*
(b) Pneumonia pathogen infects alveoli whereas the common cold affects nose and respiratory passage but not the lungs
(c) Pneumonia is a communicable disease whereas the common cold is a nutritional deficiency disease
(d) Pneumonia can be prevented by a live attenuated bacterial vaccine whereas the common cold has no effective vaccine

25. Which one of the following statements is correct with respect to immunity?
(a) Preformed antibodies need to be injected to treat the bite by a viper snake.
(b) The antibodies against small pox pathogen are produced by T – lymphocytes.
(c) Antibodies are protein molecules, each of which has four light chains.
(d) Rejection of a kidney graft is the function of B-lymphocytes.

26. Which of the following pairs contains an infections and a non-infectious disease respectively?
(a) Typhoid and AIDS
(b) AIDS and Cancer
(c) Pneumonia and malaria
(d) Cancer and malaria

27. The comon cold is caused by
(a) Rhino viruses
(b) *Streptococcus pneumoniae*
(c) *Salmonella typhimurium*
(d) *Plasmodium vivax*

28. Elephantiasis, a chronic inflammation that results in gross deformities is caused by
(a) *Ascaris* (b) *E.coli*
(c) *Wuchereria* (d) *Trichophyton*

29. Match Column-I with Column-II and select the correct answer from codes given below.

	Column-I		Column-II
A.	Sporozoites	(I)	Infectious form
B.	Filariasis	(II)	Aedes mosquitoes
C.	Typhoid	(III)	Wuchereria
D.	Chikungunya	(IV)	Widal test

(a) A-(IV), B-(II), C-(I), D-(III)
(b) A-(III), B-(IV), C-(II), D-(I)
(c) A-(II), B-(III), C-(I), D-(IV)
(d) A-(I), B-(III), C-(IV), D-(II)

30. Hepatitis B is transmitted through
(a) sneezing (b) female Anopheles
(c) coughing (d) blood transfusions

31. Which of the following is the bacterial disease in humans?
(a) Dysentery (b) Malaria
(c) Plague (d) Both (a) and (c)

32. The first line of defence in the immune system is provident by
(a) skin and mucous membrane
(b) inflammatory response
(c) the complement system
(d) none of these

33. The most abundant antiody produced against allergens
(a) lgE (b) lgA
(c) lgG (d) lgM

RESPONSE GRID					
	22. ⓐⓑⓒⓓ	23. ⓐⓑⓒⓓ	24. ⓐⓑⓒⓓ	25. ⓐⓑⓒⓓ	26. ⓐⓑⓒⓓ
	27. ⓐⓑⓒⓓ	28. ⓐⓑⓒⓓ	29. ⓐⓑⓒⓓ	30. ⓐⓑⓒⓓ	31. ⓐⓑⓒⓓ
	32. ⓐⓑⓒⓓ	33. ⓐⓑⓒⓓ			

Space for Rough Work

34. An auto-immune disease is
(a) SCID
(b) rheumatoid arthritis
(c) myasthenia gravis
(d) both (b) and (c)

35. The primary lymphoid organs are
(a) spleen and thymus
(b) bone marrow and thymus
(c) bone marrow and lymph node
(d) thymus and MALT

36. Vaccine against polio viruses is an example of
(a) auto-immunization
(b) passive immunization
(c) active immunization
(d) simple immunization

37. Which of the following is celebrated as 'World AIDS Day'?
(a) 31st March (b) 1st March
(c) 1st December (d) 31st December

38. Which of the following approaches are used for the treatment of cancer?
(a) Gene therapy and immunotherapy
(b) Surgery
(c) Radiotherapy and Chemotherapy
(d) All of these

39. Which of these is a member of the group of chemicals whose chemical structure is given below?

[Chemical structure with OH, O, H labels]

(a) Marijuana (b) Hashish
(c) Ganja (d) All of these

40. Which drug is being excessively taken by some sports persons nowadays?
(a) Opioids
(b) Barbiturates
(c) Cannabinoids
(d) Lysergic acid diethyl amides (LSD)

41. Take the odd one out
(a) Rabies, Influenza, AIDS
(b) Amoebiasis, Giardiasis, Trypanosomiasis
(c) Taeniasis, Ascariasis, Elephantiasis
(d) Cancer, Tuberculosis, Tetanus

42. Small proteins produced by vertebrate cells in response to viral infections inhibiting viral multiplication are known as
(a) Lipoproteins (b) Immuglobulins
(c) Interferons (d) Antitoxins

43. Which one of the following acts as a physiological barrier to the entry of micro-organisms in human body ?
(a) Epithelium of urogenital tract
(b) Tears
(c) Monocytes
(d) Skin

44. The treatment of snake-bite by antivenine is an example of
(a) Artificially acquired active immunity
(b) Artificially acquired passive immunity
(c) Naturally acquired passive immunity
(d) Specific natural immunity

45. The drug useful to increase cardiovascular effects in human beings is
(a) Cocaine (b) Barbiturate
(c) Benzodiazepine (d) Insulin

RESPONSE GRID					
	34. ⓐⓑⓒⓓ	35. ⓐⓑⓒⓓ	36. ⓐⓑⓒⓓ	37. ⓐⓑⓒⓓ	38. ⓐⓑⓒⓓ
	39. ⓐⓑⓒⓓ	40. ⓐⓑⓒⓓ	41. ⓐⓑⓒⓓ	42. ⓐⓑⓒⓓ	43. ⓐⓑⓒⓓ
	44. ⓐⓑⓒⓓ	45. ⓐⓑⓒⓓ			

BIOLOGY CHAPTERWISE SPEED TEST-88			
Total Questions	45	Total Marks	180
Attempted		Correct	
Incorrect		Net Score	
Cut-off Score	48	Qualifying Score	55
Success Gap = Net Score – Qualifying Score			
Net Score = (Correct × 4) – (Incorrect × 1)			

Space for Rough Work

BIOLOGY

Strategies for Enchancement in Food Production

Speed TEST 89

Chapter-wise

No. of Questions	Maximum Marks	Time
45	180	1 Hour

GENERAL INSTRUCTIONS

- This test contains 45 MCQ's. For each question only one option is correct. Darken the correct circle/ bubble in the Response Grid provided on each page.
- You have to evaluate your Response Grids yourself with the help of solutions provided at the end of this book.
- Each correct answer will get you 4 marks and 1 mark shall be deduced for each incorrect answer. No mark will be given/ deducted if no bubble is filled. Keep a timer in front of you and stop immediately at the end of 60 min.
- The sheet follows a particular syllabus. Do not attempt the sheet before you have completed your preparation for that syllabus.
- After completing the sheet check your answers with the solution booklet and complete the Result Grid. Finally spend time to analyse your performance and revise the areas which emerge out as weak in your evaluation.

1. Parthenocarpic tomato fruits can be produced by
   (a) treating the plants with low concentrations of gibberellic acid and auxins
   (b) raising the plants from vernalized seeds
   (c) treating the plants with phenylmercuric acetate
   (d) removing androecium of flowers before pollen grains are released
2. The technique of obtaining large number of plantlets by tissue culture method is called
   (a) Plantlet culture
   (b) Organ culture
   (c) Micropropagation
   (d) Macropropagation
3. Breeding of crops with high levels of minerals, vitamins and proteins is called
   (a) Somatic hybridisation
   (b) Biofortification
   (c) Biomagnification
   (d) Micropropagation
4. Jaya and Ratna developed for green revolution in India are the varieties of
   (a) maize (b) rice
   (c) wheat (d) bajra
5. Which one of the following pesticides is banned now a-days?
   (a) DDT (b) Eldrin
   (c) Aldrin (d) Toxaphene
6. Which one of the following is an exotic Indian fish ?
   (a) *Catla catla*
   (b) *Heteropneustes fossilis*
   (c) *Cyprinus carpio*
   (d) *Labeo rohita*

RESPONSE GRID	1. ⓐⓑⓒⓓ 2. ⓐⓑⓒⓓ 3. ⓐⓑⓒⓓ 4. ⓐⓑⓒⓓ 5. ⓐⓑⓒⓓ 6. ⓐⓑⓒⓓ

Space for Rough Work

7. Consider the following statements concerning food chains :
(i) Removal of 80% tigers from an area resulted in greatly increased growth of vegetation
(ii) Removal of most of the carnivores resulted in an increased population of deers
(iii) The length of food chains is generally limited to 3-4 trophic levels due to energy loss
(iv) The length of food chains may vary from 2 to 8 trophic levels
Which two of the above statements are correct?
(a) (ii) and (iii) (b) (iii) and (iv)
(c) (i) and (iv) (d) (i) and (ii)

8. Which one is a neem product used as insect repellent?
(a) Azadirachtin (b) Rotenone
(c) Parathione (d) Endrin

9. Bull semen for the purpose of artificial insemination is stored in
(a) Ice (b) Liquid oxygen
(c) Liquid nitrogen (d) Liquid CO_2

10. The 'Mule' is the result of
(a) Inbreeding depression
(b) Out breeding
(c) Cross breeding
(d) Inter-specific hybridization

11. In live stock breeding experiments the following stage is transferred to surrogate mothers
(a) Unfertilized eggs
(b) Fertilized eggs
(c) 8 to 32 celled embryo
(d) Frozen semen

12. The animal husbandry deals with the care, breeding and management of
(a) Domesticated animals
(b) Fishes
(c) Honey bees and silk worms
(d) All of these

13. Which of the following has been recently used for increasing productivity of super milk cows?
(a) Artificial insemination by a pedigree bull only
(b) Superovulation of a high production cow only
(c) Embryo transplantation only
(d) A combination of superovulation, artificial insemination and embryo transplantation into a 'carrier cow' (surrogate mother)

14. Which one of the following statements is correct in relation to honey bees?
(a) *Apis indica* is the largest wild honey bee in India
(b) Honey is predominantly sucrose and arabinose
(c) Beewax is a waste product of honey bees
(d) Communication in honey bees was discovered by Karl Von Frisch

15. 'Inland fishery' refers to
(a) Culturing fish in fresh water
(b) Trapping and capturing fishes from sea coast
(c) Deep sea fishing
(d) Extraction of oil from fishes

16. Which of the following combinations is generally recommended for composite fish farming in India?
(a) *Catla, Labeo, Cirrhinus*
(b) *Catla, Cyprinus, Clarias*
(c) *Clarias, Channa, Cyprinus*
(d) *Cirrhinus, Cyprinus, Channa*

17. Hinny is a hybrid of male
(a) Horse and female donkey
(b) Donkey and female horse
(c) Goat and female lamb
(d) Sheep and female goat.

18. When cross is made between two species of the same genus, then the cross is known as
(a) intraspecific hybridization
(b) interspecific hybridization
(c) intergeneric hybridization
(d) intervarietal hybridization

19. Which of the following is a viral disease of poultry birds?
(a) Anthrax (b) Ranikhet
(c) Coccidiosis (d) None of these

RESPONSE GRID					
	7. ⓐⓑⓒⓓ	8. ⓐⓑⓒⓓ	9. ⓐⓑⓒⓓ	10. ⓐⓑⓒⓓ	11. ⓐⓑⓒⓓ
	12. ⓐⓑⓒⓓ	13. ⓐⓑⓒⓓ	14. ⓐⓑⓒⓓ	15. ⓐⓑⓒⓓ	16. ⓐⓑⓒⓓ
	17. ⓐⓑⓒⓓ	18. ⓐⓑⓒⓓ	19. ⓐⓑⓒⓓ		

Space for Rough Work

20. Which one of the following processes of breeding increases homozygosity?
(a) Inbreeding
(b) Out breeding
(c) Cross breeding
(d) Inter-specific breeding

21. The most popular breed of fowl in India is
(a) White leg horn (b) Aseel
(c) Plymouth (d) Langshan

22. Murrah, Mehsana, Jaffarbadi are breeds of
(a) Buffalo (b) Cow
(c) Cattle (d) Horse

23. Consumption of which one of the following foods can prevent the kind of blindness associated with vitamin 'A' deficiency ?
(a) '*Flavr Savr*' tomato
(b) Canolla
(c) Golden rice
(d) Bt-Brinjal

24. Golden rice is a transgenic crop of the future with the following improved trait :
(a) insect resistance
(b) high lysine (essential amino acid) content
(c) high protein content
(d) high vitamin-A content

25. Use of transgenic plants as biological factories for the production of special chemicals is called–
(a) Molecular farming (b) Molecular genetics
(c) Molecular mapping (d) Dry farming

26. Main objective of production/use of herbicide resistant GM crops is to
(a) eliminate weeds from the field without the use of manual labour
(b) eliminate weeds from the field without the use of herbicides
(c) encourage eco-friendly herbicides
(d) reduce herbicide accumulation in food articles for health safety

27. In order to obtain virus- free plants through tissue culture, the best method is
(a) protoplast culture (b) embryo rescue
(c) anther culture (d) meristem culture

28. A collection of plants and seeds having diverse alleles of all the genes of a crop is called
(a) herbarium (b) germplasm
(c) gene library (d) genome

29. Which one of the following is a wrong matching?
(a) Somatic hybridization - Fusion of two diverse cells
(b) Vector DNA -Site for t-RNA synthesis
(c) Micropropagation - *in vitro* production of plants in large numbers
(d) Callus - Unorganised mass of cell produced in tissue culture

30. In tissue culture roots can be induced by
(a) no cytokinin and only auxins.
(b) higher concentration cytokinin and lower concentration auxins.
(c) lower concentration of cytokinin and higher concentration of auxins.
(d) only cytokinin and no auxins.

31. Three crops that contribute maximum to global food grain production are
(a) Wheat, rice and maize
(b) Wheat, rice and barley
(c) Wheat, maize and sorghum
(d) Rice, maize and sorghum

32. Himgiri developed by hybridisation and selection for disease resistance against rust pathogens is a variety of
(a) chilli (b) maize
(c) sugarcane (d) wheat

33. Bee dances are meant for
(a) Courtship (b) Communication
(c) Recreation (d) Instinct

34. Artificial insemination involves
(a) super ovulation (b) semen collection
(c) egg collection (d) embryo collection

RESPONSE GRID					
	20. ⓐⓑⓒⓓ	21. ⓐⓑⓒⓓ	22. ⓐⓑⓒⓓ	23. ⓐⓑⓒⓓ	24. ⓐⓑⓒⓓ
	25. ⓐⓑⓒⓓ	26. ⓐⓑⓒⓓ	27. ⓐⓑⓒⓓ	28. ⓐⓑⓒⓓ	29. ⓐⓑⓒⓓ
	30. ⓐⓑⓒⓓ	31. ⓐⓑⓒⓓ	32. ⓐⓑⓒⓓ	33. ⓐⓑⓒⓓ	34. ⓐⓑⓒⓓ

Space for Rough Work

35. The term "breed" refers to
(a) a group of animals not related by descent but similar in most characters
(b) a group of animals related by descent and similar in most characters
(c) a group of animals related by descent but have almost different characteristics
(d) a group of animals neither related by descent nor have similar characteristics.

36. What strategy would you suggest if a person wants to evolve a pureline in an animal?
(a) Cross-breeding (b) Inbreeding
(c) Out-breeding (d) Artificial insemination

37. Select the incorrect statement from the following.
(a) Apiculture provides additional income generating industry to the farmers.
(b) Bee keeping is labour intensive process.
(c) Bee venom is used to cure certain diseases like gout and arthritis.
(d) Honey is used as laxative, antiseptic and sedative.

38. Germplasm collection is the collection of
(a) germ cells
(b) semens
(c) plants/seeds with all the diverse alleles for all genes
(d) egg cells

39. Which of the following diseases is caused by virus?
(a) Tobacco mosaic (b) Late blight of potato
(c) Turnip mosaic (d) Both (a) and (c)

40. Single cell protein can be obtained from
(a) bacteria (b) algae
(c) fungi (d) all of these

41. Meristem culture is used
(a) to produce disease free plants
(b) in germplasm conservation
(c) in rapid clonal multiplication
(d) all of these

42. A plant cell without cell wall is called
(a) proplast (b) protoplast
(c) nucleoplasm (d) explant

43. Refer the given figures and answer the questions.

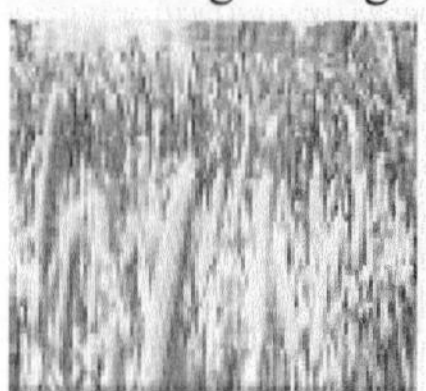 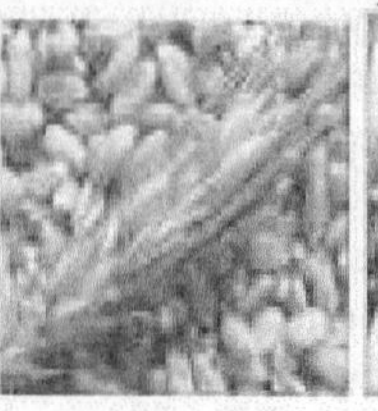 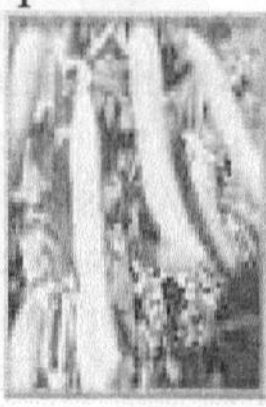

Which of the following statements is correct regarding the above figures?
(i) These are all Indian hybrid crops of low yielding varieties.
(ii) These are all Indian hybrid crops of high yielding varieties.
(iii) The production of the above crops led to dramatic increase in food production.
(iv) These crops are produced as a result of various plants breeding technique.
(a) (i), (ii), and (iii) (b) (ii), (iii) and (iv)
(c) (iii) and (iv) only (d) (i) and (iii) only

44. Match Column - I with Column - II

	Column-I		Column-II
A.	Hybrid variety	(I).	X-ray
B.	Mutation	(II).	Allopolyploidy
C.	Pure line	(III).	F_1 generation
D.	*Triticale*	(IV).	Selection in self pollinated crops
		(V).	Genetic engineering

(a) A-(III); B-(II); C-(I); D-(IV)
(b) A-(III); B-(I); C-(IV); D-(II)
(c) A-(I); B-(III); C-(IV); D-(II)
(d) A-(II); B-(I); C-(III); D-(IV)

45. Farmers in a particular region were concerned that pre-mature yellowing of leaves of a pulse crop might cause decrease in the yield. Which treatment could be most beneficial to obtain maximum seed yield ?
(a) Treatment of the plants with cytokinins along with a small dose of nitrogenous fertilizer
(b) Removal of all yellow leaves and spraying the remaining green leaves with 2, 4, 5- trichlorophenoxy acetic acid
(c) Application of iron and magnesium to promote synthesis of chlorophyll
(d) Frequent irrigation of the crop

RESPONSE GRID				
35. ⓐⓑⓒⓓ	36. ⓐⓑⓒⓓ	37. ⓐⓑⓒⓓ	38. ⓐⓑⓒⓓ	39. ⓐⓑⓒⓓ
40. ⓐⓑⓒⓓ	41. ⓐⓑⓒⓓ	42. ⓐⓑⓒⓓ	43. ⓐⓑⓒⓓ	44. ⓐⓑⓒⓓ
45. ⓐⓑⓒⓓ				

BIOLOGY CHAPTERWISE SPEED TEST-89			
Total Questions	45	Total Marks	180
Attempted		Correct	
Incorrect		Net Score	
Cut-off Score	55	Qualifying Score	60
Success Gap = Net Score – Qualifying Score			
Net Score = (Correct × 4) – (Incorrect × 1)			

Space for Rough Work

BIOLOGY

Microbes in Human Welfare

Speed TEST 90

Chapter-wise

No. of Questions	Maximum Marks	Time
45	180	1 Hour

GENERAL INSTRUCTIONS

- This test contains 45 MCQ's. For each question only one option is correct. Darken the correct circle/ bubble in the Response Grid provided on each page.
- You have to evaluate your Response Grids yourself with the help of solutions provided at the end of this book.
- Each correct answer will get you 4 marks and 1 mark shall be deduced for each incorrect answer. No mark will be given/ deducted if no bubble is filled. Keep a timer in front of you and stop immediately at the end of 60 min.
- The sheet follows a particular syllabus. Do not attempt the sheet before you have completed your preparation for that syllabus.
- After completing the sheet check your answers with the solution booklet and complete the Result Grid. Finally spend time to analyse your performance and revise the areas which emerge out as weak in your evaluation.

1. Select the correct statement from the following.
   (a) Biogas is produced by the activity of aerobic bacteria on animal waste
   (b) *Methanobacterium* is an aerobic bacterium found in rumen of cattle
   (c) Biogas, commonly called gobar gas, is pure methane
   (d) Activated sludge-sediment in settlement tanks of sewage treatment plant is a rich source of aerobic bacteria
2. Which one thing is not true about antibiotics?
   (a) The term "antibiotic" was coined by Selman Waksman in 1942
   (b) First antibiotic was discovered by Alexander Flemming
   (c) Each antibiotic is effective only against one particular kind of germ
   (d) Some persons can be allergic to a particular antibiotic
3. *Monascus purpureus* is a yeast used commercially in the production of :
   (a) ethanol
   (b) streptokinase for removing clots from the blood vessels.
   (c) citric acid
   (d) blood cholesterol lowering statins
4. A common biocontrol agent for the control of plant diseases is
   (a) Baculovirus (b) *Bacillus thuringiensis*
   (c) *Glomus* (d) *Trichoderma*
5. Continuous addition of sugars in 'fed batch' fermentation is done to:
   (a) produce methane (b) obtain antibiotics
   (c) purify enzymes (d) degrade sewage

RESPONSE GRID 1. ⓐⓑⓒⓓ 2. ⓐⓑⓒⓓ 3. ⓐⓑⓒⓓ 4. ⓐⓑⓒⓓ 5. ⓐⓑⓒⓓ

Space for Rough Work

6. Streptomycin is obtained from
   (a) *Streptomyces griseus*
   (b) S. *aureofaciens*
   (c) S. *venezuelae*
   (d) S. *ramosus*
7. For biogas production besides dung an extensive use of which weed is recommended in our country–
   (a) *Mangifera indica*
   (b) *Hydrilla*
   (c) *Eicchornia crassipes*
   (d) *Solanum*
8. Chloramphenicol and erythromycin (broad spectrum antibiotics) are produced by
   (a) *Streptomyces* (b) *Nitrobacter*
   (c) *Rhizobium* (d) *Penicillium*
9. Which one of the microorganism is used for production of citric acid in industries ?
   (a) *Lactobacillus bulgaricus*
   (b) *Penicillium citrinum*
   (c) *Aspergillus niger*
   (d) *Rhizopus nigricans*
10. A genetically engineered bacteria used for clearing oil spills is :
    (a) *Escherichia coli*
    (b) *Bacillus subtilis*
    (c) *Agrobacterium tumifaciens*
    (d) *Pseudomonas putida*
11. Human insulin is being commercially produced from a transgenic species of
    (a) *Escherichia* (b) *Mycobacterium*
    (c) *Rhizobium* (d) *Saccharomyces*
12. Which one of the following is not used in organic farming?
    (a) *Glomus* (b) Earthworm
    (c) *Oscillatoria* (d) Snail
13. What is mode of bacterial resistance against antibiotics ?
    (a) Development of thick mucilaginous layer
    (b) Alteration of cell membrane
    (c) Mutation in bacteria
    (d) All the above
14. Which one of the following is a wrong matching of a microbe and its industrial product, while the remaining three are correct ?
    (a) Yeast - statins
    (b) *Acetobacter aceti* - acetic acid
    (c) *Clostridium butylicum* - lactic acid
    (d) *Aspergillus niger* - citric acid
15. During anaerobic digestion of organic waste, such as in producing biogas, which one of the following is left undegraded ?
    (a) Lipids (b) Lignin
    (c) Hemi-cellulose (d) Cellulose
16. Rennin used in cheese industry is –
    (a) Antibiotic (b) Enzyme
    (c) Alkaloid (d) Inhibitor
17. Vitamin B_{12} is formed during fermentation of
    (a) *Ashloya gossipii*
    (b) *Rhizopus stalonifer*
    (c) *Propionibacteria*
    (d) *Saccharomyces cerevisiae*
18. The term "antibiotic" was coined by –
    (a) Edward Jenner (b) Louis Pasteur
    (c) Selman Waksman (d) Alexander Flemming
19. Which one of the following micro-organisms is used for production of citric acid in industries?
    (a) *Penicillium citrinum*
    (b) *Aspergillus niger*
    (c) *Rhizopus nigricans*
    (d) *Lactobacillus bulgaris*
20. Streptokinase which is used as a 'clot buster' obtained from
    (a) *Streptococcus* (b) *Staphylococcus*
    (c) *Lactobacillus* (d) *Saccharomyces*

RESPONSE GRID					
	6. ⓐⓑⓒⓓ	7. ⓐⓑⓒⓓ	8. ⓐⓑⓒⓓ	9. ⓐⓑⓒⓓ	10. ⓐⓑⓒⓓ
	11. ⓐⓑⓒⓓ	12. ⓐⓑⓒⓓ	13. ⓐⓑⓒⓓ	14. ⓐⓑⓒⓓ	15. ⓐⓑⓒⓓ
	16. ⓐⓑⓒⓓ	17. ⓐⓑⓒⓓ	18. ⓐⓑⓒⓓ	19. ⓐⓑⓒⓓ	20. ⓐⓑⓒⓓ

Space for Rough Work

21. Baculoviruses are excellent candidates for
(a) species-specific narrow spectrum pesticidal applications.
(b) species-specific broad spectrum pesticidal applications.
(c) species-specific narrow spectrum insecticidal applications.
(d) species-specific broad spectrum insecticidal applications.

22. Farmers have reported over 50% higher yields of rice by using the biofertilizer
(a) *Azolla pinnata*
(b) *Cyanobacteria*
(c) *Legume-Rhizobium* symbiosis
(d) Mycorrhiza

23. Microbes are present in
(a) soil (b) thermal vents
(c) polluted water (d) all of these

24. Which of the following microbes is a proteinacious infectious agent?
(a) Fungi (b) Prions
(c) Bacteria (d) Protozoa

25. Probiotics are
(a) cancer inducing microbes
(b) new kind of food allergens
(c) live microbial food supplement
(d) safe antibiotics

26. *Saccharomyces cerevisiae* is a yeast commercially used in
(a) citric acid
(b) ethanol
(c) baking
(d) streptokinase for removing clots from blood vessels

27. The masses of bacteria held together by slime and fungal filaments to form mesh like structures are called as
(a) primary sludge (b) flocs
(c) activated sludge (d) anaerobic sludge

28. The purpose of biological treatment of waste water is to
(a) reduce BOD
(b) increase BOD
(c) reduce sedimentation
(d) increase sedimentation

29. These bacteria grow anaerobically on cellulosic material, produce large amount of methane along with CO_2 and H_2, and are collectively called as methanogen. Examples of such bacteria are
(a) *Methanobacterium*
(b) *Methanobrevibacter*
(c) *Methanococcus*
(d) All of these

30. Biogas is produced by
(a) aerobic breakdown of biomass
(b) anaerobic breakdown of biomass
(c) with the help of methanogenic bacteria
(d) both (b) and (c)

31. Match Column-I with Column-II and select the correct answer from the codes given below.

	Column-I		Column-II
A.	*Trichoderma*	(I)	Nitrification
B.	*Streptomyces*	(II)	Biocontrol agent
C.	*Nitrosomonas*	(III)	Lactic acid
D.	*Lactobacillus*	(IV)	Source of antibiotic

(a) A-(II), B-(III), C-(IV), D-(I)
(b) A-(II), B-(IV), C-(I), D-(III)
(c) A-(III), B-(I), C-(II), D-(IV)
(d) A-(IV), B-(II), C-(I), D-(III)

32. Organic farming does not include
(a) green manures (b) chemical fertilizers
(c) farmyard manures (d) compost

33. The symbiotic association between fungi and roots of higher plants is referred to as
(a) lichen (b) Mycorrhiza
(c) biofertilizer (d) biocontrol agent

34. Which of the following options includes biofertilizers?
(a) Cowdung manure and farmyard waste
(b) A quick growing crop ploughed back into the field
(c) Nostoc, Oscillatoria
(d) All of these

RESPONSE GRID					
	21. ⓐⓑⓒⓓ	22. ⓐⓑⓒⓓ	23. ⓐⓑⓒⓓ	24. ⓐⓑⓒⓓ	25. ⓐⓑⓒⓓ
	26. ⓐⓑⓒⓓ	27. ⓐⓑⓒⓓ	28. ⓐⓑⓒⓓ	29. ⓐⓑⓒⓓ	30. ⓐⓑⓒⓓ
	31. ⓐⓑⓒⓓ	32. ⓐⓑⓒⓓ	33. ⓐⓑⓒⓓ	34. ⓐⓑⓒⓓ	

Space for Rough Work

35. Yeast *Saccharomyces cervisiae* is used in the industrial production of
(a) butanol (b) citric acid
(c) tetracycline (d) ethanol

36. In cheese manufacture, the micro-organisms are used for
(a) the souring of milk only
(b) the ripening only
(c) development of resistance to spoilage
(d) Both (a) and (b)

37. Brewer's yeast lack
(a) diastase and amylase (b) amylase only
(c) diastase only (d) maltose

38. Baggasse is related to the manufacture of
(a) cinchonidine (b) cellulose materials
(c) resin (d) cane sugar

39. Which of the following bacteria is used for the production of butanol and acetone from starch ?
(a) *Lactobacillus bulgaricus*
(b) *Clostridium acetobutylicum*
(c) *Streptococcum thermophilus*
(d) Both (a) and (c)

40. Which bacterium helps in the production of 'Swiss cheese'?
(a) *Propionibacterium sharmanii*
(b) *Trichoderma polysporum*
(c) *Saccharomyces cerevisiae*
(d) *Aspergillus niger*

41. Statins, a bioactive molecule, inhibiting the enzyme responsible for synthesis of
(a) carbohydrate (b) protein
(c) vitamins (d) cholestrol

42. Gallic acid is obtained from
(a) *Pseudomonas species*
(b) *Penicillium purpurogenum*
(c) *Aspergillus niger*
(d) *Streptomyces species*

43. The diagram below shows a typical biogas plant. With few structure labelled as A, B and C. Identify A, B and C.

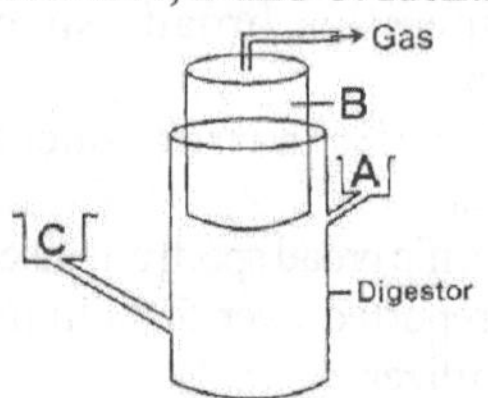

(a) A – Sludge, B – Methane, Oxygen, C – Dung, water
(b) A – Sludge, B – Methane, Carbon dioxide, C– Dung, water
(c) A – Sludge, B – Ethylin, Carbon dioxide, C – Dung, water
(d) A – Sludge, B – Methane, Carbon dioxide, C – Sewage

44. Match column-I with column-II and choose the correct option

	Column-I		Column-II
A.	Statins	I.	Yeast
B.	Ethanol	II.	Blood-cholesterol lowering agent
C.	Dung	III.	Insect-resistant plant
D.	Bt-cotton	IV.	Biogas

(a) A-II; B-I; C-IV; D-III
(b) A-III; B-IV; C-I; D-II
(c) A-I; B-II; C-III; D-IV
(d) A-IV; B- II; C-I; D-III

45. Which one of the following statement regarding BOD is true?
(a) The greater the BOD of waste water, more is its polluting potential.
(b) The greater the BOD of waste water, less is its polluting potential.
(c) The lesser the BOD of waste water, more is its polluting potential.
(d) The lesser the BOD of waste water, less is its polluting potential.

RESPONSE GRID				
35. ⓐⓑⓒⓓ	36. ⓐⓑⓒⓓ	37. ⓐⓑⓒⓓ	38. ⓐⓑⓒⓓ	39. ⓐⓑⓒⓓ
40. ⓐⓑⓒⓓ	41. ⓐⓑⓒⓓ	42. ⓐⓑⓒⓓ	43. ⓐⓑⓒⓓ	44. ⓐⓑⓒⓓ
45. ⓐⓑⓒⓓ				

BIOLOGY CHAPTERWISE SPEED TEST-90			
Total Questions	45	Total Marks	180
Attempted		Correct	
Incorrect		Net Score	
Cut-off Score	45	Qualifying Score	60
Success Gap = Net Score – Qualifying Score			
Net Score = (Correct × 4) – (Incorrect × 1)			

Space for Rough Work

BIOLOGY

Biotechnology: Principles and Processes

Speed TEST 91

Chapter-wise

No. of Questions	Maximum Marks	Time
45	180	1 Hour

GENERAL INSTRUCTIONS

- This test contains 45 MCQ's. For each question only one option is correct. Darken the correct circle/ bubble in the Response Grid provided on each page.
- You have to evaluate your Response Grids yourself with the help of solutions provided at the end of this book.
- Each correct answer will get you 4 marks and 1 mark shall be deduced for each incorrect answer. No mark will be given/ deducted if no bubble is filled. Keep a timer in front of you and stop immediately at the end of 60 min.
- The sheet follows a particular syllabus. Do not attempt the sheet before you have completed your preparation for that syllabus.
- After completing the sheet check your answers with the solution booklet and complete the Result Grid. Finally spend time to analyse your performance and revise the areas which emerge out as weak in your evaluation.

1. The linking of antibiotic resistance gene with the plasmid vector became possible with
   (a) DNA ligase
   (b) Endonucleases
   (c) DNA polymerase
   (d) Exonucleases
2. DNA or RNA segment tagged with a radioactive molecule is called
   (a) Vector (b) Probe
   (c) Clone (d) Plasmid
3. Restriction endonucleases are enzymes which
   (a) make cuts at specific positions within the DNA molecule
   (b) recognize a specific nucleotide sequence for binding of DNA ligase
   (c) restrict the action of the enzyme DNA polymerase
   (d) remove nucleotides from the ends of the DNA molecule
4. Agarose extracted from sea weeds finds use in :
   (a) Spectrophotometry
   (b) Tissue culture
   (c) PCR
   (d) Gel electrophoresis
5. PCR and Restriction Fragment Length Polymorphism are the methods for :
   (a) Study of enzymes
   (b) Genetic transformation
   (c) DNA sequencing
   (d) Genetic Fingerprinting
6. 'Cloning' is meant for/to
   (a) production of HGH gene in *E. coli*
   (b) preserve the genotype of organism
   (c) replace the original gene
   (d) All of the above
7. Which one of the following is used as vector for cloning genes into higher organisms?
   (a) Baculovirus
   (b) *Salmonella typhimurium*
   (c) *Rhizopus nigricans*
   (d) Retrovirus

RESPONSE GRID	
	1. ⓐⓑⓒⓓ 2. ⓐⓑⓒⓓ 3. ⓐⓑⓒⓓ 4. ⓐⓑⓒⓓ 5. ⓐⓑⓒⓓ
	6. ⓐⓑⓒⓓ 7. ⓐⓑⓒⓓ

Space for Rough Work

8. The figure below is the diagrammatic representation of the *E.Coli* vector pBR 322. Which one of the given options correctly identifies its certain component (s) ?

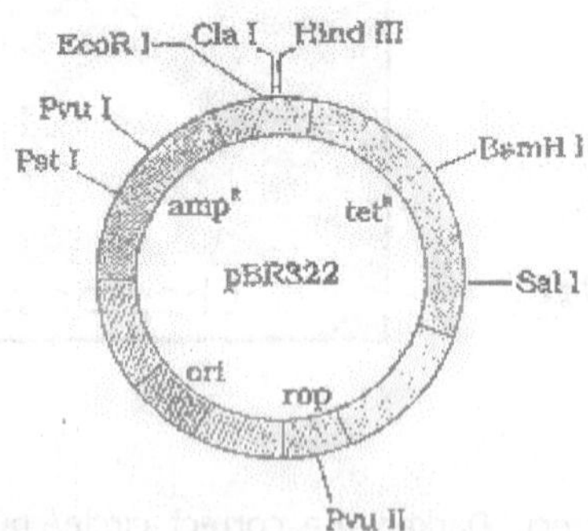

(a) ori - original restriction enzyme
(b) rop-reduced osmotic pressure
(c) Hind III, EcoRI - selectable markers
(d) amp^R, tet^R - antibiotic resistance genes

9. Electroporation procedure involves
(a) fast passage of food through sieve pores in phloem elements with the help of electric stimulation.
(b) opening of stomatal pores during night by artificial light.
(c) making transient pores in the cell membrane to introduce gene constructs.
(d) purification of saline water with the help of a membrane system.

10. What is the first step in the Southern blot technique?
(a) Denaturation of DNA on the gel for hybridization with specific probe.
(b) Production of a group of genetically identical cells.
(c) Digestion of DNA by restriction enzyme.
(d) Denaturation of DNA from a nucleated cell such as the one from the scene of crime.

11. The polymerase chain reaction (PCR) technology was discovered by
(a) Karry Mullis (b) Saiki *et al*
(c) Craig Venter (d) Maxam and Gilbert

12. For transformation, micro-particles coated with DNA to be bombarded with gene gun are made up of :
(a) Silver or Platinum
(b) Platinum or Zinc
(c) Silicon or Platinum
(d) Gold or Tungsten

13. Plasmid used to construct the first recombinant DNA was isolated from which bacterium species?
(a) *Escherichia coli*
(b) *Salmonella typhimurium*
(c) *Agrobacterium tumefaciens*
(d) *Thermus aquaticus*

14. Genetic engineering is possible because
(a) we can cut DNA at specific sites by restriction endonucleases
(b) restriction endonucleases purified from virus can be used in bacteria
(c) the phenomenon of transduction in bacteria is well understood
(d) we can seen DNA by electron microscope

15. Gel electrophoresis is a
(a) technique of separation of charged molecules under the influence of magnetic field
(b) technique of incorporation of DNA molecules into the cell through transient pores made due to electrical impulses
(c) technique of separation of DNA fragments through the pores of agarose gel under the influence of electric field
(d) technique of separation and purification of gene products.

16. In recombinant DNA technology, the term vector refers to
(a) the enzyme that cuts DNA into restriction fragments
(b) the sticky end of a DNA fragment
(c) a plasmid used to transfer DNA into a living cell
(d) a DNA fragment which carries only ori gene

17. In agarose gel electrophoresis
(a) DNA migrates towards the negative electrode
(b) supercoiled plamids migrate slower than their nicked counterparts
(c) larger molecules migrate faster than smaller molecules
(d) ethidium bromide can be used to visualize the DNA

18. Which of the following is based upon the principle of antigen-antibody interaction?
(a) PCR (b) ELISA
(c) R DNA technology (d) RNA

19. Two microbes found to be very useful in genetic engineering are
(a) *Vibrio cholerae* and a tailed bacteriophage
(b) *Diplococcus* sp. and *Pseudomonas* sp.
(c) Crown gall bacterium and *Caenorhabditis elegans*
(d) *Escherichia coli* and *Agrobacterium tumefaciens*

RESPONSE GRID	8. ⓐⓑⓒⓓ	9. ⓐⓑⓒⓓ	10. ⓐⓑⓒⓓ	11. ⓐⓑⓒⓓ	12. ⓐⓑⓒⓓ
	13. ⓐⓑⓒⓓ	14. ⓐⓑⓒⓓ	15. ⓐⓑⓒⓓ	16. ⓐⓑⓒⓓ	17. ⓐⓑⓒⓓ
	18. ⓐⓑⓒⓓ	19. ⓐⓑⓒⓓ			

Space for Rough Work

20. The figure below shows three steps (A, B, C) of Polymerase Chain Reaction (PCR). Select the option giving correct identification together with what it represents?

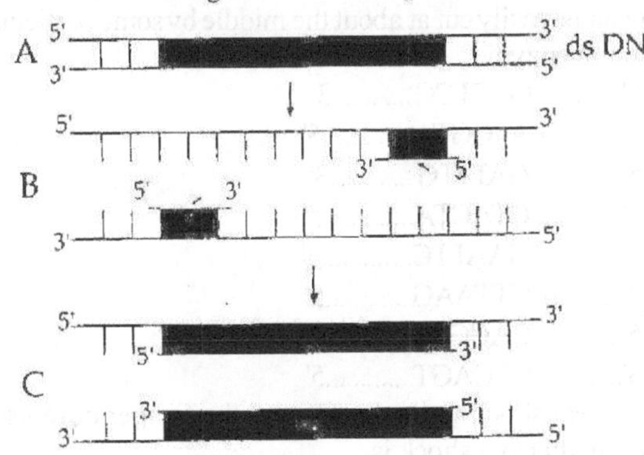

(a) B - Denaturation at a temperature of about 98°C separating the two DNA strands.
(b) A - Denaturation at a temperature of about 50°C.
(c) C - Extension in the presence of heat stable DNA polymerase.
(d) A - Annealing with two sets of primers.

21. Biolistics (gene-gun) is suitable for
(a) DNA finger printing
(b) Disarming pathogen vectors
(c) Transformation of plant cells
(d) Constructing recombinant DNA by joining with vectors

22. Baculoviruses are excellent candidates for
(a) species-specific narrow spectrum pesticidal applications.
(b) species-specific broad spectrum pesticidal applications.
(c) species-specific narrow spectrum insecticidal applications.
(d) species-specific broad spectrum insecticidal applications.

23. Which of the following technique is used for the separation of DNA fragments ?
(a) Gel electrophoresis (b) Chromatography
(c) Transformation (d) Transduction

24. Plasmids are suitable vectors for gene cloning because
(a) these are small circular DNA molecules which can integrate with host chromosomal DNA.
(b) these are small circular DNA molecules with their own replication origin site.
(c) these can shuttle between prokaryotic and eukaryotic cells.
(d) these often carry antibiotic resistance genes.

25. The term "competent" refers to
(a) increasing the competition between cells
(b) making cells impermeable for DNA
(c) increasing the efficiency with which DNA enters the bacterium through pores in its cell wall
(d) making cells permeable for divalent cations

26. The correct sequence of different steps of polymerase chain reaction is
(a) Annealing → Denaturation → Extension
(b) Denaturation → Extension → Annealing
(c) Denaturation → Annealing → Extension
(d) Extension → Denaturation → Annealing

27. Eukaryotic genes do not function properly when cloned into a bacterial cell, because
(a) of high pH present in bacterial cells
(b) of inability to excise introns and destruction by bacterial restriction enzymes
(c) of inappropriate insertion of genes
(d) both (a) and (b).

28. Which structure involved in genetic engineering?
(a) Plastid (b) Plasmid
(c) Codon (d) None of these

29. *Ti*-plasmid used in genetic engineering has been modified by
(a) adding tumour forming genes.
(b) deleting tumour forming genes.
(c) adding genes for endonucleases.
(d) deleting genes for endonucleases.

30. Which of the following technique is used for the detection of RNA fragments ?
(a) Northern blotting (b) Chromatography
(c) Transformation (d) Transduction

31. Which of these is not correctly matched ?
(a) Gene gun—biolistic gun
(b) Plasmids—extrachromosomal DNA
(c) DNA ligase—Biological scissors
(d) Bacteriophages—viruses.

32. Polyethylene glycol method is used for
(a) biodiesel production
(b) seedless fruit production
(c) energy production from sewage
(d) gene transfer without a vector

RESPONSE GRID					
	20. ⓐⓑⓒⓓ	21. ⓐⓑⓒⓓ	22. ⓐⓑⓒⓓ	23. ⓐⓑⓒⓓ	24. ⓐⓑⓒⓓ
	25. ⓐⓑⓒⓓ	26. ⓐⓑⓒⓓ	27. ⓐⓑⓒⓓ	28. ⓐⓑⓒⓓ	29. ⓐⓑⓒⓓ
	30. ⓐⓑⓒⓓ	31. ⓐⓑⓒⓓ	32. ⓐⓑⓒⓓ		

Space for Rough Work

33. Which of the following is a molecular scissors?
(a) *Eco*RI (b) *Hind* III
(c) *Bam* H II (d) All of these

34. Rennin used in cheese industry is
(a) antibiotic (b) alkaloid
(c) enzyme (d) inhibitor

35. The primary reason why the same basic techniques can be used to analyze the DNA from species as diverse as bacteria and humans is that
(a) all cells are identical.
(b) every organism has the same amount of DNA.
(c) the DNA sequences of all organisms are the same.
(d) DNA has a consistent structure in all organisms.

36. Which of the following is a plasmid?
(a) pBR 322 (b) *Bam H* I
(c) *Sal* I (d) *Eco R*I

37. There is a restriction endonuclease called *Eco*RI. What does *.co* part in it stand for ?
(a) Colon (b) Coelom
(c) Coenzyme (d) *coli*

38. Restriction endonuclease - *Hind* II always cuts DNA molecules at a particular point by recognizing a specific sequence of
(a) six base pairs. (b) five base pairs.
(c) four base pairs. (d) seven base pairs.

39. Which of the following enzyme is used in case of fungus to cause release of DNA along with other macromolecules ?
(a) Lysozyme (b) Cellulase
(c) Chitinase (d) Amylase

40. Match Column I with Column II and identify the correct option.

	Column - I		Column - II
A.	Primers	I.	PCR
B.	Separation and purification of products	II.	C_2H_5OH
C.	Precipitation of DNA	III.	Uptake of foreign DNA by bacterium
D.	Transformation	IV.	Down stream processing

(a) A-IV; B-I; C-II; D-III
(b) A-II; B-I; C-IV; D-III
(c) A-IV; B-I; C-III; D-II
(d) A-I; B-IV; C-II; D-III

41. Which one of the following palindromic base sequences in DNA can be easily cut at about the middle by some particular restriction enzyme?
(a) 5'............CGTTCG............3'
3'............ATGGTA............5'
(b) 5'............GATATG............3'
3'............CTACTA............5'
(c) 5'............GAATTC............3'
3'............CTTAAG............5'
(d) 5'............CACGTA............3'
3'............CTCAGT............5'

42. During heat shock to the bacterium, the temperature used for giving thermal shock is
(a) 52°C (b) 100°C
(c) liquid nitrogen (d) 42°C

43. Stirred-tank bioreactors have been designed for
(a) addition of preservatives to the product.
(b) purification of the product.
(c) ensuring anaerobic conditions in the culture vessel.
(d) availability of oxygen throughout the process.

44. After completion of biosynthetic stage, the product has to be subjected through a series of processes before it is ready to marketing as a finished product. This series of processes is called
(a) upstream processing (b) downstream processing
(c) elution (d) insertional inactivation

45. Which of the following is not necessary to execute a polymerase chain reaction successfully?
(a) All four DNA bases
(b) Short DNA base primers
(c) DNA polymerase
(d) DNA library

RESPONSE GRID					
	33. ⓐⓑⓒⓓ	34. ⓐⓑⓒⓓ	35. ⓐⓑⓒⓓ	36. ⓐⓑⓒⓓ	37. ⓐⓑⓒⓓ
	38. ⓐⓑⓒⓓ	39. ⓐⓑⓒⓓ	40. ⓐⓑⓒⓓ	41. ⓐⓑⓒⓓ	42. ⓐⓑⓒⓓ
	43. ⓐⓑⓒⓓ	44. ⓐⓑⓒⓓ	45. ⓐⓑⓒⓓ		

BIOLOGY CHAPTERWISE SPEED TEST-91			
Total Questions	45	Total Marks	180
Attempted		Correct	
Incorrect		Net Score	
Cut-off Score	48	Qualifying Score	60
Success Gap = Net Score – Qualifying Score			
Net Score = (Correct × 4) – (Incorrect × 1)			

Space for Rough Work

BIOLOGY

Biotechnology and its Applications

Speed TEST 92 Chapter-wise

No. of Questions	Maximum Marks	Time
45	180	1 Hour

GENERAL INSTRUCTIONS

- This test contains 45 MCQ's. For each question only one option is correct. Darken the correct circle/ bubble in the Response Grid provided on each page.
- You have to evaluate your Response Grids yourself with the help of solutions provided at the end of this book.
- Each correct answer will get you 4 marks and 1 mark shall be deduced for each incorrect answer. No mark will be given/ deducted if no bubble is filled. Keep a timer in front of you and stop immediately at the end of 60 min.
- The sheet follows a particular syllabus. Do not attempt the sheet before you have completed your preparation for that syllabus.
- After completing the sheet check your answers with the solution booklet and complete the Result Grid. Finally spend time to analyse your performance and revise the areas which emerge out as weak in your evaluation.

1. Silencing of mRNA has been used in producing transgenic plants resistant to:
   (a) bollworms (b) nematodes
   (c) white rusts (d) bacterial blights
2. Important objective of biotechnology in agriculture section is –
   (a) To produce pest resistant varieties of plants
   (b) To increase the nitrogen content
   (c) To decrease the seed number
   (d) To increase the plant weight
3. Tobacco plants resistant to a nematode have been developed by the introduction of DNA that produced (in the host cells)
   (a) both sense and anti-sense RNA
   (b) a particular hormone
   (c) an antifeedant
   (d) a toxic protein
4. Which one of the following techniques made it possible to genetically engineered living organism ?
   (a) Recombinant DNA techniques
   (b) X-ray diffraction
   (c) Heavier isotope labelling
   (d) Hybridization
5. Consider the following four statements
   (i) The first transgenic buffalo, Rosie produced milk which was human alpha-lactal albumin enriched.
   (ii) Restriction enzymes are used in isolation of DNA from other macro-molecules.
   (iii) Downstream processing is one of the steps of R-DNA technology.
   (iv) Disarmed pathogen vectors are also used in transfer of R-DNA into the host.
   Which are the two statements incorrect?
   (a) Statement (ii) and (iii)
   (b) Statement (iii) and (iv)
   (c) Statement (i) and (iii)
   (d) Statement (i) and (ii)

RESPONSE GRID	1. ⓐⓑⓒⓓ	2. ⓐⓑⓒⓓ	3. ⓐⓑⓒⓓ	4. ⓐⓑⓒⓓ	5. ⓐⓑⓒⓓ

Space for Rough Work

6. cDNA probes are copied from the messenger RNA molecules with the help of –
(a) Restriction enzymes
(b) Reverse transcriptase
(c) DNA polymerase
(d) Adenosine deaminase

7. In history of biology, human genome project led to the development of :
(a) biotechnology (b) biomonitoring
(c) bioinformatics (d) biosystematics

8. Dolly sheep was obtained by –
(a) Cloning the udder cell (somatic cell) fused with enucleated oocyte
(b) Cloning of gametes
(c) Tissue culture
(d) None of the above

9. Which of the following forms the basis of DNA Finger printing?
(a) The relative proportions of purines and pyrimidines in DNA.
(b) Satellite DNA occurring as highly repeated short DNA segments.
(c) The relative difference in the DNA occurrence in blood, skin and saliva.
(d) The relative amount of DNA in the ridges and grooves of the fingerprints.

10. The genetically-modified (GM) brinjal in India has been developed for:
(a) insect-resistance
(b) enhancing shelf life
(c) enhancing mineral content
(d) drought-resistance

11. Which of the following statement(s) is/are true ?
(i) Biowar is the use of biological weapons against humans and /or their crops and animals.
(ii) Bioethics is the unauthorized use of bioresources and traditional knowledge related to bioresources for commercial benefits.
(iii) Biopatent is exploitation of bioresources of other nations without proper authorisation.
(a) (ii) only (b) (i) only
(c) (i) and (ii) only (d) (i) and (iii) only

12. Which of the following statements is/are correct with regard to the disadvantages of GM crops?
(a) GM crops can affect human health by causing allergic reactions.
(b) Transgenes in commercial crops can endanger native species e.g., the Bt toxin gene expressed in pollen might endanger pollinators like honeybees.
(c) Production of GM crops causes damage to the natural environment and is always costly.
(d) All of these

13. Which of the following genes were introduced in cotton to protect it from cotton bollworms?
(a) Cry Ac and Cry ab
(b) Bt Ac and Bt Ab
(c) Cry IAc and Cry II Ab
(d) Nif genes

14. Hirudin is
(a) a protein produced by *Hordeum vulgare*, which is rich in lysine
(b) a toxic molecuel isolated from *Gossypium hirsutum*, which reduces human fertility
(c) a protein produced from transgenic *Brassica napus* which prevents blood clotting
(d) an antibiotic produced by a genetically engineered bacterium *Escherichia coli*.

15. Early detection of a disease is possible by
(a) PCR
(b) Gene therapy
(c) recombination DNA technology ad ELISA
(d) both (a) and (c)

16. Gene therapy can be referred to as
(a) pre-clinical testing for inherited diseases in new-borns\
(b) treatment of diseases caused by genetic defect
(c) genetic engineering using rDNA technology
(d) cancer treatment using in vitro cultured stem cells

17. Rules of conduct that may be used to regulate our activities in relation to the biological world is called
(a) bioethics (b) biowar
(c) biopatent (d) biopiracy

18. *Flavr Savr* is the transgenic variety of
(a) cotton (b) rice
(c) tomato (d) potato

19. Biopiracy is related to
(a) Traditional knowledge
(b) Biomolecules and regarding bioresources genes isolated from bioresources
(c) Bioresources
(d) All of the above

RESPONSE GRID					
	6. ⓐⓑⓒⓓ	7. ⓐⓑⓒⓓ	8. ⓐⓑⓒⓓ	9. ⓐⓑⓒⓓ	10. ⓐⓑⓒⓓ
	11. ⓐⓑⓒⓓ	12. ⓐⓑⓒⓓ	13. ⓐⓑⓒⓓ	14. ⓐⓑⓒⓓ	15. ⓐⓑⓒⓓ
	16. ⓐⓑⓒⓓ	17. ⓐⓑⓒⓓ	18. ⓐⓑⓒⓓ	19. ⓐⓑⓒⓓ	

Space for Rough Work

20. Genetically engineered bacteria have been used in commercial production of
(a) thyroxine (b) human insulin
(c) testosterone (d) penicillin

21. Golden rice is a promising transgenic crop, when released for cultivation, it will help in
(a) producing petrol like fuel from rice.
(b) alleviation of vitamin A.
(c) pest resistance.
(d) herbicide tolerance.

22. Chloramphenicol and erythromycin (broad spectrum antibiotics) are produced by
(a) *Streptomyces* (b) *Nitrobacter*
(c) *Rhizobium* (d) *Penicillium*

23. The transgenic animals are those which have
(a) foreign DNA in some cells.
(b) foreign DNA in all of their cells.
(c) foreign RNA in all of their cells.
(d) Both (a) and (c).

24. The transgenic plants are the plants having
(a) no gene.
(b) genes in transposition.
(c) genes with no function to perform.
(d) genes of an other organism.

25. Recombinant DNA technology can be used to produce quantities of biologically active form of which one of the following products in *E.coli*?
(a) Luteinizing hormone (b) Ecdyson
(c) Rifamycin (d) Interferon

26. Which of the following combinations of risk are associated with genetically modified food ?
I. Toxicity
II. Allergic reaction
III. Antibiotic resistance in micro-organisms present in alimentary canal. –
(a) I and II (b) I, II and III
(c) I and III (d) II and III

27. Cheese and Yogurt are products obtained by
(a) distillation (b) pasteurization
(c) fermentation (d) dehydration

28. Main objective of producing herbicide resistant GM crops is
(a) encourage ecofriendly herbicides.
(b) reduce herbicide accumulation in food articles for health safety.
(c) eliminate weeds from fields without the use of manual labour.
(d) eliminate weeds from the fields without the use of herbicides.

29. Which one of the following is the correctly matched pair of a product and the microorganism responsible for it ?
(a) Ethyl alcohol- Yeast
(b) Acetic acid- *Lactobacillus*
(c) Cheese - *Nitrobacter*
(d) Curd - *Azotobacter*

30. Humulin is
(a) A form of chitin
(b) A powerful antibiotic
(c) A new digestive enzyme
(d) Human insulin

31. A genetically engineered micro-organism used successfully in bioremediation of oil spills is a species of
(a) *Pseudomonas* (b) *Trichoderma*
(c) *Xanthomonas* (d) *Bacillus*

32. Prenatal screening in humans, AIDS virus testing in humans, and genetic engineering for protection against insect attack in plants all
(a) are types of gene therapy.
(b) are examples of the application of r-DNA technology.
(c) require use of the same restriction enzyme.
(d) are carried out using gene guns.

33. Genetically engineered bovine growth hormone (BGH), which is highly effective for improving overall growth and milk production in cattle, remains a hotly debated issue because
(a) BGH is clearly hazardous to human health.
(b) BGH is an environmental hazard.
(c) BGH could drive traditional family farmers out of business.
(d) scientists remain unconvince d that BGH really works.

34. DNA vaccines are
(a) mixture of hormones (b) recombinant vaccines
(c) synthetic vaccines (d) pure DNA or RNA

35. Toxic component of *Bacillus thuringiensis* is protein. Commercial preparation of *Bacillus thuringiensis* consists of mixture of spores, cry protein and inert carrier. *Bt* stands for *Bacillus thuringiensis* for in popular crop of *Bt* cotton. *Tricoderma* is used in biocontrol of fungal pathogen because it has capacity to secrete the enzyme
(a) DNAase (b) RNAase
(c) Chitinase (d) Cry protein

RESPONSE GRID				
20. ⓐⓑⓒⓓ	21. ⓐⓑⓒⓓ	22. ⓐⓑⓒⓓ	23. ⓐⓑⓒⓓ	24. ⓐⓑⓒⓓ
25. ⓐⓑⓒⓓ	26. ⓐⓑⓒⓓ	27. ⓐⓑⓒⓓ	28. ⓐⓑⓒⓓ	29. ⓐⓑⓒⓓ
30. ⓐⓑⓒⓓ	31. ⓐⓑⓒⓓ	32. ⓐⓑⓒⓓ	33. ⓐⓑⓒⓓ	34. ⓐⓑⓒⓓ
35. ⓐⓑⓒⓓ				

Space for Rough Work

36. GEAC stands for
(a) Genome Engineering Action Committee
(b) Ground Environment Action Committee
(c) Genetic Engineering Approval Committee
(d) Genetic and Environment Approval committee

37. A transgenic food crop'which may help in solving the problem of night blindness in developing countries is
(a) *Flavr Savr* tomatoes (b) Starlink maize
(c) *Bt* Soybean (d) Golden rice

38. Some of the characteristics of Bt cotton are:
(a) long fibre and resistance to aphids
(b) medium yield, long fibre and resistance to beetle pests
(c) high yield and production of toxic protein crystals which kill dipteran pests

39. It is sometimes necessary to genetically engineered mammalian cells to produce proteins because they
(a) can produce larger quantities of protein than bacteria.
(b) can read eukaryotic genes and bacteria cannot.
(c) can add sugars to make glycoproteins and bacteria cannot.
(d) are easier to grow than bacteria.

40. Which one of the following is commonly used in transfer of foreign DNA into crop plants?
(a) *Meloidogyne incognita*
(b) *Agrobacterium tumefaciens*
(c) *Penicillium expansum*
(d) *Trichoderma harzianum*

41. α-I antitrypsin is
(a) an antacid
(b) an enzyme
(c) used to treat arthritis
(d) used to treat emphysema

42. Which one of the following genes is defective in patients suffering from severe combined immuno-deficiency syndrome (SCID) ?
(a) RNAase
(b) ADA
(c) Ribonucleotide reductase
(d) DNAase

43. Which one of the following option is incorrect?
(a) The majority of baculoviruses used as biological control agents are in the genus Nucleopolyhedrovirus.
(b) Nucleopolyhedrovirus are excellent model for broad-spectrum insecticidal applications.
(c) Nucleopolyhedrovirus have no negative impacts on plants, mammals, birds, fish or even on non-target insects.
(d) This is especially desirable when beneficial insects are being conserved to aid in an overall IPM programme.

44. Select the correct set of the names for A, B, C and D.

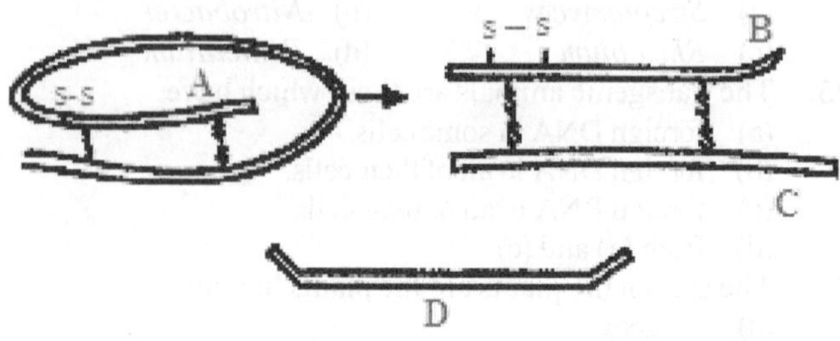

	A	B	C	D
(a)	Proinsulin	B-peptide	A-peptide	Insulin
(b)	Proinsulin	A-peptide	B-Peptide	Free C-Peptide
(c)	Proinsulin	A-peptide	B-peptide	Insulin
(d)	Proinsulin	B-Peptide	A-peptide	Free C-Peptide

45. Match the Column I with Column II and choose the correct option.

	Column I		Column II
A.	Golden rice	I.	Increased shelf life
B.	Flavr Savr tomato	II.	HGH
C.	Mouse	III.	Vitamin A
D.	Transgenic pig	IV.	Organ transplantation

(a) A-III; B-I; C-II; D-IV
(b) A-II; B-I; C-III; D-IV
(c) A-II; B-III; C-I; D-IV
(d) A-IV; B-I; C-II; D-III

RESPONSE GRID					
	36. ⓐⓑⓒⓓ	37. ⓐⓑⓒⓓ	38. ⓐⓑⓒⓓ	39. ⓐⓑⓒⓓ	40. ⓐⓑⓒⓓ
	41. ⓐⓑⓒⓓ	42. ⓐⓑⓒⓓ	43. ⓐⓑⓒⓓ	44. ⓐⓑⓒⓓ	45. ⓐⓑⓒⓓ

BIOLOGY CHAPTERWISE SPEED TEST-92			
Total Questions	45	Total Marks	180
Attempted		Correct	
Incorrect		Net Score	
Cut-off Score	40	Qualifying Score	55
Success Gap = Net Score – Qualifying Score			
Net Score = (Correct × 4) – (Incorrect × 1)			

Space for Rough Work

BIOLOGY

Organisms and Populations

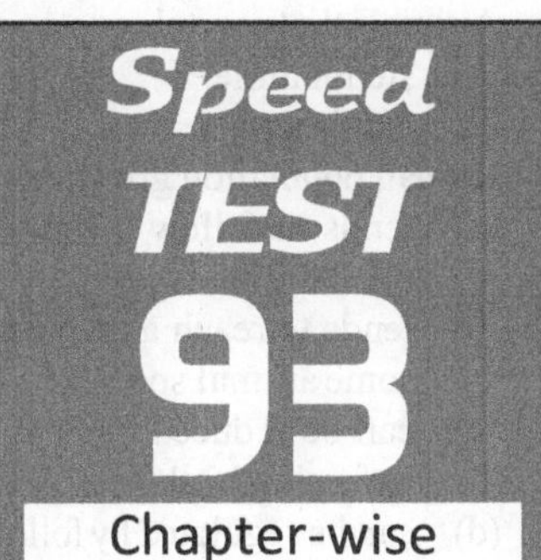

No. of Questions	Maximum Marks	Time
45	180	1 Hour

GENERAL INSTRUCTIONS

- This test contains 45 MCQ's. For each question only one option is correct. Darken the correct circle/ bubble in the Response Grid provided on each page.
- You have to evaluate your Response Grids yourself with the help of solutions provided at the end of this book.
- Each correct answer will get you 4 marks and 1 mark shall be deduced for each incorrect answer. No mark will be given/ deducted if no bubble is filled. Keep a timer in front of you and stop immediately at the end of 60 min.
- The sheet follows a particular syllabus. Do not attempt the sheet before you have completed your preparation for that syllabus.
- After completing the sheet check your answers with the solution booklet and complete the Result Grid. Finally spend time to analyse your performance and revise the areas which emerge out as weak in your evaluation.

1. Which part of the world has a high density of organisms?
(a) Grasslands
(b) Savannahs
(c) Deciduous forests
(d) Tropical rain forests

2. Competition for light, nutrients and space is most severe between
(a) closely related organism growing in different habitats
(b) closely related organisms growing in the same habitat
(c) distantly related organisms growing in the same habitat
(d) distantly related organisms growing in different habitats

3. A mutually beneficial association necessary for survival of both partners is
(a) mutualism/symbiosis (b) commensalism
(c) amensalism (d) both (a) and (b)

4. Praying mantis is a good example of
(a) warning colouration
(b) social insects
(c) camouflage
(d) mullerian mimicry

5. In increasing order of organizational complexity, which one of the following is the correct sequence?
(a) Population, species, community, ecosystem
(b) Population, variety, species, ecosystem
(c) Population, ecosystem, species, community
(d) Species, variety, ecosystem, community

6. Keystone species in an ecosystem are those
(a) present in maximum number
(b) that are most frequent
(c) attaining a large biomass
(d) contributing to ecosystem properties

7. Niche overlap indicates
(a) two different parasites on the same host
(b) sharing of one or more resources between the two species
(c) mutualism between two species
(d) active cooperation between two species

RESPONSE GRID	
	1. ⓐⓑⓒⓓ 2. ⓐⓑⓒⓓ 3. ⓐⓑⓒⓓ 4. ⓐⓑⓒⓓ 5. ⓐⓑⓒⓓ
	6. ⓐⓑⓒⓓ 7. ⓐⓑⓒⓓ

Space for Rough Work

8. Animals that can tolerate a narrow range of salinity are
(a) stenohaline (b) euryhaline
(c) anadromous (d) catadromous

9. Human population growth in India
(a) tends to follow a sigmoid curve as in case of many other animal species
(b) tends to reach a zero population growth as in case of some animal species
(c) can be reduced by permitting natural calamities and enforcing birth control measures
(d) can be regulated by following the national programme of family planning

10. Consider the following four conditions (i) - (iv) and select the correct pair of them as adaptation to environment in desert lizards.
The conditions :
(i) Burrowing in soil to escape high temperature
(ii) Losing heat rapidly from the body during high temperature
(iii) Bask in sun when temperature is low
(iv) Insulating body due to thick fatty dermis
(a) (iii), (iv) (b) (i)
(c) (iii), (ii), (iv) (d) (i), (ii)

11. A force acting against achievement of highest possible level of population growth is
(a) Carrying capacity
(b) Environment resistance
(c) Population pressure
(d) Saturation level

12. Natality is the characteristic of a population which means
(a) the total number of individuals present per unit area at a given time
(b) the increase in number of individuals in a population under given environmental conditions
(c) loss of individuals due to death in a population under given environmental conditions
(d) the movement of individuals into and out of population

13. The number of births per thousand people in the population is expressed as :
(a) Reproduction rate (b) Conception rate
(c) Crude birth rate (d) Growth rate

14. What type of human population is represented by the following age pyramid?

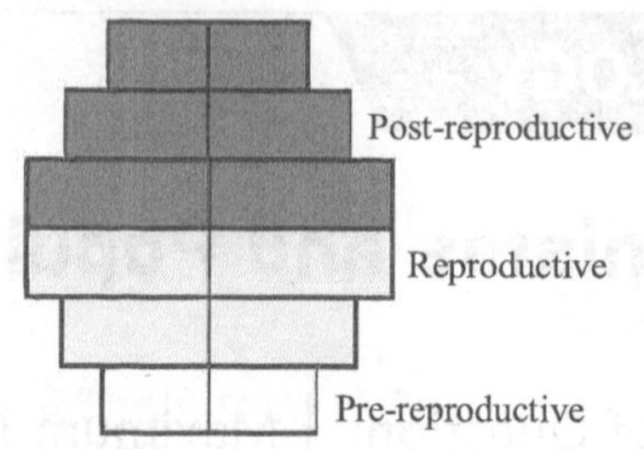

(a) Vanishing population
(b) Stable population
(c) Declining population
(d) Expanding population

15. The logistic population growth is expressed by the equation:
(a) $dt/dN = Nr\left(\frac{K-N}{K}\right)$
(b) $dN/dt = rN\left(\frac{K-N}{K}\right)$
(c) $dN/dt = rN$
(d) $dN/dt = rN\left(\frac{N-K}{N}\right)$

16. What is the best pH of soil for cultivation of plants ?
(a) 3.4 – 5.4 (b) 6.5 – 7.5
(c) 4.5 – 8.5 (d) 5.6 – 6.5

17. The maintenance of internal favourable conditions, by a self-regulated mechanism, inspite of the fact that there are changes in the environment, is known as
(a) entropy (b) enthalpy
(c) steady state (d) homeostasis

18. Two different species cannot live for long duration in the same niche or habitat. This law is
(a) Allen's law
(b) Gause's hypothesis
(c) Dollo's rule
(d) Weisman's theory

19. One of the important consequences of geographical isolation is
(a) preventing speciation
(b) speciation through reproductive isolation
(c) random creation of new species
(d) no change in the isolated fauna.

RESPONSE GRID					
	8. ⓐⓑⓒⓓ	9. ⓐⓑⓒⓓ	10. ⓐⓑⓒⓓ	11. ⓐⓑⓒⓓ	12. ⓐⓑⓒⓓ
	13. ⓐⓑⓒⓓ	14. ⓐⓑⓒⓓ	15. ⓐⓑⓒⓓ	16. ⓐⓑⓒⓓ	17. ⓐⓑⓒⓓ
	18. ⓐⓑⓒⓓ	19. ⓐⓑⓒⓓ			

Space for Rough Work

20. Which one of the following areas in India, is a hotspot of biodiversity?
(a) Eastern Ghats (b) Gangetic Plain
(c) Sunderbans (d) Western Ghats

21. A taxon facing an extremely high risk of extinction in wild in the immediate future is called :
(a) critical endangered
(b) endangered
(c) vulnerable
(d) extinct in wild

22. The species that invade a bare area are called
(a) keystone species (b) extinct species
(c) pioneer species (d) rare species

23. Several plant and animal species present together at a place constitute a
(a) genus (b) population
(c) biome (d) community

24. Deserts, rainforests, tundra, etc. are example of
(a) community (b) biome
(c) ecosystem (d) population

25. Life is sustainable with water only because
(a) it makes 90% of the protoplasm
(b) translocation of nutrients inside the body occurs with the help of water
(c) water loss in form of sweating and transpiration helps to maintain body temperature
(d) all of these

26. Which of the following algae are found in deepest ocean waters?
(a) Red algae (b) Yellow algae
(c) Green algae (d) Brown algae

27. When organisms change their location to escape from harsh environment, it is called as
(a) hibernation (b) vernalization
(c) migration (d) aestivation

28. Species interaction with negative influence on both is referred to as
(a) amensalism (b) mutualism
(c) commensalism (d) competition

29. Total number of individual of a species per unit area and per unit time is called
(a) population size
(b) population density
(c) demography
(d) population dyamics.

30. In a life table, the number of individuals alive at the begining of the 1st year to 2nd year interval is 800. During this interval, 200 individuals die. The death rate for this interval is
(a) 0.25 (b) 200
(c) 800 (d) 0.2

31. Which one of the following is the most productive ecosystem?
(a) Temperate forest (b) Grassland
(c) Desert (d) Tropical rain forest

32. Pedology is the study of –
(a) Locomotion of animals
(b) Rocks
(c) Soil
(d) Reproduction

33. Sequence of humification and mineralisation is-
(a) Dead organic matter $\rightarrow$ Litter $\rightarrow$ Duff $\rightarrow$ Humus $\rightarrow$ Minerals
(b) Humus $\rightarrow$ Minerals $\rightarrow$ Litter $\rightarrow$ Duff
(c) Minerals $\rightarrow$ Humus $\rightarrow$ Litter $\rightarrow$ Duff
(d) Dead organic matter $\rightarrow$ Duff $\rightarrow$ Litter $\rightarrow$ Minerals $\rightarrow$ Humus

34. Soil is composed of –
(a) Mineral + Water + Air
(b) Mineral + Organic matter + Water
(c) Mineral + Organic matter + Air + Water
(d) Organic matter + Water

35. Who employed the term ecology to study plants ?
(a) Haeckel (b) Odum
(c) Warming (d) Dudgeon

36. Biotic factors are –
(a) Chemical factors of soil which effect life
(b) Physical factors of soil which effect life
(c) All living organisms which influence other organisms
(d) Atmospheric factors which influence life

RESPONSE GRID					
	20. ⓐⓑⓒⓓ	21. ⓐⓑⓒⓓ	22. ⓐⓑⓒⓓ	23. ⓐⓑⓒⓓ	24. ⓐⓑⓒⓓ
	25. ⓐⓑⓒⓓ	26. ⓐⓑⓒⓓ	27. ⓐⓑⓒⓓ	28. ⓐⓑⓒⓓ	29. ⓐⓑⓒⓓ
	30. ⓐⓑⓒⓓ	31. ⓐⓑⓒⓓ	32. ⓐⓑⓒⓓ	33. ⓐⓑⓒⓓ	34. ⓐⓑⓒⓓ
	35. ⓐⓑⓒⓓ	36. ⓐⓑⓒⓓ			

Space for Rough Work

37. The age of pyramid with broad base indicates
(a) High percentage of young individuals
(b) Low percentage of young individuals
(c) High percentage of old individuals
(d) Low percentage of old individuals

38. Permafrost is the most distinctive feature of
(a) Taiga (b) Temperate grasslands
(c) Tundra (d) Pacific northwest

39. Which statement does not reflect a reason why grasses predominate in savannas ?
(a) There are few native herbivores in this biome.
(b) Grasses grow well in fine, sandy soils.
(c) The above ground portions of grass plants die during dry seasons.
(d) The deep roots of the grasses can survive many months of drought.

40. Desert regions are characterized by ___ centimeters of rainfall per year.
(a) less than 5 (b) less than 15
(c) less than 25 (d) over 50

41. To avoid summer - related problems such as heat and dessication fish undergoes
(a) hibernation (b) diapause
(c) aestivation (d) none of these

42. Seals have a thick layer of fat (blubber) below their skin that acts as an
(a) thermostat (b) capacitor
(c) resistor (d) insulator

43. Match the following

	Population		Example
A.	Predation	I.	*Cuscuta* and hedge plants
B.	Commensalism	II.	*Balanus* and *Chathamalus*
C.	Parasitism	III.	Cactus and moth
D.	Competition	IV.	Orchid and mango

(a) A-III; B-IV; C-I; D-II
(b) A-IV; B-III; C-II; D-I
(c) A-I; B-III; C-II; D-IV
(d) A-III; B-IV; C-II; D-I

44. The density of a population in a given habitat during a given period, fluctuates due to changes in four basic processes On this basis choose the correct option to fill up A and B boxes in the given diagram.

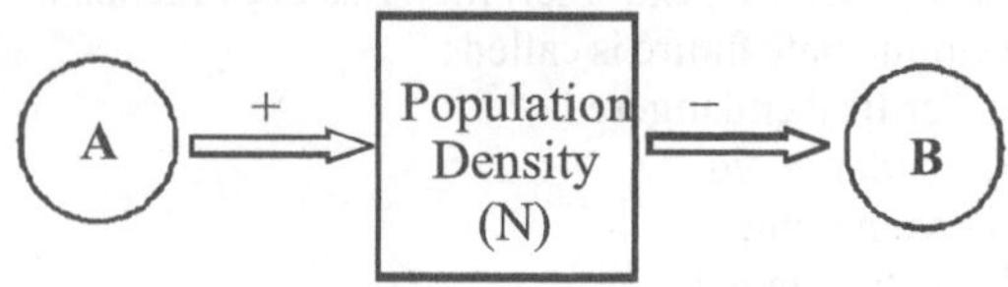

(a) A = Natality + Immigration, B = Mortality + Emigration
(b) A = Natality + Mortality, B = Immigration + Emigration
(c) A = Birth rate + Death rate, B = Mortality + Emigration
(d) A = Natality + Emigration, B = Mortality + Immigration

45. In laboratory experiments, two species of the protist *Paramecium* were grown alone and in the presence of the other species. The following graphs show growth of species 1 (left) and species 2 (right), both along and when in mixed culture.

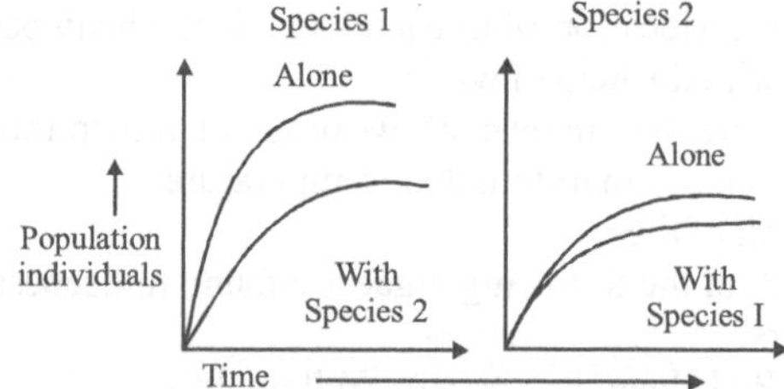

Interpretation of these graphs shows that
(a) competitive exclusion occurred in these experiments.
(b) both species are affected by interspecific competition but species 1 is less affected.
(c) both species are affected by interspecific competition but species 2 is less affected.
(d) both species are affected equally by interspecific competition.

RESPONSE GRID				
37. ⓐⓑⓒⓓ	38. ⓐⓑⓒⓓ	39. ⓐⓑⓒⓓ	40. ⓐⓑⓒⓓ	41. ⓐⓑⓒⓓ
42. ⓐⓑⓒⓓ	43. ⓐⓑⓒⓓ	44. ⓐⓑⓒⓓ	45. ⓐⓑⓒⓓ	

BIOLOGY CHAPTERWISE SPEED TEST-93

Total Questions	45	Total Marks	180
Attempted		Correct	
Incorrect		Net Score	
Cut-off Score	40	Qualifying Score	55
Success Gap = Net Score – Qualifying Score			
Net Score = (Correct × 4) – (Incorrect × 1)			

Space for Rough Work

BIOLOGY

Ecosystem

Speed TEST 94

Chapter-wise

No. of Questions	Maximum Marks	Time
45	180	1 Hour

GENERAL INSTRUCTIONS

- This test contains 45 MCQ's. For each question only one option is correct. Darken the correct circle/ bubble in the Response Grid provided on each page.
- You have to evaluate your Response Grids yourself with the help of solutions provided at the end of this book.
- Each correct answer will get you 4 marks and 1 mark shall be deduced for each incorrect answer. No mark will be given/ deducted if no bubble is filled. Keep a timer in front of you and stop immediately at the end of 60 min.
- The sheet follows a particular syllabus. Do not attempt the sheet before you have completed your preparation for that syllabus.
- After completing the sheet check your answers with the solution booklet and complete the Result Grid. Finally spend time to analyse your performance and revise the areas which emerge out as weak in your evaluation.

1. Deep black soil is productive due to high proportion of
   (a) sand and zinc (b) gravel and calcium
   (c) clay and humus (d) silt and earthworm
2. Which one of the following statements is correct for secondary succession ?
   (a) It begins on a bare rock
   (b) It occurs on a deforested site
   (c) It follows primary succession
   (d) It is similar to primary succession except that it has a relatively fast pace
3. The zone of atmosphere that lies near the ground is
   (a) troposphere (b) stratosphere
   (c) homosphere (d) ionosphere
4. Food chain in which micro-organisms breakdown the food formed by primary producers is
   (a) parasitic food chain (b) detritus food chain
   (c) consumer food chain (d) predator food chain
5. Which of the following pairs is a sedimentary type of biogeochemical cycle?
   (a) Oxygen and nitrogen
   (b) Phosphorus and sulphur
   (c) Phosphorus and nitrogen
   (d) Phosphorus and carbon dioxide
6. Mass of living matter at a trophic level in an area at any time is called
   (a) standing crop (b) detritus
   (c) humus (d) standing state
7. If we completely remove the decomposers from an ecosystem, its functioning will be adversely affected because
   (a) energy flow will be blocked
   (b) herbivores will not receive solar energy
   (c) mineral movement will be blocked
   (d) rate of decomposition will be very high
8. Humus is essential for plant growth because:
   (a) it is rich in nutrients and increases the water holding capacity of soil
   (b) it increases aeration of soil
   (c) it increases porocity of soil
   (d) All of the above

RESPONSE GRID					
	1. ⓐⓑⓒⓓ	2. ⓐⓑⓒⓓ	3. ⓐⓑⓒⓓ	4. ⓐⓑⓒⓓ	5. ⓐⓑⓒⓓ
	6. ⓐⓑⓒⓓ	7. ⓐⓑⓒⓓ	8. ⓐⓑⓒⓓ		

Space for Rough Work

9. The rate at which light energy is converted to the chemical energy of organic molecules in the ecosystem is
(a) net primary productivity
(b) gross primary productivity
(c) net secondary productivity
(d) gross secondary productivity

10. An ecosystem which can be easily damaged but can recover after some time if damaging effect stops will be having
(a) low stability and high resilience
(b) high stability and low resilience
(c) low stability and low resilience
(d) high stability and high resilience

11. Both hydrarch and xerarch successions lead to:
(a) medium water conditions
(b) xeric conditions
(c) highly dry conditions
(d) excessive wet conditions

12. Which of the following ecosystems has highest rate of gross primary production?
(a) Grasslands
(b) Mangroves
(c) Coral reefs
(d) Equatorial rain forest

13. Largest amount of fresh water is found in
(a) lakes and streams
(b) underground
(c) polar ice caps and glaciers
(d) rivers

14. Which one of the following is not a function of an ecosystem?
(a) Energy flow (b) Decomposition
(c) Productivity (d) Stratification

15. Ecosystem is
(a) always open
(b) always closed
(c) both open and closed depending upon community
(d) both open and closed depending upon biomass

16. Transition zone between two vegetations is
(a) ecotone (b) ecotype
(c) ecocline (d) ecosystem

17. Which one of the following statement is correct?
(a) Warm and moist environment favour decomposition whereas low temperature and anaerobiosis inhibit decomposition
(b) Warm and moist environment inhibit decomposition whereas low temperature and anaerobiosis favour decomposition
(c) Warm and anaerobiosis favour decomposition as well as low temperature favours decomposition
(d) Warm and low temperature inhibit decomposition whereas anaerobiosis favours decomposition

18. ______ is the rate of production of organic matter by consumers.
(a) Primary productivity
(b) Secondary productivity
(c) Net primary productivity
(d) Gross primary productivity

19. Which of the following is not a characteristic of humus?
(a) It is rich in organic matter such as lignin and cellulose.
(b) It is collodial in nature and serves as a reservoir of nutrients.
(c) It is highly resistant to microbial action and undergoes slow decomposition.
(d) It is further degraded by the process of humification.

20. Percentage of photosynthetically active radiation (PAR) in the incident solar radiation is
(a) 1 - 5% (b) 2 - 10%
(c) less than 50 % (d) approx. 100%

21. Which one of the following animals may occupy more than one trophic levels in the same ecosystem at the same time?
(a) Sparrow (b) Lion
(c) Goat (d) Frog

22. In lithosere, foliose lichens make the conditions favourable for the growth of
(a) crustose lichens (b) mosses
(c) annual grasses (d) perennial grasses

23. Which one of the following is not one of the three aspects studied in biogeochemical cycling?
(a) The nature and size of natural reservoir
(b) The rate of movement between reservoirs
(c) How different biogeochemical cycles interact
(d) How new species create their own biogeochemical cycles

RESPONSE GRID					
	9. ⓐⓑⓒⓓ	10. ⓐⓑⓒⓓ	11. ⓐⓑⓒⓓ	12. ⓐⓑⓒⓓ	13. ⓐⓑⓒⓓ
	14. ⓐⓑⓒⓓ	15. ⓐⓑⓒⓓ	16. ⓐⓑⓒⓓ	17. ⓐⓑⓒⓓ	18. ⓐⓑⓒⓓ
	19. ⓐⓑⓒⓓ	20. ⓐⓑⓒⓓ	21. ⓐⓑⓒⓓ	22. ⓐⓑⓒⓓ	23. ⓐⓑⓒⓓ

Space for Rough Work

24. The largest ecosystem of the world is-
(a) Forests (b) Grasslands
(c) Great lakes (d) Oceans

25. Which of the following is a man made artificial ecosystem?
(a) Grassland ecosystem
(b) Agro ecosystem
(c) Ecosystem of artificial lakes and dams
(d) Forest ecosystem

26. What is the annual net primary productivity of whole biosphere?
(a) 170 billion tons (dry weight) of organic matter
(b) 165 billion tons (dry weight) of organic matter
(c) 160 billion tons (dry weight) of organic matter
(d) 155 billion tons (dry weight) of organic matter

27. Select the formula for ecological efficiency
(a) $\frac{\text{Gross primary productivity} \times 100}{\text{Incident total solar radiation}}$
(b) $\frac{\text{Food primary assimilated} \times 100}{\text{Food energy ingested}}$
(c) $\frac{\text{Net primary productivity} \times 100}{\text{Gross primary productivity}}$
(d) $\frac{\text{Energy in biomass production at a trophic level} \times 100}{\text{Energy in biomass production at previous trophic level}}$

28. Vegetation of a geographic region with low rainfall, high temperature, loose and sandy soil is of the type called:
(a) grassland (b) scrub forest
(c) xerophytic (d) evergreen tropical forest

29. Which one is nature's cleaner ?
(a) Consumers
(b) Producers
(c) Decomposers and scavengers
(d) Symbionts

30. Which one of the following statement is correct?
(a) Decomposition rate is slower if detritus is rich in lignin and chitin, and quicker, if detritus is rich in nitrogen and water - soluble substances like sugars.
(b) Decomposition rate is slower if detritus is rich in nitrogen and water - soluble substances like sugars, and quicker, if detritus is rich in lignin and chitin.
(c) Decomposition rate is slower if detritus is rich in cellulose, and quicker, if detritus is rich in phosphorus.
(d) Decomposition rate is quicker if detritus is rich in lignin, and quicker, if detritus is rich in sulphur.

31. What are the two most important climatic factors that regulate decomposition through their effects on soil microbes ?
(a) Temperature and rainfall
(b) Temperature and soil - moisture
(c) Temperature and humidity
(d) Temperature and pressure

32. Which of the following process helps in nutrient conservation?
(a) Mineralisation (b) Immobilisation
(c) Leaching (d) Nitrification

33. Bacteria and fungi in a forest ecosystem are generally
(a) Producers
(b) Decomposers
(c) Primary consumers
(d) Secondary consumers

34. Which one of the following is not a gaseous biogeochemical cycle in ecosystem ?
(a) Sulphur cycle (b) Phosphorus cycle
(c) Nitrogen cycle (d) Carbon cycle

35. In grass-deer-tiger food chain, grass biomass is one tonne. The tiger biomass shall be
(a) 100 kg (b) 10 kg
(c) 200 kg (d) 1 kg

36. The early settlers on a barren area (rock) are
(a) Ferns (b) Mosses
(c) Lichens (d) Diatoms

37. A community which starts succession in a habitat is
(a) Pioneer community (b) Seral community
(c) Biotic community (d) Ecosere

38. Last stabilised community in a plant succession is known as
(a) Seral community (b) Pioneer community
(c) Ecosere (d) Climax community

39. Identification and enumeration of plant and animal species of an ecosystem gives its
(a) productivity (b) stratification
(c) species composition (d) all of these

RESPONSE GRID					
	24. ⓐⓑⓒⓓ	25. ⓐⓑⓒⓓ	26. ⓐⓑⓒⓓ	27. ⓐⓑⓒⓓ	28. ⓐⓑⓒⓓ
	29. ⓐⓑⓒⓓ	30. ⓐⓑⓒⓓ	31. ⓐⓑⓒⓓ	32. ⓐⓑⓒⓓ	33. ⓐⓑⓒⓓ
	34. ⓐⓑⓒⓓ	35. ⓐⓑⓒⓓ	36. ⓐⓑⓒⓓ	37. ⓐⓑⓒⓓ	38. ⓐⓑⓒⓓ
	39. ⓐⓑⓒⓓ				

Space for Rough Work

40. Which of the following factors influence communities ?
(i) Climate
(ii) Species interaction
(iii) Feeding relationships among organisms
(iv) Succession
(a) (i) and (iii) (b) (i) and (iv)
(c) (i), (ii) and (iii) (d) All of these

41. Grasslands can support greater grazing rates by herbivores than forests because
(a) net production of grassland is greater.
(b) more of the grassland is above the ground.
(c) grasslands receive more sunlight.
(d) grasslands produce less woody plant tissue.

42. Given below is an imaginary pyramid of numbers. What could be one of the possibilities about certain organisms at some of the different levels ?

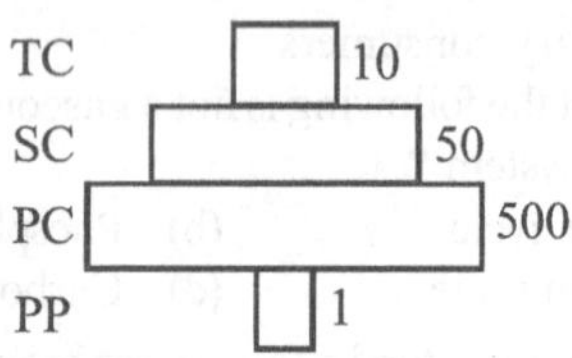

(a) Level PC is "insects" and level SC is "small insectivorous birds".
(b) Level PP is "phytoplanktons" in sea and "whale" is on top level TC.
(c) Level PP is "peepal trees" and the level SC is "sheep".
(d) Level PC is "rats" and level SC is "cats".

43. The given diagram shows (I, II, III, and IV) the flow of materials between different trophic levels. Which arrow is incorrect?

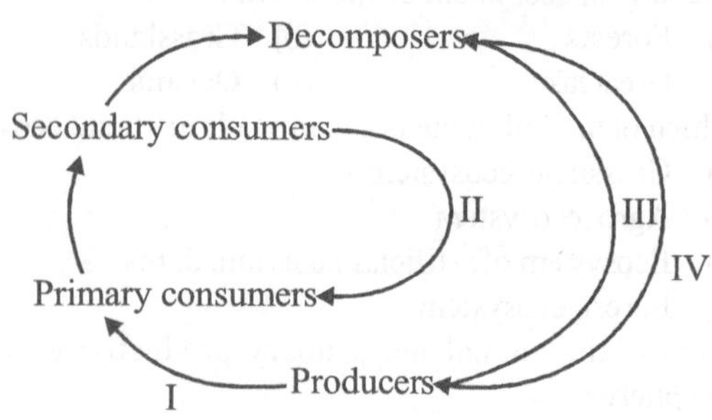

(a) I (b) II
(c) III (d) IV

44. Match the following and choose the correct option.

	Column - I		Column - II
A.	Presence of 3-4 storey of plants grown in a forest	I.	Blue-green algae
B.	A biome having grasses with scattered trees	II.	Stratification
C.	Man made ecosystem	III.	Savannah
D.	Pioneer in hydrosere	IV.	Dam

(a) A – III; B – II; C – IV; D – I
(b) A – III; B – I; C – IV; D – II
(c) A – I; B – III; C – II; D – IV
(d) A – II; B – III; C – IV; D – I

45. The correct order of the process of decomposition is
(a) Catabolism → Fragmentation → Leaching → Humification → Mineralization
(b) Catabolism → Fragmentation → Humification → Leaching → Mineralization
(c) Fragmentation → Humification → Catabolism → Leaching → Mineralization
(d) Fragmentation → Leaching → Catabolism → Humification → Mineralization

RESPONSE GRID	40. ⓐⓑⓒⓓ	41. ⓐⓑⓒⓓ	42. ⓐⓑⓒⓓ	43. ⓐⓑⓒⓓ	44. ⓐⓑⓒⓓ
	45. ⓐⓑⓒⓓ				

BIOLOGY CHAPTERWISE SPEED TEST-94			
Total Questions	45	Total Marks	180
Attempted		Correct	
Incorrect		Net Score	
Cut-off Score	50	Qualifying Score	70
Success Gap = Net Score – Qualifying Score			
Net Score = (Correct × 4) – (Incorrect × 1)			

Space for Rough Work

BIOLOGY

Biodiversity and its Conservation

Speed TEST 95

Chapter-wise

No. of Questions	Maximum Marks	Time
45	180	1 Hour

GENERAL INSTRUCTIONS

- This test contains 45 MCQ's. For each question only one option is correct. Darken the correct circle/ bubble in the Response Grid provided on each page.
- You have to evaluate your Response Grids yourself with the help of solutions provided at the end of this book.
- Each correct answer will get you 4 marks and 1 mark shall be deduced for each incorrect answer. No mark will be given/ deducted if no bubble is filled. Keep a timer in front of you and stop immediately at the end of 60 min.
- The sheet follows a particular syllabus. Do not attempt the sheet before you have completed your preparation for that syllabus.
- After completing the sheet check your answers with the solution booklet and complete the Result Grid. Finally spend time to analyse your performance and revise the areas which emerge out as weak in your evaluation.

1. Which one of the following is not included under *in-situ* conservation ?
(a) Botanical garden
(b) Biosphere reserve
(c) National park
(d) Sanctuary

2. Biodiversity Act of India was passed by the parliament in the year
(a) 1992 (b) 1996
(c) 2000 (d) 2002

3. Biodiversity of a geographical region represents
(a) endangered species found in the region.
(b) the diversity in the organisms living in the region.
(c) genetic diversity present in the dominant species of the region.
(d) species endemic to the region.

4. Which animal has become extinct from India?
(a) Snow Leopard (b) Hippopotamus
(c) Wolf (d) Cheetah

5. Which of the following is considered a hot-spot of biodiversity in India ?
(a) Indo-Gangetic Plain (b) Eastern Ghats
(c) Aravalli Hills (d) Western Ghats

6. Which group of vertebrates comprises the highest number of endangered species ?
(a) Birds (b) Mammals
(c) Fishes (d) Reptiles

7. One of endangered species of Indian medicinal plants is that of
(a) *Ocimum* (b) Garlic
(c) *Nepenthes* (d) *Podophyllum*

8. Which one of the following is the correct matched pair of an endangered animal and National Park ?
(a) Rhinoceros - Kaziranga National Park
(b) Wild Ass - Dudhwa National Park
(c) Great Indian - Keoladeo National Park Bustard
(d) Lion - Corbett National Park

RESPONSE GRID					
	1. ⓐⓑⓒⓓ	2. ⓐⓑⓒⓓ	3. ⓐⓑⓒⓓ	4. ⓐⓑⓒⓓ	5. ⓐⓑⓒⓓ
	6. ⓐⓑⓒⓓ	7. ⓐⓑⓒⓓ	8. ⓐⓑⓒⓓ		

Space for Rough Work

9. The area where wild populations, traditional life styles and genetic resources are protected is :
(a) Core Zone
(b) Buffer Zone
(c) Biosphere reserve
(d) Manipulation Zone

10. Which one of the following species of plant is considered as the world's most problematic aquatic weed?
(a) *Lantana*
(b) *Eichhornia*
(c) *Parthenium* (carrot grass)
(d) Brown algae

11. Which one of the following is not observed in biodiversity hotspots ?
(a) Endemism
(b) Accelerated species loss
(c) Lesser inter-specific competition
(d) Species richness

12. Which one of the following shows maximum genetic diversity in India ?
(a) Groundnut (b) Rice
(c) Maize (d) Mango

13. Study the four statements (i–iv) given below and select the two correct ones out of them:
(i) A lion eating a deer and a sparrow feeding on grain are ecologically similar in being consumers
(ii) Predator star fish *Pisaster* helps in maintaining species diversity of some invertebrates
(iii) Predators ultimately lead to the extinction of prey species
(iv) Production of chemicals such as nicotine, strychnine by the plants are metabolic disorders

The two correct statements are:
(a) (ii) and (iii) (b) (iii) and (iv)
(c) (i) and (iv) (d) (i) and (ii)

14. Reason of diversity in living beings is due to
(a) mutation
(b) long term evolutionary change
(c) gradual change
(d) short term evolutionary change

15. Which of the following is a reason for the greater biological diversity of tropical regions?
(a) Tropical latitudes have remained almost undisturbed for millions of years.
(b) Tropical environments are less seasonal, relatively more constant and predictable.
(c) More solar energy is available in the tropics resulting inhigh productivity.
(d) All of these.

16. An exotic species that is introduced to a new area, spreads rapidly and eliminates native species is called
(a) immigrant species
(b) invasive species
(c) *Eicchornia crasspies*
(d) all of these

17. Characters of stable community are
(a) it should not show too much variations in year-to-year productivity.
(b) it must be resistant to occasional natural or man-made disturbances.
(d) it should be resistant to invasions by alien species.
(d) All of these

18. What is the decreasing order of numbr of animals species as far as India is concerned?
(a) Mammals, Aves, Reptiles, Amphibians
(b) Aves, Reptiles, Mammals, Amphibians
(c) Mammals, Reptiles, Amphibians, Aves
(d) Reptiles, Amphibians, Mammals, Aves

19. Organization responsible for maintaning Red Data Book is
(a) IUCN (b) WWF
(c) CITES (d) IBWL

RESPONSE GRID					
	9. ⓐⓑⓒⓓ	10. ⓐⓑⓒⓓ	11. ⓐⓑⓒⓓ	12. ⓐⓑⓒⓓ	13. ⓐⓑⓒⓓ
	14. ⓐⓑⓒⓓ	15. ⓐⓑⓒⓓ	16. ⓐⓑⓒⓓ	17. ⓐⓑⓒⓓ	18. ⓐⓑⓒⓓ
	19. ⓐⓑⓒⓓ				

Space for Rough Work

20. Which option correctly describes are equations for curves A and B, in the given graph of species - area relationhip?

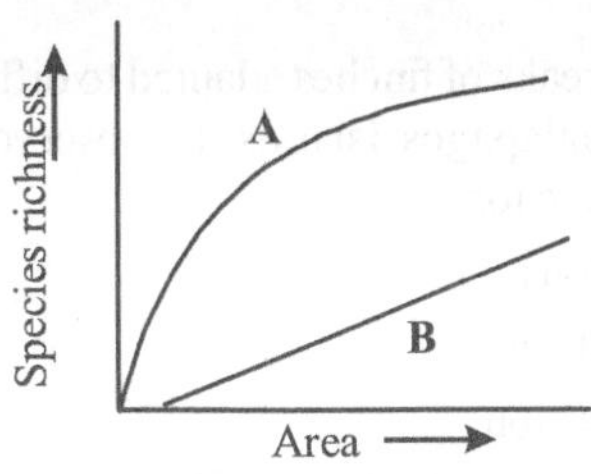

	A	B
(a)	$S = CA^Z$	$\text{Log } S = \text{Log } C + Z \text{ Log } A$
(b)	$\text{Log } S = \text{Log } C + Z \text{ Log } A$	$S = CA^Z$
(c)	$\text{Log } C = \text{Log } S + Z \text{ log } A$	$S = CA^Z$
(d)	$S = CA^Z$	$\text{Log } C = \text{Log } S + Z \text{ Log } A$

21. Genetic variations affect the productionof the drug reserpine in the medicinal plant *Rauwolfia vomitoria* growing in different Himalayan ranges. What kind of diversity does it indicate?
(a) Species diversity
(b) Genetic diversity
(c) Ecological diversity
(d) None of these

22. Keystone species deserve protection because these
(a) are capable of surviving in hash environmental conditions
(b) indicate the presence of certain minerals in the soil
(c) have become rare due to overexploitation
(d) play an important role in supporting other species.

23. In a National Park, protection is provided to
(a) flora and fauna (b) entire ecosystem
(c) fauna only (d) flora only

24. Which of thse organisms are protected by people of 'Bishnoi' community of Rajasthan?
(a) *Prosopis cineraria* (b) Black buck
(c) Bhojpatra (d) Both (a) and (b).

25. Which o the following statements regarding biodiversity hot spots are incorrect?
(i) High endemism
(ii) High levels of species richness.
(iii) Total number is 34 in the world.
(iv) Five of these occur in India.
(v) High alien species invasions.
(vi) Cover less than 2% of the earth's land area; but if properly conserved, they can reduce extinctions by about 30%.
(a) (i), (ii), (iii) (b) (i), (ii), (iii), (iv)
(c) (iv), (v), (vi) (d) (i), (ii), (iv)

26. Ex situ conservation is used for the conservation of
(a) all plants
(b) all animals
(c) threatened animals and plants
(d) both (a) and (b).

27. _______ National Park was the first National Park of India.
(a) Jim Corbett (b) Nanda Devi
(c) Kaziranga (d) Jaldapara

28. First 'Earth Summit' for 'Convention on Biological Diversity' (CBD) was held at
(a) Johannesberg (2002), S. Africa
(b) Rio de Janeiro (1992' Brazil
(c) Dehradun (1992), India
(d) New York (2000), U.S.A.

29. *Antilopa carvicapra*/Black Buck is –
(a) Vulnerable (b) Endangered
(c) Critically endangered (d) Extinct in the wild

30. Alpha diversity is present –
(a) Within community (b) Between community
(c) Ranges of communities (d) All of the above

31. Biodiversity is determined by –
(a) Number of individuals in an area
(b) Species richness
(c) Evenness
(d) Both (b) and (c)

RESPONSE GRID					
	20. ⓐⓑⓒⓓ	21. ⓐⓑⓒⓓ	22. ⓐⓑⓒⓓ	23. ⓐⓑⓒⓓ	24. ⓐⓑⓒⓓ
	25. ⓐⓑⓒⓓ	26. ⓐⓑⓒⓓ	27. ⓐⓑⓒⓓ	28. ⓐⓑⓒⓓ	29. ⓐⓑⓒⓓ
	30. ⓐⓑⓒⓓ	31. ⓐⓑⓒⓓ			

Space for Rough Work

32. Which of the following species is endangered ?
(a) *Panthera leo perrica* (b) *Pythan molurus*
(c) *Chelonia mydas* (d) *Pallas siberian crane*

33. Decrease in species diversity in tropical countries is mainly due to –
(a) Urbanisation (b) Pollution
(c) Deforestation (d) Soil erosion

34. Which of the following animal has become almost extinct in India ?
(a) Wolf (b) Rhinoceros
(c) Hippopotamus (d) Cheetah

35. Those species whose populations have been seriously depleted and whose ultimate security is not assured are known as –
(a) Threatened species (b) Endangered species
(c) Vulnerable species (d) Rare species

36. Which of the following is threatened by illegal trade in wildlife products?
(a) Nile perch (b) Elephants
(c) Key deer (d) Galapagos tortoises

37. Humans have altered _____ of Earth's land surface.
(a) very little (b) about 25%
(c) about 50% (d) about 80%

38. Which endangered animal is the source of world's finest, lightest, warmest and most expensive wool-the shahtoosh ?
(a) Nilgai (b) Cheetal
(c) Kashmiri Goat (d) Chiru

39. Which of the following is the most serious threat to biodiversity?
(a) Competition from exotic species
(b) Commercial harvesting
(c) Habitat destruction
(d) Overexploitation

40. Diversity in the type of breaks of finches adapted to different feeding habits on the Galapagos Islands, as observed by Darwin, provides evidence for
(a) intraspecific variations.
(b) intraspecific competition.
(c) interspecific competition.
(d) origin of species by natural selection.

41. Which of the following is not a step in understanding biodiversity ?
(a) Naming the species
(b) Looking at other related species
(c) Assessing the species geographic range
(d) Quantifying the species genome

42. Diversity of habitat over the total landscape is called
(a) β diversity (b) γ diveristy (gamma)
(c) landscape diversity (d) ecosystem diversity

43. The term hot spot for high diversity ecological regions was coined by –
(a) IUCN (b) Myers
(c) Odum (d) Kormandy

44. Following arrangement is correct from the point of view of decreasing biodiversity in angiosperms (N), fungi (F), pteridophytes (P) and algae(A)
(a) N>F>P>A (b) N>F>A>P
(c) F>N>P>A (d) F>N>A>P

45. The number of plant species recorded from India, is
(a) 30,000 (b) 45,000
(c) 70,000 (d) 90,000

RESPONSE GRID					
	32. ⓐⓑⓒⓓ	33. ⓐⓑⓒⓓ	34. ⓐⓑⓒⓓ	35. ⓐⓑⓒⓓ	36. ⓐⓑⓒⓓ
	37. ⓐⓑⓒⓓ	38. ⓐⓑⓒⓓ	39. ⓐⓑⓒⓓ	40. ⓐⓑⓒⓓ	41. ⓐⓑⓒⓓ
	42. ⓐⓑⓒⓓ	43. ⓐⓑⓒⓓ	44. ⓐⓑⓒⓓ	45. ⓐⓑⓒⓓ	

BIOLOGY CHAPTERWISE SPEED TEST-95			
Total Questions	45	Total Marks	180
Attempted		Correct	
Incorrect		Net Score	
Cut-off Score	50	Qualifying Score	60
Success Gap = Net Score – Qualifying Score			
Net Score = (Correct × 4) – (Incorrect × 1)			

Space for Rough Work

BIOLOGY

Environmental Issues

Speed TEST 96

Chapter-wise

No. of Questions	Maximum Marks	Time
45	180	1 Hour

GENERAL INSTRUCTIONS

- This test contains 45 MCQ's. For each question only one option is correct. Darken the correct circle/ bubble in the Response Grid provided on each page.
- You have to evaluate your Response Grids yourself with the help of solutions provided at the end of this book.
- Each correct answer will get you 4 marks and 1 mark shall be deduced for each incorrect answer. No mark will be given/ deducted if no bubble is filled. Keep a timer in front of you and stop immediately at the end of 60 min.
- The sheet follows a particular syllabus. Do not attempt the sheet before you have completed your preparation for that syllabus.
- After completing the sheet check your answers with the solution booklet and complete the Result Grid. Finally spend time to analyse your performance and revise the areas which emerge out as weak in your evaluation.

1. Acid rains are produced by
   (a) excess emissions of NO_2 and SO_2 from burning fossil fuels
   (b) excess production of NH_3 by industry and coal gas
   (c) excess release of carbon monoxide by incomplete combustion
   (d) excess formation of CO_2 by combustion and animal respiration
2. DDT residues are rapidly passed through food chain causing biomagnification because DDT is
   (a) moderately toxic
   (b) non-toxic to aquatic animals
   (c) water soluble
   (d) lipo soluble
3. Which of these is a pollution related to occupational health hazard disease ?
   (a) Pneumoconiosis (b) Asthma
   (c) Flurosis (d) Silicosis
4. Secondary sewage treatment is mainly a
   (a) physical process (b) mechanical process
   (c) chemical process (d) biological process
5. Biochemical Oxygen Demand *(BOD)* in a river water
   (a) has no relationship with concentration of oxygen in the water.
   (b) gives a measure of *Salmonella* in the water.
   (c) increases when sewage gets mixed with river water.
   (d) remains unchanged when algal bloom occurs.
6. Today, concentration of green house gases is high because of
   (a) Use of refrigerator
   (b) Increased combustion of oil and coal
   (c) Deforestation
   (d) All the above
7. The electrostatic precipitator is used for removing particulate matter from
   (a) Exhaust of the thermal power plant
   (b) Exhaust from the automobiles
   (c) Industrial effluents
   (d) Kitchen waste

RESPONSE GRID					
	1. ⓐⓑⓒⓓ	2. ⓐⓑⓒⓓ	3. ⓐⓑⓒⓓ	4. ⓐⓑⓒⓓ	5. ⓐⓑⓒⓓ
	6. ⓐⓑⓒⓓ	7. ⓐⓑⓒⓓ			

Space for Rough Work

8. Photochemical smog formed in congested metropolitan cities mainly consists of
(a) Ozone, peroxyacetyl nitrate and NOX
(b) Smoke, peroxyacetyl nitrate and SO_2
(c) Hydrocarbons, SO_2 and CO_2
(d) Hydrocarbon, ozone and SOX

9. Ozone hole means
(a) hole in the ozone layer in stratosphere.
(b) decrease in the thickness of ozone in the stratosphere.
(c) decrease in concentration of ozone in trophosphere.
(d) increase in the concentration of ozone in trophosphere.

10. A lake near a village suffered heavy mortality of fishes within a few days. Consider the following reasons for this.
(i) Lots of urea and phosphate fertilizer were used in the crops in the vicinity
(ii) The area was sprayed with DDT by an aircraft
(iii) The lake water turned green and stinky
(iv) Phytoplankton populations in the lake declined initially thereby greatly reducing photosynthesis.
(a) (i) and (iii) (b) (i), (ii) and (iv)
(c) (iii) and (iv) (d) (ii), (iii) and (iv)

11. Wildlife is destroyed most when
(a) there is lack of proper care
(b) mass scale hunting for foreign trade
(c) its natural habitat is destroyed
(d) natural calamity occurs

12. The 'Earth Summit' held at Rio de Janerio in 1992 resulted into
(a) Compilation of Red list
(b) Establishment of Biosphere Reserves
(c) Convention on Biodiversity
(d) Development of Hot Spots of Biodiversity

13. Which one of the following expanded forms of the following acronyms is correct?
(a) IPCC= International Panel for Climate Change
(b) UNEP= United Nations Environmental Policy
(c) EPA= Environmental Pollution Agency
(d) IUCN= International Union for Conservation of Nature and Natural Resources

14. Photochemical smog pollution does not contain
(a) Nitrogen dioxide
(b) Carbon dioxide
(c) PAN (peroxy acetyl nitrate)
(d) Ozone

15. When huge amount of sewage is dumped into a river, its B.O.D. will
(a) increase (b) decrease
(c) sharply decrease (d) remain unchanged

16. Which of the following statements is correct?
(a) Primary pollutants are more harmful than secondary pollutants.
(b) Primary pollutants and secondary pollutants are equally harmful.
(c) Secondary pollutants are more harmful than primary pollutants.
(d) DDT is a secondary pollutant

17. Which one of the following statements is incorrect regarding Bhopal gas tragedy?
(a) Methyl isocyanate gas leakage took place
(b) Thousands of human beings died
(c) Radioactive fall out engulfed Bhopal
(d) It took place in the night of December 2/3, 1984

18. Lichens are the indicators of
(a) water pollution
(b) air pollution
(c) soil pollution
(d) all of these.

19. Noise pollution may cause nervousness and irritability by stimulating the secretion of
(a) thyroid hormone
(b) adernaline hormone
(c) parathyroid hormone
(d) none of these

20. Atmospheric pollutant is –
(a) 0.0034% CO_2 (b) 0.034% CO_2
(c) 0.34% CO_2 (d) 3.4% CO_2

RESPONSE GRID					
	8. ⓐⓑⓒⓓ	9. ⓐⓑⓒⓓ	10. ⓐⓑⓒⓓ	11. ⓐⓑⓒⓓ	12. ⓐⓑⓒⓓ
	13. ⓐⓑⓒⓓ	14. ⓐⓑⓒⓓ	15. ⓐⓑⓒⓓ	16. ⓐⓑⓒⓓ	17. ⓐⓑⓒⓓ
	18. ⓐⓑⓒⓓ	19. ⓐⓑⓒⓓ	20. ⓐⓑⓒⓓ		

Space for Rough Work

21. Given pie-diagram represents the relative contribution of various GHGz to total global warming. Select the correct statement(s) regarding A, B and C.

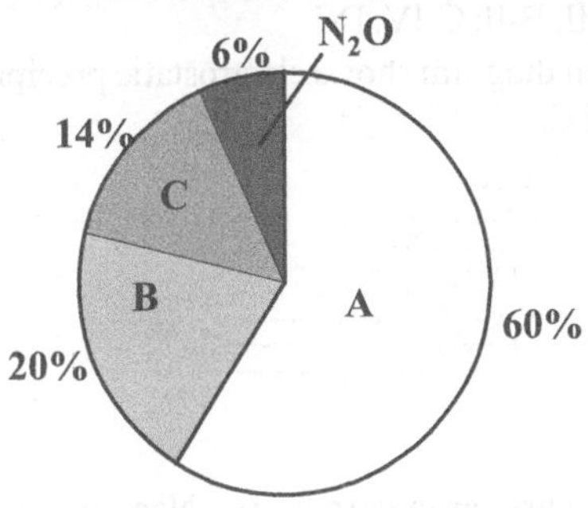

(a) A is the gas which is produced during the combustion of fossil fuels.
(b) B are the chemicals which are used as coolants in refrigerators
(c) C is the gas which is the major constituent of biogas
(d) All of these

22. Which of the following can cause DNA damage and mutations in humans?
(a) Absorption of UV-A and UV-B
(b) Absorption of UV-B
(c) Absorption of UV-A
(d) Absorption of UV-A and UV-C

23. Which of the following statements is not correct regarding jhum cultivation?
(a) It is also called as shifting cultivation and has resulted in deforestation
(b) It helps in increasing crop yield to a considerable extent.
(c) A time-gap of several years is required for the recovery of the land after cultivation.
(d) It involves cutting down of trees of the forest, burning of the plant remains and then using the land for farming.

24. Which of the following statement is incorrect ?
(a) Carbon monoxide is the major environment pollutant
(b) All pollutants are not waste
(c) Nitrogen and magnesium can pollute water
(d) Lichens are affected by sulphur

25. Noise pollution is created if noise is in excess to –
(a) 70-75 dB (b) 50-60 dB
(c) 80-99 dB (d) 40-65 dB

26. Which of the following does not cause pollution ?
(a) Thermal power project (b) Steel power plant
(c) Automobiles (d) Hydro electric project

27. Eutrophication causes reduction in
(a) dissolved CO_2 (b) dissolved O_2
(c) dissolved nutrients (d) none of the above

28. It is said, the Taj Mahal may be destroyed due to
(a) Flood in Yamuna river
(b) Decomposition of marble as a result of high temperature
(c) Air pollutants released from oil refinery of Mathura
(d) All of the above

29. The scrubber is used mainly to remove the following gas/es from the exhaust after spraying water/ lime
(a) CO_2 (b) SO_2
(c) O_2 & N_2 (d) CO & CO_2

30. Volcano is ____________ source of pollution.
(a) artificial (b) natural
(c) Both (a) and (b) (d) man-made

31. Montreal Protocol was called to check emission of
(a) e-wastes (b) UV radiation
(c) CFCs (d) All of these

32. Which of the following is normally not an atmosphere pollutant ?
(a) CO_2 (b) SO_2
(c) Hydrogen (d) CO

33. Which of the following is not properly matched
(a) Formaldehyde - carcinogenic
(b) Sulphur dioxide - respiratory problems
(c) Nitrogen oxide - brown air
(d) Mean annual temperature - 25° C

34. Cleaning Environment with biological options such as microbes and plants is called
(a) Bioremediation (b) Biotechnology
(c) Biowarfare (d) Incineration

35. The 'Jhum cultivation' in India is practiced in
(a) North- East states (b) South–West coast
(c) South- East coast (d) Gangetic plain

36. Why is the concentration of ozone is less over the north and south poles ?
(a) CFCs accumulate only in area where the air is cold
(b) CFC use is highest in these areas
(c) CFCs stick to frozen water vapour and are able to act catalysts
(d) UV rays are stronger in the atmosphere

RESPONSE GRID				
21. ⓐⓑⓒⓓ	22. ⓐⓑⓒⓓ	23. ⓐⓑⓒⓓ	24. ⓐⓑⓒⓓ	25. ⓐⓑⓒⓓ
26. ⓐⓑⓒⓓ	27. ⓐⓑⓒⓓ	28. ⓐⓑⓒⓓ	29. ⓐⓑⓒⓓ	30. ⓐⓑⓒⓓ
31. ⓐⓑⓒⓓ	32. ⓐⓑⓒⓓ	33. ⓐⓑⓒⓓ	34. ⓐⓑⓒⓓ	35. ⓐⓑⓒⓓ
36. ⓐⓑⓒⓓ				

Space for Rough Work

37. The waste water from Industries may contain toxic heavy metals having density of more than
(a) 5 g / cm^3 (b) 10 g /cm^3
(c) 2 g /cm^3 (d) 15 g /cm^3

38. DDT causes egg shell thinning in birds because it inhibits
(a) calmodulin (b) calcium ATPase
(c) magnesium ATPase (d) carbonic anhydrase

39. FOAM (Friends of the Arcata Marsh) is a group of citizens responsible for the integrated process of
(a) reducing eutrophication
(b) sewage and water treatment
(c) radio- active waste treatment
(d) minimizing global warming

40. Without Green house effect the average temperature of earth surface would have been
(a) 18 °C (b) 8°C
(c) – 8°C (d) –18°C

41. Read the following statements.
A lake near a village suffered heavy mortality of fishes within a few days. Consider the following reasons for this;
(i) Lots of urea and phosphate fertilizer were used in the crops in the vicinity.
(ii) The area was sprayed with DDT by an aircraft.
(iii) The lake water turned green and stinky.
(iv) Phytoplankton populations in the lake declined intially thereby greatly reducing photosynthesis.
Which two of the above were the main causes of fish mortality in the lake ?
(a) (i) and (iii) (b) (i) and (ii)
(c) (ii) and (iii) (d) (iii) and (iv)

42. Match column-I with column-II and select the correct option.

	Column-I		Column-II
A.	Catalytic converter	I.	Particulate matter
B.	Electrostatic precipitator	II.	Carbon monoxide and nitrogen oxides
C.	Earmuffs	III.	High noise level
D.	Land fills	IV.	Solid wastes

(a) A-I; B-II; C-III; D-IV
(b) A-II; B-I; C-III; D-IV
(c) A-IV; B-III; C-II; D-I
(d) A-III; B-II; C-IV; D-I

43. The given diagram shows electrostatic precipitator. Identify A, B and C.

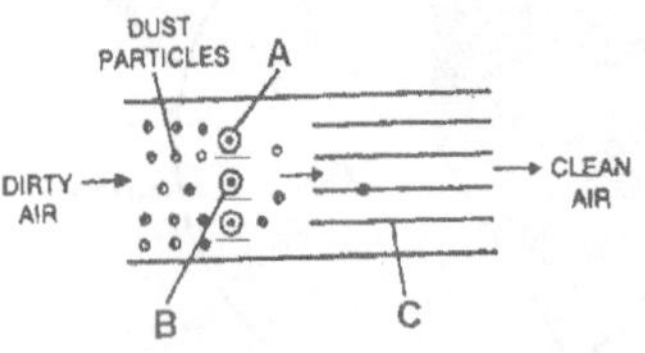

(a) A - Discharge corona, B - Negatively charged wire, C - Collection plate grounded
(b) A - Discharge corona, B - Positively charged wire, C - Collection plate grounded
(c) A - Discharge corona, B - Negatively charged wire, C - Collection plate burnt
(d) A - Uncharge corona, B - Positively charged wire, C - Collection plate never grounded

44. Which of the following statements is/are correct about 'Eco San' toilets?
(a) It is a sustainable system for handling human excreta or faecal matter by using dry 'composting toilets'.
(b) These are very useful for the rural areas where sewer systems are not possible.
(c) These toilets are hygienic, efficient, practical & most effective for the disposal of human waste.
(d) All of the above

45. Algal blooms impart a distinct colour to water due to
(a) their pigments.
(b) excretion of coloured substances.
(c) formation of coloured chemicals in water facilitated by physiological degradation of algae.
(d) absorption of light by algal cell wall.

RESPONSE GRID					
	37. ⓐⓑⓒⓓ	38. ⓐⓑⓒⓓ	39. ⓐⓑⓒⓓ	40. ⓐⓑⓒⓓ	41. ⓐⓑⓒⓓ
	42. ⓐⓑⓒⓓ	43. ⓐⓑⓒⓓ	44. ⓐⓑⓒⓓ	45. ⓐⓑⓒⓓ	

BIOLOGY CHAPTERWISE SPEED TEST-96			
Total Questions	45	Total Marks	180
Attempted		Correct	
Incorrect		Net Score	
Cut-off Score	40	Qualifying Score	60
Success Gap = Net Score – Qualifying Score			
Net Score = (Correct × 4) – (Incorrect × 1)			

Space for Rough Work

PHYSICS

Full Syllabus Test-1

Speed TEST 97 Subject-wise

No. of Questions	Maximum Marks	Time
45	180	1 Hour

GENERAL INSTRUCTIONS

- This test contains 45 MCQ's. For each question only one option is correct. Darken the correct circle/ bubble in the Response Grid provided on each page.
- You have to evaluate your Response Grids yourself with the help of solutions provided at the end of this book.
- Each correct answer will get you 4 marks and 1 mark shall be deduced for each incorrect answer. No mark will be given/ deducted if no bubble is filled. Keep a timer in front of you and stop immediately at the end of 60 min.
- The sheet follows a particular syllabus. Do not attempt the sheet before you have completed your preparation for that syllabus.
- After completing the sheet check your answers with the solution booklet and complete the Result Grid. Finally spend time to analyse your performance and revise the areas which emerge out as weak in your evaluation.

1. The electric field is given by $\vec{E} = \frac{A}{x^3}\hat{i} + By\hat{j} + Cz^2\hat{k}$. The SI units of A, B and C are respectively: [here x, y, z are in m]
(a) $\frac{Nm^3}{C}$, V/m^2, N/m^2-C (b) V-m^2, V/m, N/m^2-C
(c) V/m^2, V/m, N-C/m^2 (d) V/m, N-m^3/C, N-C/m

2. The acceleration versus time graph for a particle moving along a straight line is shown in the figure. If the particle starts from rest at $t = 0$, then its speed at $t = 30$ sec will be

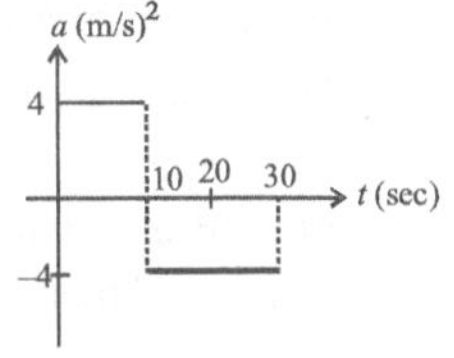

(a) 20 m/sec (b) 0 m/sec
(c) – 40 m/sec. (d) 40 m/sec.

3. A body of mass 5 kg falls from a height of 20 metres on the ground and it rebounds to a height of 0.2 m. If the loss in potential energy is used up by the body, then what will be the temperature rise?
(specific heat of material = 0.09 cal gm^{-1} °C^{-1})
(a) 0°C (b) 4°C (c) $\frac{8}{33}$°C (d) $\frac{11}{32}$°C

4. A monoatomic gas at 77°C is compressed adiabatically to $\frac{125}{343}$ of its original volume. The rise in temperature will be
(a) 186 K (b) 235 K (c) 336 K (d) 586 K

5. A man projects a coin upwards from the gate of a uniformly moving train. The path of coin for the man will be
(a) parabolic (b) inclined straight line
(c) vertical straight line (d) horizontal straight line

6. What is the disintegration constant of radon, if the number of its atoms diminishes by 18% in 24 h?
(a) $2.1 \times 10^{-3}\ s^{-1}$ (b) $2.1 \times 10^{-4}\ s^{-1}$
(c) $2.1 \times 10^{-5}\ s^{-1}$ (d) $2.1 \times 10^{-6}\ s^{-1}$

7. The refractive index of water measured by the relation $\mu = \frac{\text{real depth}}{\text{apparent depth}}$ is found to have values of 1.34, 1.38, 1.32 and 1.36; the mean value of refractive index with percentage error is
(a) $1.35 \pm 1.48\%$ (b) $1.35 \pm 0\%$
(c) $1.36 \pm 6\%$ (d) $1.36 \pm 0\%$

8. If the magnetic dipole moment of an atom of diamagnetic material, paramagnetic material and ferromagnetic material are denoted by μ_d, μ_p and μ_f respectively, then
(a) $\mu_d = 0$ and $\mu_p \neq 0$ (b) $\mu_d \neq 0$ and $\mu_p = 0$
(c) $\mu_p = 0$ and $\mu_f \neq 0$ (d) $\mu_d \neq 0$ and $\mu_f \neq 0$

RESPONSE GRID					
	1. ⓐⓑⓒⓓ	2. ⓐⓑⓒⓓ	3. ⓐⓑⓒⓓ	4. ⓐⓑⓒⓓ	5. ⓐⓑⓒⓓ
	6. ⓐⓑⓒⓓ	7. ⓐⓑⓒⓓ	8. ⓐⓑⓒⓓ		

Space for Rough Work

9. A car runs at a constant speed on a circular track of radius 100 m, taking 62.8 seconds in every circular loop. The average velocity and average speed for each circular loop respectively, is

(a) 0, 10 m/s (b) 10 m/s, 10 m/s
(c) 10 m/s, 0 (d) 0, 0

10. A mass is tied to a string and rotated in a vertical circle, the minimum velocity of the body at the top is

(a) $\sqrt{gr}$ (b) g/r (c) $\left(\frac{g}{r}\right)^{3/2}$ (d) gr

11. Power dissipated across the 8Ω resistor in the circuit shown here is 2 watt. The power dissipated in watt across the 3Ω resistor is

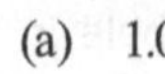

(a) 1.0
(b) 0.5
(c) 3.0
(d) 2.0

12. The energy of hydrogen atom in the 5th orbit is E, then the energy in the 7th orbit is

(a) $\frac{27}{8}E$ (b) $\frac{49}{25}E$ (c) $\frac{25}{49}E$ (d) $\frac{5E}{7}$

13. Two identical particles move towards each other with velocity 2v and 5v respectively. The velocity of centre of mass is

(a) 5v/2 (b) 9v/5 (c) 3v/2 (d) v/8

14. The mass number of He is 4 and that for sulphur is 32. The radius of sulphur nuclei is larger than that of helium by

(a) $\sqrt{8}$ (b) 4 (c) 2 (d) 8

15. According to Newton's law of cooling, the rate of cooling of a body is proportional to $(\Delta\theta)^n$, where $\Delta\theta$ is the difference of the temperature of the body and the surroundings, then n is equal to

(a) two (b) three (c) four (d) one

16. A body having initial velocity of 10 m/s moving on a rough surface comes to rest after moving 50 m. What is coefficient of friction between the body and surface? ($g = 10\ m/s^2$)

(a) 0.5 (b) 0.2 (c) 0.3 (d) 0.1

17. The separation between successive fringes in a double slit arrangement is x. If the whole arrangement is dipped under water what will be the new fringe separation? [The wavelenght of light being used is 5000 Å]

(a) 1.5x (b) x (c) 0.75x (d) 2x

18. A thin, metallic spherical shell contains a charge Q on it. A point charge q is placed at the cente of the shell and another charge q_1 is placed outside it as shown in figure. All the three charges are positive. The force on the charge at the centre is

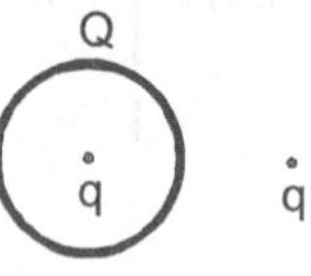

(a) towards left (b) towards right
(c) upward (d) zero

19. A charge q is moving with a velocity v parallel to a magnetic field B. Force on the charge due to magnetic field is

(a) qvB (b) qB/v (c) zero (d) Bv/q

20. A bucket full of hot water is kept in a room and it cools from 75°C to 70°C in T_1 minutes, from 70°C to 65°C in T_2 minutes and from 65°C to 60°C in T_3 minutes. Then

(a) $T_1 = T_2 = T_3$ (b) $T_1 < T_2 < T_3$
(c) $T_1 > T_2 > T_3$ (d) $T_1 < T_2 > T_3$

21. In uniform circular motion, the velocity vector and acceleration vector are

(a) perpendicular to each other
(b) in same direction
(c) in opposite direction
(d) not related to each other

22. The current in a coil of L = 40 mH is to be increased uniformly from 1A to 11A in 4 milli sec. The induced e.m.f. will be

(a) 100V (b) 0.4V (c) 440V (d) 40V

23. Two capacitors when connected in series have a capacitance of 3 μF, and when connected in parallel have a capacitance of 16 μF. Their individual capacities are

(a) 1 μF, 2 μF (b) 6 μF, 2 μF
(c) 12 μF, 4 μF (d) 3 μF, 16 μF

24. The weight of a body will be the least at

(a) poles (b) equator
(c) at height equal to R (d) centre of the earth

RESPONSE GRID				
9. ⓐⓑⓒⓓ	10. ⓐⓑⓒⓓ	11. ⓐⓑⓒⓓ	12. ⓐⓑⓒⓓ	13. ⓐⓑⓒⓓ
14. ⓐⓑⓒⓓ	15. ⓐⓑⓒⓓ	16. ⓐⓑⓒⓓ	17. ⓐⓑⓒⓓ	18. ⓐⓑⓒⓓ
19. ⓐⓑⓒⓓ	20. ⓐⓑⓒⓓ	21. ⓐⓑⓒⓓ	22. ⓐⓑⓒⓓ	23. ⓐⓑⓒⓓ
24. ⓐⓑⓒⓓ				

Space for Rough Work

25. When a tuning fork produces sound waves in air, which one of the following is same in the material of tuning fork as well as in air?
(a) Wavelength (b) Frequency
(c) Velocity (d) Amplitude

26. The fermi energy for a substance is
(a) independent of T
(b) directly proportional to $\sqrt{T}$
(c) directly proportional to T
(d) directly proportional to T^2

27. ABC is a triangular plate of uniform thickness. The sides are in the ratio shown in the figure. I_{AB}, I_{BC} and I_{CA} are the moments of inertia of the plate about AB, BC and CA as axes respectively. Which one of the following relations is correct?

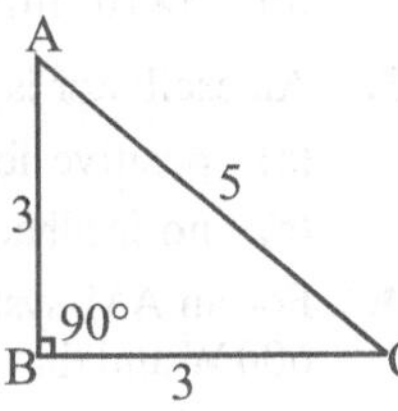

(a) $I_{AB} > I_{BC}$ (b) $I_{BC} > I_{AB}$
(c) $I_{AB} + I_{BC} = I_{CA}$ (d) I_{CA} is maximum

28. Consider the following statement:
When jumping from some height, you should bend your knees as you come to rest, instead of keeping your legs stiff. Which of the following relations can be useful in explaining the statement? Where symbols have their usual meanings.
(a) $\Delta\vec{p}_1 = -\Delta\vec{p}_2$ (b) $\Delta E = \Delta(PE + KE) = 0$
(c) $\vec{F}\Delta t = m\Delta\vec{v}$ (d) $\Delta x \propto \Delta F$

29. The amplitude of magnetic field of an electromagnetic wave is 2×10^{-7}T. It's electric field amplitude if the wave is travelling in free space is
(a) $6\,Vm^{-1}$ (b) $60\,Vm^{-1}$
(c) $10/6\,Vm^{-1}$ (d) None of these

30. The magnetic flux density B at a distance r from a long straight wire carrying a steady current varies with distance r as

(a) 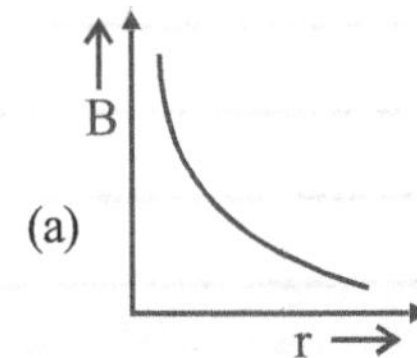

(b) 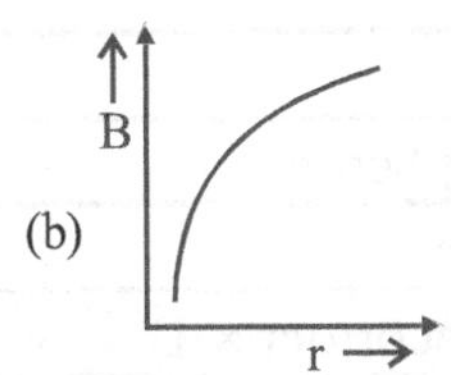

(c) 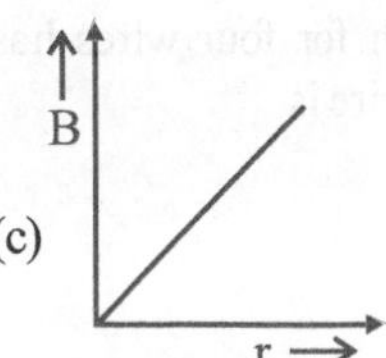

(d) 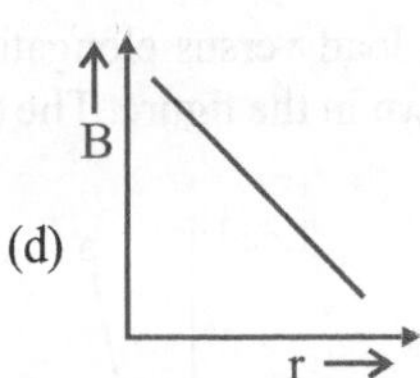

31. A metal piece is heated upto T° abs. The temperature of the surrounding is t° abs. The heat in the surrounding due to radiation is proportional to
(a) $(T-T)^4$ (b) $T^4 - t^4$ (c) $(T-t)^{1/4}$ (d) $T^2 - t^2$

32. Given, ${}_a\mu_g = \frac{3}{2}$, ${}_a\mu_w = \frac{4}{3}$, if a convex lens of focal length 10 cm is placed in water, then its focal length in water is
(a) equal to 40 cm (b) equal to 20 cm
(c) equal to 10 cm (d) None of these

33. If an alternating current is flowing in a spring, then the spring will be changing
(a) in a straight line (b) periodically
(c) elliptically (d) first (c) then (a)

34. The unit vector along 2i – 3j + k is
(a) $\frac{2i-3j+k}{\sqrt{14}}$ (b) $\frac{2i-3j+k}{5}$
(c) $\frac{2i-3j+k}{\sqrt{15}}$ (d) None of these

35. An iron rod of length 2m and cross-sectional area of 50 mm^2 is stretched by 0.5 mm, when a mass of 250 kg is hung from its lower end. Young's modulus of iron rod is
(a) $19.6\times10^{20}\,N/m^2$ (b) $19.6\times10^{18}\,N/m^2$
(c) $19.6\times10^{10}\,N/m^2$ (d) $19.6\times10^{15}\,N/m^2$

36. A particle of mass 1 kg is moving in S.H.M. with an amplitude 0.02 and a frequency of 60 Hz. The maximum force acting on the particle is
(a) $144\,\pi^2$ (b) $188\,\pi^2$
(c) $288\,\pi^2$ (d) None of these

37. According to Maxwell's hypothesis, a changing electirc field gives rise to
(a) an e.m.f (b) magnetic field
(c) electric current (d) pressure gradient.

RESPONSE GRID					
	25. ⓐⓑⓒⓓ	26. ⓐⓑⓒⓓ	27. ⓐⓑⓒⓓ	28. ⓐⓑⓒⓓ	29. ⓐⓑⓒⓓ
	30. ⓐⓑⓒⓓ	31. ⓐⓑⓒⓓ	32. ⓐⓑⓒⓓ	33. ⓐⓑⓒⓓ	34. ⓐⓑⓒⓓ
	35. ⓐⓑⓒⓓ	36. ⓐⓑⓒⓓ	37. ⓐⓑⓒⓓ		

Space for Rough Work

38. The load versus elongation graph for four wires has been shown in the figure. The thinest wire is

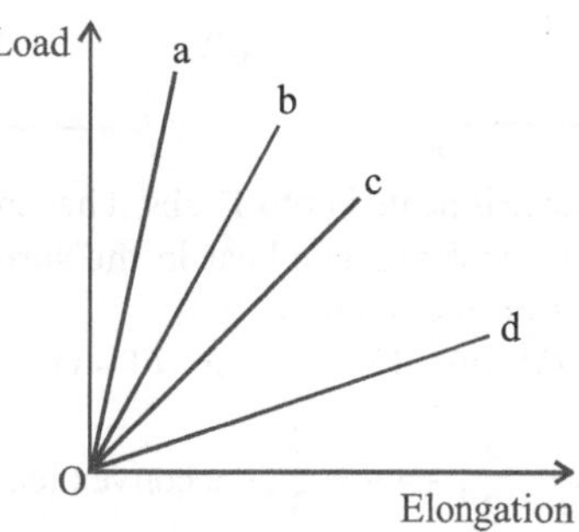

(a) a (b) b (c) c (d) d

39. A ray of light is incident on the surface of separation of a medium with the velocity of light at an angle 45° and is refracted in the medium at an angle 30°. Velocity of light in the medium will be (velocity of light in air = 3×10^8 m/s)

(a) 3.8×10^8 m/s (b) 3.38×10^8 m/s

(c) 2.12×10^8 m/s (d) 1.56×10^8 m/s

40. The rain drops are in spherical shape due to

(a) residual pressure (b) thrust on drop

(c) surface tension (d) viscosity

41. A dip circle is so set that its needle moves freely in the magnetic meridian. In this position, the angle of dip is 40°. Now the dip circle is rotated so that the plane in which the needle moves makes an angle of 30° with the magnetic meridian. In this position, the needle will dip by an angle

(a) 40° (b) 30°

(c) more than 40° (d) less than 40°

42. If the critical angle for total internal reflection from a medium to vacuum is 30°. Then velocity of light in the medium is

(a) 1.5×10^8 m/s (b) 2×10^8 m/s

(c) 3×10^8 m/s (d) 0.75×10^8 m/s

43. An oscillator is nothing but an amplifier with

(a) positive feedback (b) large gain

(c) no feedback (d) negative feedback

44. For an AM-system the total power of modulated signal is 600 W and that of carrier is 400 W, the modulation index is

(a) 0.25 (b) 0.36 (c) 0.54 (d) 1

45. The drift current in a p-n junction is

(a) from the n-side to the p-side

(b) from the p-side to the n-side

(c) from the n-side to the p-side if the junction is forward-baised and in the opposite direction if it is reverse biased

(d) from the p-side to the n-side if the junction is forward-baised and in the opposite direction if it is reverse-baised

RESPONSE GRID	
38. ⓐⓑⓒⓓ 39. ⓐⓑⓒⓓ 40. ⓐⓑⓒⓓ 41. ⓐⓑⓒⓓ 42. ⓐⓑⓒⓓ	
43. ⓐⓑⓒⓓ 44. ⓐⓑⓒⓓ 45. ⓐⓑⓒⓓ	

SUBJECTWISE SPEED TEST-97 - PHYSICS			
Total Questions	45	Total Marks	180
Attempted		Correct	
Incorrect		Net Score	
Cut-off Score	30	Qualifying Score	45
Success Gap = Net Score – Qualifying Score			
Net Score = (Correct × 4) – (Incorrect × 1)			

Space for Rough Work

CHEMISTRY

Full Syllabus Test-1

Speed TEST 98

Subject-wise

No. of Questions	Maximum Marks	Time
45	180	1 Hour

GENERAL INSTRUCTIONS

- This test contains 45 MCQ's. For each question only one option is correct. Darken the correct circle/ bubble in the Response Grid provided on each page.
- You have to evaluate your Response Grids yourself with the help of solutions provided at the end of this book.
- Each correct answer will get you 4 marks and 1 mark shall be deduced for each incorrect answer. No mark will be given/ deducted if no bubble is filled. Keep a timer in front of you and stop immediately at the end of 60 min.
- The sheet follows a particular syllabus. Do not attempt the sheet before you have completed your preparation for that syllabus.
- After completing the sheet check your answers with the solution booklet and complete the Result Grid. Finally spend time to analyse your performance and revise the areas which emerge out as weak in your evaluation.

1. A hydrocarbon A on chlorination gives B which on heating with alcoholic potassium hydroxide changes into another hydrocarbon C. The latter decolourises Baeyer's reagent and on ozonolysis forms formaldehyde only. A is
(a) Ethane (b) Butane
(c) Methane (d) Ethene

2. What is the IUPAC name of the compound ?

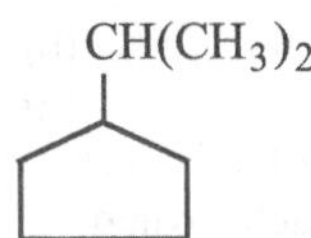

(a) 1, 1 – dimethyl – 1 – cyclopentyl methane
(b) 2 – cyclopentyl propane
(c) 1 – (1 – methyl) ethyl cyclopentane
(d) Cumene.

3. Which one of the following complexes is not expected to exhibit isomerism?
(a) $[Ni(en)_3]^{2+}$ (b) $[Ni(NH_3)_4(H_2O)_2]^{2+}$
(c) $[Pt(NH_3)_2Cl_2]$ (d) $[Ni(NH_3)_2Cl_2]$

4. The increasing order of the rate of HCN addition to compound A – D is
(A) HCHO (B) CH_3COCH_3
(C) $PhCOCH_3$ (D) PhCOPh
(a) D < C < B < A (b) C < D < B < A
(c) A < B < C < D (d) D < B < C < A

5. Phosphorus pentachloride dissociates as follows, in a closed reaction vessel
$PCl_5(g) \rightleftharpoons PCl_3(g) + Cl_2(g)$
If total pressure at equilibrium of the reaction mixture is P and degree of dissociation of PCl_5 is x, the partial pressure of PCl_3 will be
(a) $\left(\frac{x}{x-1}\right)P$ (b) $\left(\frac{x}{1-x}\right)P$ (c) $\left(\frac{x}{x+1}\right)P$ (d) $\left(\frac{2x}{1-x}\right)P$

6. Which of the following will not show cis-trans isomerism?
(a) $CH_3-CH=CH-CH_3$
(b) $CH_3-CH_2-CH=CH-CH_2-CH_3$
(c) $CH_3-C(CH_3)=CH-CH_2-CH_3$
(d) $CH_3-CH(CH_3)-CH=CH-CH_2-CH_3$

7. Point out the false statement
(a) Brownian movement and Tyndall effect are shown by colloidal systems.
(b) Gold number is a measure of the protective power of a lyophillic colloid.
(c) The colloidal solution of a liquid in liquid is called gel.
(d) Hardy - Schulze rule is related with coagulation.

RESPONSE GRID	
	1. ⓐⓑⓒⓓ 2. ⓐⓑⓒⓓ 3. ⓐⓑⓒⓓ 4. ⓐⓑⓒⓓ 5. ⓐⓑⓒⓓ
	6. ⓐⓑⓒⓓ 7. ⓐⓑⓒⓓ

Space for Rough Work

8. P_A and P_B are the vapour pressure of pure liquid components, A and B, respectively of an ideal binary solution. If X_A represents the mole fraction of component A, the total pressure of the solution will be.
(a) $P_A + X_A(P_B - P_A)$ (b) $P_A + X_A(P_A - P_B)$
(c) $P_B + X_A(P_B - P_A)$ (d) $P_B + X_A(P_A - P_B)$

9. In which one of the following species the central atom has the type of hybridization which is not the same as that present in the other three?
(a) SF_4 (b) I_3^- (c) $SbCl_5^{2-}$ (d) PCl_5

10. Which of following compound is hemiacetal?
(a) 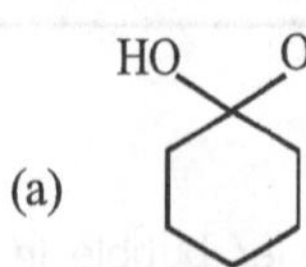

(b) O OH
(c) H OH O
(d) all of these

11. What products are expected from the disproportionation reaction of hypochlorous acid?
(a) HCl and Cl_2O (b) HCl and $HClO_3$
(c) $HClO_3$ and Cl_2O (d) $HClO_2$ and $HClO_4$

12. Which one of the following reactions does not form gaseous product?
(a) $PbO_2 + H_2O_2$
(b) Acidified $KMnO_4 + H_2O_2$
(c) Pbs + H_2O_2
(d) $Cl_2 + H_2O_2$

13. An antibiotic contains nitro group attached to aromatic nucleus. It is
(a) penicillin (b) streptomycin
(c) tetracycline (d) chloramphenicol

14. An ionic compound has a unit cell consisting of A ions at the corners of a cube and B ions on the centres of the faces of the cube. The empirical formula for this compound would be
(a) A_3B (b) AB_3 (c) A_2B (d) AB

15. In a reaction, when the concentration of reactant is increased two times, the increase in rate of reaction was four times. Order of reaction is :
(a) zero (b) 1 (c) 2 (d) 3

16. The cell reaction $Cu + 2Ag^+ \rightarrow Cu^{2+} + Ag$ is best represented by
(a) $Cu(s)\,|\,Cu^{2+}(aq)\,||\,Ag^+(aq)\,|\,Ag(s)$
(b) $Pt\,|\,Cu^{2+}\,||\,Ag^+(aq)\,|\,Ag(s)$
(c) $Cu^{2+}\,|\,Cu\,||\,Pt\,|\,Ag$
(d) None of the above representations

17. Chlorine is liberated when we heat
(a) $KMnO_4 + NaCl$ (b) $K_2Cr_2O_7 + MnO_2$
(c) $Pb(NO_3)_2 + MnO_2$ (d) $K_2Cr_2O_7 + HCl$

18. According to kinetic theory of gases, for a diatomic molecule
(a) the pressure exerted by the gas is proportional to mean velocity of the molecule
(b) the pressure exerted by the gas is proportional to the root mean velocity of the molecule
(c) the root mean square velocity of the molecule is inversely proportional to the temperature
(d) the mean translational kinetic energy of the molecule is proportional to the absolute temperature.

19. Larger number of oxidation states are exhibited by the actinoids than those by the lanthanoids, the main reason being
(a) 4*f* orbitals more diffused than the 5*f* orbitals
(b) lesser energy difference between 5*f* and 6*d* than between 4*f* and 5*d* orbitals
(c) more energy difference between 5*f* and 6*d* than between 4*f* and 5*d* orbitals
(d) more reactive nature of the actinoids than the lanthanoids

20. Which one of the following arrangements does not give the correct picture of the trends indicated against it ?
(a) $F_2 > Cl_2 > Br_2 > I_2$: Oxidizing power
(b) $F_2 > Cl_2 > Br_2 > I_2$: Electron gain enthalpy
(c) $F_2 > Cl_2 > Br_2 > I_2$: Bond dissociation energy
(d) $F_2 > Cl_2 > Br_2 > I_2$: Electronegativity.

21. The process of converting hydrated alumina into anhydrous alumina is called
(a) roasting (b) smelting
(c) dressing (d) calcination

22. The rate constant of a reaction becomes equal to the pre-exponential factor when
(a) the absolute temperature is zero
(b) the activation energy is infinity
(c) the absolute temperature is infinity
(d) the temperature in Celsius is zero.

23. Which one of the following cyano complexes would exhibit the lowest value of paramagnetic behaviour ?
(a) $[Co(CN)_6]^{3-}$ (b) $[Fe(CN)_6]^{3-}$
(c) $[Mn(CN)_6]^{3-}$ (d) $[Cr(CN)_6]^{3-}$
(At. no : Cr = 24, Mn = 25, Fe = 26, Co = 27)

RESPONSE GRID					
	8. ⓐⓑⓒⓓ	9. ⓐⓑⓒⓓ	10. ⓐⓑⓒⓓ	11. ⓐⓑⓒⓓ	12. ⓐⓑⓒⓓ
	13. ⓐⓑⓒⓓ	14. ⓐⓑⓒⓓ	15. ⓐⓑⓒⓓ	16. ⓐⓑⓒⓓ	17. ⓐⓑⓒⓓ
	18. ⓐⓑⓒⓓ	19. ⓐⓑⓒⓓ	20. ⓐⓑⓒⓓ	21. ⓐⓑⓒⓓ	22. ⓐⓑⓒⓓ
	23. ⓐⓑⓒⓓ				

Space for Rough Work

24. On the basis of the following thermochemical data : $(\Delta_f G^\circ H^+(aq) = 0)$

$H_2O(l) \rightarrow H^+(aq) + OH^-(aq); \Delta H = 57.32\text{ kJ}$

$$H_2(g) + \frac{1}{2}O_2(g) \longrightarrow H_2O(l);\ \Delta H = -286.20\text{ kJ}$$

The value of enthalpy of formation of OH^- ion at 25° C is:
(a) –228.88 kJ (b) +228.88 kJ
(c) –343.52 kJ (d) –22.88 kJ

25. In which of the following pair both the species have sp^3 hybridization?
(a) H_2S, BF_3 (b) SiF_4, BeH_2
(c) NF_3, H_2O (d) NF_3, BF_3

26. What is the product of the following reaction ?

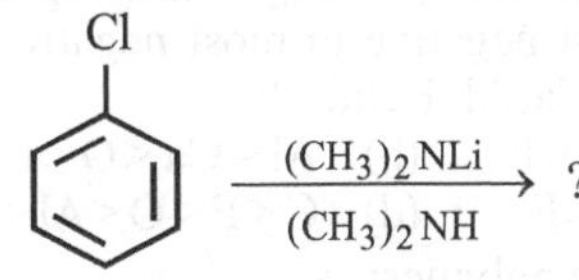

(a) N, N-dimethylaniline
(b) phenyllithium (C_6H_5Li)
(c) *para*-chloro-N, N-dimethylaniline
(d) *meta*-chloro-N, N-dimethylaniline

27. From amongst the following alcohols the one that would react fastest with conc. HCl and anhydrous $ZnCl_2$, is
(a) 2-Butanol (b) 2- Methylpropan-2-ol
(c) 2-Methylpropanol (d) 1- Butanol

28. Number of moles of MnO_4^- required to oxidize one mole of ferrous oxalate completely in acidic medium will be :
(a) 0.6 moles (b) 0.4 moles
(c) 7.5 moles (d) 0.2 moles

29. Which of the following practices will not come under green chemistry?
(a) If possible, making use of soap made of vegetable oils instead of using synthetic detergents.
(b) Using H_2O_2 for bleaching purpose instead of using chlorine based bleaching agents.
(c) Using bicycle for travelling small distances instead of using petrol/diesel based vehicles.
(d) Using plastic cans for neatly storing substances.

30. The following alcohol is treated with conc. H_2SO_4, the major product obtained is

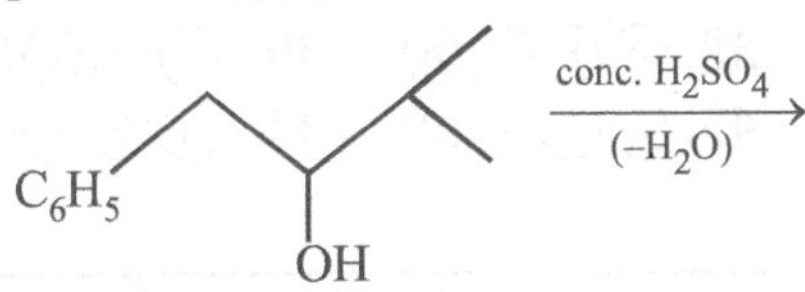

(a)
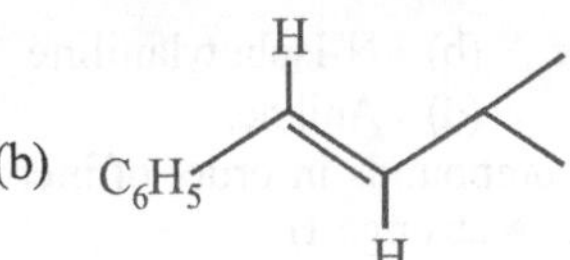

(b)
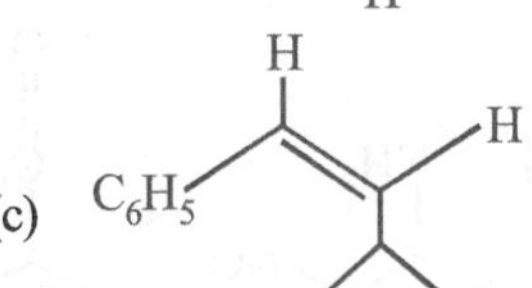

(c) C_6H_5 H H

31. The strength in volumes of a solution containing 30.36 g/L of H_2O_2 is
(a) 10V (b) 5V
(c) 20V (d) None of these

32. The position of some metals in the electrochemical series in decreasing electropositive character is given as Mg > Al > Zn > Cu > Ag. What will happen, if a copper spoon is used to stir a solution of aluminium nitrate ?
(a) The spoon will get coated with Al
(b) An alloy of Cu and Al is formed
(c) The solution becomes blue
(d) There is no reaction

33. Which of the following graph correspond to one node

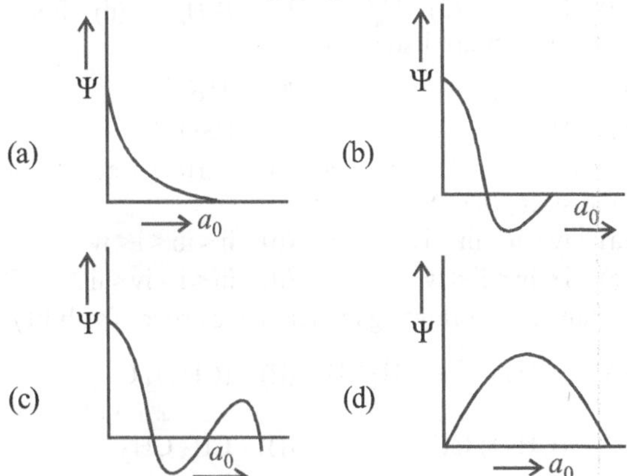

34. Arrange the following ions in the order of decreasing X – O bond length, where X is the central atom
(a) $ClO_4^-, SO_4^{2-}, PO_4^{3-}, SiO_4^-$
(b) $SiO_4^{4-}, PO_4^{3-}, SO_4^{2-}, ClO_4^-$
(c) $SiO_4^{4-}, PO_4^{3-}, ClO_4^-, SO_4^{2-}$
(d) $SiO_4^{4-}, SO_4^{2-}, PO_4^{3-}, ClO_4^-$

RESPONSE GRID

24. ⓐⓑⓒⓓ 25. ⓐⓑⓒⓓ 26. ⓐⓑⓒⓓ 27. ⓐⓑⓒⓓ 28. ⓐⓑⓒⓓ
29. ⓐⓑⓒⓓ 30. ⓐⓑⓒⓓ 31. ⓐⓑⓒⓓ 32. ⓐⓑⓒⓓ 33. ⓐⓑⓒⓓ
34. ⓐⓑⓒⓓ

Space for Rough Work

35. The reaction of benzyl chloride with sodium cyanide followed by reduction with hydrogen in the presence of nickel gives
(a) β-Phenylethylamine (b) N-Isobutylaniline
(c) Benzylamine (d) Aniline.

36. Arrange the following compounds in order of increasing basic strength. (weakest → strongest)

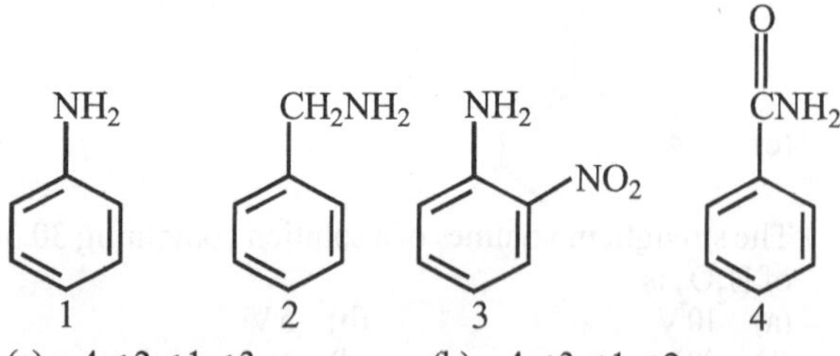

(a) 4<2<1<3 (b) 4<3<1<2
(c) 4<1<3<2 (d) 2<1<3<4

37. Which of the nitrogen of histidine is first protonated ?

$$\text{Imidazole ring with } ^{\beta}N \text{ and } ^{\alpha}NH\text{, side chain } -CH_2\overset{\overset{+}{N}H_3}{C}HCOO^-$$

(a) α (b) β (c) both (d) None

38. Which of the following structure is similar to graphite?
(a) B (b) B_4C (c) B_2H_6 (d) BN

39. Four species are listed below:
i. HCO_3^- ii. H_3O^+
iii. HSO_4^- iv. HSO_3F
Which one of the following is the correct sequence of their acid strength?
(a) iv<ii<iii<i (b) ii<iii<i<iv
(c) i<iii<ii<iv (d) iii<i<iv<ii

40. Arrange the following in increasing order of stability
(A) $(CH_3)_2\overset{+}{C}-CH_2CH_3$ (B) $(CH_3)_3\overset{+}{C}$
(C) $(CH_3)_2\overset{+}{C}H$ (D) $CH_3\overset{+}{C}H_2$
(E) $\overset{+}{C}H_3$
(a) E<D<C<B<A (b) E<D<C<A<B
(c) D<E<C<A<B (d) A<E<D<C<B

41. An organic compound A upon reacting with NH_3 gives B. On heating B gives C. C in presence of KOH reacts with Br_2 to given $CH_3CH_2NH_2$. A is :
(a) CH_3COOH (b) $CH_3CH_2CH_2COOH$
(c) $CH_3-\underset{CH_3}{\underset{|}{C}H}-COOH$ (d) CH_3CH_2COOH

42. The order of ionisation potential between He^+ ion and H-atom (both species are in gaseous state) is:
(a) I. P. (He^+) = I.P. (H) (b) I. P. (He^+) < I.P. (H)
(c) I. P. (He^+) > I.P. (H) (d) cannot be compared

43. Which one of the following arrangements represents the correct order of least negative to most negative electron gain enthalpy for C, Ca, Al, F and O?
(a) Ca<Al<C<O<F (b) Al<Ca<O<C<F
(c) Al<O<C<Ca<F (d) C<F<O<Al<Ca

44. The monomer of the polymer;

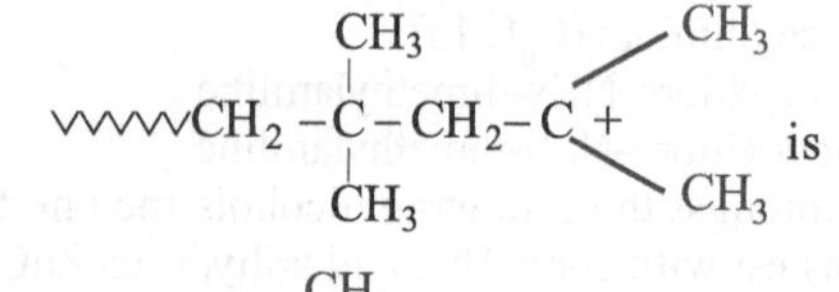

is

(a) $H_2C=C(CH_3)_2$ (b) $CH_3CH=CHCH_3$
(c) $CH_3CH=CH_2$ (d) $(CH_3)_2C=C(CH_3)_2$

45. The rate of diffusion of SO_2, CO_2, PCl_3 and SO_3 are in the following order
(a) $PCl_3 > SO_3 > SO_2 > CO_2$
(b) $CO_2 > SO_2 > PCl_3 > SO_3$
(c) $SO_2 > SO_3 > PCl_3 > CO_2$
(d) $CO_2 > SO_2 > SO_3 > PCl_3$

RESPONSE GRID					
	35. ⓐⓑⓒⓓ	36. ⓐⓑⓒⓓ	37. ⓐⓑⓒⓓ	38. ⓐⓑⓒⓓ	39. ⓐⓑⓒⓓ
	40. ⓐⓑⓒⓓ	41. ⓐⓑⓒⓓ	42. ⓐⓑⓒⓓ	43. ⓐⓑⓒⓓ	44. ⓐⓑⓒⓓ
	45. ⓐⓑⓒⓓ				

SUBJECTWISE SPEED TEST-98 - CHEMISTRY			
Total Questions	45	Total Marks	180
Attempted		Correct	
Incorrect		Net Score	
Cut-off Score	30	Qualifying Score	40
Success Gap = Net Score – Qualifying Score			
Net Score = (Correct × 4) – (Incorrect × 1)			

Space for Rough Work

BIOLOGY

Full Syllabus Test-1

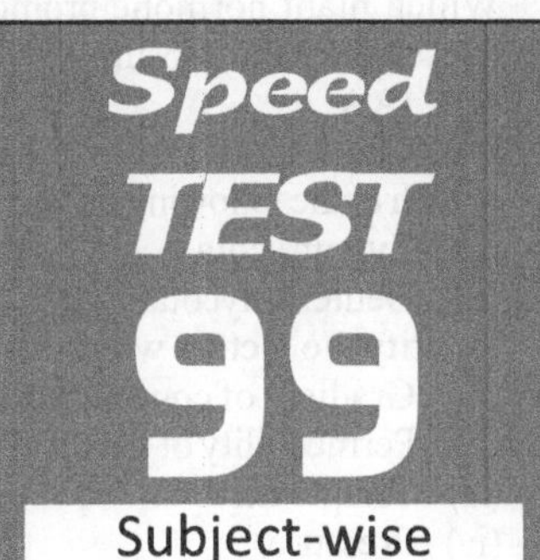

No. of Questions	Maximum Marks	Time
90	360	1 Hour

GENERAL INSTRUCTIONS

- This test contains 90 MCQ's. For each question only one option is correct. Darken the correct circle/ bubble in the Response Grid provided on each page.
- You have to evaluate your Response Grids yourself with the help of solutions provided at the end of this book.
- Each correct answer will get you 4 marks and 1 mark shall be deduced for each incorrect answer. No mark will be given/ deducted if no bubble is filled. Keep a timer in front of you and stop immediately at the end of 60 min.
- The sheet follows a particular syllabus. Do not attempt the sheet before you have completed your preparation for that syllabus.
- After completing the sheet check your answers with the solution booklet and complete the Result Grid. Finally spend time to analyse your performance and revise the areas which emerge out as weak in your evaluation.

1. The sum total of chemical reactions occurring in our body is called
   (a) Metabolism (b) Homeostasis
   (c) Irritability (d) Catabolism
2. An important criterion for modern day classification is
   (a) Resemblances in morphology
   (b) Anatomical and physiological traits
   (c) Breeding habits
   (d) Presence or absence of notochord
3. In which of the following, all listed genera belong to the same class of Algae?
   (a) *Chara, Fucus, Polysiphonia*
   (b) *Volvox, Spirogyra, Chlamydomonas*
   (c) *Porphyra, Ectocarpus, Ulothrix*
   (d) *Sargassum, Laminaria, Gracillaria*
4. In class Phaeophyceae, the plant body is usually attached to the substratum by a _____(A)_____ and has a stalk, the _____(B)_____ and leaf like photosynthetic organ the _____(C)_____.
   (a) A – holdfast, B – stipe, C – frond
   (b) A – stipe, B – holdfast, C – frond
   (c) A – frond, B – stipe, C – holdfast
   (d) A – stipe, B – frond, C – holdfast
5. The region of the stem where leaves are born are called ____________ while ___________ are the portions between two ______________ .
   (a) nodes, nodes, internodes
   (b) nodes, internodes, nodes
   (c) internodes, nodes, nodes
   (d) nodes, internodes, internodes
6. Which option is correctly matched with the diagrams?

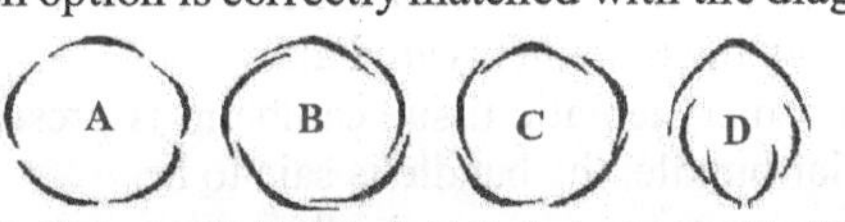

   (a) A-Valvate, B-Twisted, C-Imbricate, D-Vexillary
   (b) A-Vexillary, B-Valvate, C-Twisted, D-Imbricate
   (c) A-Imbricate, B-Vexillary, C-Valvate, D-Twisted
   (d) A-Twisted, B-Imbricate, C-Vexillary, D-Valvate
7. Plant cells that are photosynthetically active are found in the ___________ layer of leaf and are ___________cells.
   (a) epidermis, parenchymatous
   (b) mesophyll, parenchymatous
   (c) mesophyll, sclerenchymatous
   (d) aerenchyma, collenchymatous
8. Which of the following statements is/are true?
   (i) Uneven thickening of cell wall is characteristic of sclerenchyma.
   (ii) Periblem forms the cortex of the stem and the root.
   (iii) Tracheids are the chief water transporting elements in gymnosperms.
   (iv) Companion cell is devoid of nucleus at maturity.
   (v) The commercial cork is obtained from *Quercus suber.*
   (a) (i) and (iv) (b) (ii) and (v)
   (c) (iii) and (iv) (d) (ii), (iii) and (v)

RESPONSE GRID					
	1. ⓐⓑⓒⓓ	2. ⓐⓑⓒⓓ	3. ⓐⓑⓒⓓ	4. ⓐⓑⓒⓓ	5. ⓐⓑⓒⓓ
	6. ⓐⓑⓒⓓ	7. ⓐⓑⓒⓓ	8. ⓐⓑⓒⓓ		

Space for Rough Work

9. Which plant hormone promotes seed, bud dormancy and causes stomatal closure ?
(a) IAA (b) Abscisic acid
(c) GA_1 (d) Cytokinin

10. Which of the following divisions of fungi includes club fungi?
(a) Zygomycota (b) Ascomycota
(c) Deuteromycota (d) Basidiomycota

11. Identify the factors which affect the rate of diffusion.
(i) Gradient of concentration.
(ii) Permeability of the membrane.
(iii) Temperature.
(iv) Pressure.
(v) Size of diffusing material.
(a) (i), (iii) and (iv) (b) (i) and (v)
(c) All of these (d) Only (v) is correct

12. What is the number and positions of insertions of flagella in class Rhodophyceae?
(a) 2 – 8, equal, apical (b) 2, unequal, lateral
(c) 2 – 6, equal, lateral (d) Absent

13. In biological taxonomy, a ________ is a comprehensive treatment of a taxon.
(a) flora (b) manuals
(c) monograph (d) monogram

14. **Statement 1 :** A simple leaf has undivided lamina.
Statement 2 : Leaves showing pinnate and palmate venations have various type of incisions.
(a) Statement-1 is True, Statement-2 is True, Statement-2 is a correct explanation for Statement-1
(b) Statement-1 is True, Statement-2 is True, Statement-2 is NOT a correct explanation for Statement-1
(c) Statement-1 is True, Statement-2 is False
(d) Both the Statements are False

15. When a meristematic tissue cambium is present inside a vascular bundle, the bundle is said to be
(a) conjoint (b) open
(c) closed (d) collateral

16. Which one does not differ between a C_3 and a C_4 plant?
(i) Initial CO_2 acceptor
(ii) Extent of photorespiration
(iii) Enzyme catalyzing reaction that fixes CO_2
(iv) Presence of Calvin cycle
(v) Leaf anatomy
(a) (i) and (v) (b) Only (iv)
(c) (ii) and (iii) (d) Only (ii)

17. Identify the following figures.

A B C

(a) A – *Euglena*, B – *Paramecium*, C – *Agaricus*
(b) A – *Euglena*, B – *Planaria*, C – *Agaricus*
(c) A – *Planaria*, B – *Paramecium*, C – *Agaricus*
(d) A – *Euglena*, B – *Paramecium*, C – *Aspergillus*

18. Nuclear DNA exists as a complex of proteins called ______ that condenses into ______ during cellular division.
(a) chromosomes, chromatin
(b) chromatids, chromosomes
(c) chromophores, chromatin
(d) chromatin, chromosomes

19. The flower is the reproductive unit in the ________ meant for ____________ reproduction.
(a) angiosperms and sexual
(b) gymnosperms and sexual
(c) algae and asexual
(d) pteridophytes and asexual

20. R.Q. for glucose (Carbohydrates) is
(a) 1 (b) 0.5
(c) 2 (d) 0.05

21. Which one is the correct option for the labelled diagrams A, B, C and D ?

Satellite
Secondary constriction
Short arm
Shorter arm
Centromere
Centromere
Centromere
Long arm
Longer arm
A B C D

(a) A – Telocentric chromosome, B – Acrocentric chromosome, C – Submetacentric chromosome, D – Metacentric chromosome
(b) A – Acrocentric chromosome, B – Telocentric chromosome, C – Metacentric chromosome, D – Submetacentric chromosome
(c) A – Submetacentric chromosome, B – Metacentric chromosome, C – Telocentric chromosome, D – Acrocentric chromosome
(d) A – Metacentric chromosome, B – Submetacentric chromosome, C– Acrocentric chromosome, D – Telocentric chromosome

22. **Match column-I with column-II and choose the correct option.**

Column-I	**Column-II**
A. Algae	I. *Solanum tuberosum*
B. Fungi	II. *Equisetum*
C. Angiosperm	III. *Cycas*
D. Pteridophyte	IV. *Chlamydomonas*
E. Gymnosperm	V. *Rhizopus*

(a) A → V; B → IV; C → I; D → II; E → III
(b) A → IV; B → V; C → I; D → II; E → III
(c) A → IV; B → I; C → V; D → II; E → III
(d) A → IV; B → I; C → V; D → III; E → II

RESPONSE GRID					
	9. ⓐⓑⓒⓓ	10. ⓐⓑⓒⓓ	11. ⓐⓑⓒⓓ	12. ⓐⓑⓒⓓ	13. ⓐⓑⓒⓓ
	14. ⓐⓑⓒⓓ	15. ⓐⓑⓒⓓ	16. ⓐⓑⓒⓓ	17. ⓐⓑⓒⓓ	18. ⓐⓑⓒⓓ
	19. ⓐⓑⓒⓓ	20. ⓐⓑⓒⓓ	21. ⓐⓑⓒⓓ	22. ⓐⓑⓒⓓ	

Space for Rough Work

23. In animals, glucose is stored as ________ while in plants stored as ____________.
(a) cellulose, starch (b) starch, glycogen
(c) cellulose, glycogen (d) glycogen, starch

24. Vessels are absent in
(a) teak wood (b) shisham wood
(c) Pinus wood (d) sal wood

25. Identify the phases from the graph given below that shows the change in DNA content during various phases (A to D) of mitotic cell cycle.

DNA content (4C, 2C) vs *Time*; phases A, B, C, D

	A	B	C	D
(a)	G_2	G_1	S	M
(b)	G_2	S	G_1	M
(c)	G_1	S	G_2	M
(d)	M	G_1	S	G_2

26. Match column-I with column-II and Column-IIII and choose the correct option.

	Column-I (Element)		Column-II (Function)		Column-III (Deficiency Symptom)
A.	Calcium	I.	Required for ionic-balance.	(i)	Grey blot on leaves.
B.	Boron	II.	Essential for constitution of nucleic acid	(ii)	Fruit-yield decreases.
C.	Phosphorus	III.	Required for absorption of calcium.	(iii)	Red blots on leaves.
D.	Chlorine	IV.	Required to activate respiratory enzyme.	(iv)	Fruit-size diminishes.
E.	Manganese	V.	Required for synthesis of bipolar spindle.	(v)	Young root tip begin to die.

(a) A → I-iv; B → II-v; C → III-iii; D → IV-i; E → V-ii
(b) A → V-v; B → IV-iv; C → III-i; D → II-iii; E → I-ii
(c) A → IV-iii; B → I-iv; C → V-v; D → III-ii; E → II-i
(d) A → V-v; B → III-iv; C → II-iii; D → I-ii; E → IV-i

27. Match column-I with column-II and choose the correct option.

Column-I		Column-II	
A.	Transpiration	I.	Uses energy to pump molecules against a concentration gradient.
B.	Guttation	II.	Active absorption of water.
C.	Exudation	III.	Loss of water vapour from plant parts.
D.	Active transport	IV.	Loss of liquid water from leaves.
		V.	Loss of water from injured plant parts.

(a) A → I; B → II; C → III; D → V
(b) A → II; B → I; C → IV; D → III
(c) A → III; B → IV; C → V; D → I
(d) A → IV; B → V; C → II; D → III

28. The genetically-modified (GM) brinjal in India has been developed for
(a) insect-resistance
(b) enhancing shelf life
(c) enhancing mineral content
(d) drought-resistance

29. Match column-I with column-II and choose the correct option.

	Column-I		Column-II
A.	Radial vascular bundle	I.	*Cucurbita pepo*
B.	Collateral vascular bundle	II.	*Dracaena*
C.	Bicollateral vascular bundle	III.	Roots of angiosperms
D.	Amphicribral vascular bundle	IV.	Sunflower stem
E.	Amphivasal vascular bundle	V.	Fern

(a) A → III; B → IV; C → I; D → V; E → II
(b) A → II; B → III; C → I; D → V: E → IV
(c) A → III; B → IV; C → V; D → I: E → II
(d) A → III; B → I; C → II; D → IV; E → V

30. How many different kinds of gametes will be produced by a plant having the genotype AABbCC ?
(a) Four (b) Nine
(c) Two (d) Three

31. Acid rain is caused due to increase in concentration of (in atmosphere)
(a) SO_2 and NO_2 (b) CO and CO_2
(c) CO and SO_3 (d) O_3 and dust

32. Which of the following is considered a hot-spot of biodiversity in India ?
(a) Indo-Gangetic Plain (b) Eastern Ghats
(c) Aravalli Hills (d) Western Ghats

33. Measuring Biochemical Oxygen Demand (BOD) is a method used for
(a) estimating the amount of organic matter in sewage water.
(b) working out the efficiency of oil driven automobile engines.
(c) measuring the activity of *Saccharomyces cerevisiae* in producing curd on a commercial scale.
(d) working out the efficiency of RBCs about their capacity to carry oxygen.

RESPONSE GRID

23. ⓐⓑⓒⓓ 24. ⓐⓑⓒⓓ 25. ⓐⓑⓒⓓ 26. ⓐⓑⓒⓓ 27. ⓐⓑⓒⓓ
28. ⓐⓑⓒⓓ 29. ⓐⓑⓒⓓ 30. ⓐⓑⓒⓓ 31. ⓐⓑⓒⓓ 32. ⓐⓑⓒⓓ
33. ⓐⓑⓒⓓ

Space for Rough Work

34. Function of companion cells is
(a) providing energy to sieve elements for active transport
(b) providing water to phloem
(c) loading of sucrose into sieve elements by passive transport
(d) loading of sucrose into sieve elements

35. Which one of the following ecosystem types has the highest annual net primary productivity?
(a) Tropical deciduous forest
(b) Temperate evergreen forest
(c) Temperate deciduous forest
(d) Tropical rain forest

36. The impacts of loss of biodiversity include
(i) Decrease in plant production.
(ii) Lowered resistance to environmental perturbation
(iii) Increased variability in ecosystem processes like water use, pest/disease cycle, plants productivity.
(iv) None of these
(a) (i) and (ii) (b) (i), (ii), and (iii)
(c) (ii) and (iii) (d) Only (iv)

37. **Statement 1 :** DNA is associated with proteins.
Statement 2 : DNA binds around histone proteins that form a pool and the entire structure is called a nucleosome.
(a) Statement-1 is True, Statement-2 is True, Statement-2 is a correct explanation for Statement-1
(b) Statement-1 is True, Statement-2 is True, Statement-2 is NOT a correct explanation for Statement-1
(c) Statement-1 is True, Statement-2 is False
(d) Both the statements are False

38. What will happen if decomposers are removed from the ecosystem?
(a) Energy cycle is stopped
(b) Mineral cycle is stopped
(c) Consumers cannot absorb solar energy
(d) Rate of decomposition of mineral increases

39. The formula for exponential population growth is
(a) $dN/rN = dt$ (b) $rN / dN = dt$
(c) $dN / dt = rN$ (d) $dt / dN = rN$

40. Osmotic pressure of a solution is
(a) greater than pure solvent.
(b) less than pure solvent.
(c) equal to pure solvent.
(d) less than or greater than pure solvent.

41. *Himgiri* developed by hybridisation and selection for disease resistance against rust pathogens is a variety of
(a) Chilli (b) Maize
(c) Sugarcane (d) Wheat

42. The age of pyramid with broad base indicates
(a) High percentage of young individuals
(b) Low percentage of young individuals
(c) High percentage of old individuals
(d) Low percentage of old individuals

43. Match column-I with column-II and choose the correct option.

	Column-I		Column-II
A.	Auxin	I.	Herring sperm DNA
B.	Cytokinin	II.	Inhibitor of growth
C.	Gibberellin	III.	Apical dominance
D.	Ethylene	IV.	Epinasty
E.	Abscisic acid	V.	Induces amylase synthesis

(a) A → III; B → I; C → V; D → IV; E → II
(b) A → IV; B → V; C → I; D → III; E → II
(c) A → II; B → I; C → V; D → III; E → IV
(d) A → III; B → I; C → V; D → II; E → IV

44. Which of the following statement(s) is/are false?
(i) Pollen grains represent immature male gametophyte.
(ii) In angiosperms partially developed male gametophytes are pollinated.
(iii) Generative cell is siponogenous while vegetative cell is spermatogenous.
(iv) Formation and differentiation of pollen grains is called microsporogenesis.
(v) Pollen grains of some plants produce severe allergy and respiratory or bronchial diseases.
(vi) Pollen grains are poor in nutrients.
(a) (i) and (vi) (b) (iii) and (vi)
(c) (iv) and (v) (d) (v) and (vi)

45. **Statement 1 :** In case of vegetatively propagated crops, pure-line selection is not required.
Statement 2 : Hybrid vigour is mostly used in vegetatively propagated plants.
(a) Statement-1 is True, Statement-2 is True, Statement-2 is a correct explanation for Statement-1
(b) Statement-1 is True, Statement-2 is True, Statement-2 is NOT a correct explanation for Statement-1
(c) Statement-1 is True, Statement-2 is False
(d) Both the Statements are False.

46. The practical purpose of classification of living organisms is to
(a) explain the origin of living organsims
(b) trace the evolution of living organsims
(c) name the living organisms
(d) facilitate identification of unknown organisms

47. Which one of the following animals is correctly matched with its particular named taxonomic category?
(a) Tiger - *tigris*, the species
(b) Cuttle fish - mollusca, a class
(c) Humans - primata, the family
(d) Housefly - musca, an order

RESPONSE GRID					
	34. ⓐⓑⓒⓓ	35. ⓐⓑⓒⓓ	36. ⓐⓑⓒⓓ	37. ⓐⓑⓒⓓ	38. ⓐⓑⓒⓓ
	39. ⓐⓑⓒⓓ	40. ⓐⓑⓒⓓ	41. ⓐⓑⓒⓓ	42. ⓐⓑⓒⓓ	43. ⓐⓑⓒⓓ
	44. ⓐⓑⓒⓓ	45. ⓐⓑⓒⓓ	46. ⓐⓑⓒⓓ	47. ⓐⓑⓒⓓ	

Space for Rough Work

48. Glucagon is secreted by
(a) β (beta) cells of islets of langerhans
(b) α (alpha) cells of islets of langerhans
(c) β cells of pancreas
(d) Adrenal cortex

49. Choose the correct names of the different bacteria according to their shapes.

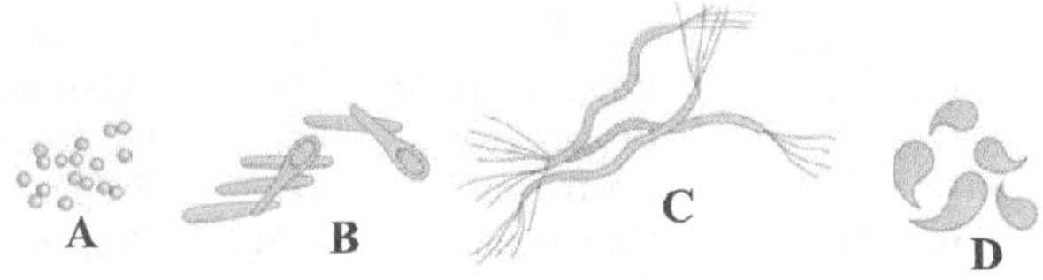

(a) A – Cocci, B – Bacilli, C – Spirilla, D – Vibrio
(b) A – Bacilli, B – Cocci, C – Spirilla, D – Vibrio
(c) A – Spirilla, B – Bacilli, C – Cocci, D – Vibrio
(d) A – Spirilla, B – Vibrio, C – Cocci, D – Bacilli

50. Which of following is not a protein hormone ?
(a) Relaxin (b) HCG
(c) Placental lactogen (d) Estradiol

51. Match column-I with column-II and choose the correct option.

Column-I (Epithelial tissue)	Column-II (Location)
A. Cuboidal	I. Epidermis of skin
B. Ciliated	II. Inner lining of blood vessels
C. Columnar	III. Inner surface of gall bladder
D. Squamous	IV. Inner lining of fallopian tube
E. Keratinized squamous	V. Lining of pancreatic duct

(a) A → V; B → IV; C → II; D → III; E → I
(b) A → III; B → IV; C → V; D → II; E → I
(c) A → V; B → IV; C → III; D → II; E → I
(d) A → III; B → IV; C → V; D → I; E → II

52. Chloramphenicol and Erythromycin (broad spectrum antibiotics) are produced by
(a) *Streptomyces* (b) *Nitrobacter*
(c) *Rhizobium* (d) *Penicillium*

53. Which one of the following statements about Human sperm is correct?
(a) Acrosome has a conical pointed structure used for piercing and penetrating the egg, resulting in fertilisation.
(b) The sperm lysins in the acrosome dissolve the egg envelope facilitating fertilisation.
(c) Acrosome serves as a sensory structure leading the sperm towards the ovum.
(d) Acrosome serves no particular function.

54. **Statement 1 :** Sponges belong to Porifera.
Statement 2 : Sponges have canal system.
(a) Statement-1 is True, Statement-2 is True, Statement-2 is a correct explanation for Statement-1
(b) Statement-1 is True, Statement-2 is True, Statement-2 is NOT a correct explanation for Statement-1
(c) Statement-1 is True, Statement-2 is False
(d) Both the Statements are False

55. Which one of the following organisms may respire in the absence of oxygen ?
(a) *Azotobacter* (b) *Clostridium*
(c) *Rhizobium* (d) *Lactobacillus*

56. Vectors include
(a) bacterial and plant plasmids
(b) viruses
(c) artificial chromosomes
(d) All of the above

57. Which of the following is not a step in understanding Biodiversity ?
(a) Naming the species
(b) Looking at other related species
(c) Assessing the species geographic range
(d) Quantifying the species genome

58. Which is part of pectoral girdle?
(a) Glenoid cavity (b) Sternum
(c) Ilium (d) Acetabulum

59. Which one of the following is a wrong matching of a microbe and its industrial product, while the remaining three are correct?
(a) Yeast - Statins
(b) *Acetobacter aceti* - Acetic acid
(c) *Clostridium butylicum* - Lactic acid
(d) *Aspergillus niger* - Citric acid

60. Which of the following is false about Columnar epithelium?
(i) It is made of tall and slender cells.
(ii) Free surface may have microvilli.
(iii) They are found in stomach and intestine and help in secretion and absorption.
(iv) Ciliated epithelium is mainly present in hollow structure like bronchioles and fallopian tubes/ products.
(v) They have apical nuclei.
(a) Only (i) (b) Only (iv)
(c) (ii) and (iv) (d) (ii) and (iii)

61. Select the correct statement from the ones given below.
(a) Barbiturates when given to criminals make them tell the truth.
(b) Morphine is often given to persons who have undergone surgery as a pain killer.
(c) Chewing tobacco lowers blood pressure and heart rate.
(d) Cocaine is given to patients after surgery as it stimulates recovery.

RESPONSE GRID					
	48. ⓐⓑⓒⓓ	49. ⓐⓑⓒⓓ	50. ⓐⓑⓒⓓ	51. ⓐⓑⓒⓓ	52. ⓐⓑⓒⓓ
	53. ⓐⓑⓒⓓ	54. ⓐⓑⓒⓓ	55. ⓐⓑⓒⓓ	56. ⓐⓑⓒⓓ	57. ⓐⓑⓒⓓ
	58. ⓐⓑⓒⓓ	59. ⓐⓑⓒⓓ	60. ⓐⓑⓒⓓ	61. ⓐⓑⓒⓓ	

62. The cell junctions called tight, adhering and gap junctions are found in
(a) muscular tissue (b) connective tissue
(c) epithelial tissue (d) neural tissue

63. Which of the following is a pair of viral diseases?
(a) Common cold, AIDS
(b) Dysentery, Common cold
(c) Typhoid, Tuberculosis
(d) Ringworm, AIDS

64. The part of the virus which gives to it the hereditary feature, is
(a) capsid (b) capsomere
(c) nucleic acid (d) None of these

65. A population of organisms has a gene for which there are two alleles, D and d. The allele frequency of D = 0.8. If this population satisfies all five of the Hardy-Weinberg conditions, what are the genotype frequencies that are expected in the next generation?
(a) DD = 0.04; Dd = 0.32; dd = 0.64
(b) DD = 0.64; Dd = 0.32; dd = 0.64
(c) DD = 0.04; Dd = 0.64; dd = 0.32
(d) DD = 0.64; Dd = 0.32; dd = 0.04

66. Which of the following organs can be called as a sort of "Blood bank" ?
(a) Lungs (b) Heart
(c) Liver (d) Spleen

67. Which one of the following groups of animals is Bilaterally symmetrical and Triploblastic?
(a) Aschelminthes (Round worms)
(b) Ctenophores
(c) Sponges
(d) Coelenterates (Cnidarians)

68. Haemophilia is more commonly seen in human males than in human females because
(a) a greater proportion of girls die in infancy.
(b) this disease is due to a Y-linked recessive mutation.
(c) this disease is due to an X-linked recessive mutation.
(d) this disease is due to an X-linked dominant mutation.

69. Which of the following statement is wrong about Chylomicrons?
(i) Chylomicrons are produced in the epithelial cells of small intestine.
(ii) It contains triglycerides, cholesterol and phospholipids.
(iii) It is protein coated small vesicles.
(iv) Chylomicrons are released from the epithelial cell into lacteals.
(a) (i) and (iv) (b) (ii) and (iii)
(c) (i), (ii), (iii) and (iv) (d) None of these

70. The following graph of relative concentrations of the four hormones present in the blood plasma of a woman during her menstrual cycle. Identify the hormones.

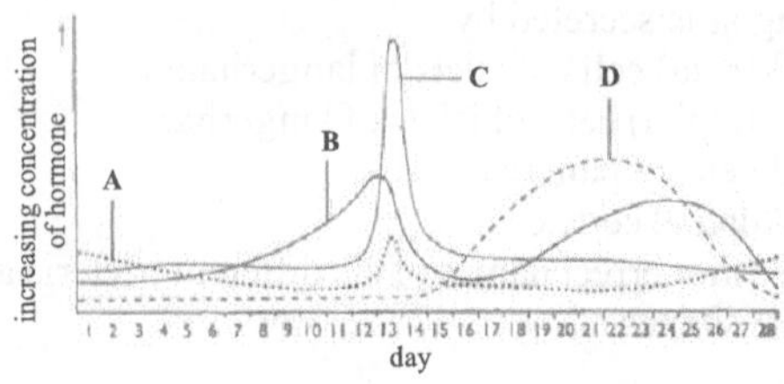

	A	B	C	D
(a)	FSH	Progesterone	LH	Oestrogen
(b)	LH	Progesterone	FSH	Oestrogen
(c)	FSH	Oestrogen	LH	Progesterone
(d)	LH	Oestrogen	FSH	Progesterone

71. Animal A and B show symmetry

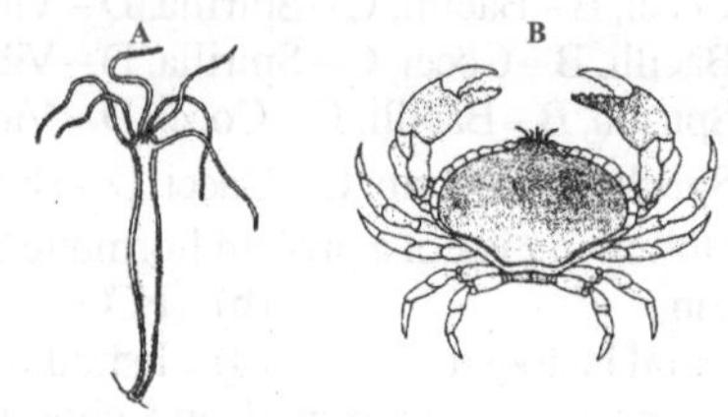

(a) Bilateral, Asymetrical
(b) Radial, Bilateral
(c) Bilateral, Bilateral
(d) Radial, Radial

72. Which of the following pair(s) is/are correct?
(a) Semicircular canal - Balancing
(b) Cochlea - Hearing
(c) Utriculus & sacculus - Balancing & hearing
(d) All of the above

73. The Ribosomes are made up of
(a) DNA + Protein (b) RNA + Protein
(c) DNA + RNA (d) None of these

74. Match column-I with column-II and choose the correct option.

	Column-I		Column-II
A.	Pinna	I.	Collects vibrations in the air which produces sound
B.	Ear canal	II.	Passage for sound wave from pinna to ear drum
C.	Tympanic membrane	III.	Transfers sound wave to ear ossicles
D.	Ear Ossicles	IV.	Increases the efficiency of transmission of sound waves to the innear ear
E.	Cochlea	V.	Has hearing receptors
F.	Eustachian tube	VI.	Equalizes the pressure on both sides of ear drum

(a) A → I; B → II; C → III; D → IV; E → V; F → VI
(b) A → I; B → VI; C → V; D → IV; E → III; F → II
(c) A → I; B → II; C → IV; D → III; E → V; F → VI
(d) A → I; B → VI; C → V; D → IV; E → III; F → II

RESPONSE GRID				
62. ⓐⓑⓒⓓ	63. ⓐⓑⓒⓓ	64. ⓐⓑⓒⓓ	65. ⓐⓑⓒⓓ	66. ⓐⓑⓒⓓ
67. ⓐⓑⓒⓓ	68. ⓐⓑⓒⓓ	69. ⓐⓑⓒⓓ	70. ⓐⓑⓒⓓ	71. ⓐⓑⓒⓓ
72. ⓐⓑⓒⓓ	73. ⓐⓑⓒⓓ	74. ⓐⓑⓒⓓ		

Space for Rough Work

75. Air is breathed through
(a) Trachea — lungs — larynx — pharynx — alveoli
(b) Nose — larynx — pharynx — bronchus — alveoli — bronchioles
(c) Nostrils — pharynx — larynx — trachea — bronchi — bronchioles — alveoli
(d) Nose — mouth — lungs

76. Match column-I with column-II and choose the correct option.

	Column-I		Column-II
A.	Limbless reptiles	I.	Elephant
B.	Jawless vertebrates	II.	Lamprey
C.	Flightless bird	III.	Ichthiophis
D.	Largest terrestrial animal	IV.	Ostrich
E.	Blind worm	V.	Cobra
		VI.	Penguin

(a) A → II; B → V; C → IV; D → I; E → III
(b) A → V; B → II; C → IV; D → I; E → III
(c) A → V; B → II; C → I; D → VI; E → III
(d) A → V; B → VI; C → II; D → VI; E → III

77. Match column-I with column-II and choose the correct option.

	Column-I		Column-II
A.	Tidal volume	I.	2500 to 3000 ml
B.	Inspiratory reserve volume	II.	1000 ml of air
C.	Expiratory reserve	III.	500 ml of air
D.	Residual volume	IV.	3400 to 4800 ml of air
E.	Vital capacity	V.	1200 ml of air

(a) A→ III; B→ IV; C→ II; D→ I; E→ V
(b) A→ III; B→ I; C→ II; D→ V; E→ IV
(c) A→ III; B→ I; C→ IV; D→ V; E→ IV
(d) A→ IV; B→ IV; C→ II; D→ I; E→ III

78. In the diagram of excretory system of humna beings given below, different parts have been indicated by alphabets; choose the answer in which these alphabets have been correctly matched with the parts which they represent

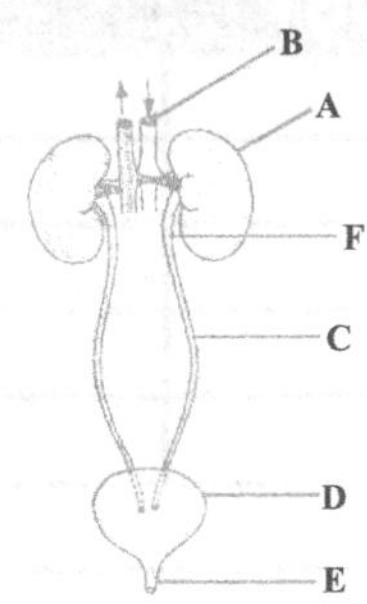

(a) A = Kidney, B = Abdominal aorta, C = Ureters, D = Urinary bladder, E = Urethra, F = Renal pelvis
(b) A = Kidney, B = Abdominal aorta, C = Urethra, D = Urinary bladder, E = Ureters , F = Renal pelvis
(c) A = Kidney, B = Renal pelvis, C = Urethra, D = Urinary bladder, E = Ureters, F = Abdominal aorta
(d) A = Kidney, B = Abdominal aorta, C = Urethra, D = Urinary bladder, E = Renal pelvis, F = Ureters

79. Given below is the diagrammatic representation of one of the categories of small molecular weight organic compounds in the living tissues. Identify the category shown and the one blank component "X" in it.

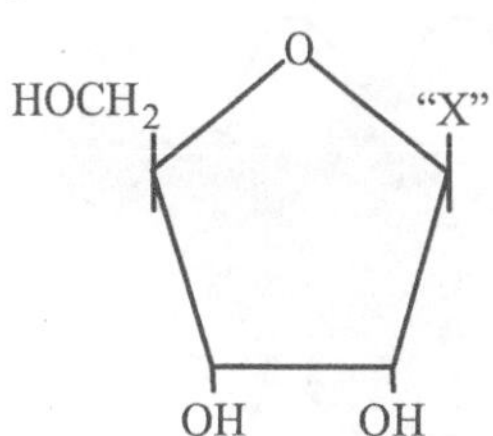

	Category	Component
(a)	Cholesterol	Guanine
(b)	Amino acid	NH_2
(c)	Nucleotide	Adenine
(d)	Nucleoside	Uracil

80. Which of the following is totally reabsorbed in renal tubules ?
(a) Na (b) K
(c) H_2O (d) $C_6H_{12}O_6$

81. In a standard ECG which one of the following alphabets is the correct representation of the respective activity of the human heart?
(a) S - start of systole
(b) T - end of diastole
(c) P - depolarisation of the atria
(d) R - repolarisation of ventricles

82. At metaphase of mitosis, each chromosome consists of _________ chromatid(s) _________ centromere(s) _______ kenetochore(s) and _______ molecules of DNA
(a) 2, 1, 2, 2 (b) 2, 2, 2, 2
(c) 2, 1, 1, 1 (d) 2, 1, 2, 1

83. Function of Gall bladder is
(a) storage of bile (b) formation of enzymes
(c) synthesis of bile (d) formation of bile salts

84. The technique called Gamete Intrafallopian Transfer (GIFT) is recommended for those females
(a) who cannot produce an ovum.
(b) who cannot retain the foetus inside uterus.
(c) whose cervical canal is too narrow to allow passage for the sperms.
(d) who cannot provide suitable environment for fertilisation.

RESPONSE GRID					
	75. ⓐⓑⓒⓓ	76. ⓐⓑⓒⓓ	77. ⓐⓑⓒⓓ	78. ⓐⓑⓒⓓ	79. ⓐⓑⓒⓓ
	80. ⓐⓑⓒⓓ	81. ⓐⓑⓒⓓ	82. ⓐⓑⓒⓓ	83. ⓐⓑⓒⓓ	84. ⓐⓑⓒⓓ

Space for Rough Work

85. Following is the figure of actin (thin) filaments. Identify A, B and C.

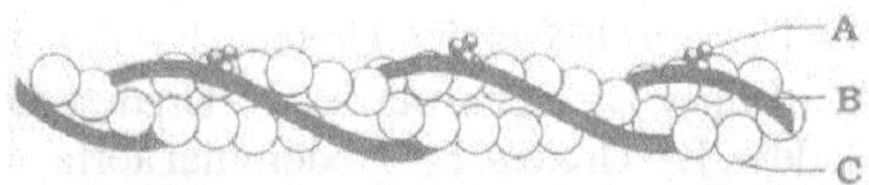

(a) A-Tropomyosin, B-Troponin, C-F-actin
(b) A-Troponin, B-Myosin, C-Tropomyosin
(c) A-Troponin, B-Tropomyosin, C-Myosin
(d) A-Troponin, B-Tropomyosin, C-F-actin

86.

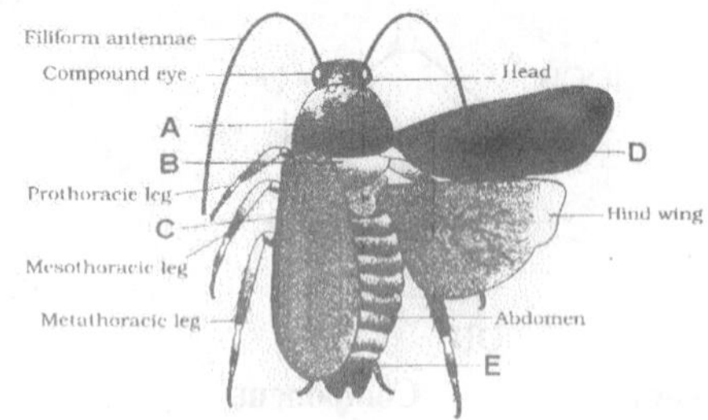

Identify A to E.
(a) A- Pronotum, B-Mesothorax, C-Metathorax, D-Tegmina, E-Pleura
(b) A- Pronotum, B-Mesothorax, C-Metathorax, D-Tegmina, E-Sterna
(c) A- Pronotum, B-Mesothorax, C-Metathorax, D-Tegmina, E-Anal cerci
(d) A- Pronotum, B-Mesothorax, C-Metathorax, D-Tegmina, E-Anal style

87. Match column-I with column-II and choose the correct option.

Column-I	**Column - II**
A. Somatostain	I. Pineal gland
B. Melatonin	II. Corpus luteum
C. Aldosterone	III. Placenta
D. Progesterone	IV. Adrenal cortex
E. hCG	V. Islet of Langerhans
	VI. Adenohypophysis

(a) A→ V; B→ I; C→ VI; D→ III; E→ II
(b) A→ I; B→ II; C→ IV; D→ III; E→ V
(c) A→ II; B→ VI; C→ IV; D→ V; E→ III
(d) A→ V; B→ I; C→ IV; D→ II; E→ III

88. **Statememt 1 :** Chiasmata is formed during diplotene.
Statememt 2 : Chiasmata are formed due to deposition of nucleoproteins.
(a) Statement-1 is True, Statement-2 is True, Statement-2 is a correct explanation for Statement-1
(b) Statement-1 is True, Statement-2 is True, Statement-2 is NOT a correct explanation for Statement-1
(c) Statement-1 is True, Statement-2 is False
(d) Both the Statements are False.

89. The primary reason why the same basic techniques can be used to analyze the DNA from species as diverse as bacteria and humans is that
(a) all cells are identical.
(b) every organism has the same amount of DNA.
(c) the DNA sequences of all organisms are the same.
(d) DNA has a consistent structure in all organisms.

90. Which one of the following statement is true?
(a) The greater the BOD of waste water, more is its polluting potential.
(b) The greater the BOD of waste water, less is its polluting potential.
(c) The lesser the BOD of waste water, more is its polluting potential.
(d) The lesser the BOD of waste water, less is its polluting potential.

RESPONSE GRID	85. ⓐⓑⓒⓓ	86. ⓐⓑⓒⓓ	87. ⓐⓑⓒⓓ	88. ⓐⓑⓒⓓ	89. ⓐⓑⓒⓓ
	90. ⓐⓑⓒⓓ				

SUBJECTWISE SPEED TEST-99 - BIOLOGY			
Total Questions	90	Total Marks	360
Attempted		Correct	
Incorrect		Net Score	
Cut-off Score	55	Qualifying Score	85
Success Gap = Net Score – Qualifying Score			
Net Score = (Correct × 4) – (Incorrect × 1)			

Space for Rough Work

Full Test-1

Speed TEST 100

Full Syllabus

No. of Questions	Maximum Marks	Time
180	**720**	**3 Hours**

GENERAL INSTRUCTIONS

- This test contents 180 MCQ's :
  - **Physics (180 marks)** : Question No. 1 to 45 are of **4 marks** each.
  - **Chemistry (180 marks)** : Question No. 46 to 90 are of **4 marks** each.
  - **Biology (360 marks)** : Question No. 91 to 180 are of **4 marks** each.
- Darken the correct circle/ bubble in the Response Grid provided at the end of this test.
- You have to evaluate your Response Grids yourself with the help of solutions provided at the end of this book.
- Each correct answer will get you 4 marks and 1 mark shall be deduced for each incorrect answer. No mark will be given/ deducted if no bubble is filled. Keep a timer in front of you and stop immediately at the end of 3 hours.
- After completing the sheet check your answers with the solution booklet and complete the Result Grid. Finally spend time to analyse your performance and revise the areas which emerge out as weak in your evaluation.

PHYSICS

DIRECTIONS : There are 45 multiple choice questions numbered 1 to 45. Each question has 4 choices (a), (b), (c) and (d), out of which ONLY ONE is correct.

1. An automobile travelling with a speed of 60 km/h, can brake to stop within a distance of 20m. If the car is going twice as fast i.e., 120 km/h, the stopping distance will be

(a) 60m (b) 40m (c) 20m (d) 80m

2. Out of the following quantities, which one has dimensions different from the remaining three?

(a) Energy per unit volume
(b) Force per unit area
(c) Product of voltage and charge per unit volume
(d) Angular momentum

3. A sphere of radius *r* and mass *m* has a velocity v_0 directed to the left and no angular velocity as it is placed on a belt moving to the right with a constant velocity v_1. If after sliding on the belt the sphere is to have no linear velocity relative to the ground as it starts rolling on the belt without sliding. In terms of v_1, the velocity v_0 is

(a) $v_0 = \frac{2}{5}v_1$

(b) $v_0 = \frac{3}{5}v_1$

(c) $v_0 = \frac{1}{5}v_1$

(d) $v_0 = 3v_1$

4. Three concentric spherical shells have radii a, b and c (a < b < c) and have surface charge densities σ, $-\sigma$ and σ respectively. If V_A, V_B and V_C denotes the potentials of the three shells, then for c = a + b, we have

(a) $V_C = V_B \neq V_A$ (b) $V_C \neq V_B \neq V_A$
(c) $V_C = V_B = V_A$ (d) $V_C = V_A \neq V_B$

5. A body of mass M is kept on a rough horizontal surface (friction coefficient μ). A person is trying to pull the body by applying a horizontal force but the body is not moving. The force by the surface on the body is F, then

(a) $F = Mg$ (b) $F = \mu Mg$

(c) $Mg \le F \le Mg\sqrt{1+\mu^2}$ (d) $Mg \ge F \ge Mg\sqrt{1+\mu^2}$

6. The ratio between the values of acceleration due to gravity at a height 1 km above and at a depth of 1 km below the Earth's surface is (radius of Earth is R)

(a) $\frac{R-2}{R-1}$ (b) $\frac{R}{R-1}$ (c) $\frac{R-2}{R}$ (d) 1

7. The moment of inertia of a body about a given axis is 1.2 kg/m^2. Initially, the body is at rest. In order to produce a rotational kinetic energy of 1500 joule, an angular acceleration of 25 $radian/sec^2$ must be applied about that axis for a duration of

(a) 4 seconds (b) 2 seconds
(c) 8 seconds (d) 10 seconds

8. A metal ball of mass 2 kg moving with a velocity of 36 km/h has a head on collision with a stationary ball of mass 3 kg. If after the collision, the two balls move together, the loss in kinetic energy due to collision is

(a) 140 J (b) 100 J (c) 60 J (d) 40 J

9. The length of a given cylindrical wire is increased by 100%. Due to the consequent decrease in diameter the change in the resistance of the wire will be

(a) 200% (b) 100% (c) 50% (d) 300%

10. A ball is dropped on a floor and bounces back to a height somewhat less than the original height. Which of the curves depicts its motion correctly?

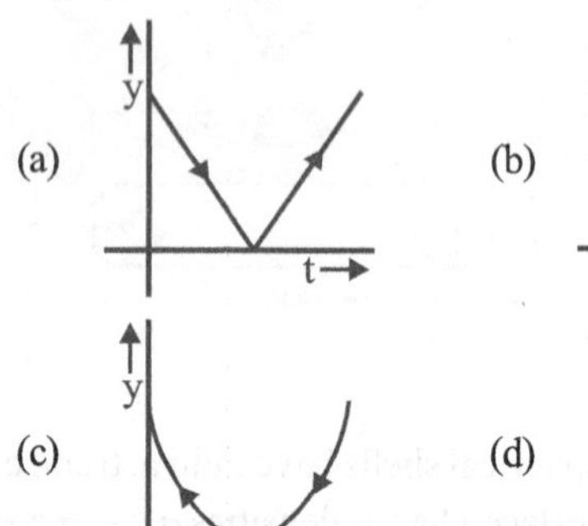

11. Two particles A and B of mass m each and moving with velocity v, hit the ends of a rigid bar of the same mass m and length l simultaneously and stick to the bar as shown in the figure. The bar is kept on a smooth horizontal plane. The linear and angular speed of the system (bar + particle) after the collision are

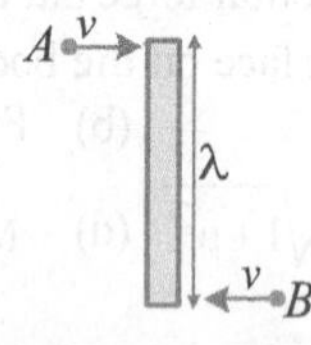

(a) $v_{cm}=0, \omega=\frac{12\,v}{7\,l}$ (b) $v_{cm}=0, \omega=\frac{4v}{l}$

(c) $v_{cm}=0, \omega=\frac{5v}{l}$ (d) $v_{cm}=0, \omega=\frac{v}{5l}$

12. When the angular velocity of a uniformly rotating body is increased thrice, the resultant force applied to it increases by 60 N. If mass of body = 3 kg, the initial and final accelerations are

(a) $2.5\ m/s^2, 7.5\ m/s^2$ (b) $7.5\ m/s^2, 22.5\ m/s^2$
(c) $5\ m/s^2, 45\ m/s^2$ (d) $2.5\ m/s^2, 22.5\ m/s^2$

13. The escape velocity of a rocket launched from the surface of the earth

(a) depends on the mass of rocket
(b) depends on the mass of planet towards which, it is moving
(c) does not depend on the mass of earth
(d) does not depend on the mass of rocket

14. A conducting circular loop is placed in a uniform magnetic field, B = 0.025 T with its plane perpendicular to the loop. The radius of the loop is made to shrink at a constant rate of 1 mm s^{-1}. The induced e.m.f. when the radius is 2 cm, is

(a) $2\pi\mu V$ (b) $\pi\mu V$ (c) $\frac{\pi}{2}\mu V$ (d) $2\mu V$

15. In the P-V diagram shown, the gas does 5J of work along isothermal ab and 4J along adiabatic bc. What is the change in the internal energy of the gas if the gas traverse the straight path from a to c?

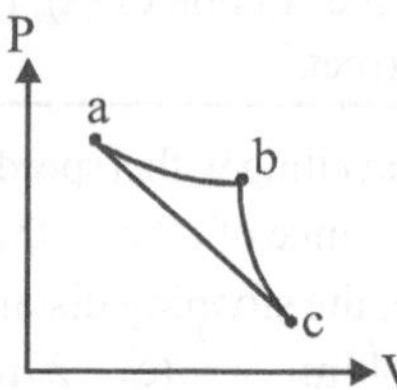

(a) 1J (b) – 4J (c) 5J (d) 9J

16. In the given figure, which of the following is reversed biased?

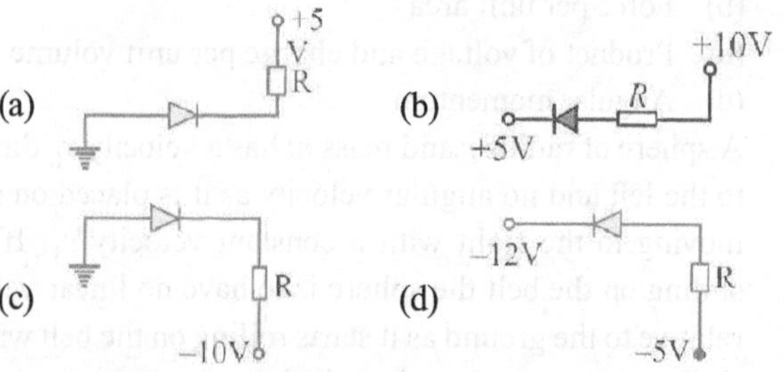

17. A solid substance is at 30°C and heat energy is supplied to it at a constant rate. Then temperature versus time graph is as shown in the figure. The substance is in liquid state for the portion (of the graph)

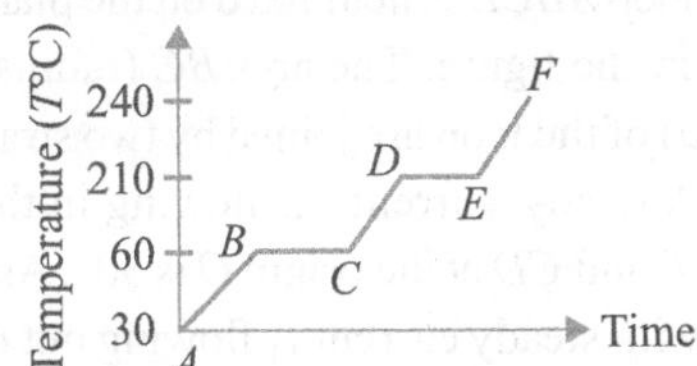

(a) BC (b) CD (c) ED (d) EF

18. The sunlight reaches us as white light and not as its components because
(a) air medium is dispersive
(b) air medium is non-dispersive
(c) air medium scatter the sunlight
(d) air medium absorbs the sunlight

19. In a room where the temperature is 30°C, a body cools from 61°C to 59°C in 4 minutes. The time (in minutes) taken by the body to cool from 51°C to 49°C will be :
(a) 8 (b) 5 (c) 6 (d) 4

20. A transistor is operated in common emitter configuration at constant collector voltage $V_c = 1.5$V such that a change in the base current from 100 μA to 150 μA produces a change in the collector current from 5 mA to 10 mA. The current gain (β) is
(a) 75 (b) 100 (c) 50 (d) 67

21. The intensity of gamma radiation emitted from a given source is I. On passing through 36 mm of lead, it is reduced to $\frac{I}{8}$. The thickness of lead which will reduce the intensity to $\frac{I}{2}$ will be
(a) 9mm (b) 6mm (c) 12mm (d) 18mm

22. A particle executing simple harmonic motion has a kinetic energy $K_0 \cos^2 \omega t$. The maximum values of the potential energy and the total energy are respectively
(a) $K_0/2$ and K_0 (b) K_0 and $2K_0$
(c) K_0 and K_0 (d) 0 and $2K_0$

23. A sonometer wire supports a 4 kg load and vibrates in fundamental mode with a tuning fork of frequency 416 Hz. The length of the wire between the bridges is now doubled. In order to maintain fundamental mode, the load should be changed to
(a) 1 kg (b) 2 kg (c) 4 kg (d) 16 kg

24. The value of power factor in a circuit connected to an A.C. is
(a) unity when the circuit contians an ideal inductance only
(b) unity when the circuit contians an ideal resistance only
(c) zero when the circuit contains an ideal resistance only
(d) unity when the circuit contains an ideal capacitance only

25. Taking the internal resistance of the battery negligible, the steady state current in the 2Ω resistor shown in the figure will be

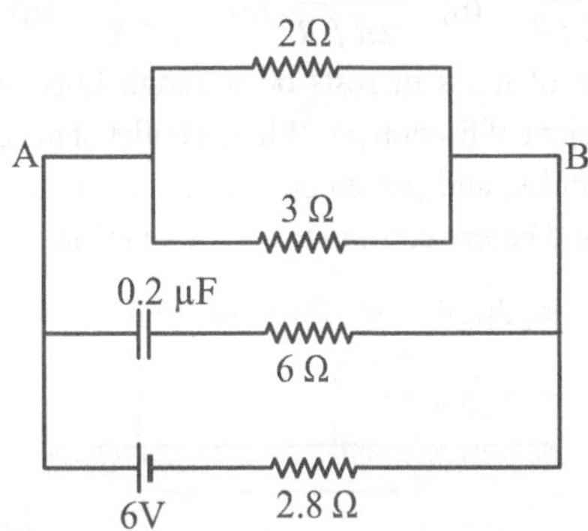

(a) 1.8 A (b) 2.9 A (c) 0.9 A (d) 2.8 A

26. Tension in the cable supporting an elevator, is equal to the weight of the elevator. From this, we can conclude that the elevator is going up or down with a
(a) uniform velocity (b) uniform acceleration
(c) variable acceleration (d) either (b) or (c)

27. A projectile is thrown in the upward direction making an angle of 60° with the horizontal direction with a velocity of 147 m s^{-1}. The time after which its inclination with the horizontal is 45°, is
(a) 15 s (b) 10.98 s (c) 5.49 s (d) 2.745 s

28. Two short bar magnets of length 1 cm each have magnetic moments 1.20 Am^2 and 1.00 Am^2 respectively. They are placed on a horizontal table parallel to each other with their N poles pointing towards the South. They have a common magnetic equator and are separated by a distance of 20.0 cm. The value of the resultant horizontal magnetic induction at the mid-point O of the line joining their centres is close to (Horizontal component of earth's magnetic induction is 3.6×10^{-5} Wb/m^2)
(a) 3.6×10^{-5} Wb/m^2 (b) 2.56×10^{-4} Wb/m^2
(c) 3.50×10^{-4} Wb/m^2 (d) 5.80×10^{-4} Wb/m^2

Space for Rough Work

29. The supply voltage to room is 120V. The resistance of the lead wires is 6Ω. A 60 W bulb is already switched on. What is the decrease of voltage across the bulb, when a 240 W heater is switched on in parallel to the bulb?

(a) zero (b) 2.9 Volt
(c) 13.3 Volt (d) 10.04 Volt

30. A thin ring of radius R meter has charge q coulomb uniformly spread on it. The ring rotates about its axis with a constant frequency of f revolutions/s. The value of magnetic induction in Wb/m^2 at the centre of the ring is

(a) $\frac{\mu_0 q f}{2\pi R}$ (b) $\frac{\mu_0 q}{2\pi f R}$ (c) $\frac{\mu_0 q}{2 f R}$ (d) $\frac{\mu_0 q f}{2R}$

31. A block of mass m rests on a rough horizontal surface (Coefficient of friction μ). When a bullet of mass m/2 strikes horizontally, and get embedded in it, the block moves a distance d before coming to rest. The initial velocity of the bullet is $k\sqrt{2\mu g d}$, then the value of k is

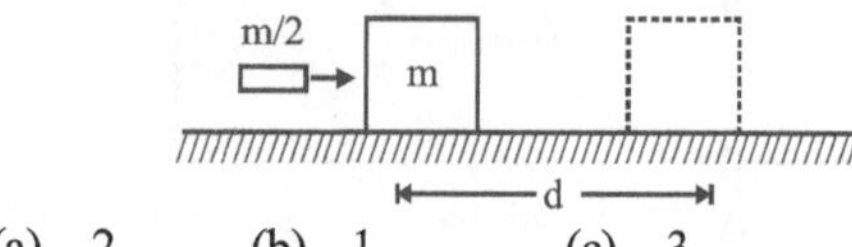

(a) 2 (b) 1 (c) 3 (d) 5

32. The magnetic field of earth at the equator is approximately 4×10^{-5} T. The radius of earth is 6.4×10^6 m. Then the dipole moment of the earth will be nearly of the order of:

(a) 10^{23} A m^2 (b) 10^{20} A m^2
(c) 10^{16} A m^2 (d) 10^{10} A m^2

33. A galvanometer of resistance 50 Ω is connected to battery of 3V along with a resistance of 2950 Ω in series. A full scale deflection of 30 divisions is obtained in the galvanometer. In order to reduce this deflection to 20 divisions, the resistance in series should be

(a) 5050 Ω (b) 5550 Ω (c) 6050 Ω (d) 4450 Ω

34. An inductor of inductance L = 400 mH and resistors of resistance $R_1 = 2\Omega$ and $R_2 = 2\Omega$ are connected to a battery of emf 12 V as shown in the figure.

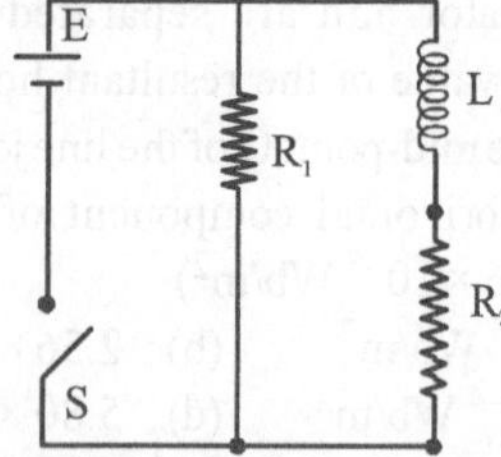

The internal resistance of the battery is negligible. The switch S is closed at $t = 0$. The potential drop across L as a function of time is

(a) $\frac{12}{t}e^{-3t}$ V (b) $6(1-e^{-t/0.2})$V
(c) $12e^{-5t}$ V (d) $6e^{-5t}$ V

35. A current loop $ABCD$ is held fixed on the plane of the paper as shown in the figure. The arcs BC (radius = b) and DA (radius = a) of the loop are joined by two straight wires AB and CD. A steady current I is flowing in the loop. Angle made by AB and CD at the origin O is 30°. Another straight thin wire with steady current I_1 flowing out of the plane of the paper is kept at the origin.

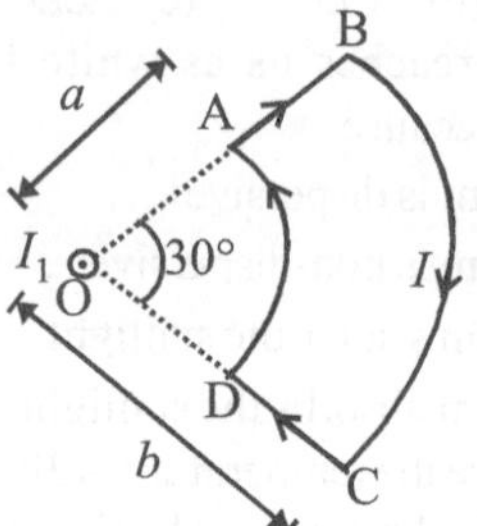

The magnitude of the magnetic field (B) due to the loop $ABCD$ at the origin (O) is :

(a) $\frac{\mu_0 I(b-a)}{24ab}$

(b) $\frac{\mu_0 I}{4\pi}\left[\frac{b-a}{ab}\right]$

(c) $\frac{\mu_0 I}{4\pi}[2(b-a)+\pi/3(a+b)]$

(d) zero

36. A polished metal plate with a rough black spot on it is heated to about 1400 K and quickly taken into a dark room. Which one of the following statements will be true?

(a) The spot will appear brighter than the plate
(b) The spot will appear darker than the plate
(c) The spot and plate will appear equally bright
(d) The spot and the plate will not be visible in the dark room

37. The angular dispersion produced by a prism

(a) increases if the average refractive index increases
(b) increases if the average refractive index decreases
(c) remains constant whether the average refractive index increases or decreases
(d) has no relation with average refractive index.

38. The tempertaure of equal masses of three different liquids A, B and C are 12°C, 19°C and 28°C respectively. The temperature when A and B are mixed is 16°C and when B and C are mixed is 23°C. The temperature when A and C are mixed is

(a) 18.2°C (b) 22°C (c) 20.2°C (d) 25.2°C

39. Two sources of light of wavelengths 2500 Å and 3500 Å are used in Young's double slit expt. simultaneously. Which orders of fringes of two wavelength patterns coincide?
(a) 3rd order of 1st and 5th of the 2nd
(b) 7th order of 1st and 5th order of 2nd
(c) 5th order of 1st and 3rd order of 2nd
(d) 5th order of 1st and 7th order of 2nd

40. An ideal gas is initially at P_1, V_1 is expanded to P_2, V_2 and then compressed adiabatically to the same volume V_1 and pressure P_3. If W is the net work done by the gas in complete process, which of the following is true ?
(a) $W > 0; P_3 > P_1$ (b) $W < 0; P_3 > P_1$
(c) $W > 0; P_3 < P_1$ (d) $W < 0; P_3 < P_1$

41. A photoelectric surface is illuminated successively by monochromatic light of wavelength λ and $\frac{\lambda}{2}$. If the maximum kinetic energy of the emitted photoelectrons in the second case is 3 times that in the first case, the work function of the surface of the material is :
(h = Planck's constant, c = speed of light)
(a) $\frac{hc}{\lambda}$ (b) $\frac{2hc}{\lambda}$ (c) $\frac{hc}{3\lambda}$ (d) $\frac{hc}{2\lambda}$

42. An ideal gas confined in an isolated closed chamber. As the gas undergoes an adiabatic expansion, the average time of collision between molecules increases as V^q, where V is the volume of the gas. The value of q is : $\left(\gamma = \frac{C_p}{C_v}\right)$
(a) $\frac{\gamma+1}{2}$ (b) $\frac{\gamma-1}{2}$ (c) $\frac{3\gamma+5}{6}$ (d) $\frac{3\gamma-5}{6}$

43. Which logic gate is represented by the following combination of logic gates

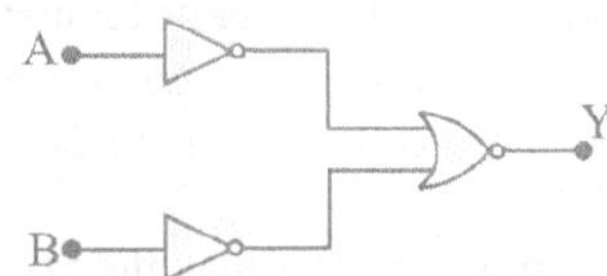

(a) OR (b) NAND (c) AND (d) NOR

44. If T is the surface tension of a liquid, the energy needed to break a liquid drop of radius R into 64 drops is
(a) $6\pi R^2 T$ (b) $\pi R^2 T$
(c) $12\pi R^2 T$ (d) $8\pi R^2 T$

45. In the Bohr model an electron moves in a circular orbit around the proton. Considering the orbiting electron to be a circular current loop, the magnetic moment of the hydrogen atom, when the electron is in n^{th} excited state, is :
(a) $\left(\frac{e}{2m}\right)\frac{n^2 h}{2\pi}$ (b) $\left(\frac{e}{m}\right)\frac{nh}{2\pi}$
(c) $\left(\frac{e}{2m}\right)\frac{nh}{2\pi}$ (d) $\left(\frac{e}{m}\right)\frac{n^2 h}{2\pi}$

CHEMISTRY

DIRECTIONS : There are 45 multiple choice questions numbered 46 to 90. Each question has 4 choices (a), (b), (c) and (d), out of which ONLY ONE is correct.

46. A hydrocarbon A on chlorination gives B which on heating with alcoholic potassium hydroxide changes into another hydrocarbon C. The latter decolourises Baeyer's reagent and on ozonolysis forms formaldehyde only. A is
(a) Ethane (b) Butane
(c) Methane (d) Ethene

47. The IUPAC name of the compound having the molecular formula $Cl_3C{-}CH_2CHO$ is
(a) 3, 3, 3- Trichloropropanal
(b) 1, 1, 1- Trichloropropanal
(c) 2, 2, 2- Trichloropropanal
(d) Chloral

48. Which one of the following complexes is not expected to exhibit isomerism?
(a) $[Ni(en)_3]^{2+}$
(b) $[Ni(NH_3)_4(H_2O)_2]^{2+}$
(c) $[Pt(NH_3)_2Cl_2]$
(d) $[Ni(NH_3)_2Cl_2]$

49. The increasing order of the rate of HCN addition to compound A – D is
(A) HCHO (B) CH_3COCH_3
(C) $PhCOCH_3$ (D) PhCOPh
(a) D<C<B<A (b) C<D<B<A
(c) A<B<C<D (d) D<B<C<A

50. Phosphorus pentachloride dissociates as follows, in a closed reaction vessel
$$PCl_5(g) \rightleftharpoons PCl_3(g) + Cl_2(g)$$
If total pressure at equilibrium of the reaction mixture is P and degree of dissociation of PCl_5 is x, the partial pressure of PCl_3 will be
(a) $\left(\frac{x}{x-1}\right)P$ (b) $\left(\frac{x}{1-x}\right)P$
(c) $\left(\frac{x}{x+1}\right)P$ (d) $\left(\frac{2x}{1-x}\right)P$

Space for Rough Work

51. Which of the following will not show cis-trans isomerism?

(a) $CH_3-CH=CH-CH_3$

(b) $CH_3-CH_2-CH=CH-CH_2-CH_3$

(c) $CH_3-C(CH_3)=CH-CH_2-CH_3$

(d) $CH_3-CH(CH_3)-CH=CH-CH_2-CH_3$

52. Point out the false statement

(a) Brownian movement and Tyndall effect are shown by colloidal systems.

(b) Gold number is a measure of the protective power of a lyophillic colloid.

(c) The colloidal solution of a liquid in liquid is called gel.

(d) Hardy - Schulze rule is related with coagulation.

53. P_A and P_B are the vapour pressure of pure liquid components, A and B, respectively of an ideal binary solution. If X_A represents the mole fraction of component A, the total pressure of the solution will be.

(a) $P_A+X_A(P_B-P_A)$ (b) $P_A+X_A(P_A-P_B)$

(c) $P_B+X_A(P_B-P_A)$ (d) $P_B+X_A(P_A-P_B)$

54. In which one of the following species the central atom has the type of hybridization which is not the same as that present in the other three?

(a) SF_4 (b) I_3^- (c) $SbCl_5^{2-}$ (d) PCl_5

55. A strong base can abstract an α -hydrogen from :

(a) alkene (b) amine

(c) ketone (d) alkane

56. What products are expected from the disproportionation reaction of hypochlorous acid?

(a) HCl and Cl_2O (b) HCl and $HClO_3$

(c) $HClO_3$ and Cl_2O (d) $HClO_2$ and $HClO_4$

57. Which one of the following pairs of substances on reaction will not evolve H_2 gas?

(a) Iron and H_2SO_4(aq)

(b) Iron and steam

(c) Copper and HCl(g)

(d) Sodium and ethyl alchohol

58. An antibiotic contains nitro group attached to aromatic nucleus. It is

(a) penicillin (b) streptomycin

(c) tetracycline (d) chloramphenicol

59. An ionic compound has a unit cell consisting of A ions at the corners of a cube and B ions on the centres of the faces of the cube. The empirical formula for this compound would be

(a) A_3B (b) AB_3

(c) A_2B (d) ABl

60. In a reaction, when the concentration of reactant is increased two times, the increase in rate of reaction was four times. Order of reaction is :

(a) zero (b) 1

(c) 2 (d) 3

61. The cell reaction $Cu+2Ag^+ \rightarrow Cu^{2+}+Ag$ is best represented by

(a) $Cu(s) | Cu^{2+}(aq) || Ag^+(aq) | Ag(s)$

(b) $Pt | Cu^{2+} || Ag^+(aq) | Ag(s)$

(c) $Cu^{2+} | Cu || Pt | Ag$

(d) None of the above representations

62. Chlorine is liberated when we heat

(a) $KMnO_4+NaCl$ (b) $K_2Cr_2O_7+MnO_2$

(c) $Pb(NO_3)_2+MnO_2$ (d) $K_2Cr_2O_7+HCl$

63. According to kinetic theory of gases, for a diatomic molecule

(a) the pressure exerted by the gas is proportional to mean velocity of the molecule

(b) the pressure exerted by the gas is proportional to the root mean velocity of the molecule

(c) the root mean square velocity of the molecule is inversely proportional to the temperature

(d) the mean translational kinetic energy of the molecule is proportional to the absolute temperature.

64. Larger number of oxidation states are exhibited by the actinoids than those by the lanthanoids, the main reason being

(a) 4*f* orbitals more diffused than the 5*f* orbitals

(b) lesser energy difference between 5*f* and 6*d* than between 4*f* and 5*d* orbitals

(c) more energy difference between 5*f* and 6*d* than between 4*f* and 5*d* orbitals

(d) more reactive nature of the actinoids than the lanthanoids

65. Which one of the following arrangements does not give the correct picture of the trends indicated against it ?

(a) $F_2>Cl_2>Br_2>I_2$: Oxidizing power

(b) $F_2>Cl_2>Br_2>I_2$: Electron gain enthalpy

(c) $F_2>Cl_2>Br_2>I_2$: Bond dissociation energy

(d) $F_2>Cl_2>Br_2>I_2$: Electronegativity.

Space for Rough Work

66. The process of converting hydrated alumina into anhydrous alumina is called
(a) roasting (b) smelting
(c) dressing (d) calcination

67. The rate constant of a reaction becomes equal to the pre-exponential factor when

(a) the absolute temperature is zero
(b) the activation energy is infinity
(c) the absolute temperature is infinity
(d) the temperature in Celsius is zero.

68. Which one of the following cyano complexes would exhibit the lowest value of paramagnetic behaviour ?

(a) $[Co(CN)_6]^{3-}$ (b) $[Fe(CN)_6]^{3-}$

(c) $[Mn(CN)_6]^{3-}$ (d) $[Cr(CN)_6]^{3-}$

(At. No : Cr = 24, Mn = 25, Fe = 26, Co = 27)

69. On the basis of the following thermochemical data : $(\Delta_f G^\circ H^+(aq) = 0)$

$H_2O(l) \rightarrow H^+(aq) + OH^-(aq); \Delta H = 57.32 kJ$

$$H_2(g) + \frac{1}{2}O_2(g) \longrightarrow H_2O(l); \ \Delta H = -286.20 kJ$$

The value of enthalpy of formation of OH^- ion at 25° C is:
(a) –228.88 kJ (b) +228.88 kJ
(c) –343.52 kJ (d) –22.88 kJ

70. In which of the following pair both the species have sp^3 hybridization?
(a) H_2S, BF_3 (b) SiF_4, BeH_2
(c) NF_3, H_2O (d) NF_3, BF_3

71. What is the product of the following reaction ?

Chlorobenzene (Cl on benzene ring) $\xrightarrow[(CH_3)_2NH]{(CH_3)_2NLi}$?

(a) N, N-dimethylaniline
(b) phenyllithium (C_6H_5Li)
(c) *para*-chloro-N, N-dimethylaniline
(d) *meta*-chloro-N, N-dimethylaniline

72. From amongst the following alcohols the one that would react fastest with conc. HCl and anhydrous $ZnCl_2$, is
(a) 2-Butanol (b) 2- Methylpropan-2-ol
(c) 2-Methylpropanol (d) 1- Butanol

73. Number of moles of MnO_4^- required to oxidize one mole of ferrous oxalate completely in acidic medium will be :
(a) 0.6 moles (b) 0.4 moles
(c) 7.5 moles (d) 0.2 moles

74. Which of the following practices will not come under green chemistry?
(a) If possible, making use of soap made of vegetable oils instead of using synthetic detergents.
(b) Using H_2O_2 for bleaching purpose instead of using chlorine based bleaching agents.
(c) Using bicycle for travelling small distances instead of using petrol/ diesel based vehicles.
(d) Using plastic cans for neatly storing substances.

75. Sodium phenoxide when heated with CO_2 under pressure at 125°C yields a product which on acetylation produces C

$C_6H_5ONa + CO_2 \xrightarrow[5\text{ Atm}]{125^\circ} B \xrightarrow[Ac_2O]{H^+} C$

The major product C would be

(a) Benzene ring with $OCOCH_3$ and ortho $COOH$
(b) Benzene ring with OH, $COCH_3$ (ortho) and $COCH_3$ (para to OH)
(c) Benzene ring with OH and ortho $COOCH_3$
(d) Benzene ring with $OCOCH_3$ and meta $COOH$

76. The strength in volumes of a solution containing 30.36 g/L of H_2O_2 is
(a) 10 V (b) 5 V
(c) 20 V (d) None of these

77. The position of some metals in the electrochemical series in decreasing electropositive character is given as Mg > Al > Zn > Cu > Ag. What will happen, if a copper spoon is used to stir a solution of aluminium nitrate ?
(a) The spoon will get coated with Al
(b) An alloy of Cu and Al is formed
(c) The solution becomes blue
(d) There is no reaction

78. Which of the following graph correspond to one node

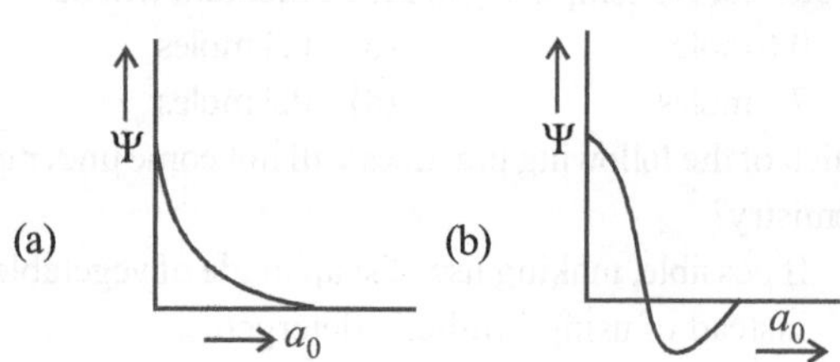

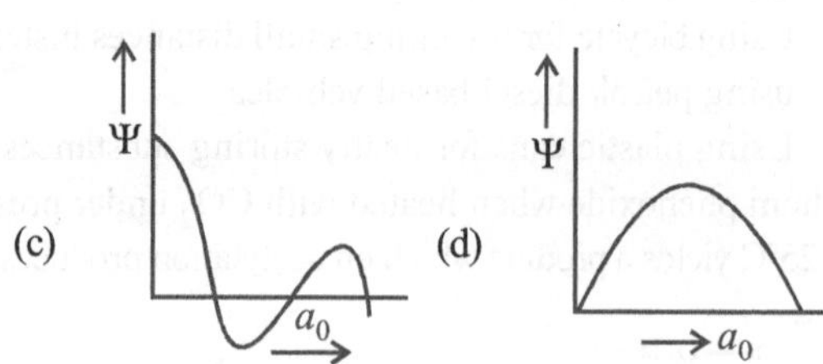

79. Which of the following substances has the greatest ionic character ?

(a) Cl_2O (b) NCl_3 (c) $PbCl_2$ (d) $BaCl_2$

80. The reaction of benzyl chloride with sodium cyanide followed by reduction with hydrogen in the presence of nickel gives

(a) β-Phenylethylamine (b) N-Isobutylaniline
(c) Benzylamine (d) Aniline.

81. F–C_6H_4–NO_2 $\xrightarrow[\text{DMF, }\Delta]{(CH_3)_2\ddot{N}H}$ (A) $\xrightarrow{Zn/HCl}$ (B)

(B) is –

(a) $H_2\ddot{N}$–C_6H_4–$N(CH_3)_2$

(b) H_2N–C_6H_4–NH_2

(c) O_2N–C_6H_4–$N(CH_3)(NH_2)$

(d) O_2N–C_6H_4–NH_2

82. Which one of the following statements is correct?

(a) All amino acids except lysine are optically active
(b) All amino acids are optically active
(c) All amino acids except glycine are optically active
(d) All amino acids except glutamic acids are optically active

83. Which of the following structure is similar to graphite?

(a) B (b) B_4C
(c) B_2H_6 (d) BN

84. Four species are listed below:

i. HCO_3^- ii. H_3O^+
iii. HSO_4^- iv. HSO_3F

Which one of the following is the correct sequence of their acid strength?

(a) iv<ii<iii<i (b) ii<iii<i<iv
(c) i<iii<ii<iv (d) iii<i<iv<ii

85. Arrange the following in increasing order of stability

(A) $(CH_3)_2\overset{\oplus}{C}-CH_2CH_3$ (B) $(CH_3)_3\overset{\oplus}{C}$
(C) $(CH_3)_2\overset{\oplus}{CH}$ (D) $CH_3\overset{\oplus}{CH_2}$
(E) $\overset{\oplus}{CH_3}$

(a) E<D<C<B<A (b) E<D<C<A<B
(c) D<E<C<A<B (d) A<E<D<C<B

86. An organic compound A upon reacting with NH_3 gives B. On heating B gives C. C in presence of KOH reacts with Br_2 to given $CH_3CH_2NH_2$. A is :

(a) CH_3COOH (b) $CH_3CH_2CH_2COOH$
(c) $CH_3-CH(CH_3)-COOH$ (d) CH_3CH_2COOH

87. The ratio of ionization energy of H and Be^{3+} is

(a) 1 : 1 (b) 1 : 3
(c) 1 : 9 (d) 1 : 16

88. Which is the correct order of electronegativity ?

(a) F>N<O>C (b) F>N>O>C
(c) F>N>O<C (d) F<N<O=C

89. **Statement-1 :** Teflon has high thermal stability and chemical inertness.

Statement-2 : Teflon is a thermoplastic.

(a) Statement-1 is true, Statement-2 is true, Statement-2 is a correct explanation for Statement -1
(b) Statement-1 is true, Statement-2 is true ; Statement-2 is NOT a correct explanation for Statement-1
(c) Statement-1 is true, Statement-2 is false
(d) Statement-1 is false, Statement-2 is true

90. The rate of diffusion of SO_2, CO_2, PCl_3 and SO_3 are in the following order
(a) $PCl_3 > SO_3 > SO_2 > CO_2$
(b) $CO_2 > SO_2 > PCl_3 > SO_3$
(c) $SO_2 > SO_3 > PCl_3 > CO_2$
(d) $CO_2 > SO_2 > SO_3 > PCl_3$

BIOLOGY

DIRECTIONS : There are 90 multiple choice questions numbered 91 to 180. Each question has 4 choices (a), (b), (c) and (d), out of which ONLY ONE is correct.

91. Select the correct statement
(a) Phosphorus cycle is an example of gaseous nutrient cycle
(b) The pyramid of biomass in sea is generally inverted
(c) By the process of humification, soluble inorganic nutrients go down into the soil horizon
(d) A given organism may not occupy more than one trophic level simultaneously

92. Select the wrong statement
(a) Human insulin is being commercially produced from a transgenic species of Escherichia coli
(b) Bt toxin genes Cry 1 Ac control the corn borer
(c) Human protein, alpha-1 -antitrypsin is used to treat emphysema
(d) The first transgenic cow, Rosie, produced alpha lactalbumin, enriched milk

93. Consider the following statements with respect to angiosperms
(A) The male sex organ in a flower is the stamen
(B) The anthers following mitosis produce pollen grains
(C) In an embryosac, the primary endosperm nucleus (PEN) is diploid
(D) After double fertilization the ovules develop into seeds and ovaries develop into fruit.

Of the above statements
(a) (C) and (D) are correct
(b) (A) and (B) are correct
(c) (A) and (C) are correct
(d) (A) and (D) are correct

94. Which of the following secondary metabolites belong to the group drugs?
I. Morphine II. Curcumin III. Codeine IV. Vinblastine V. Abrin
(a) I and II only (b) I and V only
(c) II and III only (d) II and IV only

95. FAD is electron acceptor in the citric acid cycle during the oxidation of
(a) Malic acid to oxaloacetic acid
(b) Succinic acid to malic acid
(c) Citric acid to alpha-ketoglutaric acid
(d) Alpha-ketoglutaric acid to succinic acid

96. Match the Column I with that of Column II and choose the correct combination from the options given

	Column I - Essential elements		Column II - Deficiency causes
A.	N, K, Mg, S, Fe, Mn, Zn, and Mo	I.	Inhibit cell division
B.	N, K, S and Mo	II.	Necrosis
C.	Ca, Mg, Cu and K	III.	Delay in flowering
D.	N, S and Mo	IV.	Chlorosis

(a) A–IV ; B–III ; C–II; D–I
(b) A–I ; B–II ; C–III; D–IV
(c) A–IV ; B–I ; C–II; D–III
(d) A–II ; B–III ; C–IV; D–I

97. DNA replicates semi-conservatively was first shown in
(a) *Vicia faba*
(b) *E. coli*
(c) *Streptococcus pneumoniae*
(d) *Drosophila*

98. The precursor of eukaryotic mRNA is
(a) hnRNA (b) tRNA
(c) rRNA (d) snRNA

99. The entry of food into the larynx is prevented by
(a) Mitral valve (b) Diaphragm
(c) Epiglottis (d) Hyoid

100. Covered smut of barley is caused by
(a) *Ustilago hordei*
(b) *Tilletia caries*
(c) *Ustilago nuda*
(d) *Colletotrichum falcatum*

101. Which of the following is not matched correctly?
(a) *Anabaena* - Cyanobacteria
(b) *Amoeba* - Protozoa
(c) *Gonyaulax* - Dinoflagellates
(d) *Albugo* - Chrysophytes

102. In gymnosperms, the pollen chamber represents
(a) a cell in the pollen grain in which the sperms are formed
(b) a cavity in the ovule in which pollen grains are stored after pollination
(c) an opening in the mega gametophyte through which the pollen tube approaches the egg
(d) the microsporangium in which pollen grains develop

103. Iodine is obtained from
(a) *Laminaria* (b) *Chlorella*
(c) *Polysiphonia* (d) *Porphyra*

104. Secondary body cavity with segmented mesodermal lining is called
(a) haemocoel (b) neurocoel
(c) true coelom (d) pseudocoelom

105. Pneumatic bones are expected to be found in
(a) house lizard (b) flying fish
(c) pigeon (d) tadpole of frog

106. Mark the correct statement for monosaccharides.
(a) Monosaccharides with 5 carbon atoms are smallest carbohydrates
(b) Pentose sugar ribose is rarely found in animal cells
(c) All hexoses are aldoses except fructose
(d) The most important sugar occurring in animals is cellulose

107. Fill in the blanks and select the correct option w.r.t. Meiosis.
I. The beginning of _A_ is recognized by the _B_ of the synaptonemal complex.
II. Crossing over between homologous chromosomes is completed by the end of _C_ .
III. _D_ begins with simultaneous splitting of the centromere of each chromosome.
(a) A-Diplotene B-Formation C-Pachytene D-Anaphase-I
(b) A-Diplotene B-Dissolution C-Pachytene D-Anaphase-II
(c) A-Diplotene B-Dissolution C-Diakinesis D-Anaphase-I
(d) A-Pachytene B-Dissolution C-Diplotene D-Diakinesis

108. Match the following w.r.t. shape of chromosome at anaphase of mitosis

	Column - I		Column - II
A.	Acrocentric	I.	I-shaped
B.	Sub-metacentric	II.	J-shaped
C.	Telocentric	III.	V-shaped
D.	Metacentric	IV.	L-shaped

(a) A–II ; B–I ; C–III; D–IV
(b) A–I ; B–II ; C–III; D–IV
(c) A–II ; B–III ; C–IV; D–I
(d) A–II ; B–IV ; C–I; D–III

109. Fill in the blanks and choose the correct option.
(i) According to most accepted model of ascent of sap, water column is _(A)_ in xylem.
(ii) Loss of water in liquid phase from leaf tips is known as _(B)_ .
(iii) Water is absorbed along with mineral solutes by the _(C)_ purely by diffusion.
(a) (A) Pulled, (B) Guttation, (C) Root hair
(b) (B) Transpiration, (C) Root nodules, (A) Root hair
(c) (A) Pushed, (B) Transpiration, (C) Pulled
(d) (B) Guttation, (C) Root cap, (A) pushed

110. Cyanide blocks respiratory pathway between
(a) Complex III and IV
(b) Complex II and III
(c) Complex I and II
(d) Complex IV and O_2

111. Find the incorrect match w.r.t. protein synthesis.
(a) m RNA – Codons
(b) r RNA – Catalytic role during translation
(c) UTR – Only at 3' end
(d) t RNA – Transfers amino acids

112. Interferons are glycoproteins which are ______ and are considered to be a part of ______
(a) Anti-fungal, second line of defence
(b) Anti-viral, physiological barriers
(c) Anti-viral, non specific immunity
(d) Anti-viral, specific immunity

113. In plant breeding programme, which of the following process is crucial to the success of the breeding objective and requires careful scientific evaluation of the progeny?
(a) Cross hybridisation
(b) Testing release and commercialisation of new cultivars
(c) Collection of plants
(d) Selection and testing of superior recombinants

114. Ganga Action Plan was initiated by
(a) Ministry of Environment and Forests
(b) South Asia Co-operative Environment Programme
(c) United Nations Environment Programme
(d) Environmental Protection Agency (EPA)

115. Consider the following four statements (A–D) related to organic farming and select the correct option stating true (T) and false (F). The statements are
A. Uses chemical fertilizers containing organic compounds only
B. Produces food crops rich in organic compounds but poor in minerals
C. No need to use chemical fertilizers and pesticides
D. Use biofertilizers that enrich the nutrient quality in the soil.

	A	B	C	D
(a)	F	F	F	T
(b)	T	F	T	F
(c)	F	F	T	T
(d)	F	T	T	T

116. The mode of nutrition present in *Euglena* is referred to as
(a) Osmotrophy (b) Mixotrophy
(c) Phototrophy (d) Chemotrophy

Space for Rough Work

117. Which one of the following feature/event in pteridophytes is a precursor to the seed habit that considered an important step in evolution?
(a) Steler system
(b) Oogamous reproduction
(c) Development of cone
(d) Heterospory

118. Key evolutionary advances of the flatworms are bilateral symmetry and
(a) a one-way digestive tract
(b) a body cavity
(c) Internal organs
(d) Intracellular digestion

119. Type of venation in cucumber and banana is respectively
(a) reticulate and furcate
(b) reticulate and parallel
(c) parallel and reticulate
(d) furcate and parallel

120. A. The vascular bundles are absent in veins
B. The veins vary in thickness in the reticulate venation of the dicot leaves
C. Spongy parenchyma is located on adaxial surface of monocot leaf
Which of the above statement(s) is/are correct?
(a) A & C are correct
(b) B & C are incorrect
(c) Only C is incorrect
(d) Only B is correct

121. Choose the wrong statement regarding urine formation
(a) Filtration is non-selective process performed by glomerulus
(b) The glomerular capillary blood pressure causes filtration of blood through three layers
(c) GFR in a healthy individual is approximately 125ml/min
(d) The ascending limb of the Henle's loop is permeable to water but allows transport of electrolytes actively or passively

122. The skeletal muscle fibre is a 'syncytium', which means it is
(a) multinucleated
(b) made up of many proteins
(c) long and slender
(d) swollen in the middle with tapered ends

123. The projecting ridge in ampulla of semi-circular canals in ear is called
(a) Succus entericus (b) Maccula
(c) Otolith (d) Crista ampullaris

124. Function of the somatostatin is to
(a) stimulate pituitary synthesis and release gonadotropins
(b) inhibit the release of gonadotropins from pituitary
(c) stimulate pituitary and promotes the secretion of growth hormone
(d) inhibit the release of growth hormone from the pituitary

125. Which of the following statements regarding cyclic flow of electrons during light reactions is **false**?
(a) This process takes place in the stromal lamella
(b) ATP synthesis takes place
(c) NADPH + H^+ is synthesized
(d) Takes place only when light of wavelength beyond 680 nm is available for excitation

126. The term 'keel' is used for special type of
(a) sepals (b) petals
(c) stamens (d) carpels

127. In dicotyledonous roots, the initiation of lateral roots takes place in
(a) endodermal cells (b) cortical cells
(c) epidermal cells (d) pericycle cells.

128. Read the following statements and choose the correct option.
A. Blood cells secrete fibres of structural proteins called collagen or elastin.
B. Neuroglial cells protect and support the nephrons.
C. Osteocytes are present in spaces called lacunae.
D. Striated muscle fibres are bundled together in a parallel fashion.
E. Biceps are involuntary and striated.
(a) C and D alone are wrong
(b) B and D alone are wrong
(c) A and C alone are wrong
(d) A, B and E alone are wrong

129. Select the matched ones.
(a) Amyloplasts - store proteins
(b) Mitochondrion - 'powerhouse' of the cell
(c) Stroma - chlorophyll pigment
(d) Axoneme - 9 + 2 array
(a) (a) and (c) only (b) (b), (c) and (d) only
(c) (c) and (d) only (d) (b) and (d) only

130. Match the protein with its function and choose the right option.

Protein	Function
(A) Collagen	(i) Glucose transport
(B) Trypsin	(ii) Hormone
(C) Insulin	(iii) Intercellular ground substance
(D) GLUT-4	(iv) Enzyme

(a) A-(iii), B-(iv), C-(ii), D-(i)
(b) A-(iv), B- (i), C-(ii), D-(iii)
(c) A-(ii), B-(iv), C-(i), D-(iii)
(d) A-(iii), B-(iv), C-(i), D-(ii)

131. Select the matched ones.
(i) Guttation - water loss in its liquid phase
(ii) Adhesion - mutual attraction between water molecules
(iii) Imbibition - absorption of water by dry wood
(iv) Hypotonic solution - cells shrink
(a) (i), (ii) and (iii) only
(b) (ii) and (iv) only
(c) (i) and (iii) only
(d) (ii), (iii) and (iv) only

132. Find out the correct option w.r.t. the human dentition.
(a) Ameloblasts – Secrete the major portion of tooth, i.e., enamel
(b) Odontoblast – ectodermal in origin
(c) Enamel – soft living tissue of the body
(d) Crown – Forms the hard chewing surface of the teeth, helps in mastication of food

133. The ejection of stomach contents through the mouth is controlled by neural centres present in
(a) Cerebrum (b) Cerebellum
(c) Pons (d) Medulla

134. Progressive degeneration of skeletal muscle is mostly due to genetic disorder of
(a) Tetany (b) Gouty arthritis
(c) Myasthenia gravis (d) Muscular dystrophy

135. Which of the pair is not a correct match?
(a) Iris – Accommodation
(b) Retina – Screen to form image
(c) Scotopic vision – Rods
(d) Ciliary body – Form aqueous humour

136. Cortisol is
A. Anti-inflammatory hormone
B. Stress hormone
C. Immunosuppressive hormone
D. Hyperglycaemic hormone
(a) Only A, B and C are correct
(b) A, B, C and D are correct
(c) Only A is correct
(d) Only A and B are correct

137. During biofortification, breeding for improved nutritional quality is undertaken with objective of improving all, except
(a) Micronutrient content
(b) Protein quality
(c) Vitamin quality
(d) Oil quality

138. Technique used to transfer ssDNA from gel to nitrocellulose membrane is called as
(a) Northern blotting
(b) Western blotting
(c) Southern blotting
(d) Gel electrophoresis

139. Micro-injection is a method used to
(a) produce sticky ends of DNA
(b) provide protection against pathogen
(c) purify the DNA
(d) inject recombinant DNA into the nucleus of an animal cell

140. The sticky ends of a fragmented DNA molecule are made of
(a) calcium salts (b) endonuclease enzyme
(c) unpaired bases (d) methyl groups

141. Which of the following is required to perform polymerase chain reaction?
(a) Primers, dNTPs and DNA polymerase
(b) DNA, $CaCl_2$ and nuclease
(c) Mg^{+2}, DNA
(d) Both (a) and (c)

142. Choose odd w.r.t. collenchyma.
(a) Found in hypodermis of dicot stem
(b) Living mechanical tissue
(c) Absent in monocots
(d) Thickening of wall is due to deposition of cellulose and lignin

143. How many given below meristems are examples of lateral meristems?
Cylindrical meristems, Apical meristem, Fasciular meristem, Axillary meristem, Interfascicular cambium, Intercalary meristem and Cork cambium.
(a) Three (b) Four
(c) Five (d) Six

144. One hormone hastens the maturity period in juvenile conifers, a second hormone controls xylem differentiation while the third increases the tolerance of plants to various stresses and they are respectively
(a) Auxin, Gibberellin and Cytokinin
(b) Gibberellin, Auxin and Cytokinin
(c) Gibberellin, Auxin and Ethylene
(d) Gibberellin, Auxin and ABA

145. The ozone hole over Antarctica develops each year between
(a) Late December and early February
(b) Late February and early April
(c) Late April and early June
(d) Late August and early October

146. Match Column I with Column II and select the correct option

	Column I		Column II
A.	Ascomycetes	I.	*Ustilago*
B.	Phycomycetes	II.	*Saccharomyces*
C.	Basidiomycetes	III.	*Trichoderma*
D.	Deuteromycetes	IV.	*Albugo*

(a) A–II ; B–I ; C–IV; D–III
(b) A–IV ; B–III ; C–II; D–I
(c) A–II ; B–IV ; C–I; D–III
(d) A–III ; B–IV ; C–I; D–II

147. Which of the following are heterosporous pteridophytes?
I. *Lycopodium* II. *Selaginella*
III. *Equisetum* IV. *Salvinia*
(a) I and II only (b) II and III only
(c) II and IV only (d) II and IV only

148. If an inheritable mutation is observed in a population at high frequency, it is referred as
(a) DNA polymorphism
(b) Expressed sequence tag
(c) Sequence annotation
(d) Linkage

Space for Rough Work

149. To generate pressure gradients to facilitate expiration and inspiration, the human body uses the intercostal muscles and
(a) alveolar sacs
(b) bronchi
(c) primary, secondary and tertiary bronchioles
(d) diaphragm

150. Identify the correct statement regarding cardiac activity
(a) Normal activities of the human heart is regulated intrinsically hence it is neurogenic
(b) A special neural centre in the medulla oblongata can moderate the cardiac function through the CNS
(c) Parasympathetic neural signals increase the rate of heart beat
(d) Adrenal medullary hormones can increase cardiac output

151. Find the **wrongly** matched pair
(a) Endemism - species confined to one region and not found anywhere else
(b) *In situ* conservation - IVFD
(c) Alien species to India - *Clarias gariepinus*
(d) Lungs of the planet - Amazon Rain Forest

152. Match Column I with Column II and choose the correct option.

	Column I		Column II
A.	breeding crops with higher levels of nutrients	I.	Totipotency
B.	plant grown from hybrid protoplast	II.	Micropropagation
C.	producing a large number of plants through tissue culture	III.	Somaclone
D.	capacity to generate a whole plant from an explant	IV.	Somatic hybrid
E.	Plants genetically identical to the original plant	V.	Biofortification

(a) A – V; B – IV; C – II; D – I; E–III
(b) A – I; B – III; C – V; D – IV; E–II
(c) A – V; B – II; C – I; D – IV; E–III
(d) A – III; B – I; C – V; D – IV; E–II

153. Match Column I with Column II and choose the correct answer.

	Column I		Column II
A.	Sponges	I.	Incomplete digestive system
B.	Coelenterates	II.	Cellular level of organization
C.	Annelids	III.	Radial symmetry
D.	Platyhelminthes	IV.	Pseudocoelomate
E.	Aschelminthes	V.	Metamerism

(a) A – III; B – IV; C – I; D – II; E–V
(b) A – V; B – III; C – IV; D – I; E–II
(c) A – II; B – III; C – V; D – I; E–IV
(d) A – I; B – II; C – III; D – IV; E–V

154. Choose the **wrong** statement
(a) In grasshopper, besides autosomes males have only one X-chromosome, whereas females have a pair of X-chromosomes
(b) In XY type of sex determination, both males and females have same number of chromosomes
(c) In *Drosophila*, males have one X and one Y chromosome, whereas females have a pair of X-chromosome besides autosomes
(d) In birds, females have one Z and one W chromosomes, whereas males have a pair of Z chromosomes besides autosomes

155. Secretion of pancreatic juice is stimulated by
(a) gastrin (b) secretin
(c) enterogasteron (d) enterokinase

156. Choose the correct statement
(a) Non myelinated nerve fibres are found in spinal and cranial nerves.
(b) Retina has multipolar neurons.
(c) Electrical synapses are commonly present in humans.
(d) Impulse transmission across an electrical synapse is faster than across a chemical synapse.

157. Which of the following hormones have antagonistic (opposing) effects?
(a) Thyroxine and calcitonin
(b) Insulin and glucagon
(c) Growth hormone and epinephrine
(d) ACTH and glucocorticoids

158. Number of chromosomes in an angiospermic plant is 14, then the number of chromosomes in synergid cells will be
(a) 14 (b) 7
(c) 28 (d) 21

159. Match the items in column I with those in column II and chose the correct answer.

	Column I		Column II
A.	Small opening of ovule	I.	Funicle
B.	Stalk of ovule	II.	Integuments
C.	Protective envelopes of ovule	III.	Chalaza
D.	Junction part of ovule and stalk	IV	Hilum
E.	Basal part of the ovule	V.	Micropyle

(a) A – V; B – I; C – II; D – IV; E–III
(b) A – I; B – III; C – II; D – IV; E–V
(c) A – III; B – I; C – II; D – IV; E–V
(d) A – IV; B – I; C – V; D – II; E–III

Space for Rough Work

160. During embryonic development endoskeleton and muscle develop from which germinal layer?
(a) Ectoderm (b) Endoderm
(c) Mesoderm (d) Blastopore

161. Match list I with list II and choose the correct answer

	List I		List II
A.	Hypothalamus	I.	Sperm lysins
B.	Acrosome	II.	Estrogen
C.	Graafian follicle	III.	Relaxin
D.	Leydig cells	IV.	GnRH
E.	Parturition	V.	Testosterone

(a) A – IV, B – I, C – II, D – III, E – V
(b) A – II, B – I, C – IV, D – III, E – V
(c) A – II, B – I, C – V, D – IV, E – III
(d) A – IV, B – I, C – II, D – V, E – III

162. Which of the following statements is incorrect?
(a) Osmoconformers are able to maintain osmotic concentration of their cells by either physiological or behavioural means.
(b) Most vertebrates, except the birds and mammals are unable to thermoregulate.
(c) Success of mammals is mainly due to their ability to thermoregulate and live comfortably whether they are in Antarctica or in Sahara desert.
(d) None of these

163. Archaebacteria that flourish in temperature above 100°C have special ______ molecules that do not coagulate at high temperatures and remain functional.
(a) carbohydrate (b) ester
(c) protein (d) fat

164. The age structure of a population influences population growth because
(a) younger females have more offsprings than do older females
(b) different age groups have different reproductive capabilities
(c) more is the number of immature individuals, slower is the growth of population
(d) a shorter generation time results in slower population growth

165. The following figure given below is a diagrammatic representation of organismic response to abiotic factors. What do (a), (b) and (c) represent respectively?

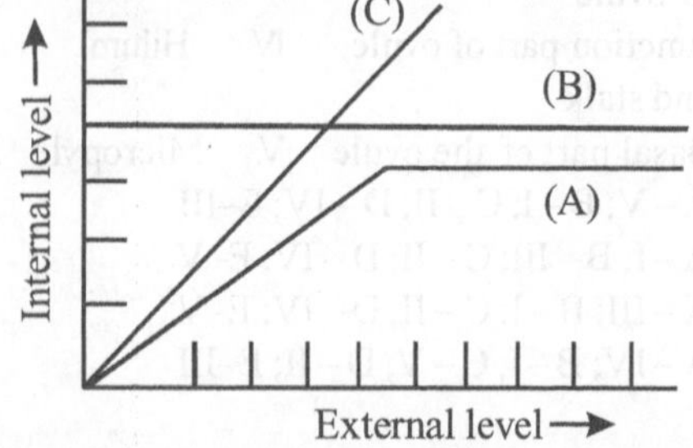

(a) (A) Conformers (B) Regulators (C) Partial regulators
(b) (A) Regulators (B) Partial regulators (C) Conformers
(c) (A) Partial regulators (B) Regulators (C) Conformers
(d) (A) Partial regulators (B) Conformers (C) Regulators

166. The hormone releasing IUD is
(a) LNG20
(b) Lippes loop
(c) CuT
(d) Multiload 375

167. Read the statements regarding a stable community and choose the correct option
(a) must be resistant to occasional disturbances
(b) should show much variation in productivity from year to year
(c) must be resistant to invasions by alien species
(a) (a) and (b) are correct
(b) (a), (b) and (c) are correct
(c) (a) only is correct
(d) (a) and (c) are correct

168. The cytokine barrier among these is
(a) Polymorphonuclear neutrophil
(b) Monocyte
(c) NK cell
(d) Interferon

169. Read the statements regarding echinoderms and choose the correct option
(a) All are marine with organ system level of organisation
(b) Adults are bilaterally symmetrical
(c) They are dioecious
(d) Fertilisation is internal and indirect development is observed
(e) Triploblastic and acoelomate animals
(a) (a) and (c) are correct
(b) (e) alone is correct
(c) (a), (c) and (e) are correct
(d) (a) and (e) are correct

170. The number of cells in mature female and male gametophyte in angiosperms is ______ and ______ respectively.
(a) 8, 1 (b) 7, 4
(c) 7, 3 (d) 8, 2

171. Arrange the following terms in the correct developmental sequence in flowering plants.

A.	Sperms	B.	Heart-shaped embryo
C.	Syngamy	D.	Microspore mother cell
E.	Sporic meiosis	F.	Globular embryo

(a) E, D, A, C, F, B (b) D, E, A, C, F, B
(c) D, E, A, C, B, F (d) E, D, A, C, B, F

172. The most common mode of entry of pollen tube into ovule is
(a) Chalazogamy (b) Xenogamy
(c) Porogamy (d) Basigamy

Space for Rough Work

173. Which of the following is wrongly matched?
(a) AIH – Semen collected from donor is artificially introduced into vagina or uterus of female.
(b) IVF – Fertilisation takes place outside female's body in a dish in a laboratory.
(c) ZIFT – Embryo upto 8 blastomeres is transferred into fallopian tube
(d) GIFT – Ovum collected from donor is transferred into another female

174. During parturition
(a) There is increase in estrogen to progesterone ratio
(b) Prostaglandin level falls
(c) Relaxin promotes contraction of uterine muscles
(d) Cervical mucus plug strengthens by progesterone activity

175. Match the columns and select correct option.

	Column - I		Column - II
A.	Down's syndrome	I.	Holandric trait
B.	Porcupine skin	II.	Autosomal recessive
C.	Alkaptonuria	III.	X-linked trait
D.	Haemophilia	IV.	Trisomy

(a) A – IV; B – I; C – II; D – III
(b) A – III; B – IV; C – II; D – I
(c) A – III; B – II; C – IV; D – I
(d) A – I; B – II; C – III; D – IV

176. Choose the odd option w.r.t. sickle cell anaemia.
(a) It is a result of transversion
(b) Heterozygous (Hb^A Hb^S) are carrier of the disease
(c) It is due to point mutation
(d) GTG in the coding strand is replaced by GAG

177. Normal visioned male marries a carrier female for colour blindness then
(a) All sons will be colour blind, daughters will be normal.
(b) 50% daughters are colour blind carriers.
(c) Both the sons and daughters will be colour blind.
(d) A male offspring has 50% chance of active disease.

178. Unwinding of DNA creates tension which is released by enzyme
(a) Pyrophosphatase (b) Primase
(c) Helicase (d) Topoisomerase

179. Consider the following statements regarding transformation experiment
A. DNAase inhibits transformation
B. It proved that DNA is the genetic material in virus
C. Avery, MacLeod and MacCarty used protease, RNAase and DNAse enzymes
D. It was performed on Streptococcus pneumoniae by F. Griffith
(a) B & D (b) Only A
(c) A, C & D (d) A, B & C

180. Match the columns and choose the correct combination

	Column - I		Column - II
A.	Non sense codon	I.	UUU
B.	Ambiguous codon	II.	UGG
C.	Codon for tryptophan	III.	GUG
D.	Phenylalanine codon	IV.	UAG

(a) A – II; B – III; C – IV; D – I
(b) A – II; B – III; C – I; D – IV
(c) A – IV; B – III; C – II; D – I
(d) A – IV; B – III; C – I; D – II

FULL SYLLABUS SPEED TEST-100			
Total Questions	180	Total Marks	720
Attempted		Correct	
Incorrect		Net Score	
Cut-off Score	135	Qualifying Score	100
Success Gap = Net Score – Qualifying Score			
Net Score = (Correct × 4) – (Incorrect × 1)			

Space for Rough Work

Response Grid

PHYSICS

1. (a)(b)(c)(d) 2. (a)(b)(c)(d) 3. (a)(b)(c)(d) 4. (a)(b)(c)(d) 5. (a)(b)(c)(d)
6. (a)(b)(c)(d) 7. (a)(b)(c)(d) 8. (a)(b)(c)(d) 9. (a)(b)(c)(d) 10. (a)(b)(c)(d)
11. (a)(b)(c)(d) 12. (a)(b)(c)(d) 13. (a)(b)(c)(d) 14. (a)(b)(c)(d) 15. (a)(b)(c)(d)
16. (a)(b)(c)(d) 17. (a)(b)(c)(d) 18. (a)(b)(c)(d) 19. (a)(b)(c)(d) 20. (a)(b)(c)(d)
21. (a)(b)(c)(d) 22. (a)(b)(c)(d) 23. (a)(b)(c)(d) 24. (a)(b)(c)(d) 25. (a)(b)(c)(d)
26. (a)(b)(c)(d) 27. (a)(b)(c)(d) 28. (a)(b)(c)(d) 29. (a)(b)(c)(d) 30. (a)(b)(c)(d)
31. (a)(b)(c)(d) 32. (a)(b)(c)(d) 33. (a)(b)(c)(d) 34. (a)(b)(c)(d) 35. (a)(b)(c)(d)
36. (a)(b)(c)(d) 37. (a)(b)(c)(d) 38. (a)(b)(c)(d) 39. (a)(b)(c)(d) 40. (a)(b)(c)(d)
41. (a)(b)(c)(d) 42. (a)(b)(c)(d) 43. (a)(b)(c)(d) 44. (a)(b)(c)(d) 45. (a)(b)(c)(d)

CHEMISTRY

46. (a)(b)(c)(d) 47. (a)(b)(c)(d) 48. (a)(b)(c)(d) 49. (a)(b)(c)(d) 50. (a)(b)(c)(d)
51. (a)(b)(c)(d) 52. (a)(b)(c)(d) 53. (a)(b)(c)(d) 54. (a)(b)(c)(d) 55. (a)(b)(c)(d)
56. (a)(b)(c)(d) 57. (a)(b)(c)(d) 58. (a)(b)(c)(d) 59. (a)(b)(c)(d) 60. (a)(b)(c)(d)
61. (a)(b)(c)(d) 62. (a)(b)(c)(d) 63. (a)(b)(c)(d) 64. (a)(b)(c)(d) 65. (a)(b)(c)(d)
66. (a)(b)(c)(d) 67. (a)(b)(c)(d) 68. (a)(b)(c)(d) 69. (a)(b)(c)(d) 70. (a)(b)(c)(d)
71. (a)(b)(c)(d) 72. (a)(b)(c)(d) 73. (a)(b)(c)(d) 74. (a)(b)(c)(d) 75. (a)(b)(c)(d)
76. (a)(b)(c)(d) 77. (a)(b)(c)(d) 78. (a)(b)(c)(d) 79. (a)(b)(c)(d) 80. (a)(b)(c)(d)
81. (a)(b)(c)(d) 82. (a)(b)(c)(d) 83. (a)(b)(c)(d) 84. (a)(b)(c)(d) 85. (a)(b)(c)(d)
86. (a)(b)(c)(d) 87. (a)(b)(c)(d) 88. (a)(b)(c)(d) 89. (a)(b)(c)(d) 90. (a)(b)(c)(d)

BIOLOGY

91. (a)(b)(c)(d) 92. (a)(b)(c)(d) 93. (a)(b)(c)(d) 94. (a)(b)(c)(d) 95. (a)(b)(c)(d)
96. (a)(b)(c)(d) 97. (a)(b)(c)(d) 98. (a)(b)(c)(d) 99. (a)(b)(c)(d) 100. (a)(b)(c)(d)
101. (a)(b)(c)(d) 102. (a)(b)(c)(d) 103. (a)(b)(c)(d) 104. (a)(b)(c)(d) 105. (a)(b)(c)(d)
106. (a)(b)(c)(d) 107. (a)(b)(c)(d) 108. (a)(b)(c)(d) 109. (a)(b)(c)(d) 110. (a)(b)(c)(d)
111. (a)(b)(c)(d) 112. (a)(b)(c)(d) 113. (a)(b)(c)(d) 114. (a)(b)(c)(d) 115. (a)(b)(c)(d)
116. (a)(b)(c)(d) 117. (a)(b)(c)(d) 118. (a)(b)(c)(d) 119. (a)(b)(c)(d) 120. (a)(b)(c)(d)
121. (a)(b)(c)(d) 122. (a)(b)(c)(d) 123. (a)(b)(c)(d) 124. (a)(b)(c)(d) 125. (a)(b)(c)(d)
126. (a)(b)(c)(d) 127. (a)(b)(c)(d) 128. (a)(b)(c)(d) 129. (a)(b)(c)(d) 130. (a)(b)(c)(d)
131. (a)(b)(c)(d) 132. (a)(b)(c)(d) 133. (a)(b)(c)(d) 134. (a)(b)(c)(d) 135. (a)(b)(c)(d)
136. (a)(b)(c)(d) 137. (a)(b)(c)(d) 138. (a)(b)(c)(d) 139. (a)(b)(c)(d) 140. (a)(b)(c)(d)
141. (a)(b)(c)(d) 142. (a)(b)(c)(d) 143. (a)(b)(c)(d) 144. (a)(b)(c)(d) 145. (a)(b)(c)(d)
146. (a)(b)(c)(d) 147. (a)(b)(c)(d) 148. (a)(b)(c)(d) 149. (a)(b)(c)(d) 150. (a)(b)(c)(d)
151. (a)(b)(c)(d) 152. (a)(b)(c)(d) 153. (a)(b)(c)(d) 154. (a)(b)(c)(d) 155. (a)(b)(c)(d)
156. (a)(b)(c)(d) 157. (a)(b)(c)(d) 158. (a)(b)(c)(d) 159. (a)(b)(c)(d) 160. (a)(b)(c)(d)
161. (a)(b)(c)(d) 162. (a)(b)(c)(d) 163. (a)(b)(c)(d) 164. (a)(b)(c)(d) 165. (a)(b)(c)(d)
166. (a)(b)(c)(d) 167. (a)(b)(c)(d) 168. (a)(b)(c)(d) 169. (a)(b)(c)(d) 170. (a)(b)(c)(d)
171. (a)(b)(c)(d) 172. (a)(b)(c)(d) 173. (a)(b)(c)(d) 174. (a)(b)(c)(d) 175. (a)(b)(c)(d)
176. (a)(b)(c)(d) 177. (a)(b)(c)(d) 178. (a)(b)(c)(d) 179. (a)(b)(c)(d) 180. (a)(b)(c)(d)

Full Test-2

Speed TEST 101

Full Syllabus

No. of Questions	Maximum Marks	Time
180	720	3 Hours

GENERAL INSTRUCTIONS

- This test contents 180 MCQ's :
  - **Physics (180 marks)** : Question No. 1 to 45 are of **4 marks** each.
  - **Chemistry (180 marks)** : Question No. 46 to 90 are of **4 marks** each.
  - **Biology (360 marks)** : Question No. 91 to 180 are of **4 marks** each.
- Darken the correct circle/ bubble in the Response Grid provided at the end of this test.
- You have to evaluate your Response Grids yourself with the help of solutions provided at the end of this book.
- Each correct answer will get you 4 marks and 1 mark shall be deduced for each incorrect answer. No mark will be given/ deducted if no bubble is filled. Keep a timer in front of you and stop immediately at the end of 3 hours.
- After completing the sheet check your answers with the solution booklet and complete the Result Grid. Finally spend time to analyse your performance and revise the areas which emerge out as weak in your evaluation.

PHYSICS

DIRECTIONS : There are 45 multiple choice questions numbered 1 to 45. Each question has 4 choices (a), (b), (c) and (d), out of which ONLY ONE is correct.

1. Two concentric shells having radii R and $2R$, charges q_1 and q_2 and potentials 3 V and V respectively. Now outer shell is earthed, then

(a) Potential difference between shell increases

(b) Potential difference between shell decreases

(c) Potential of inner shell will become 2 V

(d) Potential of common centre will become 2.5 V

2. A thermodynamic process is shown in the figure. In the process AB 500 J of heat are added and in process BD, 150 J of heat are added. The change in the internal energy in the process ABD is :

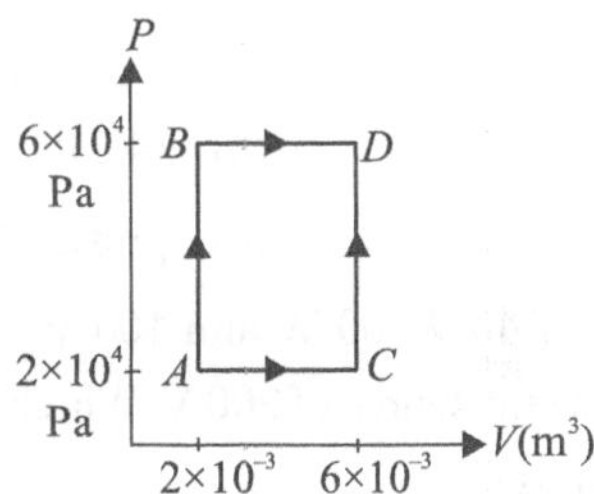

(a) 890 J (b) 410 J (c) 650 J (d) 240 J

3. The density of a material in CGS system is $4 g/cm^3$. In a system of units in which unit of length is 10 cm and unit of mass is 100 g, the value of density of material will be

(a) 0.4 (b) 40 (c) 400 (d) 0.04

4. At what altitude will the value of the acceleration due to gravity be half of its value at the surface of the earth? (R = radius of earth)

(a) $\frac{R}{2}$ (b) $\frac{R}{\sqrt{2}}$

(c) $(\sqrt{2}+1)R$ (d) $(\sqrt{2}-1)R$

Space for Rough Work

5. Water falls from a height of 60 m at the rate of 15 kg/s to operate a turbine. The losses due to frictional force are 10% of energy. How much power is generated by the turbine?($g = 10\ m/s^2$)

(a) 8.1 kW (b) 10.2 kW (c) 12.3 kW (d) 7.0 kW

6. A circular disc with a groove along its diameter is placed horizontally. A block of mass 1 kg is placed as shown. The coefficient of friction between the block and all the surfaces of groove in contact is $\mu = 2/5$. The disc has an acceleration of 25 m/s². The acceleration of the block with respect to disc is $\left(\cos\theta = \frac{4}{5}\right), \left(\sin\theta = \frac{3}{5}\right)$

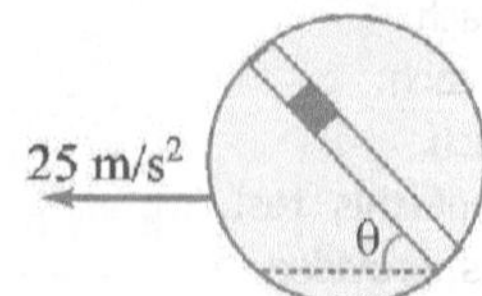

(a) $10\ m/s^2$ (b) $8\ m/s^2$ (c) $5\ m/s^2$ (d) zero

7. In a photo-emissive cell, with exciting wavelength λ, the fastest electron has speed v. If the exciting wavelength is changed to $\frac{3\lambda}{4}$, the speed of the fastest emitted electron will be

(a) $(3/4)^{1/2}.v$ (b) $(4/3)^{1/2}.v$

(c) less than $(4/3)^{1/2}.v$ (d) greater than $(4/3)^{1/2}.v$

8. Three bulbs of 40 W, 60 W and 100 W are connected in series to a current source of 200 V. Which of the following statements is true ?

(a) 40 W bulb glows brightest

(b) 60 W bulb glows brightest

(c) 100 W bulb glows brightest

(d) All bulbs glow with same brightness

9. If the moment of inertia of a disc about an axis tangential and parallel to its surface be I, then what will be the moment of inertia about the axis tangential but perpendicular to the surface?

(a) $\frac{6}{5}I$ (b) $\frac{3}{4}I$ (c) $\frac{3}{2}I$ (d) $\frac{5}{4}I$

10. A cyclic process $ABCD$ is shown in the P-V diagram. Which of the following curves represent the same process?

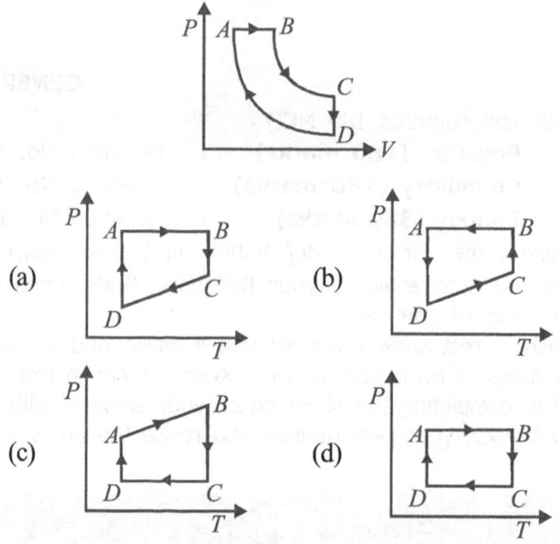

11. An uncharged metal ball is placed in the uniform electric field of a plane capacitor. Which of following correctly represents the field lines on the ball ?

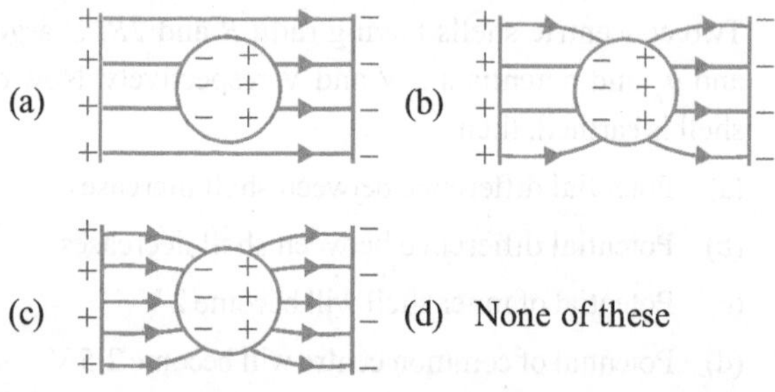

(d) None of these

12. A 12.5 eV electron beam is used to bombard gaseous hydrogen at room temperature. It will emit :
(a) 2 lines in the Lyman series and 1 line in the Balmar series
(b) 3 lines in the Lyman series
(c) 1 line in the Lyman series and 2 lines in the Balmar series
(d) 3 lines in the Balmer series

13. A boat takes two hous to travel 8 km and back in still water. If the velocity of water is 4 km/h, the time taken for going upstream 8 km and coming back is
(a) 2 hr (b) 2hr 40 min
(c) 1hr 20 min (d) 2 hr 30 min

14. If an ideal junction diode is connected as shown, then the value of the current I is
(a) 0.013 A
(b) 0.02 A
(c) 0.01 A
(d) 0.1 A

+3 V 200 Ω +1 V

15. If the time period t of a drop of liquid of density d, radius r, vibrating under surface tension s is given by the formula $t = \sqrt{d^a r^b s^c}$ and if a = 1, c = –1, then b is
(a) 1 (b) 2 (c) 3 (d) 4

16. A simple pendulum attached to the ceiling of a stationary lift has a time period T. The distance y covered by the lift moving upwards varies with time t as $y = t^2$ where y is in metres and t in seconds. If $g = 10\ m/s^2$, the time period of pendulum will be
(a) $\sqrt{\frac{4}{5}}T$ (b) $\sqrt{\frac{5}{6}}T$ (c) $\sqrt{\frac{5}{4}}T$ (d) $\sqrt{\frac{6}{5}}T$

17. A paper, with two marks having separation d, is held normal to the line of sight of an observer at a distance of 50m. The diameter of the eye-lens of the observer is 2 mm. Which of the following is the least value of d, so that the marks can be seen as separate ? (The mean wavelength of visible light may be taken as 5000 Å)
(a) 1.25m (b) 12.5 cm (c) 1.25 cm (d) 2.5mm

18. In the network shown, each resistance is equal to R. The equivalent resistance between A and D is
(a) R
(b) $\frac{2}{3}R$
(c) $\frac{3}{7}R$
(d) $\frac{8}{15}R$

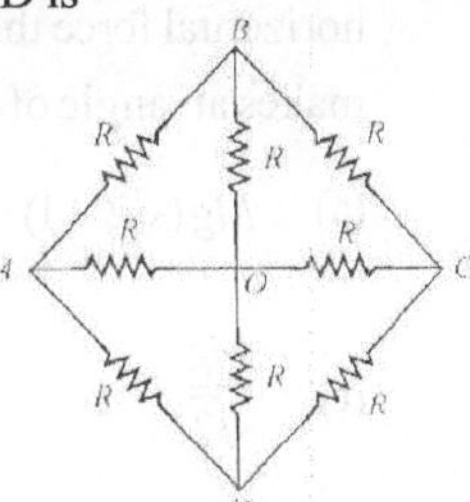

19. A charged particle *q* is placed at the centre *O* of a cube of length *L* (*ABCDEFGH*). Another same charge *q* is placed at a distance *L* from *O*. Then the electric flux through *ABCD* is

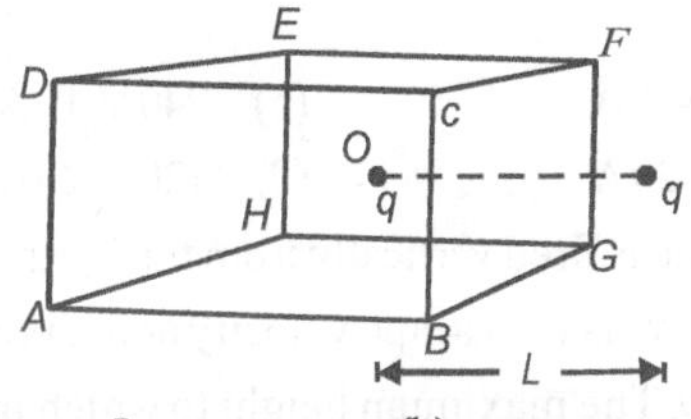

(a) $q/4\pi\epsilon_0 L$ (b) zero
(c) $q/2\pi\epsilon_0 L$ (d) $q/3\pi\epsilon_0 L$

20. Four mole of hydrogen, two mole of helium and one mole of water vapour form an ideal gas mixture. What is the molar specific heat at constant pressure of mixture?
(a) $\frac{16}{7}R$ (b) $\frac{7}{16}R$ (c) R (d) $\frac{23}{7}R$

21. The equivalent capacitance between *A* and *B* is

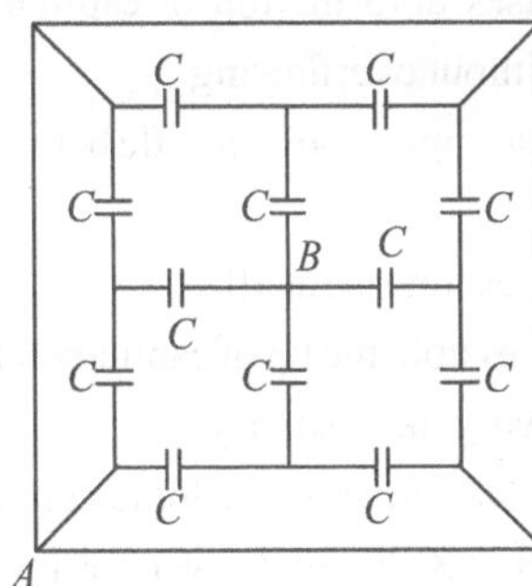

(a) $\frac{4C}{3}$ (b) $\frac{8C}{3}$ (c) 12C (d) $\frac{5C}{12}$

22. A mass of M kg is suspended by a weightless string. The horizontal force that is required to displace it until the string makes an angle of 45° with the initial vertical direction is

(a) $Mg(\sqrt{2}+1)$ (b) $Mg\sqrt{2}$

(c) $\frac{Mg}{\sqrt{2}}$ (d) $Mg(\sqrt{2}-1)$

23. The primary winding of a transformer has 100 turns and its secondary winding has 200 turns. The primary is connected to an A.C. supply of 120 V and the current flowing in it is 10 A. The voltage and the current in the secondary winding are

(a) 240 V, 5 A (b) 240 V, 10 A

(c) 60 V, 20 A (d) 120 V, 20 A

24. A projectile is fired vertically from the Earth with a velocity kv_e where v_e is the escape velocity and k is a constant less than unity. The maximum height to which projectile rises, as measured from the centre of Earth, is

(a) $\frac{R}{k}$ (b) $\frac{R}{k-1}$ (c) $\frac{R}{1-k^2}$ (d) $\frac{R}{1+k^2}$

25. Water rises to a height 'h' in a capillary tube. If the length of capaillary tube above the surface of water is made less than 'h' then :

(a) water rises upto the top of capillary tube and stays there without overflowing

(b) water rises upto a point a little below the top and stays there

(c) water does not rise at all.

(d) water rises upto the tip of capillary tube and then starts overflowing like fountain.

26. The circuit diagram shows a logic combination with the states of outputs X, Y and Z given for inputs P, Q, R and S all at state 1. When inputs P and R change to state 0 with inputs Q and S still at 1, the states of outputs X, Y and Z change to

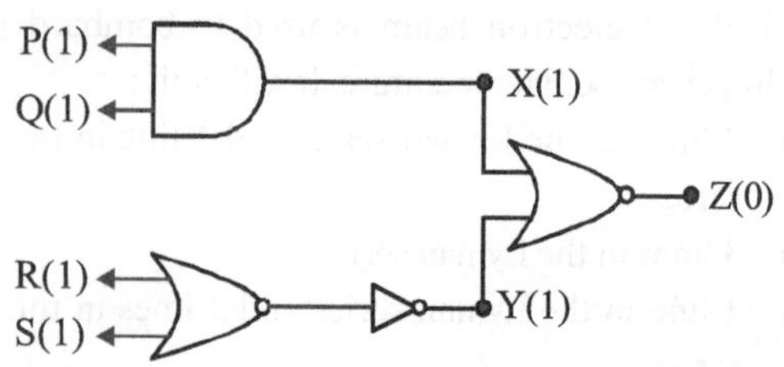

(a) 1, 0, 0 (b) 1, 1, 1 (c) 0, 1, 0 (d) 0, 0, 1

27. The self inductance of a long solenoid cannot be increased by

(a) increasing its area of cross section

(b) increasing its length

(c) changing the medium with greater permeability

(d) increasing the current through it

28. A car moving on a horizontal road may be thrown out of the road in taking a turn

(a) by the gravitational force

(b) due to the lack of proper centripetal force

(c) due to the rolling frictional force between the tyre and road

(d) due to the reaction of the ground

29. If T_1 and T_2 are the time-periods of oscillation of a simple pendulum on the surface of earth (of radius R) and at a depth d, then d is equal to

(a) $\left(1-\frac{T_1^2}{T_2^2}\right)R$ (b) $\left(1-\frac{T_2^2}{T_1^2}\right)R$

(c) $\left(1-\frac{T_1}{T_2}\right)R$ (d) $\left(1-\frac{T_2}{T_1}\right)R$

30. Which of the following is more close to a black body?

(a) black board paint (b) green leaves

(c) black holes (d) red roses

31. A circular coil of radius 6 cm and 20 turns rotates about its vertical diameter with an angular speed of 40 rad s^{-1} in a uniform horizontal magnetic field of magnitude 2×10^{-2} T. If the coil form a closed loop of resistance 8Ω, then the average power loss is

(a) 2.07×10^{-3} W (b) 1.23×10^{-3} W

(c) 3.14×10^{-3} W (d) 1.80×10^{-3} W

Space for Rough Work

32. For an angle of incidence θ on an equilateral prism of refractive index $\sqrt{3}$, the ray refracted is parallel to the base inside the prism. The value of θ is

(a) 30° (b) 45° (c) 60° (d) 75°

33. A closely wound solenoid of 2000 turns and area of cross-section 1.5×10^{-4} m^2 carries a current of 2.0 A. It suspended through its centre and perpendicular to its length, allowing it to turn in a horizontal plane in a uniform magnetic field 5×10^{-2} tesla making an angle of 30° with the axis of the solenoid. The torque on the solenoid will be:

(a) 3×10^{-2} N-m (b) 3×10^{-3} N-m

(c) 1.5×10^{-3} N-m (d) 1.5×10^{-2} N-m

34. A body weighs 72 N on the surface of the earth. What is the gravitational force on it due to earth at a height equal to half the radius of the earth from the surface?

(a) 32 N (b) 28 N (c) 16 N (d) 72 N

35. The length of a metal is ℓ_1 when the tension in it is T_1 and is ℓ_2 when the tension is T_2. The original length of the wire is

(a) $\frac{\ell_1 + \ell_2}{2}$ (b) $\frac{\ell_1 T_2 + \ell_2 T_1}{T_1 + T_2}$

(c) $\frac{\ell_1 T_2 - \ell_2 T_1}{T_2 - T_1}$ (d) $\sqrt{T_1 T_2 \ell_1 \ell_2}$

36. An ideal gas has temperature T_1 at the initial state i shown in the P-V diagram. The gas has a higher temperature T_2 at the final states a and b, which it can reach the paths shown. The change in entropy is

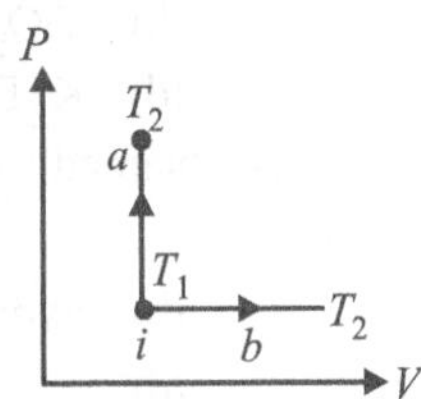

(a) greatest in a (b) greatest in b

(c) same in a and b (d) cannot be said

37. A proton carrying 1 MeV kinetic energy is moving in a circular path of radius R in uniform magnetic field. What should be the energy of an α-particle to describe a circle of same radius in the same field?

(a) 2 MeV (b) 1 MeV

(c) 0.5 MeV (d) 4 MeV

38. The rate of steady volume flow of water through a capillary tube of length 'l' and radius 'r' under a pressure difference of P is V. This tube is connected with another tube of the same length but half the radius, in series. Then the rate of steady volume flow through them is (The pressure difference across the combination is P)

(a) $\frac{V}{16}$ (b) $\frac{V}{17}$

(c) $\frac{16V}{17}$ (d) $\frac{17V}{16}$

39. A container is filled with water ($\mu = 1.33$) upto a height of 33.25 cm. A concave mirror is placed 15 cm above the water level and the image of an object placed at the bottom is formed 25 cm below the water level. The focal length of the mirror is

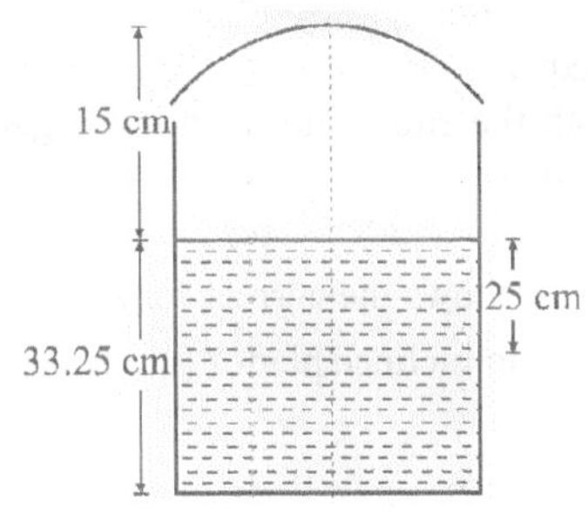

(a) 10 cm (b) 15 cm

(c) 18.30 cm (d) 25 cm

40. A solid cube and a solid sphere of the same material have equal surface area. Both are at the same temperture 120°C, then

(a) both the cube and the sphere cool down at the same rate
(b) the cube cools down faster than the sphere
(c) the sphere cools down faster than the cube
(d) whichever is having more mass will cool down faster

41. A current carrying loop in the form of a right angle isosceles triangle ABC is placed in a uniform magnetic field acting along AB. If the magnetic force on the arm BC is F, what is the force on the arm AC?

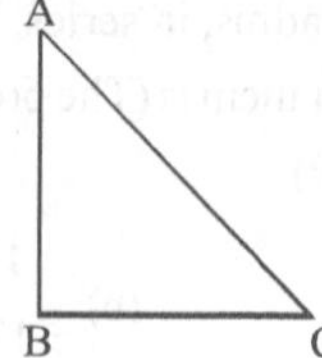

(a) $-\sqrt{2}\,\vec{F}$ (b) $-\vec{F}$ (c) $\vec{F}$ (d) $\sqrt{2}\,\vec{F}$

42. A radioactive element forms its own isotope after 3 consecutive disintegrations. The particles emitted are

(a) 3 β–particles
(b) 2 β–particles and 1 α–particle
(c) 3 β–particles and 1 α–particle
(d) 2 α–particles and 1 β–particle.

43. The fundamental frequency of a closed organ pipe of length 20 cm is equal to the second overtone of an organ pipe open at both the ends. The length of organ pipe open at both the ends is

(a) 100 cm (b) 120 cm (c) 140 cm (d) 80 cm

44. Which figure shows the correct force acting on the body sliding down an inclined plane? (m → mass, f_s → force of friction)

(a) 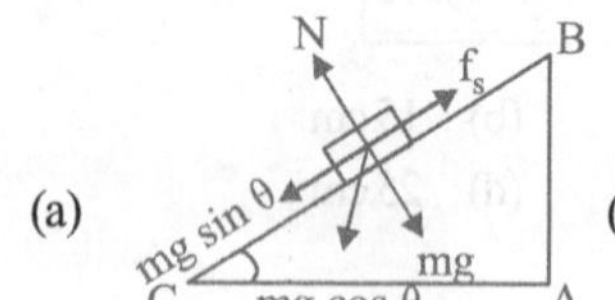

(b) 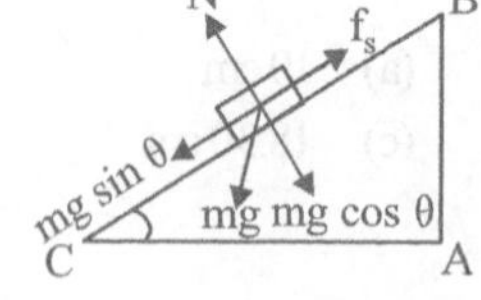

(c) N, B, mg sin θ, f_s, mg mg cos θ, C, A

(d) N, B, mgsinθ, f_s, mg mg cos θ, C, A

45. Forward biasing is that in which applied voltage

(a) increases potential barrier
(b) cancels the potential barrier
(c) is equal to 1.5 volt
(d) decreases potential barrier

CHEMISTRY

DIRECTIONS : There are 45 multiple choice questions numbered 46 to 90. Each question has 4 choices (a), (b), (c) and (d), out of which ONLY ONE is correct.

46. 100 ml O_2 and H_2 kept at same temperature and pressure. What is true about their number of molecules

(a) $N_{O_2} > N_{H_2}$ (b) $N_{O_2} < N_{H_2}$
(c) $N_{O_2} = N_{H_2}$ (d) $N_{O_2} + N_{H_2} = 1$ mole

47. How many joules of heat are absorbed when 70.0 grams of water is completely vaporised at its boiling point?

(a) 23,352 (b) 7,000
(c) 15,813 (d) 158,200

48. Faraday's laws of electrolysis will fail when

(a) temperature is increased
(b) inert electrodes are used
(c) a mixture of electrolytes is used
(d) in none of the above cases

49. The titanium (atomic number = 22) compound that does not exist is

(a) TiO (b) TiO_2
(c) K_2TiF_6 (d) K_2TiO_4

50. Iso-butyl bromide may be obtained from iso-butylene and HBr in the presence of

(a) peroxide (b) hydroquinone
(c) diphenylamine (d) All of these

Space for Rough Work

51. A sequence of how many nucleotides in messenger RNA makes a codon for an amino acid?
(a) Three (b) Four
(c) One (d) Two

52. $FeS_2 + O_2 \rightarrow Fe_2O_3 + SO_2$
In the above equation, the number of electrons lost by one molecule of FeS_2 are –
(a) 6 (b) 2
(c) 1 (d) 11

53. The enthalpies of formation of Al_2O_3 and Cr_2O_3 are –1596 kJ and –1134 kJ respectively. ΔH for the reaction
$2Al + Cr_2O_3 \rightarrow 2Cr + Al_2O_3$ is
(a) –2730 kJ (b) –462 kJ
(c) –1365 kJ (d) +2730 kJ

54. An electrochemical cell is set up as follows :
Pt (H_2, 1 atm)/0.1 M HCl/0.1 M acetic acid/(H_2, 1 atm) Pt
EMF of this cell will not be zero because
(a) the temperature is constant
(b) the pH of 0.1 M HCl and 0.1 M acetic acid is not the same
(c) acids used in the two compartments are different
(d) EMF of a cell depends on molarities of the acids used

55. Which of the following oxides is amphoteric in character?
(a) SnO_2 (b) SiO_2
(c) CO_2 (d) CaO

56. Match List - I (substances) with List - II (processes) employed in the manufacture of the substances and select the correct option.

List - I Substances	List - II Processes
(A) Sulphuric acid	(i) Haber's process
(B) Steel	(ii) Bessemer's process
(C) Sodium hydroxide	(iii) Leblanc process
(D) Ammonia	(iv) Contact process

Options:

	(A)	(B)	(C)	(D)
(a)	(iv)	(ii)	(iii)	(i)
(b)	(i)	(iv)	(ii)	(iii)
(c)	(i)	(ii)	(iii)	(iv)
(d)	(iv)	(iii)	(ii)	(i)

57. The IUPAC name of the compound $CH_3CH{=}CHC{\equiv}CH$ is
(a) Pent-l-yn-3-ene (b) Pent-4-yn-2-ene
(c) Pent-3-en-1-yne (d) Pent-2-en-4-yne

58. Butter of tin is
(a) $SnCl_4.6H_2O$ (b) $SnCl_4.4H_2O$
(c) $SnCl_4.5H_2O$ (d) $SnCl_4.2H_2O$

59. In lime kiln, the reversible reaction
$CaCO_3 (s) \rightleftharpoons CaO (s) + CO_2 (g)$
proceeds to completion because
(a) of high temperature (b) CO_2 escaped out
(c) CaO is removed (d) of low temperature

60. Rate of a reaction can be expressed by following rate expression
Rate = k[Average]^2 [B], if concentration of A is increased by 3 times, and concentration of B is increased by 2 times, how many times rate of reaction increases?
(a) 9 times (b) 27 times
(c) 18 times (d) 8 times

61. In nucleophilic substitution reaction, order of halogens as incoming (attacking) nucleophile is :
$I^- < Br^- < Cl^-$
The order of halogens as departing nucleophile should be :
(a) $Br^- > I^- > Cl^-$ (b) $I^- > Br^- > Cl^-$
(c) $Cl^- > Br^- > I^-$ (d) $Cl^- > I^- > Br^-$

62. Glycerol on heating with oxalic acid at 110°C gives
(a) ethanol (b) ethanal
(c) ether (d) formic acid

63. Electrolytic reduction of nitrobenzene in weakly acidic medium gives
(a) N-Phenylhydroxylamine
(b) Nitrosobenzene
(c) Aniline
(d) *p*-Hydroxyaniline

64. In the presence of cobalt chloride ($CoCl_2$), bleaching powder decomposes to form
(a) $CaCO_3$ and O_3 (b) ClO_2 and CaO
(c) Cl_2O and CaO (d) $CaCl_2$ and O_2

65. $\bar{C}H_2-\underset{\underset{O}{||}}{C}-CH_3$ and $CH_2=\underset{\underset{:\ddot{O}:^{-}}{|}}{C}-CH_3$ are
(a) resonating structures (b) tautomers
(c) geometrical isomers (d) optical isomers

66. The reaction $L \longrightarrow M$ is started with 10.0 g of L. After 30 and 90 minutes 5.0 g and 1.25 g of L respectively are left. The order of the reaction is
(a) 0 (b) 1
(c) 2 (d) 3

67. The outer orbitals of C in ethene molecule can be considered to be hybridized to give three equivalent sp^2 orbitals. The total number of sigma (σ) and pi (π) bonds in ethene molecule is
(a) 1 sigma (σ) and 2 pi (π) bonds
(b) 3 sigma (σ) and 2 pi (π) bonds
(c) 4 sigma (σ) and 1 pi (π) bonds
(d) 5 sigma (σ) and 1 pi (π) bonds

68. **Statement-1 :** Tropylium cation is aromatic in nature

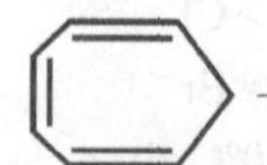

Statement-2 : The only property that determines its aromatic behaviour is its planar structure.
(a) Statement-1 is True, Statement-2 is True, Statement-2 is a correct explanation for Statement-1
(b) Statement-1 is True, Statement-2 is True ; Statement-2 is NOT a correct explanation for Statement-1
(c) Statement-1 is True, Statement-2 is False
(d) Statement-1 is False, Statement-2 is True

69. The reaction of $C_6H_5CH=CHCHO$ with $NaBH_4$ gives
(a) $C_6H_5CH_2CH_2CH_2OH$ (b) $C_6H_5CH=CHCH_2OH$
(c) $C_6H_5CH_2CH_2CHO$ (d) $C_6H_5CH_2CHOHCH_3$

70. Fractional distillation of coal-tar produces the following fractions. Phenol is the main component of which fraction?
(a) Light oil (b) Middle oil
(c) Heavy oil (d) Green oil

71. If one end of a piece of a metal is heated the other end becomes hot after some time. This is due to
(a) Energised electrons moving to the other part of the metal
(b) resistance of the metal
(c) mobility of atoms, in the metal
(d) minor perturbation in the energy of atoms.

72. Which inert gas show abnormal behaviour on liquefaction
(a) Xe (b) He (c) Ar (d) Kr

73. An organometallic compound amongst the following is
(a) Ferrocene
(b) Diethyl zinc
(c) Tetraethyl lead (TEL)
(d) All of these

74. Which of the following cannot be formed ?
(a) He^{2+} (b) He^{+} (c) He (d) He_2

75. Which of the following is not a characteristic of interstitial compounds of transition elements?
(a) The formulae of these compounds do not correspond to any normal oxidation state
(b) They have melting points higher than those of pure elements
(c) They are very hard and some compounds approach diamond in hardness
(d) They are insulators in contrast to the transition metals

76. **Statement-1 :** The drugs which act on the central nervous system and help in reducing anxiety are called antibiotics.
Statement-2 : Penicillin is an antibiotic.
(a) Statement-1 is true, Statement-2 is true, Statement-2 is a correct explanation for Statement-1
(b) Statement-1 is true, Statement-2 is true ; Statement-2 is NOT a correct explanation for Statement-1
(c) Statement-1 is true, Statement-2 is false
(d) Statement-1 is false, Statement-2 is true

77. Which observation(s) reflect(s) colligative properties?
(i) a 0.5 m NaBr solution has a higher vapour pressure than a 0.5 m $BaCl_2$ solution at the same temperature
(ii) pure water freezes at the higher temperature than pure methanol
(iii) a 0.1 m NaOH solution freezes at a lower temperature than pure water
Choose the correct answer from the codes given below
(a) (i), (ii) and (iii) (b) (i) and (ii)
(c) (ii) and (iii) (d) (i) and (iii)

78. In the commercial electrochemical process for aluminium extraction the electrolyte used is
(a) $Al(OH)_3$ in NaOH solution
(b) An aqueous solution of $Al_2(SO_4)_3$
(c) A molten mixture of Al_2O_3 and Na_3AlF_6
(d) A molten mixture of Al_2O_3 and $Al(OH)_3$

79. Aryl halides do not undergo nucleophilic substitution reactions under ordinary conditions because
1. approach of nucleophile is retarded
2. carbon carrying halogen atom is sp^3 hybridised
3. the substrate molecule is destabilised due to resonance
4. partial double bond character between carbon and halogen
(a) 2 and 4 only (b) 1 and 4 only
(c) 2 and 3 only (d) 2, 3 and 4 only

80. According to kinetic theory of gases, for a diatomic molecule
(a) the pressure exerted by the gas is proportional to mean velocity of the molecule
(b) the pressure exerted by the gas is proportional to the root mean velocity of the molecule
(c) the root mean square velocity of the molecule is inversely proportional to the temperature
(d) the mean translational kinetic energy of the molecule is proportional to the absolute temperature.

81. The absolute enthalpy of neutralisation of the reaction:
$MgO(s) + 2HCl(aq) \longrightarrow MgCl_2(aq) + H_2O(l)$ will be:
(a) -57.33 kJ mol^{-1}
(b) greater than -57.33 kJ mol^{-1}
(c) less than -57.33 kJ mol^{-1}
(d) 57.33 kJ mol^{-1}

82. Which of the following electrolytes is least effective in coagulating ferric hydroxide solution?
(a) KBr (b) K_2SO_4
(c) K_2CrO_4 (d) $K_4[Fe(CN)_6]$

83. Estimation of calcium and magnesium is done by
(a) EDTA (b) oxalate
(c) Phosphate (d) none of these

84. Which of the following is colourless in water?
(a) Ti^{3+} (b) V^{3+}
(c) Cu^{3+} (d) Sc^{3+}

85. Which is a polymer of three different monomers ?
(a) ABS (b) SBR
(c) NBR (d) Nylon-26

86. Which of the following element is extracted commercially by the electrolysis of an aqueous solution of its compound?
(a) Chlorine (b) Bromine
(c) Sodium (d) Aluminium

87. Correct order of stability is :
(a) cis -2- butene > 1-butene > trans -2-butene
(b) trans-2-butene > cis-2-butene > 1-butene
(c) 1-butene > cis-2-butene > trans-2- butene
(d) cis-2-butene > trans-2-butene > 1-butene

88. Which of the following is the incorrect statement?
(a) NaCl has 6 : 6 coordination and CsCl has 8 : 8 coordination.
(b) In Na_2O each oxide ion is coordinated by 8Na^+ ions and each Na^+ ion by 4 oxide ions
(c) NaCl structure transform to CsCl structure on heating
(d) In CaF_2 structure each F^- ion is coordinated by 4 Ca^{2+} and vice-versa.

89. The property which distinguishes formic acid from acetic acid is
(a) only ammonium salt of formic acid on heating gives amide
(b) when heated with alcohol/H_2SO_4 only acetic acid forms ester
(c) only acetic acid forms salts with alkali
(d) only formic acid reduces Fehling's solution

Space for Rough Work

90. Phenol on reaction with Br_2 in non-polar aprotic solvent furnishes
(a) 2, 4, 6-Tribromophenol (b) *p*-Bromophenol
(c) *o- and p*-Bromophenol (d) *m*-Bromophenol

BIOLOGY

DIRECTIONS : There are 90 multiple choice questions numbered 91 to 180. Each question has 4 choices (a), (b), (c) and (d), out of which ONLY ONE is correct.

91. Early and late blight of potato are caused respectively by
(a) *Fusarium* and *Claviceps*
(b) *Gibberella* and *Penicillium*
(c) *Aspergillus* and *Ustilago*
(d) None of the above

92. The green alga rich in proteins used as food supplements even by space travellers is
(a) *Chlamydomonas* (b) *Spirogyra*
(c) *Spirulina* (d) *Chlorella*

93. Which of the following pteridophytes is heterosporous in nature?
(a) *Psilotum* (b) *Adiantum*
(c) *Equisetum* (d) *Salvinia*

94. Which of the following does not have an excretory system?
(a) *Myxine* (b) *Carcharodon*
(c) *Balanoglossus* (d) *Asterias*

95. The flightless bird among the following is
(a) *Columba* (b) *Neophron*
(c) *Struthio* (d) *Corvus*

96. When tripalmitin is used as a substrate in respiration, the R.Q. is
(a) >1 (b) 1.0
(c) 0.9 (d) 0.7

97. Select the activities associated with gibberellins.
(A) Apical dominance (B) Good herbicides
(C) Promotes bolting (D) Delay senescence
(E) Stimulates closure of stomata
(a) (A) and (B) only (b) (B) and (C) only
(c) (B) and (D) only (d) (C) and (D) only

98. Much developed larynx of human male is called
(a) Aristole's lantern (b) Syrinx
(c) Adam's apple (d) Muller's organ

99. The layer of cells that secrete enamel of tooth is
(a) dentoblast (b) ameloblast
(c) osteoblast (d) odontoblast

100. Dead space air in man is
(a) 500 ml (b) 150 ml
(c) 250 ml (d) 1.5 L

101. Human chorionic gonadotropin is secreted by
(a) chorion (b) amnion
(c) corpus luteum (d) placenta

102. What is the function of copper-T ?
(a) Checks mutation
(b) Stops fertilization
(c) Stops zygote formation
(d) Stops oblituation of blastocoel

103. The most important component of the oral contraceptive pills is
(a) progesterone (b) growth hormone
(c) thyroxine (d) luteinising hormone

104. A woman with two genes (one on each X-chromosome) for haemophilia and one gene for color blindness on the X-chromosome marries a normal man. How will the progeny be?
(a) All sons and daughters are haemophilic and colorblind
(b) Haemophilic and colorblind daughters
(c) 50% haemophilic, colorblind sons and 50% haemophilic sons
(d) 50% haemophilic daughters and 50% colorblind daughters

105. X linked recessive gene is
(a) always expressed in male
(b) always expressed in female
(c) lethal
(d) sub-lethal

106. Read the given statements and select the incorrect ones.
(i) Sporophyte in mosses is more elaborate than that in liverworts.
(ii) *Salivinia* is homosporous
(iii) Life-cycle in all spermatophytes is diplontic
(iv) In *Cycas*, male cones and megasporophylls are borne on the same trees
(a) (i) and (ii) (b) (i) and (iii)
(c) (ii) and (iv) (d) (iii) and (iv)

107. Read the following statements and select the incorrect ones.
(i) Circulatory system in arthropods is of closed type.
(ii) Parapodia in annelids help in swimming.
(iii) Phylum Mollusca is the second largest animal phylum.
(iv) Aschelminthes are dioecious.
(a) (i) and (iii) only (b) (i) only
(c) (iii) only (d) (iii) and (iv) only

Space for Rough Work

108. Which one of the following groups of animal is correctly matched with its characteristic feature without any exception?
(a) Reptilia : possess 3-chambered heart with an incompletely divided ventricle
(b) Chordata : possess a mouth with an upper and a lower jaw
(c) Chondrichthyes : possess cartilaginous endoskeleton
(d) Mammalia : give birth to young ones

109. Match Column-I with Column-II and select the correct option from the codes given below.

	Column-I		**Column-II**
A.	Vessels	I.	Cells are living with thin cellulosic cell walls
B.	Tracheids	II.	Cells possess highly thickened walls with obliterated central lumen
C.	Xylem fibres	III.	Individual members are interconnected through perforations in their common walls
D.	Xylem parenchyma	IV.	Elongated tube-like cells with thick, lignified walls and tapering ends

(a) A – IV; B – III; C – II; D – I
(b) A – III; B – IV; C – II; D – I
(c) A – II; B – IV; C – III; D – I
(d) A – IV; B – II; C – III; D – I

110. Three types of tissue system have been recognized in plants on the basis of their functions. Select the correct option regarding this.
(a) Epidermal tissue system consists of epidermis and epidermal appendages, which provide protection to the internal tissues.
(b) All tissues except epidermis and vascular bundles constitute the ground tissue, which forms the major part of a plant's body.
(c) Vascular tissue system consists of complex tissues i.e., xylem and phloem.
(d) All of these

111. AIDS is characterized by
(a) decrease in the number of killer T-cells
(b) decrease in the number of supressor T-cells
(c) decrease in the number of helper T-cells
(d) increase in the number of helper T-cells

112. Holstein-Friesian, Brown Swiss and Jersey are all well known
(a) exotic breeds of cow
(b) exotic breeds of goat
(c) exotic breeds of poultry
(d) animal husbandry scientists

113. Which of the following statement is/are not correct for single cell protein (SCP)?
(i) The biomass is obtained from unicellular microorganisms only
(ii) It provides a protein rich supplement
(iii) SCP can be produced by using bacteria and algae but not fungi
(iv) It helps to minimise environmental pollution
(v) SCP has to be processed before use
(a) (i), (iii) and (iv) (b) (iii) only
(c) (iv) only (d) (i) and (iii)

114. Which one of the following combinations of organisms are responsible for the formation and flavour of yoghurt?
(a) *Lactobacillus bulgaricus* and *Streptococcus thermophilus*
(b) *Rhizobium meliloti* and *Azotobacter*
(c) *Bacillus subtilis* and *Escherichia coli*
(d) *Bacillus megathermus* and *Xanthomonas* species

115. India relishes a history of religious and cultural traditions which emphasized the protection of nature. In many cultures, tracts of forest were set aside, all the trees and wildlife within were venerated and given total protection. Such areas are referred to as
(a) hot spots (b) ethical groves
(c) sacred groves (d) protected areas

116. Amrita Devi Bishnoi Wildlife Protection Award is for the individuals or communities from rural areas that have shown extraordinary courage in
(a) reducing environmental pollution
(b) reducing globar warming
(c) protecting wildlife
(d) reforestration in deforested area

117. How many of the given features are associated with keys? Couplet, Quick referral system, Ex-situ Conservation, Analytics, Preservation of specimen, Lead
(a) Four (b) Three
(c) Five (d) Six

118. Structural and functional feature of fungi in endomycorrhiza is
(a) Hartig net (b) Mantle
(c) Extracellular sheath (d) Arbuscule

Space for Rough Work

119. Which of the following group of animal have a partially open, fluid filled body cavity which develop from the first formed embryonic cavity blastocoel?
(a) Flatworms (b) Earthworms
(c) Roundworms (d) Shipworms

120. Ephyra is the stage in the life cycle of
(a) *Physalia* (b) *Obelia*
(c) *Aurelia* (d) sea anemone

121. Aril is the edible part of
(a) apple (b) litchi
(c) banana (d) mango.

122. Which of the following is the characteristic feature of androecium of *Pisum sativum?*
(a) Ten stamens, diadelphous and dithecous anther.
(b) Five stamens, diadelphous and monothecous anther.
(c) Five stamens, epipetalous and dithecous anther.
(d) Six stamens, epipetalous and dithecous anther.

123. Alburnum is otherwise known as
(a) periderm (b) sapwood
(c) heart wood (d) bark

124. Which of the following is not a part of epidermal tissue system?
(a) Companion cells (b) Trichomes
(c) Root hair (d) Guard cells

125. In earthworms setae are present in all segments except
(a) first and the last segments
(b) first segment and the clitellum
(c) first segment
(d) clitellum and last segments

126. Which of the following enzymes has heme as a prosthetic group?
(i) Catalase
(ii) Carboxypeptidase
(iii) Succinic dehydrogenase
(iv) Peroxidase
(a) (i) only (b) (i) & (ii)
(c) (iii) & (iv) (d) (i) & (iv)

127. Colchicine prevents the mitosis of cells at which of the following stage ?
(a) Anaphase (b) Metaphase
(c) Prophase (d) Interphase

128. Select the correct events leading to the opening of the stomata
(A) decline in guard cell solutes
(B) lowering of osmotic potential of guard cells
(C) rise in potassium levels in guard cells
(D) movement of water from neighbouring cells into guard cells
(E) guard cells becoming flaccid
(a) A and E only (b) B, C and D only
(c) A, C and D only (d) B, D and E only

129. DCMU
(a) inhibits PS-I
(b) inhibits PS-II
(c) destroys chloroplast
(d) inhibits oxidative phosphorylation

130. A bird excretes nitrogenous waste materials in the form of
(a) uric acid (b) ammonia
(c) urea (d) amino acids

131. The joint between atlas and axis is called
(a) pivot joint (b) hinge joint
(c) saddle joint (d) angular joint

132. Fenestra ovalis is the opening of –
(a) Cranium (b) Tympanum
(c) Tympanic cavity (d) Brain

133. Autonomic nervous system affects
(a) reflex actions (b) sensory organs
(c) internal organ (d) None of these

134. The order of the three layers of cells in the retina of human eye from inside to outside is
(a) bipolar cells, photoreceptor cells, ganglion cells
(b) ganglion cells, rods, cones
(c) ganglion cells, bipolar cells, photoreceptor cells
(d) photoreceptor cells, ganglion cells, bipolar cells

135. The contraction of gall bladder is due to
(a) gastrin (b) secretin
(c) cholecystokinin (d) enterogastrone

136. The hormone which regulates sleep-wake cycle in man is
(a) oxytocin (b) vasopressin
(c) thyroxine (d) thyrocalcitonin

137. What is common between vegetative reproduction and apomixis?
(a) Both are applicable to only dicot plants
(b) Both bypass the flowering phase
(c) Both occur round the year
(d) Both produces progeny identical to the parent

138. Double fertilization occurs in
(a) *Riccia* (b) *Pteridium*
(c) *Cycas* (d) *Capsella*

Space for Rough Work

139. Which of these is a condition that makes flowers invariably autogamous?
(a) Dioecy (b) Self-incompatibility
(c) Cleistogamy (d) Xenogamy

140. Accessory sexual character in female is promoted by
(a) androgen (b) progesterone
(c) estrogen (d) testosterone

141. In Morgan's experiments on linkage, the percentage of white eyed, miniature winged recombinants in F_2 generation is
(a) 1.3 (b) 37.2
(c) 62.8 (d) 73.2

142. When yellow round heterozygous pea plants are self-fertilized, the frequency of occurrence of RrYY genotype among the offsprings is
(a) 9/26 (b) 3/16
(c) 2/16 (d) 1/16

143. If percentage of cytosine is 18%, then percentage of adenine will be
(a) 32% (b) 64%
(c) 36% (d) 23%.

144. Which of the following codons has no tRNA?
(a) UAA (b) UAU
(c) UGU (d) UGC

145. During Meselson and Stahl's experiments, heavy DNA was distinguished from normal DNA by centrifugation in
(a) CsOH gradient (b) $^{14}NH_4Cl$
(c) $^{35}SO_2$ (d) CsCl gradient

146. In *lac* operon, the genes *a, i, y* and *z* code respectively for
(a) respressor protein, permease, β-galactosidase, transacetylase
(b) transacetylase, permease, β-galactosidase, repressor protein
(c) permease, transacetylase, repressor protein, β-galactosidase
(d) transacetylase, repressor protein, permease, β-galactosidase

147. Presence of tail in a child is an example of
(a) atavism (b) divergent evolution
(c) convergent evolution (d) mutation

148. *Yersinia pestis* is responsible for
(a) syphilis (b) whooping cough
(c) plague (d) leprosy

149. Morphine, which is used as an analgesic is obtained from
(a) *Chinchona*
(b) *Papaver somniferum officinalis*
(c) *Taxus brevifolia*
(d) *Berberis nilghiriensis*

150. Which of the following is the pair of biofertilizers?
(a) *Azolla* and Blue green algae
(b) *Nostoc* and legume
(c) *Rhizobium* and grasses
(d) *Salmonella* & *E. coli*

151. ELISA is used to detect viruses where the key reagent is
(a) DNA probe (b) RNAse
(c) alkaline phosphatase (d) catalase

152. Restriction endonuclease - Hind II always cuts DNA molecules at a particular point by recognizing a specific sequence of
(a) Six base pairs. (b) Five base pairs.
(c) Four base pairs. (d) Seven base pairs.

153. The formula for exponential population growth is
(a) dN/rN = dt (b) rN / dN = dt
(c) dN / dt = rN (d) dt / dN = rNV

154. Animals from colder climates generally have smaller limbs. This is called
(a) Niche rule (b) Allen's rule
(c) Ehrlich rule (d) None of these.

155. In an ecosystem, keystone are those which
(a) are most frequent
(b) are present in maximum number
(c) attain a large biomass
(d) contribute to ecosystem properties

156. Which of the following statements is incorrect regarding enzymatic activity?
(a) It increases with increase in substrate concentration upto the saturation point.
(b) It is highest at optimum pH value.
(c) It initially decreases with increase in pH value.
(d) It initially increases with increase in temperature and then decreases.

157. Effective filtration pressure in glomerulus is caused due to
(a) powerful pumping action of the heart
(b) secretion of adrenaline
(c) afferent arteriole is slightly larger than efferent arteriole
(d) vacuum develops in proximal convoluted tubule and sucks the blood

158. Refer the given statements.
(i) Outer exine is made up of sporopollenin.
(ii) Inner intine is pecto-cellulosic in nature.
(iii) Generative cell is bigger and contains abundant food reserve.
(iv) Vegetative cell is small and floats in the cytoplasm of the generative cell.

Which of the given statements are not true regarding structure of pollen grain?
(a) (i) and (ii) (b) (ii) and (iii)
(c) (iii) and (iv) (d) (i) and (iv)

Space for Rough Work

159. Identify the parts labelled as A, B, C and D in the given figure and select the correct option from the codes given below.

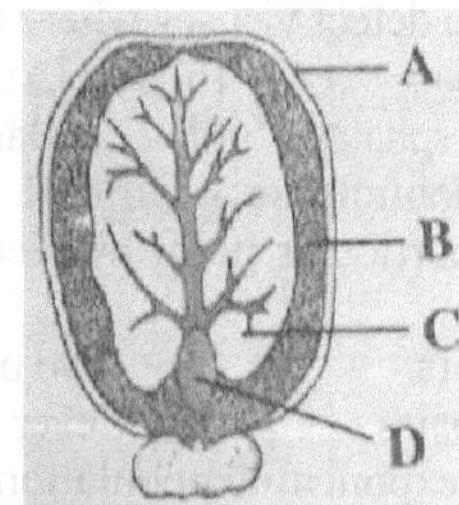

	A	B	C	D
(a)	Seed coat	Scutellum	Epicotyl	Hypocotyl
(b)	Seed coat	Scutellum	Hypocotyl	Epicotyl
(c)	Seed coat	Cotyledon	Endosperm	Hypocotyl
(d)	Seed coat	Endosperm	Cotyledon	Hypocotyl

160. The third stage of parturition is called "after-birth". In this stage
(a) excessive bleeding occurs
(b) foetus is born and cervix and vagina contraction to normal condition happens
(c) foetus is born and contraction of uterine wall prevents excessive bleeding
(d) placenta is expelled out

161. If map distance between genes P and Q is 4 units, between P and R is 11 units, and between Q and R is 7 units, the order of genes on the linkage map can be traced as follows.

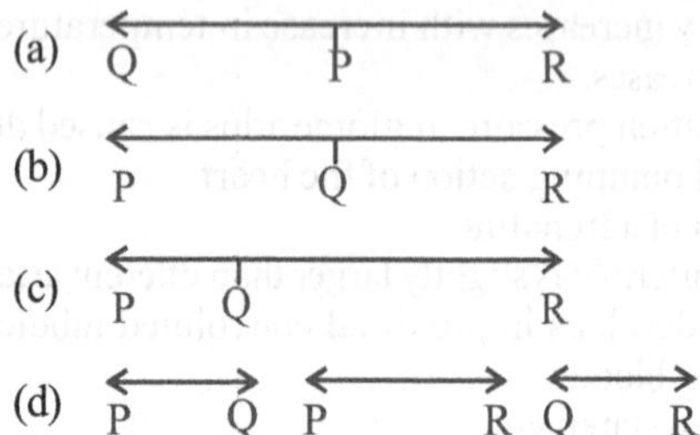

162. Which of the following statements regarding 'human genome' is incorrect?
(a) Human genome consists of 3×10^9 bp and about 20,500 genes.
(b) The average gene size is 3000 bp and dystophin is the largest known human gene.
(c) Chromosome 1 contains maximum (2968) number of genes and the Y-chromosome has the least (231) number of genes.
(d) Repeated (or repetitive) sequences are not present in human genome.

163. In a mRNA molecule, untranslated regions (UTRs) are present at
(a) 5' - end (before start codon)
(b) 3' - end (after stop codon)
(c) both (a) and (b)
(d) no UTRs present in mRNA

164. Statins used for lowering blood-cholesterol level are extracted from
(a) algae (b) bacteria
(c) viruses (d) yeast

165. One of the key factors, which makes the plasmid the vector in genetic engineering is
(a) its resistance to antibiotics
(b) its resistance to restriction enzymes
(c) its ability to carry a foreign gene
(d) its ability to cause infection in the host

166. Primers are
(a) chemically synthesized oligonucleotides that are complementary to the regions of DNA
(b) chemically synthesized oligonucleotides that are not complementary to the regions of DNA
(c) chemically synthesized, autonomously replicating circular DNA molecules
(d) specific sequences present on recombinant DNA

167. Which of the following statements regarding the structure of proinsulin and mature insulin are not correct?
(a) Proinsulin is made up of three polypeptide chains – A, B and C.
(b) C - polypeptide chain with 33 amino acids is removed prior to insulin formation.
(c) Mature insulin is made up of 51 amino acids arranged in two polypeptide chains – A and B.
(d) Polypeptide chains A and B are interconnected by only one S – S linkage.

168. Kangaroo and desert rat that live in conditions of water scarcity are capable of meeting all their water requirements by
(a) having a thick coat to minimise evaporative desiccation
(b) oxidizing stored fat to produce water as by product
(c) producing very concentrated urine and solid faeces
(d) all of these

169. The exotic species, which when introduced in India became notorious weed(s), is/are
(a) *Lantana camara*
(b) *Eicchornia crassipes*
(c) *Parthenium hysterophorus*
(d) all of these

Space for Rough Work

170. The diversity of organisms sharing the same habitat or community is termed as
(a) alpha diversity (b) beta diversity
(c) gamma diversity (d) delta diversity

171. Select correct statements for non-vascular archegoniates.
A. Independent sporophyte & gametophyte
B. Dependent sporophyte
C. Multicellular independent gametophyte
D. Many neck canal cells in female sex organ
E. Homosporous and mitospores are formed
(a) B, C, D (b) A, C, D
(c) B, C, E (d) A, D, E

172. Which of the following statements is wrong regarding model of plasma membrane given by S.J. Singer and G.L. Nicolson?
(a) The quasi-fluid nature of protein enables lateral movement of lipids
(b) The integral proteins are partially or totally buried in the membrane
(c) Protein icebergs in sea of lipids
(d) Phosphoglycerides are present in lipid component

173. Which of the following events listed below, is not observed during mitosis?
(a) Movements of centrioles to opposite poles
(b) Chromatin condensation
(c) Appearance of recombination nodule
(d) Appearance of chromosomes with two chromatids joined together at the centromere

174. During fat absorption, a very small protein coated fat globules called chylomicron is formed in
(a) Lumen of intestine
(b) Intestinal cell
(c) Lymph vessel
(d) Blood stream

175. Which of the following will be the cardiac output (in L/min) of the heart that has stroke volume 0.07 L and is beating at the rate of 75/min?
(a) 52.5 (b) 5.25
(c) 0.52 (d) 0.052

176. Milk formative hormone is
(a) Prolactin (b) Melatonin
(c) Oxytocin (d) Pitressin

177. All of the following changes occur during contraction of a muscle fibre except one
(a) Width of A-band and I-band remain same
(b) Actin filament slides over the myosin filaments
(c) Length of actin and myosin filaments remain same
(d) Width of H-zone decreases

178. In phloem
A. Transport of sugar is essentially unidirectional
B. Sap mainly consists of water and sucrose
C. Loading and unloading of sugar is passive process
D. Translocation from source to sink occurs by mass flow
(a) A and C are incorrect
(b) Only D is correct
(c) A and B are correct
(d) B and C are incorrect

179. Which of the following elements can become toxic at higher concentration?
(a) S (b) Mn
(c) N (d) K

180. How many ATP are produced by substrate level phosphorylation from one molecule of PGAL if it is oxidised completely during aerobic respiration?
(a) 2 (b) 3
(c) 6 (d) 4

FULL SYLLABUS SPEED TEST-101

Total Questions	180	Total Marks	720
Attempted		Correct	
Incorrect		Net Score	
Cut-off Score	140	Qualifying Score	190
Success Gap = Net Score – Qualifying Score			
Net Score = (Correct × 4) – (Incorrect × 1)			

Space for Rough Work

Response Grid

PHYSICS

1. (a)(b)(c)(d)	2. (a)(b)(c)(d)	3. (a)(b)(c)(d)	4. (a)(b)(c)(d)	5. (a)(b)(c)(d)
6. (a)(b)(c)(d)	7. (a)(b)(c)(d)	8. (a)(b)(c)(d)	9. (a)(b)(c)(d)	10. (a)(b)(c)(d)
11. (a)(b)(c)(d)	12. (a)(b)(c)(d)	13. (a)(b)(c)(d)	14. (a)(b)(c)(d)	15. (a)(b)(c)(d)
16. (a)(b)(c)(d)	17. (a)(b)(c)(d)	18. (a)(b)(c)(d)	19. (a)(b)(c)(d)	20. (a)(b)(c)(d)
21. (a)(b)(c)(d)	22. (a)(b)(c)(d)	23. (a)(b)(c)(d)	24. (a)(b)(c)(d)	25. (a)(b)(c)(d)
26. (a)(b)(c)(d)	27. (a)(b)(c)(d)	28. (a)(b)(c)(d)	29. (a)(b)(c)(d)	30. (a)(b)(c)(d)
31. (a)(b)(c)(d)	32. (a)(b)(c)(d)	33. (a)(b)(c)(d)	34. (a)(b)(c)(d)	35. (a)(b)(c)(d)
36. (a)(b)(c)(d)	37. (a)(b)(c)(d)	38. (a)(b)(c)(d)	39. (a)(b)(c)(d)	40. (a)(b)(c)(d)
41. (a)(b)(c)(d)	42. (a)(b)(c)(d)	43. (a)(b)(c)(d)	44. (a)(b)(c)(d)	45. (a)(b)(c)(d)

CHEMISTRY

46. (a)(b)(c)(d)	47. (a)(b)(c)(d)	48. (a)(b)(c)(d)	49. (a)(b)(c)(d)	50. (a)(b)(c)(d)
51. (a)(b)(c)(d)	52. (a)(b)(c)(d)	53. (a)(b)(c)(d)	54. (a)(b)(c)(d)	55. (a)(b)(c)(d)
56. (a)(b)(c)(d)	57. (a)(b)(c)(d)	58. (a)(b)(c)(d)	59. (a)(b)(c)(d)	60. (a)(b)(c)(d)
61. (a)(b)(c)(d)	62. (a)(b)(c)(d)	63. (a)(b)(c)(d)	64. (a)(b)(c)(d)	65. (a)(b)(c)(d)
66. (a)(b)(c)(d)	67. (a)(b)(c)(d)	68. (a)(b)(c)(d)	69. (a)(b)(c)(d)	70. (a)(b)(c)(d)
71. (a)(b)(c)(d)	72. (a)(b)(c)(d)	73. (a)(b)(c)(d)	74. (a)(b)(c)(d)	75. (a)(b)(c)(d)
76. (a)(b)(c)(d)	77. (a)(b)(c)(d)	78. (a)(b)(c)(d)	79. (a)(b)(c)(d)	80. (a)(b)(c)(d)
81. (a)(b)(c)(d)	82. (a)(b)(c)(d)	83. (a)(b)(c)(d)	84. (a)(b)(c)(d)	85. (a)(b)(c)(d)
86. (a)(b)(c)(d)	87. (a)(b)(c)(d)	88. (a)(b)(c)(d)	89. (a)(b)(c)(d)	90. (a)(b)(c)(d)

BIOLOGY

91. (a)(b)(c)(d)	92. (a)(b)(c)(d)	93. (a)(b)(c)(d)	94. (a)(b)(c)(d)	95. (a)(b)(c)(d)
96. (a)(b)(c)(d)	97. (a)(b)(c)(d)	98. (a)(b)(c)(d)	99. (a)(b)(c)(d)	100. (a)(b)(c)(d)
101. (a)(b)(c)(d)	102. (a)(b)(c)(d)	103. (a)(b)(c)(d)	104. (a)(b)(c)(d)	105. (a)(b)(c)(d)
106. (a)(b)(c)(d)	107. (a)(b)(c)(d)	108. (a)(b)(c)(d)	109. (a)(b)(c)(d)	110. (a)(b)(c)(d)
111. (a)(b)(c)(d)	112. (a)(b)(c)(d)	113. (a)(b)(c)(d)	114. (a)(b)(c)(d)	115. (a)(b)(c)(d)
116. (a)(b)(c)(d)	117. (a)(b)(c)(d)	118. (a)(b)(c)(d)	119. (a)(b)(c)(d)	120. (a)(b)(c)(d)
121. (a)(b)(c)(d)	122. (a)(b)(c)(d)	123. (a)(b)(c)(d)	124. (a)(b)(c)(d)	125. (a)(b)(c)(d)
126. (a)(b)(c)(d)	127. (a)(b)(c)(d)	128. (a)(b)(c)(d)	129. (a)(b)(c)(d)	130. (a)(b)(c)(d)
131. (a)(b)(c)(d)	132. (a)(b)(c)(d)	133. (a)(b)(c)(d)	134. (a)(b)(c)(d)	135. (a)(b)(c)(d)
136. (a)(b)(c)(d)	137. (a)(b)(c)(d)	138. (a)(b)(c)(d)	139. (a)(b)(c)(d)	140. (a)(b)(c)(d)
141. (a)(b)(c)(d)	142. (a)(b)(c)(d)	143. (a)(b)(c)(d)	144. (a)(b)(c)(d)	145. (a)(b)(c)(d)
146. (a)(b)(c)(d)	147. (a)(b)(c)(d)	148. (a)(b)(c)(d)	149. (a)(b)(c)(d)	150. (a)(b)(c)(d)
151. (a)(b)(c)(d)	152. (a)(b)(c)(d)	153. (a)(b)(c)(d)	154. (a)(b)(c)(d)	155. (a)(b)(c)(d)
156. (a)(b)(c)(d)	157. (a)(b)(c)(d)	158. (a)(b)(c)(d)	159. (a)(b)(c)(d)	160. (a)(b)(c)(d)
161. (a)(b)(c)(d)	162. (a)(b)(c)(d)	163. (a)(b)(c)(d)	164. (a)(b)(c)(d)	165. (a)(b)(c)(d)
166. (a)(b)(c)(d)	167. (a)(b)(c)(d)	168. (a)(b)(c)(d)	169. (a)(b)(c)(d)	170. (a)(b)(c)(d)
171. (a)(b)(c)(d)	172. (a)(b)(c)(d)	173. (a)(b)(c)(d)	174. (a)(b)(c)(d)	175. (a)(b)(c)(d)
176. (a)(b)(c)(d)	177. (a)(b)(c)(d)	178. (a)(b)(c)(d)	179. (a)(b)(c)(d)	180. (a)(b)(c)(d)

HINTS & SOLUTIONS (PHYSICS – Chapter-wise Tests)

Speed Test-1

1. **(b)** In CGS system,

$$d = 4\frac{g}{cm^3}$$

The unit of mass is 100g and unit of length is 10 cm, so

$$\text{density} = \frac{4\left(\frac{100g}{100}\right)}{\left(\frac{10}{10}cm\right)^3}$$

$$= \frac{\left(\frac{4}{100}\right)}{\left(\frac{1}{10}\right)^3}\frac{(100g)}{(10cm)^3}$$

$$= \frac{4}{100}\times(10)^3\cdot\frac{100g}{(10cm)^3}$$

$= 40$ unit

2. **(a)** $T = P^a D^b S^c$

$M^0L^0T^1 = (ML^{-1}T^{-2})^a (ML^{-3})^b (MT^{-2})^c$

$= M^{a+b+c} L^{-a-3b} T^{-2a-2c}$

Applying principle of homogeneity

$a + b + c = 0;\ -a - 3b = 0;\ -2a - 2c = 1$

on solving, we get $a = -3/2$, $b = 1/2$, $c = 1$

3. **(a)** Number of significant figures in 23.023 = 5

Number of significant figures in 0.0003 = 1

Number of significant figures in $2.1 \times 10^{-3} = 2$

4. **(a)** $Y = \frac{\text{Stress}}{\text{Strain}} = \frac{\text{Force / Area}}{\text{Dimensionless}} \Rightarrow Y = \text{Pressure.}$

5. **(d)** For angular momentum, the dimensional formula is $[ML^2T^{-1}]$. For other three, it is $[ML^2T^{-2}]$.

6. **(c)** $\frac{\Delta P}{P}\times 100 = \frac{\Delta F}{F}\times 100 + 2\frac{\Delta \ell}{\ell}\times 100 = 4\% + 2\times 2\%$

$= 8\%$

7. **(d)** Conductance,

$$G = \frac{1}{\text{resistance}} = \text{mho}(\Omega^{-1}) \text{ or siemen (S)}$$

8. **(d)** $F \propto v \Rightarrow F = kv \Rightarrow [k] = \left[\frac{F}{v}\right] = \left[\frac{MLT^{-2}}{LT^{-1}}\right] = [ML^0T^{-1}]$

9. **(c)** $\frac{0.2}{25}\times 100 = 0.8\,\%$

10. **(c)** Weber is the unit of magnetic flux in S.I. system.

1 Wb(S.I unit) = 10^8 maxwell

11. **(b)** Solar constant = energy/area/time

$$= \frac{ML^2T^{-2}}{L^2T} = [M^1T^{-3}].$$

12. **(b)** $b = \lambda_m T = LK = [M^0 L^1 T^0 K^1]$

13. **(d)** Let unit 'u' related with e, a_0, h and c as follows.

$$[u] = [e]^a [a_0]^b [h]^c [C]^d$$

Using dimensional method,

$[M^{-1}L^{-2}T^{+4}A^{+2}] = [A^1T^1]^a[L]^b[ML2T^{-1}]^c[LT^{-1}]^d$

$[M^{-1}L^{-2}T^{+4}A^{+2}] = [M^c L^{b+2c+d} T^{a-c-d} A^a]$

$a = 2,\ b = 1,\ c = -1,\ d = -1$

$$\therefore\ u = \frac{e^2 a_0}{hc}$$

14. **(c)** From $F = \frac{1}{4\pi\varepsilon_0}\frac{e^2}{r^2}$.

$$\therefore\ \frac{e^2}{\varepsilon_0} = 4\pi F r^2 \text{ (dimensionally)}$$

$$\frac{e^2}{\varepsilon_0 hc} = \frac{4\pi Fr^2}{hc} = \frac{(MLT^{-2})L^2}{ML^2T^{-1}[LT^{-1}]} = [M^0 L^0 T^0 A^0],$$

$\frac{e^2}{\varepsilon_0 hc}$ is called fine structure constant & has value $\frac{1}{137}$.

15. **(d)** $\text{Density} = \frac{\text{Mass}}{\text{Volume}}$

$$\rho = \frac{M}{L^3} \qquad \therefore\ \frac{\Delta\rho}{\rho} = \frac{\Delta M}{M} + 3\frac{\Delta L}{L}$$

% error in density = % error in Mass + 3 (% error in length]

$= 4 + 3(3) = 13\%$

16. **(d)** Poisson's ratio is a unitless quantity.

17. **(d)** Dimensionally $\varepsilon_0 L$ = Capacitance (c)

$$\therefore\ \varepsilon_0 L\frac{\Delta V}{\Delta t} = \frac{C\Delta V}{\Delta t} = \frac{q}{\Delta t} = I$$

18. **(c)** $\frac{\Delta V}{V} = 3\frac{\Delta r}{r}$ or $6\% = 3\frac{\Delta r}{r}$ or $\frac{\Delta r}{r} = 2\%$

Now surface area $s = 4\pi r^2$ or $\log s = \log 4\pi + 2\log r$

$$\therefore\ \frac{\Delta s}{s} = 2\frac{\Delta r}{r} = 2\times 2\% = 4\%.$$

19. **(d)** Let $(M) = V^a F^b E^c$

Putting the dimensions of V, F and E, we have

$(M) = (LT^{-1})^a \times (MLT^{-2})^b \times (ML^2T^{-2})^c$

or $M^1 = M^{b+c} L^{a+b+2c} T^{-a-2b-2c}$

Equating the powers of dimensions, we have

$b + c = 1$
$a + b + 2c = 0; \quad -a - 2b - 2c = 0$
which give $a = -2, b = 0$ and $c = 1$.
Therefore $(M) = (V^{-2} F^0 E)$.

20. (d) Number of significant figures in multiplication is three, corresponding to the minimum number
$107.88 \times 0.610 = 65.8068 = 65.8$

21. (d) A quantity which has dimensions and a constant value is called dimensional constant. Therefore, gravitational constant (G) is a dimensional constant.

22. (a) $\dfrac{[ML^2T^{-2}][ML^2T^{-1}]^2}{[M^5][M^{-1}L^3T^{-2}]^2} = [M^0L^0T^0] = \text{angle}.$

23. (a) The mean value of refractive index,

$$\mu = \frac{1.34 + 1.38 + 1.32 + 1.36}{4} = 1.35$$

and

$$\Delta\mu = \frac{|(1.35 - 1.34)| + |(1.35 - 1.38)| + |(1.35 - 1.32)| + |(1.35 - 1.36)|}{4} = 0.02$$

Thus $\dfrac{\Delta\mu}{\mu} \times 100 = \dfrac{0.02}{1.35} \times 100 = 1.48$

24. (c) $\dfrac{eV}{T} = \dfrac{W}{T} = \dfrac{PV}{T} = R$

and $\dfrac{R}{N} =$ Boltzmann constant.

25. (b) Mobility $\mu = \dfrac{\text{drift velocity } V_d}{\text{electric field } E} = \dfrac{(ms^{-1})}{(Vm^{-1})} = \dfrac{m^2 s^{-3}}{V}$

$$\left(\because \text{Volt} = V = \frac{\text{joule(J)}}{\text{coulomb(C)}}\right)$$

$$= \frac{m^2 s^{-1} C}{J} = \frac{m^2 s^{-1} As}{kg\, m^2 s^{-2}} [\text{Coulomb}, c = As]$$

$= kg^{-1} s^2 A = M^{-1} T^2 A$

26. (a)

27. (b) $v = k \lambda^a \rho^b g^c$

$[M^0 LT^{-1}] = L^a (ML^{-3})^b (LT^{-2})^c$

$= M^b L^{a-3b+c} T^{-2c}$

$\therefore \; b = 0; \; a - 3b + c = 1$

$-2c = -1 \Rightarrow c = 1/2 \qquad \therefore \; a = \dfrac{1}{2}$

$v \propto \lambda^{1/2} \rho^0 g^{1/2}$ or $v^2 \propto \lambda g$

28. (b) $[\text{momentum}] = [M][L][T^{-1}] = [MLT^{-1}]$

Planck's constant $= \dfrac{E}{\nu} = \dfrac{[M][LT^{-1}]^2}{T^{-1}} = ML^2T^{-1}$

29. (d) Let dimensions of length is related as,

$$L = [c]^x [G]^y \left[\frac{e^2}{4\pi\varepsilon_0}\right]^z$$

$$\frac{e^2}{4\pi\varepsilon_0} = ML^3T^{-2}$$

$L = [LT^{-1}]^x [M^{-1}L^3T^{-2}]^y [ML^3T^{-2}]^z$

$[L] = [L^{x+3y+3z} M^{-y+z} T^{-x-2y-2z}]$

Comparing both sides

$-y + z = 0 \Rightarrow y = z$ ...(i)

$x + 3y + 3z = 1$ ...(ii)

$-x - 4z = 0 \quad (\because y = z)$ ...(iii)

From (i), (ii) & (iii)

$z = y = \dfrac{1}{2}, \; x = -2$

Hence, $L = c^{-2}\left[G \cdot \dfrac{e^2}{4\pi\varepsilon_0}\right]^{1/2}$

30. (c) Impulse = change in momentum

31. (c) We know that $\dfrac{Q^2}{2C}$ is energy of capacitor so it represent the dimension of energy $= [ML^2T^{-2}]$.

32. (b) Let $M = p^n v^m$

$ML^{-2}T^{-1} = (ML^{-1}T^{-2})^n (LT^{-1})^m$

$= M^n L^{-n+m} T^{-2n-m}$

$\therefore \; n = 1; \; -n + m = -2$

$\therefore \; m = -2 + n = -2 + 1 = -1 \qquad \therefore \; m = -n$

33. (c) $I = AT^2 e^{-B/kT}$

Dimensions of $A = I/T^2$; Dimensions of $B = kT$

($\because$ power of exponential is dimensionless)

$AB^2 = \dfrac{I}{T^2}(kT)^2 = Ik^2$

34. (a) $\eta = \dfrac{p(r^2 - x^2)}{4vl} = \dfrac{[ML^{-1}T^{-2}][L^2]}{[LT^{-1}][L]} = [ML^{-1}T^{-1}]$

35. (a) The unit of λ, x and A are the same

36. (c) $L + B = 2.331 + 2.1 \cong 4.4$ cm

Since minimum significant figure is 2.

37. (c) Given, $x = \cos(\omega t + kx)$

$(\omega t + kx)$ is an angle and hence it is a dimension less quantity.

$[(\omega t + kx)] = [M^0L^0T^0]$

or $[\omega t] = [M^0L^0T^0]$

$$[\omega] = \frac{[M^0L^0T^0]}{[T]} = [M^0L^0T^{-1}]$$

38. (c) $10\,VD = 9MD, \; 1VD = \dfrac{9}{10}MD$

Vernier constant = 1 MD − 1 VD

$$= \left(1 - \frac{9}{10}\right)MD = \frac{1}{10}MD = \frac{1}{10} \times \frac{1}{2} = 0.05\,\text{mm}$$

39. (c) $[\text{Energy density}] = \frac{[\text{Work done}]}{[\text{Volume}]}$

$$= \frac{ML^2T^{-2}}{L^3} = ML^{-1}T^{-2}$$

$$[\text{Young's Modulus}] = \left[\frac{F}{A} \times \frac{l}{\Delta l}\right]$$

$$= \frac{MLT^{-2}}{L^2} \cdot \frac{L}{L} = [ML^{-1}T^{-2}]$$

40. (b) As $\frac{a}{V^2} = P$

$$\therefore\ a = PV^2 = \frac{\text{dyne}}{\text{cm}^2}(\text{cm}^3)^2 = \text{dyne cm}^4$$

41. (a) Reyonld's constant is a pure number, hence it has no dimensions.

42. (d) $\omega k = \frac{1}{T} \times \frac{1}{L} = [L^{-1}\,T^{-1}]$

The dimensions of the quantities in a, b, c are of velocity $[LT^{-1}]$

43. (a) M = Pole strength × length
= amp – metre × metre = amp – metre^2

44. (b) According to the question.

$$t = (90 \pm 1) \text{ or, } \frac{\Delta t}{t} = \frac{1}{90}$$

$$l = (20 \pm 0.1) \text{ or, } \frac{\Delta l}{l} = \frac{0.1}{20}$$

$$\frac{\Delta g}{g}\% = ?$$

As we know,

$$t = 2\pi\sqrt{\frac{l}{g}}$$

$$\Rightarrow\quad g = \frac{4\pi^2 l}{t^2}$$

$$\text{or,}\quad \frac{\Delta g}{g} = \pm\left(\frac{\Delta l}{l} + 2\frac{\Delta t}{t}\right)$$

$$= \left(\frac{0.1}{20} + 2 \times \frac{1}{90}\right)$$

$$= 0.027$$

$$\therefore\quad \frac{\Delta g}{g}\% = 2.7\%$$

45. (a) Dimension of magnetic flux
= Dimension of voltage × Dimension of time
= $[ML^2T^{-3}A^{-1}]\,[T] = [ML^2T^{-2}A^{-1}]$

$$\because \text{Voltage} = \frac{\text{work}}{\text{charge}}$$

Speed Test-2

1. (a) Acceleration of the particle $a = 2t - 1$
The particle retards when acceleration is opposite to velocity.
$\Rightarrow a.v < 0 \Rightarrow (2t-1)(t^2 - t) < 0 \Rightarrow t(2t-1)(t-1) < 0$
Now t is always positive
$\therefore (2t-1)(t-1) < 0$

or $2t - 1 < 0$ and $t - 1 > 0 \Rightarrow t < \frac{1}{2}$ and $t > 1$.

This is not possible
or $2t - 1 > 0$ & $t - 1 < 0 \Rightarrow 1/2 < t < 1$

2. (b) $x = \alpha t^3$ and $y = \beta t^3$

$v_x = \frac{dx}{dt} = 3\alpha t^2$ and $v_y = \frac{dy}{dt} = 3\beta t^2$

$\therefore v = \sqrt{v_x^2 + v_y^2} = \sqrt{9\alpha^2 t^4 + 9\beta^2 t^4}$

$= 3t^2\sqrt{\alpha^2 + \beta^2}$

3. (d) Average speed$=\frac{\text{Total distance travelled}}{\text{Total time taken}}$

$= \frac{x}{\frac{2x/5}{v_1} + \frac{3x/5}{v_2}} = \frac{5v_1v_2}{3v_1 + 2v_2}$

4. (a) Instantaneous speed is the distance being covered by the particle per unit time at the given instant. It is equal to the magnitude of the instantaneous velocity at the given instant.

5. (a) $v = \alpha\sqrt{x}$, $\frac{dx}{dt} = \alpha\sqrt{x} \Rightarrow \frac{dx}{\sqrt{x}} = \alpha\, dt$

$\int_0^x \frac{dx}{\sqrt{x}} = \alpha\int_0^t dt$

$\left[\frac{2\sqrt{x}}{1}\right]_0^x = \alpha[t]_0^t$

$\Rightarrow 2\sqrt{x} = \alpha t \Rightarrow x = \frac{\alpha^2}{4}t^2$

6. (c) $\frac{1}{2}(1+4)\times 4 - \frac{1}{2}\times 1\times 2 - \frac{1}{2}\times 3\times 4 = 3\text{ m}$

7. (b) The distance travel in nth second is
$S_n = u + ½(2n-1)a$ ....(1)
so distance travel in tth & (t+1)th second are
$S_t = u + ½(2t-1)a$ ....(2)
$S_{t+1} = u + ½(2t+1)a$ ....(3)
As per question,
$S_t + S_{t+1} = 100 = 2(u + at)$ ....(4)
Now from first equation of motion the velocity, of particle after time t, if it moves with an accleration a is
$v = u + at$ ....(5)
where u is initial velocity
So from eq(4) and (5), we get v = 50 cm/sec.

8. (d) Relative speed of police with respect to thief
= 10 – 9 = 1 m/s
Instantaneous separation = 100 m

$\text{Time} = \frac{\text{Distance}}{\text{Velocity}} = \frac{100}{1} = 100\text{sec}.$

9. (d) $x = \frac{a}{b}(1 - e^{-b\times\frac{1}{b}}) = \frac{a}{b}(1 - e^{-1}) = \frac{a}{b}(1 - \frac{1}{e})$

$= \frac{a}{b}\frac{(e-1)}{e} = \frac{a}{b}\frac{(2.718-1)}{2.718} = \frac{a}{b}\frac{(1.718)}{2.718} = 0.637\frac{a}{b} \simeq \frac{2}{3}a/b$

velocity $v = \frac{dx}{dt} = ae^{-bt}$, $v_0 = a$

accleration $a = \frac{dv}{dt} = -abe^{-bt}$ & $a_0 = -ab$

At $t = 0$, $x = \frac{a}{b}(1-1) = 0$ and

At $t = \frac{1}{b}$, $x = \frac{a}{b}(1 - e^{-1}) = \frac{a}{b}(1 - \frac{1}{e}) = \frac{2}{3}a/b$

At $t = \infty$, $x = \frac{a}{b}$

It cannot go beyond this, so point $x > \frac{a}{b}$ is not reached by the particle.

At $t = 0, x = 0$, at $t = \infty$, $x = \frac{a}{b}$, therefore the particle does not come back to its starting point at $t = \infty$.

10. (d) Ist part: u = 0, t = 5s, v = 108 km/hr = 30 m/s
$v = u + at \Rightarrow 30 = 0 + a\times 5 \Rightarrow a = 6\text{ m/s}^2$

$s = ut + \frac{1}{2}at^2 = 0\times 5 + \frac{1}{2}\times 6\times 5^2 = 75\text{ m}$

IIIrd part: s = 45m, u = 30m/s, v = 0

$a = \frac{v^2 - u^2}{2s} = \frac{-30\times 30}{2\times 45} = -10\text{m/s}^2$

$v = u + at \Rightarrow 0 = 30 - 10\times t \Rightarrow t = 3\text{s}$
IInd part :
$s = s_1 + s_2 + s_3$
$395 = 75 + s_2 + 45 \Rightarrow s_2 = 275\text{ m}$

$t = \frac{275}{30} = 9.16 = 9.2\text{s}.$

Total time taken = (5 + 9.2 + 3) sec = 17.2 sec

11. (a) $\frac{dv}{dt} = -kv^3$ or $\frac{dv}{v^3} = -k\, dt$

Integrating we get, $-\frac{1}{2v^2} = -kt + c$ ...(1)

At $t = 0, v = v_0$ $\therefore -\frac{1}{2v_0^2} = c$

Putting in (1)

$$-\frac{1}{2v^2} = -kt - \frac{1}{2v_0^2} \text{ or } \frac{1}{2v_0^2} - \frac{1}{2v^2} = -kt$$

$$\text{or } \left[\frac{1}{2v_0^2} + kt\right] = \frac{1}{2v^2} \text{ or } \left[1 + 2v_0^2\,kt\right] = \frac{v_0^2}{v^2}$$

$$\text{or } v^2 = \frac{v_0^2}{1 + 2v_0^2\,kt} \text{ or } v = \frac{v_0}{\sqrt{1 + 2v_0^2\,kt}}$$

12. (c) We know that, $v = \frac{dx}{dt} \Rightarrow dx = v\,dt$

Integrating, $\int_0^x dx = \int_0^t v\,dt$

or $x = \int_0^t (v_0 + gt + ft^2)\,dt$

$$= \left[v_0 t + \frac{gt^2}{2} + \frac{ft^3}{3}\right]_0^t$$

or, $x = v_0 t + \frac{gt^2}{2} + \frac{ft^3}{3}$

At $t = 1$, $x = v_0 + \frac{g}{2} + \frac{f}{3}$.

13. (c) Let man will catch the bus after 't' sec. So he will cover distance ut.

Similarly, distance travelled by the bus will be $\frac{1}{2}at^2$

For the given condition

$ut = 45 + \frac{1}{2}at^2 = 45 + 1.25t^2$ [As a = 2.5 m/s²]

$\Rightarrow u = \frac{45}{t} + 1.25t$

To find the minimum value of u $\frac{du}{dt} = 0$

so we get t = 6 sec then,

$u = \frac{45}{6} + 1.25 \times 6 = 7.5 + 7.5 = 15$ m/s

14. (b) For the body starting from rest

$x_1 = 0 + \frac{1}{2}at^2$

$\Rightarrow x_1 = \frac{1}{2}at^2$

For the body moving with constant speed

$x_2 = vt$

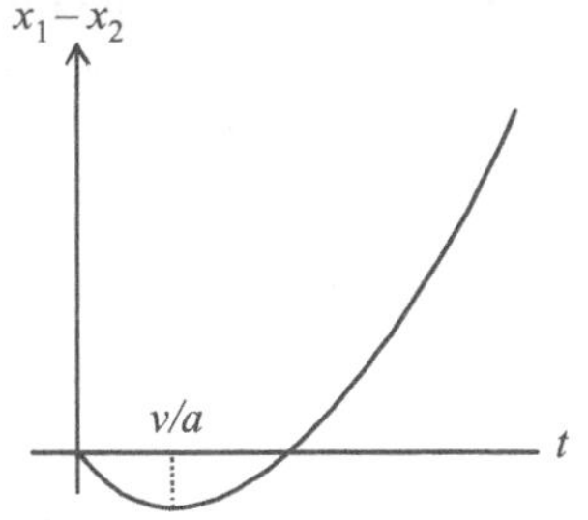

$\therefore\ x_1 - x_2 = \frac{1}{2}at^2 - vt$

at $t = 0, x_1 - x_2 = 0$

For $t < \frac{v}{a}$; the slope is negative

For $t = \frac{v}{a}$; the slope is zero

For $t > \frac{v}{a}$; the slope is positive

These characteristics are represented by graph (b).

15. (d) The stone reaches its maximum height after time t_1 given by

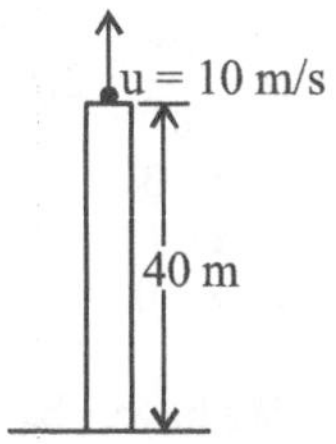

$t_1 = \frac{u}{g}$ ($\because v = u - gt$)

$= \frac{10}{10} = 1$ sec

Again it reaches to its initial position in 1 sec and falls with same initial speed of 10 m/s.

Let t_2 be the time taken to reach the ground, then

$v_{ground} = u + gt_2$

But $v_{ground}^2 = u^2 + 2gh$

$= (10)^2 + 2 \times 10 \times 40 = 900$

$\Rightarrow v_{ground} = \sqrt{900} = 30$ m/s

$\therefore\ t_2 = \frac{v_{ground} - u}{g} = \frac{30 - 10}{10} = 2$ sec.

$\therefore$ Total required time $= (1 + 1 + 2)$ sec $= 4$ sec

16. (b)

$$L = \frac{1}{2}gt^2 - \frac{1}{2}g(t - T)^2$$

$$\Rightarrow t = \frac{T}{2} + \frac{L}{gt}.$$

17. (b) $S = AB = \frac{1}{2}g t_1^2 \Rightarrow 2S = AC = \frac{1}{2}g(t_1 + t_2)^2$

and $3S = AD = \frac{1}{2}g(t_1 + t_2 + t_3)^2$

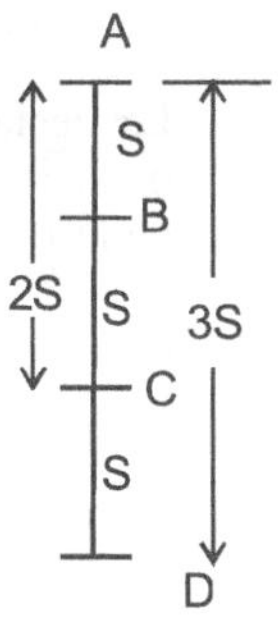

$t_1 = \sqrt{\frac{2S}{g}}$

$t_1 + t_2 = \sqrt{\frac{4S}{g}}$, $t_2 = \sqrt{\frac{4S}{g}} - \sqrt{\frac{2S}{g}}$

$t_1 + t_2 + t_3 = \sqrt{\frac{6S}{g}}$

$t_3 = \sqrt{\frac{6S}{g}} - \sqrt{\frac{4S}{g}}$

$t_1 : t_2 : t_3 :: 1 : (\sqrt{2} - 1) : (\sqrt{3} - \sqrt{2})$

18. (c) Height of tap = 5m and (g) = 10 m/sec².

For the first drop,

$5 = ut + \frac{1}{2}gt^2 = (0 \times t) + \frac{1}{2} \times 10t^2 = 5t^2$ or $t^2 = 1$ or $t = 1$.

It means that the third drop leaves after one second of the first drop. Or, each drop leaves after every 0.5 sec. Distance covered by the second drop in 0.5 sec

$= ut + \frac{1}{2}gt^2 = (0 \times 0.5) + \frac{1}{2} \times 10 = (0.5)^2 = 1.25m$.

Therefore, distance of the second drop above the ground $= 5 - 1.25 = 3.75$ m.

19. (c) $\because t = \sqrt{x} + 3$

$\Rightarrow \sqrt{x} = t - 3 \Rightarrow x = (t-3)^2$

$v = \frac{dx}{dt} = 2(t-3) = 0$

$\Rightarrow t = 3$

$\therefore x = (3-3)^2$

$\Rightarrow x = 0.$

20. (c) We have, $S_n = u + \frac{a}{2}(2n-1)$

or $65 = u + \frac{a}{2}(2 \times 5 - 1)$

or $65 = u + \frac{9}{2}a$ .....(1)

Also, $105 = u + \frac{a}{2}(2 \times 9 - 1)$

or $105 = u + \frac{17}{2}a$ .....(2)

Equation (2) – (1) gives,

$40 = \frac{17}{2}a - \frac{9}{2}a = 4a$ or $a = 10\ m/s^2$.

Substitute this value in (1) we get,

$u = 65 - \frac{9}{2} \times 10 = 65 - 45 = 20\ m/s$

$\therefore$ The distance travelled by the body in 20 s is,

$s = ut + \frac{1}{2}at^2 = 20 \times 20 + \frac{1}{2} \times 10 \times (20)^2$

$= 400 + 2000 = 2400$ m.

21. (d) Speed, $u = 60 \times \frac{5}{18}\ m/s = \frac{50}{3}\ m/s$

$d = 20m,\ u' = 120 \times \frac{5}{18} = \frac{100}{3}\ m/s$

Let declaration be a then $(0)^2 - u^2 = -2ad$

or $u^2 = 2ad$ ...(1)

and $(0)^2 - u'^2 = -2ad'$

or $u'^2 = 2ad'$ ...(2)

(2) divided by (1) gives,

$4 = \frac{d'}{d} \Rightarrow d' = 4 \times 20 = 80m$

22. (b) $8 = a\,t_1$ and $0 = 8 - a\,(4 - t_1)$

or $t_1 = \frac{8}{a}\ \therefore\ 8 = a\left(4 - \frac{8}{a}\right)$

$8 = 4a - 8$ or $a = 4$ and $t_1 = 8/4 = 2$ sec

Now, $s_1 = 0 \times 2 + \frac{1}{2} \times 4(2)^2$ or $s_1 = 8\,m$

$s_2 = 8 \times 2 - \frac{1}{2} \times 4 \times (2)^2$ or $s_2 = 8\,m$

$\therefore\ s_1 + s_2 = 16$ m

23. (d)

24. (a) $x = \frac{1}{t+5}$

$\therefore\ v = \frac{dx}{dt} = \frac{-1}{(t+5)^2}$

$\therefore\ a = \frac{d^2x}{dt^2} = \frac{2}{(t+5)^3} = 2x^3$

Now $\frac{1}{(t+5)} \propto v^{\frac{1}{2}}$

$\therefore\ \frac{1}{(t+5)^3} \propto v^{\frac{3}{2}} \propto a$

25. (d)

B (v = 0)
4 sec | 4 sec
(2 sec) A | C
(t = 0) D

As the time taken from D to A = 2 sec.
and D → A → B → C = 10 sec (given).
As ball goes from B → C (u = 0, t = 4 sec)
$v_c = 0 + 4g$.

As it moves from C to D, $s = ut + \frac{1}{2}gt^2$

$s = 4g \times 2 + \frac{1}{2}g \times 4 = 10$ g.

26. (d) $y = \frac{1}{2}g(n+1)^2 - \frac{1}{2}gn^2$

$= \frac{g}{2}[(n+1)^2 - n^2] = \frac{g}{2}(2n+1)$ ......(i)

Also, $h = \frac{g}{2}(2n-1)$ ......(ii)

From (i) and (ii)

$y = h + g$

27. (b) The stone rises up till its vertical velocity is zero and again reached the top of the tower with a speed u (downward). The speed of the stone at the base is 3u.

u ↑ –
+ ↓ v, g, h

Hence $(3u)^2 = (-u)^2 + 2gh$ or $h = \frac{4u^2}{g}$

28. **(b)** $x = 40 + 12t - t^3$

$$v = \frac{dx}{dt} = 12 - 3t^2$$

For $v = 0$; $t = \sqrt{\frac{12}{3}} = 2$ sec

So, after 2 seconds velocity becomes zero.
Value of x in 2 secs $= 40 + 12 \times 2 - 2^3$
$= 40 + 24 - 8 = 56$ m

29. **(b)** The slope of v-t graph is constant and velocity decreasing for first half. It is positive and constant over next half.

30. **(c)** Here, $f = f_0\left(1 - \frac{t}{T}\right)$ or, $\frac{dv}{dt} = f_0\left(1 - \frac{t}{T}\right)$

or, $dv = f_0\left(1 - \frac{t}{T}\right) dt$

$$\therefore v = \int dv = \int \left[f_0\left(1 - \frac{t}{T}\right)\right] dt$$

or, $v = f_0\left(t - \frac{t^2}{2T}\right) + C$

where C is the constant of integration.
At $t = 0$, $v = 0$.

$$\therefore 0 = f_0\left(0 - \frac{0}{2T}\right) + C \Rightarrow C = 0$$

$$\therefore v = f_0\left(t - \frac{t^2}{2T}\right)$$

If $f = 0$, then

$$0 = f_0\left(1 - \frac{t}{T}\right) \Rightarrow t = T$$

Hence, particle's velocity in the time interval $t = 0$ and $t = T$ is given by

$$v_x = \int_{t=0}^{t=T} dv = \int_{t=0}^{T} \left[f_0\left(1 - \frac{t}{T}\right)\right] dt$$

$$= f_0\left[\left(t - \frac{t^2}{2T}\right)\right]_0^T$$

$$= f_0\left(T - \frac{T^2}{2T}\right) = f_0\left(T - \frac{T}{2}\right)$$

$$= \frac{1}{2} f_0 T.$$

31. **(a)** Using $v^2 = u^2 - 2gh$ i.e., $h = \frac{u^2 - v^2}{2g}$,

$$AB = \frac{\left(\frac{u}{2}\right)^2 - \left(\frac{u}{3}\right)^2}{2g}$$

and $BC = \frac{\left(\frac{u}{3}\right)^2 - \left(\frac{u}{4}\right)^2}{2g}$

C	u/4 ↑
B	u/3 ↑
A	u/2 ↑
O	u ↑

$$\therefore \frac{AB}{BC} = \frac{\left(\frac{u}{2}\right)^2 - \left(\frac{u}{3}\right)^2}{\left(\frac{u}{3}\right)^2 - \left(\frac{u}{4}\right)^2} = \frac{\left(\frac{1}{2}\right)^2 - \left(\frac{1}{3}\right)^2}{\left(\frac{1}{3}\right)^2 - \left(\frac{1}{4}\right)^2} = \frac{20}{7}$$

32. **(a)** Velocity of boat $= \frac{8+8}{2} = 8\,\text{km h}^{-1}$

Velocity of water $= 4\,\text{km h}^{-1}$

$$t = \frac{8}{8-4} + \frac{8}{8+4} = \frac{8}{3}\text{h} = 160 \text{ minutes}$$

33. **(b)** $v_{av} = \frac{x + 2x + 3x}{t_1 + t_2 + t_3}$

$t_1 = \frac{2x}{v_{max}}$, $t_2 = \frac{2x}{v_{max}}$, $t_3 = \frac{6x}{v_{max}}$

$$v_{av} = \frac{6x\, v_{max}}{10x}$$

$$\frac{v_{av}}{v_{max}} = \frac{3}{5}$$

34. **(b)** No external force is acting, therefore,
$50u + 0.5 \times 2 = 0$
where u is the velocity of man.

$$u = -\frac{1}{50}\,\text{ms}^{-1}$$

Negative sign of u shows that man moves upward.
Time taken by the stone to reach the ground

$$= \frac{10}{2} = 5\text{S}$$

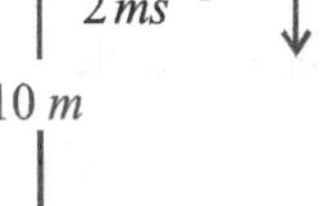

Distance moved by the man

$$= 5 \times \frac{1}{50} = 0.1\text{m}$$

$\therefore$ when the stone reaches the floor, the distance of the man above floor = 10.1 m

35. **(a)** Use $\vec{v}_{AB} = \vec{v}_A - \vec{v}_B$.

36. **(c)** Downward motion

$$v^2 - 0^2 = 2 \times 9.8 \times 5$$

$\Rightarrow v=\sqrt{98}=9.9$

Also for upward motion

$0^2-u^2=2\times(-9.8)\times 1.8$

$\Rightarrow u=\sqrt{3528}=5.94$

Fractional loss $=\dfrac{9.9-5.94}{9.9}=0.4$

37. **(c)** Distance travelled by the stone in the last second is

$\dfrac{9h}{25}=\dfrac{g}{2}(2t-1)\quad (\because u=0)$ ...(i)

Distance travelled by the stone in t s is

$h=\dfrac{1}{2}gt^2\quad$ (using $s=ut+\dfrac{1}{2}at^2$) ...(ii)

Divide (i) by (ii), we get

$\dfrac{9}{25}=\dfrac{(2t-1)}{t^2}$

$9t^2=50t-25,\ 9t^2-50t+25=0$

Solving, we get

$t=5s$ or $t=\dfrac{5}{9}s$

Substituting $t=5s$ in (ii), we get

$h=\dfrac{1}{2}\times 9.8\times(5)^2=122.5\text{ m}$

38. **(b)** $y\propto t^2; v\text{-}\propto t'; a\propto t^{\circ}$

39. **(b)** Average velocity for the second half of the distance is

$=\dfrac{v_1+v_2}{2}=\dfrac{4+8}{2}=6\,ms^{-1}$

Given that first half distance is covered with a velocity of $6ms^{-1}$. Therefore, the average velocity for the whole time of motion is $6ms^{-1}$

40. **(b)** Bullet will take $\dfrac{100}{1000}=0.1$ sec to reach target.

During this period vertical distance (downward) travelled by the bullet

$=\dfrac{1}{2}gt^2=\dfrac{1}{2}\times 10\times(0.1)^2=0.05\text{m}=5\text{cm}$

So the gun should be aimed 5 cm above the target.

41. **(c)** The distance covered in n^{th} second is

$S_n=u+\dfrac{1}{2}(2n-1)a$

where u is initial velocity & a is acceleration

then $26=u+\dfrac{19a}{2}$ ....(1)

$28=u+\dfrac{21a}{2}$ ....(2)

$30=u+\dfrac{23a}{2}$ ....(3)

$32=u+\dfrac{25a}{2}$ ....(4)

From eqs. (1) and (2) we get u = 7m/sec, a=2m/sec^2

$\therefore$ The body starts with initial velocity u =7m/sec and moves with uniform acceleration a = 2m/sec^2

42. **(a)** $8=\dfrac{x}{t_1},\ 12=\dfrac{x}{t_2}$

$\bar{v}=\dfrac{2x}{t_1+t_2}=\dfrac{2x}{\dfrac{x}{8}+\dfrac{x}{12}}=\dfrac{2\times 8\times 12}{12+8}=9.6\text{ ms}^{-1}$

43. **(b)** Distance = Area under v – t graph $=A_1+A_2+A_3+A_4$

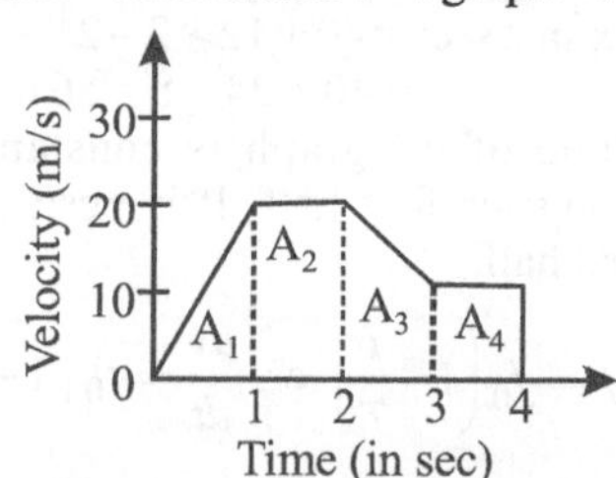

$=\dfrac{1}{2}\times 1\times 20+(20\times 1)+\dfrac{1}{2}(20+10)\times 1+(10\times 1)$

$=10+20+15+10=55\text{ m}$

44. **(a)** $\because\ h=\dfrac{1}{2}gt^2$

$\therefore\ h_1=\dfrac{1}{2}g(5)^2=125$

$h_1+h_2=\dfrac{1}{2}g(10)^2=500$

$\Rightarrow h_2=375$

$h_1+h_2+h_3=\dfrac{1}{2}g(15)^2=1125$

$\Rightarrow h_3=625$

$h_2=3h_1,\ h_3=5h_1$

or $h_1=\dfrac{h_2}{3}=\dfrac{h_3}{5}$

45. **(d)** Distance from A to $B=S=\dfrac{1}{2}ft_1^2$

Distance from B to $C=(ft_1)t$

Distance from C to $D=\dfrac{u^2}{2a}=\dfrac{(ft_1)^2}{2(f/2)}=ft_1^2=2S$

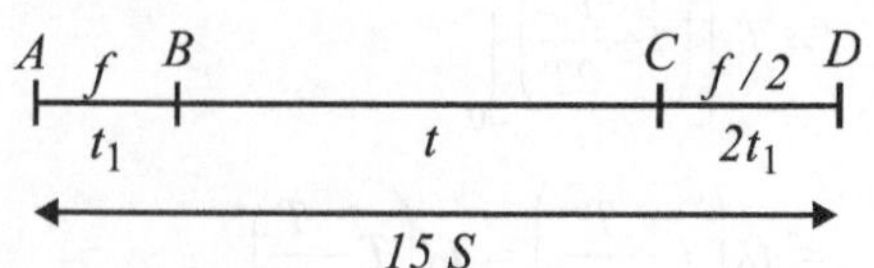

$\Rightarrow S+ft_1t+2S=15S$

$\Rightarrow ft_1t=12S$ .... (i)

$\dfrac{1}{2}ft_1^2=S$ .... (ii)

Dividing (i) by (ii), we get $t_1=\dfrac{t}{6}$

$\Rightarrow S=\dfrac{1}{2}f\left(\dfrac{t}{6}\right)^2=\dfrac{ft^2}{72}$

Speed Test-3

1. **(b)** $\vec{u} = \hat{i} + 2\hat{j} = u_x\hat{i} + u_y\hat{j} \Rightarrow u\cos\theta = 1,\ u\sin\theta = 2$

$$y = x\tan\theta - \frac{1}{2}\frac{gx^2}{u_x^2}$$

$$\therefore\ y = 2x - \frac{1}{2}gx^2 = 2x - 5x^2$$

2. **(c)** $500\cos\theta = 250 \Rightarrow \cos\theta = \frac{1}{2}$

or $\theta = 60°$.

3. **(c)** As time periods are equal therefore ratio of angular speeds will be 1 : 1. $\left(\omega = \frac{2\pi}{T}\right)$.

4. **(d)**

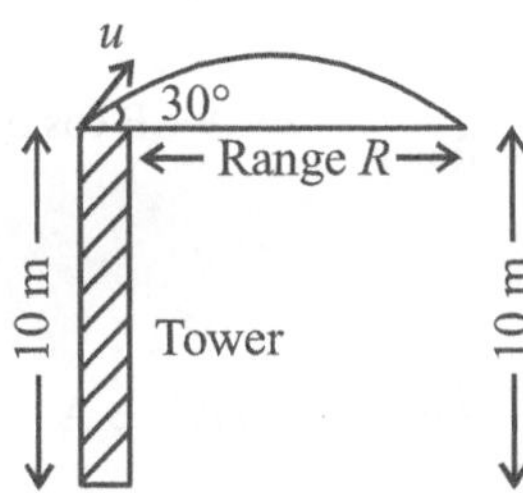

From the figure it is clear that range is required

$$R = \frac{u^2\sin 2\theta}{g} = \frac{(10)^2\sin(2\times 30°)}{10} = 5\sqrt{3} = 8.66\text{ m}$$

5. **(a)** Horizontal component of velocity $v_x = 500$ m/s and vertical component of velocity while striking the ground.

$u_v = 0 + 10 \times 10 = 100$ m/s

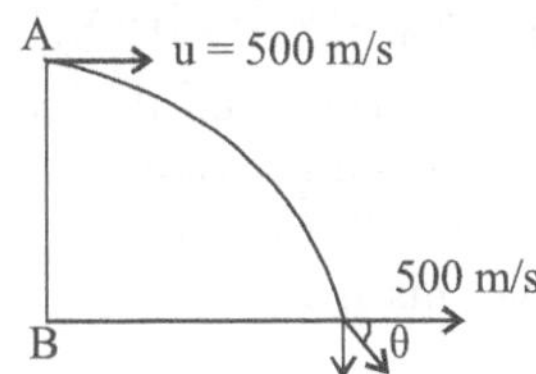

$\therefore$ Angle with which it strikes the ground

$$\theta = \tan^{-1}\left(\frac{u_v}{u_x}\right) = \tan^{-1}\left(\frac{100}{500}\right) = \tan^{-1}\left(\frac{1}{5}\right)$$

6. **(b)**

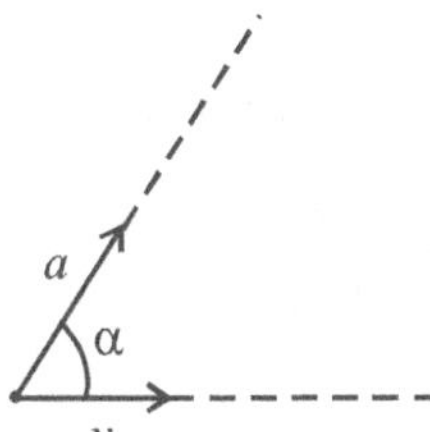

The velocity of first particle, $v_1 = v$

The velocity of second particle, $v_2 = at$

Relative velocity, $\vec{v}_{12} = \vec{v}_1 - \vec{v}_2$

or $v_{12}^2 = v^2 + (at)^2 - 2v(at\cos\alpha)$

For least value of relative velocity, $\frac{dv_{12}}{dt} = 0$

or $\frac{d}{dt}\left[v^2 + a^2t^2 - 2vat\cos\alpha\right] = 0$

or $0 + a^2 \times 2t - 2va\cos\alpha = 0$

or $t = \frac{v\cos\alpha}{a}$

7. **(d)** $t = \frac{2u\sin 30°}{g\cos 30°} = \frac{2(10)(1/2)}{10(\sqrt{3}/2)} = \frac{2}{\sqrt{3}}$ sec

$$R = 10\cos 30°\, t - \frac{1}{2}\, g\sin 30°\, t^2$$

$$= \frac{10\sqrt{3}}{2}\left(\frac{2}{\sqrt{3}}\right) - \frac{1}{2}(10)\left(\frac{1}{2}\right)\frac{4}{3} = 10 - \frac{10}{3} = \frac{20}{3}\text{ m}$$

8. **(b)** $\overline{AB} = (4\hat{i} + 5\hat{j} + 6\hat{k}) - (3\hat{i} + 4\hat{j} + 5\hat{k}) = \hat{i} + \hat{j} + \hat{k}$

$\overline{CD} = (4\hat{i} + 6\hat{j}) - (7\hat{i} + 9\hat{j} + 3\hat{k}) = 3\hat{i} - 3\hat{j} + 3\hat{k}$

$\overline{AB}$ and $\overline{CD}$ are parallel, because its cross-product is 0.

9. **(c)** Here v = 0.5 m/sec. u = ?

so $\sin\theta = \frac{u}{v} \Rightarrow \frac{u}{.5} = \frac{1}{2}$ or $u = 0.25\text{ ms}^{-1}$

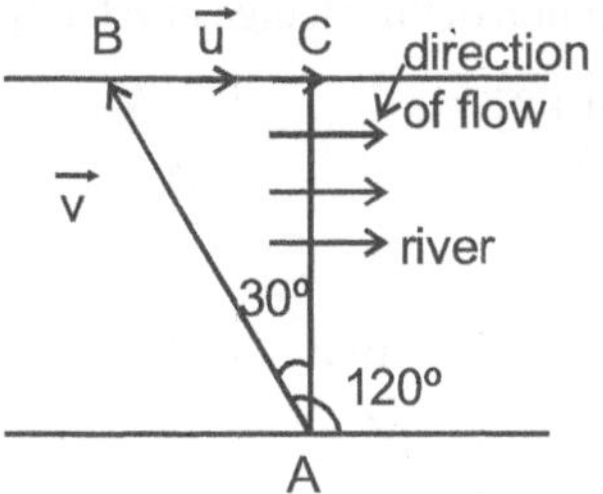

10. **(d)** Max. height = $H = \frac{v^2\sin^2(90-\theta)}{2g}$ .....(i)

Time of flight, $T = \frac{2v\sin(90-\theta)}{g}$ ...(ii)

From (i), $\frac{v\cos\theta}{g} = \sqrt{\frac{2H}{g}}$

From (ii), $T = 2\sqrt{\frac{2H}{g}} = \sqrt{\frac{8H}{g}}$

Vertical
v
θ
Horizontal

11. (c) Yes, the person can catch the ball when horizontal velocity is equal to the horizontal component of ball's velocity, the motion of ball will be only in vertical direction with respect to person for that,

$$\frac{v_o}{2} = v_o \cos\theta \text{ or } \theta = 60°$$

12. (b) Two vectors are

$\vec{A} = \cos\omega t\hat{i} + \sin\omega t\hat{j}$

$\vec{B} = \cos\frac{\omega t}{2}\hat{i} + \sin\frac{\omega t}{2}\hat{j}$

For two vectors $\vec{A}$ and $\vec{B}$ to be orthogonal A.B = 0

$\vec{A}.\vec{B} = 0 = \cos\omega t.\cos\frac{\omega t}{2} + \sin\omega t.\sin\frac{\omega t}{2}$

$= \cos\left(\omega t - \frac{\omega t}{2}\right) = \cos\left(\frac{\omega t}{2}\right)$

So, $\frac{\omega t}{2} = \frac{\pi}{2}$ $\quad\therefore t = \frac{\pi}{\omega}$

13. (a) $\vec{v_1} = 50 \text{ km h}^{-1}$ due North;

$\vec{v_2} = 50 \text{ km h}^{-1}$ due West. Angle between $\vec{v_1}$ and $\vec{v_2} = 90°$

$-\vec{v_1} = 50 \text{ km h}^{-1}$ due South

∴ Change in velocity

$= |\vec{v_2} - \vec{v_1}| = |\vec{v_2} + (-\vec{v_1})|$

$= \sqrt{v_2^2 + v_1^2} = \sqrt{50^2 + 50^2} = 70.7$ km/h

The direction of this change in velocity is in South-West.

14. (b) $\vec{v} = 6\hat{i} + 8\hat{j}$

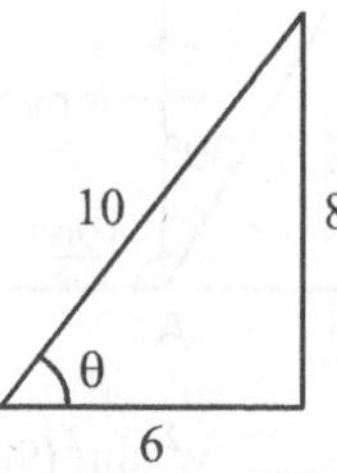

Comparing with $\vec{v} = v_x\hat{i} + v_y\hat{j}$, we get

$v_x = 6\text{ms}^{-1}$ and $v_y = 8 \text{ ms}^{-1}$

Also, $v^2 = v_x^2 + v_y^2 = 36 + 64 = 100$

or $v = 10 \text{ ms}^{-1}$

$\sin\theta = \frac{8}{10}$ and $\cos\theta = \frac{6}{10}$

$R = \frac{v^2 \sin 2\theta}{g} = \frac{2v^2 \sin\theta\cos\theta}{g}$

$R = 2 \times 10 \times 10 \times \frac{8}{10} \times \frac{6}{10} \times \frac{1}{10} = 9.6$ m

15. (d) $s = t^3 + 5$

$\Rightarrow$ velocity, $v = \frac{ds}{dt} = 3t^2$

Tangential acceleration $a_t = \frac{dv}{dt} = 6t$

Radial acceleration $a_c = \frac{v^2}{R} = \frac{9t^4}{R}$

At $t = 2s$, $a_t = 6 \times 2 = 12$ m/s²

$a_c = \frac{9 \times 16}{20} = 7.2$ m/s²

∴ Resultant acceleration

$= \sqrt{a_t^2 + a_c^2} = \sqrt{(12)^2 + (7.2)^2} = \sqrt{144 + 51.84}$

$= \sqrt{195.84} = 14$ m/s²

16. (b) $\frac{B}{2} = \sqrt{A^2 + B^2 + 2AB\cos\theta}$ ...... (i)

$\therefore \quad \tan 90° = \frac{B\sin\theta}{A + B\cos\theta} \Rightarrow A + B\cos\theta = 0$

$\therefore \quad \cos\theta = -\frac{A}{B}$

Hence, from (i) $\frac{B^2}{A} = A^2 + B^2 - 2A^2 \Rightarrow A = \sqrt{3}\frac{B}{2}$

$\Rightarrow \cos\theta = -\frac{A}{B} = -\frac{\sqrt{3}}{2} \quad \therefore \theta = 150°$

17. (b) Suppose velocity of rain

$\vec{v}_R = v_x\hat{i} - v_y\hat{j}$

and the velocity of the man

$\vec{v}_m = u\hat{i}$

∴ Velocity of rain relative to man

$\vec{v}_{Rm} = \vec{v}_R - \vec{v}_m = (v_x - u)\hat{i} - v_y\hat{j}$

According to given condition that rain appears to fall vertically, so $(v_x - u)$ must be zero.

∴ $v_x - u = 0$ or $v_x = u$

When he doubles his speed,

$\vec{v}'_m = 2u\hat{i}$

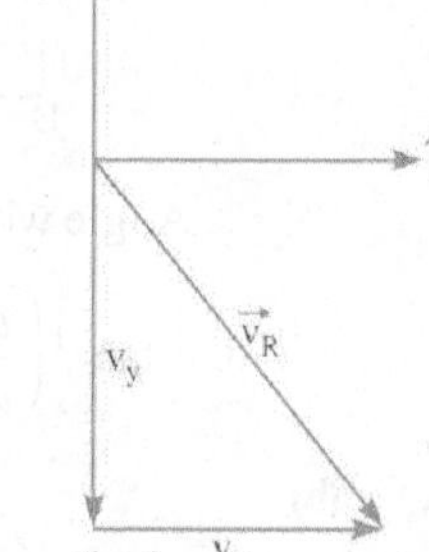

Now $\vec{v}_{Rm} = \vec{v}_R - \vec{v}'_m$

$= (v_x\hat{i} - v_y\hat{j}) - (2u\hat{i})$

$= (v_x - 2u)\hat{i} - v_y\hat{j}$

The $\vec{v}_{Rm}$ makes an angle θ with the vertical

$\tan\theta = \frac{x - \text{componend of } \vec{v}_{Rm}}{y - \text{componend of } \vec{v}_{Rm}}$

$= \frac{(v_x - 2u)}{-v_y}$

$= \frac{u - 2u}{-v_y}$

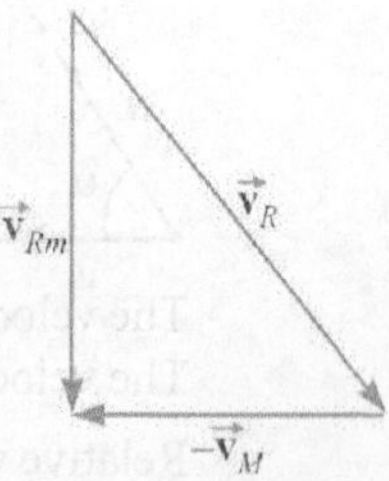

which gives

$$v_y = \frac{u}{\tan\theta}$$

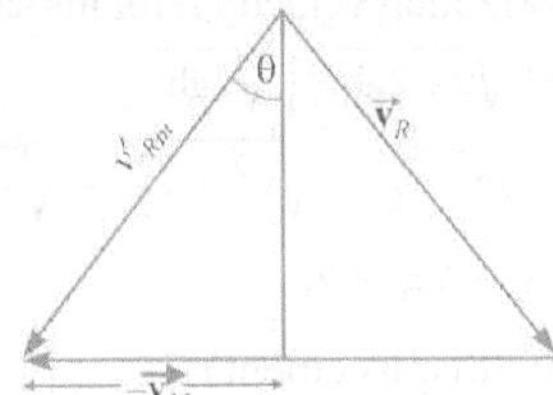

Thus the velocity of rain

$$\vec{\mathbf{v}}_R = v_x\hat{\mathbf{i}} - v_y\hat{\mathbf{i}}$$

$$= u\hat{\mathbf{i}} - \frac{u}{\tan\theta}\hat{\mathbf{j}}.$$

18. **(c)** For projectile A

Maximum height, $H_A = \dfrac{u_A^2 \sin^2 45°}{2g}$

For projectile B

Maximum height, $H_B = \dfrac{u_B^2 \sin^2 \theta}{2g}$

As we know, $H_A = H_B$

$$\frac{u_A^2 \sin^2 45°}{2g} = \frac{u_B^2 \sin^2 \theta}{2g}$$

$$\frac{\sin^2\theta}{\sin^2 45°} = \frac{u_A^2}{u_B^2}$$

$$\sin^2\theta = \left(\frac{u_A}{u_B}\right)^2 \sin^2 45°$$

$$\sin^2\theta = \left(\frac{1}{\sqrt{2}}\right)^2\left(\frac{1}{\sqrt{2}}\right)^2 = \frac{1}{4}$$

$$\sin\theta = \frac{1}{2} \Rightarrow \theta = \sin^{-1}\left(\frac{1}{2}\right) = 30°$$

19. **(a)** The angle for which the ranges are same is complementary.
Let one angle be θ, then other is $90° - \theta$

$$T_1 = \frac{2u\sin\theta}{g}, T_2 = \frac{2u\cos\theta}{g}$$

$$T_1T_2 = \frac{4u^2\sin\theta\cos\theta}{g} = 2R \quad \left(\because R = \frac{u^2\sin^2\theta}{g}\right)$$

Hence it is proportional to R.

20. **(c)** When particle thrown in vertically downward direction with velocity u then final velocity at the ground level

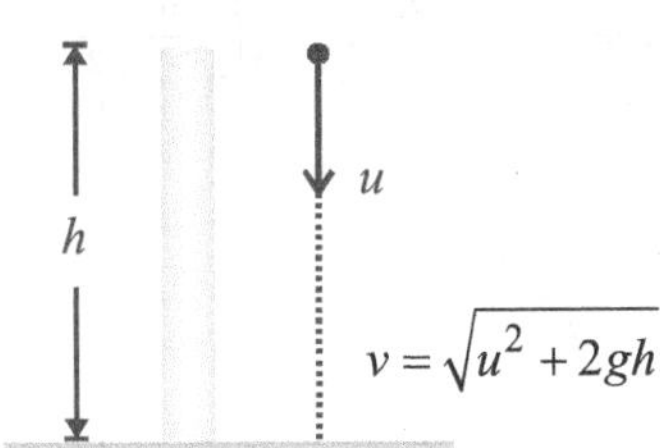

$$v^2 = u^2 + 2gh \;\therefore\; v = \sqrt{u^2 + 2gh}$$

Another particle is thrown horizontally with same velocity then velocity of particle at the surface of earth.

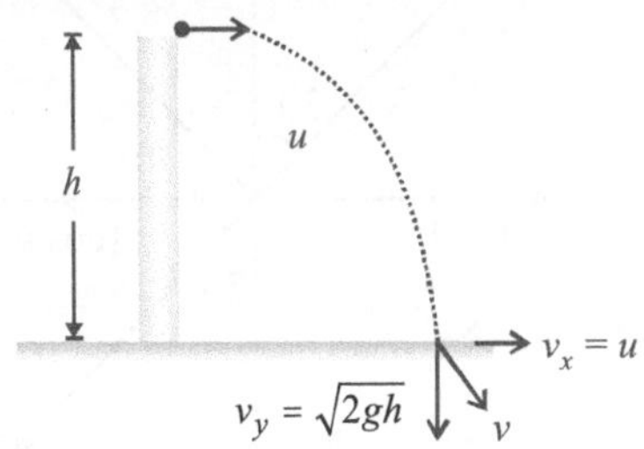

Horizontal component of velocity $v_x = u$

$\therefore$ Resultant velocity, $v = \sqrt{u^2 + 2gh}$

For both the particles, final velocities when they reach the earth's surface are equal.

21. **(b)** $\hat{r} = 0.5\hat{i} + 0.8\hat{j} + c\hat{k}$

$$|\hat{r}| = 1 = \sqrt{(0.5)^2 + (0.8)^2 + c^2}$$

$$(0.5)^2 + (0.8)^2 + c^2 = 1$$

$$c^2 = 0.11 \Rightarrow c = \sqrt{0.11}$$

22. **(c)** The pilot will see the ball falling in straight line because the reference frame is moving with the same horizontal velocity but the observer at rest will see the ball falling in parabolic path.

23. **(a)** R = 2H (given)

We know, $R = 4H\cot\theta \Rightarrow \cot\theta = \dfrac{1}{2}$

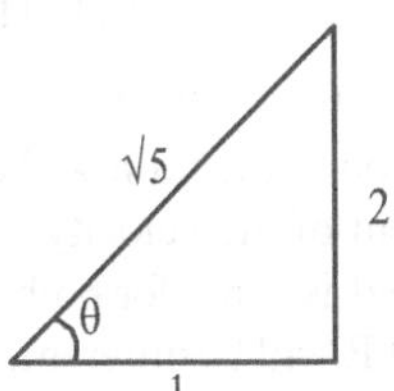

From triangle we can say that $\sin\theta = \dfrac{2}{\sqrt{5}}, \cos\theta = \dfrac{1}{\sqrt{5}}$

$\therefore$ Range of projectile $R = \dfrac{2v^2\sin\theta\cos\theta}{g}$

$$= \frac{2v^2}{g} \times \frac{2}{\sqrt{5}} \times \frac{1}{\sqrt{5}} = \frac{4v^2}{5g}$$

24. **(a)** Note that the given angles of projection add upto 90°. For complementary angles of projection $(45° + \alpha)$ and $(45° - \alpha)$ with same initial velocity u, range R is same.

$$\theta_1 + \theta_2 = (45° + \alpha) + (45° - \alpha) = 90°$$

So, the ratio of horizontal ranges is 1 : 1.

25. **(a)** The components of 1 N and 2N forces along + x axis = 1 cos 60° + 2 sin 30°

$$= 1 \times \frac{1}{2} + 2 \times \frac{1}{2} = \frac{1}{2} + 1 = \frac{3}{2} = 1.5\text{N}$$

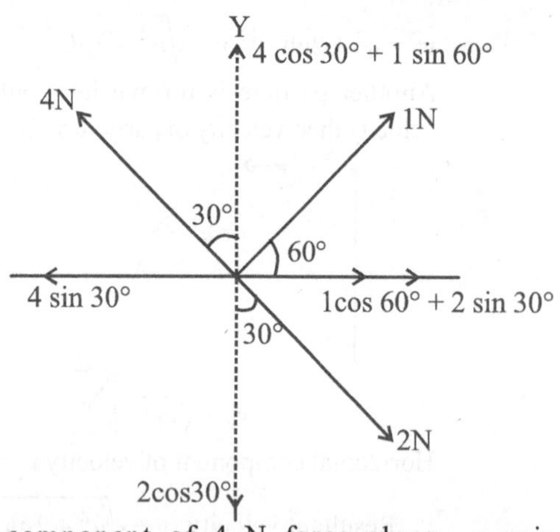

The component of 4 N force along –x-axis $= 4 \sin 30° = 4 \times \frac{1}{2} = 2\text{N}$.

Therefore, if a force of 0.5N is applied along + x-axis, the resultant force along x-axis will become zero and the resultant force will be obtained only along y-axis.

26. **(d)** $F_x = \frac{dp_x}{dt} = -2\sin\theta.$

Similarly, $F_y = \frac{dp_y}{dx} = 2\cos\theta.$

Angle θ between two vectors

$$\cos\theta = \frac{F_x p_x + F_y p_y}{|\vec{F}||\vec{p}|}$$

$$= \frac{(-2\sin\theta)(2\cos\theta) + (2\cos\theta)(2\sin\theta)}{|\vec{F}||\vec{p}|}$$

$$\Rightarrow \cos\theta = 0 \Rightarrow \theta = 90°$$

27. **(a)** The motion of the train will affect only the horizontal component of the velocity of the ball. Since, vertical component is same for both observers, the y_m will be same, but R will be different.

28. **(d)** As body covers equal angle in equal time intervals. Its angular velocity and hence magnitude of linear velocity is constant.

29. **(a)** **For A:** It goes up with velocity u will it reaches its maximum height (i.e. velocity becomes zero) and comes back to O and attains velocity u.

Using $v^2 = u^2 + 2as \Rightarrow v_A = \sqrt{u^2 + 2gh}$

u
O
$u = v_x$
u
h
v_B v_A
$u = v_x$ $V_c = \sqrt{v_x^2 + v_y^2}$
v_C

For B, going down with velocity u

$$\Rightarrow v_B = \sqrt{u^2 + 2gh}$$

For C, horizontal velocity remains same, i.e. u. Vertical velocity $= \sqrt{0 + 2gh} = \sqrt{2gh}$

The resultant $v_C = \sqrt{v_x^2 + v_y^2} = \sqrt{u^2 + 2gh}$.

Hence $v_A = v_B = v_C$

30. **(d)** $\vec{v}_{av} = \frac{\Delta\vec{r}\text{ (displacement)}}{\Delta t\text{ (time taken)}}$

$$= \frac{(13-2)\hat{i} + (14-3)\hat{j}}{5-0} = \frac{11}{5}(\hat{i} + \hat{j})$$

31. **(c)** Position vector

$\vec{r} = \cos wt\ \hat{x} + \sin\omega t\ \hat{y}$

$\therefore$ Velocity, $\vec{v} = -\omega\sin\omega t\ \hat{x} + \omega\cos\omega t\ \hat{y}$ and acceleration,

$\vec{a} = -\omega^2\cos\omega t\ \hat{x} + \omega\sin\omega t\ \hat{y} = -\omega 2\ \vec{r}$

$\vec{r} \cdot \vec{v} = 0$ hence $\vec{r} \perp \vec{v}$ and

$\vec{a}$ is directed towards the origin.

32. **(d)**

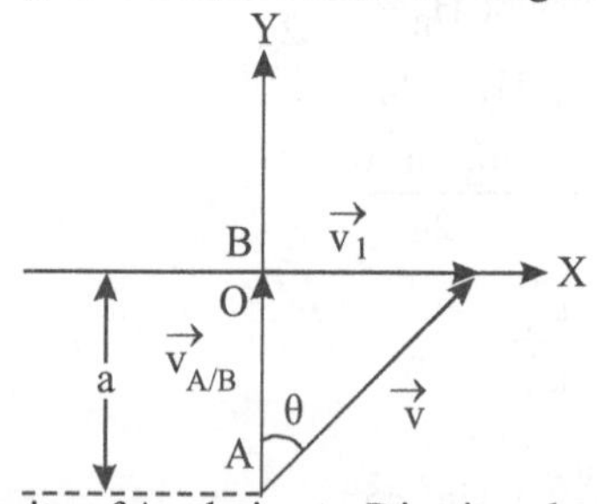

Velocity of A relative to *B* is given by

$$\vec{v}_{A/B} = \vec{v}_A - \vec{v}_B = \vec{v} - \vec{v}_1 \quad ....(1)$$

By taking x-components of equation (1), we get

$$0 = v\sin\theta - v_1 \Rightarrow \sin\theta = \frac{v_1}{v} \quad ....(2)$$

By taking *Y*-components of equation (1), we get

$$v_y = v\cos\theta \quad .....(3)$$

Time taken by boy at *A* to catch the boy at *B* is given by

$$t = \frac{\text{Relative displacement along Y - axis}}{\text{Relative velocity along Y - axis}}$$

$$= \frac{a}{v\cos\theta} = \frac{a}{v.\sqrt{1-\sin^2\theta}} = \frac{a}{v.\sqrt{1-\left(\frac{v_1}{v}\right)^2}}$$

[From equation (1)]

$$= \frac{a}{v.\sqrt{\frac{v^2 - v_1^2}{v^2}}} = \frac{a}{\sqrt{v^2 - v_1^2}} = \sqrt{\frac{a^2}{v^2 - v_1^2}}$$

33. **(b)** $H = \frac{u^2\sin^2 45°}{2g} = \frac{u^2}{4g}$ ...(1)

$$R = \frac{u^2 \sin 90°}{g} = \frac{u^2}{g}$$

$$\therefore \frac{R}{2} = \frac{u^2}{2g} \quad ...(2)$$

$$\therefore \tan\alpha = \frac{H}{R/2}$$

$$= \frac{\frac{u^2}{4g}}{\frac{u^2}{2g}} = \frac{1}{2} \qquad \therefore \alpha = \tan^{-1}\left(\frac{1}{2}\right)$$

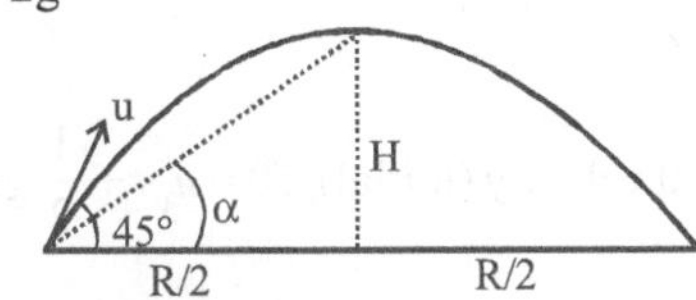

34. (b) Here, $x = 4\sin(2\pi t)$ ...(*i*)

$y = 4\cos(2\pi t)$ ...(*ii*)

Squaring and adding equation (*i*) and (*ii*)

$x^2 + y^2 = 4^2 \Rightarrow R = 4$

Motion of the particle is circular motion, acceleration vector is along $-\vec{R}$ and its magnitude $= \frac{v^2}{R}$

Velocity of particle, $v = \omega R = (2\pi)(4) = 8\pi$

35. (d) $|\vec{A}+\vec{B}|^2 = |\vec{A}-\vec{B}|^2$

$|\vec{A}+\vec{B}|^2 = |\vec{A}|^2 + |\vec{B}|^2 + 2\vec{A}.\vec{B} = A^2 + B^2 + 2AB\cos\theta$

$|\vec{A}-\vec{B}|^2 = |\vec{A}|^2 + |\vec{B}|^2 - 2\vec{A}.\vec{B}$

$= A^2 + B^2 - 2AB\cos\theta$

So, $A^2 + B^2 + 2AB\cos\theta$
$= A^2 + B^2 - 2AB\cos\theta$

$4AB\cos\theta = 0 \Rightarrow \cos\theta = 0$

$\therefore \theta = 90°$

So, angle between A & B is 90°.

36. (b) $\vec{v} = 6\hat{i} + 8\hat{j}$

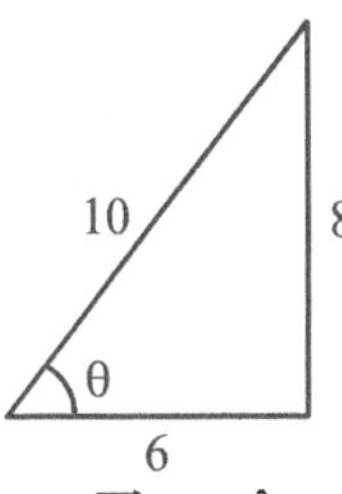

Comparing with $\vec{v} = v_x\hat{i} + v_y\hat{j}$, we get

$v_x = 6\,ms^{-1}$ and $v_y = 8\,ms^{-1}$

Also, $v^2 = v_x^2 + v_y^2 = 36 + 64 = 100$

or $v = 10\ ms^{-1}$

$\sin\theta = \frac{8}{10}$ and $\cos\theta = \frac{6}{10}$

$$R = \frac{v^2 \sin 2\theta}{g} = \frac{2v^2 \sin\theta\cos\theta}{g}$$

$$R = 2\times10\times10\times\frac{8}{10}\times\frac{6}{10}\times\frac{1}{10} = 9.6\,m$$

37. (a) Range of a projectile is maximum when it is projected at an angle of 45° and is given by

$R_{max} = \frac{u^2}{g}$, where u is the velocity of projection

$\Rightarrow R = \frac{u^2}{g} \qquad \therefore u^2 = Rg \quad ...(i)$

Now, to hit a target at a distance (R/2) from the gun, we must have

$\frac{R}{2} = \frac{u^2 \sin 2\theta}{g}$, where θ is the angle of projection.

$\Rightarrow \frac{R}{2} = \frac{Rg\sin 2\theta}{g}$; from (i)

$\Rightarrow \sin 2\theta = \frac{1}{2} \Rightarrow \sin 2\theta = \sin 30°$

$\Rightarrow 2\theta = 30° \quad \therefore \theta = 15°$

38. (a) Distance covered in one circular loop $= 2\pi r$
$= 2\times3.14\times100 = 628$ m

Speed $= \frac{628}{62.8} = 10$ m/sec

Displacement in one circular loop = 0

Velocity $= \frac{0}{\text{time}} = 0$

39. (a) $\overrightarrow{PQ} + \overrightarrow{QR} = \overrightarrow{PR}$

$\therefore \overrightarrow{QR} = \vec{b}' - \vec{b}$

R, $\vec{b}'$, θ, P, $\vec{b}$, Q

Now $|\vec{b}' - \vec{b}|^2 = (\vec{b}' - \vec{b}).(\vec{b}' - \vec{b})$

$= b'^2 - 2bb'\cos\theta + b^2$

$= 2b^2(1-\cos\theta) \qquad [\because b' = b]$

$\vec{b}' - \vec{b} = \sqrt{2}b\sqrt{1-\cos\theta}$

$= \sqrt{2}b\left(\sqrt{2}\sin\frac{\theta}{2}\right) = 2b\sin\frac{\theta}{2}$

40. (a) $H_1 = \frac{u^2\sin^2\theta}{2g}$

and $H_2 = \frac{u^2\sin^2(90°-\theta)}{2g} = \frac{u^2\cos^2\theta}{2g}$

$H_1H_2 = \frac{u^2\sin^2\theta}{2g}\times\frac{u^2\cos^2\theta}{2g} = \frac{(u^2\sin 2\theta)^2}{16g^2} = \frac{R^2}{16}$

$\therefore R = 4\sqrt{H_1H_2}$

41. (c) $\vec{P}$ = vector sum $= \vec{A} + \vec{B}$

$\vec{Q}$ = vector differences $= \vec{A} - \vec{B}$

Since $\vec{P}$ and $\vec{Q}$ are perpendicular

$\therefore \vec{P}.\vec{Q}=0$

$\Rightarrow (\vec{A}+\vec{B}).(\vec{A}-\vec{B})=0 \Rightarrow A^2=B^2 \Rightarrow |A|=|B|$

42. (b) $y=bx^2$

Differentiating w.r.t to t an both sides, we get

$$\frac{dy}{dx}=b2x\frac{dx}{dt}$$

$v_y=2bxv_x$

Again differentiating w.r.t to t on both sides we get

$$\frac{dv_y}{dt}=2bv_x\frac{dx}{dt}+2bx\frac{dv_x}{dt}=2bv_x^2+0$$

[$\frac{dv_x}{dt}=0$, because the particle has constant acceleration along y-direction]

Now, $\frac{dv_y}{dt}=a=2bv_x^2$;

$$v_x^2=\frac{a}{2b}$$

$$v_x=\sqrt{\frac{a}{2b}}$$

43. (a) Arc length = radius × angle

So, $|\vec{B}-\vec{A}|=|\vec{A}|\Delta\theta$

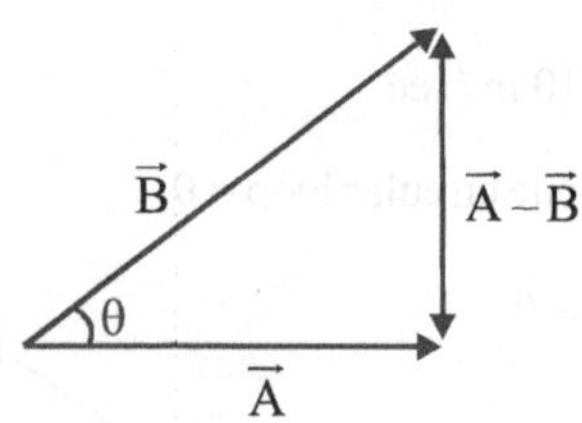

44. (c) Speed, V = constant (from question)

Centripetal acceleration,

$$a=\frac{V^2}{r}$$

ra = constant

Hence graph (c) correctly describes relation between acceleration and radius.

45. (c) From question,

Horizontal velocity (initial),

$$u_x=\frac{40}{2}=20\,\text{m/s}$$

Vertical velocity (initial), $50=u_y t+\frac{1}{2}gt^2$

$\Rightarrow \quad u_y\times 2+\frac{1}{2}(-10)\times 4$

or, $\quad 50=2u_y-20$

or, $\quad u_y=\frac{70}{2}=35\,\text{m/s}$

$\therefore \quad \tan\theta=\frac{u_y}{u_x}=\frac{35}{20}=\frac{7}{4}$

$\Rightarrow \quad$ Angle $\theta=\tan^{-1}\frac{7}{4}$

Speed Test-4

1. **(d)** Here $m = 0.5$ kg ; $u = -10$ m/s; $t = 1/50$ s ; $v = +15$ ms^{-1}
Force $= m(v-u)/t = 0.5(10+15)\times 50 = 625$ N

2. **(b)**

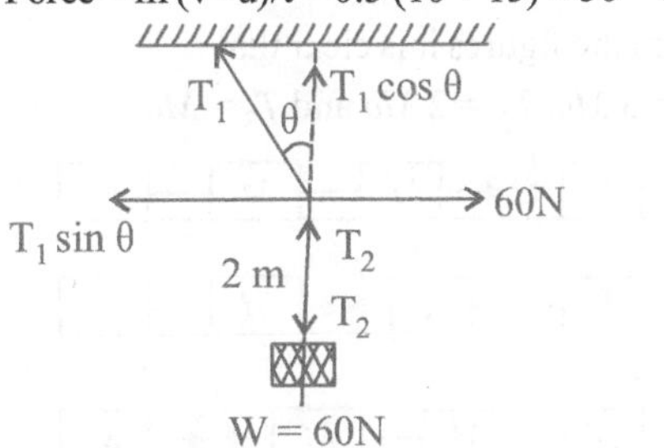

In eqbm $T_1 \cos\theta = T_2 = 60$N. ...(1)
$T_1 \sin\theta = 60$ N ...(2)
$\therefore$ $\tan\theta = 1$
$\theta = 45°$.

3. **(d)** Mass of rocket (m) = 5000 Kg
Exhaust speed (v) = 800 m/s
Acceleration of rocket (a) = 20 m/s^2
Gravitational acceleration (g) = 10 m/s^2
We know that upward force
$F = m(g+a) = 5000(10+20)$
$= 5000 \times 30 = 150000$ N.
We also know that amount of gas ejected

$$\left(\frac{dm}{dt}\right) = \frac{F}{v} = \frac{150000}{800} = 187.5 \text{ kg/s}$$

4. **(b)** (i) If a body is moved up an inclined plane, then the work done against friction will be zero as there is no friction. But work must be done against gravity. So this statement is incorrect.
(ii) This statement is correct, because moving vehicles are stopped by air friction only.
(iii) The normal reaction acting on a body on an inclined plane is given by,
$R = mg\cos\theta$
Where θ is the angle of inclination.
As θ increases, $\cos\theta$ decreases and hence R decreases. So this statement is incorrect.
(iv) The applied force needed to rub the duster upward,

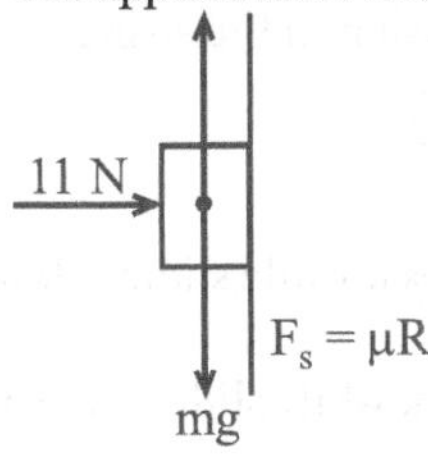

$F_{applied} = mg + \mu R = 0.5\times 10 + 0.5\times 11$
$= 5 + 5.5 = 10.5$ N
$\therefore$ The work done in rubbing it upward through a distance of 10 cm,

$W = F_{applied} \times d = 10.5 \times 0.10 = 1.05$ J
Hence this statement is incorrect.

5. **(b)** Momentum $P = mv = m\sqrt{2gh}$
($\because v^2 = u^2 + 2gh$; Here $u = 0$)
When stone hits the ground momentum
$$P = m\sqrt{2gh}$$
when same stone dropped from $2h$ (100% of initial) then momentum
$$P' = m\sqrt{2g(2h)} = \sqrt{2}P$$
Which is changed by 41% of initial.

6. **(c)** Change in momentum along the wall
$= mv\cos 60° - mv\cos 60° = 0$
Change in momentum perpendicular to the wall
$= mv\sin 60° - (-mv\sin 60°) = 2mv\sin 60°$
$$\therefore \text{Applied force} = \frac{\text{Change in momentum}}{\text{Time}}$$
$$= \frac{2\,mv\sin 60°}{0.20}$$
$$= \frac{2\times 3\times 10\times\sqrt{3}}{2\times 20} = 50\times 3\sqrt{3}$$
$$= 150\sqrt{3} \text{ newton}$$

7. **(b)**

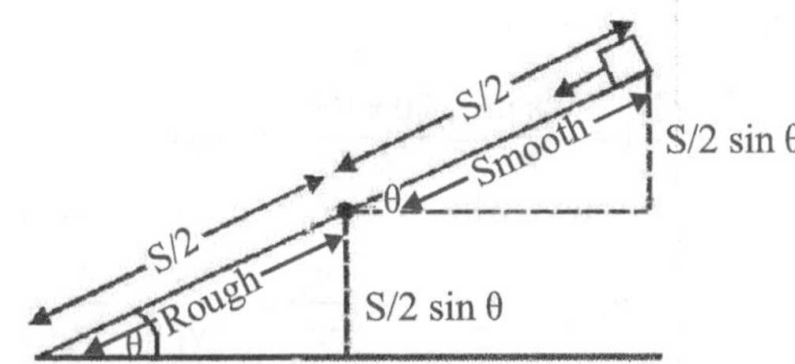

For upper half of inclined plane
$v^2 = u^2 + 2a\,S/2 = 2(g\sin\theta)\,S/2 = gS\sin\theta$
For lower half of inclined plane
$0 = u^2 + 2g(\sin\theta - \mu\cos\theta)\,S/2$
$\Rightarrow -gS\sin\theta = gS(\sin\theta - \mu\cos\theta)$
$\Rightarrow 2\sin\theta = \mu\cos\theta$
$$\Rightarrow \mu = \frac{2\sin\theta}{\cos\theta} = 2\tan\theta$$

8. **(c)** Forces acting on the block are as shown in the fig. Normal reaction N is provided by the force $m\alpha$ due to acceleration α

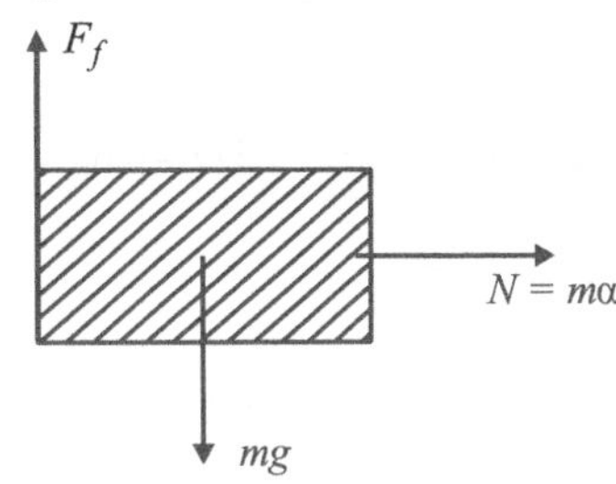

$\therefore$ $N = m\alpha$

For the block not to fall, frictional force, $F_f \geq mg$

$\Rightarrow$ $\mu N \geq mg$

$\Rightarrow$ $\mu m\alpha \geq mg$

$\Rightarrow$ $\alpha \geq g/\mu$

9. **(b)** $v = \sqrt{gr} = \sqrt{10 \times 40} = 20 \text{ m s}^{-1}$

10. **(a)**

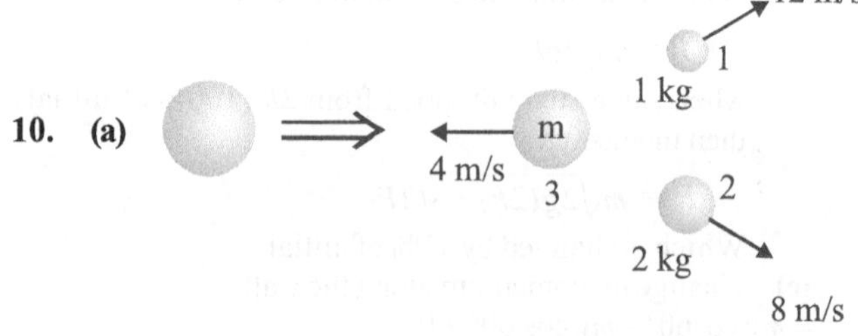

According to conservation of linear momentum

$$P_3 = \sqrt{p_1^2 + p_2^2}$$

$$\Rightarrow m \times 4 = \sqrt{(1 \times 12)^2 + (2 \times 8)^2} = 20 \Rightarrow m = 5 \text{ kg.}$$

11. **(c)** Let T be the tension in the branch of a tree when monkey is descending with acceleration a. Then mg – T = ma; and T = 75% of weight of monkey

$$= \left(\frac{75}{100}\right)mg = \left(\frac{1}{4}\right)mg \text{ or } a = \frac{g}{4}.$$

12. **(d)** $v = u - at \Rightarrow t = \frac{u}{a}$ [As v = 0]

$$t = \frac{u \times m}{F} = \frac{30 \times 1000}{5000} = 6 \text{sec}$$

13. **(c)** Applying law of conservation of linear momentum

$$m_1 v_1 + m_2 v_2 = 0, \frac{m_1}{m_2} = -\frac{v_2}{v_1} \text{ or } \frac{v_1}{v_2} = -\frac{m_2}{m_1}$$

14. **(a)** The frictional force acting on M is μmg

$$\therefore \text{Acceleration} = \frac{\mu mg}{M}$$

15. **(c)** $\frac{dM}{dt} = 0.1$ kg/s, $v_{gas} = 50$ m/s,

Mass of the rocket = 2 kg. Mv = constant

$$-v\frac{dM}{dt} + M\frac{dv}{dt} = 0 \;.\; \therefore \; \frac{dv}{dt} = \frac{1}{M}v\frac{dM}{dt}$$

$$\Rightarrow \text{Acceleration} = \frac{1}{2} \times 50 \times 0.1 = 2.5 \text{ m/s}^2$$

16. **(a)** Coefficient of static friction,

$$\mu_s = \tan 30° = \frac{1}{\sqrt{3}} = 0.577 \cong 0.6$$

$$S = ut + \frac{1}{2}at^2$$

$$4 = \frac{1}{2}a(4)^2 \Rightarrow a = \frac{1}{2} = 0.5$$

[$\because$ s = 4m and t = 4s given]

$$a = g\sin\theta - \mu_k(g)\cos\theta$$

$$\Rightarrow \mu_k = \frac{0.9}{\sqrt{3}} = 0.5$$

17. **(c)** All blocks will move with the same aceleration Let it be a. Then

$$F = 4Ma \Rightarrow a = \frac{F}{4M}$$

From the figures it is clear that

$T_1 = 3\,Ma$, $T_2 = 2\,Ma$ and $T_3 = Ma$

F ← M —T₁— M — M — M

F ← M — M —T₂— M — M

F ← M — M — M —T₃— M

Putting the value of a, we get

$$T_1 = \frac{3}{4}F,\; T_2 = \frac{F}{2} \text{ and } T_3 = \frac{F}{4}$$

18. **(c)** Maximum force by surface when friction works

$$F = \sqrt{f^2 + R^2} = \sqrt{(\mu R)^2 + R^2} = R\sqrt{\mu^2 + 1}$$

Minimum force = R when there is no friction

Hence ranging from R to $R\sqrt{\mu^2 + 1}$ [where, R = mg]

19. **(c)** Motion with constant momentum along a straight line. According to Newton's second law rate of change of momentum is directly proportional to force applied.

20. **(b)** For the motion of both the blocks

$m_1 a = T - \mu_k m_1 g$

$m_2 g - T = m_2 a$

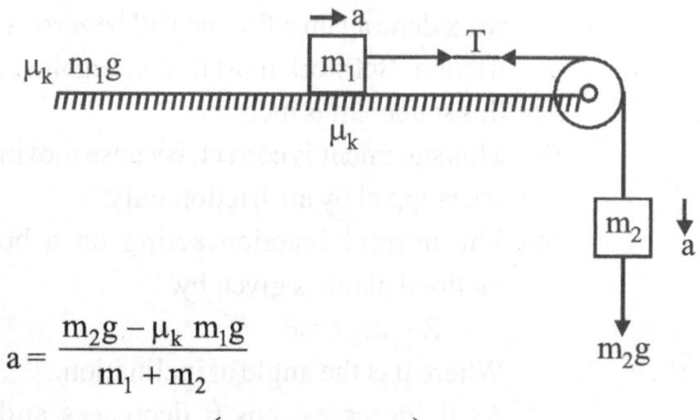

$$a = \frac{m_2 g - \mu_k m_1 g}{m_1 + m_2}$$

$$m_2 g - T = (m_2)\left(\frac{m_2 g - \mu_k m_1 g}{m_1 + m_2}\right)$$

solving we get tension in the string

$$T = \frac{m_1 m_2 (1 + \mu_k) g}{m_1 + m_2}$$

21. **(d)** Acceleration of block while sliding down upper half = $g\sin\phi$;

retardation of block while sliding down lower half = $-(g\sin\phi - \mu g\cos\phi)$

For the block to come to rest at the bottom, acceleration in I half = retardation in II half.

$$g\sin\phi = -(g\sin\phi - \mu g\cos\phi)$$

$$\Rightarrow \mu = 2\tan\phi$$

22. (d) The particle is moving in circular path

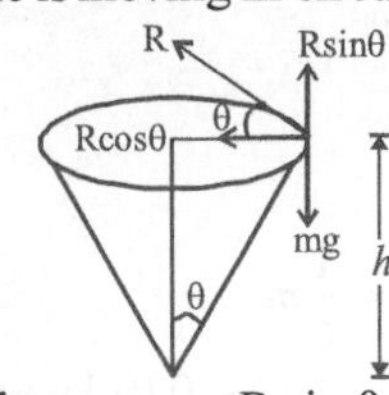

From the figure, mg = R sin θ ... (i)

$$\frac{mv^2}{r} = R\cos\theta \quad \text{... (ii)}$$

From equations (i) and (ii) we get

$$\tan\theta = \frac{rg}{v^2} \text{ but } \tan\theta = \frac{r}{h}$$

$$\therefore h = \frac{v^2}{g} = \frac{(0.5)^2}{10} = 0.025\text{m} = 2.5\text{cm}$$

23. (b) By spitting or sneezing we get a momentum in opposite direction which will help us in getting off the plane. In all other cases we will slip on ice as there is no friction.

24. (a) Force required to just move a body (F) = force due to static friction = μ_s mg

When body moves with a constant acceleration (a) then

$F - f_k = ma$, where f_k is the force of kinetic friction = μ_k mg

$$\therefore a = \frac{F - f_k}{m} = \frac{F - f_k}{m} = \frac{\mu_s mg - \mu_k mg}{m}$$

$$= (\mu_s - \mu_k)g = (0.75 - 0.5)g = \frac{g}{4}.$$

25. (c) Considering the two masses and the rope a system, then

Initial net force $= [25 - (15+5)]g = 5g$

Final net force $= [(25+5) - 15]g = 15\text{ g}$

$\Rightarrow$ (acceleration)$_{final}$ = 3 (acceleration)$_{initial}$

26. (c)

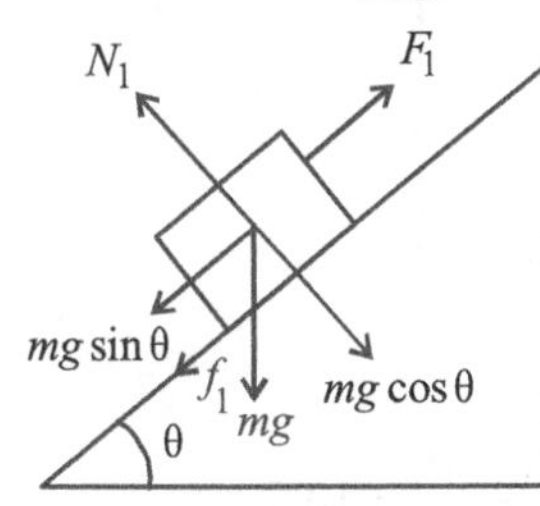

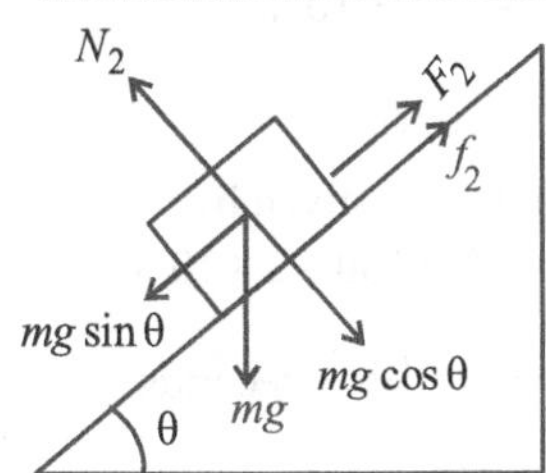

For the upward motion of the body

$$mg\sin\theta + f_1 = F_1$$

or, $F_1 = mg\sin\theta + \mu mg\cos\theta$

For the downward motion of the body,

$$mg\sin\theta - f_2 = F_2$$

or $F_2 = mg\sin\theta - \mu mg\cos\theta$

$$\therefore \frac{F_1}{F_2} = \frac{\sin\theta + \mu\cos\theta}{\sin\theta - \mu\cos\theta}$$

$$\Rightarrow \frac{\tan\theta + \mu}{\tan\theta - \mu} = \frac{2\mu + \mu}{2\mu - \mu} = \frac{3\mu}{\mu} = 3$$

27. (b) Considering the equilibrium of B

$-m_B g + T = m_B a$

Since the block A slides down with constant speed.

a = 0.

Therefore $T = m_B g$

Considering the equilibrium of A, we get

$10a = 10g\sin 30° - T - \mu N$

where $N = 10g\cos 30°$

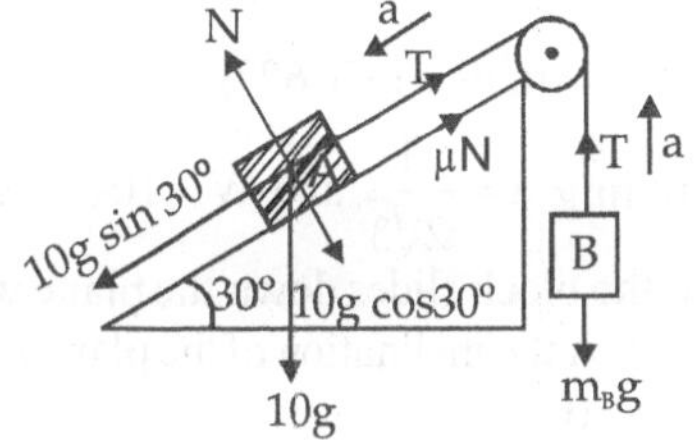

$$\therefore 10a = \frac{10}{2}g - T - \mu \times 10g\cos 30°$$

but a = 0, $T = m_B g$

$$0 = 5g - m_B g - \frac{0.2\sqrt{3}}{2} \times 10 \times g$$

$\Rightarrow m_B = 3.268 \approx 3.3$ kg

28. (a) When tension in the cable is equal to the weight of cable, the system is in equilibrium. It means the system is at rest or moving with uniform velocity.

29. (c) Tension at the highest point

$$T_{top} = \frac{mv^2}{r} - mg = 2mg \quad (\because v_{top} = \sqrt{3gr})$$

Tension at the lowest point

$T_{bottom} = 2mg + 6mg = 8mg$

$$\therefore \frac{T_{top}}{T_{bottom}} = \frac{2mg}{8mg} = \frac{1}{4}.$$

30. (d) When brakes are on, the wheels of the cycle will slide on the road instead of rolling there. It means the sliding friction will come into play instead of rolling friction. The value of sliding friction is more than that of rolling friction.

31. (a) When car moves towards right with acceleration a then due to pseudo force the plumb line will tilt in backward direction making an angle θ with vertical

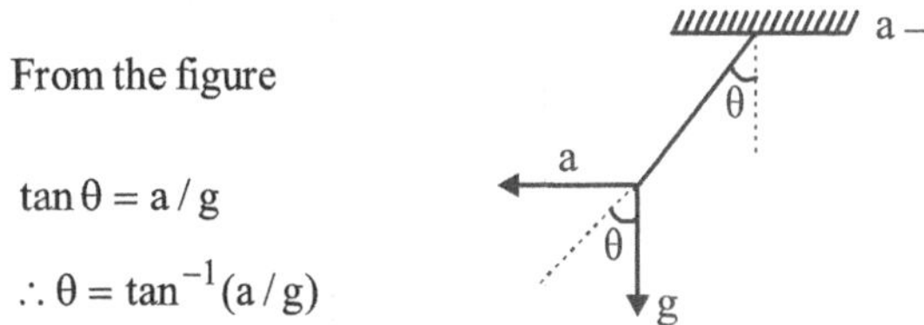

From the figure

$\tan\theta = a/g$

$\therefore \theta = \tan^{-1}(a/g)$

32. **(b)** See fig.

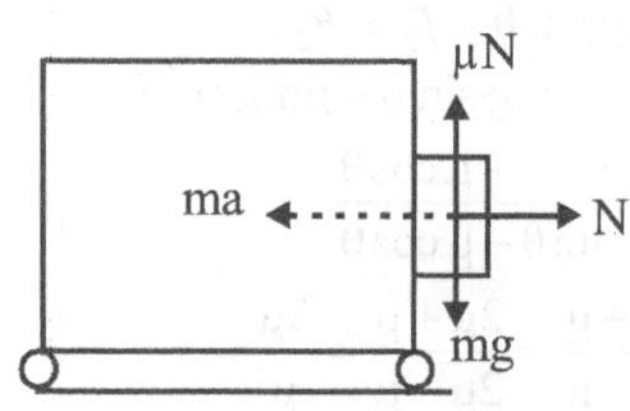

If a = acceleration of the cart, then N = ma

$\therefore$ μN = mg or μ ma = mg or a = g/μ

33. **(a)**

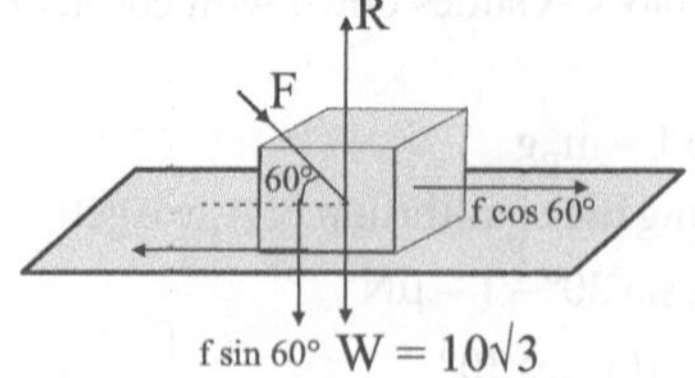

$f = \mu R$

$F\cos 60° = \mu(W + F\sin 60°)$

Substituing $\mu = \dfrac{1}{2\sqrt{3}}$ and $W = 10\sqrt{3}$ we get F = 20 N

34. **(d)** When the block slides down the plane with a constant speed, then the inclination of the plane is equal to angle of repose (θ).
Coeff. of friction = tan of the angle of repose = tan θ.

35. **(d)** Writing free body-diagrams for m & M,

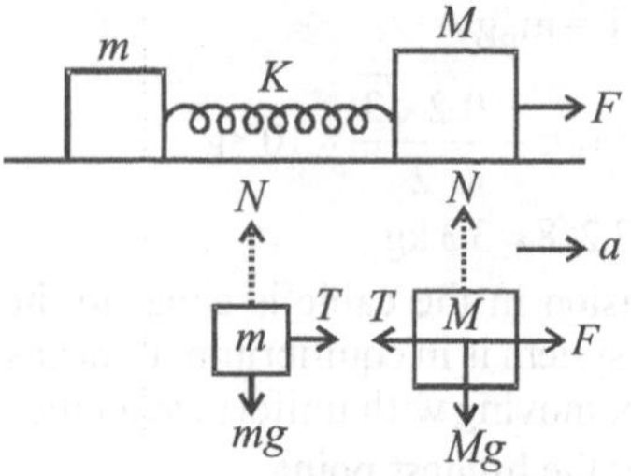

we get $T = ma$ and $F - T = Ma$
where T is force due to spring
$\Rightarrow F - ma = Ma$ or, $F = Ma + ma$

$\therefore\ a = \dfrac{F}{M+m}$.

Now, force acting on the block of mass m is

$ma = m\left(\dfrac{F}{M+m}\right) = \dfrac{mF}{m+M}$

36. **(a)** At limiting equilibrium, μ = tan θ

$\tan\theta = \mu = \dfrac{dy}{dx} = \dfrac{x^2}{2}$ (from question)

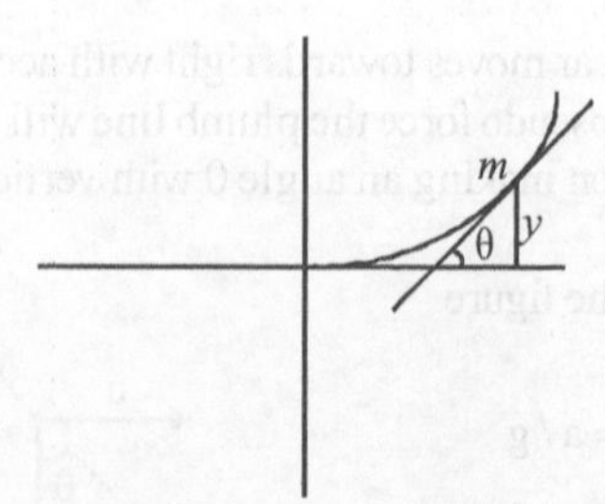

$\because$ Coefficient of friction μ = 0.5

$\therefore\quad 0.5 = \dfrac{x^2}{2}$

$\Rightarrow\quad x = \pm 1$

Now, $y = \dfrac{x^3}{6} = \dfrac{1}{6}m$

37. **(a)** As the ball, m = 10 g = 0.01 kg rebounds after striking the wall
$\therefore$ Change in momentum = $mv - (-mv) = 2mv$
Inpulse = Change in momentum = $2mv$

$\therefore\ v = \dfrac{\text{Impulse}}{2m} = \dfrac{0.54\text{ N s}}{2 \times 0.01\text{ kg}} = 27\text{ m s}^{-1}$

38. **(b)** From the F.B.D.
N = mg cos θ
F = ma = mg sin θ – μN
$\Rightarrow$ a = g(sin θ – μ cos θ)

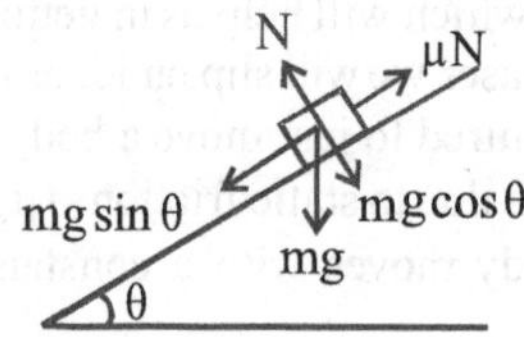

Now using, $v^2 - u^2 = 2as$

or, $v^2 = 2 \times g(\sin\theta - \mu\cos\theta)\ell$
(ℓ = length of incline)

or, $v = \sqrt{2g\ell(\sin\theta - \mu\cos\theta)}$

39. **(a)** During collision of ball with the wall horizontal momentum changes (vertical momentum remains constant)

$\therefore\quad F = \dfrac{\text{Change in horizontal momentum}}{\text{Time of contact}}$

$= \dfrac{2P\cos\theta}{0.1} = \dfrac{2mv\cos\theta}{0.1}$

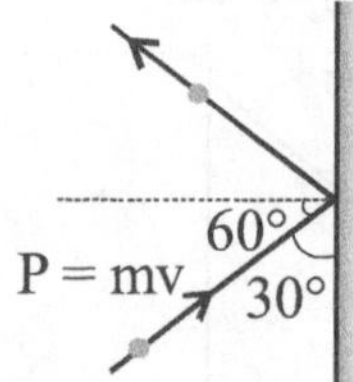

$= \dfrac{2 \times 0.1 \times 10 \times \cos 60°}{0.1} = 10\text{N}$

40. **(d)** Given $F = 600 - (2 \times 10^5 t)$
The force is zero at time t, given by
$0 = 600 - 2 \times 10^5 t$

$\Rightarrow\quad t = \dfrac{600}{2 \times 10^5} = 3 \times 10^{-3}$ seconds

$\therefore$ Impulse $= \int_0^t F dt = \int_0^{3\times10^{-3}} (600 - 2 \times 10^5 t)\, dt$

$$= \left[600t - \frac{2\times10^5 t^2}{2}\right]_0^{3\times10^{-3}}$$

$$= 600\times3\times10^{-3} - 10^5(3\times10^{-3})^2$$

$$= 1.8 - 0.9 = 0.9\text{Ns}$$

41. **(d)** According to question, two stones experience same centripetal force

i.e. $F_{C_1} = F_{C_2}$

or, $\frac{mv_1^2}{r} = \frac{2mv_2^2}{(r/2)}$ or, $V_1^2 = 4V_2^2$

So, $V_1 = 2V_2$ i.e., $n = 2$

42. **(b)** $T_1 = m(g+a) = 0.1(10+5) = 1.5N$

$T_2 = m(g-a) = 0.1(10-5) = 0.5N$

$\Rightarrow T_1 - T_2 = (1.5 - 0.5)N = 1N$

43. **(d)** As shown in the figure, the three forces are represented by the sides of a triangle taken in the same order. Therefore the resultant force is zero. $\vec{F}_{net} = m\vec{a}$. Therefore acceleration is also zero i.e., velocity remains unchanged.

44. **(b)** Rate of flow of water will depend on the net acceleration due to gravity.

When the lift is moving upward with acceleration a,

$g'_u = g + a$

When the lift is moving downward with acceleration on a, $g'_d = g - a$

$\therefore\ g'_u > g > g'_d \quad \therefore R_u > R_0 > R_d$

45. **(d)** According to law of conservation of momentum the third piece has momentum

$= 1\times -(3\hat{i} + 4\hat{j})$ kg ms^{-1}

Impulse = Average force × time

$\Rightarrow$ Average force $= \frac{\text{Impulse}}{\text{time}}$

$= \frac{\text{Change in momentum}}{\text{time}} = \frac{-(3\hat{i}+4\hat{j})\text{kg ms}^{-1}}{10^{-4}\text{s}}$

Speed Test-5

1. **(b)** $k = 5 \times 10^3$ N/m

$$W = \frac{1}{2}k\left(x_2^2 - x_1^2\right) = \frac{1}{2}\times 5\times 10^3\left[(0.1)^2 - (0.05)^2\right]$$

$$= \frac{5000}{2}\times 0.15\times 0.05 = 18.75 \text{ Nm}$$

2. **(a)** Given: Mass of particle, $M = 10\text{g} = \frac{10}{1000}$ kg

radius of circle R = 6.4 cm

Kinetic energy E of particle = 8×10^{-4}J

acceleration a_t = ?

$$\frac{1}{2}mv^2 = E$$

$$\Rightarrow \frac{1}{2}\left(\frac{10}{1000}\right)v^2 = 8\times 10^{-4}$$

$$\Rightarrow v^2 = 16\times 10^{-2}$$

$$\Rightarrow v = 4\times 10^{-1} = 0.4 \text{ m/s}$$

Now, using

$v^2 = u^2 + 2a_t s$ $\qquad$ $(s = 4\pi R)$

$$(0.4)^2 = 0^2 + 2a_t\left(4\times\frac{22}{7}\times\frac{6.4}{100}\right)$$

$$\Rightarrow a_t = (0.4)^2\times\frac{7\times 100}{8\times 22\times 6.4} = 0.1 \text{ m/s}^2$$

3. **(b)** We know that $F \times v$ = Power

$\therefore F\times v = c$ where c = constant

$$m\frac{dv}{dt}\times v = c \qquad \left(\because F = ma = \frac{mdv}{dt}\right)$$

$$m\int_0^v v\,dv = c\int_0^t dt \qquad \Rightarrow \frac{1}{2}mv^2 = ct$$

$$v = \sqrt{\frac{2c}{m}}\times t^{1/2}$$

$$\frac{dx}{dt} = \sqrt{\frac{2c}{m}}\times t^{1/2} \quad \text{where } v = \frac{dx}{dt}$$

$$\int_0^x dx = \sqrt{\frac{2c}{m}}\times\int_0^t t^{1/2}dt$$

$$x = \sqrt{\frac{2c}{m}}\times\frac{2t^{3/2}}{3} \Rightarrow x \propto t^{3/2}$$

4. **(a)** When ball collides with the ground it loses its 50% of energy

$$\therefore \frac{KE_f}{KE_i} = \frac{1}{2} \Rightarrow \frac{\frac{1}{2}mV_f^2}{\frac{1}{2}mV_i^2} = \frac{1}{2}$$

$$\text{or } \frac{V_f}{V_i} = \frac{1}{\sqrt{2}}$$

$$\text{or, } \frac{\sqrt{2gh}}{\sqrt{v_0^2 + 2gh}} = \frac{1}{\sqrt{2}}$$

$$\text{or, } 4gh = v_0^2 + 2gh$$

$$\therefore v_0 = 20\text{ms}^{-1}$$

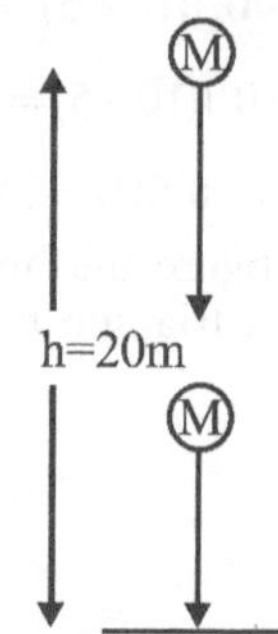

5. **(c)** As the cord is trying to hold the motion of the block, work done by the cord is negative.

$$W = -M(g-a)d = -M\left(g - \frac{g}{4}\right)d = \frac{-3Mgd}{4}$$

6. **(b)** According to principle of conservation of energy Loss in potential energy = Gain in kinetic energy

$$\Rightarrow mgh = \frac{1}{2}mv^2 \Rightarrow v = \sqrt{2gh}$$

If h_1 and h_2 are initial and final heights, then

$$v_1 = \sqrt{2gh_1}, v_2 = \sqrt{2gh_2}$$

Loss in velocity

$$\Delta v = v_1 - v_2 = \sqrt{2gh_1} - \sqrt{2gh_2}$$

$\therefore$ Fractional loss in velocity

$$= \frac{\Delta v}{v_1} = \frac{\sqrt{2gh_1} - \sqrt{2gh_2}}{\sqrt{2gh_1}} = 1 - \sqrt{\frac{h_2}{h_1}}$$

$$= 1 - \sqrt{\frac{1.8}{5}} = 1 - \sqrt{0.36} = 1 - 0.6 = 0.4 = \frac{2}{5}$$

7. **(a)** As $u_2 = 0$ and $m_1 = m_2$, therefore from

$m_1 u_1 + m_2 u_2 = m_1 v_1 + m_2 v_2$ we get $u_1 = v_1 + v_2$

$$\text{Also, } e = \frac{v_2 - v_1}{u_1} = \frac{v_2 - v_1}{v_2 + v_1} = \frac{1 - v_1/v_2}{1 + v_1/v_2},$$

$$\text{which gives } \frac{v_1}{v_2} = \frac{1-e}{1+e}$$

8. (d) As we know power $P = \frac{dw}{dt}$

$\Rightarrow \quad w = Pt = \frac{1}{2}mv^2$

So, $v = \sqrt{\frac{2Pt}{m}}$

Hence, acceleration $a = \frac{dv}{dt} = \sqrt{\frac{2P}{m}} \cdot \frac{1}{2\sqrt{t}}$

Therefore, force on the particle at time 't'

$$= ma = \sqrt{\frac{2Km^2}{m}} \cdot \frac{1}{2\sqrt{t}} = \sqrt{\frac{Km}{2t}} = \sqrt{\frac{mK}{2}}\, t^{-1/2}$$

9. (b) $x = \frac{t^3}{3} \Rightarrow \frac{dx}{dt} = \frac{3t^2}{3} = t^2 \quad \Rightarrow v = t^2$

when, $t = 2$ sec, $v = t^2 = (2)^2 = 4$ m/s

Work done = K.E. acquired $= \frac{1}{2}mv^2$

$$= \frac{1}{2} \times (2) \times (4)^2 = 16\,J$$

10. (b) For elastic collision in one dimension

$$v_1 = \frac{2m_2u_2}{m_1 + m_2} + \frac{(m_1 - m_2)u_1}{(m_1 + m_2)}$$

As mass 2m, is at rest, So $u_2 = 0$

$$\Rightarrow \quad v_1 = \frac{(8m - 2m)u}{8m + 2m} = \frac{3}{5}u$$

Final energy of sphere = $(K.E.)_f$

$$= \frac{1}{2}(8m)\left(\frac{3u}{5}\right)^2 = \frac{1}{2}(8m)u^2 \times \left(\frac{3}{5}\right)^2$$

$$= \frac{9}{25}E = 0.36\,E$$

11. (b) As we know work done in stretching spring

$$w = \frac{1}{2}kx^2$$

where k = spring constant
x = extension

Case (a) If extension (x) is same,

$$W = \frac{1}{2}K\,x^2$$

So, $W_P > W_Q \qquad (\because K_P > K_Q)$

Case (b) If spring force (F) is same $W = \frac{F^2}{2K}$

So, $W_Q > W_P$

12. (b) If the particle is released at the origin, it will try to go in the direction of force. Here $\frac{dU}{dx}$ is positive and hence force is negative, as a result it will move towards –ve x-axis.

13. (c) The potential energy of a spring is given by,

$$U = \frac{1}{2}kx^2 \Rightarrow 10\,J = \frac{1}{2}ks^2 \qquad \text{.... (i)}$$

The potential energy stored when stretched

through$(2s) = \frac{1}{2}k(2s^2) = \frac{1}{2}ks^2 \times 4$

Substituting from (i)
P.E. = 40 J.
But to increase 's' to '2s', the work done
= 40 – 10 = 30 J.

14. (b) Power $= \frac{\text{Work done}}{\text{Time}} = \frac{\frac{1}{2}m\left(v^2 - u^2\right)}{t}$

$$P = \frac{1}{2} \times \frac{2.05 \times 10^6 \times \left[(25)^2 - (5^2)\right]}{5 \times 60}$$

$P = 2.05 \times 10^6$ W = 2.05 MW

15. (b) Work done = Area under F-x graph
= area of rectangle ABCD + area of rectangle LCFE
+ area of rectangle GFIH + area of triangle IJK

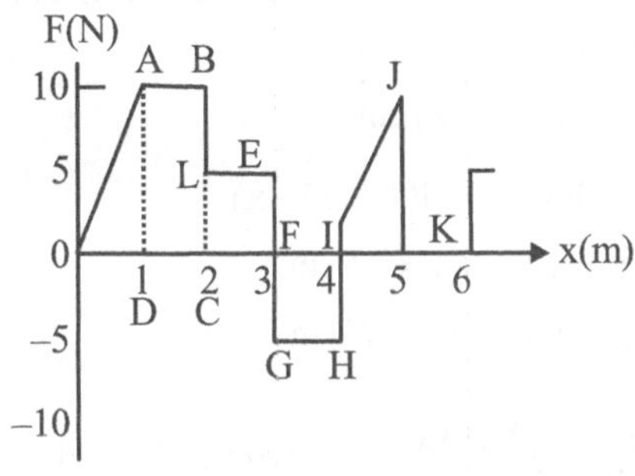

$= (2–1)\times(10–0) + (3–2)\,(5–0)\;(4–3)(–5–0)$

$+\frac{1}{2}(5-4)(10-0) = 15\,J$

16. (c)

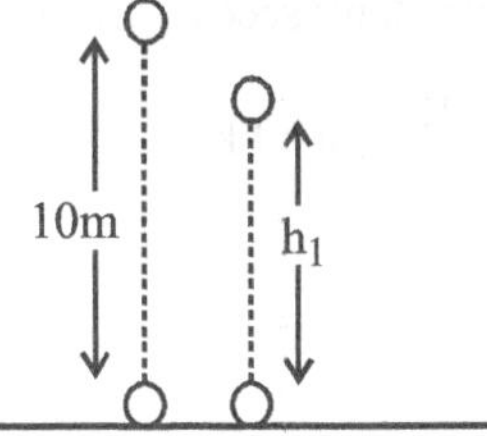

Just before impact, energy
E = mgh = 10mg ....(1)
Just after impact

$$E_1 = mgh - \frac{25}{100}mgh = 0.75\,mgh$$

Hence, $mgh_1 = E_1$ (from given figure)

$mgh_1 = 0.75\, mg(10)$

$h_1 = 7.5m$

17. (d) When C strikes A

$\frac{1}{2}mv_0^2 = \frac{1}{2}mv'^2 + \frac{1}{2}kx_0^2$ (v' = velocity of A)

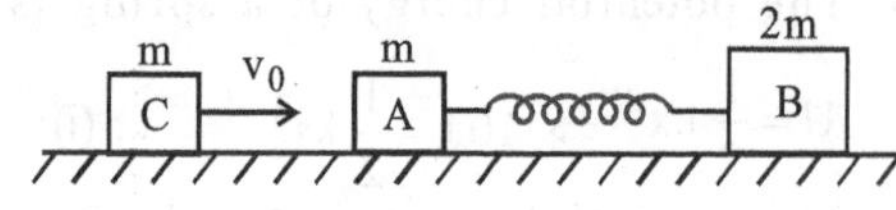

$kx_0^2 = m(v_0^2 - v'^2)$ .... (i)

$\frac{1}{2}2mv'^2 = \frac{1}{2}kx_0^2$

(When A and B Block attains K.E.)

$\therefore \quad \frac{1}{2}kx_0^2 = mv'^2$ .... (ii)

From (i) and (ii),

$$kx_0^2 = mv_0^2 - mv'^2 = mv_0^2 - \frac{k}{2}x_0^2$$

$$\Rightarrow kx_0^2 + \frac{k}{2}x_0^2 = mv_0^2$$

$$\frac{3}{2}kx_0^2 = mv_0^2 \therefore k = \frac{2}{3}m\frac{v_0^2}{x_0^2}$$

18. (a) Given : $k_A = 300\,N/m, \; k_B = 400\,N/m$

Let the combination of springs is compressed by force F. Spring A is compressed by x. Therefore compression in spring B

$x_B = (8.75 - x)$ cm

$F = 300 \times x = 400(8.75 - x)$

Solving we get, x = 5 cm

$x_B = 8.75 - 5 = 3.75\,cm$

$$\frac{E_A}{E_B} = \frac{\frac{1}{2}k_A(x_A)^2}{\frac{1}{2}k_B(x_B)^2} = \frac{300 \times (5)^2}{400 \times (3.75)^2} = \frac{4}{3}$$

19. (d) Given force $\vec{F} = 2t\hat{i} + 3t^2\hat{j}$

According to Newton's second law of motion,

$$m\frac{d\vec{v}}{dt} = 2t\hat{i} + 3t^2\hat{j} \quad (m = 1\,kg)$$

$$\Rightarrow \int_0^{\vec{v}} d\vec{v} = \int_0^t (2t\hat{i} + 3t^2\hat{j})dt$$

$$\Rightarrow \vec{v} = t^2\hat{i} + t^3\hat{j}$$

Power $P = \vec{F} \cdot \vec{v} = (2t\hat{i} + 3t^2\hat{j}) \cdot (t^2\hat{i} + t^3\hat{j})$

$= (2t^3 + 3t^5)W$

20. (a) According to conservation of linear momentum,

$M_bV_b = M_{bl}V_{bl} + M_bV_b^1$ ....(i)

where v_b is velocity of bullet before collision v_b^1 velocity of bullet after collision and v_{bl} is the velocity of block.

K.E. of block = P.E. of block

$\frac{1}{2}M_{bl}V_{bl}^2 = M_{bl}\,gh$ (h = 0.2m)

Solving we get $V_{bl} = 2ms^{-1}$

Now from eq (i)

$20 \times 10^{-3} \times 600 = 4 \times 2 + 20 \times 10^{-3}\, V_b^1$

Solving we get $V_b^1 = 200$ m/s

21. (d) $\sin\theta = \frac{1}{x}$

From free body diagram of the body

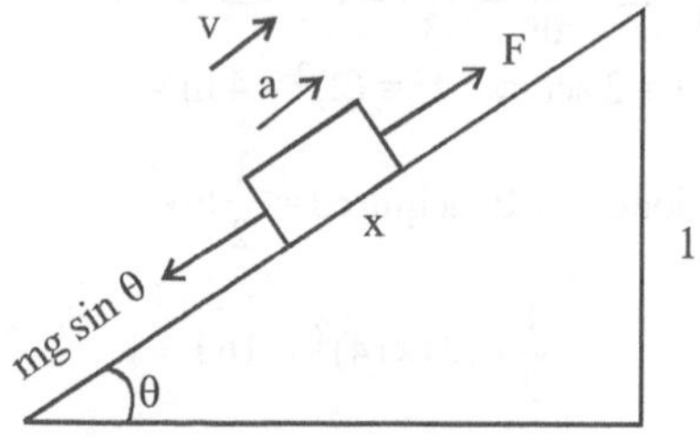

$F - mg\sin\theta = ma$

$F = m(g\sin\theta + a) = m\left(\frac{g}{x} + a\right)$ .... (1)

Displacement of the body till its velocity reaches v

$v^2 = 0 + 2as \Rightarrow s = \frac{v^2}{2a}$

Now, work done = F s cos 0° $= \frac{m}{x}(g + ax) \times \frac{v^2}{2a}$

$= \frac{mv^2}{2ax}(g + ax)$

22. (c) $t_{AB} = \sqrt{\frac{2h}{g}}$

$t_{BC} + t_{CB} = 2\sqrt{\frac{2h_1}{g}}$

$= 2\sqrt{\frac{2e^2h}{g}} = 2e\sqrt{\frac{2h}{g}}$

$t_{BD} + t_{DB} = 2e^2\sqrt{\frac{2h}{g}}$

$\therefore$ Total time taken by the body in coming to rest

$$= \sqrt{\frac{2h}{g}} + 2e\sqrt{\frac{2h}{g}} + 2e^2\sqrt{\frac{2h}{g}} + ...$$

$$= \sqrt{\frac{2h}{g}} + 2e\sqrt{\frac{2h}{g}}\,[1 + e + e^2 + ...]$$

$$= \sqrt{\frac{2h}{g}} + 2e\sqrt{\frac{2h}{g}} \times \frac{1}{1-e} = \sqrt{\frac{2h}{g}}\left[\frac{1+e}{1-e}\right] = t\left(\frac{1+e}{1-e}\right)$$

23. (a) Velocity is maximum when K.E. is maximum

For minimum. P.E.,

$$\frac{dV}{dx} = 0 \Rightarrow x^3 - x = 0 \Rightarrow x = \pm 1$$

$$\Rightarrow \text{Min. P.E.} = \frac{1}{4} - \frac{1}{2} = -\frac{1}{4} \text{ J}$$

$$\text{K.E.}_{(max.)} + \text{P.E.}_{(min.)} = 2 \text{ (Given)}$$

$$\therefore \text{K.E.}_{(max.)} = 2 + \frac{1}{4} = \frac{9}{4}$$

$$\text{K.E.}_{max.} = \frac{1}{2}mv_{max.}^2$$

$$\Rightarrow \frac{1}{2} \times 1 \times v_{max.}^2 = \frac{9}{4} \Rightarrow v_{max.} = \frac{3}{\sqrt{2}}$$

24. (a) Given, h = 60m, g = 10 ms^{-2},

Rate of flow of water = 15 kg/s

∴ Power of the falling water

= 15 kgs^{-1} × 10 ms^{-2} × 60 m = 900 watt.

Loss in energy due to friction

$$= 9000 \times \frac{10}{100} = 900 \text{ watt.}$$

∴ Power generated by the turbine

= (9000 – 900) watt = 8100 watt = 8.1 kW

24. (b) Let initial velocity of the bullet be v.

By linear momentum conservation

$$\frac{m}{2}v = \left(\frac{m}{2} + m\right) v_1$$

(v_1 = combined velocity)

$$v_1 = \frac{v}{3} \qquad \text{....(1)}$$

retardation = μg

$$0 = \left(\frac{v}{3}\right)^2 - 2\mu gd \Rightarrow v = 3\sqrt{2\mu gd}$$

25. (c) Force constant of a spring

$$k = \frac{F}{x} = \frac{mg}{x} = \frac{1\times10}{2\times10^{-2}} \Rightarrow k = 500N/m$$

Increment in the length = 60 – 50 = 10 cm

$$U = \frac{1}{2}kx^2 = \frac{1}{2}500\left(10\times10^{-2}\right)^2 = 2.5J$$

26. (b) Constant power of car $P_0 = F.v = ma.v$

$$P_0 = m\frac{dv}{dt}.v$$

$P_0 dt = mvdv$ Integrating

$$P_0 t = \frac{mv^2}{2}$$

$$v = \sqrt{\frac{2P_0 t}{m}}$$

∵ P_0, m and 2 are constant

$$\therefore \quad v \propto \sqrt{t}$$

27. (a) $x = 3t - 4t^2 + t^3$

$$\frac{dx}{dt} = 3 - 8t + 3t^2$$

$$\text{Acceleration} = \frac{d^2x}{dt^2} = -8 + 6t$$

Acceleration after 4 sec

= –8 + 6 × 4 = 16 ms^{-2}

Displacement in 4 sec

= 3 × 4 – 4 × 4^2 + 4^3 = 12 m

∴ Work = Force × displacement

= Mass × acc. × disp.

= 3 × 10^{-3} × 16 × 12 = 576 mJ

28. (c) $K_i = \frac{1}{2}m_1u_1^2,$

$$K_f = \frac{1}{2}m_1v_1^2, v_1 = \frac{m_1 - m_2}{m_1 + m_2}u_1$$

Fractional loss

$$\frac{K_i - K_f}{K_i} = \frac{\frac{1}{2}m_1u_1^2 - \frac{1}{2}m_1v_1^2}{\frac{1}{2}m_1u_1^2}$$

$$= 1 - \frac{v_1^2}{u_1^2} = 1 - \frac{(m_1 - m_2)^2}{(m_1 + m_2)^2} = \frac{4m_1m_2}{(m_1 + m_2)^2}$$

$$(m_2 = m;\ m_1 = nm); \qquad = \frac{4n}{(1+n)^2}$$

Energy transfer is maximum when $K_f = 0$

$$\frac{4n}{(1+n)^2} = 1 \Rightarrow 4n = 1 + n^2 + 2n \Rightarrow n^2 + 1 - 2n = 0$$

$$(n-1)^2 = 0 \qquad n = 1 \text{ ie. } m_2 = m,\ m_1 = m$$

Transfer will be maximum when both masses are equal and one is at rest.

29. (a) For inelastic collision, linear momentum is conserved

$$\Rightarrow mv_1 = 2mv_2 \Rightarrow v_2 = \frac{v_1}{2}$$

Loss in K.E. = Gain in P.E.

$$= \frac{1}{2}mv_1^2 - \frac{1}{2}(2m)v_2^2 = 2mgh$$

$$\Rightarrow 4\text{ mgh} = mv_1^2 - \frac{mv_1^2}{2} = \frac{mv_1^2}{2} = \frac{mv^2}{2}$$

$$\Rightarrow h = \frac{v^2}{8g}$$

30. (c) Volume of water to raise = 22380 l = $22380\times10^{-3}m^3$

$$P=\frac{mgh}{t}=\frac{V\rho gh}{t}\Rightarrow t=\frac{V\rho gh}{P}$$

$$t=\frac{22380\times10^{-3}\times10^{3}\times10\times10}{10\times746}=15 \text{ min}$$

31. (b) $E=\frac{p^2}{2m}$

or, $E_1=\frac{p_1^2}{2m_1}, E_2=\frac{p_2^2}{2m_2}$

or, $m_1=\frac{p_1^2}{2E_1}, m_2=\frac{p_2^2}{2E_2}$

$m_1>m_2\Rightarrow\frac{m_1}{m_2}>1$

$\therefore \frac{p_1^2E_2}{E_1p_2^2}>1\Rightarrow\frac{E_2}{E_1}>1 \quad [\because p_1=p_2]$

or, $E_2>E_1$

32. (d) From, F = ma

$$a=\frac{F}{m}=\frac{0.1x}{10}=0.01x=V\frac{dV}{dx}$$

So, $\int_{V_1}^{V_2}VdV=\int_{20}^{30}\frac{x}{100}dx$

$$-\frac{V^2}{2}\bigg|_{V_1}^{V_2}=\frac{x^2}{200}\bigg|_{20}^{30}=\frac{30\times30}{200}-\frac{20\times20}{200}$$

$=4.5-2=2.5$

$=\frac{1}{2}m\left(V_2^2-V_1^2\right)=10\times2.5\text{ J}=-25\text{J}$

Final K.E.

$=\frac{1}{2}mV_2^2=\frac{1}{2}mV_1^2-25=\frac{1}{2}\times10\times10\times10-25$

$=500-25=475$ J

33. (c) Friction is a non-conservative force. Work done by a non-conservative force over a closed path is not zero.

34. (b) $F=\frac{12}{100}\times1000\times10\text{ N}=1200\text{ N}$

$P=Fv=1200\text{ N}\times15\text{ ms}^{-1}=18\text{ kW}.$

35. (c) When the ball is released from the top of tower then ratio of distances covered by the ball in first, second and third second

$h_I:h_{II}:h_{III}=1:3:5$: [Because $h_n\propto(2n-1)$]

$\therefore$ Ratio of work done $mgh_I:mgh_{II}:mgh_{III}=1:3:5$

36. (c) m_2 m_1

Ⓑ→ v Ⓐ

$u=0$

conservation of linear momentum along x-direction

$m_2v=m_1v_x \Rightarrow \frac{m_2v}{m_1}=v_x$

along y-direction

$m_2\times\frac{v}{2}=m_1v_y \Rightarrow v_y=\frac{m_2v}{2m_1}$

Note: Let A moves in the direction, which makes an angle θ with initial direction i.e.

$$\tan\theta=\frac{v_y}{v_x}=\frac{m_2v}{2m_1}\Big/\frac{m_2v}{m_1}$$

$$\tan\theta=\frac{1}{2}$$

$\Rightarrow \quad \theta=\tan^{-1}\left(\frac{1}{2}\right)$ to the x-axis.

37. (b) Let the block compress the spring by x before stopping.

Kinetic energy of the block = (P.E of compressed spring) + work done against friction.

$\frac{1}{2}\times2\times(4)^2=\frac{1}{2}\times10{,}000\times x^2+15\times x$

$10{,}000x^2+30x-32=0$

$\Rightarrow 5000x^2+15x-16=0$

$\therefore \; x=\frac{-15\pm\sqrt{(15)^2-4\times(5000)(-16)}}{2\times5000}$

$=0.055\text{m}=5.5\text{cm}.$

38. (a) Amount of water flowing per second from the pipe

$=\frac{m}{time}=\frac{m}{\ell}\cdot\frac{\ell}{t}=\left(\frac{m}{\ell}\right)v$

Power = K.E. of water flowing per second

$=\frac{1}{2}\left(\frac{m}{\ell}\right)v\cdot v^2$

$=\frac{1}{2}\left(\frac{m}{\ell}\right)v^3$

$=\frac{1}{2}\times100\times8=400\,W$

39. (b) Mass of over hanging chain $m'=\frac{4}{2}\times(0.6)$kg

Let at the surface PE = 0

C.M.of hanging part = 0.3 m below the table

$U_i=-m'gx=-\frac{4}{2}\times0.6\times10\times0.30$

$\Delta U=m'gx=3.6\text{J}$ = Work done in putting the entire chain on the table.

40. (d)

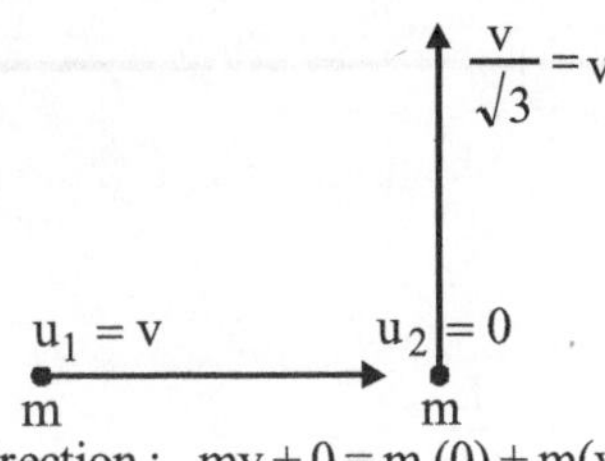

In x-direction : $mv + 0 = m(0) + m(v_2)_x$

In y-direction : $0 + 0 = m\left(\frac{v}{\sqrt{3}}\right) + m(v_2)_y$ is

$\Rightarrow (v_2)_y = \frac{v}{\sqrt{3}}$ and $(v_2)_x = v$

$\therefore \; v_2 = \sqrt{\left(\frac{v}{\sqrt{3}}\right)^2 + v^2}$

$\Rightarrow \; v_2 = \sqrt{\frac{v^2}{3} + v^2} = v\sqrt{\frac{4}{3}} = \frac{2v}{\sqrt{3}}$

Alternative method : In x-direction,
$mv = mv_1 \cos\theta$ ...(1)
where v_1 is the velocity of second mass
In y-direction,

$0 = \frac{mv}{\sqrt{3}} - mv_1 \sin\theta$

or $m_1 v_1 \sin\theta = \frac{mv}{\sqrt{3}}$ ...(2)

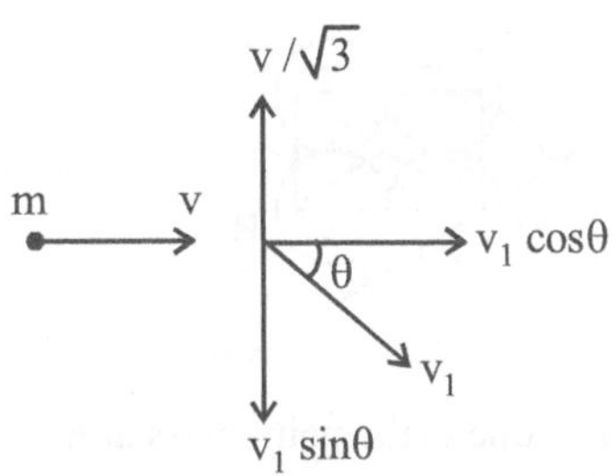

Squaring and adding eqns. (1) and (2)

$v_1^2 = v^2 + \frac{v^2}{\sqrt{3}} \Rightarrow v_1 = \frac{2}{\sqrt{3}} v$

41. (b)

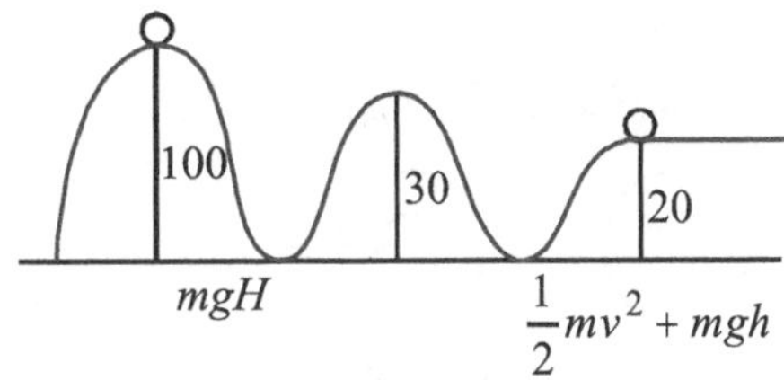

Using conservation of energy,

$m(10 \times 100) = m\left(\frac{1}{2}v^2 + 10 \times 20\right)$

or $\frac{1}{2}v^2 = 800$ or $v = \sqrt{1600} = 40$ m/s

42. (b)

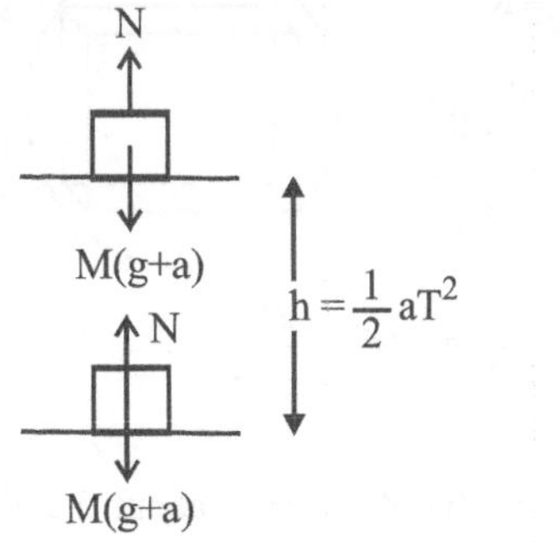

Work done by normal reaction

$= Nh = M(g+a)\frac{1}{2}aT^2 = \frac{1}{2}M(g+a)aT^2$

43. (c) Applying W-E theorem on the block for any compression x :

$W_{ext} + W_g + W_{spring} = \Delta KE$

$\Rightarrow \; Fx + 0 - \frac{1}{2}Kx^2 = \frac{1}{2}mv^2$

$\Rightarrow$ KE vs x is inverted parabola.

44. (d) $K.E. = \frac{1}{2}mv^2$

Further, $v^2 = u^2 + 2as = 0 + 2ad = 2ad$
$= 2(F/m)d$

Hence, $K.E. = \frac{1}{2}m \times 2(F/m)d = Fd$

or, K.E. acquired = Work done
$= F \times d =$ constant.
i.e., it is independent of mass m.

45. (a) Gravitational potential energy of ball gets converted into elastic potential energy of the spring.

$mg(h+d) = \frac{1}{2}kd^2$

Net work done $= mg(h+d) - \frac{1}{2}kd^2 = 0$

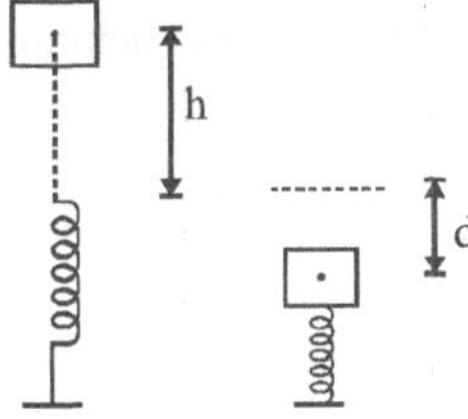

Speed Test-6

1. (a) Here $a = \frac{2}{\sqrt{3}}R$

Now, $\frac{M}{M'} = \frac{\frac{4}{3}\pi R^3}{a^3}$

$= \frac{\frac{4}{3}\pi R^3}{\left(\frac{2}{\sqrt{3}}R\right)^3} = \frac{\sqrt{3}}{2}\pi.\ \ M' = \frac{2M}{\sqrt{3}\pi}$

Moment of inertia of the cube about the given axis,

$$I = \frac{M'a^2}{6} = \frac{\frac{2M}{\sqrt{3}\pi} \times \left(\frac{2}{\sqrt{3}}R\right)^2}{6} = \frac{4MR^2}{9\sqrt{3}\pi}$$

2. (d) Initially centre of mass is at the centre. When sand is poured it will fall and again after a limit, centre of mass will rise.

3. (a) Does not shift as no external force acts. The centre of mass of the system continues its original path. It is only the internal forces which comes into play while breaking.

4. (d) Let the mass of loop P (radius = r) = m
So, the mass of loop Q (radius = nr) = nm

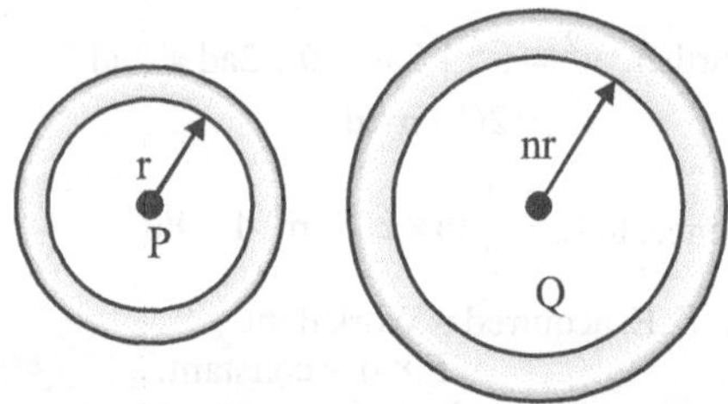

Moment of inertia of loop P, $I_P = mr^2$
Moment of inertia of loop Q, $I_Q = nm(nr)^2 = n^3mr^2$

$\therefore \frac{I_Q}{I_P} = n^3 = 8 \Rightarrow n = 2$

5. (d) When the ball is hit by a cue, the linear impulse imparted to the ball = change in momentum = mv_0

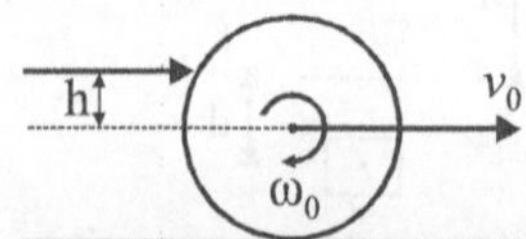

Angular momentum = Moment of momentum

$I\omega_0 = (mv_0)h$

$\frac{2}{5}mr^2\omega_0 = mv_0h$ or $\omega_0 = \frac{5v_0h}{2r^2}$

6. (d)

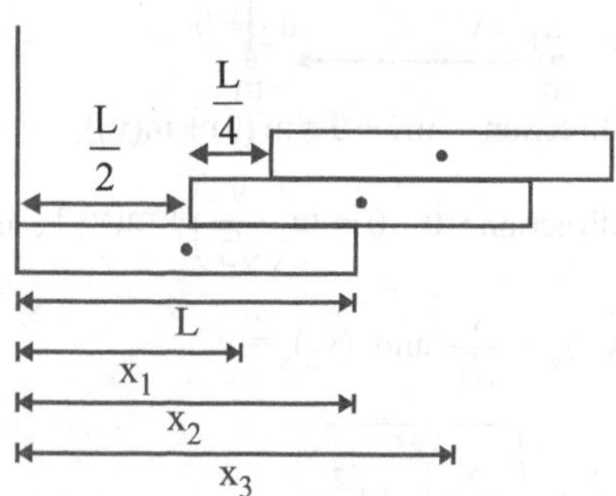

$x_1 = \frac{L}{2},\ x_2 = L,\ x_3 = \frac{5L}{4}$

$\therefore X_{CM} = \frac{m_1x_1 + m_2x_2 + m_3x_3}{m_1 + m_2 + m_3}$

$= \frac{M \times \frac{L}{2} + M \times L + M \times \frac{5L}{4}}{M + M + M}$

$= \frac{\frac{11}{4}ML}{3M} = \frac{11L}{12}$

7. (c)

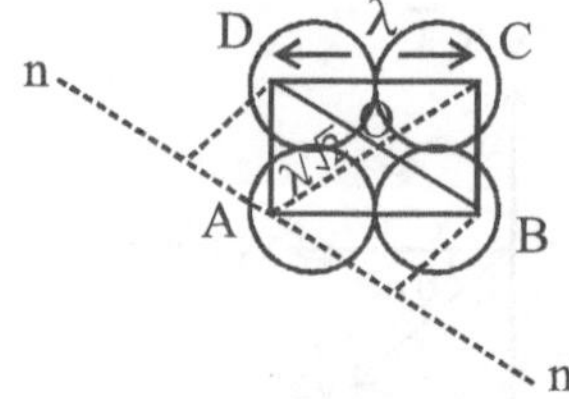

$I_{nn'}$ = M.I due to the point mass at B + M.I due to the point mass at D + M.I due to the point mass at C.

$$I_{nn'} = 2 \times m\left(\frac{\ell}{\sqrt{2}}\right)^2 + m(\sqrt{2}\ell)^2$$

$$= m\ell^2 + 2m\ell^2 = 3m\ell^2$$

8. (c)

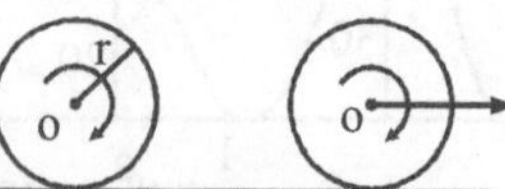

From conservation of angular momentum about any fix point on the surface,

$mr^2\omega_0 = 2mr^2\omega$

$\Rightarrow \omega = \omega_0/2 \Rightarrow v = \frac{\omega_0 r}{2}$ $[\because v = r\omega]$

9. (d) Initial position of cm $= \frac{m_2\ell}{m_1 + m_2}$

Also $x_{cm} = \frac{m_1\Delta x_1 + m_2\Delta x_2}{m_1+m_2} = \frac{m_1 v_0 t + 0}{m_1+m_2}$

$\therefore$ final position $= \frac{m_2\ell}{m_1+m_2} + \frac{m_1 v_0 t}{m_1+m_2}$

10. (a) Here, $L = 1.8\text{ kg m}^2\text{ s}^{-1}, M = 1.5\text{ kg}$, $\omega = 0.3\text{ rad s}^{-1}$
Angular momentum, $L = I\omega$
$L = k^2 M\omega$ $\quad (\because I = MK^2)$
or $1.8 = k^2 \times 1.5 \times (0.3)$

$\Rightarrow k^2 = \frac{1.8}{1.5 \times 0.3} = 4$

$\Rightarrow k = 2\text{ m}.$

11. (b) $\vec{\tau} = \vec{r} \times \vec{F} \Rightarrow \vec{r}\cdot\vec{\tau} = 0 \quad \vec{F}\cdot\vec{\tau} = 0$

Since, $\vec{\tau}$ is perpendicular to the plane of $\vec{r}$ and $\vec{F}$, hence the dot product of $\vec{\tau}$ with $\vec{r}$ and $\vec{F}$ is zero.

12. (c)

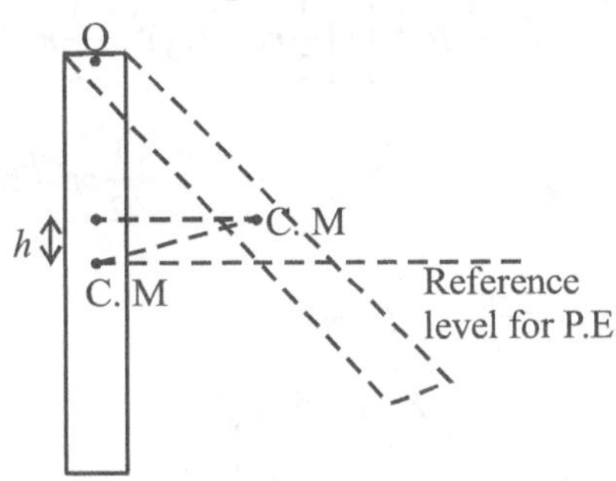

The moment of inertia of the rod about O is $\frac{1}{3}m\ell^2$.
The maximum angular speed of the rod is when the rod is instantaneously vertical. The energy of the rod in this condition is $\frac{1}{2}I\omega^2$ where I is the moment of inertia of the rod about O. When the rod is in its extreme portion, its angular velocity is zero momentarily. In this case, the energy of the rod is mgh where h is the maximum height to which the centre of mass (C.M) rises

$\therefore mgh = \frac{1}{2}I\omega^2 = \frac{1}{2}\left(\frac{1}{3}ml^2\right)\omega^2$

$\Rightarrow h = \frac{\ell^2\omega^2}{6g}$

13. (b)

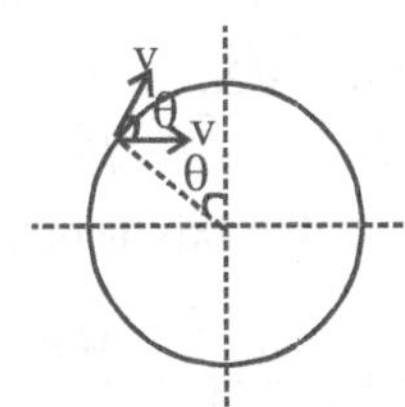

$v_R = \sqrt{v^2 + v^2 + 2v^2\cos\theta} = \sqrt{2v^2(1+\cos\theta)}$

$= 2v\cos\frac{\theta}{2}$

14. (b) $K.E_{rotational} = \frac{1}{2}I\omega^2$

$= \frac{1}{2}\frac{2}{5}\omega r^2 d^2 \left(\because I_{\text{Solid sphere}} = \frac{2}{5}mr^2\right)$

$K.E_{translational} = \frac{1}{2}mv^2$

$\therefore \frac{K.E_{rotational}}{K.E_{translational}} = \frac{2}{5}$

Hence option (b) is correct

15. (c) Kinetic energy $_{(rotational)}$ $K_R = \frac{1}{2}I\omega^2$

Kinetic energy $_{(translational)}$ $K_T = \frac{1}{2}Mv^2$ $\quad (v = R\omega)$

M.I.$_{(initial)}$ $I_{ring} = MR^2$; $\omega_{initial} = \omega$

M.I.$_{(new)}$ $I'_{(system)} = MR^2 + 2mR^2$

$\omega'_{(system)} = \frac{M\omega}{M+2m}$

Solving we get loss in K.E.

$= \frac{Mm}{(M+2m)}\omega^2R^2$

16. (b) For no angular acceleration $\tau_{net} = 0$
$\Rightarrow F_1 \times 5 = F_2 \times 30$ (given $F_2 = 4N$) $\Rightarrow F_1 = 24N$

17. (c) For toppling $Mg\frac{L}{2} = F_1 \times h$

For sliding
$\mu Mg = F_2$
For sliding to occur first
$F_1 > F_2$

or $\frac{mgL}{2} > \mu Mg$ or $L > 2\mu h$

h L L/2 Mg

18. (a)

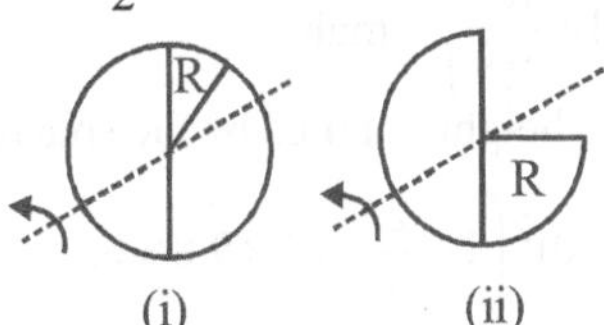

Moment of inertia of a ring about a given axis is $I = MR^2$

Mass of the remaining portion of the ring $= \frac{3M}{4}$

Moment of inertia of the remaining portion of the ring about a given axis is

$I' = \frac{3}{4}MR^2$

Given $I' = kMR^2$

$\therefore$ $k = 3/4$.

19. (b) Applying angular momentum conservation

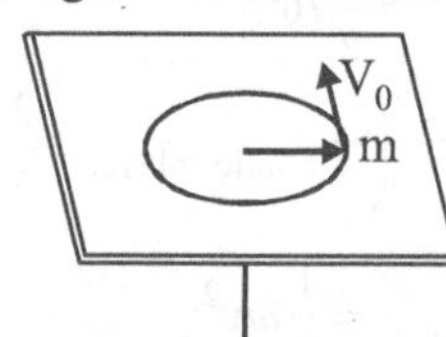

$mV_0R_0 = (m)(V^1)\left(\frac{R_0}{2}\right)$

$\therefore \quad v^1 = 2V_0$

Therefore, new KE $= \frac{1}{2}m(2V_0)^2 = 2mv_0^2$

20. (c) If rotation axis is passing through its middle point & is $\perp$ to its plane, then moment of inertia about YY' is

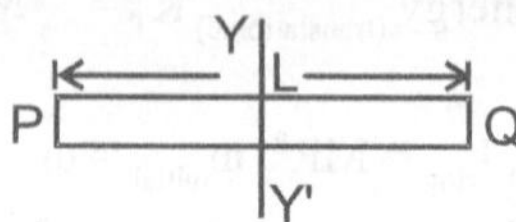

$I = \frac{ML^2}{12}$ where M = volume × density = (L×A)×ρ

so $I = \frac{L^3 A\rho}{12}$

so rotational K.E $= \frac{1}{2}I\omega^2 = \frac{L^3 A\rho\omega^2}{24}$

21. (c) If a body rolls on a horizontal surface, it possesses both translational and rotational kinetic energies. The net kinetic energy is given by

$K_{net} = \frac{1}{2}mv^2\left(1+\frac{K^2}{R^2}\right),$

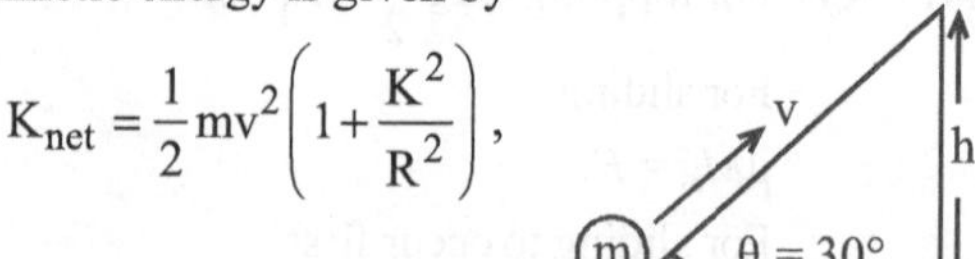

where K is the radius of gyration.
So from law of conservation of energy,

$\frac{1}{2}mv^2\left(1+\frac{K^2}{R^2}\right) = mgh,$

where h is the height attained by the sphere.

i.e., $\frac{1}{2}\times 2\times(10)^2\left(1+\frac{2}{5}\right) = 2\times 9.8\times h.$

i.e., $\frac{1}{2}\times 100\times\left(\frac{7}{5}\right) = 9.8h$

or $h = \frac{700}{98} = 7.1m$

22. (c) After collision velocity of COM of *A* becomes zero and that of *B* becomes equal to initial velocity of COM of *A*. But angular velocity of *A* remains unchanged as the two spheres are smooth.

23. (b) M.I. of disc $= \frac{1}{2}MR^2 = \frac{1}{2}M\left(\frac{M}{\pi t\rho}\right) = \frac{1}{2}\frac{M^2}{\pi t\rho}$

$\left(\text{As } \rho = \frac{M}{\pi R^2 t} \text{ Therefore } R^2 = \frac{M}{\pi t\rho}\right)$

If mass and thickness are same then, $I \propto \frac{1}{\rho}$

$\therefore \frac{I_1}{I_2} = \frac{\rho_2}{\rho_1} = \frac{3}{1}$

24. (c)

When the system is released, heavier mass move downward and the lighter one upward. Thus, centre of mass will move towards the heavier mass with acceleration

$a = \left(\frac{3m - m}{3m + m}\right)g = \frac{g}{2}$

25. (c) $K = K_{ring} + K_{particles}$

$= \left[\frac{1}{2}mv_0^2 + \frac{1}{2}I\omega^2\right] + \left[\frac{1}{2}m(\sqrt{2}v_0)^2 + \frac{1}{2}m(2v_0)^2 + \frac{1}{2}m(\sqrt{2}v_0)^2 + 0\right]$

Also $\omega = \frac{v_0}{R}$, $I = mR^2$

$\therefore \quad K = 5mv_0^2$

26. (d) $I_{nn'} = \frac{1}{12}M(a^2 + a^2) = \frac{Ma^2}{6}$

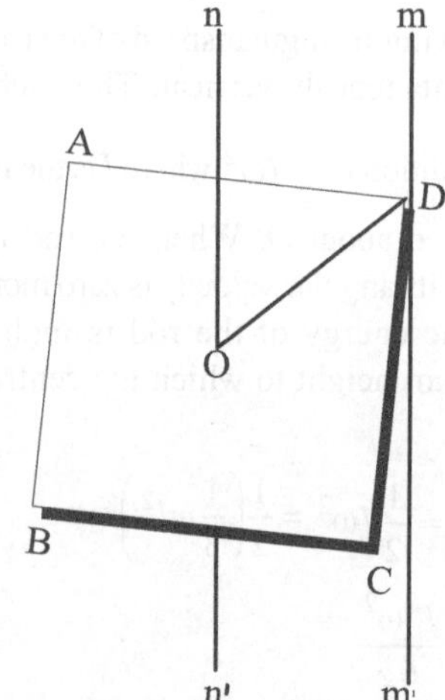

Also, $DO = \frac{DB}{2} = \frac{\sqrt{2}a}{2} = \frac{a}{\sqrt{2}}$

According to parallel axis theorem

$I_{mm'} = I_{nn'} + M\left(\frac{a}{\sqrt{2}}\right)^2 = \frac{Ma^2}{6} + \frac{Ma^2}{2}$

$= \frac{Ma^2 + 3Ma^2}{6} = \frac{2}{3}Ma^2$

27. **(a)** From law of conservation of angular momentum,

$I\omega = I'\omega'$

Given $I' = I/n$

$\therefore \quad \omega' = n\omega \quad$ or $\quad \omega' \propto n$

28. **(b)**

29. **(d)** Melting of ice produces water which will spread over larger distance away from the axis of rotation. This increases the moment of inertia so angular velocity decreases

30. **(c)** $I_p = \frac{mr^2}{2} + 2\left[\frac{mr^2}{2} + m(2r)^2\right] + \left[\frac{mr^2}{2} + m(2r)^2\right]$

$+ \left[\frac{mr^2}{2} + (2r)^2\right] + 2\left[\frac{mr^2}{2} + m(2\sqrt{3}r)^2\right]$

$= \frac{111}{2}mr^2$

31. **(d)** $0 = \frac{m_1(-x_1) + m_2x_2}{m_1 + m_2}$

$\therefore \quad m_1x_1 = m_2x_2$

$x_1 - d \quad x_2 - d'$

d   d'

m_1 O m_2

Now, $0 = \frac{-m_1(x_1 - d) + m_2(x_2 - d)}{m_1 + m_2}$

$0 = m_1(d - x_1) + m_2(x_2 - d')$

$\Rightarrow 0 = m_1d - m_1x_1 + m_2x_2 - m_2d'$

$\therefore \; d' = \frac{m_1}{m_2}d$

32. **(c)** This is a torque problem. While the fulcrum can be placed anywhere, placing it at the far right end of the bar eliminated cable B from the calculation. There are now only two forces acting on the bar ; the weight that produces a counterclockwise rotation and the tension in cable A that produces a clockwise rotation. Since the bar is in equilibrium, these two torques must sum to zero.

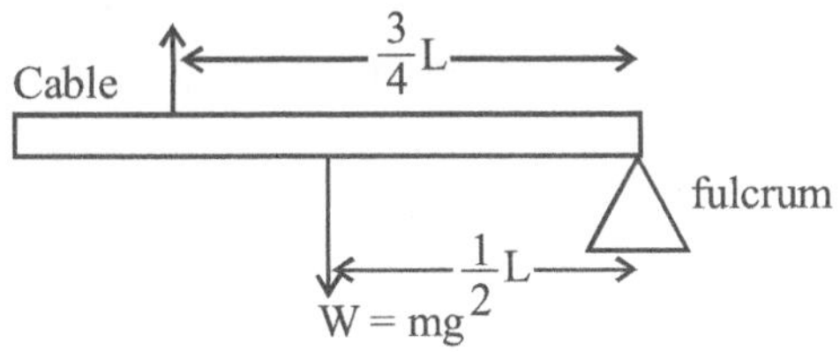

$\Sigma\tau = T_A(3/4L) - Mg(1/2L) = 0$

Therefore

$T_A = (MgL/2)/(3L/4) = (MgL/2)(4/3L) = 2Mg/3$

33. **(b)** Couple produces purely rotational motion.

34. **(a)**

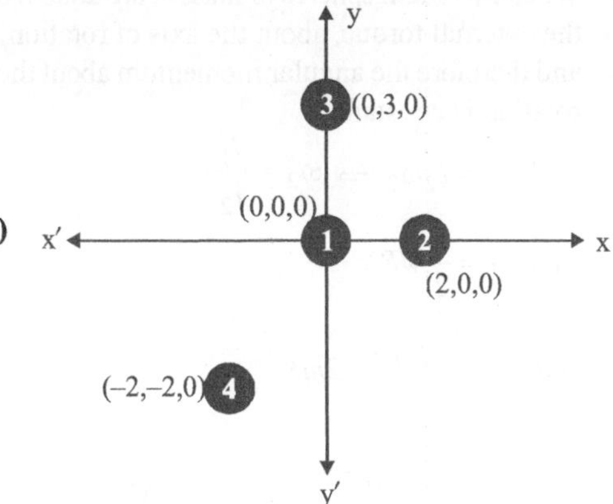

$I_1 = I_2 = 0$, because these particles are placed on x-axis

The M.I. of system about x-axis, $= I_1 + I_2 + I_3 + I_4$

$= 0 + 0 + 3 \times (3)^2 + 4 \times (-2)^2 = 27 + 16 = 43$ kg – m²

35. **(b)**

36. **(b)** $I = 1.2$ kg m², $E_r = 1500$ J,

$\alpha = 25$ rad/sec², $\omega_1 = 0$, $t = ?$

As $E_r = \frac{1}{2}I\omega^2$, $\omega = \sqrt{\frac{2E_r}{I}} = \sqrt{\frac{2 \times 1500}{1.2}} = 50$ rad / sec

From $\omega_2 = \omega_1 + \alpha t$

$50 = 0 + 25t, \quad \therefore \; t = 2$ seconds

37. **(b)** Since no external torque act on gymnast, so angular momentum ($L = I\omega$) is conserved. After pulling her arms & legs, the angular velocity increases but moment of inertia of gymnast, decreases in such a way that angular momentum remains constant.

38. **(b)** The *M.I.* about the axis of rotation is not constant as the perpendicular distance of the bead with the axis of rotation increases.

Also since no external torque is acting.

$\therefore \tau_{ext} = \frac{dL}{dt} \Rightarrow L = \text{constant} \Rightarrow I\omega = \text{constant}$

Since, *I* increases, ω decreases.

39. **(c)**

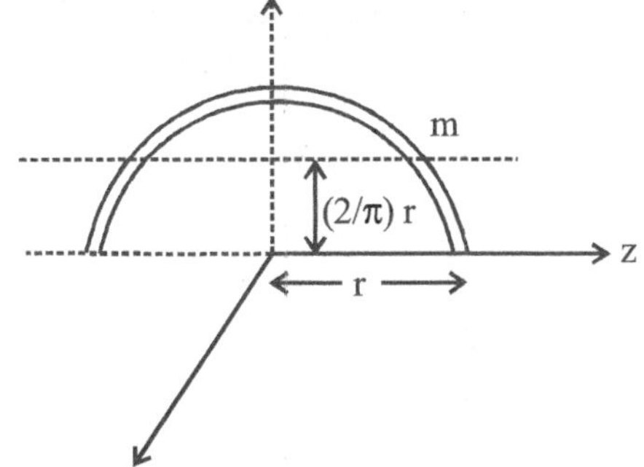

Moment of inertia about z-axis, $I_z = mr^2$

(about centre of mass)

Applying parallel axes theorem,

$I_z = I_{cm} + mk^2$

$I_{cm} = I_z - m\left(\frac{2}{\pi}r\right)^2 = mr^2 - \frac{m4r^2}{\pi^2} = mr^2\left(1 - \frac{4}{\pi^2}\right)$

i.e., $k = 4$

40. (c) When two small spheres of mass m are attached gently, the external torque, about the axis of rotation, is zero and therefore the angular momentum about the axis of rotation is constant.

$\therefore\ I_1\omega_1 = I_2\omega_2 \Rightarrow \omega_2 = \frac{I_1}{I_2}\omega_1$

Here $I_1 = \frac{1}{2}MR^2$

and $I_2 = \frac{1}{2}MR^2 + 2mR^2$

$$\therefore\ \omega_2 = \frac{\frac{1}{2}MR^2}{\frac{1}{2}MR^2 + 2mR^2} \times \omega_1 = \frac{M}{M+4m}\omega_1$$

41. (b) $Tr = \frac{mr^2}{2}\alpha_1$ .... (1)

$Tr = \frac{mr^2}{2}\alpha$ .... (2)

$\alpha_1 = \alpha$ .... (3)

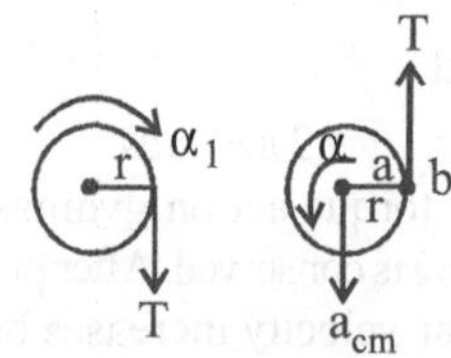

Acceleration of point b = acceleration of point a

$r\alpha_1 = a_{cm} - r\alpha$ .... (4)

Hence, $2r\alpha = a_{cm}$

42. (c) $X_{C.M.} = \frac{1\times0+2\times2+3\times0+4\times2+5\times1}{1+2+3+4+5}$

$= \frac{4+8+5}{15} = \frac{17}{15} = 1.1$

$Y_{C.M} = \frac{1\times0+2\times0+3\times2+4\times2+5\times1}{1+2+3+4+5}$

$= \frac{6+8+5}{15} = 1.3$

43. (d) $I_{AX} = m(AB)^2 + m(OC)^2 = m\ell^2 + m(\ell\cos60^\circ)^2$
$= m\ell^2 + m\ell^2/4 = 5/4\, m\ell^2$

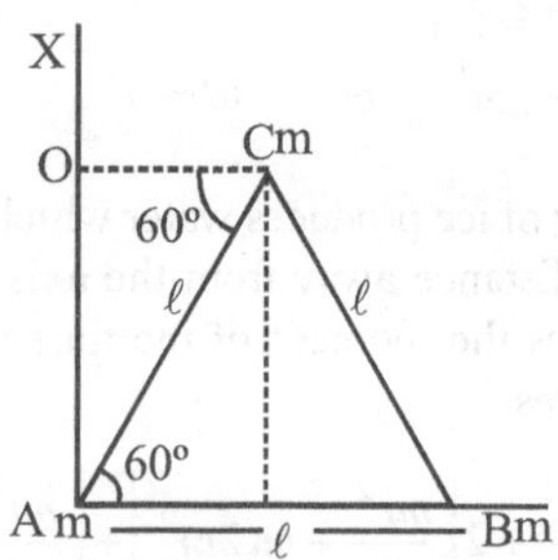

44. (c) Angle turned in three seconds, $\theta_{3s} = 2\pi \times 10 = 20\pi$ rad.

From $\theta = \omega_0 t + \frac{1}{2}\alpha t^2 \Rightarrow 20\pi = 0 + \frac{1}{2}\alpha \times (3)^2$

$\Rightarrow \alpha = \frac{40\pi}{9}$ rad/s^2

Now angle turned in 6 sec from the starting

$\theta_{6s} = \omega_0 t + \frac{1}{2}\alpha t^2 = 0 + \frac{1}{2}\times\left(\frac{40\pi}{9}\right)\times(6)^2 == 80\pi$ rad

$\therefore$ Angle turned between $t = 3$s to $t = 6$s

$\theta_{last\ 3s} = \theta_{6s} - \theta_{3s} = 80\pi - 20\pi = 60\pi$

Number of revolutions $= \frac{60\pi}{2\pi} = 30$.

45. (c) $a = \frac{f}{m} = \mu g$

and $\alpha = \frac{fR}{I} = \frac{\mu mgR}{\frac{2}{5}mR^2} = \frac{5}{2}\frac{\mu g}{R}$

Now $v = 0 + at$

and $\omega' = \omega - \alpha t$

Also $\omega' = \frac{v}{R}$

After solving above equations, we get $\omega' = \frac{2\omega}{7}$

Speed Test-7

1. (a) The escape velocity on the earth is defined as

$$v_e = \sqrt{2g_eR_e}$$

Where R_e & g_e are the radius & acceleration due to gravity of earth.

Now for planet $g_P=2g_e$, $R_P=R_e/4$

$$\text{So } v_P = \sqrt{2g_PR_P} = \sqrt{2\times 2g_e \times R_e/4} = \frac{v_e}{\sqrt{2}}$$

2. (c) Applying conservation of energy principle, we get

$$\frac{1}{2}mk^2v_e^2 - \frac{GMm}{R} = -\frac{GMm}{r}$$

$$\Rightarrow \frac{1}{2}mk^2\frac{2GM}{R} - \frac{GMm}{R} = -\frac{GMm}{r}$$

$$\Rightarrow \frac{k^2}{R} - \frac{1}{R} = -\frac{1}{r} \Rightarrow \frac{1}{r} = \frac{1}{R} - \frac{k^2}{R}$$

$$\Rightarrow \frac{1}{r} = \frac{1}{R}(1-k^2) \Rightarrow r = \frac{R}{1-k^2}$$

3. (d) The gravitational force due to the whole sphere at A point is

$$F_1 = \frac{GM_em_o}{(2R)^2}$$, where m_0 is the assumed rest mass at point A.

In the second case, when we made a cavity of radius (R/2), then gravitational force at point A is

$$F_2 = \frac{GM_em_o}{(R+R/2)^2} \qquad \therefore F_2/F_1 = 1/9$$

4. (c) According to Kepler's law of period $T^2 \propto R^3$

$$\frac{T_1^2}{T_2^2} = \frac{R_1^3}{R_2^3} = \frac{(6R)^3}{(3R)^3} = 8$$

$$\frac{24\times 24}{T_2^2} = 8$$

$$T_2^2 = \frac{24\times 24}{8} = 72 = 36\times 2$$

$$T_2 = 6\sqrt{2}$$

5. (d) Total energy $= -KE = \frac{PE}{2}$

$$KE = \frac{1}{2}mv^2$$

$$\therefore \text{ Total energy} = -\frac{1}{2}mv^2$$

6. (a) The force of attraction between sphere and shaded position $dF = GM\frac{\left(\frac{m}{l}dx\right)}{x^2}$

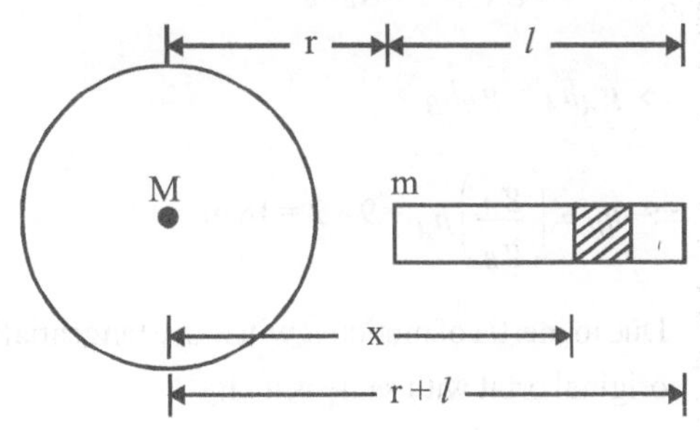

$$F = \int_r^{r+l}\frac{GMm}{lx^2}dx = \frac{GMm}{l}\int_r^{r+l}\frac{1}{x^2}dx$$

$$= \frac{GMm}{l}\int_r^{r+l}x^{-2}dx = \frac{GMm}{l}\left[\frac{x^{-2+1}}{-2+1}\right]_r^{r+l}$$

$$= -\frac{GMm}{l}\left[x^{-1}\right]_r^{r+l} = -\frac{GMm}{l}\left[\frac{1}{x}\right]_r^{r+l} = \frac{GMm}{r(r+l)}$$

7. (b) $F = \frac{k}{R} = \frac{Mv^2}{R}$. Hence $v \propto R^0$

8. (d) $\frac{mv^2}{(R+x)} = \frac{GmM}{(R+x)^2}$ also $g = \frac{GM}{R^2}$

$$\therefore \frac{mv^2}{(R+x)} = m\left(\frac{GM}{R^2}\right)\frac{R^2}{(R+x)^2}$$

$$\therefore \frac{mv^2}{(R+x)} = mg\frac{R^2}{(R+x)^2}$$

$$\therefore v^2 = \frac{gR^2}{R+x} \Rightarrow v = \left(\frac{gR^2}{R+x}\right)^{1/2}$$

9. (b) $v = \frac{3}{4}v_e$

$$K.E. = \frac{1}{2}mv^2 = \frac{1}{2}m\left(\frac{3}{4}v_e\right)^2 = \frac{9}{32}mv_e^2$$

$$= \frac{9}{32}m\left(\frac{2GM}{R}\right)$$

$$K.E. = \frac{9}{16}\frac{GMm}{R}\ ;\ P.E. = -\frac{GMm}{R}$$

$$\text{Total energy} = K.E. + P.E. = -\frac{7}{16}\frac{GMm}{R}$$

Let the height above the surface of earth be h, then

$$P.E. = -\frac{GMm}{h}$$

$$-\frac{7}{16}\frac{GMm}{R} = -\frac{GMm}{h} \quad \therefore h = \frac{16R}{7}$$

10. (a) When closer to the sun, velocity of planet will be greater. So time taken in covering a given area will be less.

11. (c) Applying conservation of total mechanical energy principle

$$\frac{1}{2}mv^2 = mg_A h_A = mg_B h_B$$

$$\Rightarrow g_A h_A = g_B h_B$$

$$\Rightarrow h_B = \left(\frac{g_A}{g_B}\right) h_A = 9 \times 2 = 18\,\text{m}$$

12. (b) Due to inertia of motion it will move tangentially to the original orbit with same velocity.

13. (a) $F \propto xM \times (1-x)M = xM^2(1-x)$

For maximum force, $\frac{dF}{dx} = 0$

$$\Rightarrow \frac{dF}{dx} = M^2 - 2xM^2 = 0 \Rightarrow x = 1/2$$

14. (c) Mass of the satellite = m and height of satellite from earth (h) = 6.4×10^6 m.

We know that gravitational potential energy of the satellite at height

$$h = -\frac{GM_e m}{R_e + h} = -\frac{gR_e^2 m}{2R_e} = -\frac{gR_e m}{2} = -0.5\,mgR_e$$

(where, $GM_e = gR_e^2$ and $h = R_e$)

15. (d) Acceleration due to gravity on earth's surface

$$g = G\frac{M}{R^2}$$

This implies that as radius decreases, the acceleration due to gravity increases.

$$\frac{\Delta g}{g} = -2\frac{\Delta R}{R} \quad \text{But} \quad \frac{\Delta R}{R} = -1\%$$

('–' sign is due to shrinking of earth)

$$\therefore \quad \frac{\Delta g}{g} = -2 \times (-1\%) = 2\%$$

16. (a) According to kepler's law of area

$$\frac{dA}{dt} = \frac{L}{2m}$$

For central forces, torque = 0

$\therefore$ L = constant

$$\therefore \quad \frac{dA}{dt} = \text{constant}$$

17. (b) Potential energy of particle at the centre of square

$$= -4\left(\frac{GMm}{\frac{a}{\sqrt{2}}}\right)$$

$$\therefore -4\left(\frac{GMm}{a/\sqrt{2}}\right) + \frac{1}{2}mv^2 = 0 \Rightarrow v^2 = \frac{8\sqrt{2}\,GM}{a}$$

18. (c) The potential energy for a conservative force is defined as

$$F = \frac{-dU}{dr} \quad \text{or} \quad U = -\int_{\infty}^{r} \vec{F}.d\vec{r} \quad \text{......(i)}$$

$$\text{or } U_r = \int_{\infty}^{r} \frac{GM_1M_2}{r^2}\,dr = \frac{-GM_1M_2}{r} \quad \text{......(ii)}$$

$(\because U_\infty = 0)$

If we bring the mass from the infinity to the centre of earth, then we obtain work, 'so it has negative (gravitational force do work on the object) sign & potential energy decreases. But if we bring the mass from the surface of earth to infinite, then we must do work against gravitational force & potential energy of the mass increases.

Now in equation (i) if $F = \frac{GM_1M_2}{r^{5/2}}$ instead of

$F = \frac{GM_1M_2}{r^2}$ then

$$U_r = \int_{\infty}^{r} \frac{GM_1M_2}{r^{5/2}}\,dr = \frac{-2}{3}\frac{GM_1M_2}{r^{3/2}}$$

$$\Rightarrow U_r \propto \frac{1}{r^{+3/2}}$$

19. (b) As we know, the minimum speed with which a body is projected so that it does not return back is called escape speed.

$$V_e = \sqrt{\frac{2GM}{r}} = \sqrt{\frac{2GM}{R+h}} = \sqrt{\frac{2GM}{4R}}$$

$$= \left(\frac{GM}{2R}\right)^{\frac{1}{2}} \quad (\because h = 3R)$$

20. (a) Acceleration due to gravity at a height h above the earth's surface is

$$g_h = g\left(1 - \frac{2h}{R}\right)$$

Acceleration due to gravity at a depth d below the earth's surface is

$$g_d = g\left(1 - \frac{d}{R}\right)$$

$$\text{Now, } \frac{g_h}{g_d} = \frac{\left(1-\frac{2h}{R}\right)}{\left(1-\frac{d}{R}\right)} = \frac{(R-2h)}{(R-d)}$$

As h = 1 km, d = 1 km

$$\therefore \quad \frac{g_h}{g_d} = \frac{R-2}{R-1}$$

21. (a) At the surface of earth, the value of $g = 9.8 m/sec^2$. If we go towards the centre of earth or we go above the surface of earth, then in both the cases the value of g decreases.

Hence $W_1 = mg_{mine}$, $W_2 = mg_{sea\ level}$, $W_3 = mg_{moun}$

So $W_1 < W_2 > W_3$ (g at the sea level = g at the suface of earth)

22. (d) Time period does not depend upon the mass of satellite

23. (a) $T = \dfrac{2\pi r}{v_0} = \dfrac{2\pi r}{(gR^2/r)^{1/2}} = \dfrac{2\pi r^{3/2}}{\sqrt{gR^2}} = \dfrac{2\pi}{\omega}$

Hence, $r^{3/2} = \dfrac{\sqrt{gR^2}}{\omega}$ or $r^3 = \dfrac{gR^2}{\omega^2}$

or, $r = (gR^2/\omega^2)^{1/3}$

24. (b) $g' = g - \omega^2 R\cos^2\lambda$

To make effective acceleration due to gravity zero at equator $\lambda = 0$ and $g' = 0$

$\therefore 0 = g - \omega^2 R \Rightarrow \omega = \sqrt{\dfrac{g}{R}} = \dfrac{1}{800}\dfrac{rad}{s}$

25. (a) $mg = 72$ N (body weight on the surface)

$g = \dfrac{GM}{R^2}$

At a height $H = \dfrac{R}{2}$,

$g' = \dfrac{GM}{\left(R + \dfrac{R}{2}\right)^2} = \dfrac{4\ GM}{9\ R^2}$

Body weight at height $H = \dfrac{R}{2}$,

$mg' = m \times \dfrac{4}{9}\dfrac{GM}{R^2}$

$= m \times \dfrac{4}{9} \times g = \dfrac{4}{9} mg$

$= \dfrac{4}{9} \times 72 = 32$ N

26. (c) At a height h,

$g' = g\dfrac{R^2}{(R+h)^2} \Rightarrow mg' = mg\left(\dfrac{R}{R+h}\right)^2$

$\Rightarrow W' = W\left(\dfrac{R}{R+h}\right)^2$

Here, h = R/2

$\therefore W' = \dfrac{4}{9}W$

27. (c) Gravitational P.E. = m × gravitational potential U = mV, so the graph of U will be same as that of V for a spherical shell.

28. (c) Applying the properties of ellipse, we have

$\dfrac{2}{R} = \dfrac{1}{r_1} + \dfrac{1}{r_2} = \dfrac{r_1 + r_2}{r_1 r_2}$

Instant position of satellite
Sun
R
major axis
r_1 r_2

$R = \dfrac{2 r_1 r_2}{r_1 + r_2}$

29. (c) In a circular or elliptical orbital motion, torque is always acting parallel to displacement or velocity. So, angular momentum is conserved. In attractive field, potential energy is negative. Kinetic energy changes as velocity increase when distance is less. So, option (c) is correct.

30. (a) Here, $v = \sqrt{\dfrac{2GM}{R}}$ and $kv = \sqrt{\dfrac{2GM}{R+R}}$.

Solving $k = \dfrac{1}{\sqrt{2}}$

31. (a) $g = \dfrac{G(2M)}{(2R)^2} = \dfrac{GM}{2R^2}$

From $h = \dfrac{1}{2}gt^2$ $[\because U = 0]$

$t = \sqrt{\dfrac{2h}{g}} = 2\sqrt{\dfrac{hR^2}{GM}}$

32. (b) $P.E. = \int_{R_0}^{R} \dfrac{GMm}{r^2} dr = -GMm\left[\dfrac{1}{R} - \dfrac{1}{R_0}\right]$

The K.E. acquired by the body at the surface $= \dfrac{1}{2}mv^2$

$\therefore \dfrac{1}{2}mv^2 = -GMm\left[\dfrac{1}{R} - \dfrac{1}{R_0}\right]$

$v = \sqrt{2GM\left(\dfrac{1}{R_0} - \dfrac{1}{R}\right)}$

33. (b) $\dfrac{mv^2}{R} = \dfrac{k}{R^2}$ or $mv^2 = \dfrac{k}{R}$

Kinetic energy $= \dfrac{1}{2}mv^2 = \dfrac{k}{2R}$

In case of satellites P.E = – 2 K.E

and T.E = P. E + K. E

Total energy $= \dfrac{k}{2R} - \dfrac{k}{R} = -\dfrac{k}{2R}$

34. (d) Variation of g with altitude is,

$g_h = g\left[1 - \dfrac{2h}{R}\right]$;

variation of g with depth is,

$$g_d = g\left[1 - \frac{d}{R}\right]$$

Equating g_h and g_d, we get $d = 2h$

35. (a) The total momentum will be zero and hence velocity will be zero just after collisiion. The pull of earth will make it fall down.

36. (b) Loss in potential energy = Gain in kinetic energy

$$-\frac{GMm}{R} - \left(-\frac{3}{2}\frac{GMm}{R}\right) = \frac{1}{2}mv^2$$

$$\Rightarrow \frac{GMm}{2R} = \frac{1}{2}mv^2 \Rightarrow v = \sqrt{\frac{GM}{R}} = \sqrt{gR}$$

37. (d)

38. (b) $g \propto \frac{1}{R^2}$

R decreasing g increase hence, curve b represents correct variation.

39. (d) Angular momentum, $L = I\omega$; moment of inertia of sphere along the axis passing through centre of mass,

$$I = \frac{2}{5}MR^2 \text{ and } \omega = \frac{2\pi}{T}.$$

Putting these values, $L = \frac{4\pi\, MR^2}{5T}$

40. (c) $T = 2\pi\sqrt{\frac{(R+h)^3}{GM}}$

$$T_1 = 2\pi\sqrt{\frac{R^3}{GM}},\quad T_2 = 2\pi\sqrt{\frac{(1.01R)^3}{GM}}$$

$$\frac{T_2 - T_1}{T_1} \times 100 = 1.5\%$$

41. (a) The gravitational potential at the centre of uniform spherical shell is equal to the gravitational potential at the surface of shell i.e.,

$V = \frac{-GM}{a}$, where a is radius of spherical shell

Now, if the shell shrinks then its radius decrease then density increases, but mass is constant. so from above expression if a decreases, then V increases.

42. (b) $g' = g\left(1 - \frac{d}{R}\right) \Rightarrow \frac{g}{n} = g\left(1 - \frac{d}{R}\right)$

$$\Rightarrow d = \left(\frac{n-1}{n}\right)R$$

43. (d) $E_{earth} = E_{moon}$

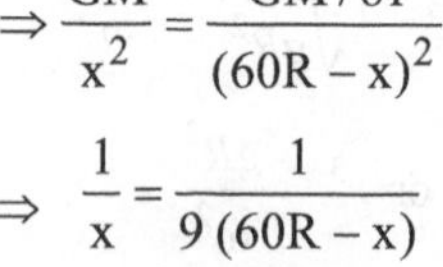

$$\Rightarrow \frac{GM}{x^2} = \frac{GM/81}{(60R - x)^2}$$

$$\Rightarrow \frac{1}{x} = \frac{1}{9(60R - x)}$$

$\Rightarrow x = 54$ R from centre of earth.

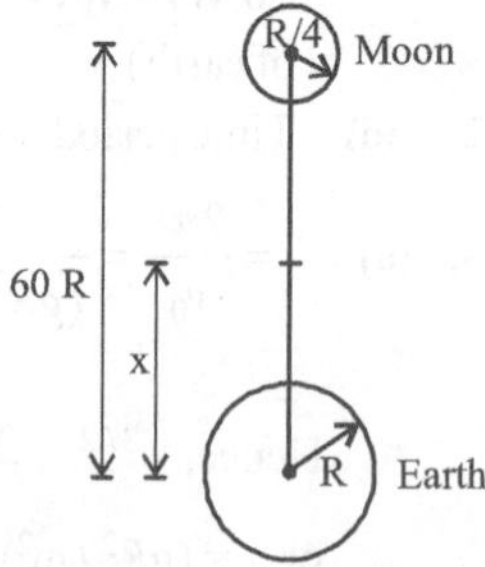

44. (b) Acceleration due to gravity at lattitude' λ ' is given by

$$g_\lambda = g_e - R_e\omega^2\cos^2\lambda$$

At equator, $\lambda = 90° \Rightarrow \cos\lambda = \cos 90° = 0$

or $g_\lambda = g_e = g$ (as given in question)

At 30°, $g_{30} = g - R\omega^2\cos^2 30 = g - \frac{3}{4}R\omega^2$

or, $g - g_{30} = \frac{3}{4}R\omega^2$

45. (a) As we know,

Gravitational potential energy $= \frac{-GMm}{r}$

and orbital velocity, $v_0 = \sqrt{GM/R+h}$

$$E_f = \frac{1}{2}mv_0^2 - \frac{GMm}{3R} = \frac{1}{2}m\frac{GM}{3R} - \frac{GMm}{3R}$$

$$= \frac{GMm}{3R}\left(\frac{1}{2} - 1\right) = \frac{-GMm}{6R}$$

$$E_i = \frac{-GMm}{R} + K$$

$$E_i = E_f$$

Therefore minimum required energy, $K = \frac{5GMm}{6R}$

Speed Test-8

1. (c) We know that Young's modulus

$$Y = \frac{F}{\pi r^2} \times \frac{L}{\ell}$$

Since Y, F are same for both the wires, we have,

$$\frac{1}{r_1^2}\frac{L_1}{\ell_1} = \frac{1}{r_2^2}\frac{L_2}{\ell_2}$$

or, $$\frac{\ell_1}{\ell_2} = \frac{r_2^2 \times L_1}{r_1^2 \times L_2} = \frac{(D_2/2)^2 \times L_1}{(D_1/2)^2 \times L_2}$$

or, $$\frac{\ell_1}{\ell_2} = \frac{D_2^2 \times L_1}{D_1^2 \times L_2} = \frac{D_2^2}{(2D_2)^2} \times \frac{L_2}{2L_2} = \frac{1}{8}$$

So, $\ell_1 : \ell_2 = 1 : 8$

2. (a) From the graph, it is clear that for the same value of load, elongation is maximum for wire *OA*. Hence *OA* is the thinnest wire among the four wires.

3. (b) Small amount of work done in extending the spring by *dx* is

$dW = k\,x\,dx$

$$\therefore W = k\int_{0.05}^{0.15} x\,dx$$

$$= \frac{800}{2}\left[(0.15)^2 - (0.05)^2\right]$$

$= 400\,[(0.15 + 0.05)(0.15 - 0.05)]$

$= 400 \times 0.2 \times 0.1 = 8\text{ J}$

4. (c) Using the usual expression for the Young's modulus, the force constant for the wire can be written as $k = \frac{F}{\Delta l} = \frac{YA}{L}$ where the symbols have their usual meanings. Now the two wires together will have an effective force constant $\left[\frac{k_1 k_2}{k_1 + k_2}\right]$. Substituting the corresponding lengths and the Young's moduli we get the answer.

5. (b) Compressibility of water,

$K = 45.4 \times 10^{-11}\text{ Pa}^{-1}$

density of water $P = 10^3\text{ kg/m}^3$

depth of ocean, $h = 2700$ m

We have to find $\frac{\Delta V}{V} = ?$

As we know, compressibility,

$$K = \frac{1}{B} = \frac{(\Delta V/V)}{P}\ (P = \rho g h)$$

So, $(\Delta V/V) = K\rho g h$

$= 45.4 \times 10^{-11} \times 10^3 \times 10 \times 2700$

$= 1.2258 \times 10^{-2}$

6. (a) Young's modulus $Y = \frac{W}{A}\cdot\frac{l}{\Delta l}$

$$\frac{W_1}{Y_1} = \frac{W_2}{Y_2}$$

[$\because$ A, l, Δl same for both brass and steel]

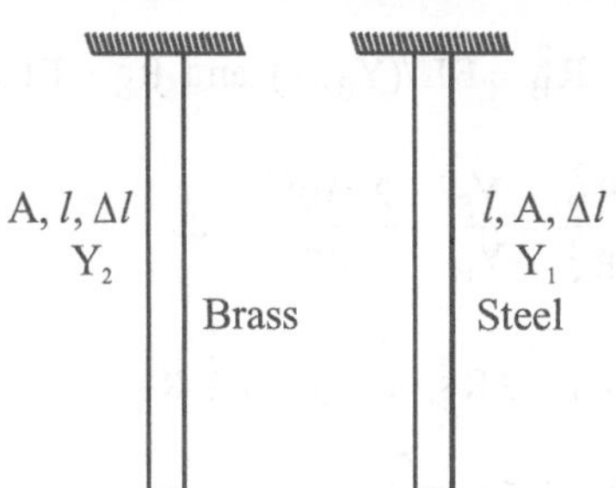

$$\frac{W_1}{W_2} = \frac{Y_1}{Y_2} = 2 \quad [Y_{steel}/Y_{brass} = 2 \text{ given}]$$

7. (b) Solids are least compressible whereas gases are highly compressible.

8. (d) $Y_c \times (\Delta L_c / L_c) = Y_s \times (\Delta L_s / L_s)$

$$\Rightarrow 1\times 10^{11} \times \left(\frac{1\times 10^{-3}}{1}\right) = 2\times 10^{11} \times \left(\frac{\Delta L_s}{0.5}\right)$$

$$\therefore \Delta L_s = \frac{0.5 \times 10^{-3}}{2} = 0.25\text{ mm}$$

Therefore, total extension of the composite wire = $\Delta L_c + \Delta L_s$

$= 1\text{ mm} + 0.25\text{ mm} = 1.25\text{ mm}$

9. (b) Bulk modulus $B = \frac{-P}{(\Delta V/V)} = \frac{-PV}{\Delta V}$ ....(1)

and $\Delta V = \gamma V \Delta T = 3\alpha.V.T$ or $\frac{-V}{\Delta V} = \frac{1}{3\alpha.T.}$ ...(2)

From eqs. (1) and (2), $B = P/(3\alpha.T)$ or $T = \frac{P}{3\alpha B}$

10. (a) When same stress is applied at two different temperatures, the increase in length is more at higher temperature. Thus $T_1 > T_2$.

11. (c) According to questions,

$$\frac{\ell_s}{\ell_b} = a,\ \frac{r_s}{r_b} = b,\ \frac{y_s}{y_b} = c,\ \frac{\Delta\ell s}{\Delta\ell_b} = ?$$

As, $y = \frac{F\ell}{A\Delta\ell} \Rightarrow \Delta\ell = \frac{F\ell}{Ay}$

$$\Delta\ell_s = \frac{3mg\ell_s}{\pi r_s^2 . y_s} \quad [\because F_s = (M + 2M)g]$$

$$\Delta\ell_b = \frac{2Mg\ell_b}{\pi r_b^2 \cdot y_b} \quad [\because F_b = 2Mg]$$

$$\therefore \frac{\Delta\ell_s}{\Delta\ell_b} = \frac{\dfrac{3Mg\ell_s}{\pi r_s^2 \cdot y_s}}{\dfrac{2Mg.\ell_b}{\pi r_b^2 \cdot y_b}} = \frac{3a}{2b^2 c}$$

12. (b) We know that $Y = FL/\pi r^2 \ell$ or $r^2 = FL/(Y\pi\ell)$

$$\therefore \quad R_B^2 = FL/(Y_B \pi\ell) \text{ and } R_S^2 = FL/(Y_S \pi\ell)$$

$$\text{or } \frac{R_B^2}{R_S^2} = \frac{Y_S}{Y_B} = \frac{2\times10^{10}}{10^{10}} = 2$$

$$\text{or } R_B^2 = 2R_S^2 \text{ or } R_B = \sqrt{2}\, R_S$$

$$\therefore R_S = R_B/\sqrt{2}$$

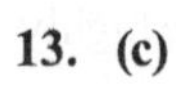
13. (c)

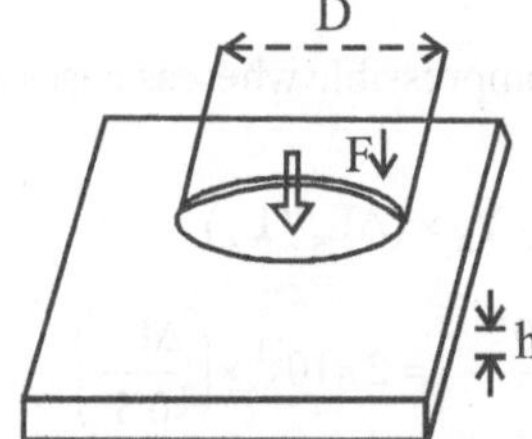

Shearing strain is created along the side surface of the punched disk. Note that the forces exerted on the disk are exerted along the circumference of the disk, and the total force exerted on its center only.
Let us assume that the shearing stress along the side surface of the disk is uniform, then

$$F = \int_{\text{surface}} dF_{max} = \int_{\text{surface}} \sigma_{max} dA = \sigma_{max} \int_{\text{surface}} dA$$

$$= \int \sigma_{max} . A = \sigma_{max} . 2\pi\left(\frac{D}{2}\right)h$$

$$= 3.5\times10^8 \times\left(\frac{1}{2}\times10^{-2}\right)\times0.3\times10^{-2}\times2\pi$$

$$= 3.297\times10^4 \simeq 3.3\times10^4 \text{N}$$

14. (d) Bulk modulus is given by, $k = \dfrac{F/A}{\Delta V/V}$

$$= \frac{mg}{A\left(\dfrac{\Delta V}{V}\right)} = \frac{h\rho g}{\left(\dfrac{\Delta V}{V}\right)}, \quad \left(\because \rho = \frac{m}{V}, V = A\times h\right)$$

Given, $h = 400$ m, $\dfrac{\Delta V}{V} = \dfrac{0.2}{100}$

and $\rho = 1\times 10^3$ kg/m^3

$$\therefore k = \frac{400\times10^3\times9.8}{0.2/100} = 196\times10^7 \text{N m}^{-2}$$

$$k = 1.96\times10^9 \text{N m}^{-2}.$$

15. (a) $C_1 = \dfrac{\pi\eta(r_2^4 - r_1^4)}{2\ell}, C_2 = \dfrac{\pi\eta r^4}{2\ell}$

Initial volume = Final volume

$$\therefore \pi[r_2^2 - r_1^2]\ell\rho = \pi r^2 \ell\rho$$

$$\Rightarrow r^2 = r_2^2 - r_1^2 \Rightarrow r^2 = (r_2 + r_1)(r_2 - r_1)$$

$$\Rightarrow r^2 = (8.02 + 7.98)(8.02 - 7.98)$$

$$\Rightarrow r^2 = 16\times0.04 = 0.64 \text{ cm} \Rightarrow r = 0.8 \text{ cm}$$

$$\therefore \frac{C_1}{C_2} = \frac{r_2^4 - r_1^4}{r^4} = \frac{[8.02]^4 - [7.98]^4}{[0.8]^4}$$

16. (c)

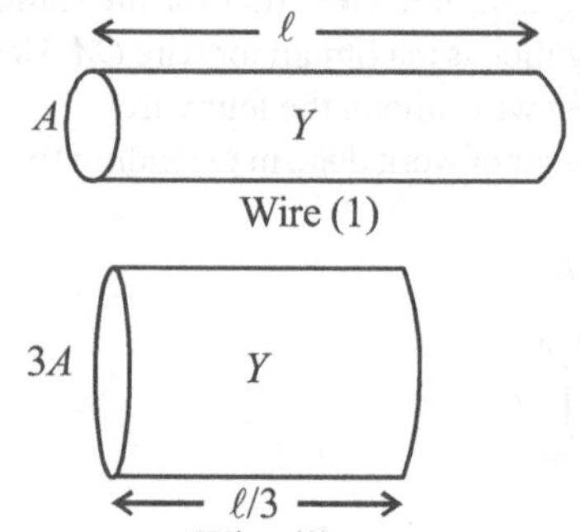

As shown in the figure, the wires will have the same Young's modulus (same material) and the length of the wire of area of cross-section $3A$ will be $\ell/3$ (same volume as wire 1).
For wire 1,

$$Y = \frac{F/A}{\Delta x/\ell} \quad \text{...(i)}$$

For wire 2,

$$Y = \frac{F'/3A}{\Delta x/(\ell/3)} \quad \text{...(ii)}$$

From (i) and (ii), $\dfrac{F}{A}\times\dfrac{\ell}{\Delta x} = \dfrac{F'}{3A}\times\dfrac{\ell}{3\Delta x} \Rightarrow F' = 9F$

17. (c) Poisson's ratio, $\sigma = \dfrac{\text{lateral strain }(\beta)}{\text{longitudinal strain }(\alpha)}$

For material like copper, $\sigma = 0.33$
And, $y = 3k(1 - 2\sigma)$

Also, $\dfrac{9}{y} = \dfrac{1}{k} + \dfrac{3}{n}$

$y = 2n(1 + \sigma)$
Hence, $n < y < k$

18. (b) Stress = 1 kg wt/mm^2 = 9.8 N/mm^2
= 9.8 × 10^6 N/m^2.

$$Y = 1\times10^{11}\,N/m^2, \quad \frac{\Delta\ell}{\ell}\times100 = ?$$

$$Y = \frac{\text{Stress}}{\text{Strain}} = \frac{\text{Stress}}{\Delta\ell/\ell}$$

$$\therefore \frac{\Delta\ell}{\ell} = \frac{\text{Stress}}{Y} = \frac{9.8\times10^6}{1\times10^{11}}$$

$$\frac{\Delta\ell}{\ell}\times100 = 9.8\times10^{-11}\times100\times10^6$$

$= 9.8 \times 10^{-3} = 0.0098$ %

19. (d) $W_1 = \frac{1}{2}kx^2$

and $W_2 = \frac{1}{2}k(x+y)^2$

$$\therefore \quad W = W_2 - W_1 = \frac{1}{2}k(x+y)^2 - \frac{1}{2}kx^2$$

$$= \frac{1}{2}ky(2x+y)$$

20. (c) Here, $k_Q = \frac{k_P}{2}$

According to Hooke's law

$\therefore$ $F_p = -k_p x_p$

$$F_Q = -k_Q x_Q \Rightarrow \frac{F_P}{F_Q} = \frac{k_P\,x_P}{k_Q\,x_Q}$$

$F_p = F_Q$ [Given]

$$\therefore \quad \frac{x_P}{x_Q} = \frac{k_Q}{k_P} \quad ...(i)$$

Energy stored in a spring is $U = \frac{1}{2}kx^2$

$$\therefore \quad \frac{U_P}{U_Q} = \frac{k_P x_P^2}{k_Q x_Q^2} = \frac{k_P}{k_Q}\times\frac{k_Q^2}{k_P^2} = \frac{1}{2} \qquad \left[\because k_Q = \frac{k_P}{2}\right]$$

$$\Rightarrow \quad U_P = \frac{U_Q}{2} = \frac{E}{2} \qquad [\therefore U_Q = E]$$

21. (a) Young's modulus $Y = \frac{\text{stress}}{\text{strain}}$

stress = Y × strain

Stress in steel wire = Applied pressure

Pressure = stress = Y × strain

Strain $= \frac{\Delta L}{L} = \alpha\,\Delta T$ (As length is constant)

$= 2 \times 10^{11} \times 1.1 \times 10^{-5} \times 100 = 2.2 \times 10^8$ Pa

22. (b) Let T be the tension in the ring, then

$$Y = \frac{T.2\pi r}{A.2\pi(R-r)} = \frac{T r}{A(R-r)} \quad \therefore \quad T = \frac{YA(R-r)}{r}$$

23. (a) Ratio of radii $r_1 : r_2 = 1:2$

Ratio of area, $A_1 : A_2 = \pi r_1^2 : \pi r_2^2$

$A_1 : A_2 = 1 : 4$

Now, Stress$_1$: Stress$_2$ = 4 : 1

So, Strain$_1$: Strain$_2$ = 4 : 1

$$\therefore \quad \frac{l_1}{l_2} = \frac{4}{1} \Rightarrow 4l_2 = l_1 = 8$$

$\therefore$ $l_2 = 2$ mm

Increase in length of B is 2 mm.

24. (b) $\frac{dV}{V} = (1+2\sigma)\frac{dL}{L}$

$$\frac{dV}{V} = 2\times2\times10^{-3} = 4\times10^{-3}$$

$$\left[\because \sigma = 0.5 = \frac{1}{2}\right]$$

$\therefore$ Percentage change in volume = 4 × 10^{-1} = 0.4%

25. (b) $r\theta = \ell\phi \Rightarrow \phi = \frac{r\theta}{\ell} = \frac{6\text{mm}\times30°}{1\text{m}} = 0.18°$

26. (d) Bulk modulus $B = \frac{|-dp|}{\left|\left(\frac{dV}{V}\right)\right|}$

$\therefore$ Pressure, $dp = B\left(\frac{\Delta V}{V}\right)$

27. (a) Given: $F = 100$ kN $= 10^5$ N

$Y = 2 \times 10^{11}$ Nm^{-2}

$\ell_0 = 1.0$ m

radius r = 10 mm = 10^{-2} m

From formula, $Y = \frac{\text{Stress}}{\text{Strain}}$

$$\Rightarrow \quad \text{Strain} = \frac{\text{Stress}}{Y} = \frac{F}{AY}$$

$$= \frac{10^5}{\pi r^2 Y} = \frac{10^5}{3.14\times10^{-4}\times2\times10^{11}}$$

$$= \frac{1}{628}$$

Therefore % strain $= \frac{1}{628}\times100 = 0.16\%$

28. (c)

For a beam, the depression at the centre is given by,

$$\delta = \left(\frac{fL}{4Ybd^3}\right)$$

[f, L, b, d are constants for a particular beam]

i.e. $\delta \propto \frac{1}{Y}$

29. (b) $K = \frac{F}{x} = \frac{4 \times 9.8}{2 \times 10^{-2}} = 19.6 \times 10^2$

Work done $= \frac{1}{2} \times 19.6 \times 10^2 \times (0.05)^2 = 2.45 J$

30. (c) If ℓ is the original length of wire, then change in length of first wire, $\Delta \ell_1 = (\ell_1 - \ell)$

change in length of second wire, $\Delta \ell_2 = (\ell_2 - \ell)$

Now, $Y = \frac{T_1}{A} \times \frac{\ell}{\Delta \ell_1} = \frac{T_2}{A} \times \frac{\ell}{\Delta \ell_2}$

or $\frac{T_1}{\Delta \ell_1} = \frac{T_2}{\Delta \ell_2}$ or $\frac{T_1}{\ell_1 - \ell} = \frac{T_2}{\ell_2 - \ell}$

or $T_1 \ell_2 - T_1 \ell = T_2 \ell_1 - \ell T_2$ or $\ell = \frac{T_2 \ell_1 - T_1 \ell_2}{T_2 - T_1}$

31. (a) $\delta = \frac{W\ell^3}{3YI}$, where W = load, ℓ = length of beam and I is geometrical moment of inertia for rectangular beam,

$I = \frac{bd^3}{12}$ where b = breadth and d = depth

For square beam b = d

$\therefore I_1 = \frac{b^4}{12}$

For a beam of circular cross-section, $I_2 = \left(\frac{\pi r^4}{4}\right)$

$\therefore \quad \delta_1 = \frac{W\ell^3 \times 12}{3Yb^4} = \frac{4W\ell^3}{Yb^4}$ (for sq. cross section)

and $\delta_2 = \frac{W\ell^3}{3Y(\pi r^4/4)} = \frac{4W\ell^3}{3Y(\pi r^4)}$

(for circular cross-section)

Now $\frac{\delta_1}{\delta_2} = \frac{3\pi r^4}{b^4} = \frac{3\pi r^4}{(\pi r^2)^2} = \frac{3}{\pi}$

($\because b^2 = \pi r^2$ i.e., they have same cross-sectional area)

32. (a) Compressibility $= \frac{1}{\text{Bulk modulus}}$

As bulk modulus is least for ethanol (0.9) and maximum for mercury (25) among ehtanol, mercury and water.

Hence compression in volume $\frac{\Delta V}{V}$

Ethanol > Water > Mercury

33. (c) The given graph does not obey Hooke's law. and there is no well defined plastic region. So the graph represents elastomers.

34. (a) $U/\text{volume} = \frac{1}{2} Y \times \text{strain}^2 = 3600 \text{ J m}^{-3}$

[Strain = 0.06×10^{-2}]

35. (d) Potential energy per unit volume of the wire is given by :

$u = \frac{1}{2} \frac{(\text{Stress})^2}{\text{Young's modulus}} = \frac{1}{2} \frac{S^2}{Y}$

As stress, $S = \frac{\text{Force}}{\text{Area}}$

$\therefore \frac{S_1}{S_2} = \left(\frac{F_1}{F_2}\right)\left(\frac{A_2}{A_1}\right)$

As $F_1 = F_2$ (Given)

$\therefore \frac{S_1}{S_2} = \left(\frac{F_1}{F_2}\right)\left(\frac{A_2}{A_1}\right) = \left(\frac{A_2}{A_1}\right)$ ..(i)

The two wires are of the same material, therefore their Young's moduli will be same i.e., $Y_1 = Y_2$

$\therefore \frac{u_1}{u_2} = \left(\frac{S_1}{S_2}\right)^2 = \left(\frac{A_2}{A_1}\right)^2$

$= \left(\frac{\pi\left(\frac{d_2}{2}\right)^2}{\pi\left(\frac{d_1}{2}\right)^2}\right)^2 = \left[\left(\frac{d_2}{d_1}\right)^2\right]^2$

$= \left(\frac{d_2}{d_1}\right)^4 = \left(\frac{2}{1}\right)^4 = \frac{16}{1} \quad \left(\because \frac{d_1}{d_2} = \frac{1}{2} \text{ (Given)}\right)$

36. (b) Using Hooke's law, $F = kx$ we can write

$4 = k(a - \ell_0)$ ...(i)

and $5 = k(b - \ell_0)$ ...(ii)

If ℓ be the length under tension 9N, then

$9 = k(\ell - \ell_0)$ ...(iii)

After solving above equations, we get

$\ell = (5b - 4a)$.

37. (b) $F = Y \times A \times \frac{l}{L} \Rightarrow F \propto r^2$ (*Y, l* and and *L* are constant)

If diameter is made four times then force required will be 16 times, i.e., 16×10^3 N

38. (c) Young's modulus of elasticity is

$Y = \frac{F/A}{\Delta L/L}$

$\therefore \Delta L = \frac{FL}{AY}$

So, $\Delta L \propto \frac{L}{A}$

$\therefore \frac{\Delta L_2}{\Delta L_1} = \frac{L_2}{L_1} \times \frac{A_1}{A_2} = \frac{2}{1} \times \frac{2}{1} = 4$

$\Delta L_2 = 4 \times \Delta L_1 = 4 \times 1 = 4$ cm

39. (a) $y = \frac{F/A}{\Delta l/l} = \frac{F}{A} \cdot \frac{l}{\Delta l}$

$= \frac{20 \times 1}{10^{-6} \times 10^{-4}} = 2 \times 10^{11} \text{Nm}^{-2}$

40. (d) $K = \frac{\Delta P}{\Delta V/V} = \frac{h\rho g}{\Delta V/V} = \frac{200 \times 10^3 \times 10}{0.1/100} = 2 \times 10^9$

41. (d) Bulk Modulus $= \frac{dp}{\frac{dv}{v}}$

$dp = h\rho g = 200 \times 10^3 \times 9.8$

$\frac{dv}{v} = \frac{0.1}{100}$

Bulk modulus $= \frac{200 \times 10^3 \times 9.8}{0.1/100} = 19.6 \times 10^8 \text{N/m}^2$

42. (c)

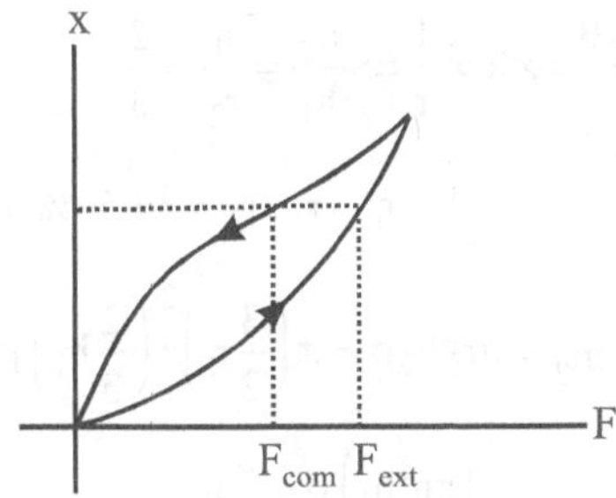

From the figure, it is clear that
$F_{com} < F_{ext.}$

43. (d) $\frac{\Delta r/r}{\Delta l/l} = 0.5 = \frac{1}{2}, \frac{\Delta r}{r} = \frac{1}{2}\frac{\Delta l}{l}$

44. (b) As $Y = \frac{\frac{F}{A}}{\frac{\Delta l}{l}} \Rightarrow \Delta l = \frac{Fl}{AY}$

But $V = Al$ so $A = \frac{V}{l}$

Therefore $\Delta l = \frac{Fl^2}{VY} \propto l^2$

Hence graph of Δl versus l^2 will give a straight line.

45. (b) $K = \frac{F}{x} = \frac{4 \times 9.8}{2 \times 10^{-2}} = 19.6 \times 10^2$

Work done $= \frac{1}{2} \times 19.6 \times 10^2 \times (0.05)^2 = 2.45\,J$

Speed Test-9

1. **(a)** Bulk modulus,

$$B = -\frac{\Delta P}{\left(\frac{\Delta V}{V_0}\right)} \Rightarrow \Delta V = -V_0 \frac{\Delta P}{B}$$

or $V - V_0 = -V_0 \frac{\Delta P}{B}$ (Here V_0 = volume at the surface and V = volume at the depth)

or $V = V_0 - V_0 \frac{\Delta P}{B} \Rightarrow V = V_0\left(1 - \frac{\Delta P}{B}\right)$

$\therefore$ Density, $\rho' = \frac{m}{V} = \frac{m}{V_0\left(1 - \frac{\Delta P}{B}\right)}$

$$= \frac{m}{\frac{m}{\rho}\left(1 - \frac{nP_0 - P_0}{B}\right)} \quad (\because \Delta P = nP_0 - P_0)$$

$$\rho' = \frac{\rho B}{B - (n-1)P_0}$$

2. **(c)** Velocity of ball when it strikes the water surface

$v = \sqrt{2gh}$ ...(i)

Terminal velocity of ball inside the water

$v = \frac{2}{9} r^2 g \frac{(\rho - 1)}{\eta}$ ...(ii)

Equation (i) and (ii) we get $\sqrt{2gh} = \frac{2}{9}\frac{r^2 g}{\eta}(\rho - 1)$

$$\Rightarrow h = \frac{2}{81} r^4 \left(\frac{\rho - 1}{\eta}\right)^2 g$$

3. **(b)**

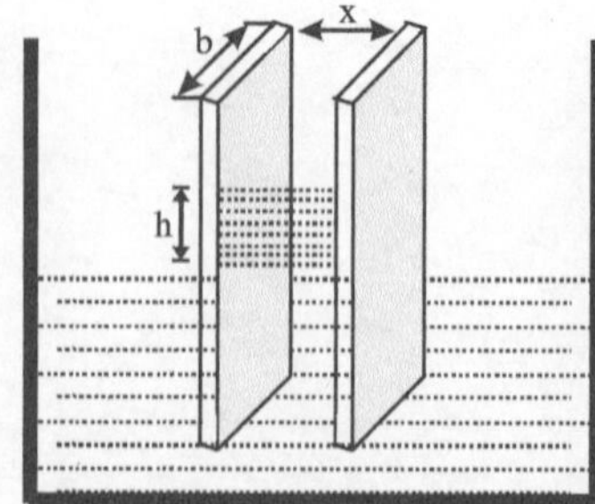

Let the width of each plate is b and due to surface tension liquid will rise upto height h then upward force due to surface tension.

= 2Tbcosθ ...(i)

Weight of the liquid rises in between the plates

= Vdg = (bxh)dg ...(ii)

Equating (i) and (ii) we get, 2T cosθ = xhdg

$$\therefore h = \frac{2T\cos\theta}{xdg}$$

4. **(b)** The theorem of continuity is valid.

$\therefore A_1 v_1 \rho = A_2 v_2 \rho$ as the density of the liquid can be taken as uniform.

A_1 A_2

$\therefore A_1 v_1 = A_2 v_2$

$\Rightarrow$ Smaller the area, greater the velocity.

5. **(c)** $P_a + \frac{1}{2}\rho_1 v_1^2 + 0 = P_a + \frac{1}{2}\rho_2 v_2^2 + (\rho_1 g h_1 + \rho_2 g h_2)$

As $v_2 << v_1$, $\therefore v_1 = \sqrt{2g(h_1 + h_2)\left(\frac{\rho_2}{\rho_1}\right)}$.

6. **(c)** $h = \frac{2T\cos\theta}{r\rho g} \Rightarrow h \propto \frac{1}{r} \Rightarrow \frac{h_2}{h_1} = \frac{r_1}{r_2} = \frac{2}{3}$

$\left(\because r_1 = r,\ r_2 = r + 50\% \text{ of } r = \frac{3}{2}r\right)$

New mass $m_2 = \pi r_2^2 h_2 \rho = \pi\left(\frac{3}{2}r_1\right)^2\left(\frac{2}{3}h_1\right)\rho$

$= \frac{3}{2}\left(\pi r_1^2 h_1\right)\rho = \frac{3}{2}m$

7. **(a)** When a body falls through a viscous liquid, its velocity increases due to gravity but after some time its velocity becomes uniform because of viscous force becoming equal to the gravitational force. Viscous force itself is a variable force which increases as velocity increases, so curve (a) represents the correct alternative.

8. **(c)** Sum of volumes of 2 smaller drops = Volume of the bigger drop

$2.\frac{4}{3}\pi r^3 = \frac{4}{3}\pi R^3 \Rightarrow R = 2^{1/3} r$

Surface energy = $T.4\pi R^2$

$= T4\pi 2^{2/3} r^2 = T.2^{8/3}\pi r^2$.

9. **(c)** Angle of contact θ

$\cos\theta = \frac{T_{SA} - T_{SL}}{T_{LA}}$

when water is on a waxy or oily surface

$T_{SA} < T_{SL}$ cos θ is negative i.e., $90° < \theta < 180°$

i.e., angle of contact θ increases

And for $\theta > 90°$ liquid level in capillary tube fall. i.e., h decreases

10. **(a)** $F = 6\pi\eta r v$

$= 6 \times 3.14 \times (8 \times 10^{-5}) \times 0.03 \times 100$

$= 4.52 \times 10^{-3}$ dyne

11. **(a)** Velocity of water from hole = $v_1 = \sqrt{2gh}$

Velocity of water from hole B

$v_2 = \sqrt{2g(H_0 - h)}$

Time of reaching the ground from hole B

$t_1 = \sqrt{2(H_0 - h)/g}$

Time of reaching the ground from hole A

$t_2 = \sqrt{2h/g}$

12. (a) Fluid resistance is given by $R = \dfrac{8\eta L}{\pi r^4}$

When two capillary tubes of same size are joined in parallel, then equivalent fluid resistance is

$$R_S = R_1 + R_2 = \frac{8\eta L}{\pi R^4} + \frac{8\eta \times 2L}{\pi (2R)^4} = \left(\frac{8\eta L}{\pi R^4}\right) \times \frac{9}{8}$$

$$\text{Rate of flow} = \frac{P}{R_S} = \frac{\pi P R^4}{8\eta L} \times \frac{8}{9} = \frac{8}{9}X \quad \left[\text{as } X = \frac{\pi P R^4}{8\eta L}\right]$$

13. (b) The candle floats on the water with half its length above and below water level. Let its length be 10 cm with 5 cm below the surface and 5 cm above it. If its length is reduced to 8 cm, it will have 4 cm above water surface. So we see tip going down by 1 cm.

∴ rate of fall of tip = 1 cm/hour.

14. (a) Inside pressure must be $\dfrac{4T}{r}$ greater than outside pressure in bubble.

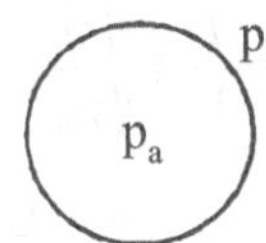

This excess pressure is provided by charge on bubble.

$$\frac{4T}{r} = \frac{\sigma^2}{2\varepsilon_0}; \quad \frac{4T}{r} = \frac{Q^2}{16\pi^2 r^4 \times 2\varepsilon_0} \quad \left[\sigma = \frac{Q}{4\pi r^2}\right]$$

$$Q = 8\pi r\sqrt{2rT\varepsilon_0}$$

15. (a) Because film tries to cover minimum surface area.

16. (d)

17. (a) The condition for terminal speed (v_t) is

Weight = Buoyant force + Viscous force

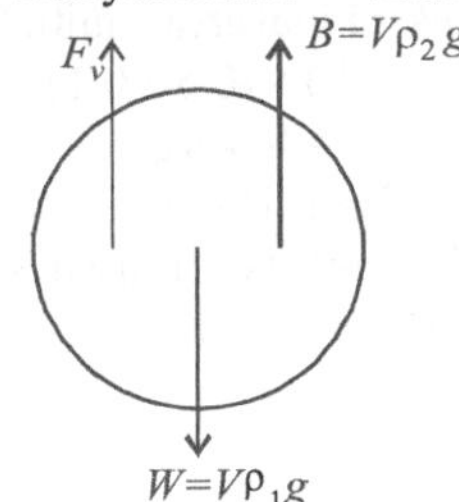

$$\therefore V\rho_1 g = V\rho_2 g + kv_t^2 \qquad \therefore v_t = \sqrt{\frac{Vg(\rho_1 - \rho_2)}{k}}$$

18. (d) According to Bernoulli's theorem, when velocity of liquid flow increases, the pressure decreases.

19. (c) Wetability of a surface by a liquid primarily depends on angle of contact between the surface and liquid. If angle of contact is acute liquids wet the solid and vice-versa.

20. (a) dv = 8 cm/s and dx = 0.1 cm

$$\text{Velocity gradient} = \frac{dv}{dx} = \frac{8}{0.1} = 80/\text{s}.$$

21. (a) Terminal velocities of rain drops are proportional to square of their radii.

Terminal velocity of a body is given by

$$v_T = \frac{2R^2}{9\eta}(d - \sigma)g. \text{ or, } V \propto R^2$$

22. (b)

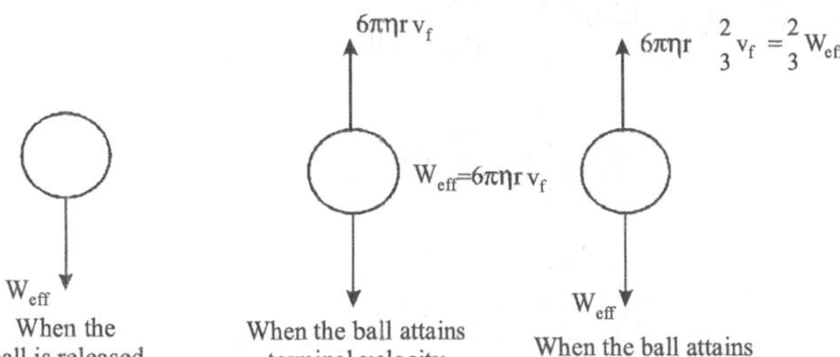

When the ball is just released, the net force on ball is W_{eff} (= mg – buoyant force)

The terminal velocity v_f of the ball is attained when net force on the ball is zero.

∴ Viscous force $6\pi\eta r\, v_f = W_{eff}$

When the ball acquires $\frac{2}{3}$rd of its maximum velocity v_f

the viscous force is $= \frac{2}{3}W_{eff}$

Hence net force is $W_{eff} - \frac{2}{3}W_{eff} = \frac{1}{3}W_{eff}$

∴ required acceleration is a/3

23. (a) $(2\pi r_1 + 2\pi r_2)\sigma = mg$

$$\left[2\pi \times \frac{8.7}{2} + 2\pi \times \frac{8.5}{2}\right]\sigma = 3.97 \times 980$$

$$\Rightarrow \sigma = 72 \text{ dyne cm}^{-1}$$

24. (b) Over a small temperature ranges, S.T. of water decreases linearly with rise of temperature.

25. (c) Volume of air bubble $V = \frac{4}{3}\pi r^3$

We get, $V \propto r^3$

If r is 2 times, V becomes 8 times at the surface of lake.

Pressure at the surface of lake is given by

P_1 = 1 atmosphere, $V_1 = 8V$

⇒ P_1 = Hdg where, d = density of water

Pressure at the bottom of lake,

P_2 = Pressure of atmosphere + Pressure of water

P_2 = Hdg + hdg = (H + h) dg where, h = depth of lake

Let final volume, $V_2 = V$.

Because temperature is constant, hence from Boyle's law

$P_1V_1 = P_2V_2 \Rightarrow Hdg \times 8V = (H+h)dg \times V \Rightarrow h = 7H.$

26. (c)

27. (b) Volume of first piece of metal = $\frac{32}{8} = 4\,\text{cm}^3$

Upthrust = 4 gf

Effective weight = (32 – 4) gf = 28 gf

If m be the mass of second body, volume of second body is $\frac{m}{5}$

Now, $28 = m - \frac{m}{5} \Rightarrow m = 35$ g

28. (b) $g_{\text{eff.}} = 12\ \text{m/s}^2$, $= \frac{\rho_m}{\rho_w} = \frac{4}{10}$

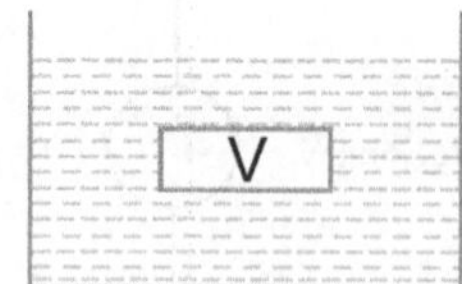

$$a = \frac{V\rho_w \times 12 - V\rho_m \times 12}{V\rho_m} = 18\,\text{m/s}^2$$

$1 = \frac{1}{2} \times 18\,t^2,\ t = \frac{1}{3}$ s.

29. (b) Due to increase in velocity, pressure will be low above the surface of water.

30. (c) If ρ is the density of the ball and ρ′ that of the another ball, *m* for the balls are the same, but $r' = 2r$

$\therefore mg = 6\pi r\eta v$ (by Stoke's law)

or, $6\pi r\eta v = 6\pi 2r\eta v'$ So, $v' = \frac{v}{2}$

31. (d) As we know,

Pressure P = Vdg

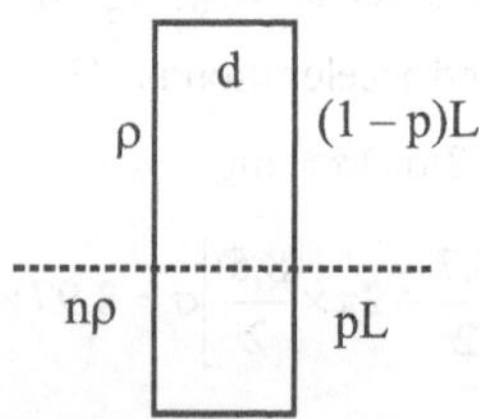

Here, LA d g = (pL) A (nρ)g + (1 – p)LA ρ g

$\Rightarrow$ d = (1 – p)ρ + pn ρ = [1 + (n – 1)p]ρ

32. (d) At equilibrium, weight of the given block is balanced by force due to surface tension, i.e.,

2L. S = W

or $S = \frac{W}{2L} = \frac{1.5\times10^{-2}\,N}{2\times0.3\,m} = 0.025\,Nm^{-1}$

33. (a)

34. (d) $T_1 + T\cos(\pi - \theta) = T_2$

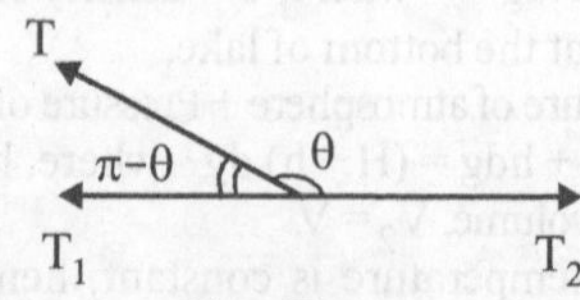

$\therefore \cos(\pi - \theta) = \frac{T_2 - T_1}{T}$

$\therefore -\cos\theta = \frac{T_2 - T_1}{T}$

$\therefore \cos\theta = \frac{T_1 - T_2}{T}$

35. (a) Let L = PQ = length of rod

$\therefore$ SP = SQ = $\frac{L}{2}$

Weight of rod, W = A*l*ρg.

Acting at point S

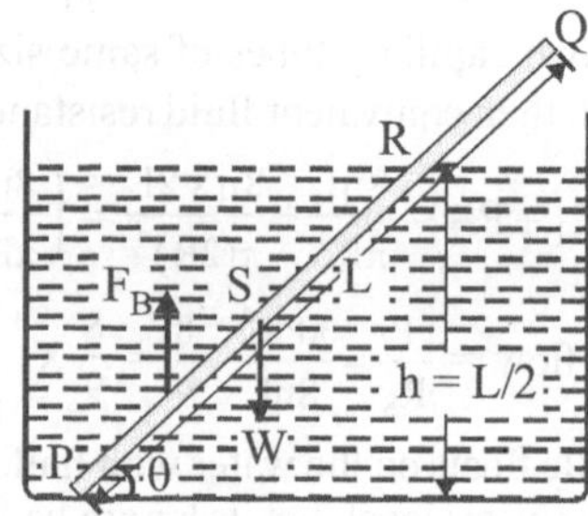

And force of buoyancy,

$F_B = Al\rho_0 g$. [*l* = PR]

Which acts at mid-point of PR.

For rotational equilibrium.

$$Al\rho_0 g \times \frac{\ell}{2}\cos\theta = AL\rho g \times \frac{L}{2}\cos\theta$$

$$\Rightarrow \frac{l^2}{L^2} = \frac{\rho}{\rho_0} \Rightarrow \frac{l}{L} = \sqrt{\frac{\rho}{\rho_0}}$$

From figure, $\sin\theta = \frac{h}{l} = \frac{L}{2l} = \frac{1}{2}\sqrt{\frac{\rho_0}{\rho}}$

36. (b) Terminal velocity, $v_0 = \frac{2\,r^2(\rho - \rho_0)g}{9\eta}$

$$= \frac{2\times(2\times10^{-3})^2\times(8-1.3)\times10^3\times9.8}{9\times0.83} = 0.07\ \text{ms}^{-1}$$

37. (c) Work done = Surface tension × increase in area of the film

W = S × ΔA

Increase in area = Final area – initial area

= 10 × (0.5 + 0.1) – 10 × 0.5 = 1 cm²

$\therefore$ W = 72 × 2 × 1 = 144 erg

[$\because$ There are 2 free surfaces; $\therefore$ ΔA = 2 × 1].

38. (b) Waterproofing agents are used so that the material does not get wet. This means angle of contact is obtuse.

39. (c)

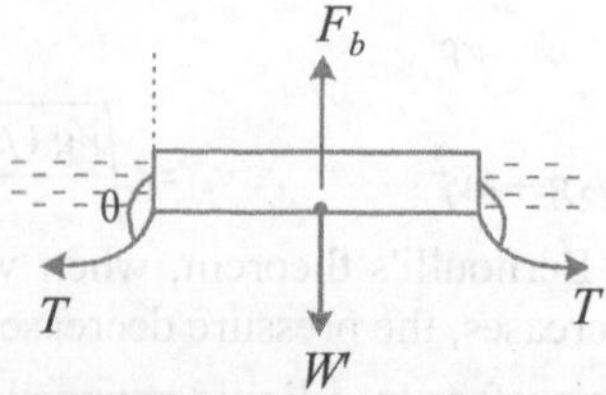

For floating disc, $F_{\text{net}} = 0$

or $F_b + 2\pi rT\cos\theta = W'$

or $W + 2\pi rT\cos\theta = W'$

40. **(b)**

41. **(d)** From the figure it is clear that liquid 1 floats on liquid 2. The lighter liquid floats over heavier liquid. Therefore we can conclude that $\rho_1 < \rho_2$
Also $\rho_3 < \rho_2$ otherwise the ball would have sink to the bottom of the jar.
Also $\rho_3 > \rho_1$ otherwise the ball would have floated in liquid 1. From the above discussion we conclude that

$$\rho_1 < \rho_3 < \rho_2.$$

42. **(a)** When the bubble gets detached,
Buoyant force = force due to surface tension

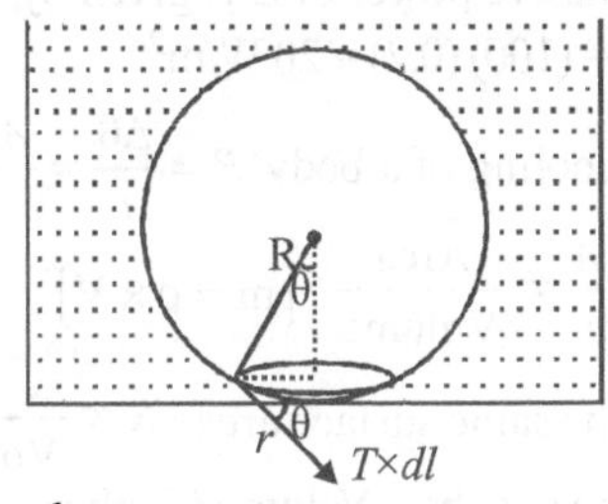

Force due to excess pressure = upthrust

Access pressure in air bubble $= \dfrac{2T}{R}$

$$\frac{2T}{R}(\pi r^2) = \frac{4\pi R^3}{3}\rho_w g$$

$$\Rightarrow r^2 = \frac{2R^4\rho_w g}{3T} \Rightarrow r = R^2\sqrt{\frac{2\rho_w g}{3T}}$$

43. **(b)** Bernoulli's theorem.

44. **(a)** Inflow rate of volume of the liquid = Outflow rate of volume of the liquid

$$\pi R^2 V = n\pi r^2 (v) \Rightarrow v = \frac{\pi R^2 V}{n\pi r^2} = \frac{VR^2}{nr^2}$$

45. **(c)** $T \times 2\pi r + mg = F_b$

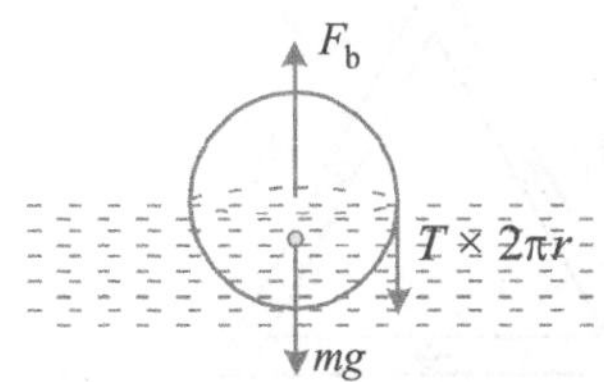

or $\quad T \times 2\pi r + \rho\frac{4}{3}\pi r^3 g = \left[\dfrac{\frac{4}{3}\pi r^3}{2}\right]\sigma g$

$$\therefore \quad r = \sqrt{\frac{3T}{g(2\rho - \sigma)}}$$

Speed Test-10

1. (a) $E = \frac{S}{S_0}\sigma T^4 = \frac{4\pi r^2}{4\pi R^2}\sigma T^4$

$= \sigma \frac{r^2}{R^2} T^4$

2. (c)

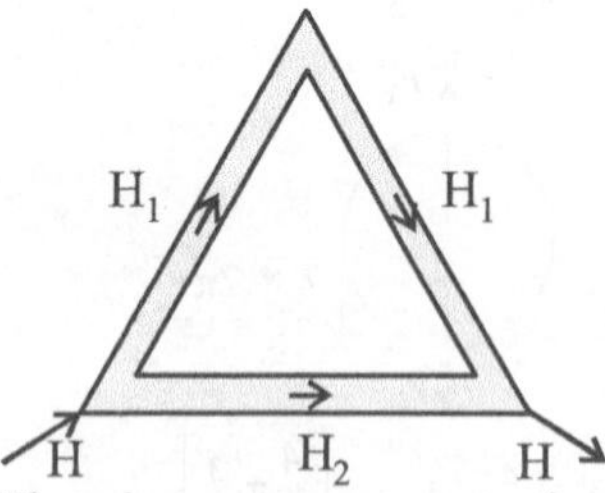

The given arrangement of rods can be redrawn as follows

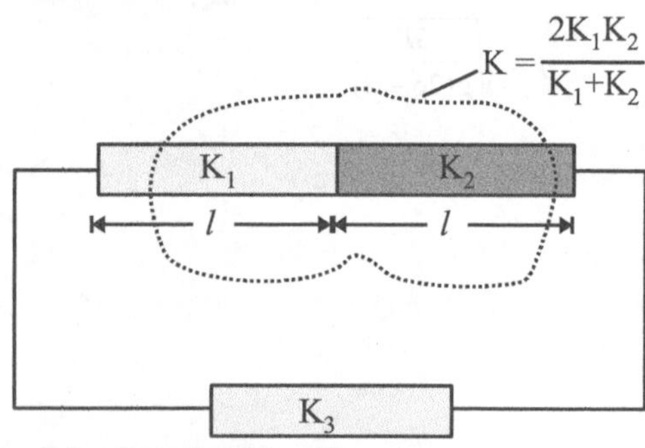

It is given that $H_1 = H_2$

$$\Rightarrow \frac{KA(\theta_1 - \theta_2)}{2l} = \frac{K_3 A(\theta_1 - \theta_2)}{l} \Rightarrow K_3 = \frac{K}{2} = \frac{K_1 K_2}{K_1 + K_2}$$

3. (c) $Q = mc\Delta T$

$Q = mc\,(T - T_0)$ ......(i)

$Q = Kt$ whereas K is heating rate

$\therefore$ from 50 to boiling temperature, T increases linearly.

At vaporization, equation is $Q = mL$

so, temperature remains constant till vaporisation is complete

After that, again Eqn (i) is followed and temperature increases linearly

4. (b) At constant temperature molar heat capacity

$$C_T = \frac{\Delta Q}{n\Delta T}$$

T is const. $\Rightarrow \Delta T = 0$

$$\therefore \quad C_T = \frac{\Delta Q}{0} = \infty$$

5. (d) Required work = energy released

Here, $Q = \int mc\, dT$

$$= \int_{20}^{4} 0.1 \times 32 \times \left(\frac{T^3}{400^3}\right) dT \approx 0.002\,\text{kJ}.$$

Therefore, required work = 0.002 kJ

6. (b) Since, e = a = 0.2

Since a = (1 – r – t) = 0.2 for the body B

Thus emissive power of B is given by,

$E = a E_b = (100)\,(0.2) = 20\ \text{W/m}^2$

7. (b) Rate of cooling of a body $R = \frac{\Delta\theta}{t} = \frac{A\varepsilon\sigma(T^4 - T_0^4)}{mc}$

$\Rightarrow R \propto \frac{A}{m} \propto \frac{\text{Area}}{\text{Volume}}$ $[m = \rho \times V]$

$\Rightarrow$ For the same surface area. $R \propto \frac{1}{\text{Volume}}$

$\because$ Volume of cube < Volume of sphere

$\Rightarrow R_{\text{cube}} > R_{\text{Sphere}}$ i.e., cube, cools down with faster rate.

8. (b) From question,

$\Delta\rho = (998 - 992)\ \text{kg/m}^3 = 6\ \text{kg/m}^3$

$\rho = \frac{998 + 992}{2}\ \text{kg/m}^3 = 995\ \text{kg/m}^3$

$\rho = \frac{m}{V}$

$\Rightarrow \frac{\Delta\rho}{\rho} = -\frac{\Delta V}{V} \quad \Rightarrow \left|\frac{\Delta\rho}{\rho}\right| = \left|\frac{\Delta V}{V}\right|$

$\therefore$ Coefficient of volume expansion of water,

$$\frac{1}{V}\frac{\Delta V}{\Delta t} = \frac{1}{\rho}\frac{\Delta\rho}{\Delta t} = \frac{6}{995 \times 20} \approx 3 \times 10^{-4}\,/\,°\text{C}$$

9. (a) $E = \frac{F/A}{\Delta l/l} = \frac{\text{stress}}{\text{strain}}$ where $\Delta\ell = (\ell' - \ell) = \ell\alpha t$ so $F = EA\alpha t$

10. (c)

11. (a) $F = Y\alpha t A$ or $F \propto \alpha$

($\because$ Y t A is same for both copper and iron)

or $F_C \propto \alpha_C$ and $F_I \propto \alpha_I$

$$\therefore \quad \frac{F_C}{F_I} = \frac{3/2}{1} = \frac{3}{2}$$

12. (c) According to question only one-quarter of the heat produced by falling piece of ice is absorbed in the melting of ice.

i.e., $\frac{mgh}{4} = mL$

$$\Rightarrow \quad h = \frac{4L}{g} = \frac{4 \times 3.4 \times 10^5}{10} = 136\ \text{km}.$$

13. (d) $W = W_1 - W_2 = mgh - mgh' = mg\,(h - h')$

$= 5 \times 10\ (20 - 0.2) = 5 \times 10 \times 19.8$

$= 5 \times 198 = 990$ joule

This energy is converted into heat when the ball strikes the earth. Heat produced is

$$Q = \frac{990}{4.2} \text{ calorie}$$

$$\Delta T = \frac{Q}{mc} = \frac{99 \times 100}{42 \times 5000 \times 0.09} = \frac{11}{32} \text{ °C}$$

14. (b) Let the angle subtended by the arc formed be θ. Then

$$\theta = \frac{\ell}{r} \text{ or } \theta = \frac{\Delta \ell}{\Delta r} = \frac{\ell_2 - \ell_1}{r_1 - r_2}$$

$$\therefore \theta = \frac{\ell(\alpha_2 - \alpha_1)\Delta T}{t} \text{ or } \frac{\ell}{r} = \frac{\ell(\alpha_2 - \alpha_1)\Delta T}{t}$$

So, $r = \frac{t}{(\alpha_2 - \alpha_1)\Delta T}$

15. (d)

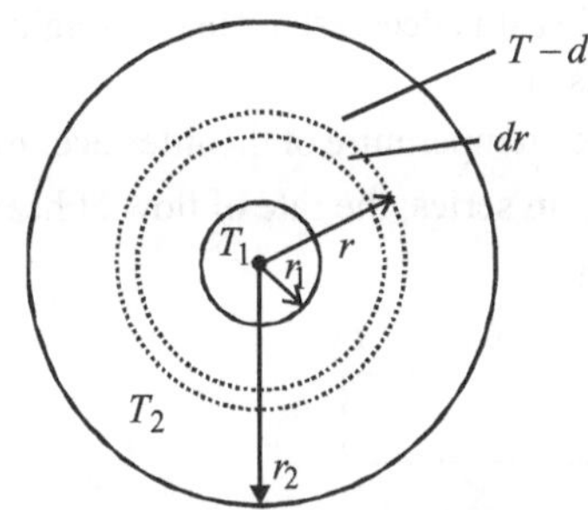

Consider a shell of thickness (dr) and of radius (r) and let the temperature of inner and outer surfaces of this shell be T and $(T - dT)$ respectively.

$\frac{dQ}{dt}$ = rate of flow of heat through it

$$= \frac{KA[(T - dT) - T]}{dr} = \frac{-KAdT}{dr}$$

$$= -4\pi K r^2 \frac{dT}{dr} \qquad (\because A = 4\pi r^2)$$

To measure the radial rate of heat flow, integration technique is used, since the area of the surface through which heat will flow is not constant.

$$\text{Then, } \left(\frac{dQ}{dt}\right)\int_{r_1}^{r_2} \frac{1}{r^2} dr = -4\pi K \int_{T_1}^{T_2} dT$$

$$\frac{dQ}{dt}\left[\frac{1}{r_1} - \frac{1}{r_2}\right] = -4\pi K\left[T_2 - T_1\right]$$

$$\text{or } \frac{dQ}{dt} = \frac{-4\pi K r_1 r_2 (T_2 - T_1)}{(r_2 - r_1)}$$

$$\therefore \frac{dQ}{dt} \propto \frac{r_1 r_2}{(r_2 - r_1)}$$

16. (a) According to Newton's law of cooling if temperature difference between body & surrounding is large, then rate of cooling is also fast hence curve A shows correct behaviour.

17. (a) Among glass, wood and metals, metals expand more for same rise in temperature.

18. (b) According to Wein's law $\lambda_m \propto \frac{1}{T}$ and from the figure

$(\lambda_m)_1 < (\lambda_m)_3 < (\lambda_m)_2$ therefore $T_1 > T_3 > T_2$.

19. (a) Moment of inertia of a rod,

$$I = \frac{1}{12} ML^2$$

Differentiating w.r.t. to ΔL, we get

$$\frac{\Delta I}{\Delta L} = \frac{1}{12} \times 2ML$$

$$\Delta I = \frac{1}{12} 2ML\Delta L \qquad \therefore \frac{\Delta I}{I} = 2\frac{\Delta L}{L}$$

As we know, $\Delta L = L\alpha\Delta t$ or $\frac{\Delta L}{L} = \alpha\Delta t$

Substituting the value $\frac{\Delta L}{L}$, we get

$$\frac{\Delta I}{I} = 2\alpha\Delta t$$

20. (c) The lengths of each rod increases by the same amount

$$\therefore \Delta\ell_a = \Delta\ell_s \Rightarrow \ell_1\alpha_a t = \ell_2\alpha_s t$$

$$\Rightarrow \frac{\ell_2}{\ell_1} = \frac{\alpha_a}{\alpha_s} \Rightarrow \frac{\ell_2}{\ell_1} + 1 = \frac{\alpha_a}{\alpha_s} + 1$$

$$\Rightarrow \frac{\ell_2 + \ell_1}{\ell_1} = \frac{\alpha_a + \alpha_s}{\alpha_s} \Rightarrow \frac{\ell_1}{\ell_1 + \ell_2} = \frac{\alpha_s}{\alpha_a + \alpha_s}$$

21. (a) According to Kirchhoff law, good absorbers are good emitters. Since black spot is good absorber so it is also a good emitter & will be brighter than plate.

22. (a) From Wein's displacement law

$\lambda_m \times T = \text{constant}$

P – max. intensity is at violet

$\Rightarrow \lambda_m$ is minimum $\Rightarrow$ temp maximum

R – max. intensity is at green

$\Rightarrow \lambda_m$ is moderate $\Rightarrow$ temp moderate

Q – max. intensity is at red $\Rightarrow \lambda_m$ is maximum $\Rightarrow$ temp. minimum i.e., $T_p > T_R > T_Q$

23. (c)

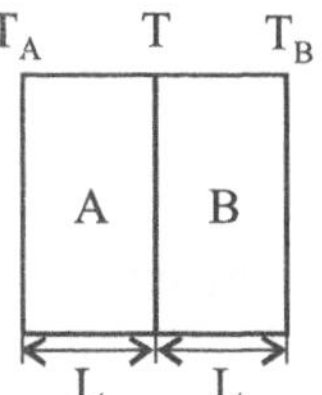

Let T be temperature of the junction

Here, $K_A = 2K_B$, $T - T_B = 50K$

At the steady state,

$$H_A = H_B$$

$$\therefore \frac{K_A A(T_A - T)}{L} = \frac{K_B A(T - T_B)}{L}$$

$$2K_B(T_A - T) = K_B(T - T_B)$$

$$T_A - T = \frac{T - T_B}{2}$$

$$= \frac{50K}{2} = 25K$$

24. (b)

25. (a) Suppose, height of liquid in each arm before rising the temperature is l.

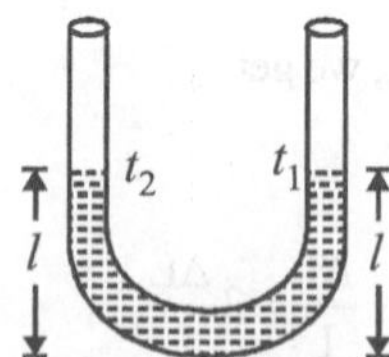

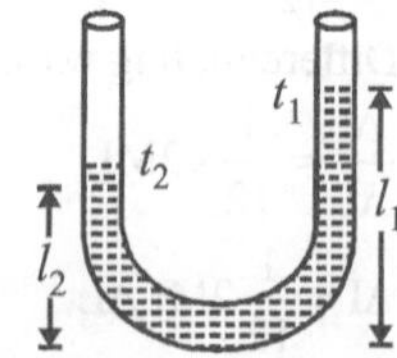

With temperature rise height of liquid in each arm increases *i.e.* $l_1 > l$ and $l_2 > l$

Also $l = \frac{l_1}{1+\gamma t_1} = \frac{l_2}{1+\gamma t_2}$

$$\Rightarrow l_1 + \gamma l_1 t_2 = l_2 + \gamma l_2 t_1 \Rightarrow \gamma = \frac{l_1 - l_2}{l_2 t_1 - l_1 t_2}.$$

26. (a) The rate of heat loss per unit area due to radiation $= \varepsilon\sigma(T^4 - T_0^4)$
$= 0.6 \times 5.67 \times 10^{-8}[(400)^4 - (300)^4] = 595 \text{ Jm}^{-2}\text{s}^{-1}$.

27. (d) According to Wein's displacement law, product of wavelength belonging to maximum intensity and temperature is constant i.e., $\lambda_m T$ = constant.

28. (c) According to Newton's law of cooling, the temperature goes on decreasing with time non-linearly.

29. (d) $t \propto \frac{\ell}{A}$, $t' \propto \frac{2\ell}{A/2}$

$$\frac{t'}{t} = 4\frac{\ell / A}{\ell / A}$$

$t' = 4 \times t$

$3/t' = 48s$

30. (a) In series, equivalent thermal conductivity

$$K_{eq} = \frac{2K_1K_2}{K_1 + K_2}$$

or, $K_{eq} = \frac{2 \times K \times 2K}{K + 2K} = \frac{4}{3}K$

31. (c) $Q = -KA\left(\frac{d\theta}{dx}\right) \times t$

32. (c) Using Wein's law, $\lambda_m T$ = constant

$$\lambda_1 T_1 = \lambda_2 T_2$$

$$\lambda_2 = \lambda_1 \frac{T_1}{T_2}$$

$$\lambda_2 = \frac{\lambda_0 T}{2T} = \frac{\lambda_0}{2}$$

33. (b) Total power radiated by Sun $= \sigma T^4 \times 4\pi R^2$
The intensity of power at earth's surface

$$= \frac{\sigma T^4 \times 4\pi R^2}{4\pi r^2}$$

Total power received by Earth

$$= \frac{\sigma T^4 R^2}{r^2}(\pi r_0^2)$$

34. (c) The upthrust is given by $\frac{4}{3}\pi R_t^3 \rho g$

Here $R_t^3 = R_0^3(1 + \gamma_m t)$ and $\rho_t = \rho_0/(1 + \gamma_a t)$

So, the upthrust at t°C is given by

$$= \frac{4}{3}\pi R_0^3(1 + \gamma_m t) \times \{\rho_0/(1 + \gamma_a t)\} g$$

As $\gamma_m < \gamma_a$, hence upthrust at t°C < upthrust at 0°C

So, the upthrust is decreased. Hence weight in liquid gets increased.

35. (d) Let T be the temperature of the interface. As the two sections are in series, the rate of flow of heat in them will be equal.

T_1 ℓ_1	ℓ_2 T_2
K_1	K_2

$$\therefore \frac{K_1A(T_1 - T)}{\ell_1} = \frac{K_2A(T - T_2)}{\ell_2},$$

where A is the area of cross-section.

or, $K_1A(T_1 - T)\ell_2 = K_2A(T - T_2)\ell_1$

or, $K_1T_1\ell_2 - K_1T\ell_2 = K_2T\ell_1 - K_2T_2\ell_1$

or, $(K_2\ell_1 + K_1\ell_2)T = K_1T_1\ell_2 + K_2T_2\ell_1$

$$\therefore T = \frac{K_1T_1\ell_2 + K_2T_2\ell_1}{K_2\ell_1 + K_1\ell_2} = \frac{K_1\ell_2T_1 + K_2\ell_1T_2}{K_1\ell_2 + K_2\ell_1}.$$

36. (d) Radius of small sphere = r
Thickness of small sphere = t
Radius of bigger sphere = 2r
Thickness of bigger sphere = t/4
Mass of ice melted = (volume of sphere) × (density of ice)
Let K_1 and K_2 be the thermal conductivities of larger and smaller sphere.
For bigger sphere,

$$\frac{K_1 4\pi(2r)^2 \times 100}{t/4} = \frac{\frac{4}{3}\pi(2r)^3\rho L}{25 \times 60}$$

For smaller sphere,

$$\frac{K_2 \times 4\pi r^2 \times 100}{t} = \frac{\frac{4}{3}\pi r^3 \rho L}{16 \times 60}$$

$$\therefore \frac{K_1}{K_2} = \frac{8}{25}$$

37. (b) According to Wein's displacement law,

$\lambda_m T = 2.88 \times 10^{-3}$

When T = 2000 K,

$\lambda_m (2000) = 2.88 \times 10^{-3}$ ....(1)

When T = 3000 K,

$\lambda'_m (3000) = 2.88 \times 10^{-3}$ ....(2)

Dividing (1) by (2),

$$\frac{2}{3}\frac{\lambda_m}{\lambda'_m} = 1 \Rightarrow \frac{\lambda_m}{\lambda'_m} = \frac{3}{2} \Rightarrow \lambda'_m = \frac{2}{3}\lambda_m$$

38. (c) AB represents latent heat of fusion

$Q_1 = mL_F$

Here, $L_F \propto$ length of line AB

CD represents latent heat of vaporization $Q_2 = mL_V$

Here, $L_V \propto$ length of line CD

$\therefore\ Q_2 = 2Q_1$ $[\because$ As CD = 2AB$]$

39. (b) Let the final temperature be *T*

Heat gained by ice $= mL + m \times s \times (T - 0)$

$= 10 \times 80 + 10 \times 1 \times T$

Heat lost by water $= 55 \times 1 \times (40 - T)$

By using law of calorimetery,

$800 + 10\,T = 55 \times (40 - T)$

$\Rightarrow T = 21.54°C = 22°C$

40. (a) According to Newton's law of cooling,

$$\frac{\theta_1 - \theta_2}{t} = K\left[\frac{\theta_1 + \theta_2}{2} - \theta_0\right]$$

where θ_0 is the surrounding temperature.

$$\therefore\ \frac{60 - 40}{7} = K\left(\frac{60 + 40}{2} - 10\right)$$

$$\Rightarrow \frac{20}{7} = 40K \Rightarrow K = \frac{1}{14}$$

$$\therefore\ \frac{40 - 28}{t} = K\left[\frac{40 + 28}{2} - 10\right] \Rightarrow \frac{12}{t} = 24K$$

$$\text{or}\ \ t = \frac{12}{24K} = \frac{12 \times 14}{24} = 7\,\text{min}$$

41. (d) $\frac{Q}{t} = K_1 A_1 \frac{d\theta}{dx} = K_2 A_2 \frac{d\theta}{dx}$

42. (c) Since specific heat $= 0.6\ kcal/g \times °C = 0.6\ cal/g \times °C$

From graph it is clear that in a minute, the temperature is raised from 0°C to 50°C.

$\Rightarrow$ Heat required for a minute $= 50 \times 0.6 \times 50 = 1500\ cal.$

Also from graph, Boiling point of wax is 200°C.

43. (b) Temperature of B will be higher because, due to expansion centre of mass B will come down same heat is supplied but in B, potential energy is decreased therefore internal energy gain will be more.

44. (d) According to the principle of calorimetry.

Heat lost = Heat gained

$mL_v + ms_w\Delta\theta = m_w s_w \Delta\theta$

$\Rightarrow m \times 540 + m \times 1 \times (100 - 80)$

$= 20 \times 1 \times (80 - 10)$

$\Rightarrow m = 2.5\,g$

Therefore total mass of water at 80°C

$= (20 + 2.5)\,g = 22.5\,g$

45. (a) Initial rate of loss of heat $= \frac{\sigma T^4 \times A_1 \times e}{\sigma T^4 \times A_2 \times e} = \frac{R_1^2}{R_2^2}$

Speed Test-11

1. **(a)** $U = a + bPV$ ......(1)

In adiabatic change,

$$dU = -dW = \frac{nR}{\gamma-1}(T_2 - T_1) = \frac{nR}{\gamma-1}(dT)$$

$$\Rightarrow U = \int dU = \frac{nR}{\gamma-1}\int dT$$

or $U = \left(\frac{nR}{\gamma-1}\right)T + a = \frac{PV}{\gamma-1} + a$ ......(2)

where a is the constant of integration.

Comparing (1) and (2), we get

$$b = \frac{1}{\gamma-1} \Rightarrow \gamma = \frac{b+1}{b}.$$

2. **(d)** For path ab : $(\Delta U)_{ab} = 7000\,J$

By using $\Delta U = \mu C_V \Delta T$

$$7000 = \mu \times \frac{5}{2}R \times 700 \Rightarrow \mu = 0.48$$

For path ca :

$(\Delta Q)_{ca} = (\Delta U)_{ca} + (\Delta W)_{ca}$ ...(i)

$\because (\Delta U)_{ab} + (\Delta U)_{bc} + (\Delta U)_{ca} = 0$

$\because 7000 + 0 + (\Delta U)_{ca} = 0 \Rightarrow (\Delta U)_{ca} = -7000\,J$ ...(ii)

Also $(\Delta W)_{ca} = P_1(V_1 - V_2) = \mu R(T_1 - T_2)$

$= 0.48 \times 8.31 \times (300 - 1000) = -2792.16\text{J}$ ...(iii)

On solving equations (i), (ii) and (iii)

$$(\Delta Q)_{ca} = -7000 - 2792.16 = -9792.16\,J \approx -9800\,J$$

3. **(c)** The efficiency (η) of a Carnot engine and the coefficient of performance (β) of a refrigerator are related as

$\beta = \frac{1-\eta}{\eta}$ Here, $\eta = \frac{1}{10}$

$$\therefore \beta = \frac{1 - \frac{1}{10}}{\left(\frac{1}{10}\right)} = 9.$$

Also, Coefficient of performance (β) is given by $\beta = \frac{Q_2}{W}$,

where Q_2 is the energy absorbed from the reservoir.

or, $9 = \frac{Q_2}{10}$ $\therefore Q_2 = 90$ J.

4. **(b)** According to first law of thermodynamics,

$\Delta Q = \Delta U + \Delta W$

ΔQ = heat absorbed by gas

ΔW = work done by gas.

$-20\text{J} = \Delta U - 8\text{J}$

$\Delta U = -12\text{J} = U_{\text{Final}} - U_{\text{initial}}$

$U_{\text{initial}} = 30\text{J}$.

$U_{\text{Final}} = 30 - 12 = 18\,\text{J}$.

5. **(a)** The volume on both sides will be so adjusted that the original pressure × volume is kept constant as the piston moves slowly (isothermal change)

$P5V = P'V'$ .... (1)

$10PV = P'V''$ .... (2)

From (1) and (2), $V'' = 2V'$

and from $V' + V'' = 6V$

$V' = 2V,\ V'' = 4V$

6. **(a)** $W_{AB} = 0$, $W_{BC} = P\Delta V = nR\Delta T = -nRT_0$

$$W_{CA} = nRT\ell n\frac{V_f}{V_i} = nR(2T_0)\ell n2$$

$$Q_{BC} = nC_p\Delta T = \left(\frac{nR\gamma}{\gamma-1}\right)T_0$$

Efficiency, $\eta = \frac{W}{Q} = \left[\frac{2\ell n2 - 1}{\gamma/(\gamma-1)}\right]$

7. **(c)** $T_1 = 273 + 27 = 300\text{K}$

$T_2 = 273 + 927 = 1200\text{K}$

For adiabatic process,

$P^{1-\gamma}\,T^{\gamma}$ = constant

$\Rightarrow P_1^{1-\gamma}T_1^{\gamma} = P_2^{1-\gamma}T_2^{\gamma}$

$$\Rightarrow \left(\frac{P_2}{P_1}\right)^{1-\gamma} = \left(\frac{T_1}{T_2}\right)^{\gamma} \Rightarrow \left(\frac{P_1}{T_2}\right)^{1-\gamma} = \left(\frac{T_2}{T_1}\right)^{\gamma}$$

$$\left(\frac{P_1}{P_2}\right)^{1-1.4} = \left(\frac{1200}{300}\right)^{1.4} \Rightarrow \left(\frac{P_1}{P_2}\right)^{-0.4} = (4)^{1.4}$$

$$\left(\frac{P_2}{P_1}\right)^{0.4} = 4^{1.4}$$

$$P_2 = P_1\,4^{\left(\frac{1.4}{0.4}\right)} = P_1\,4^{\left(\frac{7}{2}\right)}$$

$= P_1\,(2^7) = 2 \times 128 = 256$ atm

8. **(b)**

P
T_1
(V, T_1)
$(32\,V, T_2)$
T_2
$V \rightarrow$

We have, $TV^{\gamma-1}$ = constant

$\Rightarrow T_1V^{\gamma-1} = T_2(32V)^{\gamma-1}$

$\Rightarrow T_1 = (32)^{\gamma-1}.T_2$

For diatomic gas, $\gamma = \frac{7}{5}$

$\therefore \gamma - 1 = \frac{2}{5}$

$\therefore T_1 = (32)^{\frac{2}{5}} . T_2 \Rightarrow T_1 = 4T_2$

Now, efficiency $= 1 - \frac{T_2}{T_1}$

$= 1 - \frac{T_2}{4T_2} = 1 - \frac{1}{4} = \frac{3}{4} = 0.75.$

9. (d) Isobaric compression is represented by curve AO
Work done = area under AD
$= 2 \times 10^2 \times (3 - 1)$
$= 4 \times 10^2 = 400$ J.

10. (a) As $P \propto \frac{1}{V^{1.5}}$, So $PV^{1.5}$ = constant

$\therefore \gamma = 1.5$ ($\because$ Process is adiabatic)

As we know, $\frac{C_p}{C_v} = \gamma \quad \therefore \frac{C_p}{C_v} = 1.5$

11. (a) $W = \frac{nR\Delta T}{1-\gamma} \Rightarrow -146000 = \frac{1000 \times 8.3 \times 7}{1-\gamma}$

or $1 - \gamma = -\frac{58.1}{146} \Rightarrow \gamma = 1 + \frac{58.1}{146} = 1.4$

Hence the gas is diatomic.

12. (a) As, $P = \frac{1}{3}\left(\frac{U}{V}\right)$

But $\frac{U}{V} = KT^4$

So, $P = \frac{1}{3} KT^4$

or $\frac{uRT}{V} = \frac{1}{3} KT^4$ [As PV = u RT]

$\frac{4}{3}\pi R^3 T^3$ = constant

Therefore, $T \propto \frac{1}{R}$

13. (c) Heat required to change the temperature of vessel by a small amount dT

$$-dQ = mCdT$$

Total heat required

$$-Q = m\int_{20}^{4} 32\left(\frac{T}{400}\right)^3 dT = \frac{100 \times 10^{-3} \times 32}{(400)^3}\left[\frac{T^4}{4}\right]_{20}^{4}$$

$\Rightarrow Q = 0.001996$ kJ

Work done required to maintain the temperature of sink to T_2

$W = Q_1 - Q_2 = \frac{Q_1 - Q_2}{Q_2} Q_2 = \left(\frac{T_1}{T_2} - 1\right) Q_2$

$\Rightarrow W = \left(\frac{T_1 - T_2}{T_2}\right) Q_2$

For $T_2 = 20$ K

$W_1 = \frac{300 - 20}{20} \times 0.001996 = 0.028$ kJ

For $T_2 = 4$ K

$W_2 = \frac{300 - 4}{4} \times 0.001996 = 0.148$ kJ

As temperature is changing from 20k to 4 k, work done required will be more than W_1 but less than W_2.

14. (a) Initially
$V_1 = 5.6\ell, T_1 = 273K, P_1 = 1$ atm,

$\gamma = \frac{5}{3}$ (For monatomic gas)

The number of moles of gas is

$n = \frac{5.6\ell}{22.4\ell} = \frac{1}{4}$

Finally (after adiabatic compression)

$V_2 = 0.7\ell$

For adiabatic compression

$$T_1 V_1^{\gamma-1} = T_2 V_2^{\gamma-1}$$

$$\therefore T_2 = T_1\left(\frac{V_1}{V_2}\right)^{\gamma-1} = T_1\left(\frac{5.6}{0.7}\right)^{\frac{5}{3}-1}$$

$$= T_1(8)^{2/3} = 4T_1$$

We know that work done in adiabatic process is

$$W = \frac{nR\Delta T}{\gamma - 1} = \frac{9}{8} RT_1$$

15. (c) Curve A, B shows expansion. For expansion of a gas,
$W_{isothermal} > W_{adiabatic}$
$P_{isothermal} > P_{adiabatic}$
$T_{isothermal} > T_{adiabatic}$
$\Rightarrow$ Slope of curve for isothermal change < slope of curve for adiabatic change.
So, curve B shows isothermal change and curve A shows adiabatic change.

16. (a) $PV^{3/2} = K, \quad \log P + \frac{3}{2}\log V = \log K$

$\frac{\Delta P}{P} + \frac{3}{2}\frac{\Delta V}{V} = 0$

$\frac{\Delta V}{V} = -\frac{2}{3}\frac{\Delta P}{P}$ or $\frac{\Delta V}{V} = \left(-\frac{2}{3}\right)\left(\frac{2}{3}\right) = -\frac{4}{9}$

17. (a) Initially the efficiency of the engine was $\frac{1}{6}$ which increases to $\frac{1}{3}$ when the sink temperature reduces by 62° C.

$\eta = \frac{1}{6} = 1 - \frac{T_2}{T_1}$, when T_2 = sink temperature

T_1 = source temperature

$\Rightarrow T_2 = \frac{5}{6}T_1$

Secondly,

$\frac{1}{3} = 1 - \frac{T_2 - 62}{T_1} = 1 - \frac{T_2}{T_1} + \frac{62}{T_1} = 1 - \frac{5}{6} + \frac{62}{T_1}$

or, $T_1 = 62 \times 6 = 372\text{K} = 372 - 273 = 99°\text{C}$

& $T_2 = \frac{5}{6} \times 372 = 310\text{K} = 310 - 273 = 37°\text{C}$

18. (b) For an adiabatic process, the temperature-volume relationship is

$$T_1 V_1^{\gamma-1} = T_2 V_2^{\gamma-1} \Rightarrow T_1 = T_2\left(\frac{V_2}{V_1}\right)^{\gamma-1}$$

Here $\gamma = 1.4$ (for diatomic gas). $V_2 = \frac{V_1}{32}, T_1 = T_i, T_2 = aT_i$

$\therefore T_i = aT_i\left[\frac{1}{32}\right]^{1.4-1} \quad \therefore T_i = aT_i\left[\frac{1}{2^5}\right]^{0.4} = \frac{aT_i}{4}$

$\therefore$ a = 4

19. (b) In the first-case adiabatic change,

$\Delta Q = 0, \Delta W = -35$ J

From 1st law of thermodynamics,

$\Delta Q = \Delta U + \Delta W$,

or $0 = \Delta U - 35$

$\therefore \Delta U = 35$ J

In the second case

$\Delta Q = 12$ cal $= 12 \times 4.2$ J $= 50.4$ J

$\Delta W = \Delta Q - \Delta U = 50.4 - 35 = 15.4$ J

20. (a) For an adiabatic change PV^γ = constant

$P_1 V_1^\gamma = P_2 V_2^\gamma$

As molar specific heat of gas at constant volume

$C_V = \frac{3}{2}R$

$C_P = C_V + R = \frac{3}{2}R + R = \frac{5}{2}R;$

$\gamma = \frac{C_P}{C_V} = \frac{(5/2)R}{(3/2)R} = \frac{5}{3}$

$\therefore$ From eq^n. (1)

$$P_2 = \left(\frac{V_1}{V_2}\right)^\gamma P_1 = \left(\frac{6}{2}\right)^{5/3} \times 10^5 \text{ N/m}^2$$

$= (3)^{5/3} \times 10^5 = 6.19 \times 10^5$ N/m^2

Work done

$$= \frac{1}{1-(5/3)}[6.19 \times 10^5 \times 2 \times 10^{-3} - 10^{-5} \times 6 \times 10^{-3}]$$

$$= -\left[\frac{2 \times 10^2 \times 3}{2}(6.19 - 3)\right]$$

$= -3 \times 10^2 \times 3.19 = -957$ joules

[–ve sign shows external work done on the gas]

21. (b) Efficiency of Carnot engine, $\eta = 1 - \frac{T_2}{T_1}$

where T_1 and T_2 be the temperature of source and sink respectively.

$\therefore \quad \frac{T_2}{T_1} = 1 - \eta = 1 - \frac{40}{100} = \frac{60}{100} = \frac{3}{5} \quad (\because \eta = 40\%)$

$T_2 = \frac{3}{5}T_1 = \frac{3}{5} \times 500\text{ K} = 300\text{ K} \quad$ ...(i)

$(\because T_1 = 500\text{ K})$

Let T_1' be the temperature of the source for the same sink temperature when efficiency $\eta' = 50\%$

$\therefore \frac{T_2}{T_1'} = 1 - \eta' = 1 - \frac{50}{100} = \frac{1}{2}$

$T_1' = 2T_2 = 2 \times 300\text{ K} = 600\text{ K} \quad$ (Using eq. (i))

22. (b) $dW = P\Delta V = 1.01 \times 10^5 [1671 - 1] \times 10^{-6}$ Joule

$= \frac{1.01 \times 167}{4.2}$ cal.

$= 40$ cal. nearly

$\Delta Q = mL = 1 \times 540$,

$\Delta Q = \Delta W + \Delta U$

or $\Delta U = 540 - 40 = 500$ cal.

23. (c) The temperature remains unchanged therefore

$U_f = U_i$.

Also, $\Delta Q = \Delta W$.

In the first step which is isochoric, $\Delta W = 0$.

In second step, pressure $= \frac{P}{n}$. Volume V is increased from V to nV.

$\therefore \quad W = \frac{P}{n}(nV - V)$

$= PV\left(\frac{n-1}{n}\right)$

$= RT(1 - n^{-1})$

24. (b) Efficiency of carnot engine

$n = 1 - \frac{T_2}{T_1}$ i.e., $\frac{1}{10} = 1 - \frac{T_2}{T_1}$

$\Rightarrow \quad \frac{T_2}{T_1} = 1 - \frac{1}{10} = \frac{9}{10} \Rightarrow \frac{T_1}{T_2} = \frac{10}{9}$

$\therefore \quad w = Q_2\left(\frac{T_1}{T_2} - 1\right)$

i.e., $10 = Q_2\left(\frac{10}{9} - 1\right) \quad 10 = Q_2\left(\frac{1}{9}\right)$

$\Rightarrow Q_2 = 90$ J

So, 90 J heat is absorbed at lower temperature.

25. (a) $V_1 = 1\ell = 1000\ cm^3,\ P_1 = 72$ cm of Hg.
$V_2 = 900\ cm^3,\ P_2 = ?$
$\because$ The process is isothermal
$\therefore\ P_1V_1 = P_2V_2$
$72 \times 1000 = P_2 \times 900$
$P_2 = 80$ cm of Hg
$\therefore$ Stress $= P_2 - P_1 = 80 - 72 = 8$ cm of Hg.

26. (a) Process A $\rightarrow$ B occurs at constant pressure Hence work done in this process is

$$W_{AB} = PdV = P(V_2 - V_1)$$
$$= 10 \times (2-1) = 10\ J$$

Process B $\rightarrow$ C, occurs at constant volume.

Hence, $W_{BC} = 0$

Given : Q = 5 J therefore, total work done is $W_1 = 5J$

($\because \Delta U = 0$ in a cyclic process)

Therefore, we have

$$W_1 = W_{AB} + W_{BC} + W_{CA}$$

or $5J = 10\,J + 0 + W_{CA}$

$\therefore\ W_{CA} = -5$ joule

27. (d) We know that in adiabatic process,
PV^γ = constant ....(1)
From ideal gas equation, we know that
$PV = nRT$

$$V = \frac{nRT}{P} \quad ....(2)$$

Puttingt the value from equation (2) in equation (1),

$$P\left(\frac{nRT}{P}\right)^\gamma = \text{constant}$$

$P^{(1-\gamma)}\,T^\gamma$ = constant

28. (b) According to first law of thermodynamics,

$\Delta Q = \Delta U + \Delta W$
ΔQ = heat absorbed by gas
ΔW = work done by gas.
$-20J = \Delta U - 8J$
$\Delta U = -12J = U_{Final} - U_{initial}$
$U_{initial} = 30J.$
$U_{Final} = 30 - 12 = 18J.$

29. (d) Coefficient of performance,

$$Cop = \frac{T_2}{T_1 - T_2}$$

$$5 = \frac{273-20}{T_1 - (273-20)} = \frac{253}{T_1 - 253}$$

$5T_1 - (5 \times 253) = 253$
$5T_1 = 253 + (5 \times 253) = 1518$

$$\therefore T_1 = \frac{1518}{5} = 303.6$$

or, $T_1 = 303.6 - 273 = 30.6 \cong 31°C$

30. (a) $W = \dfrac{nRdT}{\gamma - 1}$ γ is minimum for a polyatomic gas

Hence, W is greatest for polyatomic gas

31. (b) Heat is extracted from the source in path DA and AB is

$$\Delta Q = \frac{3}{2}R\left(\frac{P_0V_0}{R}\right) + \frac{5}{2}R\left(\frac{2P_0V_0}{R}\right)$$

$$\Rightarrow \frac{3}{2}P_0V_0 + \frac{5}{2}2P_0V_0 = \left(\frac{13}{2}\right)P_0V_0$$

32. (d) Isochoric proceess $dV = 0$
$W = 0$ proceess 1
Isobaric : $W = P\,\Delta V = nR\Delta T$

Adiabatic $|W| = \dfrac{nR\Delta T}{\gamma - 1}$ $0 < \gamma - 1 < 1$

As workdone in case of adiabatic process is more so process 3 is adiabatic and process 2 is isobaric

33. (c) For adiabatic process, $dU = -100$ J

which remains same for other processes also.

Let C be the heat capacity of 2nd process then

$-(C)\,5 = dU + dW$

$= -100 + 25 = -75$

$\therefore\ C = 15$ J/K

34. (c) Coefficient of performance of a refrigerator,

$$\beta = \frac{Q_2}{W} = \frac{T_2}{T_1 - T_2}$$ (Where Q_2 is heat removed)

Given: $T_2 = 4°C = 4 + 273 = 277$ k
$T_1 = 30°C = 30 + 273 = 303$ k

$$\therefore\ \beta = \frac{600 \times 4.2}{W} = \frac{277}{303 - 277}$$

$\Rightarrow$ W = 236.5 joule

Power $P = \dfrac{W}{t} = \dfrac{236.5\text{joule}}{1\text{sec}} = 236.5$ watt.

35. (d) $dU = dQ - dW = (8 \times 10^5 - 6.5 \times 10^5) = 1.5 \times 10^5$ J

$dW = dQ - dU = 10^5 - 1.5 \times 10^5 = -0.5 \times 10^5\ J$

– ve sign indicates that work done on the gas is 0.5×10^5 J.

36. (d) In cyclic process, change in total internal energy is zero.

$\Delta U_{cyclic} = 0$

$$\Delta U_{BC} = nC_v\Delta T = 1 \times \frac{5R}{2}\Delta T$$

Where, C_v = molar specific heat at constant volume.
For BC, $\Delta T = -200$ K

$\therefore \quad \Delta U_{BC} = -500R$

37. **(d)** Efficiency of engine A, $\eta_1 = 1 - \frac{T}{T_1}$,

Efficiency of engine B, $\eta_2 = 1 - \frac{T_2}{T}$

Here, $\eta_1 = \eta_2$

$\therefore \quad \frac{T}{T_1} = \frac{T_2}{T} \Rightarrow T = \sqrt{T_1 T_2}$

38. **(b)** In the first process W is + ve as ΔV is positive, in the second process W is – ve as ΔV is – ve and area under the curve of second process is more

$\therefore$ Net Work < 0 and also $P_3 > P_1$.

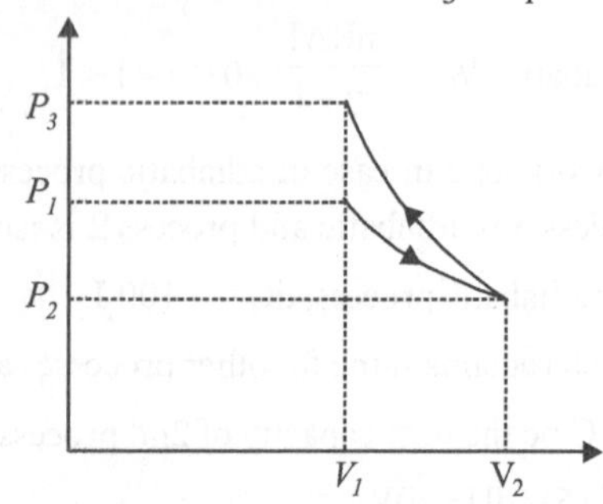

39. **(b)** Internal energy and entropy are state function, they do not depend upon path but on the state.

40. **(d)** 1st process is isothermal expansion which is only correct shown in option (d)

2nd process is isobaric compression which is correctly shown in option (d)

41. **(c)** $P_1 V_1^\gamma = P_2 V_2^\gamma$ (Adiabatic change)

$$P_2 = P_1\left(\frac{V_1}{V_2}\right)^\gamma = P_1\left(\frac{V_1}{V_1/3}\right)^\gamma = P_2(3)^\gamma$$

42. **(b)** W_{ext} = negative of area with volume-axis
W(adiabatic) > W(isothermal)

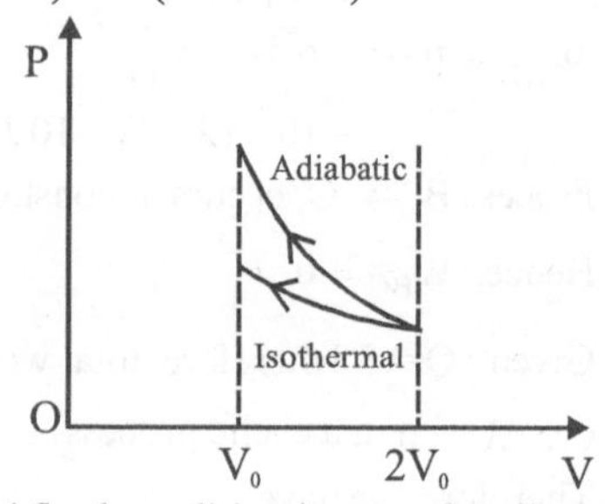

43. **(a)** Initial and final condition is same for all process

$\Delta U_1 = \Delta U_2 = \Delta U_3$

from first law of thermodynamics

$\Delta Q = \Delta U + \Delta W$

Work done

$\Delta W_1 > \Delta W_2 > \Delta W_3$ (Area of P.V. graph)

So $\Delta Q_1 > \Delta Q_2 > \Delta Q_3$

44. **(c)** $W = \frac{\pi r_1 r_2}{2} = \frac{\pi \times 1 \times 1}{2}$

$= \pi/2$ J

45. **(b)** Differentiate PV = constant w.r.t V

$\Rightarrow P\Delta V + V\Delta P = 0 \Rightarrow \frac{\Delta P}{P} = -\frac{\Delta V}{V}$

Speed Test-12

1. (d) Molar mass of the gas = 4g/mol
Speed of any quantity x

$$V=\sqrt{\frac{\gamma RT}{m}} \Rightarrow 952=\sqrt{\frac{\gamma\times 3.3\times 273}{4\times 10^{-3}}}$$

$$\Rightarrow \gamma = 1.6=\frac{16}{10}=\frac{8}{5}$$

Also, $\gamma=\frac{C_P}{C_V}=\frac{8}{5}$

So, $C_P=\frac{8\times 5}{5}=8JK^{-1}mol^{-1}$

2. (d) Since v_{rms} is doubled by increasing the temp. so by $v_{rms}=\sqrt{\frac{3KT}{m}}$, the temp. increase by four times.

Now for constant pressure $\frac{V_1}{T_1}=\frac{V_2}{T_2}$

V_1=V, T_1=T°K, T_2=4T°K, V_2=?

V_2=4V

3. (a) For mixture of gas, $C_v=\frac{n_1C_{v_1}+n_2C_{v_2}}{n_1+n_2}$

$$=\frac{4\times\frac{3}{2}R+\frac{1}{2}\times\frac{5}{2}R}{\left(4+\frac{1}{2}\right)}=\frac{6R+\frac{5}{4}R}{\frac{9}{2}}=\frac{29R\times 2}{9\times 4}=\frac{29R}{18}$$

and $C_p=\frac{n_1C_{p_1}+n_2C_{p_2}}{(n_1+n_2)}=\frac{4\times\frac{5R}{2}+\frac{1}{2}\times\frac{7R}{2}}{\left(4+\frac{1}{2}\right)}$

$$=\frac{10R+\frac{7}{4}R}{\frac{9}{2}}=\frac{47R}{18}$$

$$\therefore \frac{C_p}{C_v}=\frac{47R}{18}\times\frac{18}{29R}=1.62$$

4. (b) $\frac{P_1V_1}{T_1}=\frac{P_2V_2}{T_2}$ Here, $P_1=200kPa$

$T_1=22°C=295K$, $T_2=42°C=315K$

$$V_2=V_1+\frac{2}{100}V_1=1.02V_1$$

$$\therefore P_2=\frac{200\times 315V_1}{295\times 1.02V_1}=209.37kPa$$

5. (c) By kinetic theory of gases,
rms (root mean square) velocity of gas

$$V_{rms}=\sqrt{\frac{3RT}{M}}=\sqrt{\frac{3KT}{m}}$$

Where M and m are mol. wt and mass of gas respectively

$$V_{rms}=\sqrt{\frac{3\times 1.38\times 10^{-23}\times 273}{5\times 10^{-17}}}$$

$$=1.5\times 10^{-2} m/s=1.5 cm/s$$

6. (d) $C_p=\frac{5}{2}R$ and $C_v=\frac{3}{2}R$

We know that $Q_v=nC_v\Delta T$ and $Q_p=nC_p\Delta T$

$$\Rightarrow \frac{Q_v}{Q_p}=\frac{3}{5}.$$

Given $Q_p=207J\Rightarrow Q_v\cong 124$ J

7. (c) On giving same amount of heat at constant pressure, there is change in temperature for mono, dia and polyatomic gas.

$$(\Delta Q)_P=\mu C_p\Delta T\left(\mu=\frac{\text{No. of molecules}}{\text{Avogadro's no.}}\right)$$

or $$\Delta T\propto\frac{1}{\text{no. of molecules}}$$

8. (a) $C=C_{v\,mix}+\frac{R}{1-n}$ .....(1)

Now, $C_{vmix}=\frac{n_1C_{v1}+n_2C_{v2}}{n_1+n_2}$

$$=\frac{1\times\frac{3R}{2}+2\times\frac{5R}{2}}{1+2}=\frac{13R}{6}$$

From (1), $3R=\frac{13R}{6}+\frac{R}{1-n}\Rightarrow n=-\frac{1}{5}$

9. (a) $P=\frac{1}{3}\rho\bar{\upsilon}^2=\frac{1}{3}\times(6\times 10^{-2})\times(500)^2$

$$=5\times 10^3 N/m^2$$

10. (d) $v_{rms}=\sqrt{\frac{3kT}{m}}$ ....(1)

$v'_{rms}=\sqrt{\frac{3k\times 3T}{m}}$ ....(2)

Equ. (2) is dividing by equ. (1)

$$\frac{v'_{rms}}{v_{rms}} = \sqrt{\frac{3k.3T.m}{m.3kT}} = \sqrt{3}$$

$v'_{rms} = \sqrt{3}v_{rms}$

11. (a) $\tau = \dfrac{1}{\sqrt{2}\pi d^2\left(\dfrac{N}{V}\right)\sqrt{\dfrac{3RT}{M}}}$

$\tau \propto \dfrac{V}{\sqrt{T}}$

As, $TV^{\gamma-1} = K$
So, $\tau \propto V^{\gamma+1/2}$

Therefore, $q = \dfrac{\gamma+1}{2}$

12. (a) Volume $= \dfrac{\text{mass}}{\text{density}} = \dfrac{1}{4}\text{ m}^3$

$K.E = \dfrac{5}{2}PV = \dfrac{5}{2}\times 8\times 10^4\times\dfrac{1}{4} = 5\times 10^4 J$

13. (c) As no heat is lost,
Loss of kinetic energy = gain of internal energy of gas

$\dfrac{1}{2}mv^2 = nC_V\Delta T \Rightarrow \dfrac{1}{2}mv^2 = \dfrac{m}{M}\cdot\dfrac{R}{\gamma-1}\Delta T$

$\Rightarrow \Delta T = \dfrac{Mv^2(\gamma-1)}{2R}K$

14. (b) From graph, $T^2V = \text{const.}$ .....(1)
As we know that $TV^{\gamma-1} = \text{const}$

$\Rightarrow VT^{\frac{1}{\gamma-1}} = \text{const.}$ ....(2)

On comparing (1) and (2), we get
$\Rightarrow \gamma = 3/2$

Also $v_{rms} = \sqrt{\dfrac{3P}{\rho}}$ and $v_{sound} = \sqrt{\dfrac{P\gamma}{\rho}}$

$\Rightarrow \dfrac{v_{rms}}{v_{sound}} = \sqrt{\dfrac{3}{\gamma}} = \sqrt{2}$

15. (a) $W = \dfrac{nR\Delta T}{1-\gamma} \Rightarrow -146000 = \dfrac{1000\times 8.3\times 7}{1-\gamma}$

or $1-\gamma = -\dfrac{58.1}{146} \Rightarrow \gamma = 1+\dfrac{58.1}{146} = 1.4$
Hence the gas is diatomic.

16. (a) $C_{rms} = \sqrt{\dfrac{3RT}{M}}$

M is molecular wt.

$= \sqrt{\dfrac{3R(273+47)}{16}} = \sqrt{\dfrac{3RT}{2}}$

$\Rightarrow T = 40\text{ K}.$

17. (a) When temperature is same according to kinetic theory of gases, kinetic energy of molecules will be same.

$K.E. = \dfrac{1}{2}\times 32\times\left(\dfrac{1}{2}\right)^2 = \dfrac{1}{2}\times 2\times v^2$

RMS velocity of hydrogen molecules = 2 km/sec.

18. (a) Let T be the temperature of the mixture, then
$U = U_1 + U_2$

$\Rightarrow \dfrac{f}{2}(n_1+n_2)RT$

$= \dfrac{f}{2}(n_1)(R)(T_0) + \dfrac{f}{2}(n_2)(R)(2T_0)$

$\Rightarrow (2+4)T = 2T_0 + 8T_0\ (\because n_1 = 2, n_2 = 4)$

$\therefore T = \dfrac{5}{3}T_0$

19. (b) Coefficient of volume expansion at constant pressure is $\dfrac{1}{273}$ for all gases. The average transnational K.E. is same for molecules of all gases and for each molecules it is $\dfrac{3}{2}kT$

Mean free path $\lambda = \dfrac{kT}{\sqrt{2}\,\pi d^2 P}$ (as P decreases, λ increases)

20. (c) For a given pressure, volume will be more if temperature is more (Charle's law)

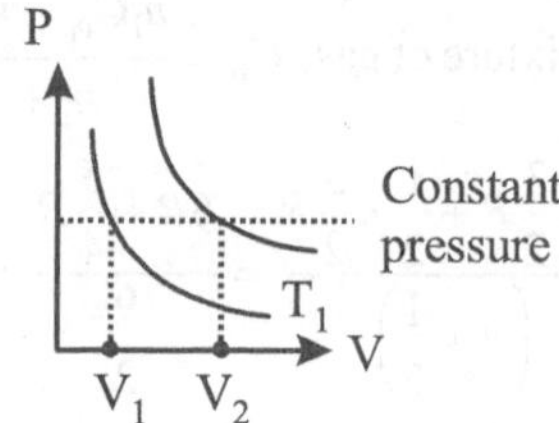

From the graph it is clear that $V_2 > V_1 \Rightarrow T_2 > T_1$

21. (a) $\dfrac{c_2}{c_1} = \sqrt{\dfrac{400}{300}} = \dfrac{2}{\sqrt{3}} \Rightarrow c_2 = \dfrac{2}{\sqrt{3}}\times 200 = \dfrac{400}{\sqrt{3}}\text{ ms}^{-1}$

22. (c) $\dfrac{PV}{T} = nR = \left(\dfrac{m}{M}\right)R$ or $\dfrac{PV}{T} = \left(\dfrac{R}{M}\right)m$

i.e., $\dfrac{PV}{T}$ versus m graph is straight line passing through origin with slope R/M, i.e. the slope depends on molecular mass of the gas M and is different for different gases.

23. (d) Molecule number ratio is $H_2 : O_2 = \dfrac{2}{3} : \dfrac{1}{3}$.

That gives $(c_{rms})^2 = 16\left(\dfrac{2}{3}\right) + 1\left(\dfrac{1}{3}\right)$ times the value for O_2.

24. (a) According to Vander Waal's equation

$P = \dfrac{nRT}{V-n\beta} - \dfrac{\alpha n^2}{V^2}$

Work done,

$$W=\int_{V_1}^{V_2} PdV = nRT\int_{V_1}^{V_2}\frac{dV}{V-n\beta}-\alpha n^2\int_{V_1}^{V_2}\frac{dV}{V^2}$$

$$=nRT\left[\log_e(V-n\beta)\right]_{V_1}^{V_2}+\alpha n^2\left[\frac{1}{V}\right]_{V_1}^{V_2}$$

$$=nRT\log_e\left(\frac{V_2-n\beta}{V_1-n\beta}\right)+\alpha n^2\left[\frac{V_1-V_2}{V_1V_2}\right]$$

25. (a) From PV = nRT

$$P_A=\frac{\rho_A M_A}{RT} \text{ and } P_B=\frac{\rho_B M_B}{RT}$$

From question,

$$\frac{P_A}{P_B}=\frac{\rho_A}{\rho_B}\frac{M_A}{M_B}=2\frac{M_A}{M_B}=\frac{3}{2}$$

So, $\frac{M_A}{M_B}=\frac{3}{4}$

26. (b) $(C_p)_{mix}=\frac{\mu_1 C_{p_1}+\mu_2 C_{p_2}}{\mu_1+\mu_2}$

$(C_{p_1}(He)=\frac{5}{2}R \text{ and } C_{p_2}(H_2)=\frac{7}{2}R)$

$(C_p)_{mix}==\frac{1\times\frac{5}{2}R+1\times\frac{7}{2}R}{1+1}$ 3R = 3 × 2 = 6 cal/mol.°C

∴ Amount of heat needed to raise the temperature from 0°C to 100°C

$(\Delta Q)_p=\mu C_p\Delta T=2\times6\times100=1200\,cal$

27. (a) 1 mole = 22.4 L at S.T.P.

$\frac{4.5g}{18g}=22.4\times\frac{4.5}{18}=5.6\,L$

28. (d) Internal energy of 2 moles of oxygen

$U_{O_2}=\mu\left(\frac{5}{2}RT\right)=2.\frac{5}{2}RT=5RT$

Internal energy of 4 moles of Argon.

$U_{Ar}=\mu\left(\frac{3}{2}RT\right)=4.\frac{3}{2}RT=6RT$

∴ Total internal energy

$U=U_{O_2}+U_{Ar}=11RT$

29. (d) $PV=\frac{m}{M}RT$

Initially, $PV=\frac{6}{M}R\times500$

Finally, $\frac{P}{2}V=\frac{(6-x)}{M}R\times300$ (if x g gas leaks out)

Hence, $2=\frac{6}{6-x}\times\frac{5}{3}$ ∴ x = 1 gram

30. (b) $\gamma=1+\frac{2}{f},\Rightarrow\gamma-1=\frac{2}{f}\Rightarrow\frac{f}{2}=\frac{1}{\gamma-1}\Rightarrow f=\frac{2}{\gamma-1}$

31. (a)

32. (a) Number of moles of first gas $=\frac{n_1}{N_A}$

Number of moles of second gas $=\frac{n_2}{N_A}$

Number of moles of third gas $=\frac{n_3}{N_A}$

If there is no loss of energy then

$P_1V_1+P_2V_2+P_3V_3=PV$

$$\frac{n_1}{N_A}RT_1+\frac{n_2}{N_A}RT_2+\frac{n_3}{N_A}RT_3=\frac{n_1+n_2+n_3}{N_A}RT_{mix}$$

$$\Rightarrow T_{mix}=\frac{n_1T_1+n_2T_2+n_3T_3}{n_1+n_2+n_3}$$

33. (d) Since it hits the plane wall parallel to *y z* – plane and it rebounds with same velocity, its *y* and *z* components of velocity do not change, but the *x*-component reverses the sign.

∴ Velocity after collision is $(-v_x, v_y \text{ and } v_z)$.

The change in momentum is

$-mv_x-mv_x=-2mv_x$

34. (c) *V* and *T* will be same for both gases.

$P_1V=\mu_1RT$ and $P_2V=\mu_2RT$

$(P_1/P_2)=\frac{5}{3}$ ∴ $\left(\frac{\mu_1}{\mu_2}\right)=\frac{5}{3}$

By definition, $\mu_1=\frac{N_1}{N_A}$ and $\mu_2=\frac{N_2}{N_A}$

∴ $\frac{N_1}{N_2}=\frac{\mu_1}{\mu_2}=\frac{5}{3}$

35. (d) $E=\frac{3}{2}\times300;\ E'=\frac{3}{2}R(600)=2E=2\times6.21\times10^{-21}$

$=12.42\times10^{-21}$ J.

$v_{rms}=\sqrt{\frac{3R\times300}{M}};\ v'_{rms}=\sqrt{\frac{3R\times600}{M}}=\sqrt{2}\,v_{rms}$

= 684.44 m/s

36. (d) Let the mass of the gas be m.

At a fixed temperature and pressure, volume is fixed.

Density of the gas, $\rho=\frac{m}{V}$

Now $\frac{\rho}{P}=\frac{m}{PV}=\frac{m}{nRT}$

$\Rightarrow\frac{m}{nRT}=x$ (By question)

$\Rightarrow xT=\text{constant}\Rightarrow x_1T_1=x_2T_2$

$$\Rightarrow x_2\Rightarrow\frac{x_1T_1}{T_2}=\frac{283}{383}x\quad\left[\begin{array}{l}\therefore\\ T_1 = 283K\\ T_2 = 383K\end{array}\right]$$

37. (b) $F=\frac{dU}{dr}=-\frac{d}{dr}\left[\frac{M}{r^3}-\frac{N}{R^{12}}\right]=-\left[\frac{-6M}{r^2}+\frac{12N}{r^{13}}\right]$

In equilibrium position, F = 0

$\therefore \quad \frac{6M}{r^2} - \frac{12N}{r^{13}} = 0$ or, $r^6 = \frac{2N}{M}$

$\therefore$ Potential energy at equilibrium position

$$U = \frac{M}{(2N/M)} = \frac{N}{(2N/M)^2} = \frac{M^2}{2N} - \frac{M^2}{4N} = \frac{M^2}{4N}$$

38. **(a)** Pressure of the gas will not be affected by motion of the system, hence by

$$v_{rms} = \sqrt{\frac{3P}{\rho}} \Rightarrow \bar{c}^2 = \frac{3P}{\rho} \Rightarrow P = \frac{1}{3}\rho\bar{c}^2$$

39. **(b)** Mean free path in a gas is 100 times the interatomic distance.

40. **(a)** $V_{rms} = \left[\frac{(2)^2 + (3)^2 + (4)^2 + (5)^2}{4}\right]^{1/2} = \sqrt{\left[\frac{54}{4}\right]}$

41. **(c)** If a gas is heated at constant volume then no work is done. The heat supplied is given by

$dQ = nC_v dT$

But $C_v = \frac{f}{2}R$ where f is the degree of freedom of the gas

$$\therefore dQ = \frac{nfRdT}{2}$$

$$= \frac{2 \times 3 \times R \times (373 - 273)}{2} = 300\,R$$

42. **(b)** For 1 molecule of a gas, $V_{rms} = \sqrt{\frac{3KT}{m}}$

where m is the mass of one molecule

For N molecule of a gas, $V_1 = \sqrt{\frac{3KT \times N}{m}}$

For 2N molecule of a gas $V_2 = \sqrt{\frac{3KT \times 2N}{(2m)}}$

$$\therefore \quad \frac{V_1}{V_2} = 1$$

43. **(c)**

44. **(c)** P-V diagram of the gas is a straight line passing through origin. Hence $P \propto V$ or PV^{-1} = constant

Molar heat capacity in the process PV^x = constant

$C = \frac{R}{\gamma - 1} + \frac{R}{1 - x}$; Here $\gamma = 1.4$ (For diatomic gas)

$$\Rightarrow C = \frac{R}{1.4 - 1} + \frac{R}{1 + 1} \Rightarrow C = 3R$$

45. **(c)** Given

$C_P - C_V = 5000$ J / mole °C ....(i)

$\frac{C_P}{C_V} = 1.6$ ....(ii)

From Equation (i) & (ii),

$$\Rightarrow \frac{C_P}{C_V} - \frac{C_V}{C_V} = \frac{5000}{C_V}$$

$$\Rightarrow 1.6 - 1 = \frac{5000}{C_V}$$

$$\Rightarrow C_V = \frac{5000}{0.6} = 8.33 \times 10^3$$

Hence $C_P = 1.6\,C_V = 1.6 \times 8.33 \times 10^3$

$C_P = 1.33 \times 10^4$

Speed Test-13

1. **(a)** For an SHM, the acceleration $a = -\omega^2 x$ where ω^2 is a constant. Therefore, $\frac{a}{x}$ is a constant. The time period T is also constant. Therefore, $\frac{aT}{x}$ is a constant.

2. **(b)** $t_1 = 2\pi\sqrt{\frac{m}{k_1}}$ or $t_1^2 = \frac{4\pi^2 m}{k_1}$ or $k_1 = \frac{4\pi^2 m}{t_1^2}$

Similarly, $k_2 = \frac{4\pi^2 m}{t_2^2}$ and $(k_1 + k_2) = \frac{4\pi^2 m}{t_0^2}$

$\therefore \frac{4\pi^2 m}{t_0^2} = \frac{4\pi^2 m}{t_1^2} + \frac{4\pi^2 m}{t_2^2}$ or $\frac{1}{t_0^2} = \frac{1}{t_1^2} + \frac{1}{t_2^2}$

3. **(b)**

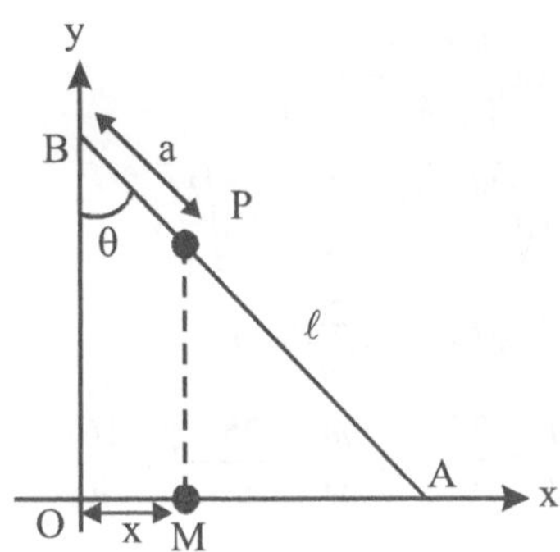

$\frac{d\theta}{dt} = 2 \therefore \theta = 2t$

Let BP = a, $\therefore$ x = OM = a sin θ = a sin (2t)

Hence M executes SHM within the given time period and its acceleration is opposite to x that means towards left.

4. **(b)** The kinetic energy of a particle executing S.H.M. is given by

$K = \frac{1}{2} ma^2 \omega^2 \sin^2 \omega t$

where, m = mass of particle
a = amplitude
ω = angular frequency
t = time

Now, average K.E. $= \langle K \rangle = \langle \frac{1}{2} m\omega^2 a^2 \sin^2 \omega t \rangle$

$= \frac{1}{2} m\omega^2 a^2 \langle \sin^2 \omega t \rangle$

$= \frac{1}{2} m\omega^2 a^2 \left(\frac{1}{2}\right) \quad \left(\because \langle \sin^2 \theta \rangle = \frac{1}{2}\right)$

$= \frac{1}{4} m\omega^2 a^2 = \frac{1}{4} ma^2 (2\pi\nu)^2 \quad (\because \omega = 2\pi\nu)$

or, $\langle K \rangle = \pi^2 ma^2 \nu^2$

5. **(a)** We know that $T = 2\pi\sqrt{\frac{M}{k}}$

From first case, $2 = 2\pi\sqrt{\frac{M}{k}}$ .... (1)

In second case, $4 = 2\pi\sqrt{\frac{M+2}{k}}$ .... (2)

From eq. (1) and eq. (2)

$\frac{4}{2} = \sqrt{\frac{M+2}{M}} \Rightarrow 4 = 1 + \frac{2}{M}$

$\frac{2}{M} = 3 \Rightarrow M = \frac{2}{3}$ kg

6. **(b)** Amplitude of a damped oscillator at any instant t is given by

$A = A_0 e^{-bt/2m}$

where A_0 is the original amplitude

From question,

When t = 2 s, $A = \frac{A_0}{3}$

$\therefore \frac{A_0}{3} = A_0 e^{-2b/2m}$

or, $\frac{1}{3} = e^{-b/m}$ ...(i)

When t = 6 s, $A = \frac{A_0}{n}$

$\therefore \frac{A_0}{n} = A_0 e^{-6b/2m}$

or, $\frac{1}{n} = e^{-3b/m} = (e^{-b/m})^3$

or, $\frac{1}{n} = \left(\frac{1}{3}\right)^3$ (Using eq. (i))

$\therefore n = 3^3$

7. **(c)** Acceleration due to gravity at a depth 'd' is given by,

$g' = g\left(1 - \frac{d}{R}\right) = g\left(\frac{R-d}{R}\right) = \frac{g}{R} y$

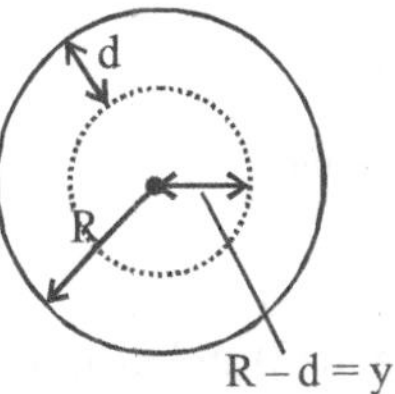

or acceleration ∝ displacement

which is the condition for SHM. So, body will oscillate simple harmonically in tunnel.

8. (c) Time to complete 1/4th oscillation is $\frac{T}{4}$ s. Time to complete $\frac{1}{8}$th vibration from extreme position is obtained from

$$y = \frac{a}{2} = a\cos\omega t = a\cos\frac{2\pi}{T}t \text{ or } t = \frac{T}{6}s$$

So time to complete 3/8th oscillation

$$= \frac{T}{4} + \frac{T}{6} = \frac{5T}{12}$$

9. (a) As we know, kinetic energy $= \frac{1}{2}m\omega^2(A^2 - x^2)$

Potential energy $= \frac{1}{2}m\omega^2x^2$

$$\therefore \frac{\frac{1}{2}m\omega^2(A^2 - x^2)}{\frac{1}{2}m\omega^2x^2} = \frac{1}{4} \Rightarrow \frac{A^2 - x^2}{x^2} = \frac{1}{4}$$

$$4A^2 - 4x^2 = x^2 \Rightarrow x^2 = \frac{4}{5}A^2 \quad \therefore x = \frac{2}{\sqrt{5}}A.$$

10. (d) $T = 2\pi\sqrt{\frac{\ell}{g}}$ and $T' = 2\pi\sqrt{\frac{1.21\ell}{g}}$

$(\because \ell' = \ell + 21\% \text{ of } \ell)$

$$\% \text{ increase} = \frac{T' - T}{T} \times 100$$

$$= \frac{\sqrt{1.21\ell} - \sqrt{\ell}}{\sqrt{\ell}} \times 100 = \left(\sqrt{1.21} - \sqrt{1}\right) \times 100$$

$$= (1.1 - 1) \times 100 = 10\%$$

11. (d) $T = 2\pi\sqrt{\frac{m}{k}}$

When a spring is cut into n parts

Spring constant for each part = nk

Here, $n = 4$

$$T_1 = 2\pi\sqrt{\frac{m}{4k}} = \frac{T}{2}$$

12. (d) $x = A\cos(\omega t + \delta)$

$y = A\cos(\omega t + \alpha)$ ....(1)

When $\delta = \alpha + \frac{\pi}{2}$

$$x = A\cos\left(\frac{\pi}{2} + \omega t + \alpha\right)$$

$x = -A\sin(\omega t + \alpha)$ ....(2)

Squaring (1) and (2) and then adding

$x^2 + y^2 = A^2[\cos^2(\omega t + \alpha) + \sin^2(\omega t + \alpha)]$

or $x^2 + y^2 = A^2$, which is the equation of a circle. The present motion is anticlockwise.

13. (a) Here,

$x = x_0\cos(\omega t - \pi/4)$

$\therefore$ Velocity, $v = \frac{dx}{dt} = -x_0\omega\sin\left(\omega t - \frac{\pi}{4}\right)$

Acceleration,

$$a = \frac{dv}{dt} = -x_0\omega^2\cos\left(\omega t - \frac{\pi}{4}\right)$$

$$= x_0\omega^2\cos\left[\pi + \left(\omega t - \frac{\pi}{4}\right)\right]$$

$$= x_0\omega^2\cos\left(\omega t + \frac{3\pi}{4}\right) \quad ...(1)$$

Acceleration, $a = A\cos(\omega t + \delta)$ ...(2)

Comparing the two equations, we get

$A = x_0\omega^2$ and $\delta = \frac{3\pi}{4}$.

14. (c) $T = 2\pi\sqrt{\frac{M}{k}}$

$$T' = 2\pi\sqrt{\frac{M + m}{k}} = \frac{5T}{3}$$

$$\therefore 2\pi\sqrt{\frac{M + m}{k}} = \frac{5}{3} \times 2\pi\sqrt{\frac{M}{k}}$$

$$M + m = \frac{25}{9} \times M$$

$$1 + \frac{m}{M} = \frac{25}{9} \Rightarrow \frac{m}{M} = \frac{25}{9} - 1 = \frac{16}{9}$$

15. (d) $A = 0.05$ m, $y = 0.01$ m

Acceleration, $a = 1.0$ m/s^2

We have, $a = -\omega^2 y$ or $|a| = \omega^2 y$

$\Rightarrow 1.0 = \omega^2 \times 0.01$

$\therefore \omega^2 = \frac{1.0}{0.01} = 100 \Rightarrow \omega = 10$

Now, time period, $T = \frac{2\pi}{\omega} = \frac{2\pi}{10} = \frac{\pi}{5}$ sec.

16. (c) We have, $U + K = E$

where, U = potential energy, K = Kinetic energy, E = Total energy.

Also, we know that, in S.H.M., when potential energy is maximum, K.E. is zero and vice-versa.

$\therefore U_{max} + 0 = E \Rightarrow U_{max} = E$

Further,

$$K.E. = \frac{1}{2}m\omega^2a^2\cos^2\omega t$$

But by question, $K.E. = K_0\cos^2\omega t$

$$\therefore K_0 = \frac{1}{2}m\omega^2a^2$$

Hence, total energy, $E = \frac{1}{2}m\omega^2a^2 = K_0$

$\therefore U_{max} = K_0$ & $E = K_0$.

17. (b) Distance covered by lift is given by
$y = t^2$
$\therefore$ Acceleration of lift upwards

$$= \frac{d^2y}{dt^2} = \frac{d}{dt}(2t) = 2\ m/s^2 = \frac{g}{5}$$

Now, $T = 2\pi\sqrt{\frac{\ell}{g}}$

$$T' = 2\pi\sqrt{\frac{\ell}{g+\frac{g}{5}}} = 2\pi\sqrt{\frac{\ell}{\frac{6}{5}g}} = \sqrt{\frac{5}{6}}T.$$

18. (d) In simple harmonic motion, starting from rest,
At $t = 0$, $x = A$
$x = A\cos\omega t$ .....(i)
When $t = \tau$, $x = A - a$
When $t = 2\tau$, $x = A - 3a$
From equation (i)
$A - a = A\cos\omega\tau$ ......(ii)
$A - 3a = A\cos 2\omega\tau$ ....(iii)
As $\cos 2\omega\tau = 2\cos^2\omega\tau - 1$ ...(iv)
From equation (ii), (iii) and (iv)

$$\frac{A-3a}{A} = 2\left(\frac{A-a}{A}\right)^2 - 1$$

$$\Rightarrow \frac{A-3a}{A} = \frac{2A^2 + 2a^2 - 4Aa - A^2}{A^2}$$

$\Rightarrow A^2 - 3aA = A^2 + 2a^2 - 4Aa$
$\Rightarrow 2a^2 = aA$
$\Rightarrow A = 2a$

$$\Rightarrow \frac{a}{A} = \frac{1}{2}$$

Now, $A - a = A\cos\omega\tau$

$$\Rightarrow \cos\omega\tau = \frac{A-a}{A}$$

$$\Rightarrow \cos\omega\tau = \frac{1}{2} \text{ or } \frac{2\pi}{T}\tau = \frac{\pi}{3}$$

$\Rightarrow T = 6\tau$

19. (b) $v_1 = \frac{dy_1}{dt} = 0.1\times 100\pi\cos\left(100\pi t + \frac{\pi}{3}\right)$

$$v_2 = \frac{dy_2}{dt} = -0.1\pi\sin\pi t = 0.1\pi\cos\left(\pi t + \frac{\pi}{2}\right)$$

$$\therefore \text{Phase diff.} = \phi_1 - \phi_2 = \frac{\pi}{3} - \frac{\pi}{2} = \frac{2\pi - 3\pi}{6} = -\frac{\pi}{6}$$

20. (c) $f_A = \frac{1}{2\pi}\sqrt{\frac{g}{L_A}}$ and $f_B = \frac{f_A}{2} = \frac{1}{2\pi}\sqrt{\frac{g}{L_B}}$

$$\therefore \frac{f_A}{f_{A/2}} = \frac{1}{2\pi}\sqrt{\frac{g}{L_A}} \times 2\pi\sqrt{\frac{L_B}{g}} \Rightarrow 2 = \sqrt{\frac{L_B}{L_A}} \Rightarrow 4 = \frac{L_B}{L_A},$$

regardless of mass

21. (d)

22. (c) Here all the three springs are connected in parallel to mass m. Hence equivalent spring constant
$k = K + K + 2K = 4K$.

23. (a) K.E. $= \frac{1}{2}m\omega^2(a^2 - x^2)$

When $x = 0$, K.E is maximum and is equal to $\frac{1}{2}m\omega^2a^2$.

24. (d) $y = 5\sin(\pi t + 4\pi)$, comparing it with standard equation

$$y = a\sin(\omega t + \phi) = a\sin\left(\frac{2\pi t}{T} + \phi\right)$$

$$a = 5m \text{ and } \frac{2\pi t}{T} = \pi t \Rightarrow T = 2\text{ sec}.$$

25. (b) $T = 2\pi\sqrt{\frac{\text{displacement}}{\text{acceleration}}} = 2\pi\sqrt{\frac{x}{zx}} = 2\pi/\sqrt{z}$

26. (b) Here, $x = 2\times 10^{-2}\cos\pi t$
Speed is given by

$$v = \frac{dx}{dt} = 2\times 10^{-2}\,\pi\sin\pi t$$

For the first time, the speed to be maximum,
$\sin\pi t = 1$ or, $\sin\pi t = \sin\frac{\pi}{2}$

$$\Rightarrow \pi t = \frac{\pi}{2} \text{ or, } t = \frac{1}{2} = 0.5\text{ sec.}$$

27. (d) $T = 2\pi\sqrt{\frac{R}{g}} = 2\pi\sqrt{\frac{64\times 10^6}{9.8}} = 2\times\frac{22}{7}\times\frac{8\times 10^3}{7\times\sqrt{2}}$

$$= \frac{\sqrt{2}\times 22\times 8\times 1000}{49\times 60}\text{ min} = 84.6\text{ min}$$

28. (a) $x = 3\sin 2t + 4\cos 2t$. From given equation

$$a_1 = 3,\ a_2 = 4, \text{ and } \phi = \frac{\pi}{2}$$

$$\therefore a = \sqrt{a_1^2 + a_2^2} = \sqrt{3^2 + 4^2} = 5$$

$$\Rightarrow v_{max} = a\omega = 5\times 2 = 10$$

29. (d) Slope of F - x curve $= -k = -\frac{80}{0.2} \Rightarrow k = 400$ N/m,

Time period, $T = 2\pi\sqrt{\frac{m}{k}} = 0.0314$ sec.

30. (b) Phase change π in 50 oscillations.
Phase change 2π in 100 oscillations.
So frequency different ~ 1 in 100.

31. (a) $T = 2\pi\sqrt{\frac{\ell}{g}}$; $2 = 2\pi\sqrt{\frac{\ell}{g}} = 2\pi\sqrt{\frac{\ell'}{(g/6)}}$

Time period will remain constant if on moon,
$\ell' = \ell/6 = 1/6$ m

32. (b) Let k be the force constant of spring of length l_2. Since $l_1 = n\,l_2$, where n is an integer, so the spring is made of $(n + 1)$ equal parts in length each of length l_2.

$\therefore \quad \frac{1}{K}=\frac{(n+1)}{k}$ or $k=(n+1)K$

The spring of length l_1 $(= n\, l_2)$ will be equivalent to n springs connected in series where spring constant

$k'=\frac{k}{n}=(n+1)K/n$ & spring constant of length ℓ_2 is $K(n+1)$.

33. (c) Given

$y = 0.2 \sin(10\pi t + 1.5\pi)\cos(10\pi t + 1.5\pi)$

We know that 2 sinA cos A = sin2A, we get

$y = 0.1 \sin 2\,(10\pi t + 1.5\pi) = 0.1 \sin(20\pi t + 3\pi)$

On comparing with wave equation

$y = a \sin(\omega t + \phi)$ we get

$\omega = 20\pi$

$T=\frac{2\pi}{\omega}=\frac{2\pi}{20\pi}=\frac{1}{10}\text{sec.}=0.1\text{sec.}$

34. (a) The displacement of a particle in S.H.M. is given by

$y = a \sin(\omega t + \phi)$

velocity $=\frac{dy}{dt}=\omega a\cos(\omega t+\phi)$

The velocity is maximum when the particle passes through the mean position i.e.,

$\left(\frac{dy}{dt}\right)_{max}=\omega a$

The kinetic energy at this instant is given by

$\frac{1}{2}m\left(\frac{dy}{dt}\right)^2_{max}=\frac{1}{2}m\omega^2 a^2=8\times10^{-3}$ joule

or $\quad \frac{1}{2}\times(0.1)\,\omega^2\times(0.1)^2=8\times10^{-3}$

Solving we get $\quad \omega = \pm 4$

Substituting the values of a, ω and ϕ in the equation of S.H.M., we get

$y = 0.1 \sin(\pm 4t + \pi/4)$ metre.

35. (d) $K.E=\frac{1}{2}k(A^2-d^2)$

and $P.E.=\frac{1}{2}kd^2$

At mean position $d = 0$. At extrement positions $d = A$

36. (b) $y=3\sin\frac{\pi}{2}(50t-x)$

$y=3\sin\left(25\pi t-\frac{\pi}{2}x\right)$ on comparing with the standard wave equation

$y = a \sin(\omega t - kx)$

Wave velocity $v=\frac{\omega}{k}=\frac{25\pi}{\pi/2}=50$ m/sec.

The velocity of particle

$v_p=\frac{\partial y}{\partial t}=75\pi\cos\left(25\pi t-\frac{\pi}{2}x\right)$

$v_{p\,max}=75\pi$

then $\frac{v_{p\max}}{v}=\frac{75\pi}{50}=\frac{3\pi}{2}$

37. (b) The equivalent situation is a series combination of two springs of spring constants k and 2k.

If k' is the equivalent spring constant, then

$k'=\frac{(k)(2k)}{3k}=\frac{2k}{3}$

$\Rightarrow T=2\pi\sqrt{\frac{3m}{2k}}$

38. (a) Time period of simple pendulum $T=2\pi\sqrt{\left(\frac{l}{g}\right)}\propto\sqrt{l}$

where l is effective length.

[i.e distance between centre of suspension and centre of gravity of bob]

Initially, centre of gravity is at the centre of sphere. When water leaks the centre of gravity goes down until it is half filled; then it begins to go up and finally it again goes at the centre. That is effective length first increases and then decreases. As $T\propto\sqrt{l}$, so time period first increases and then decreases.

39. (d) At $t = 0$, $x = 5 = \frac{A}{2}$

$\Rightarrow$ Initial phase, $\phi = 30° = \frac{\pi}{6}$

$\Rightarrow x = A\sin(\omega t + \phi)$

$=10\sin\left(\frac{2\pi}{T}t+\frac{\pi}{6}\right)=10\sin\left(\pi t+\frac{\pi}{6}\right)$

40. (b) For block A to move in S.H.M.

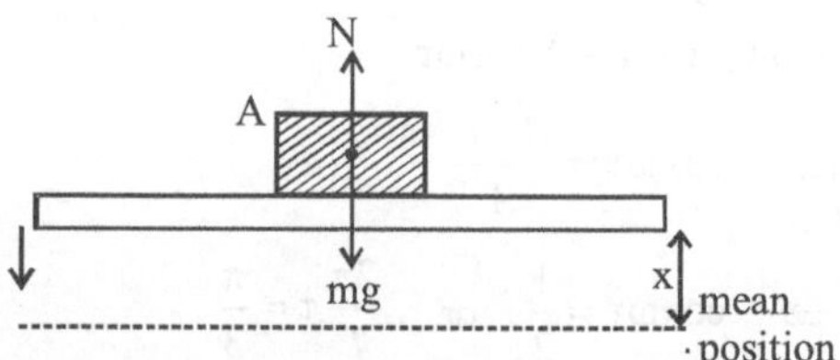

$mg - N = m\omega^2 x$

where x is the distance from mean position

For block to leave contact N = 0

$\Rightarrow mg=m\omega^2x\Rightarrow x=\frac{g}{\omega^2}$

41. (a) $t=2\pi\sqrt{\frac{\ell}{g_{eff}}}$; $t_0=2\pi\sqrt{\frac{\ell}{g}}$

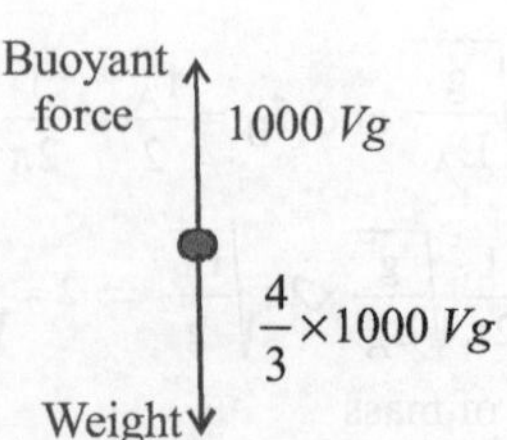

Net force $= \left(\frac{4}{3}-1\right)\times 1000\ Vg = \frac{1000}{3}Vg$

$$g_{eff} = \frac{1000\ Vg}{3\times\frac{4}{3}\times 1000V} = \frac{g}{4}$$

$$\therefore t = 2\pi\sqrt{\frac{\ell}{g/4}}$$

$t = 2t_0$

42. (a) K.E. of a body undergoing SHM is given by,

$$K.E. = \frac{1}{2}ma^2\omega^2\cos^2\omega t$$

$$T.E. = \frac{1}{2}ma^2\omega^2$$

Given K.E. = 0.75 T.E.

$$\Rightarrow 0.75 = \cos^2\omega t \Rightarrow \omega t = \frac{\pi}{6}$$

$$\Rightarrow t = \frac{\pi}{6\times\omega} \Rightarrow t = \frac{\pi\times 2}{6\times 2\pi} \Rightarrow t = \frac{1}{6}\ s$$

43. (a) Under the action of first force, $F_1 = m\omega_1^2 y$

Under the action of second force,

$F_2 = m\omega_2^2 y$

Under the action of resultant force,

$F_1 + F_2 = m\omega^2 y$

$\Rightarrow m\omega^2 y = m\omega_1^2 y + m\omega_2^2 y$

$\Rightarrow \omega^2 = \omega_1^2 + \omega_2^2$

$$\Rightarrow \left(\frac{2\pi}{T}\right)^2 = \left(\frac{2\pi}{T_1}\right)^2 + \left(\frac{2\pi}{T_2}\right)^2$$

$$\Rightarrow T = \sqrt{\frac{T_1^2T_2^2}{T_1^2+T_2^2}} = \sqrt{\frac{\left(\frac{4}{5}\right)^2\cdot\left(\frac{3}{5}\right)^2}{\left(\frac{4}{5}\right)^2+\left(\frac{3}{5}\right)^2}} = \frac{12}{25}.$$

44. (d) $F = -bV$, b depends on all the three i.e, shape and size of he block and viscosity of the medium.

45. (c) When the bob moves from maximum angular displacement θ to mean position, then the loss of gravitational potential energy is mgh where $h = l(1-\cos\theta)$

Speed Test-14

1. **(a)**

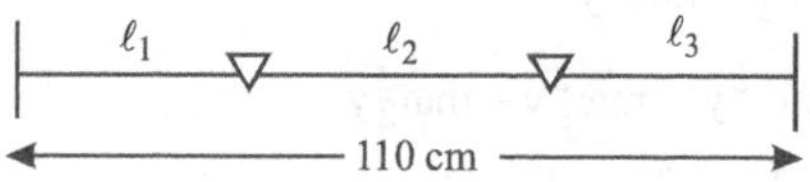

ℓ_1 | ℓ_2 | ℓ_3 — 110 cm

$n_1 : n_2 : n_3 = 3 : 2 : 1$

$n \propto \frac{1}{\ell}$

$\ell_1 : \ell_2 : \ell_3 = \frac{1}{3} : \frac{1}{2} : \frac{1}{1} = 2 : 3 : 6$

$\ell_1 + \ell_2 + \ell_3 = 110$

$\Rightarrow 2x + 3x + 6x = 110 \Rightarrow x = 10$

$\therefore$ The two bridges should be set at 2x i.e, 20 cm from one end and 6x i.e, 60 cm from the other end.

2. **(a)** Equation of the harmonic progressive wave given by : $y = a \sin 2\pi (bt - cx)$.

Here $\upsilon = b$

$k = \frac{2\pi}{\lambda} = 2\pi c$ take, $\frac{1}{\lambda} = c$

$\therefore$ Velocity of the wave $= \upsilon\lambda = b\frac{1}{c} = \frac{b}{c}$

$\frac{dy}{dt} = a\,2\pi b \cos 2\pi (bt - cx) = a\omega \cos(\omega t - kx)$

Maximum particle velocity $= a\omega = a2\pi b = 2\pi ab$

given this is $2 \times \frac{b}{c}$ i.e. $2\pi a = \frac{2}{c}$ or $c = \frac{1}{\pi a}$

3. **(c)** $y = 0.25 \sin(10\pi x - 2\pi t)$

Comparing this equation with the standard wave equation

$y = a\sin(kx - \omega t)$

We get, $k = 10\pi$

$\Rightarrow \frac{2\pi}{\lambda} = 10\pi \Rightarrow \lambda = 0.2\,m$

And $\omega = 2\pi$ or, $2\pi v = 2\pi \Rightarrow v = 1Hz$.

The sign inside the bracket is negative, hence the wave travels in + ve x- direction.

4. **(b)** Amplitude of reflected wave $= \frac{2}{3} \times 0.9 = 0.6$

It would travel along negative direction of x-axis, and on reflection at a rigid support, there occurs a phase change of π.

5. **(c)** Velocity of source $= 18\ km\ h^{-1} = 5\ m\ s^{-1}$

(i) S moves towards listener (v_S)

(ii) listener moves towards source (v_L)

$v' = \frac{v + v_L}{v - v_S} v = 280$ Hz , Beats $= v' - v = 8$.

6. **(d)** Third overtone has a frequency 7 n, which means $L = \frac{7\lambda}{4}$ = three full loops + one half loop, which would make four nodes and four antinodes.

7. **(c)** Comparing it with $y(x, t) = A\cos(\omega t + \pi/2)\cos kx$.

If $kx = \pi/2$, a node occurs ; $\therefore 10\pi x = \pi/2 \Rightarrow x = 0.05$ m

If $kx = \pi$, an antinode occurs $\Rightarrow 10\pi x = \pi$

$\Rightarrow x = 0.1$ m

Also speed of wave $\omega / k = \frac{50\pi}{10\pi} = 5 m/s$ and

$\lambda = 2\pi / k = 2\pi / 10\pi = 0.2$ m

8. **(a)** $\ell_1 + x = \frac{\lambda}{4} = 22.7$ equation (1)

$\ell_2 + x = \frac{3\lambda}{4} = 70.2$ equation (2)

$l_3 + x = \frac{5\lambda}{4}$ equation (3)

From equation (1) and (2)

$x = \frac{\ell_2 - 3\ell_1}{2} = \frac{70.2 - 68.1}{2} = \frac{2.1}{2} = 1.05$ cm

From equation (2) and (3) $\frac{\ell_3 + x}{\ell_1 + x} = 5$

$\ell_3 = 5\ell_1 + 4x = 5 \times 22.7 + 4 \times 1.05 = 117.7$ cm

9. **(d)**

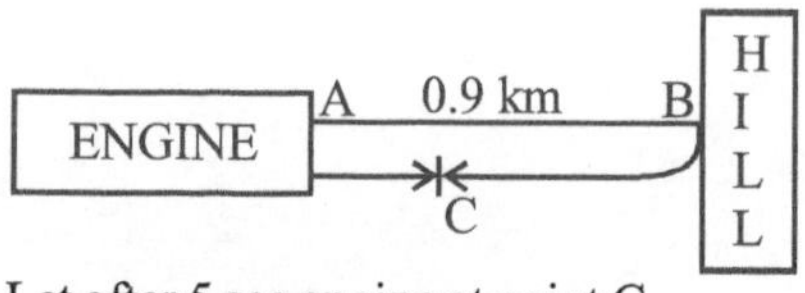

ENGINE — A — 0.9 km — B — HILL; C

Let after 5 sec engine at point C

$t = \frac{AB}{330} + \frac{BC}{330}$

$5 = \frac{0.9 \times 1000}{330} + \frac{BC}{330}$

$\therefore BC = 750\,m$

Distance travelled by engine in 5 sec $= 900\,m - 750\,m = 150\,m$

Therefore velocity of engine

$= \frac{150\,m}{5\,sec} = 30$ m/s

10. **(a)** For fundamental mode,

$f = \frac{1}{2\ell}\sqrt{\frac{T}{\mu}}$

Taking logarithm on both sides, we get

$$\log f = \log\left(\frac{1}{2\ell}\right) + \log\left(\sqrt{\frac{T}{\mu}}\right)$$

$$= \log\left(\frac{1}{2\ell}\right) + \frac{1}{2}\log\left(\frac{T}{\mu}\right)$$

$$\text{or } \log f = \log\left(\frac{1}{2\ell}\right) + \frac{1}{2}[\log T - \log \mu]$$

Differentiating both sides, we get

$$\frac{df}{f} = \frac{1}{2}\frac{dT}{T} \quad (\text{as } \ell \text{ and } \mu \text{ are constants})$$

$$\Rightarrow \frac{dT}{T} = 2 \times \frac{df}{f}$$

Here $df = 6$

$f = 600$ Hz

$$\therefore \frac{dT}{T} = \frac{2 \times 6}{600} = 0.02$$

11. (b) Frequency received by listener from the rear source,

$$n' = \frac{v-u}{v} \times n = \frac{v-u}{v} \times \frac{v}{\lambda} = \frac{v-u}{\lambda}$$

Frequency received by listener from the front source,

$$n'' = \frac{v+u}{v} \times \frac{v}{\lambda} = \frac{v+u}{\lambda}$$

No. of beats $= n'' - n'$

$$= \frac{v+u}{\lambda} - \frac{v-u}{\lambda} = \frac{v+u-v+u}{\lambda} = \frac{2u}{\lambda}$$

12. (c) $n' = n\left[\frac{v+v_0}{v}\right] = n\left[\frac{v+\frac{v}{5}}{v}\right] = n\left[\frac{6}{5}\right]$

$$\frac{n'}{n} = \frac{6}{5};\ \frac{n'-n}{n} = \frac{6-5}{5} \times 100 = 20\%$$

13. (c) In a closed organ pipe the fundamental frequency is

$$\upsilon = \frac{\upsilon}{4L}$$

$$\upsilon = \frac{320\ ms^{-1}}{4 \times 1\ m} = 80\ Hz$$

In a closed organ pipe only odd harmonics are present. So, it can resonate with 80 Hz, 240 Hz, 400 Hz, 560 Hz.

14. (b)

f (S) → 30 ms^{-1} ⇢ |f' (O)   f'' (O) → 30 ms^{-1} ← |f' (S)

f' is the apparent frequency received by an observer at the hill. f'' is the frequency of the reflected sound as heard by driver.

$$f' = \frac{v}{v-30} f,$$

$$f'' = \frac{v+30}{v} f' = \frac{v+30}{v-30} f = \frac{360}{300} \times 600$$

$= 720$ Hz

15. (d) Figure(a) represents a harmonic wave of frequency 7.0 Hz, figure (b) represents a harmonic wave of frequency 5.0 Hz. Therefore beat frequency $v_s = 7 - 5 = 2.0$ Hz.

16. (a) $\upsilon \propto \sqrt{T}$

17. (b) In fundamental mode,

$$\frac{\lambda}{2} = l \Rightarrow \lambda = 2l$$

$$\therefore f = \frac{v}{\lambda} = \frac{v}{2l} \qquad \text{.......(1)}$$

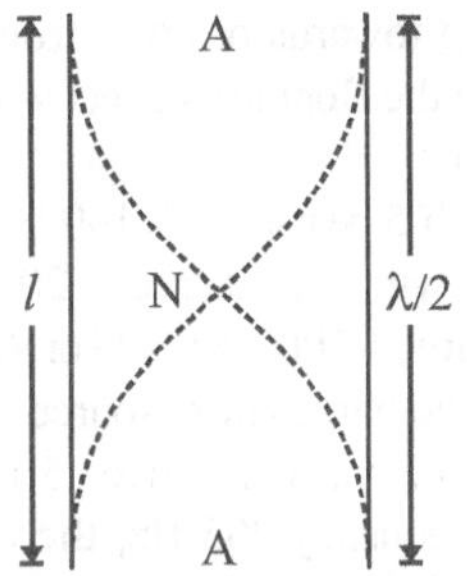

Fundamental mode

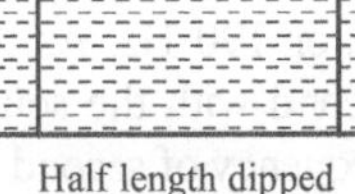

Half length dipped in water

In half length dipped in water mode,

$$\frac{l}{2} = \frac{\lambda}{4} \Rightarrow \lambda = 2l$$

$$\therefore f' = \frac{v}{\lambda} = \frac{v}{2l} = f$$

18. (a) Given wave equation is $y(x,t)$

$$= e^{\left(-ax^2+bt^2+2\sqrt{ab}\,xt\right)}$$

$$= e^{-[(\sqrt{a}x)^2+(\sqrt{b}t)^2+2\sqrt{a}x.\sqrt{b}t]}$$

$$= e^{-(\sqrt{a}x+\sqrt{b}t)^2}$$

$$= e^{-\left(x+\sqrt{\frac{b}{a}}t\right)^2}$$

It is a function of type $y = f(x+vt)$

$$\Rightarrow \text{Speed of wave} = \sqrt{\frac{b}{a}}$$

19. (c) Particle velocity

$$v = \frac{d}{dt}\left[x_0 \sin 2\pi\left(nt - \frac{x}{\lambda}\right)\right]$$

$$= 2\pi n x_0 \cos 2\pi\left(nt - \frac{x}{\lambda}\right)$$

$\therefore$ Maximum particle velocity $= 2\pi n x_0$

$$\text{Wave velocity} = \frac{\lambda}{T} = n\lambda$$

$$\text{Given, } 2\pi n x_0 = 4n\lambda \Rightarrow \lambda = \frac{2\pi n x_0}{4n} = \frac{\pi x_0}{2}$$

20. (d) As number of beats/sec = diff. in frequencies has to be less than 10, therefore $0 < (n_1 - n_2) < 10$

21. (c) Length of pipe = 85 cm = 0.85m
Frequency of oscillations of air column in closed organ pipe is given by,

$$f=\frac{(2n-1)\upsilon}{4L}$$

$$f=\frac{(2n-1)\upsilon}{4L}\le 1250$$

$$\Rightarrow \frac{(2n-1)\times 340}{0.85\times 4}\le 1250$$

$\Rightarrow 2n-1\le 12.5\approx 6$

22. (b) As the source is not moving towards or away from the observer in a straight line, so the Doppler's effect will not be observed by the observer.

23. (c) Frequency of first source with 5 beats/ sec = 100 Hz and frequency of second source with 5 beats/sec = 205 Hz. The frequency of the first source = 100 ± 5 = 105 or 95 Hz. Therefore, frequency of second harmonic of source = 210 Hz or 190 Hz. As the second harmonic gives 5 beats/ second with the sound of frequency 205 Hz, therefore, frequency of second harmonic source should be 210 Hz or frequency of source = 105 Hz.

24. (c) Pressure change will be minimum at both ends. In fact, pressure variation is maximum at $\ell/2$ because the displacement node is pressure antinode.

25. (a) $n_{Last}=n_{First}+(N-1)x$
$2n=n+(41-1)\times 5$
$\Rightarrow n_{First}=200$ Hz and $n_{Last}=400$ Hz

26. (b) Here, T = 0.05 sec, v = 300 ms^{-1}.

Now $\lambda=\frac{v}{\nu}=vT=(300\times 0.05)$m

or, $\lambda=15$ m
Phase of the point at 10 m from the source

$$=\frac{2\pi}{\lambda}\times x=\frac{2\pi}{15}\times 10=\frac{4\pi}{3}\text{rad}$$

Phase of the point at 15 m from the source

$$\frac{2\pi}{\lambda}\times x=\frac{2\pi}{15}\times 15=2\pi\,\text{rad}$$

∴ The phase difference between the points

$$=2\pi-\frac{4\pi}{3}=\frac{2\pi}{3}\text{rad}$$

27. (a) We have, $L_1=10\log\left(\frac{I_1}{I_0}\right)$; $L_2=10\log\left(\frac{I_2}{I_0}\right)$

$$\therefore L_1-L_2=10\log\left(\frac{I_1}{I_0}\right)-10\log\left(\frac{I_2}{I_0}\right)$$

or, $\Delta L=10\log\left(\frac{I_1}{I_0}\times\frac{I_0}{I_2}\right)$ or, $\Delta L=10\log\left(\frac{I_1}{I_2}\right)$

or, $20=10\log\left(\frac{I_1}{I_2}\right)$ or, $2=\log\left(\frac{I_1}{I_2}\right)$

or, $\frac{I_1}{I_2}=10^2$ or, $I_2=\frac{I_1}{100}$.

⇒ Intensity decreases by a factor 100.

28. (a) $y(x,t)=0.005\cos(\alpha x-\beta t)$ (Given)
Comparing it with the standard equation of wave
$y(x,t)=a\cos(kx-\omega t)$ we get
$k=\alpha$ and $\omega=\beta$

But $k=\frac{2\pi}{\lambda}$ and $\omega=\frac{2\pi}{T}$

$\Rightarrow \frac{2\pi}{\lambda}=\alpha$ and $\frac{2\pi}{T}=\beta$

Given that $\lambda=0.08$ m and $T=2.0$s

$\therefore \alpha=\frac{2\pi}{0.08}=25\pi$ and $\beta=\frac{2\pi}{2}=\pi$

29. (b) Equation is of stationary wave. Comparing with the standard equation

$$y=2A\sin\left(\frac{2\pi}{T}\right)t\cos\left(\frac{2\pi}{\lambda}\right)x$$

$$\frac{2\pi}{\lambda}=4.5 \text{ or } \lambda=\frac{2\pi}{4.5}=1.4\text{m}$$

30. (b) Waves are kind of disturbances which moves from one place to another without the actual physical transfer of matter of the medium as a whole. The particles of the medium only oscillate but do not travel from one place to another.
Waves transport energy and the pattern of disturbance has information that propagate from one point to another. Here, wave pattern propagates.
All our communication essentially depend on transmission of signals through the waves.

31. (b) $\frac{v}{4\ell_1}=\frac{3v}{2\ell_2}$, $\therefore \frac{\ell_1}{\ell_2}=\frac{1}{6}$

32. (c) $\omega_1=600\pi, \omega_2=604\pi,$
$f_1=300$ Hz, $f_2=302$ Hz
Beat frequency, $f_2-f_1=2$ Hz
⇒ number of beats in three seconds = 6

33. (b) Given $f_A=1800$Hz
$v_t=v$
$f_B=2150$ Hz

Reflected wave frequency received by A, $f_A'=?$
Applying doppler's effect of sound,

$$f'=\frac{v_s f}{v_s-v_t}$$

here, $v_t=v_s\left(1-\frac{f_A}{f_B}\right)$

$$=343\left(1-\frac{1800}{2150}\right)$$

$v_t=55.8372$ m/s

Now, for the reflected wave,

$$\therefore \quad f_A' = \left(\frac{v_s + v_t}{v_s - v_t}\right) f_A$$

$$= \left(\frac{343+55.83}{343-55.83}\right) \times 1800$$

$= 2499.44 \approx 2500\text{Hz}$

34. (a) Standing waves are produced when two waves propagate in opposite direction

As z_1 & z_2 are propagating in +ve x-axis & –ve x-axis

so, $z_1 + z_2$ will represent a standing wave.

35. (d) Load supported by sonometer wire = 4 kg

Tension in sonometer wire = 4 g

If μ = mass per unit length

then frequency $\upsilon = \frac{1}{2l}\sqrt{\frac{T}{\mu}}$

$$\Rightarrow \quad 416 = \frac{1}{2l}\sqrt{\frac{4g}{\mu}}$$

When length is doubled, i.e., $l' = 2l$

Let new load = L

As, $\upsilon' = \upsilon$

$$\therefore \quad \frac{1}{2l'}\sqrt{\frac{Lg}{\mu}} = \frac{1}{2l}\sqrt{\frac{4g}{\mu}}$$

$$\Rightarrow \quad \frac{1}{4l}\sqrt{\frac{Lg}{\mu}} = \frac{1}{2l}\sqrt{\frac{4g}{\mu}}$$

$\Rightarrow \sqrt{L} = 2 \times 2 \Rightarrow L = 16\,\text{kg}$

36. (b) Let the string vibrates in p loops, wavelength of the pth mode of vibration is given by

$$\lambda_p = \frac{2l}{p}$$

Given, $y = 2\sin\left(\frac{4\pi x}{15}\right)\cos(96\pi t)$

or $y = 2\left[\sin\left(\frac{4\pi x}{15} + 96\pi t\right) + \sin\left(\frac{4\pi x}{15} - 96\pi t\right)\right.$

Comparing it with standard equation, we get

$$\upsilon = \frac{96\pi}{2\pi} = 48 \text{ Hz and } k = \frac{4\pi}{15}$$

$$\frac{1}{48} = \frac{2\times 60}{p} \times \frac{4\pi}{15 \times 96\pi}$$

$\Rightarrow p = 16.$

37. (b) [Figure: string vibrating in three segments labelled l_1, l_2, l_3]

$$n = \frac{1}{2l}\sqrt{\frac{T}{m}}$$

or, $n \propto \frac{1}{l}$ or nl = constant, K

$\therefore n_1 l_1 = K,$

$n_2 l_2 = K, n_3 l_3 = K$

Also, $l = l_1 + l_2 + l_3$

or, $\frac{K}{n} = \frac{K}{n_1} + \frac{K}{n_2} + \frac{K}{n_3}$

or, $\frac{1}{n} = \frac{1}{n_1} + \frac{1}{n_2} + \frac{1}{n_3}$

38. (a) Time taken for two syllables $t = \frac{2}{5}$ sec.

$x + x = v \times t = 330 \times \frac{2}{5} \qquad \therefore x = 66\,\text{m}$

39. (a) Velocity of sound = $\sqrt{\frac{\gamma RT}{M}}$

When water vapour are represent in air average molecular weight of air decreases and hence velocity increases.

40. (b) $\frac{I_{max}}{I_{min}} = \frac{(a+b)^2}{(a-b)^2} = 49 \qquad \therefore \frac{a+b}{a-b} = 7$

$7a - 7b = a + b$ or $6a = 8b$ or $\frac{a}{b} = \frac{8}{6} = \frac{4}{3}$

41. (a) By the concept of accoustic, the observer and source are moving towards each other, each with a velocity of 18 m s^{-1}.

$$\therefore v' = \frac{330+18}{330-18} \times 1000 \approx 1115 \text{ Hz}$$

42. (c) Compare the given equation with standard form

$$y = r\sin\left[\frac{2\pi x}{\lambda} - \frac{2\pi t}{T}\right]$$

$$\frac{2\pi}{\lambda} = 3, \lambda = \frac{2\pi}{3} \text{ and } \frac{2\pi}{T} = 15$$

$$T = \frac{2\pi}{15}$$

Speed of propagation, $v = \frac{\lambda}{T} = \frac{2\pi/3}{2\pi/15} = 5$

43. (c) The contrast will be maximum, when $I_1 = I_2$ i.e. a = b. In that event, $I_{min} = (a-b)^2 = 0$, where a and b are the amplitudes of interfering waves.

44. (b) Fundamental frequency of closed organ pipe

$$V_c = \frac{V}{4l_c}$$

Fundamental frequency of open organ pipe

$$V_0 = \frac{V}{2l_0}$$

Second overtone frequency of open organ pipe $= \dfrac{3V}{2l_0}$

From question,

$$\frac{V}{4l_c} = \frac{3V}{2l_0}$$

$\Rightarrow \quad l_0 = 6l_c = 6 \times 20 = 120$ cm

45. **(b)** $y = 60\cos(180t - 6x)$ ....(1)

$\omega = 180, k = 6 \Rightarrow \dfrac{2\pi}{\lambda} = 6$

$$v = \frac{\omega}{k} = \frac{2\pi}{T} \times \frac{\lambda}{2\pi} = \frac{180}{6} = 30 \text{ m/s}$$

Differentiating (1) w.r.t. t,

$$v = \frac{dy}{dt} = -60 \times 180 \sin(180t - 6x)$$

$v_{max} = 60 \times 180$ μm/s

$= 10800$ μm/s $= 0.0108$ m/s

$$\frac{v_{max}}{v} = \frac{0.0108}{30} = 3.6 \times 10^{-4}$$

Speed Test-15

1. (a) Electric field intensity at the centre of the disc.

$E = \frac{\sigma}{2 \epsilon_0}$ (given)

Electric field along the axis at any distance x from the centre of the disc

$$E' = \frac{\sigma}{2 \epsilon_0}\left(1 - \frac{x}{\sqrt{x^2 + R^2}}\right)$$

From question, x = R (radius of disc)

$$\therefore E' = \frac{\sigma}{2 \epsilon_0}\left(1 - \frac{R}{\sqrt{R^2 + R^2}}\right)$$

$$= \frac{\sigma}{2 \epsilon_0}\left(\frac{\sqrt{2}R - R}{\sqrt{2}R}\right)$$

$$= \frac{4}{14}E$$

$\therefore$ % reduction in the value of electric field

$$= \frac{\left(E - \frac{4}{14}E\right) \times 100}{E} = \frac{1000}{14}\% \simeq 70.7\%$$

2. (a) Surface charge density $(\sigma) = \frac{\text{Charge}}{\text{Surface area}}$

So $\sigma_{inner} = \frac{-2Q}{4\pi b^2}$

and $\sigma_{Outer} = \frac{Q}{4\pi c^2}$

– Q + 2Q = Q

–2Q

a b c

+2Q

3. (a) Initial force between the two spheres carrying charge (say q) is

$F = \frac{1}{4\pi\varepsilon_0}\frac{q^2}{r^2}$ (r is the distance between them)

Further when an uncharged sphere is kept in touch with the sphere of charge q, the net charge on both become $\frac{q+0}{2} = \frac{q}{2}$. Force on the 3rd charge, when placed in center of the 1st two

r / 2 r / 2

B C A

q q / 2 q / 2

$$F_3 = \frac{1}{4\pi\varepsilon_0}\frac{q\left(\frac{q}{2}\right)}{\left(\frac{r}{2}\right)^2} - \frac{1}{4\pi\varepsilon_0}\frac{\left(\frac{q}{2}\right)^2}{\left(\frac{r}{2}\right)^2}$$

$$= \frac{1}{4\pi\varepsilon_0}\frac{q^2}{r^2}[2 - 1] = F$$

4. (d) Since electric field $\vec{E}$ decreases inside water, therefore flux $\phi = \vec{E}.\vec{A}$ also decreases.

5. (d) Unit positive charge at O will be repelled equally by three charges at the three corners of triangle. By symmetry, resultant $\vec{E}$ at O would be zero.

6. (c) When a dipole is placed in a uniform electric field, two equal and opposite forces act on it. Therefore, a torque acts which rotates the dipole.

7. (d) Force acting on the charged particle due to electric field = $q\vec{E}$

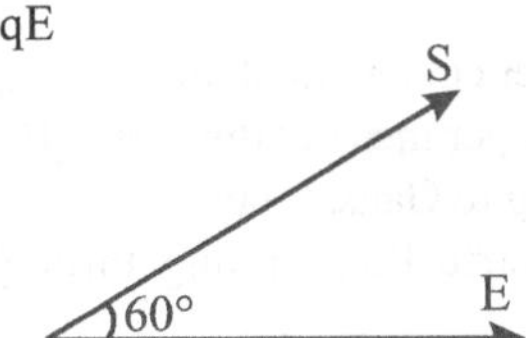

work done in moving through distance S,

$$W = q\vec{E}.\vec{S} = (qE) \times S \times \cos\theta$$

$$\therefore 10\,J = (0.5\,C) \times E \times 2\cos 60°$$

$$E = 10 \times 2 = 20\,NC^{-1} = 20\,Vm^{-1}$$

8. (c) The charged sphere is a conductor. Therefore the field inside is zero and outside it is proportional to $1/r^2$

9. (d) Since $\phi_{total} = \phi_A + \phi_B + \phi_C = \frac{q}{\varepsilon_0}$,

where q is the total charge.

As shown in the figure, flux associated with the curved surface B is $\phi = \phi_B$

Let us assume flux linked with the plane surfaces A and C be

$\phi_A = \phi_C = \phi'$

Therefore,

$$\frac{q}{\varepsilon_0} = 2\phi' + \phi_B = 2\phi' + \phi$$

$$\Rightarrow \phi' = \frac{1}{2}\left(\frac{q}{\varepsilon_0} - \phi\right)$$

10. (b) We have $E_a = \frac{2kp}{r^3}$ and $E_e = \frac{kp}{r^3}$; $\therefore E_a = 2E_e$

11. (c) Electric lines of force due to a positive charge is spherically symmetric.

All the charges are positive and equal in magnitude. So repulsion takes place. Due to which no lines of force are present inside the equilateral triangle and the resulting lines of force obtained as shown:

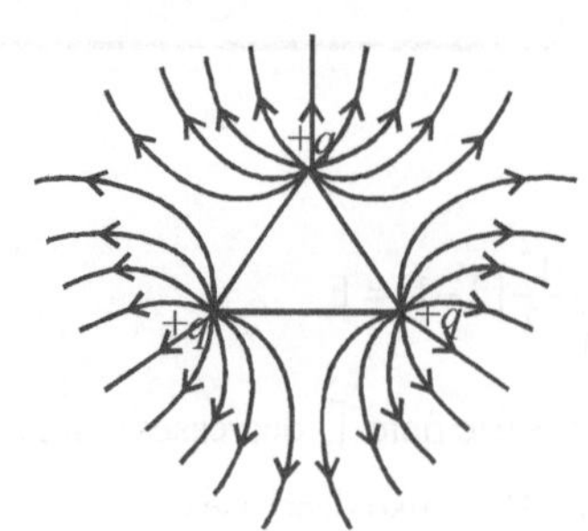

12. (a) ←a→←a→ Q_1 Q_2 Q_3

$Q_2 = -Q_3 = Q$

Force on Q_3 due to Q_2 + Force on Q_3 due to $Q_1 = 0$.

$$\frac{1}{4\pi\epsilon_0}\left(\frac{-Q^2}{a^2}\right)+\frac{1}{4\pi\epsilon_0}\frac{Q_1 Q}{4a^2}=0 \Rightarrow Q_1 = 4Q_3$$

13. (b) Charge per cm length of the wire = qC

$\therefore$ Charge per metre of the wire = 100q C

According to Gauss's law,

Total electric flux passing through the cylindrical surface

$$\phi = \frac{q_{enclosed}}{\varepsilon_0} = \frac{100q}{\varepsilon_0}$$

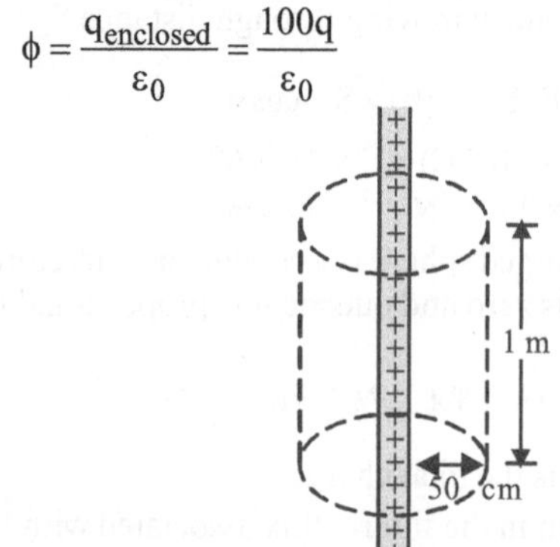

14. (c) $T_0 = 2\pi\sqrt{\frac{L}{g}}$

When the plates are charged, the net acceleration is, $g' = g + a$

$$g' = g + \frac{qE}{m} \qquad \left(a = \frac{qE}{m}\right)$$

$$\therefore \quad T = 2\pi\sqrt{\frac{L}{g+\frac{qE}{m}}}$$

$$\therefore \quad \frac{T}{T_0} = \left(\frac{g}{g+\frac{qE}{m}}\right)^{1/2}$$

15. (c) Charges (q) = 2×10^{-6} C, Distance (d) = 3 cm = 3×10^{-2} m and electric field (E) = 2×10^5 N/C. Torque (τ) = q.d.

E = $(2 \times 10^{-6}) \times (3 \times 10^{-2}) \times (2 \times 10^5)$

= 12×10^{-3} N–m.

16. (b) Net flux emmited from a spherical surface of radius a according to Gauss's theorem

$$\phi_{net} = \frac{q_{in}}{\varepsilon_0}$$

or, $(Aa)(4\pi a^2) = \frac{q_{in}}{\varepsilon_0}$

So, $q_{in} = 4\pi\varepsilon_0 A a^3$

17. (a) Since lines of force starts from A and ends at B, so A is +ve and B is –ve. Lines of forces are more crowded near A, so A > B.

18. (c) Net force on each of the charge due to the other charges is zero. However, disturbance in any direction other than along the line on which the charges lie, will not make the charges return.

19. (c)

20. (d) For distances far away from centre of dipole

$$E_{axis} = E_a = \frac{1}{4\pi\varepsilon_0}\frac{2p}{r^3}$$

$$E_{equa} = E_e = \frac{1}{4\pi\varepsilon_0}-\frac{p}{r^3}$$

$$\frac{d}{dr}(E_a) = \frac{1}{4\pi\varepsilon_0}2p\frac{d}{dr}(r^{-3})$$

$$= -6\cdot\frac{1}{4\pi\varepsilon_0}\frac{p}{r^4} \qquad \text{...(i)}$$

$$\frac{d}{dr}(E_e) = \frac{1}{4\pi\varepsilon_0}p\frac{d}{dr}(r^{-3})$$

$$= -3\frac{1}{4\pi\varepsilon_0}\frac{p}{r^4} \qquad \text{...(ii)}$$

From equation (i) and (ii) the magnitude of change in electric field w.r.t. distance is more in case of axis of dipole as compared to equatorial plane.

21. (b) 2*q* at *P*, *q* at *A*, –3*q* at *B*; ←ℓ→←*d*→

Let a charge 2*q* be placed at *P*, at a distance *l* from A where charge *q* is placed, as shown in figure. The charge 2*q* will not experience any force, when force, when force of repulsion on it due to *q* is balanced by force of attraction on it due to –3*q* at *B* where AB = *d*

$$\text{or} \quad \frac{(2q)(q)}{4\pi\varepsilon_0\ell^2} = \frac{(2q)(-3q)}{4\pi\varepsilon_0(\ell+d)^2}$$

$$(\ell + d)^2 = 3\ell^2$$

$$\text{or} \quad 2\ell^2 - 2\ell d - d^2 = 0$$

$$\therefore \quad \ell = \frac{2d \pm \sqrt{4d^2+2d^2}}{4} = \frac{d}{2} \pm \frac{\sqrt{3}d}{2}$$

$$\ell = \frac{d+\sqrt{3}d}{2}$$

22. (d) Let F be the force between Q and Q. The force between q and Q should be attractive for net force on Q to be zero. Let F' be the force between Q and q. The resultant of F' and F' is R. For equilibrium

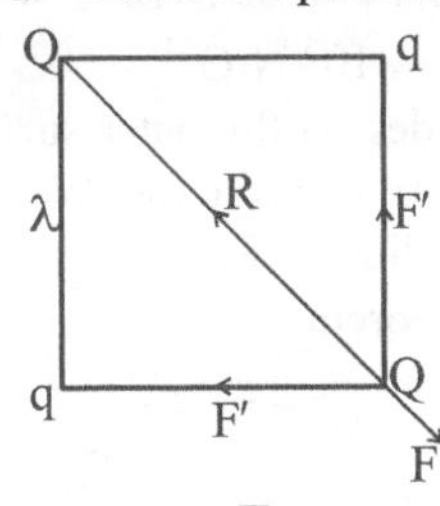

$\vec{R}+\vec{F}=0 \qquad \sqrt{2}F'=-F$

$$\sqrt{2}\times k\frac{Qq}{\ell^2}=-k\frac{Q^2}{(\sqrt{2}\ell)^2} \Rightarrow \frac{Q}{q}=-2\sqrt{2}$$

23. (b) Nuclear force binds the protons and neutrons in the nucleus of an atom.

24. (c) Net downward force on the drop $=\frac{4}{3}\pi r^3(\rho-\rho_0)g$

For equilibrium, electric force must be upwards i.e. charge on the drop is positive.

$$neE=\frac{4}{3}\pi r^3(\rho-\rho_0)g \text{ i.e. } n=\frac{4\pi r^3(\rho-\rho_0)g}{3eE}$$

25. (d) Electric flux, $\phi=EA\cos\theta$,

where θ = angle between E and normal to the surface.

Here $\theta=\frac{\pi}{2}$

$\Rightarrow \phi=0$

26. (a) Potential energy of an electric dipole in an electric field is, $U=-\vec{p}.\vec{E}$ i.e. $U=-pE\cos\theta$

For minimum U, $\theta=0°$

$\Rightarrow U_{min}=-pE\cos 0=-pE$

27. (c) Milikan demonstrated the quantisation of charge experimentally. Charge on electron $=-e=-1.6\times10^{-19}$ C. Addition of charge can occur in integral multiples of e.

28. (c) Let n be the number of electrons missing.

$$F=\frac{1}{4\pi\varepsilon_0}\cdot\frac{q^2}{d^2}$$

$$\Rightarrow q=\sqrt{4\pi\varepsilon_0 d^2F}=ne$$

$$\therefore n=\sqrt{\frac{4\pi\varepsilon_0 Fd^2}{e^2}}$$

29. (b) $F=\frac{1}{4\pi\varepsilon_0}\frac{(4q)(-4q)}{r^2}$

when C is touched with A, then charge on A & C each = 2q after that C is touched with B, charge on

$$B=\frac{2q+(-4q)}{2}=-q$$

Now, force $F'=\frac{1}{4\pi\varepsilon_0}\frac{(2q)(-q)}{r^2}\Rightarrow F'=\frac{F}{8}$

30. (a) $-eE=mg$

$$\vec{E}=-\frac{9.1\times10^{-31}\times10}{1.6\times10^{-19}}=-5.6\times10^{-11}\text{N/C}$$

31. (d) Torque, $\vec{\tau}=\vec{p}\times\vec{E}=pE\sin\theta$

$4=p\times2\times10^5\times\sin 30°$

or, $p=\frac{4}{2\times10^5\times\sin 30°}=4\times10^{-5}$ Cm

Dipole moment, $p=q\times l$

$$q=\frac{p}{l}=\frac{4\times10^{-5}}{0.02}=2\times10^{-3}\text{C}=2\text{mC}$$

32. (c) K.E. = Force × distance = qE.y

33. (d) Charge (q) = 0.2 C; Distance (d) = 2 m; Angle $\theta=60°$ and Work done (W) = 4J.

Work done in moving the charge (W)

$=F.d\cos\theta=qEd\cos\theta$

or, $E=\frac{W}{qd\cos\theta}=\frac{4}{0.2\times2\times\cos 60°}=\frac{4}{0.4\times0.5}=20$ N/C.

34. (a) $\phi=\vec{E}.\vec{A}=4\hat{i}.(2\hat{i}+3\hat{j})=8$ V-m

35. (d) The dipole is placed in a non-uniform field, therefore a force as well as a couple acts on it. The force on the negative charge is more ($F\propto E$) and is directed along negative x-axis. Thus the dipole moves along negative x-axis and rotates in an anticlockwise direction.

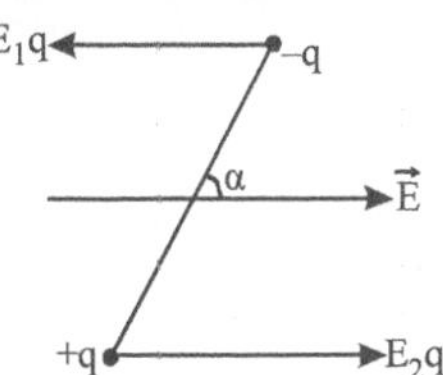

36. (b) Flux $=\vec{E}.\vec{A}$.

$\vec{E}$ is electric field vector & $\vec{A}$ is area vector.

Here, angle between $\vec{E}$ & $\vec{A}$ is 90°.

So, $\vec{E}.\vec{A}=0$; Flux = 0

37. (c) The charge on disc A is 10^{-6} μC. The charge on disc B is 10×10^{-6} μC. The total charge on both = 11 μC. When touched, this charge will be distributed equally i.e. 5.5 μC on each disc.

38. (a) According to Gauss's law total electric flux through a closed surface is $\frac{1}{\varepsilon_0}$ times the total charge inside that surface.

Electric flux, $\phi_E=\frac{q}{\varepsilon_0}$

Charge on α-particle = 2e

$$\phi_E = \frac{2e}{\varepsilon_0}$$

39. (b) It is possible to create or destroy charged particles but it is not possible to create or destroy net charge. The charge of an isolated system is conserved.

40. (a) The flux is zero according to Gauss' Law because it is a open surface which enclosed a charge q.

41. (d) By Gauss law, we know that

$\phi = \frac{q}{\varepsilon_0}$ Here, Net electric flux, $\phi = \phi_2 - \phi_1$

$$= 9 \times 10^6 - 6 \times 10^6 = \frac{q}{\varepsilon_0} \Rightarrow q = 3 \times 10^6 \times \varepsilon_0.$$

42. (d) They will not experience any force if $|\vec{F}_G| = |\vec{F}_e|$

$$\Rightarrow G\frac{m^2}{(16\times10^{-2})^2} = \frac{1}{4\pi\varepsilon_0}\cdot\frac{q^2}{(16\times10^{-2})^2} \Rightarrow \frac{q}{m} = \sqrt{4\pi\varepsilon_0 G}$$

43. (c) Here, $\ell = 2.4\ m$, $r = 4.6\ mm = 4.6 \times 10^{-3}\ m$

$q = -4.2 \times 10^{-7}$ C

Linear charge density, $\lambda = \frac{q}{\ell}$

$$= \frac{-4.2\times10^{-7}}{2.4} = -1.75\times10^{-7}\ \text{C m}^{-1}$$

Electric field, $E = \frac{\lambda}{2\pi\varepsilon_0 r}$

$$= \frac{-1.75\times10^{-7}}{2\times3.14\times8.854\times10^{-12}\times4.6\times10^{-3}}$$

$= -6.7 \times 10^5$ N C^{-1}

44. (a) Charge resides on the outer surface of a conducting hollow sphere of radius R. We consider a spherical surface of radius r < R.

By Gauss theorem

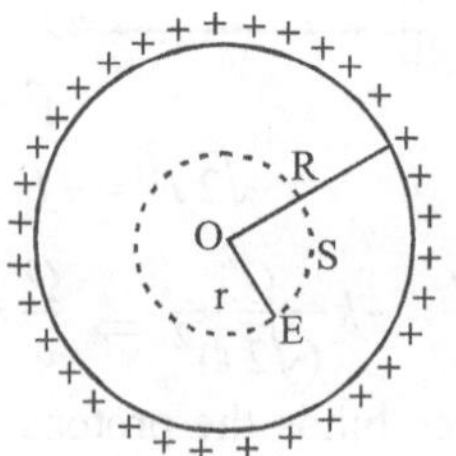

$$\int_S \vec{E}.\vec{ds} = \frac{1}{\varepsilon_0} \times \text{charge enclosed or } E \times 4\pi r^2 = \frac{1}{\varepsilon_0} \times 0$$

$\Rightarrow E = 0$

i.e electric field inside a hollow sphere is zero.

45. (c) By Gauss's theorem, $\phi = \frac{Q_{in}}{\epsilon_0}$

Thus, the net flux depends only on the charge enclosed by the surface. Hence, there will be no effect on the net flux if the radius of the surface is doubled.

Speed Test-16

1. (d) As volume remains constant, therefore,

$$\frac{4}{3}\pi R^3 = n \times \frac{4}{3}\pi r^3 \quad \therefore \quad R = n^{1/3} r.$$

New potential $= V' = \frac{nq}{4\pi\varepsilon_0 R} = \frac{nq}{4\pi\varepsilon_0 (n^{1/3} r)}$

$$= n^{2/3}\frac{q}{4\pi\varepsilon_0 r} = n^{2/3} V.$$

2. (a) $C_a = \frac{\epsilon_0 A}{d}$ and $C_b = \frac{\epsilon_0 A}{\frac{d}{2}+\frac{d}{2K}} = \frac{2\epsilon_0 A(1+K)}{d}$

and $C_c = \frac{\epsilon_0 \frac{A}{2}}{d} + \frac{\epsilon_0 \frac{A}{2}K}{d} = \frac{\epsilon_0 A}{2d}(1+K)$

or $C_b = \frac{\epsilon_0 A}{d} 2(1+K) > C_a$

or $C_c = \frac{\epsilon_0 A}{d}\frac{1+K}{2} > C_a \quad \therefore C_b$ and $C_c > C_a$

3. (c) Charges reside only on the outer surface of a conductor with cavity.

4. (b) In oil, C becomes twice, V becomes half. Therefore, $E = V/d$ becomes half.

5. (d)

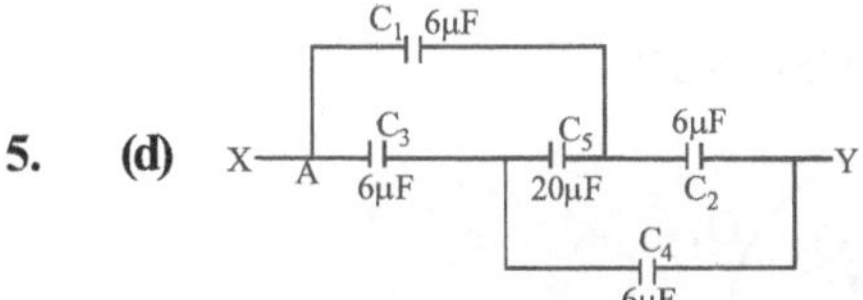

Equivalent circuit

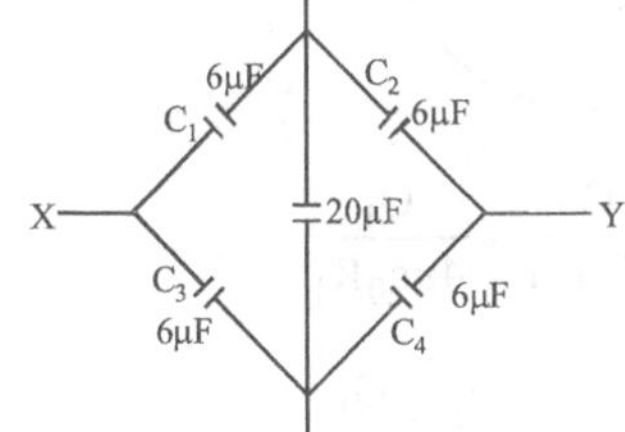

Here, $\frac{C_1}{C_3} = \frac{C_2}{C_4}$

Hence, no charge will flow through 20μF

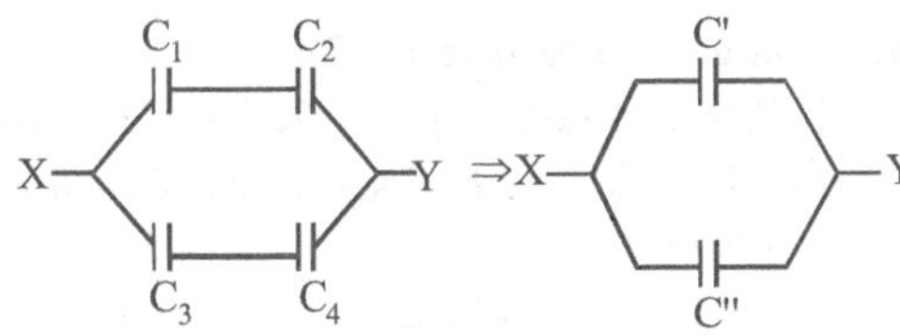

C_1 and C_2 are in series, also C_3 and C_4 are in series.

Hence, $C' = 3\ \mu F$, $C'' = 3\ \mu F$

C' and C'' are in parallel.

Hence net capacitance $= C' + C'' = 3 + 3 = 6\ \mu F$

6. (c)

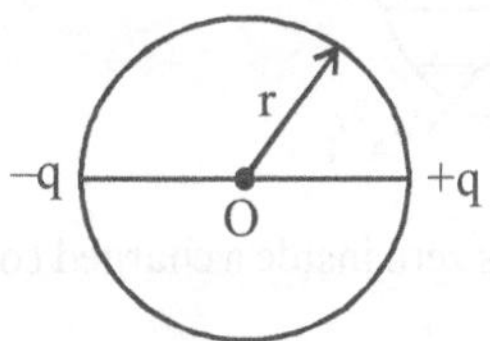

$$\frac{mv^2}{r} = \frac{kq^2}{(2r)^2}\ ;\ mv^2 = \frac{kq^2}{4r}$$

Kinetic energy of each particle

$$= \frac{1}{2}mv^2 = \frac{kq^2}{8r}$$

7. (b) It consists of two capacitors in parallel, therefore, the total capacitance is $= \frac{2\epsilon_0 A}{d}$

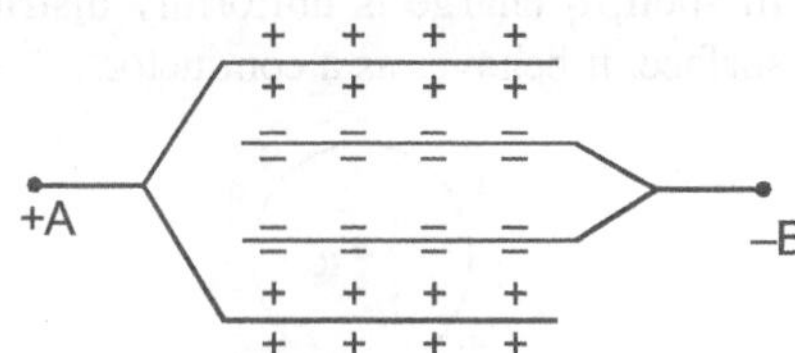

(The plates of B, having negative charge do not constitute a capacitor).

8. (a) The potential energy of a charged capacitor is given by $U = \frac{Q^2}{2C}$.

If a dielectric slab is inserted between the plates, the energy is given by $\frac{Q^2}{2KC}$, where K is the dielectric constant.

Again, when the dielectric slab is removed slowly its energy increases to initial potential energy. Thus, work done is zero.

9. (a) As $x = t\left(1-\frac{1}{K}\right)$, where x is the addition distance of plate, to restore the capacity of original value.

$$\therefore \quad 3.5\times10^{-5} = 4\times10^{-5}\left(1-\frac{1}{K}\right).$$

Solving, we get, $K = 8$.

10. (b) At. equipotential surface, the potential is same at any point i.e., $V_A = V_B$ as shown in figure. Hence no work is required to move unit change from one point to another i.e.,

$$V_A - V_B = \frac{W}{\text{unit charge}} = 0 \Rightarrow W = 0$$

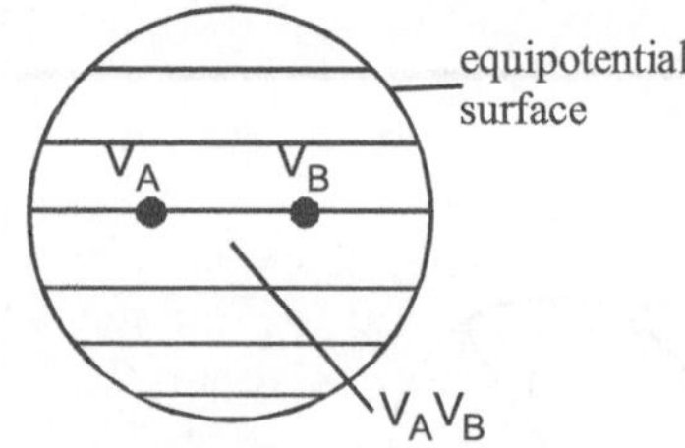

11. **(b)**
(i) Electrostatic field is zero inside a charged conductor or neutral conductor.
(ii) Electrostatic field at the surface of a charged conductor must be normal to the surface at every point.
(iii) There is no net charge at any point inside the conductor and any excess charge must reside at the surface.
(iv) Electrostatic potential is constant throughout the volume of the conductor and has the same value (as insde) on its surface.
(v) Electric field at the surface of a charged conductor is

$$\vec{E} = \frac{\sigma}{\varepsilon_0}\hat{n}$$

12. **(b)** In shell, q charge is uniformly distributed over its surface, it behaves as a conductor.

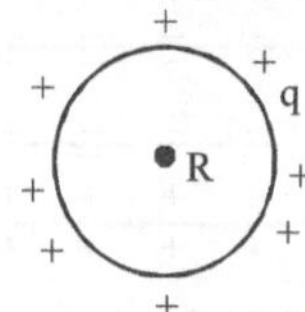

V= potential at surface $= \frac{q}{4\pi\varepsilon_0 R}$ and inside

$$V = \frac{q}{4\pi\varepsilon_0 R}$$

Because of this it behaves as an equipotential surface.

13. **(c)** Volume of big drop = 1000 × volume of each small drop

$$\frac{4}{3}\pi R^3 = 1000 \times \frac{4}{3}\pi r^3 \Rightarrow R = 10r$$

$$\because \quad V = \frac{kq}{r} \text{ and } V' = \frac{kq}{R} \times 1000$$

Total charge on one small droplet is q and on the big drop is 1000q.

$$\Rightarrow \frac{V'}{V} = \frac{1000r}{R} = \frac{1000}{10} = 100$$

$$\therefore \quad V' = 100V$$

14. **(c)** In a round trip, displacement is zero. Hence, work done is zero.

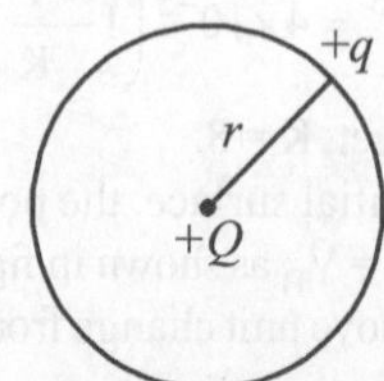

15. **(b)** The two capacitors are in parallel so

$$C = \frac{\varepsilon_0 A}{t \times 2}(k_1 + k_2)$$

16. **(d)** In equilibrium, $F = qE = (ne)\frac{V}{d} = mg$

$$n = \frac{mgd}{eV} = \frac{1.96 \times 10^{-15} \times 9.8 \times 0.02}{1.6 \times 10^{-19} \times 800} = 3$$

17. **(a)** $E = \frac{1}{2}CV^2 = \frac{1}{2} \times 1 \times 10^{-6} \times (4000)^2 = 8\,J.$

18. **(d)** As we know,

$$\text{Common potential} = \frac{\text{Total charge}}{\text{Total capacity}}$$

$Q_1 = C_0 V_1, Q_2 = 0$, therefore

$$V_2 = \frac{C_0 V_1 + 0}{C_0 + kC_0} = \frac{V_1}{1+k}$$

$$1 + k = \frac{V_1}{V_2} \text{ or } k = \frac{V_1}{V_2} - 1 = \frac{V_1 - V_2}{V_2}$$

19. **(b)** Potential difference across the branch de is 6 V. Net capacitance of de branch is 2.1 μF

So, $q = CV$

$\Rightarrow q = 2.1 \times 6\,\mu C$

$\Rightarrow q = 12.6\,\mu C$

Potential across 3 μF capacitance is

$$V = \frac{12.6}{3} = 4.2 \text{ volt}$$

Potential across 2 and 5 combination in parallel is $6 - 4.2 = 1.8\,V$

So, $q' = (1.8)(5) = 9\,\mu C$

20. **(c)**

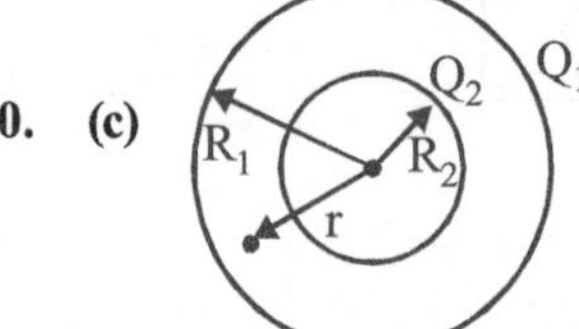

$$V_r = \frac{Q_2}{4\pi\varepsilon_0 r} + \frac{Q_1}{4\pi\varepsilon_0 R_1}$$

$$V_r = \frac{1}{4\pi\varepsilon_0}\left(\frac{Q_2}{r} + \frac{Q_1}{R_1}\right)$$

21. **(d)** $U = \frac{1}{2}QV$ = Area of triangle OAB

22. **(b)** Charge on α particle, q = 2 e.

K.E. = work done = $q \times V = 2e \times 10^6 V = 2$ MeV.

23. **(a)** Let the side length of square be '*a*' then potential at centre *O* is

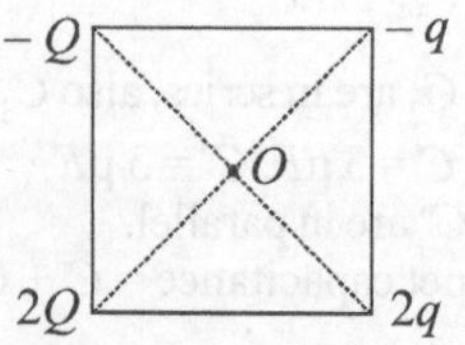

$$V=\frac{k(-Q)}{\left(\frac{a}{\sqrt{2}}\right)}+\frac{k(-q)}{\frac{a}{\sqrt{2}}}+\frac{k(2q)}{\frac{a}{\sqrt{2}}}+\frac{k(2Q)}{\frac{a}{\sqrt{2}}}=0$$

(Given)

$$=-Q-q+2q+2Q=0=Q+q=0$$
$$=Q=-q$$

24. (b) $C_0=\frac{k\epsilon_0 A}{d}$

$$C=\frac{k\epsilon_0 2}{3d}+\frac{2k\epsilon_0 A}{3d}=\frac{4}{3}\frac{k\epsilon_0 A}{d}$$

$$\therefore \frac{C}{C_0}=\frac{\frac{4}{3}\frac{k\epsilon_0 A}{d}}{\frac{k\epsilon_0 A}{d}}=\frac{4}{3}$$

25. (b) Work done = Change in energy

$$=\frac{1}{2}\left(C+\frac{C}{2}\right)V^2=\frac{1}{2}\left(\frac{3C}{2}\right)V^2=\frac{3CV^2}{4}$$

26. (a) Potential at B, V_B is maximum

$$V_B>V_C>V_A$$

As in the direction of electric field potential decreases.

27. (a) The equivalent circuit diagram as shown in the figure.

The equivalent capacitance between A and B is

$$C_{eq}=\frac{2\mu F\times 3\mu F}{2\mu F+3\mu F}+2\mu F=\frac{16}{5}\mu F$$

Total charge of the given circuit is

$$Q=\frac{16}{5}\mu F\times 5V=16\mu C$$

$$Q_1=(2\mu F)\times 5V=10\mu C$$

$\therefore$ $Q_2=Q-Q_1=16\,\mu C-10\,\mu C=6\,\mu C$

$\therefore$ Voltage between B and C is

$$V_{BC}=\frac{Q_2}{3\mu F}=\frac{6\mu C}{3\mu F}=2V$$

28. (d) Electric field

$$E=\frac{\sigma}{\varepsilon}=\frac{Q}{A\varepsilon}$$

ε of kerosine oil is more than that of air.

As ε increases, E decreases.

29. (c) When a battery across the plates of capacitor is disconnected and dielectric slab is placed in between the plates, then

(i) capacity C increases

(ii) charge q remains unchanged

(iii) potential V decreases

(iv) energy E decreases

30. (b) Electric lines of force are always perpendicular to an equipotential surface.

31. (c) All the charge given to inner sphere will pass on to the outer one. So capacitance that of outer one is $4\pi\epsilon_0 b$.

32. (a) In Ist case when capacitor C attached with battery charged with the energy.

U_1= U (stored energy on capacitor).

In IInd case after disconnect of battery similar capacitor is attached in parallel with Ist capacitor then

C_{eq}=C'=2C.

$$\text{Now, }\frac{U_1}{U_2}=\frac{\frac{1}{2}\frac{q^2}{C}}{\frac{1}{2}\frac{q^2}{C'}}=\frac{C'}{C}=\frac{2C}{C}\qquad (\because C'=2C)$$

$$U_2=\frac{U}{2}$$

33. (a) Here we have to findout the shape of equipotential surface, these surface are perpendicular to the field lines, so there must be electric field which can not be without charge.

So, the collection of charges, whose total sum is not zero, with regard to great distance can be considered as a point charge. The equipotentials due to point charge are spherical in shape as electric potential due to point charge q is given by

$$V=K_e\frac{q}{r}$$

This suggest that electric potentials due to point charge is same for all equidistant points. The locus of these equidistant points which are at same potential, form spherical surface.

The lines of field from point charge are radial. So the equipotential surface perpendicular to field lines from a sphere.

34. (c) Equipotential surfaces are normal to the electric field lines. The following figure shows the equipotential surfaces along with electric field lines for a system of two positive charges.

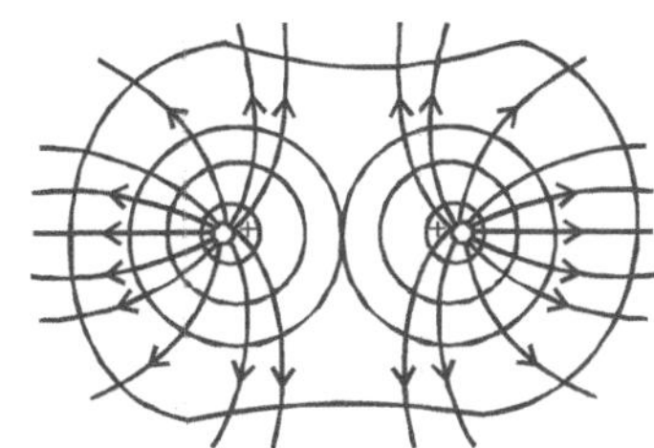

35. (c) Let plate A plate B be carrying charges Q_1 and Q_2 respectively. When they are brought closer, they induce equal and opposite charges on each other i.e. $-Q_2$ on

plate A and $-Q_1$ on plate B. Therefore, net charge on plate A = $Q_1 - Q_2$ and net charge on plate B = $-(Q_1 - Q_2)$, so the charge on the capacitor = $Q_1 - Q_2$.
∴ Potential different between the plates
$$V = \frac{Q_1 - Q_2}{C}$$

36. **(d)** $C = \frac{\epsilon_0 A}{d}$
A → common area, Here $A = A_1$

37. **(a)** The equivalent circuit is shown in figure.
$C_{AB} = 3\mu F$.

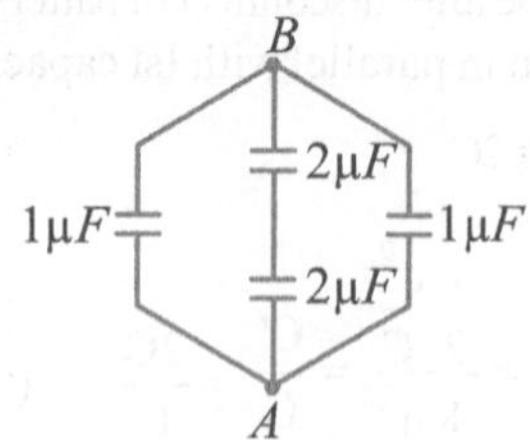

38. **(c)** If we increase the distance between the plates its capacity decreases resulting in higher potential as we know $Q = CV$. Since Q is constant (battery has been disconnected), on decreasing C, V will increase.

39. **(a)** $V = V_1 + V_2 + V_3 = \frac{1}{4\pi \epsilon_0} \cdot \frac{Q}{R} + \frac{1}{4\pi \epsilon_0}\left(\frac{-2Q}{R}\right)$
$$+ \frac{1}{4\pi \epsilon_0}\left(\frac{3Q}{R}\right) = \frac{1}{4\pi \epsilon_0}\left(\frac{2Q}{R}\right)$$

40. **(a)** As we know, $E = -\frac{dV}{dx}$
Potential at the point x = 2m, y = 2m is given by :
$$\int_0^V dV = -\int_0^{2,2} (25dx + 30dy)$$
on solving we get,
V = – 110 volt.

41. **(d)** On the equipotential surface, electric field is normal to the charged surface (where potential exists) so that no work will be done.

42. **(b)**

43. **(b)** Potential at the centre of the triangle,
$$V = \frac{\Sigma q}{4\pi\varepsilon_0 r} = \frac{2q - q - q}{4\pi\varepsilon_0 r} = 0$$
Obviously, $E \neq 0$

44. **(a)** Whenever a charge (+50 nC) is kept inside a hollow metallic spherical shell, it induces an equal and opposite charge on the inner surface and an equal and same type of charges on the outer surface.
∴ Inside, induced charge is – 50 nC and outside, +50 nC – 150 nC already present.

45. **(b)** In parallel, potential is same, say V
$$\frac{Q_1}{Q_2} = \frac{C_1 V}{C_2 V} = \frac{C_1}{C_2}$$

Speed Test-17

1. (b) $V = IR = (neAv_d)\rho\frac{\ell}{A}$

$\therefore \quad \rho = \frac{V}{V_d l n e}$

Here V = potential difference

l = length of wire

n = no. of electrons per unit volume of conductor.

e = no. of electrons

Placing the value of above parameters we get resistivity

$$\rho = \frac{5}{8\times10^{28}\times1.6\times10^{-19}\times2.5\times10^{-4}\times0.1}$$

$= 1.6 \times 10^{-5}\Omega m$

2. (d) From the curve it is clear that slopes at points *A*, *B*, *C*, *D* have following order $A > B > C > D$.

And also resistance at any point equals to slope of the *V-i* curve.

So order of resistance at three points will be

$R_A > R_B > R_C > R_D$

3. (d) From the principle of potentiometer, $V \propto l$

$\Rightarrow \frac{V}{E} = \frac{l}{L}$; where

V = emf of battery, E = emf of standard cell.

L = length of potentiometer wire

$V = \frac{El}{L} = \frac{30E}{100}$

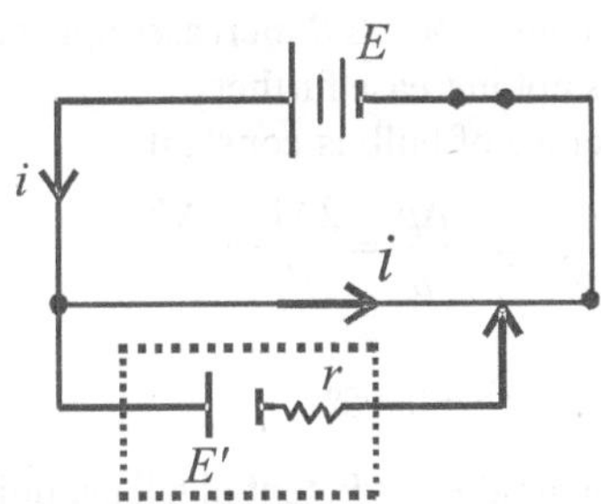

NOTE In this arrangement, the internal resistance of the battery E does not play any role as current is not passing through the battery.

4. (d) $R = \frac{\rho l}{\pi r^2}$. But $m = \pi r^2 ld \therefore \pi r^2 = \frac{m}{ld}$

$\therefore R = \frac{\rho l^2 d}{m}, \; R_1 = \frac{\rho l_1^2 d}{m_1}, \; R_2 = \frac{\rho l_2^2 d}{m_2}$

$R_3 = \frac{\rho l_3^2 d}{m_3}$

$R_1 : R_2 : R_3 = \frac{l_1^2}{m_1} : \frac{l_2^2}{m_2} : \frac{l_3^2}{m_3}$

$R_1 : R_2 : R_3 = \frac{25}{1} : \frac{9}{3} : \frac{1}{5} = 125 : 15 : 1$

5. (c) In series, $R_s = nR$

In parallel, $\frac{1}{R_p} = \frac{1}{R} + \frac{1}{R} + ...n$ terms

$\therefore R_s/R_p = n^2/1 = n^2$

6. (a) Efficiency is given by $\eta = \frac{\text{output}}{\text{input}}$

$= \frac{5\times15\times14}{10\times8\times15} = 0.875$ or 87.5%

7. (b) According to the condition of balancing

$\frac{55}{20} = \frac{R}{80} \Rightarrow R = 220\Omega$

8. (a) $J = \sigma E \Rightarrow J\rho = E$

J is current density, E is electric field

so B = ρ = resistivity.

9. (d) Kirchhoff's first law is based on conservation of charge and Kirchhoff's second law is based on conservation of energy.

10. (c) $R = \frac{\rho\ell}{A}$

When wire is cut into 4 pieces and connected in parallel.

$R_{eff.} = \frac{R}{16} \Rightarrow P_C = 16P$

$P_A : P_B : P_C : P_D = \frac{V^2}{R} : \frac{V^2}{R/4} : \frac{V^2}{R/16} : \frac{V^2}{R/2}$

11. (b) $S = \frac{I_g R}{nI_g - I_g} \Rightarrow S = \frac{I_g}{(n-1)I_g} R$

12. (d) Resistance of a conductor, $R = \frac{m}{ne^2\tau}\frac{l}{A}$

As the temperature increases, the relaxation time τ decreases because the number of collisions of electrons per second increases due to increase in thermal energy of electrons.

13. (b)

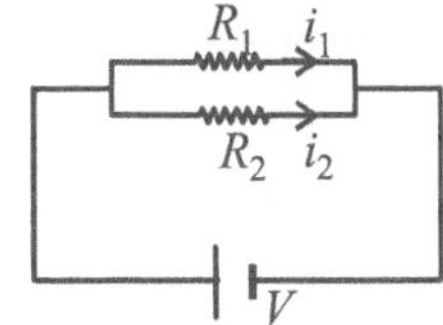

$R_1 = \frac{\rho \ell_1}{\pi r_1^2}$; $R_2 = \frac{\rho \ell_2}{\pi r_2^2}$

$i_1 R_1 = i_2 R_2$ (same potential difference)

$\therefore \frac{i_1}{i_2} = \frac{R_2}{R_1} = \frac{\ell_2}{\ell_1} \times \frac{r_1^2}{r_2^2} = \frac{3}{4} \times \frac{4}{9} = \frac{1}{3}$

14. **(c)** $\frac{R_1}{R_2} = \frac{\ell_1}{\ell_2}$ where $\ell_2 = 100 - \ell_1$

In the first case $\frac{X}{Y} = \frac{20}{80}$

In the second case

$\frac{4X}{Y} = \frac{\ell}{100 - \ell} \Rightarrow \ell = 50$

15. **(c)** Before connecting E, the circuit diagram is

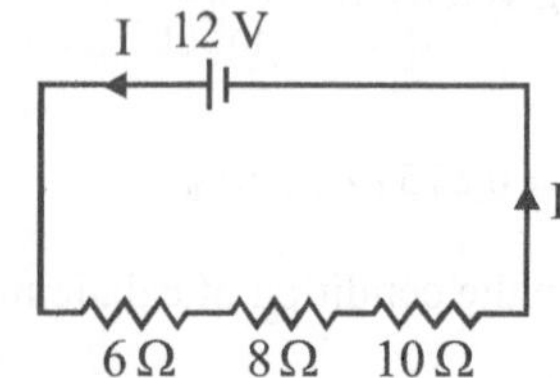

Then, $R_{eq} = 6\,\Omega + 8\,\Omega + 10\,\Omega = 24\,\Omega$

Current in the 8 Ω resistance, $I = \frac{12V}{24\Omega} = \frac{1}{2}A$

After connecting E, the current through 8 Ω is

$I = \frac{1}{2}A$

$\therefore \quad E = \frac{1}{2}A \times 8\Omega = 4V$

16. **(d)** By junction rule at point B

$-I + 1A + 2A = 0$

So, $I = 3A$

By Loop rule,

$-3 \times 2 - 1 \times 1 - E + 12 = 0$

$E = 5V$

17. **(d)** Resistance of bulb $R_b = \frac{(1.5)^2}{4.5} = 0.5\Omega$

Current drawn from battery $= \frac{E}{2.67 + 0.33} = \frac{E}{3}$

Share of bulb $= \frac{2}{3} \times \frac{E}{3} = \frac{2E}{9}$

$\therefore \left(\frac{2E}{9}\right)^2 \times 0.5 = 4.5$ or $E = 13.5$ V.

18. **(d)** The equivalent circuit is given below :

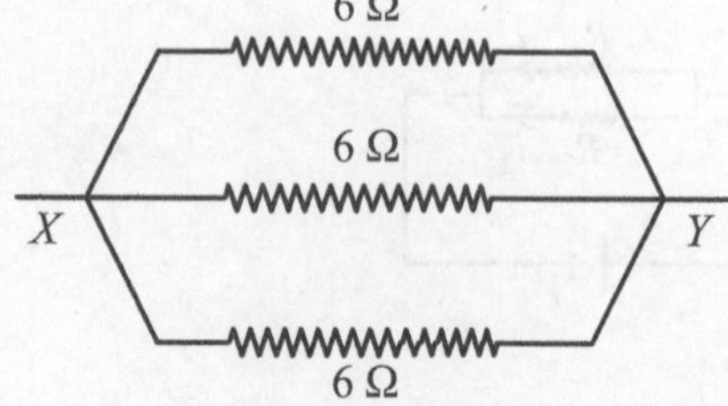

The equivalent resistance is given by

$\frac{1}{R} = \frac{1}{6} + \frac{1}{6} + \frac{1}{6} = \frac{3}{6} = \frac{1}{2}$

$\Rightarrow R_{eq} = 2\Omega$

19. **(a)** Since average drift velocity $= \frac{1}{2}\frac{eE}{m} \times (\tau)$

Now $I = NeA \times$ (avg. drift velocity)

$= \frac{Ne^2AE}{2m\ell} \times \tau = \frac{Ne^2AV}{2m\ell} \times \tau$

$R = \frac{V}{I} = \frac{2m\ell}{Ne^2\tau A}$, where N is electron density.

20. **(c)** The current through the resistance R

$I = \left(\frac{\varepsilon}{R + r}\right)$

The potential difference across R

$V = IR = \left(\frac{\varepsilon}{R + r}\right)R$

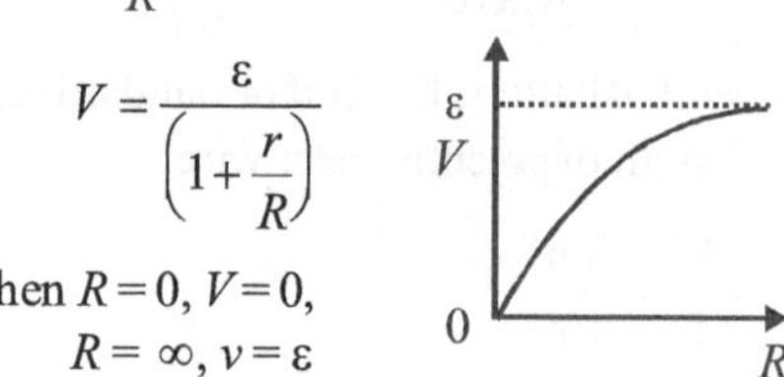

$V = \frac{\varepsilon}{\left(1 + \frac{r}{R}\right)}$

when $R = 0$, $V = 0$,

$R = \infty$, $v = \varepsilon$

Thus V increases as R increases upto certain limit, but it does not increase further.

21. **(c)** Resistance of bulb is constant

$P = \frac{V^2}{R} \Rightarrow \frac{\Delta p}{p} = \frac{2\Delta V}{V} + \frac{\Delta R}{R}$

$\frac{\Delta p}{p} = 2 \times 2.5 + 0 = 5\%$

22. **(a)** Potential gradient = Potential fall per unit length. In this case resistance of unit length.

$R = \frac{\rho l}{A} = \frac{10^{-7} \times 1}{10^{-6}} = 10^{-1}\Omega$

Potential fall across R is

$V = I.R = 0.1 \times 10^{-1} = 0.01$ volt/m.

$= 10^{-2}$ volt / m

23. **(d)** $R_1 + R_2 =$ Constant, R_1 will increase, R_2 will decrease.

$R_1\alpha\Delta T - R\beta\Delta T = 0 \Rightarrow R_1\alpha\Delta T = R_2\beta\Delta T$

$\therefore \frac{R_1}{R_2} = \frac{\beta}{\alpha}$

24. (d) Given : Number of cells, $n=5$, emf of each cell $=E$
Internal resistance of each cell $=r$
In series, current through resistance R

$$I=\frac{nE}{nr+R}=\frac{5E}{5r+R}$$

In parallel, current through resistance R

$$I'=\frac{E}{\frac{r}{n}+R}=\frac{nE}{r+nR}=\frac{5E}{r+5R}$$

According to question, $I=I'$

$$\therefore \frac{5E}{5r+5R}=\frac{5E}{r+5R} \Rightarrow 5r+R=r+5R$$

or $R=r \quad \therefore \frac{R}{r}=1$

25. (d) The total volume remains the same before and after stretching.

Therefore $A\times\ell = A'\times\ell'$

Here $\ell'=2\ell$

$$\therefore A'=\frac{A\times\ell}{\ell'}=\frac{A\times\ell}{2\ell}=\frac{A}{2}$$

Percentage change in resistance

$$=\frac{R_f-R_i}{R_i}\times100=\frac{\rho\left(\frac{\ell'}{A'}-\frac{\ell}{A}\right)}{\rho\frac{\ell}{A}}\times100$$

$$=\left[\left(\frac{\ell'}{A'}\times\frac{A}{\ell}\right)-1\right]\times100=\left[\left(\frac{2\ell}{A/2}\times\frac{A}{\ell}\right)-1\right]\times100$$

$=300\%$

26. (a) Pot. gradient $=0.2$mV/cm

$$=\frac{0.2\times10^{-3}}{10^{-2}}=2\times10^{-2}\text{V/m}$$

Emf of cell $=2\times10^{-2}\times1\text{m}=2\times10^{-2}\text{V}=0.02\text{ V}$
As per the condition of potentiometer
$0.02\,(R+490)=2\,(R)$ or $1.98\,R=9.8$

$$\Rightarrow \quad R=\frac{9.8}{1.98}=4.9\ \Omega$$

27. (d)

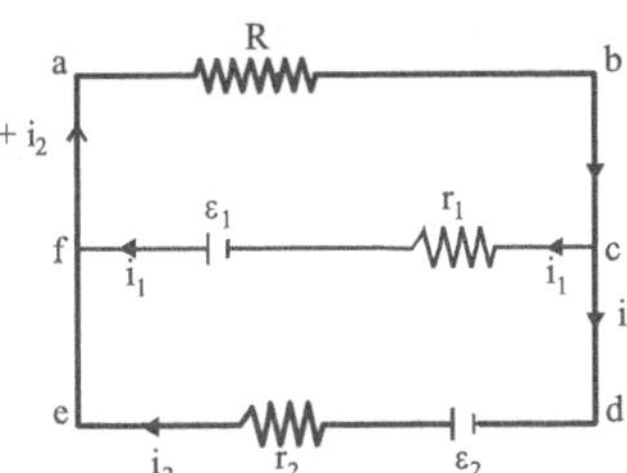

Applying Kirchhoff's rule in loop **abcfa**
$\varepsilon_1-(i_1+i_2)R-i_1\,r_1=0.$

28. (c) Total power consumed by electrical appliances in the building, $P_{total}=2500$W

Watt $=$ Volt $\times$ ampere

$\Rightarrow 2500=V\times I \Rightarrow 2500=220\,I$

$$\Rightarrow \quad I=\frac{2500}{220}=11.36\approx12\text{A}$$

(Minimum capacity of main fuse)

29. (a)

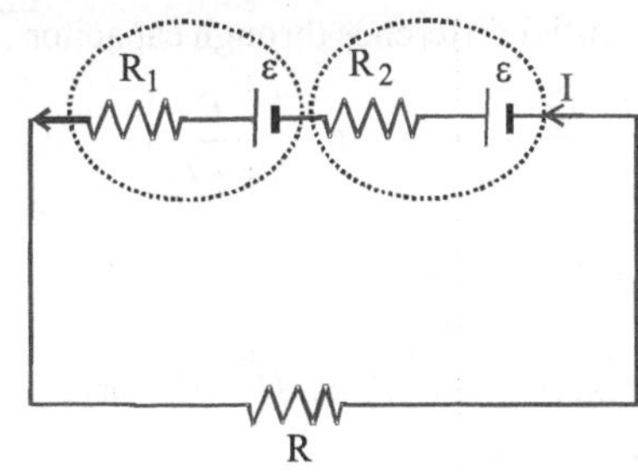

$$I=\frac{2\varepsilon}{R+R_1+R_2}$$

Potential difference across second cell

$=V=\varepsilon-iR_2=0$

$$\varepsilon-\frac{2\varepsilon}{R+R_1+R_2}.R_2=0$$

$R+R_1+R_2-2R_2=0$

$R+R_1-R_2=0$

$\therefore R=R_2-R_1$

30. (c) $R_1 \quad R_2$

Resistance of the series combination,
$S=R_1+R_2$
Resistance of the parallel combination,

$$P=\frac{R_1R_2}{R_1+R_2}$$

$$S=nP\Rightarrow R_1+R_2=\frac{n(R_1R_2)}{(R_1+R_2)}$$

$\Rightarrow (R_1+R_2)^2=nR_1R_2$
Minimum value of n is 4 for that

$(R_1+R_2)^2=4R_1R_2 \Rightarrow (R_1-R_2)^2=0$

31. (c) To convert a galvanometer into a voltmeter we connect a high resistance in series with the galvanometer. The same procedure needs to be done if ammeter is to be used as a voltmeter.

32. (c) Given, emf of cell E = 200 V
Internal resistance of cells = 1 Ω
D. C. main supply voltage V = 220 V
External resistance R = ?

$$r=\left(\frac{E-V}{V}\right)R$$

$$1=\left(\frac{20}{220}\right)\times R$$

$\therefore \quad R=11\,\Omega.$

33. (a) In steady state, flow fo current through capacitor will be zero.

Current through the circuit,

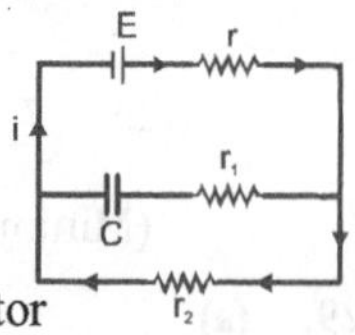

$$i = \frac{E}{r + r_2}$$

Potential difference through capacitor

$$V_c = \frac{Q}{C} = E - ir = E - \left(\frac{E}{r + r_2}\right) r$$

$$\therefore \quad Q = CE\frac{r_2}{r + r_2}$$

34. (c) $i = neAV_d$ and $V_d \propto \sqrt{E}$ (Given)

or, $i \propto \sqrt{E}$

$i^2 \propto E$

$i^2 \propto V$

Hence graph (c) correctly dipicts the *V-I* graph for a wire made of such type of material.

35. (b) Current, $I = (2.9 \times 10^{18} + 1.2 \times 10^{18}) \times 1.6 \times 10^{-19}$

$= 0.66$A towards right.

36. (a) Copper rod and iron rod are joined in series.

$$\therefore R = R_{Cu} + R_{Fe} = (\rho_1 + \rho_2)\frac{\ell}{A}$$

$$\left(\because R = \rho\frac{\ell}{A}\right)$$

From ohm's law $V = RI$

$= (1.7 \times 10^{-6} \times 10^{-2} + 10^{-5} \times 10^{-2}) \div 0.01 \times 10^{-4}$ volt

$= 0.117$ volt ($\because$ I = 1A)

37. (d) $I = \frac{E}{R + r}$, Internal resistance (r) is zero, $I = \frac{E}{R}$ = constant.

38. (b) $R_t = R_0(1 + \alpha t)$

Initially, $R_0(1 + 30\alpha) = 10\,\Omega$

Finally, $R_0(1 + \alpha t) = 11\,\Omega$

$$\therefore \frac{11}{10} = \frac{1 + \alpha t}{1 + 30\alpha}$$

or, $10 + (10 \times 0.002 \times t) = 11 + 330 \times 0.002$

or, $0.02t = 1 + 0.66 = 1.066$ or $t = \frac{1.66}{0.02} = 83°C$.

39. (b) As $P = I^2R$, so $P_1 = (1.01\,I)^2R = 1.02I^2R = 1.02P$.

It means % increase in power

$$= \left(\frac{P_1}{P} - 1\right) \times 100 = 2\%.$$

40. (b) Let I_1 be the current throug 5 Ω resistance, I_2 through (6 + 9) Ω resistance. Then as per question,

$I_1^2 \times 5 = 20$ or, $I_1 = 2$A.

Potential difference across C and D = 2 × 5 = 10V

Current $I_2 = \frac{10}{6+9} = \frac{2}{3}$A.

Heat produced per second in 2 Ω

$$= I^2R\left(\frac{8}{3}\right)^2 \times 2 = 14.2 \text{ cal/s}.$$

41. (b) $\frac{P}{Q} = \frac{R}{S}$ where $S = \frac{S_1S_2}{S_1 + S_2}$

42. (c) $R = \frac{\rho\ell_1}{A_1}$, now $\ell_2 = 2\ell_1$

$A_2 = \pi(r_2)^2 = \pi(2r_1)^2 = 4\pi r_1^2 = 4A_1$

$$\therefore \quad R_2 = \frac{\rho(2\ell_1)}{4A_1} = \frac{\rho\ell_1}{2A_1} = \frac{R}{2}$$

$\therefore$ Resistance is halved, but specific resistance remains the same.

43. (d) E = V + Ir

V = 12 − 3 = 9 volt

44. (c) $I = neAV_d$

$$V_d = \frac{I}{neA} = 5 \times 10^{-3} \text{ m/sec}$$

45. (d) Since due to wrong connection of each cell the total emf reduced to 2ε then for wrong connection of three cells the total emf will reduced to ($n\varepsilon$ – 6ε) whereas the total or equivalent resistance of cell combination will be *nr*.

Speed Test-18

1. **(a)** At a distance x consider small element of width dx. Magnetic moment of the small element is

$$dm = \frac{\left(\frac{q}{\ell}dx\right)\omega}{2\pi}.\pi x^2$$

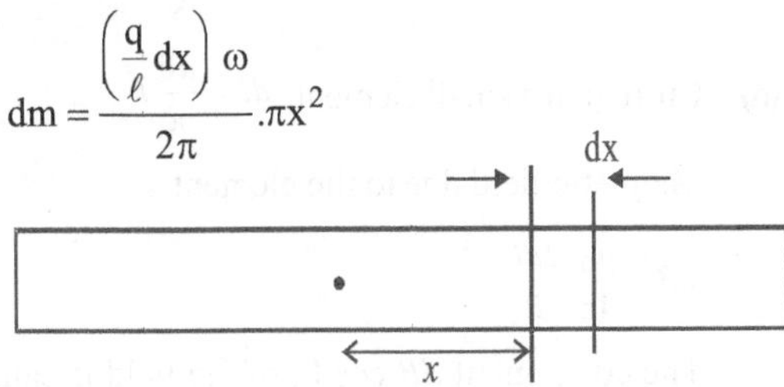

$$M = \int_{-\ell/2}^{\ell/2} \frac{q\omega}{2\ell}x^2 dx \;;\; M = \frac{q\omega\ell^2}{24} = \frac{q\pi f\ell^2}{12}$$

2. **(d)** The straight part will not contribute magnetic field at the centre of the semicircle because every element of the straight part will be 0° or 180° with the line joining the centre and the element

Due to circular portion, the field is $\frac{1}{2}\frac{\mu_0 i}{2r} = \frac{\mu_0 i}{4r}$

Hence total field at O $= \frac{\mu_0 i}{4r}$ tesla

3. **(d)** Torque on the solenoid is given by
$\tau = MB\sin\theta$
where θ is the angle between the magnetic field and the axis of solenoid.
$M = niA$
$\therefore\ \tau = niA\,B\sin 30°$

$$= 2000\times 2\times 1.5\times 10^{-4}\times 5\times 10^{-2}\times\frac{1}{2}$$

$$= 1.5\times 10^{-2}\,N-m$$

4. **(c)** Time period of cyclotron is

$$T = \frac{1}{\upsilon} = \frac{2\pi m}{eB};\; B = \frac{2\pi m}{e}\upsilon;\; R = \frac{m\upsilon}{eB} = \frac{p}{eB}$$

$$\Rightarrow\quad p = eBR = e\times\frac{2\pi m\upsilon}{e}R = 2\pi m\upsilon R$$

$$\text{K.E.} = \frac{p^2}{2m} = \frac{(2\pi m\upsilon R)^2}{2m} = 2\pi^2 m\upsilon^2 R^2$$

5. **(a)** $R_g = 50\Omega, I_g = 25\times 4\times 10^{-4}\Omega = 10^{-2}$ A
Range of V = 25 volts
$V = I_g(R_e + R_g)$

$$\therefore R_e = \frac{V}{I_g} - R_g = 2450\Omega$$

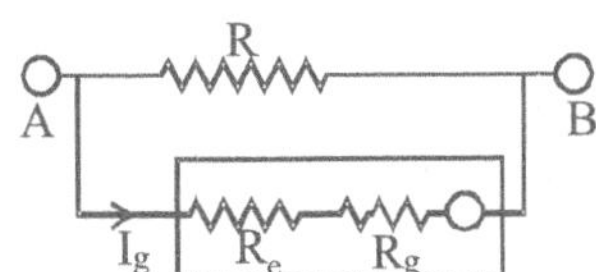

6. **(c)** $B_{axis} = \left(\frac{\mu_0 NI}{2x^3}\right)R^2$

$B \propto R^2$
So, when radius is doubled, magnetic field becomes four times.

7. **(c)** When a charged particle enters a transverse magnetic field it traverse a circular path. Its kinetic energy remains constant.

8. **(c)** K.E. of electron = 10 eV

$$\Rightarrow \frac{1}{2}mv^2 = 10\text{ eV}$$

$$\Rightarrow \frac{1}{2}(9.1\times 10^{-31})v^2 = 10\times 1.6\times 10^{-19}$$

$$\Rightarrow v^2 = \frac{2\times 10\times 1.6\times 10^{-19}}{9.1\times 10^{-31}}$$

$\Rightarrow v^2 = 3.52\times 10^{12} \Rightarrow v = 1.88\times 10^6$ m
Also we know that for circular motion

$$\frac{mv^2}{r} = Bev \Rightarrow r = \frac{mv}{Be} = 11\text{ cm}$$

9. **(d)** No magnetic force acts on the electron and force due to electric field will act opposite to its initial direction of motion. Hence its velocity decreases in magnitude.

10. **(b)** $\frac{mv^2}{r} = qvB \;\Rightarrow r = \frac{mv}{qB}$

$$\Rightarrow r_p = \frac{m_p v_p}{q_p B};$$

$$r_d = \frac{m_d v_d}{q_d B};\quad r_\alpha = \frac{m_\alpha v_\alpha}{q_\alpha B}$$

$$m_\alpha = 4m_p,\ m_d = 2m_p$$

$$q_\alpha = 2q_p,\ q_d = q_p$$

From the problem

$$E_p = E_d = E_\alpha = \frac{1}{2}m_p v_p^2$$

$$= \frac{1}{2}m_d v_d^2 = \frac{1}{2}m_\alpha v_\alpha^2$$

$$\Rightarrow v_p^2 = 2v_d^2 = 4mv_2^2$$

Thus we have, $r_\alpha = r_p < r_d$

11. **(c)** Resistance of Galvanometer,

$$G = \frac{\text{Current sensitivity}}{\text{Voltage sensitivity}} \Rightarrow G = \frac{10}{2} = 5\Omega$$

Here i_g = Full scale deflection current

$= \frac{150}{10} = 15\,mA$

V = voltage to be measured = 150 volts
(such that each division reads 1 volt)

$\Rightarrow R = \frac{150}{15\times10^{-3}} - 5 = 9995\Omega$

12. (d) Magnetic field at the centre of the current loop is

$$B = \frac{\mu_0 2\pi I}{4\pi R}$$

$$\text{or, } B = \frac{\mu_0 2\pi q\upsilon}{4\pi R}, \quad R = \frac{\mu_0 2\pi q\upsilon}{4\pi B}$$

Substituting the given values, we get

$$R = \frac{4\pi\times10^{-7}\times2\pi\times2\times10^{-6}\times6.25\times10^{12}}{4\pi\times6.28} = 1.25\,m$$

13. (b) Here, $\vec{E}$ and $\vec{B}$ are perpendicular to each other and the velocity $\vec{v}$ does not change; therefore

$qE = qvB \Rightarrow v = \frac{E}{B}$

Also,

$$\left|\frac{\vec{E}\times\vec{B}}{B^2}\right| = \frac{E\,B\sin\theta}{B^2} = \frac{E\,B\sin 90°}{B^2} = \frac{E}{B} = |\vec{v}| = v$$

14. (b) The force on the two arms parallel to the field is zero.

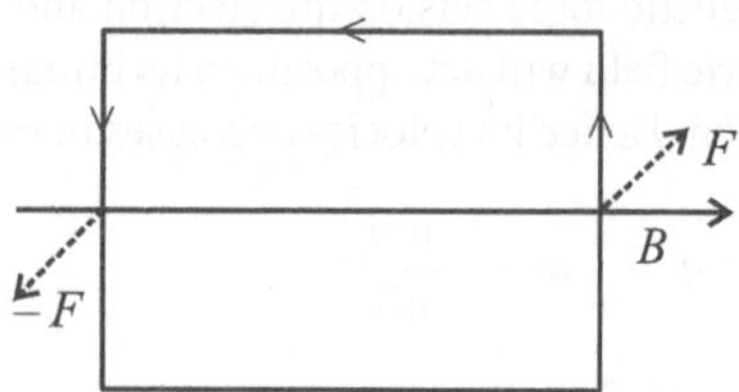

15. (d) Magnetic field at a point on the axis of a current carrying wire is always zero.

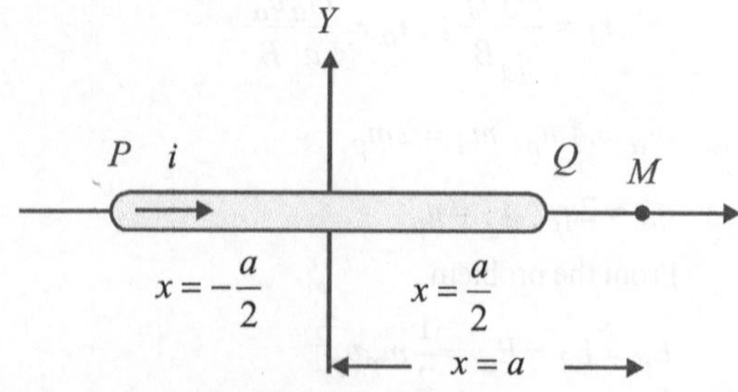

16. (b) Current carrying conductors will attract each other, while electron beams will repel each other.

17. (c) To keep the main current in the circuit unchanged, the resistance of the galvanometer should be equal to the net resistance.

$$\therefore G = \left(\frac{GS}{G+S}\right) + S'$$

$$\Rightarrow G - \frac{GS}{G+S} = S'$$

$$\therefore S' = \frac{G^2}{G+S}.$$

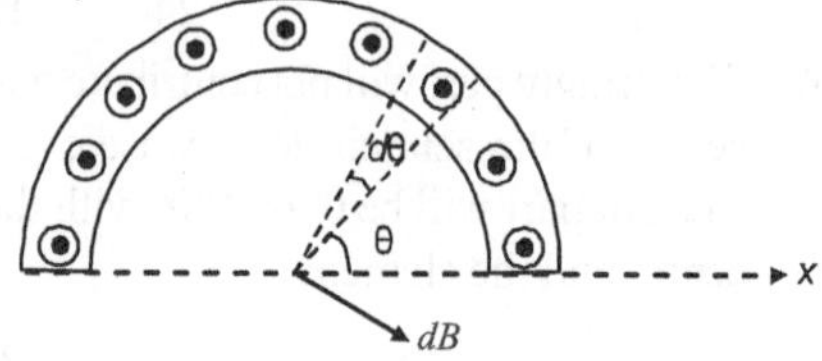

18. (d) Current in a small element, $dI = \frac{d\theta}{\pi}I$

Magnetic field due to the element

$$dB = \frac{\mu_0}{4\pi}\frac{2dI}{R}$$

The component $dB\cos\theta$, of the field is cancelled by another opposite component.

Therefore,

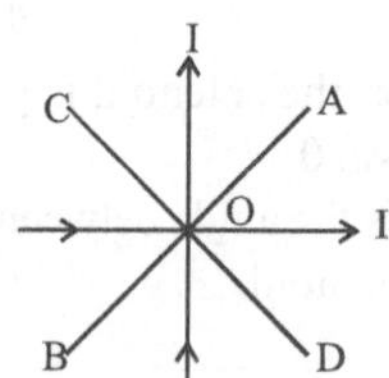

$$B_{net} = \int dB\sin\theta = \frac{\mu_0 I}{2\pi^2 R}\int_0^{\pi}\sin\theta d\theta = \frac{\mu_0 I}{\pi^2 R}$$

19. (a)

Net magnetic field on AB is zero because magnetic field due to both current carrying wires is equal in magnitude but opposite in direction.

20. (b) According to the figure the magnitude of force on the segment QM is $F_3 - F_1$ and PM is F_2.

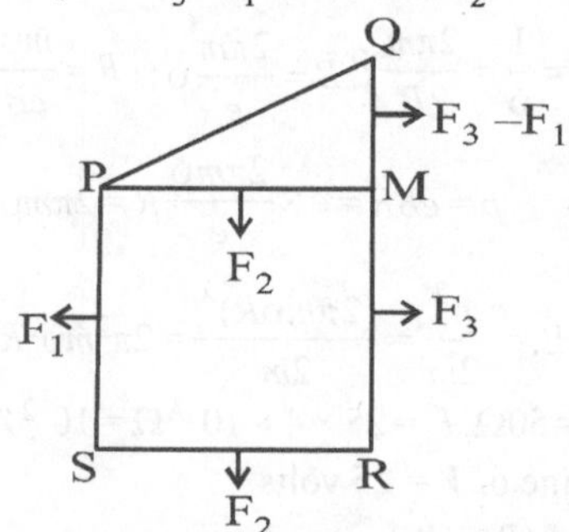

Therefore, the magnitude of the force on segment PQ is $\sqrt{(F_3 - F_1)^2 + F_2^2}$

21. (c) $B = \mu_0 ni$

$$B_1 = (\mu_0)\left(\frac{n}{2}\right)(2\,i) = \mu_0 ni = B$$

$$\Rightarrow B_1 = B$$

22. (c) The angular momentum L of the particle is given by $L = mr^2\omega$ where $\omega = 2\pi n$.

$\therefore$ Frequency $n = \dfrac{\omega}{2\pi}$; Further $i = q \times n = \dfrac{\omega q}{2\pi}$

Magnetic moment, $M = iA = \dfrac{\omega q}{2\pi} \times \pi r^2$;

$\therefore M = \dfrac{\omega q r^2}{2}$ So, $\dfrac{M}{L} = \dfrac{\omega q r^2}{2mr^2\omega} = \dfrac{q}{2m}$

23. (c) A current loop in a magnetic field is in equilibrium in two orientations one is stable and another unstable.

$\because \quad \vec{\tau} = \vec{M} \times \vec{B} = MB\sin\theta$
If $\theta = 0° \Rightarrow \tau = 0$ (stable)
If $\theta = \pi \Rightarrow \tau = 0$ (unstable)

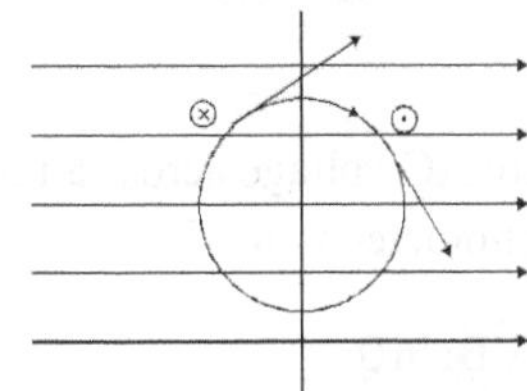

Do not experience a torque in some orientations
Hence option (c) is correct.

24. (c) $B = \dfrac{\mu_0}{4\pi}\dfrac{2i_2}{(r/2)} - \dfrac{\mu_0}{4\pi}\dfrac{2i_1}{(r/2)} = \dfrac{\mu_0}{4\pi}\dfrac{4}{r}(i_2 - i_1)$

$= \dfrac{\mu_0}{4\pi}\dfrac{4}{5}(5 - 2.5) = \dfrac{\mu_0}{2\pi}$.

25. (a) The direction of $\vec{B}$ is along $(-\hat{k})$

$\therefore$ The magnetic force

$\vec{F} = Q(\vec{v} \times \vec{B}) = Q(v\hat{i}) \times B(-\hat{k}) = QvB\hat{j}$

$\Rightarrow \vec{F}$ is along OY.

26. (a) According to Ampere's circuit law

$\oint \vec{B}.d\vec{l} = \mu_0 I_{enclosed} = \mu_0(2A - 1A) = \mu_0$

27. (a) We know that the magnetic field produced by a current carrying circular coil of radius r at its centre is

$B = \dfrac{\mu_0}{4\pi}\dfrac{I}{r} \times 2\pi$

Here $B_A = \dfrac{\mu_0}{4\pi}\dfrac{I}{R} \times 2\pi$

and $B_B = \dfrac{\mu_0}{4\pi}\dfrac{2I}{2R} \times 2\pi$

$\Rightarrow \dfrac{B_A}{B_B} = 1$

28. (b) When a charged particle enters a magnetic field at a direction perpendicular to the direction of motion, the path of the motion is circular. In circular motion the direction of velocity changes at every point (the magnitude remains constant).
Therefore, the tangential momentum will change at every point. But kinetic energy will remain constant as it is given by $\frac{1}{2}mv^2$ and v^2 is the square of the magnitude of velocity which does not change.

29. (a) $I = 50\,k$; $I_g = 20k$, where k is the figure of merit of galvanometer; $S = I_g R_g (I - I_g)$; so $12 = \dfrac{20k.R_g}{(50k - 20k)}$

On solving we get $R_g = 18\,\Omega$.

30. (d) Let I be current and l be the length of the wire.

For Ist case : $B = \dfrac{\mu_0 In}{2r} = \dfrac{\mu_0 I \times \pi}{l}$ where $2\pi r = l$

and $n = 1$

For IInd case : $l = n(2\pi r') \Rightarrow r' = \dfrac{l}{2n\pi}$

$B' = \dfrac{\mu_0 nI}{2r'} = \dfrac{\mu_0 nI}{2\dfrac{l}{2n\pi}} = \dfrac{n^2\mu_0\pi I}{l} = n^2 B$

31. (c) $B = \dfrac{\mu_0 i\, a^2}{2(x^2 + a^2)^{3/2}}$

$B' = \dfrac{\mu_0 i}{2a} = \dfrac{\mu_0 i\, a^2}{2a(x^2 + a^2)^{3/2}}\left(\dfrac{(x^2 + a^2)^{3/2}}{a^2}\right)$

$B' = \dfrac{B.(x^2 + a^2)^{3/2}}{a^3}$

Put $x = 4$ & $a = 3 \Rightarrow B' = \dfrac{54(5^3)}{3 \times 3 \times 3} = 250\mu T$

32. (a) The force acting on a charged particle in magnetic field is given by

$F = q(\vec{v} \times \vec{B})$ or $F = qvB\sin\theta$

when angle between v and B is 180°,
$F = 0$

33. (b) The force acting on electron will be perpendicular to the direction of velocity till the electron remains in the magnetic field. So the electron will follow the path as given.

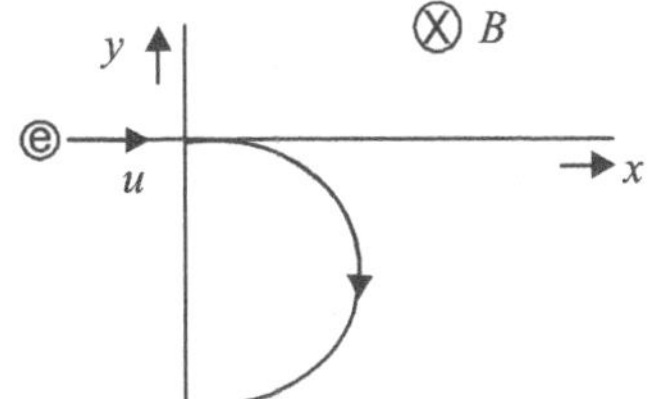

34. (c) A voltmeter is a high resistance galvanometer and is connected in parallel to circuit and ammeter is a low resitance galvanometer so if we connect high resistance in series with ammeter its resistance will be much high.

35. (d) Here, the wire does not produce any magnetic field at O because the conductor lies on the line of O. Also, the loop does not produce magnetic field at O.

36. (d) Magnetic field between the plates in this case is zero.

37. (d) For a given perimeter the area of circle is maximum. So magnetic moment of (S) is greatest.

38. (a) Lorentz force, $\vec{F} = q\{\vec{E} + (\vec{v} \times \vec{B})\}$

$$\vec{v} \times \vec{B} = \begin{vmatrix} \hat{i} & \hat{j} & \hat{k} \\ 1 & 2 & 0 \\ 5 & 3 & 4 \end{vmatrix} = 8\hat{i} - 4\hat{j} - 7\hat{k}$$

$$\vec{F} = 1(2\hat{i} - 3\hat{j} + 8\hat{i} - 4\hat{j} - 7\hat{k}) = (10\hat{i} - 7\hat{j} - 7\hat{k})$$

39. (b) Here, $R_g = 100\,\Omega$; $I_g = 10^{-5}$ A; I=1A; S = ?

$$S = \frac{I_g R_g}{I - I_g} = \frac{10^{-5} \times 100}{1 - 10^{-5}} = 10^{-3}\,\Omega \text{ in parallel}$$

40. (d)

I_1, I, F_1, F_2, F_3, F_4

$F_1 > F_2$ as $F \propto \frac{1}{d}$, and F_3 and F_4 are equal and opposite.

Hence, the net attraction force will be towards the conductor.

41. (c) $\vec{F}_1 = \vec{F}_2 = 0$

because of action and reaction pair

42. (c) As electron move with constant velocity without deflection. Hence, force due to magnetic field is equal and opposite to force due to electric field.

$$qvB = qE \Rightarrow v = \frac{E}{B} = \frac{20}{0.5} = 40 \text{ m/s}$$

43. (c)

44. (b) To measure AC voltage across a resistance a moving coil galvanometer is used.

45. (c) As $\vec{F} = q\vec{V}\vec{B}\sin\theta$

F is zero for sin 0° or sin 180° and is non-zero for angle between $\vec{V}$ and $\vec{B}$ any value other than zero and 180°.

Speed Test-19

1. (b) As the axes are perpendicular, mid point lies on axial line of one magnet and on equatorial line of other magnet.

$$\therefore\ B_1 = \frac{\mu_0}{4\pi}\frac{2M}{d^3} = \frac{10^{-7}\times 2\times 1}{1^3} = 2\times 10^{-7}$$

and $B_2 = \frac{\mu_0}{4\pi}\frac{M}{d^3} = 10^{-7}$

$\therefore$ Resultant field $= \sqrt{B_1^2 + B_2^2} = \sqrt{5}\times 10^{-7}\,T$

2. (c) Initial magnetic moment of each magnet $= m \times \ell$.
As is clear from Fig., S_1 and N_2 neutralize each other.
Effective distance between

N_1 and $S_2 = \sqrt{\ell^2 + \ell^2} = \ell\sqrt{2}$

$\therefore\ M' = m\ell\sqrt{2}$.

3. (d) As shown in the figure, the magnetic lines of force are directed from south to north inside a bar magnet.

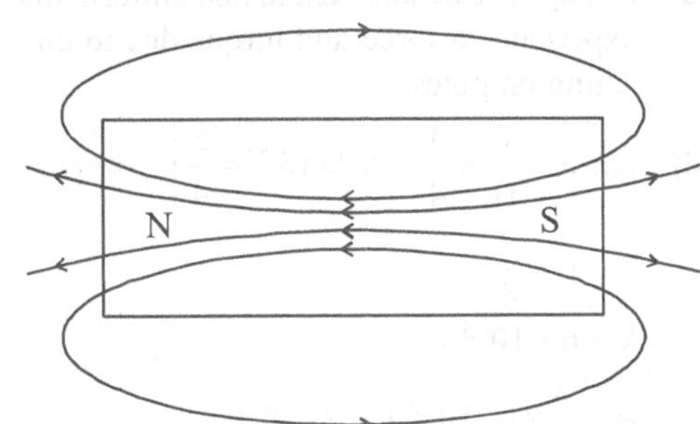

4. (b) For a diamagnetic material, the value of μ_r is less than one. For any material, the value of ϵ_r is always greater than 1.

5. (a) The time period of oscillation of a freely suspended magnet is given by

$$T = 2\pi\sqrt{\frac{I}{MH}}$$

Thus, $\frac{T}{T'} = \frac{2\pi\sqrt{\frac{I}{MH}}}{2\pi\sqrt{\frac{I}{MH'}}}$

Given, $T = 4$ sec, $T' = 2$ sec,

So, $\frac{4}{2} = \sqrt{\frac{H'}{H}}$

or $\sqrt{\frac{H'}{H}} = 2$

or $H' = 4H$

6. (b) Diamagnetic materials are repelled in an external magnetic field.
Bar *B* represents diamagnetic materials.

7. (a) The temperature above which a ferromagnetic substance becomes paramagnetic is called Curie's temperature.

8. (a) Iron is ferromagnetic.

9. (b) $\tau = MB\sin\theta$

$\tau = iAB\sin 90°$

$\therefore\ A = \frac{\tau}{iB}$

Also, A = 1/2 (BC) (AD)

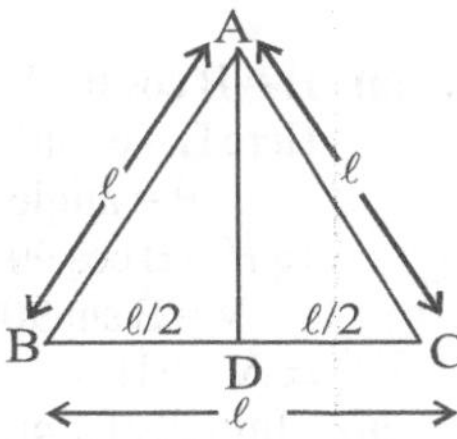

But $\frac{1}{2}(BC)(AD) = \frac{1}{2}(l)\sqrt{l^2 - \left(\frac{l}{2}\right)^2} = \frac{\sqrt{3}}{4}l^2$

$\Rightarrow\ \frac{\sqrt{3}}{4}(l)^2 = \frac{\tau}{Bi}$

$\therefore\ l = 2\left(\frac{\tau}{\sqrt{3}\,B.i}\right)^{\frac{1}{2}}$

10. (a) $M = 60\,Am^2$

$\vec{\tau} = 1.2\times 10^{-3}$ Nm, $B_H = 40\times 10^{-6}$ Wb/m^2

$\vec{\tau} = \vec{M}\times\vec{B}_H \Rightarrow \tau = MB_H\sin\theta$

$\Rightarrow 1.2\times 10^{-3} = 60\times 40\times 10^{-6}\sin\theta$

$\Rightarrow \sin\theta = \frac{1.2\times 10^{-3}}{60\times 40\times 10^{-6}} = \frac{1}{2} = \sin 30°$

$\Rightarrow \theta = 30°$

11. (b) Electro magnet should be amenable to magnetisation and demagnetization.
$\therefore$ retentivity and coercivity should be low.

12. (b) $T = 2\pi\sqrt{\frac{I}{M\times B}} = 2\pi\sqrt{\frac{I}{MB}}$ where $I = \frac{1}{12}m\ell^2$

When the magnet is cut into three pieces the pole strength will remain the same and

M.I. $(I') = \frac{1}{12}\left(\frac{m}{3}\right)\left(\frac{\ell}{3}\right)^2 \times 3 = \frac{I}{9}$

We have, Magnetic moment (*M*)
= Pole strength (*m*) × ℓ

$\therefore$ New magnetic moment,

$M' = m\times\left(\frac{\ell}{3}\right)\times 3 = m\ell = M$

$\therefore\ T' = \frac{T}{\sqrt{9}} = \frac{2}{3}s$.

13. (b) Graph [A] is for material used for making permanent magnets (high coercivity)
Graph [B] is for making electromagnets and transformers.

14. (a) The earth's core is hot and molten. Hence, convective current in earth's core is responsible for it's magnetic field.

15. (b) $T \propto \frac{1}{\sqrt{H}} \Rightarrow \frac{T_1}{T_2} = \sqrt{\frac{H_2}{H_1}} \Rightarrow \frac{2}{1} = \sqrt{\frac{H+F}{H}}$

$\Rightarrow F = 3H \, or \frac{H}{F} = \frac{1}{3}$

16. (a) H = B cos θ, V = B sin θ
Here B = earth's magnetic field
θ = angle of dip = 90° at north pole
⇒ H = B cos 90° = 0
V = B sin 90° = B
⇒ V >> H

17. (d) Initially for circular coil $L = 2\pi r$ and $M = i \times \pi r^2$

$= i \times \pi\left(\frac{L}{2\pi}\right)^2 = \frac{iL^2}{4\pi}$ ...(i)

Finally for square coil side $a = \frac{L}{4}$ and

$M' = i \times \left(\frac{L}{4}\right)^2 = \frac{iL^2}{16}$ ...(ii)

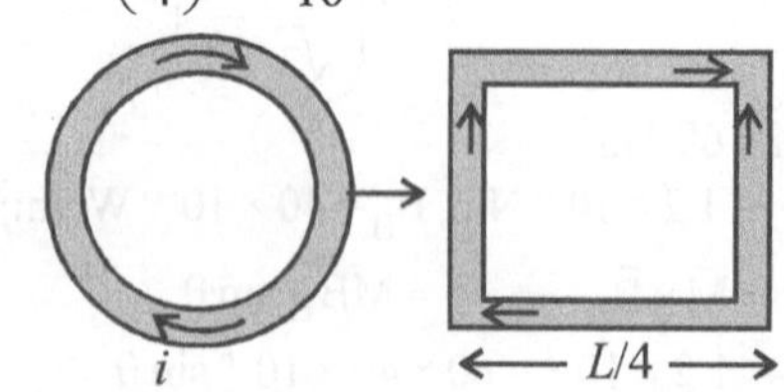

Solving equation (i) and (ii) $M' = \frac{\pi M}{4}$

18. (b) $FL = MB$ (= Torque) $\Rightarrow L = \frac{MB}{F}$

19. (a) $\chi_d < \chi_p < \chi_f$
For diamagnetic substance χ_d is small and negative (10^{-5})
For paramagnetic substances χ_p is small and positive (10^{-3} to 10^{-5})
For ferromagnetic substanes χ_f is very large (10^3 to 10^5)

20. (b) $B = \mu_0 \mu_r H \Rightarrow \mu_r \propto \frac{B}{H}$ = slope of B-H curve

According to the given graph, slope of the graph is highest at point Q.

21. (d) On increasing the temperature by 700°C, the magnetic needle is demagnetised. Therefore, the needle stops vibrating.

22. (b) $\tau = MB \sin \theta$ $(\theta = 90°)$

$\tau = MB \Rightarrow \frac{B_1}{B_2} = \frac{\tau_1}{\tau_2}$ (since magnetic moment is same)

23. (a) Magnetic field due to a bar magnet in the broad-side on position is given by

$$B = \frac{\mu_0}{4\pi} \frac{M}{\left[r^2 + \frac{\ell^2}{4}\right]^{3/2}}; M = m\ell.$$

After substituting the values and simplifying we get $B = 6 \times 1^{-5}$ A-m

24. (c) Initially magnetic moment of system

$M_1 = \sqrt{M^2 + M^2} = \sqrt{2}M$ and moment of inertia

$I_1 = I + I = 2I$.

Finally when one of the magnet is removed then

$M_2 = M$ and $I_2 = I$

So, $T = 2\pi\sqrt{\frac{I}{M B_H}}$

$\frac{T_1}{T_2} = \sqrt{\frac{I_1}{I_2} \times \frac{M_2}{M_1}} = \sqrt{\frac{2I}{I} \times \frac{M}{\sqrt{2}M}}$

$\Rightarrow T_2 = \frac{2^{5/4}}{2^{1/4}} = 2\,\text{sec}$

25. (d) A magnetic needle kept in non uniform magnetic field experience a force and torque due to unequal forces acting on poles.

26. (d) $\tan \delta = \frac{V}{H} = \frac{3}{4}$ $\left[\because \tan 37° = \frac{3}{4}\right]$

$\therefore V = \frac{3}{4} H$

$V = 6 \times 10^{-5}$ T

$H = \frac{4}{3} \times 6 \times 10^{-5}\,T = 8 \times 10^{-5}\,T$

$\therefore B_{total} = \sqrt{V^2 + H^2} = \sqrt{(36+64)} \times 10^{-5}$
$= 10 \times 10^{-5} = 10^{-4}$T.

27. (b) Ferromagnetic substance has magnetic domains whereas paramagnetic substances have magnetic dipoles which get attracted to a magnetic field. Diamagnetic substances do not have magnetic dipole but in the presence of external magnetic field due to their orbital motion of electrons these substances are repelled.

28. (d) PQ_6 corresponds to the lowest potential energy among all the configurations shown.

29. (a) $\tan \theta = \frac{V}{H}, \tan \theta' = \frac{V}{H \cos x}; \frac{\tan \theta'}{\tan \theta} = \frac{1}{\cos x}$

30. (d) In series, same current flows through two tangent galvanometers.

31. (c) Net magnetic dipole moment = $2 M \cos\frac{\theta}{2}$

As value of $\cos\frac{\theta}{2}$ is maximum in case (c) hence net magnetic dipole moment is maximum for option (c).

32. (b) Since magnetic field is in vertical direction and needle is free to totate in horizontal plane only so magnetic force cannot rotate the needle in horizontal plane so needle can stay in any position.

33. (b) Work done in rotating the magnetic dipole from position $\theta_1 = 0°$ to $\theta_2 = 180°$

$\because W = MB(\cos\theta_1 - \cos\theta_2)$

$\therefore W = MB(\cos 0° - \cos 180°) = 2MB$

34. (b) The time period of a bar magnet in a magnetic field is given by.

$$T = 2\pi\sqrt{\frac{I}{MB}};$$

Here, I = moment of inertia $\propto m$, M = moment of magnet, B = magnetic field.

$T \propto \sqrt{I} \propto \sqrt{m}$; so, T becomes twice as mass becomes four times

35. (a) Given, $B = 4 \times 10^{-5}$ T

$R_E = 6.4 \times 10^6$ m

Dipole moment of the earth M = ?

$$B = \frac{\mu_0}{4\pi}\frac{M}{d^3}$$

$$4 \times 10^{-5} = \frac{4\pi \times 10^{-7} \times M}{4\pi \times (6.4 \times 10^6)^3}$$

$\therefore$ $M \cong 10^{23}$ Am^2

36. (b) From $\mu_r = 1 + \chi_m$;

Magnetic suscaptibility, $\chi_m = \mu_r - 1$

$\chi_m = 0.075 - 1 = -0.925.$

37. (d) $\delta_1 = 40°, \delta_2 = 30°, \delta = ?$

$$\cot\delta = \sqrt{\cot^2\delta_1 + \cot^2\delta_2} = \sqrt{\cot^2 40° + \cot^2 30°}$$

$$\cot\delta = \sqrt{1.19^2 + 3} = 2.1$$

$\therefore \delta = 25°$ i.e. $\delta < 40°$.

38. (d) In magnetic dipole

Force $\propto \frac{1}{r^4}$

In the given question,

Force $\propto x^{-n}$

Hence, n = 4

39. (b) According to Curie's law, $\chi_m = \frac{\mu_0 C}{T}$

where C is Curie constant, T = temperature

$$\therefore \chi_m \alpha \frac{1}{T}$$

$$\frac{\chi_{m_1}}{\chi_{m_2}} = \frac{T_2}{T_1} = \frac{273+333}{273+30} = \frac{606}{303} = 2$$

$$\therefore \chi_{m_2} = \chi_{m_1}/2 = 0.5\chi_{m_1} = 0.5\chi\ (\because \chi_{m_1} = \chi)$$

40. (a) We know that $\mu_r = 1 + x$

$= 1 + 5500 = 5501$

$\therefore$ $\mu = \mu_r\mu_0 = (5501) \times (4\pi \times 10^{-7})$

$= 6.9 \times 10^{-3}$

41. (a) We know that $T_1 = 2\pi\sqrt{\frac{T}{MB_{H_1}}}$ ...(i)

Where $B_{H_1} = 24 \times 10^{-6}$ T

The magnetic field produced by, wire

$$B = \frac{\mu_0}{2\pi}.\frac{i}{r}$$

$$= (2 \times 10^{-7}) \times \frac{(18)}{0.20}$$

$$= 1.8 \times 10^{-6}\ \text{T}$$

Now $B_{H_2} = B_{H_1} + B = 42 \times 10^{-6}$ T

$T_2 = 2\pi\sqrt{\frac{I}{MBH_2}}$ ...(ii)

Using equations (i) and (ii), and substituting the values, we get

$T_2 = 0.076$ s

42. (a) As $BI = \mu_0 MI_M = \mu_0(I + I_M)$

Here, $I = 0$

Then $\mu_0 MI = \mu_0(I_M)$

$\Rightarrow I_M = MI = 10^5$ A

43. (a) Given $M = 8 \times 10^{22}$ Am^2

$d = R_e = 6.4 \times 10^6$m

Earth's magnetic field, $B = \frac{\mu_0}{4\pi}.\frac{2M}{d^3}$

$$= \frac{4\pi \times 10^{-7}}{4\pi} \times \frac{2 \times 8 \times 10^{22}}{(6.4 \times 10^6)^3}$$

$\cong 0.6$ Gauss

44. (c) Magnetic field in solenoid $B = \mu_0 n\, i$

$$\Rightarrow \frac{B}{\mu_0} = ni$$

(Where n = number of turns per unit length)

$$\Rightarrow \frac{B}{\mu_0} = \frac{Ni}{L}$$

$$\Rightarrow 3 \times 10^3 = \frac{100i}{10 \times 10^{-2}}$$

$\Rightarrow i = 3$A

45. (a) As length of each part also becomes half, therefore magnetic moment M = pole strength × length

$\Rightarrow \frac{1}{2} \times \frac{1}{2} = \frac{1}{4}$th i.e. M/4.

Speed Test-20

1. (b) Induced emf produced between the centre and a point on the disc is given by

$$e = \frac{1}{2}\omega BR^2$$

Putting the values,

$\omega = 60$ rad/s, $B = 0.05$ Wb/m^2

and $R = 100$ cm $= 1$m

We get $e = \frac{1}{2} \times 60 \times 0.05 \times (1)^2 = 1.5V$

2. (a) According to Faraday's law of electromagnetic induction, $\varepsilon = \frac{d\phi}{dt}$

Also, $\varepsilon = iR$

$\therefore \quad iR = \frac{d\phi}{dt} \quad \Rightarrow \quad \int d\phi = R\int idt$

Magnitude of change in flux $(d\phi) = R \times$ area under current vs time graph

or, $d\phi = 100 \times \frac{1}{2} \times \frac{1}{2} \times 10 = 250$ Wb

3. (a) If a wire, ℓ meter in length, moves perpendicular to a magnetic field of B weber/meter^2 with a velocity of v meter/second, then the e.m.f. induced in the wire is given by

$V = Bv\ell$ volt.

Here, $B = 0.30 \times 10^{-4}$ weber/meter^2,

$v = 5.0$ meter/second and $\ell = 10$ meter.

$\therefore \quad B = 0.30 \times 10^{-4} \times 5.0 \times 10 = 0.0015$ volt.

4. (d) The magnetic field is increasing in the downward direction. Therefore, according to Lenz's law, the current I_1 will flow in the direction ab and I_2 in the direction dc.

5. (a) Self inductance of a solenoid,

$$L = \frac{\mu_0 N^2 A}{l} = \frac{\mu_0 N^2 \pi r^2}{l}$$

$$\therefore \quad \frac{L_1}{L_2} = \left(\frac{r_1}{r_2}\right)^2 \left(\frac{l_2}{l_1}\right) \qquad [\because N_1 = N_2]$$

Here, $\frac{l_1}{l_2} = \frac{1}{2}, \frac{r_1}{r_2} = \frac{1}{2}$

$$\therefore \quad \frac{L_1}{L_2} = \left(\frac{1}{2}\right)^2 \left(\frac{2}{1}\right) = \frac{1}{2}$$

6. (b) $\ell = 1$m, $\omega = 5$ rad/s, $B = 0.2 \times 10^{-4} T$

$$\varepsilon = \frac{B\omega\ell}{2} = \frac{0.2 \times 10^{-4} \times 5 \times 1}{2} = 50\mu V$$

7. (c)

8. (c) Emf induced in side 1 of frame $e_1 = B_1 V\ell$

$$B_1 = \frac{\mu_0 I}{2\pi (x - a/2)}$$

Emf induced in side 2 of frame $e_2 = B_2 V\ell$

$$B_2 = \frac{\mu_0 I}{2\pi (x + a/2)}$$

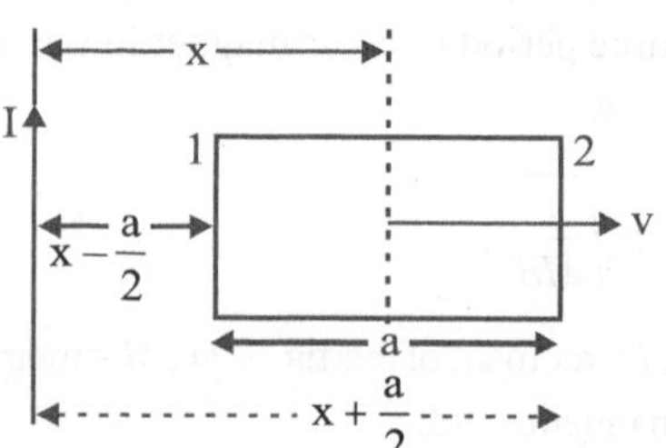

Emf induced in square frame

$e = B_1 V\ell - B_2 V\ell$

$$= \frac{\mu_0 I}{2\pi (x - a/2)} \ell v - \frac{\mu_0 I}{2\pi (x + a/2)} \ell v$$

or, $e \propto \frac{1}{(2x - a)(2x + a)}$

9. (a) When a north pole of a bar magnet moves towards the coil, the induced current in the coil flows in a direction such that the coil presents its north pole to the bar magnet as shown in figure (a). Therefore, the induced current flows in the coil in the anticlockwise direction. When a north pole of a bar magnet moves away from the coil, the induced current in the coil flows in a direction such that the coil presents its south pole to the bar magnet as shown in figure (b).

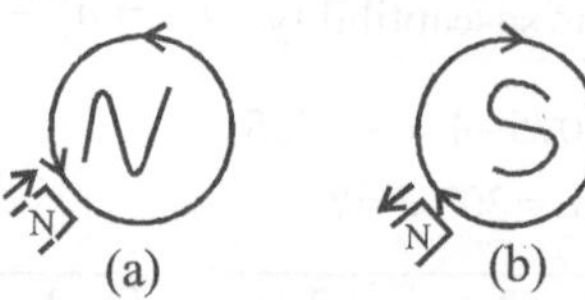

Therefore induced current flows in the coil in the clockwise direction.

10. (d) Given: $\phi = 4t^2 + 2t + 1$ wb

$$\therefore \quad \frac{d\phi}{dt} = \frac{d}{dt}(4t^2 + 2t + 1) = 8t + 2 = |\varepsilon|$$

Induced current, $I = \frac{|\varepsilon|}{R} = \frac{8t+2}{10\Omega} = \frac{8t+2}{10}$A

At t = 1 s,

$$I = \frac{8 \times 1 + 2}{10} A = 1A$$

11. (d) $M = \frac{\mu_0 N_1 N_2 A}{\ell}$

$$= \frac{4\pi \times 10^{-7} \times 300 \times 400 \times 100 \times 10^{-4}}{0.2}$$

$$M = \frac{\mu_0 N_1 N_2 A}{\ell}$$

$$= 2.4\pi \times 10^{-4}\text{H}$$

12. (d) $e = -\frac{\Delta\phi}{\Delta t} = \frac{-\Delta(LI)}{\Delta t} = -L\frac{\Delta I}{\Delta t}$

$\therefore |e| = L\frac{\Delta I}{\Delta t} \Rightarrow 8 = L \times \frac{4}{0.05}$

$\Rightarrow L = \frac{8 \times 0.05}{4} = 0.1\text{H}$

13. (c) Total number of turns in the solenoid, N = 500
Current, I = 2A.
Magnetic flux linked with each turn
$= 4 \times 10^{-3}$ Wb

As, $\phi = LI$ or $N\phi = LI \Rightarrow L = \frac{N\phi}{1}$

$= \frac{500 \times 4 \times 10^{-3}}{2}$ henry = 1 H.

14. (d) Electric field will be induced, as ABCD moves, in both *AD* and *BC*. The metallic square loop moves in its own plane with velocity *v*. A uniform magnetic field is imposed perpendicular to the plane of the square loop. *AD* and *BC* are perpendicular to the velocity as well as perpendicular to applied field so an emf is induced in both, this will cause electric fields in both.

A B
v
D C

15. (d) E.M.F. generated, $e = -\frac{d\phi}{dt} = -\frac{d(N\vec{B}.\vec{A})}{dt}$

$= -N\frac{d}{dt}(BA\cos\omega t) = NBA\omega\sin\omega t$

$\Rightarrow e_{max} = NBA\omega$

16. (c) $L = 2\text{mH}, i = t^2e^{-t}$

$E = -L\frac{di}{dt} = -L[-t^2e^{-t} + 2te^{-t}]$

when $E = 0$,

$-e^{-t}t^2 + 2te^{-t} = 0$

or, $2te^{-t} = e^{-t}t^2$

$\Rightarrow t = 2$ sec.

17. (b)

18. (b) $\frac{d\phi}{dt} = \frac{(W_2 - W_1)}{t}$ $R_{tot} = (R + 4R)\Omega = 5R\ \Omega$

$i = \frac{nd\varphi}{R_{tot}dt} = \frac{-n(W_2 - W_1)}{5Rt}$.

($\because$ W_2 & W_1 are magnetic flux)

19. (b) The individual emf produced in the coil $e = \frac{-d\phi}{dt}$

$\therefore$ The current induced will be $i = \frac{|e|}{R} \Rightarrow i = \frac{1}{R}\frac{d\phi}{dt}$

But $i = \frac{dq}{dt} \Rightarrow \frac{dq}{dt} = \frac{1}{R}\frac{d\phi}{dt} \Rightarrow \int dq = \frac{1}{R}\int d\phi \Rightarrow q = \frac{BA}{R}$

20. (c) Induced emf $= vB_H l = 1.5 \times 5 \times 10^{-5} \times 2$
$= 15 \times 10^{-5}$
$= 0.15$ mV

21. (b) $\varepsilon = \frac{d\phi}{dt} = nA\frac{dB}{dt}$

$\therefore$ $\varepsilon = 10 \times (10 \times 10^{-4})(10^4)$ [10^8 Gauss/sec $= 10^4$ T/s]

$= 100$ V.

$I = (\varepsilon/R) = (100/20) = 5$ amp.

22. (a)

W E

$\varepsilon_{ind} = Bv\ell$

$= 0.3 \times 10^{-4} \times 5 \times 20$

$= 3 \times 10^{-3}$ V $= 3$ mV.

23. (d) The self inductance of a long solenoid is given by

$L = \mu_r\mu_0 n^2 Al$

Self inductance of a long solenoid is independent of the current flowing through it.

24. (d) Here, induced e.m.f.

ω 2λ λ
dx
x

$e = \int_{2\ell}^{3\ell}(\omega x)Bdx$

$= B\omega\frac{[(3\ell)^2 - (2\ell)^2]}{2} = \frac{5B\ell^2\omega}{2}$

25. (b)

26. (b) Induced e.m.f. in the ring opposes the motion of the magnet.

27. (a)

28. (b)

29. (d) Magnetic flux, $\phi_B = BA\cos\theta$
Induced emf, $\varepsilon = BA\sin\theta$
Here, $\theta = 0°$
$\therefore$ Magnetic flux is maximum and induced emf is zero.

30. (c) e.m.f. induced $= \frac{1}{2}BR^2\omega = \frac{1}{2}BR^2(2\pi n)$

$= \frac{1}{2} \times (0.1) \times (0.1)^2 \times 2\pi \times 10 = (0.1)^2\ \pi$ volts

31. (a) $E = \frac{d}{dt}(NMI) \Rightarrow E = NM\frac{dI}{dt} \Rightarrow E = \frac{NMI}{t}$

emf induced per unit turn $= \frac{E}{N} = \frac{MI}{t}$

32. (d) According to Lenz's law, when switch is closed, the flux in the loop increases out of plane of paper, so induced current will be clockwise.

33. (a) Since $\varepsilon = -\frac{Nd\phi}{dt}$ if $\frac{d\phi}{dt}$ is fast, so ε is large.

34. (d) The e.m.f. is induced when there is change of flux. As in this case there is no change of flux, hence no e.m.f. will be induced in the wire.

35. (b) Given, $B = 0.01\ T, A = \pi R^2 = \pi \times (1\ m)^2 = \pi m^2$

$\omega = 100\ rads^{-1}$

$\therefore$ The maximum induced emf $\varepsilon_{max} = BA\omega$

$= 0.01 \times \pi \times 100\ V = \pi V$

36. (b) $e = \frac{-(\phi_2 - \phi_1)}{t} = \frac{-(0 - NBA)}{t} = \frac{NBA}{t}$

$$t = \frac{NBA}{e} = \frac{50 \times 2 \times 10^{-2} \times 10^{-2}}{0.1} = 0.1\ s$$

37. (c) $\frac{\Delta\phi}{\Delta t} = \varepsilon = iR \Rightarrow \Delta\phi = (i\Delta t)R = QR$

$$\Rightarrow Q = \frac{\Delta\phi}{R}$$

38. (d) $\phi = BA\cos\theta = 2.0 \times 0.5 \times \cos 60°$

$$= \frac{2.0 \times 0.5}{2} = 0.5 \text{ weber.}$$

39. (a) $\xi = \frac{W}{Q} \Rightarrow V = \frac{W}{Q} \Rightarrow W = QV$

40. (b) Mutual inductance depends on the relative position and orientation of the two coils.

41. (c)

42. (a) As the magnetic field increases, its flux also increases into the page and so induced current in bigger loop will be anticlockwise. i.e., from D to C in bigger loop and then from B to A in smaller loop.

43. (c) As I increases, ϕ increases

$\therefore$ I_i is such that it opposes the increases in ϕ.

Hence, ϕ decreases (By Right Hand Rule). The induced current will be counterclockwise.

44. (d) According to Faraday's law of electromagnetic induction,

Induced emf, $e = \frac{Ldi}{dt}$

$$50 = L\left(\frac{5-2}{0.1\text{sec}}\right)$$

$$\Rightarrow \quad L = \frac{50 \times 0.1}{3} = \frac{5}{3} = 1.67\ H$$

45. (d) Mutual inductance between two coil in the same plane with their centers coinciding is given by

$$M = \frac{\mu_0}{4\pi}\left(\frac{2\pi^2 R_2^2 N_1 N_2}{R_1}\right) henry.$$

Speed Test-21

1. (c) Across resistor, $I = \frac{V}{R} = \frac{100}{1000} = 0.1\,A$

At resonance,

$$X_L = X_C = \frac{1}{\omega C} = \frac{1}{200 \times 2 \times 10^{-6}} = 2500$$

Voltage across L is

$$I X_L = 0.1 \times 2500 = 250\,\text{V}$$

2. (a) The phase angle between voltage V and current I is $\pi/2$. Therefore, power factor $\cos\phi = \cos(\pi/2) = 0$. Hence the power consumed is zero.

3. (c) The current drawn by inductor and capacitor will be in opposite phase. Hence net current drawn from generator $= I_L - I_C = 0.9 - 0.4 = 0.5$ amp.

4. (c) Capacitive reactance, $X = \frac{1}{\omega C} = \frac{1}{2\pi f C}$

$$\Rightarrow X \propto \frac{1}{fC}$$

$$\therefore \frac{X'}{X} = \frac{f}{f'} \times \frac{C}{C'} = \frac{f}{2f} \times \frac{C}{2C} = \frac{1}{4} \Rightarrow X' = \frac{X}{4}$$

5. (a) The charging of inductance given by,

$$i = i_0\left(1 - e^{-\frac{Rt}{L}}\right)$$

$$\frac{i_0}{2} = i_0(1 - e^{-\frac{Rt}{L}}) \Rightarrow e^{-\frac{Rt}{L}} = \frac{1}{2}$$

Taking log on both the sides,

$$-\frac{Rt}{L} = \log 1 - \log 2$$

$$\Rightarrow t = \frac{L}{R}\log 2 = \frac{300 \times 10^{-3}}{2} \times 0.69$$

$$\Rightarrow t = 0.1 \text{ sec.}$$

6. (c) $\tan\phi = \frac{\omega L}{R} = \frac{X_L}{R}$

Given $\phi = 45°$. Hence $X_L = R$.

7. (d)

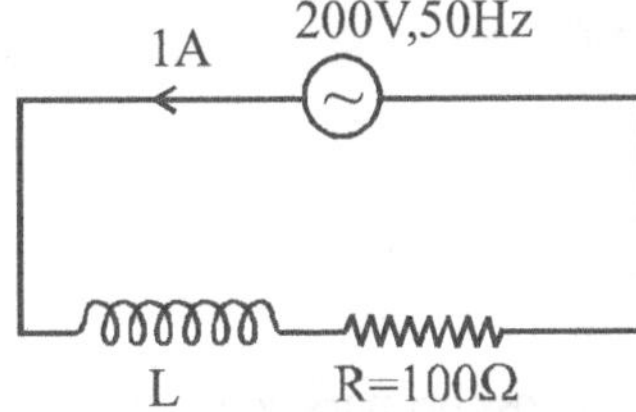

From the rating of the bulb, the resistance of the bulb can be calculated.

$$R = \frac{V_{rms}^2}{P} = 100\Omega$$

For the bulb to be operated at its rated value the rms current through it should be 1A

Also, $I_{rms} = \frac{V_{rms}}{Z}$

$$\therefore \quad 1 = \frac{200}{\sqrt{100^2 + (2\pi 50.L)^2}}$$

$$L = \frac{\sqrt{3}}{\pi}\text{H}$$

8. (a) At angular frequency ω, the current in RC circuit is given by

$$i_{max} = \frac{V_{max}}{\sqrt{R^2 + \left(\frac{1}{\omega C}\right)^2}} \quad ....(i)$$

$$\text{Also } \frac{i_{rms}}{2} = \frac{V_{rms}}{\sqrt{R^2 + \left(\frac{1}{\frac{\omega}{3}C}\right)^2}} = \frac{V_{max}}{\sqrt{R^2 + \frac{9}{\omega^2 C^2}}} \quad .....(ii)$$

From equation (i) and (ii) we get

$$3R^2 = \frac{5}{\omega^2 C^2} \Rightarrow \frac{\frac{1}{\omega C}}{R} = \sqrt{\frac{3}{5}} \Rightarrow \frac{X_C}{R} = \sqrt{\frac{3}{5}}$$

9. (c)

10. (c) Growth in current in LR_2 branch when switch is closed is given by

$$i = \frac{E}{R_2}[1 - e^{-R_2 t/L}]$$

$$\Rightarrow \frac{di}{dt} = \frac{E}{R_2}.\frac{R_2}{L}.e^{-R_2 t/L} = \frac{E}{L}e^{-\frac{R_2 t}{L}}$$

Hence, potential drop across L

$$= \left(\frac{E}{L}e^{-R_2 t/L}\right)L = Ee^{-R_2 t/L}$$

$$= 12e^{-\frac{2t}{400 \times 10^{-3}}} = 12e^{-5t}\text{V}$$

11. (a) $I = I_o\left(1 - e^{-\frac{R}{L}t}\right)$

(When current is in growth in LR circuit)

$$= \frac{E}{R}\left(1 - e^{-\frac{R}{L}t}\right) = \frac{5}{5}\left(1 - e^{-\frac{5}{10}\times 2}\right)$$

$$= (1 - e^{-1})$$

12. (d) Power, $P = I_{r.m.s} \times V_{r.m.s} \times \cos\phi$

In the given problem, the phase difference between voltage and current is $\pi/2$. Hence

$$P = I_{r.m.s} \times V_{r.m.s} \times \cos(\pi/2) = 0.$$

13. (c) When the capacitor is completely charged, the total energy in the LC circuit is with the capacitor and that energy is $E = \frac{1}{2}\frac{Q^2}{C}$

When half energy is with the capacitor in the form of electric field between the plates of the capacitor we get

$\frac{E}{2} = \frac{1}{2}\frac{Q'^2}{C}$ where Q' is the charge on one plate of the capacitor

$\therefore \frac{1}{2} \times \frac{1}{2}\frac{Q^2}{C} = \frac{1}{2}\frac{Q'^2}{C} \Rightarrow Q' = \frac{Q}{\sqrt{2}}$

14. (a) Energy stored in magnetic field $= \frac{1}{2}Li^2$

Energy stored in electric field $= \frac{1}{2}\frac{q^2}{C}$

$\therefore \frac{1}{2}Li^2 = \frac{1}{2}\frac{q^2}{C}$

Also $q = q_0 \cos \omega t$ and $\omega = \frac{1}{\sqrt{LC}}$

On solving $t = \frac{\pi}{4}\sqrt{LC}$

15. (c) The circuit will have inductive nature if

$\omega > \frac{1}{\sqrt{LC}} \left(\omega L > \frac{1}{\sqrt{LC}}\right)$

Hence (a) is false. Also if circuit has inductive nature the current will lag behind voltage. Hence (d) is also false.

If $\omega = \frac{1}{\sqrt{LC}} \left(\omega L = \frac{1}{\omega C}\right)$ the circuit will have resistance nature. Hence (b) is false.

Power factor

$$\cos\phi = \frac{R}{\sqrt{R^2 + \left(\omega L - \frac{1}{\omega C}\right)^2}} = 1 \text{ if } \omega L = \frac{1}{\omega C}$$

16. (b) $V_{rms} = \sqrt{\frac{(T/2)V_0^2 + 0}{T}} = \frac{V_0}{\sqrt{2}}$.

17. (d) Option (d) is false because the reason why the voltage leads the current is because $\frac{1}{C\omega} > L\omega$ and if the voltage lags, the inductive reactance is greater than the capacitive reactance.

18. (b) $P = \frac{1}{2}V_0 i_0 \cos\phi \Rightarrow P = P_{peak} \cdot \cos\phi$

$\Rightarrow \frac{1}{2}(P_{peak}) = P_{peak}\cos\phi \Rightarrow \cos\phi = \frac{1}{2} \Rightarrow \phi = \frac{\pi}{3}$

19. (c) $\eta = \frac{E_s I_s}{E_p I_p} \therefore \eta = \frac{110 \times 9}{220 \times 5} = 0.9 \times 100\% = 90\%$

20. (d) $V = \frac{V_0}{T/4}t \Rightarrow V = \frac{4V_0}{T}t$

$$\Rightarrow V_{rms} = \sqrt{\langle V^2 \rangle} = \frac{4V_0}{T}\sqrt{\langle t^2 \rangle} = \frac{4V_0}{T}\left\{\frac{\int_0^{T/4} t^2 dt}{\int_0^{T/4} dt}\right\}^{1/2} = \frac{V_0}{\sqrt{3}}$$

21. (a) $L = 10\text{ mHz} = 10^{-2}\text{ Hz}$
$f = 1\text{MHz} = 10^6\text{ Hz}$

$f = \frac{1}{2\pi\sqrt{LC}}$

$f^2 = \frac{1}{4\pi^2 LC}$

$\Rightarrow C = \frac{1}{4\pi^2 f^2 L} = \frac{1}{4 \times 10 \times 10^{-2} \times 10^{12}} = \frac{10^{-12}}{0.4} = 2.5\ pF$

22. (d) Current is maximum when $X_L = X_C$

$\Rightarrow \omega L = \frac{1}{\omega C} \Rightarrow \omega = \frac{1}{\sqrt{LC}} = \frac{1}{\sqrt{0.5 \times 8 \times 10^{-6}}}$

$= \frac{1}{2 \times 10^{-3}} = 500$ rad/s.

23. (a) If $\omega = 50 \times 2\pi$ then $\omega L = 20\Omega$
If $\omega' = 100 \times 2\pi$ then $\omega' L = 40\Omega$
Current flowing in the coil is

$$I = \frac{200}{Z} = \frac{200}{\sqrt{R^2 + (\omega' L)^2}} = \frac{200}{\sqrt{(30)^2 + (40)^2}}$$

$I = 4A$.

24. (a) At resonance impedance is minimum ($\because X_L = X_C$) current is maximum, because V_L and V_C are equal in magnitude
$\therefore V_{LC} = V_L - V_C = 0$
Hence, voltmeter V_2 read 0 volt.

25. (b)

26. (d) As $E_p I_p = P_i \quad \therefore I_p = \frac{P_i}{E_p} = \frac{4000}{100} = 40$ A.

27. (c) The phase angle is given by

$\tan\phi = \frac{\omega L}{R} = \frac{2\pi \times 50 \times 0.21}{12} = 5.5$

$\phi = \tan^{-1} 5.5 = 80°$

28. (c)

29. (a) Since $\frac{V_s}{V_p} = \frac{N_s}{N_p}$

Where
N_s = No. of turns across primary coil = 50
N_p = No. of turns across secondary coil = 1500

and $V_p = \frac{d\phi}{dt} = \frac{d}{dt}(\phi_0 + 4t) = 4$

$\Rightarrow V_s = \frac{1500}{50} \times 4 = 120$ V

30. (a) $\frac{E_s}{E_p} = \frac{n_s}{n_p}$ or $E_s = E_p \times \left(\frac{n_s}{n_p}\right)$

$\therefore \; E_s = 120 \times \left(\frac{200}{100}\right) = 240\,V$

$\frac{I_p}{I_s} = \frac{n_s}{n_p}$ or $I_s = I_p \left(\frac{n_p}{n_s}\right) \; \therefore \; I_s = 10\left(\frac{100}{200}\right) = 5$ amp

31. (b) $R\uparrow \Rightarrow I\downarrow \Rightarrow \frac{dI}{dt} \rightarrow (-ve) \rightarrow e = (+ve)$

$\left[\text{As } e = -L\frac{dI}{dt}\right]$

Supporting $\rightarrow I_{net} \uparrow$

32. (b) We know that, $i = i_0(1 - e^{-t/\tau})$

or $\frac{3}{4} i_0 = i_0(1 - e^{-4/\tau})$

or $e^{-4/\tau} = \frac{1}{4}$

or $e^{4/\tau} = 4$

$\therefore \; \frac{4}{\tau} = \ln 4$

or $\tau = \frac{2}{\ln 2} s$

33. (d) At resonance, $\omega L = \frac{1}{\omega C}$. The circuit behaves as if it contains R only. So, phase difference = 0
At resonance, impedance is minimum $Z_{min} = R$ and current is maximum, given by

$I_{max} = \frac{E}{Z_{min}} = \frac{E}{R}$

It is interesting to note that before resonance the current leads the applied emf, at resonance it is in phase, and after resonance it lags behind the emf. LCR series circuit is also called as acceptor circuit and parallel LCR circuit is called rejector circuit.

34. (d) Condition for which the current is maximum in a series LCR circuit is,

$\omega = \frac{1}{\sqrt{LC}}$

$1000 = \frac{1}{\sqrt{L(10 \times 10^{-6})}}$

$\Rightarrow = L = 100\,mH$

35. (c) When a circuit is broken, the induced e.m.f. is largest. So the answer is (c).

36. (b) $V = 50 \times 2 \sin 100\pi \cos 100\pi t = 50 \sin 200\pi t$
$\Rightarrow V_0 = 50\,Volts$ and $\nu = 100\,Hz$

37. (d) $V = -L\frac{di}{dt}$

Here $\frac{di}{dt}$ is + ve for $\frac{T}{2}$ time and

$\frac{di}{dt}$ is – ve for next $\frac{T}{2}$ time

38. (b) $V = V_0 \sin \omega t$
Voltage in r.m.s. value

$V_0 = \sqrt{2} \times 234\,V = 331$ volt

and $\omega t = 2\pi n t = 2\pi \times 50 \times t = 100\pi t$
Thus, the equation of line voltage is given by
$V = 331 \sin(100\,\pi\,t)$

39. (a) The resistance in the middle plays no part in the charging process of C, as it does not alter either the potential difference across the RC combination or the current through it.

40. (a) Here, $C = 100\,\mu F = 100 \times 10^{-6} F, R = 40\,\Omega$,
$V_{rms} = 110\,V, f = 60\,Hz$
Peak voltage,

$V_0 = \sqrt{2}\,.\,V_{rms} = 100\sqrt{2} = 155.54\,V$

Circuit impedance,

$Z = \sqrt{R^2 + \frac{1}{\omega^2 C^2}}$

$= \sqrt{40^2 + \frac{1}{(2 \times \pi \times 60 \times 100 \times 10^{-6})^2}}$

$= \sqrt{1600 + 703.60} = \sqrt{2303.60} = 48\,\Omega$

hence, maximum current in coil,

$I_0 = \frac{V_0}{Z} = \frac{155.54}{48} = 3.24\,A$

41. (a) Laminated core provide less area of cross-section for the current to flow. Because of this, resistance of the core increases and current decreases thereby decreasing the eddy current losses.

42. (b) $V = 200V;\; r = 10\Omega$
$R' = 10 + 100\Omega = 110\Omega$

$I = \frac{V}{R'} = \frac{220}{100} = 2A$

$P = I^2R = 4 \times 100 = 400\,W$

43. (b) For step-down transformer,

$\frac{V_P}{V_S} = \frac{I_S}{I_P} \quad \because V_P > V_S \quad \therefore I_S > I_P$

44. (b) At $t = 0$, no current will flow through L and R_1

$\therefore$ Current through battery $= \frac{V}{R_2}$

At $t = \infty$,

effective resistance, $R_{eff} = \frac{R_1 R_2}{R_1 + R_2}$

$\therefore$ Current through battery $= \frac{V}{R_{eff}}$

$= \frac{V(R_1 + R_2)}{R_1 R_2}$

45. (d) These three inductors are connected in parallel. The equivalent inductance L_p is given by

$\frac{1}{L_p} = \frac{1}{L_1} + \frac{1}{L_2} + \frac{1}{L_3} = \frac{1}{3} + \frac{1}{3} + \frac{1}{3} = \frac{3}{3} = 1$

$\therefore L_p = 1$

Speed Test-22

1. (b) ∵ The E.M. wave are transverse in nature i.e.,

$$= \frac{\vec{k}\times\vec{E}}{\mu\omega} = \vec{H} \quad \ldots(i)$$

where $\vec{H} = \frac{\vec{B}}{\mu}$

and $\frac{\vec{k}\times\vec{H}}{\omega\varepsilon} = -\vec{E} \quad \ldots(ii)$

$\vec{k}$ is $\perp$ $\vec{H}$ and $\vec{k}$ is also $\perp$ to $\vec{E}$

or In other words $\vec{X} \parallel \vec{E}$ and $\vec{k} \parallel \vec{E}\times\vec{B}$

2. (a) $E_{rms} = 720$

The average total energy density

$$= \frac{1}{2}\epsilon_0 E_0^2 = \frac{1}{2}\epsilon_0 [\sqrt{2}E_{rms}]^2 = \epsilon_0 E_{rms}^2$$

$$= 8.85\times10^{-12}\times(720)^2$$

$$= 4.58\times10^{-6}\ J/m^3$$

3. (d) $I_d = 1\ mA = 10^{-3}$ A

$C = 2\mu F = 2 \times 10^{-6}$ F

$$I_D = I_C = \frac{d}{dt}(CV) = C\frac{dV}{dt}$$

Therefore, $\frac{dV}{dt} = \frac{I_D}{C} = \frac{10^{-3}}{2\times10^{-6}} = 500\ Vs^{-1}$

Therefore, applying a varying potential difference of 500 V s^{-1} would produce a displacement current of desired value.

4. (c) $E_0 = CB_0$ and $C = \frac{1}{\sqrt{\mu_0\varepsilon_0}}$

Electric energy density $= \frac{1}{2}\varepsilon_0 E_0^2 = \mu_E$

Magnetic energy density $= \frac{1}{2}\frac{Bo^2}{\mu_0} = \mu_B$

Thus, $\mu_E = \mu_B$

Energy is equally divided between electric and magnetic field

5. (c) In an electromagnetic wave electric field and magnetic field are perpendicular to the direction of propagation of wave. The vector equation for the electric field is

$$\vec{E} = E_0 \cos\left(\omega t - \frac{2\pi}{\lambda}y\right)\hat{z}$$

6. (a) Frequency remains constant during refraction

$$v_{med} = \frac{1}{\sqrt{\mu_0 \epsilon_0 \times 4}} = \frac{c}{2}$$

$$\frac{\lambda_{med}}{\lambda_{air}} = \frac{v_{med}}{v_{air}} = \frac{c/2}{c} = \frac{1}{2}$$

∴ wavelength is halved and frequency remains unchanged.

7. (b) For electromagnetic waves we know that,

$$\frac{E}{B} = c$$

$$\therefore \frac{9\times10^{-4}}{B} = 3\times10^8\ ms^{-1}$$

$B = 3 \times 10^{-12}$ T.

8. (b) Here, $k = \frac{2\pi}{\lambda}$, $\omega = 2\pi\upsilon$

$$\therefore \frac{k}{\omega} = \frac{2\pi/\lambda}{2\pi\upsilon} = \frac{1}{\pi\upsilon} = \frac{1}{c} \quad (\because c = \upsilon\lambda)$$

where c is the speed of electromagnetic wave in vacuum. It is a constant whose value is $3 \times 10^6\ m\ s^{-1}$

9. (a) E.M. wave always propagates in a direction perpendicular to both electric and magnetic fields. So, electric and magnetic fields should be along + X– and + Y–directions respectively. Therefore, option (a) is the correct option.

10. (d) $\frac{1}{2}\varepsilon_0 E_0^2$ is electric energy density.

$\frac{B^2}{2\mu_0}$ is magnetic energy density.

So, total energy $= \frac{1}{2}\varepsilon_0 E_0^2 + \frac{B_0^2}{2\mu_0}$

11. (c) Incident momentum, $p = \frac{E}{c}$

For perfectly reflecting surface with normal incidence

$$\Delta p = 2p = \frac{2E}{c}$$

$$F = \frac{\Delta p}{\Delta t} = \frac{2E}{ct}$$

$$P = \frac{F}{A} = \frac{2E}{ctA}$$

12. (a) E_x and B_y would generate a plane EM wave travelling in z-direction, $\vec{E}$, $\vec{B}$ and $\vec{k}$ from a right handed system $\vec{k}$ is along z-axis. As $\hat{i}\times\hat{j} = \hat{k}$

$\Rightarrow E_x\hat{i}\times B_y\hat{j} = C\hat{k}$ i.e., E is along x-axis and B is along y-axis.

13. (b) From question,

$B_0 = 20\ nT = 20 \times 10^{-9}$T

($\because$ velocity of light in vacuum $C = 3 \times 10^8\ ms^{-1}$)

$\vec{E}_0 = \vec{B}_0 \times \vec{C}$

$$|\vec{E}_0| = |\vec{B}|\cdot|\vec{C}| = 20\times10^{-9}\times3\times10^8$$

$= 6$ V/m.

14. (c) Microwave oven acts on the principle of giving vibrational energy to water molecules.

15. (a) Displacement current is set up in a region where the electric field is changing with time.

16. (a) On comparing the given equation to

$\vec{E} = a_0\hat{i}\cos(\omega t - kz)$

$\omega = 6 \times 10^{8z}$,

$k = \frac{2\pi}{r} = \frac{\omega}{c}$

$k = \frac{\omega}{c} = \frac{6\times10^8}{3\times10^8} = 2\,\text{m}^{-1}$

17. (b) Displacement current, I_D = conduction current, I_C

$\therefore \frac{dq}{dt} = \frac{d}{dt}[q_0 \cos 2\pi\upsilon t] = -q_0\, 2\pi\upsilon \sin 2\pi\upsilon t$

18. (a) Momentum of light falling on reflecting surface $p = \frac{E}{C}$

As surface is perfectly reflecting so momentum reflect

$p^1 = -\frac{E}{C}$

$\frac{E}{C}$ ↓ ↑ $\frac{E}{C} = P$

So, momentum transferred

$= P - P^1 = \frac{E}{C} - \left(-\frac{E}{C}\right) = \frac{2E}{C}$

19. (d) (1) Infrared rays are used to treat muscular strain because these are heat rays.
(2) Radio waves are used for broadcasting because these waves have very long wavelength ranging from few centimeters to few hundred kilometers
(3) X-rays are used to detect fracture of bones because they have high penetrating power but they can't penetrate through denser medium like dones.
(4) Ultraviolet rays are absorbed by ozone of the atmosphere.

20. (d) Given : $\vec{B} = 1.2\times10^{-8}\hat{k}\text{T}$

$\vec{E} = ?$

From formula,

$E = Bc = (1.2\times10^{-8}\text{T})(3\times10^8\text{ms}^{-1}) = 3.6\text{ Vm}^{-1}$

$\vec{B}$ is along Z-direction and the wave propagates along X-direction. Therefore $\vec{E}$ should be along Y-direction.

Thus, $\vec{E} = 3.6\hat{j}\,\text{Vm}^{-1}$

21. (d)

22. (a) $E = \frac{hc}{\lambda} \Rightarrow \lambda = \frac{hc}{E}$

$\Rightarrow \lambda = \frac{6.6\times10^{-34}\times3\times10^8}{11\times1000\times1.6\times10^{-19}} = 12.4\text{ Å}$

Increasing order of frequency →

x-rays u-v rays visible Infrared

23. (a) Velocity of light

$C = \frac{E}{B} \Rightarrow B = \frac{E}{C} = \frac{9.3}{3\times10^8} = 3.1\times10^{-8}\text{T}$

24. (b) The average energy stored in the electric field

$U_E = \frac{1}{2}\varepsilon_0 E^2$

The average energy stored in the magnetic field $= U_B = \frac{1}{2}\frac{B^2}{\mu_0}$,

According to conservation of energy $U_E = U_B$

$\varepsilon_0\mu_0 = \frac{B^2}{E^2}$

$\frac{B}{E} = \sqrt{\varepsilon_0\mu_0} = \frac{1}{c}$

25. (b) EM waves carry momentum and hence can exert pressure on surfaces. They also transfer energy to the surface so $p \neq 0$ and $E \neq 0$.

26. (b)

27. (a) The decreasing order of the wavelengths is as given below :
microwave, infrared, ultraviolet, gamma rays.

28. (b) Infrared causes heating effect.

29. (c) Speed of EM waves in vacuum $= \frac{1}{\sqrt{\mu_0\,\varepsilon_0}}$ = constant

30. (b)

31. (a) $I_D = \varepsilon_o\, d\phi_E / dt$.

32. (d) $\nu_{\gamma\text{-rays}} > \nu_{\text{visible radiation}} > \nu_{\text{infrared}} > \nu_{\text{Radio waves}}$

33. (b)

34. (d) Wave is uv rays.

35. (b)

36. (c) Electromagnetic waves are the combination of mutually perpendicular electric and magnetic fields.

37. (b) Audible waves are not electromagnetic wave.

38. (b) Wave impedance $= Z = \sqrt{\frac{\mu_0}{\varepsilon_0}} = 376.6\ \Omega$

39. (b)

40. (b) Depends on the magnitude of frequency

41. (d) $B_0 = \frac{E_0}{c} = \frac{9\times10^3}{3\times10^8} = 3\times10^{-5}\text{T}$.

42. (d) To generate electromagnetic waves we need accelerating charge particle.

43. (d)

44. (d) For an E.M. wave power is transmitted in a direction perpendicular to both the fields.

45. (c) Speed of light of vacuum $c = \frac{1}{\sqrt{\mu_0\varepsilon_0}}$ and in another medium $v = \frac{1}{\sqrt{\mu\varepsilon}}$

$\therefore \frac{c}{v} = \sqrt{\frac{\mu\varepsilon}{\mu_0\varepsilon_0}} = \sqrt{\mu_r K} \Rightarrow v = \frac{c}{\sqrt{\mu_r K}}$.

Speed Test-23

1. (b) $\frac{1}{f_R} = (1.5-1)\left(\frac{1}{R_1} - \frac{1}{R_2}\right)$

$$\frac{1}{f_v} = (1.45-1)\left(\frac{1}{R_1} - \frac{1}{R_2}\right)$$

$$\frac{f_v}{f_R} = \frac{0.5}{0.45} = \frac{10}{9}$$

$$f_R = \frac{9}{10} f_v = \frac{9}{10} \times 20 \text{ cm} = 18 \text{ cm}.$$

2. (a) We have,

$$\mu = \frac{\sin\left(\frac{A+\delta_m}{2}\right)}{\sin\left(\frac{A}{2}\right)}$$

$$\Rightarrow \cot\frac{A}{2} = \frac{\sin\left(\frac{A+\delta_m}{2}\right)}{\sin\left(\frac{A}{2}\right)}$$

$$\text{or } \sin\frac{A}{2} \cdot \cot\frac{A}{2} = \sin\left(\frac{A+\delta_m}{2}\right)$$

$$\text{or } \sin\frac{A}{2} \cdot \frac{\cos\frac{A}{2}}{\sin\frac{A}{2}} = \sin\left(\frac{A+\delta_m}{2}\right)$$

$$\text{or } \cos\frac{A}{2} = \cos\left[\frac{\pi}{2} - \left(\frac{A+\delta_m}{2}\right)\right]$$

$$\Rightarrow \frac{A}{2} = \frac{\pi}{2} - \left(\frac{A+\delta_m}{2}\right)$$

or $A = \pi - A - \delta_m \Rightarrow \delta_m = \pi - 2A$.

3. (a) Let the distance between the lenses be d.

Then, equivalent power is

$P = P_1 + P_2 - d P_1 P_2$

Given $P_1 = P_2 = +5$ D

$\therefore \quad P = (10 - 25d)$ D

For P to be –ve,

$10 - 25d < 0 \Rightarrow d > \frac{2}{5}$ m

or, $d > 0.4$ m or $d > 40$ cm

4. (b) ${}^a\mu_g = \frac{\sin 60°}{\sin 35°}$ ... (i)

${}^a\mu_w = \frac{\sin 60°}{\sin 41°}$ ... (ii)

${}^w\mu_g = \frac{\sin 41°}{\sin\theta}$ ... (iii)

${}^a\mu_w \times {}^w\mu_g = {}^a\mu_g$

$$\frac{\sin 60°}{\sin 41°} \times \frac{\sin 41°}{\sin\theta} = \frac{\sin 60°}{\sin 35°}$$

(Using (i), (ii) and (iii))

$= \sin\theta = \sin 35° \quad \theta = 35°$

5. (d)

r

$h = 12$ cm

C

$$\sin C = \frac{1}{\mu} = \frac{1}{4/3} = \frac{3}{4}.$$

Now $\quad r = h \tan C$

$$= 12 \times \frac{3}{\sqrt{7}} = \frac{36}{\sqrt{7}} \text{ cm}$$

6. (a) $\frac{1}{f} = (\mu - 1)\left(\frac{1}{R_1} - \frac{1}{R_2}\right)$

According to Cauchy relation

$\mu = A + \frac{B}{\lambda^2} + \frac{C}{\lambda^4} \ldots$ Hence $f \propto \lambda$.

Hence, red light having maximum wavelength has maximum focal length.

$\therefore \quad f_v < f_r$ and also $F_v > F_r$ as focal length is negative for a concave lens.

7. (c) To minimise spherical aberration in a lens, the total deviation should be equally distributed over the two surfaces.

8. (d)

$f = 10$ cm

B A

–10 cm –20 cm

The focal length of the mirror

$$-\frac{1}{f} = \frac{1}{v} + \frac{1}{u}$$

For A end of the rod the image distance

When $u_1 = -20$ cm

$$\Rightarrow \frac{-1}{10} = \frac{1}{v_1} - \frac{1}{20}$$

$$\frac{1}{v_1}=\frac{-1}{10}+\frac{1}{20}=\frac{-2+1}{20}$$

$v_1=-20$ cm

For when $u_2=-30$ cm

$$\frac{1}{f}=\frac{1}{v_2}-\frac{1}{30}$$

$$\frac{1}{v_2}=\frac{-1}{10}+\frac{1}{30}=\frac{-30+10}{300}=\frac{-20}{300}$$

$v_2=-15$ cm

$L=v_2-v_1=-15-(-20)$

$L=5$ cm

9. (a) Magnification

$$=\frac{f_0}{f_e}=\frac{\text{Angle subtended by final image on the eye}}{\text{Angle subtended by the object on eye (or objective)}}$$

$$\Rightarrow \frac{0.3\text{m}}{3\text{cm}}=\frac{\beta}{0.5°}\Rightarrow\frac{30\text{ cm}}{3\text{cm}}=\frac{\beta}{0.5°}$$

$\Rightarrow \beta=5°$

10. (b) Due to difference in refractive indices images obtained will be two. Two media will form images at two different points due to difference in focal lengths.

11. (c) For reading purposes :

u = – 25 cm, v = – 50 cm, f = ?

$$\frac{1}{f}=\frac{1}{v}-\frac{1}{u}=-\frac{1}{50}+\frac{1}{25}=\frac{1}{50};$$

$$P=\frac{100}{f}=+2\text{ D}$$

For distant vision, f′ = distance of far point = –3 m

$$P=\frac{1}{f'}=-\frac{1}{3}\text{D}=-0.33\text{ D}$$

12. (a) Clearly,

$i+r+90°=180°$

$\Rightarrow i+r=90°$ ...(i)

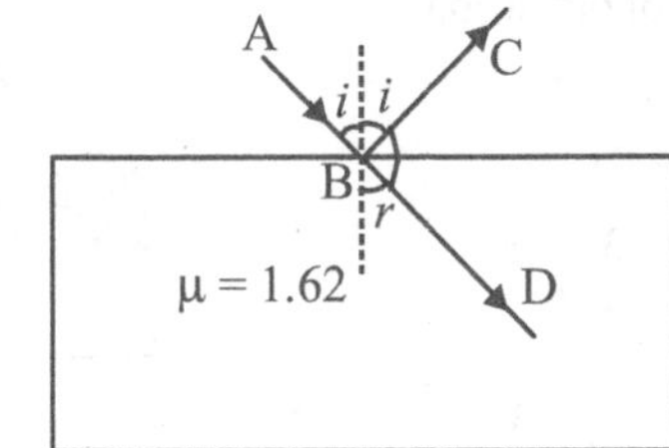

Now, $\frac{\sin i}{\sin r}=\mu$

$\Rightarrow \frac{\sin i}{\sin(90°-i)}=\mu$, from (1)

or $\frac{\sin i}{\cos i}=\mu\Rightarrow \tan i=\mu$

or $i=\tan^{-1}(\mu)$ i.e., $i=\tan^{-1}(1.62)$

13. (b) $f_0=100$ cm, $f_e=5$ cm

When final image is formed at least distance of distinct vision (d), then

$$M=\frac{f_0}{f_e}\left(1+\frac{f_e}{d}\right)=\frac{100}{5}\left(1+\frac{5}{25}\right)\quad[\because D=25\text{ cm}]$$

$$M=20\times\frac{6}{5}=24$$

14. (b) Secondary rainbow is formed by rays undergoing internal reflection twice inside the drop.

15. (b) $\tan 45°=\frac{h}{60}\Rightarrow h=60m$

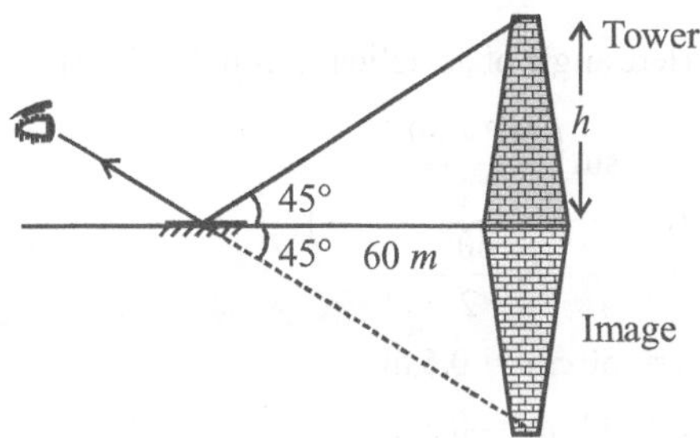

16. (c) Using, $\frac{\mu}{v}-\frac{1}{u}=\frac{\mu-1}{R}$

or $\frac{2}{v}-\frac{1}{\infty}=\frac{2-1}{R}$

$\therefore\quad v=2R$

17. (a) ${}_an_\ell=1.6,\ {}_an_w=1.33$

f = 20 cm

We have,

$$\frac{1}{f}=({}_an_\ell-1)\left(\frac{1}{R_1}-\frac{1}{R_2}\right)$$

$$\frac{1}{20}=(1.6-1)\left(\frac{1}{R_1}-\frac{1}{R_2}\right)\quad .....(1)$$

Also, $\frac{1}{f'}=({}_wn_\ell-1)\left(\frac{1}{R_1}-\frac{1}{R_2}\right)$

$$=\left(\frac{{}_an_\ell}{{}_an_w}-1\right)\left(\frac{1}{R_1}-\frac{1}{R_2}\right)$$

$$\frac{1}{f'}=\left(\frac{1.6}{1.33}-1\right)\left(\frac{1}{R_1}-\frac{1}{R_2}\right)\quad .....(2)$$

Dividing equation (1) by (2)

$$\Rightarrow \frac{f'}{20}=\frac{0.6}{(1.2-1)}$$

$$f'=\frac{0.6\times20}{0.2}=60\text{ cm.}$$

Hence it's focal length is three times longer than in air.

18. (a) $m = \frac{v_0}{|u_0|}\left(1+\frac{d}{f_e}\right) = \frac{20}{5}\left(1+\frac{20}{10}\right)$

$= 4\left(\frac{10+20}{10}\right) = \frac{4\times 30}{10} = 12$

19. (a) Given $i = 60°$

$A = \delta = e$

$\delta = i + e - A \Rightarrow \delta = i \quad (\because e = A)$

$$\mu = \frac{\sin\left(\frac{A+\delta_m}{2}\right)}{\sin\frac{A}{2}}$$

Here angle of deviation is min. ($\because i = e$)

$$\mu = \frac{\sin\left(\frac{60°+60°}{2}\right)}{\sin\frac{60°}{2}} = 1.73$$

20. (b) $u = -50\text{ cm} = -0.5\text{ m}$

$v = -30\text{ cm} = -0.3\text{ m}$

$$P = \frac{1}{f} = \frac{1}{v} - \frac{1}{u} = \frac{-1}{0.3} + \frac{1}{0.5} = \frac{-0.2}{0.15} = -1.33\text{ D}.$$

21. (b) Object distance $u = -40$ cm

Focal length $f = -20$ cm

According to mirror formula

$\frac{1}{u} + \frac{1}{v} = \frac{1}{f}$ or $\frac{1}{v} = \frac{1}{f} - \frac{1}{u}$

or $\frac{1}{v} + \frac{1}{-20} - \frac{1}{(-40)} = \frac{1}{-20} + \frac{1}{40}$

$\frac{1}{v} = \frac{-2+1}{40} = -\frac{1}{40}$ or $v = -40$ cm.

Negative sign shows that image is infront of concave mirror. The image is real.

Magnification, $m = \frac{-v}{u} = -\frac{(-40)}{(-40)} = -1$

The image is of the same size and inverted.

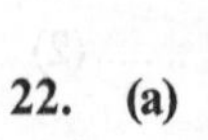

22. (a)

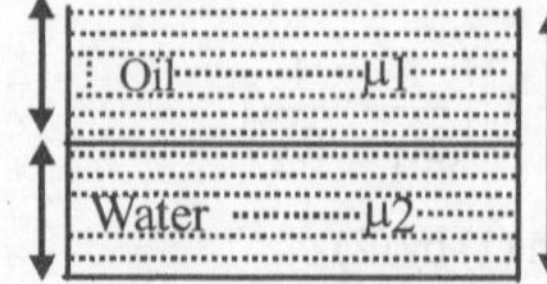

As refractive index, $\mu = \frac{\text{Real depth}}{\text{Apparent depth}}$

$\therefore$ Apparent depth of the vessel when viewed from above is

$$d_{\text{apparent}} = \frac{x}{2\mu_1} + \frac{x}{2\mu_2} = \frac{x}{2}\left(\frac{1}{\mu_1} + \frac{1}{\mu_2}\right)$$

$$= \frac{x}{2}\left(\frac{\mu_2+\mu_1}{\mu_1\mu_2}\right) = \frac{x(\mu_1+\mu_2)}{2\mu_1\mu_2}$$

23. (d) As $r_1 < i_1$ i.e., the incident ray bends towards the normal $\Rightarrow$ medium 2 is denser than medium 1.
Or $r_2 < i_1 \Rightarrow$ medium 3 is denser than medium 1.
Also, $r_2 > r_1 \Rightarrow$ medium 2 is denser than medium 3.

24. (d) Here, $v_A = 1.8 \times 10^8\text{ m s}^{-1}$
$v_B = 2.4 \times 10^8\text{ m s}^{-1}$
Light travels slower in denser medium. Hence medium A is a denser medium and medium B is a rarer medium. Here, Light travels from medium A to medium B. Let C be the critical angle between them.

$\therefore \quad \sin C = {}^A\mu_B = \frac{1}{{}^B\mu_A}$

Refractive index of medium B w.r.t. to medium A is

$${}^A\mu_B = \frac{\text{Velocity of light in medium } A}{\text{Velocity of light in medium } B} = \frac{v_A}{v_B}$$

$\therefore \quad \sin C = \frac{v_A}{v_B} = \frac{1.8\times10^8}{2.4\times10^8} = \frac{3}{4}$ or $C = \sin^{-1}\left(\frac{3}{4}\right)$

25. (a) For a thin prism, $D = (\mu - 1)A$
Since $\lambda_b < \lambda_r \Rightarrow \mu_r < \mu_b \Rightarrow D_1 < D_2$

26. (b) Difference between apparent and real depth of a pond is due to the refraction of light, not due to the total internal reflection. Other three phenomena are due to the total internal reflection.

27. (b) Using the lens formula $\frac{1}{f} = \frac{1}{v} - \frac{1}{u}$

Given $v = d$, for equal size image $|v| = |u| = d$

By sign convention $u = -d$

$\therefore \quad \frac{1}{f} = \frac{1}{d} + \frac{1}{d}$ or $f = \frac{d}{2}$

28. (a) Due to covering the reflection from lower part is not there so it makes the image less bright.

29. (b) From the fig.
Angle of deviation,

$\delta = i + e - A$

Here, $e = i$

and $e = \frac{3}{4}A$

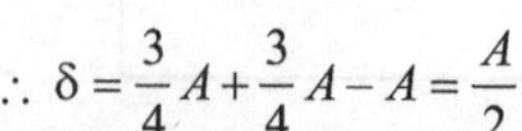

$\therefore \delta = \frac{3}{4}A + \frac{3}{4}A - A = \frac{A}{2}$

For equilateral prism, $A = 60°$

$\therefore \delta = \frac{60°}{2} = 30°$

30. (a) Power of lens, P (in dioptre)

$$= \frac{100}{\text{focal length f (in cm)}}$$

$$\therefore \quad f = \frac{100}{10} = 10 \text{ cm}$$

By lens maker's formula, $\frac{1}{f} = (\mu - 1)\left(\frac{1}{R_1} - \frac{1}{R_2}\right)$

For biconvex lens, $R_1 = +R$, and $R_2 = -R$

$$\therefore \quad \frac{1}{f} = (\mu - 1)\left(\frac{1}{R} + \frac{1}{R}\right)$$

$$\frac{1}{f} = (\mu - 1)\left(\frac{2}{R}\right)$$

$$\frac{1}{10} = (\mu - 1)\left(\frac{2}{10}\right)$$

$$(\mu - 1) = \frac{1}{2} \text{ or } \mu = \frac{1}{2} + 1 = \frac{3}{2}$$

31. **(d)** In the later case microscope will be focussed for *O'*. So, it is required to be lifted by distance *OO'*.
OO' = real depth of O – apparent depth of *O*.

Image → •*O'*
O

$$= 3 - \frac{3}{1.5} \quad \left[\mu = \frac{\text{real depth}}{\text{apparent depth}}\right]$$

$$= 3\left[\frac{1.5 - 1}{1.5}\right] = \frac{3 \times .5}{1.5} = 1 \text{ cm}$$

32. **(d)** The cause of chromatic aberration is that lens focusses different colours at different points.

33. **(c)** For the prism as the angle of incidence (i) increases, the angle of deviation (δ) first decreases goes to minimum value and then increases.

34. **(d)** $d_A : d_B = 6 : 4$
$\because$ Time taken $\propto$ thickness

and time taken $\propto \frac{1}{\text{velocity}}$

$\therefore$ Thickness $\propto \frac{1}{\text{velocity}}$

$$\therefore \quad \frac{d_A}{d_B} = \frac{v_B}{v_A}$$

Also, $\mu = \frac{c}{v} \quad \therefore \frac{\mu_A}{\mu_B} = \frac{v_B}{v_A}$

$$\therefore \quad \frac{d_A}{d_B} = \frac{\mu_A}{\mu_B} = \frac{6}{4} = \frac{3}{2} = 1.5$$

$$\therefore \quad {}_B\mu_A = 1.5$$

35. **(b)** Since $\frac{\text{Apparent depth}}{\text{Real depth}} = \frac{1}{\mu}$
$\Rightarrow$ Apparent depth = d/μ
So mark raised up = Real depth – Apparent depth

$$= d - \frac{d}{\mu} = d\left(1 - \frac{1}{\mu}\right) = \left(\frac{\mu - 1}{\mu}\right)d$$

36. **(b)** Dispersive power of a prism $\omega = \frac{\mu_V - \mu_R}{\mu_y - 1} = \frac{d\mu}{\mu - 1}$,

where $\mu = \mu_y = \frac{\mu_V + \mu_R}{2}$

37. **(a)** Considering refraction at the curved surface,
$u = -20,\ \mu_2 = 1$
$\mu_1 = 3/2,\ R = +20$

Applying $\frac{\mu_2}{v} - \frac{\mu_1}{u} = \frac{\mu_2 - \mu_1}{R}$

$$\Rightarrow \frac{1}{v} - \frac{3/2}{-20} = \frac{1 - 3/2}{20} \Rightarrow v = -10$$

i.e., 10 cm below the curved surface or 10 cm above the actual position of flower.

38. **(b)** When θ = 90° then $\frac{360}{\theta} = \frac{360}{90} = 4$

is an even number. The number of images formed is given by

$$n = \frac{360}{\theta} - 1 = \frac{360}{90} - 1 = 4 - 1 = 3$$

39. **(b)** The critical angle of incidence is that angle at which angle of refraction is 90°.

n_1
n_2
i_c

$\sin i_c = \frac{n_1}{n_2}$ where $n_2 > n_1$

As, refractive index = $\frac{\text{velocity (air)}}{\text{velocity (medium)}}$

$$\therefore \sin i_c = \frac{2.2 \times 10^8 \text{ m/sec}}{2.4 \times 10^8 \text{ m/sec}} = \frac{11}{12}$$

$$\Rightarrow i_C = \sin^{-1}\left(\frac{11}{12}\right)$$

40. **(b)** $\frac{P_a}{P_l} = \frac{\left(\frac{\mu_g}{\mu_a} - 1\right)}{\left(\frac{\mu_g}{\mu_l} - 1\right)} = \frac{+5}{-100/100} = -5$

$$-5\left(\frac{\mu_g}{\mu_l} - 1\right) = \frac{\mu_g}{\mu_a} - 1$$

$$\frac{1.5}{\mu_1}-1=\frac{-1}{5}(1.5-1)=-0.1;\ \mu_1=\frac{1.5}{0.9}=\frac{5}{3}$$

41. (d) $\sin C=\frac{1}{\mu}=\frac{1}{\sqrt{2}}$ $\therefore\ C=\sin^{-1}\left(\frac{1}{\sqrt{2}}\right)=45°$

Now $\frac{\sin C}{\sin r}=\frac{1}{\mu}$ or $\frac{\sin 45°}{\sin r}=\frac{1}{\sqrt{2}}$

$\sin r=1$ or $r=90°$

42. (d)

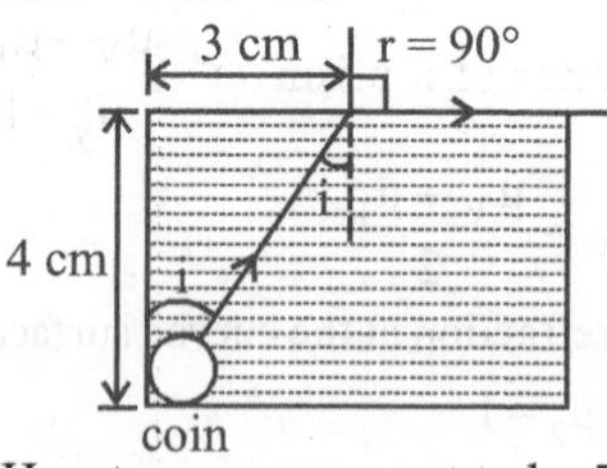

Hypotenuse comes out to be 5 cm.

Since, $\frac{1}{\mu}=\frac{\sin i}{\sin 90°}$

$\mu=\frac{1}{\sin i}=\frac{5}{3}$

Speed, $v=\frac{c}{\mu}=\frac{3\times10^8}{5/3}=1.8\times10^8$ m/s

43. (a)

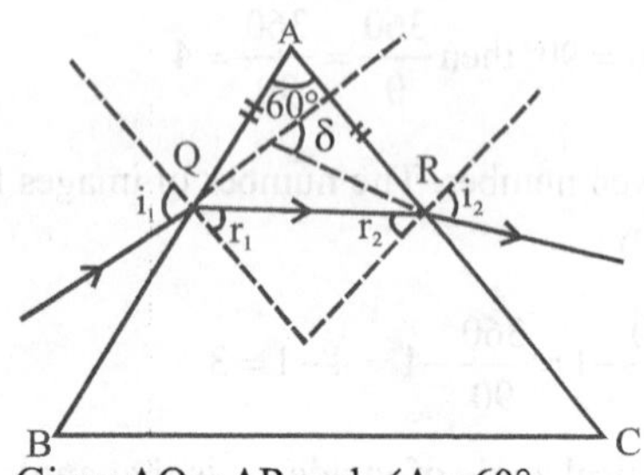

Given AQ = AR and $\angle A=60°$

$\therefore\ \angle AQR=\angle ARQ=60°$

$\therefore\ r_1=r_2=30°$

Applying Snell's law on face AB.

$\sin i_1=\mu\sin r_1$

$\Rightarrow\ \sin i_1=\sqrt{3}\sin 30°=\sqrt{3}\times\frac{1}{2}=\frac{\sqrt{3}}{2}$

$\therefore\ i_1=60°$

Similarly, $i_2=60°$

In a prism, deviation

$\delta=i_1+i_2-A=60°+60°-60°=60°$

44. (a) $\frac{1}{f}=\left(\frac{\mu_g}{\mu_m}-1\right)\left(\frac{1}{R_1}-\frac{1}{R_2}\right)$

If $\mu_g=\mu_m$, then $\frac{1}{f}=(1-1)\left(\frac{1}{R_1}-\frac{1}{R_2}\right)$

$\Rightarrow\ \frac{1}{f}=0$

$$\boxed{f=\frac{1}{0}=\infty}$$

This implies that the liquid must have refractive index equal to glass.

45. (b) Minimum deviation of the prism when it is dipped in water $=\delta_m'=({}_w\mu_g-1)A$

$$=\left(\frac{{}_a\mu_g}{{}_a\mu_\omega}-1\right)A=\left(\frac{\frac{3}{2}}{\frac{4}{3}}-1\right)A=\frac{1}{8}A$$

Minimum deviation of the prism with respect to air

$$=\delta_m=(\mu-1)A=\left(\frac{3}{2}-1\right)A=\frac{1}{2}A$$

$$\frac{\delta_m'}{\delta_m}=\frac{\frac{1}{8}A}{\frac{1}{2}A}=\frac{1}{4}$$

Speed Test-24

1. **(b)** For path difference λ, phase

difference $= 2\pi\left(Q = \frac{2\pi}{\lambda}x = \frac{2\pi}{\lambda}.\lambda = 2\pi\right)$

$\Rightarrow I = I_0 + I_0 + 2I_0 \cos 2\pi$

$\Rightarrow I = 4I_0 \qquad (\because \cos 2\pi = 1)$

For $x = \frac{\lambda}{4}$, phase difference $= \frac{\pi}{2}$

$\therefore I' = I_1 + I_2 + 2\sqrt{I_1}\sqrt{I_2}\cos\frac{\pi}{2}$

If $I_1 = I_2 = I_0$ then $I' = 2I_0 = 2.\frac{I}{4} = \frac{I}{2}$

2. **(c)** Here Angle of incidence, i = 57
tan 57° = 1.54
$u_{glass} = \tan i$
It means, Here Brewster's law is followed and the reflected ray is completely polarised.
Now, when reflected ray is analysed through a polaroid then intensity of light is given by malus law.
i.e. $I = I_0 \cos^2\theta$
on rotating polaroid 'θ' changes. Due to which intensity first decreases and then increases.

3. **(b)** Let nth fringe of 2500 Å coincide with (n – 2)th fringe of 3500Å.

∴ 3500 (n – 2) = 2500 × n
1000 n = 7000, n = 7

∴ 7th order fringe of 1st source will coincide with 5th order fringe of 2nd source.

4. **(a)** When incident wavefronts passes through a prism, then lower portion of wavefront (B) is delayed resulting in a tilt. So, time taken by light to reach *A*' from *A* is equal to the time taken to reach *B*' from *B*.

5. **(b)** ${}^a\mu_g = \tan\theta_P$ where θ_P = polarising angle.
or, ${}^a\mu_g = \tan 60°$

or, $\frac{c}{v_g} = \sqrt{3}$

or, $v_g = \frac{c}{\sqrt{3}} = \frac{3\times10^8}{\sqrt{3}} = \sqrt{3}\times10^8\,ms^{-1}$

6. **(c)** Angular width $= \frac{\lambda}{d} = 10^{-3}$ (given)

∴ No. of fringes within 0.12° will be

$n = \frac{0.12\times2\pi}{360\times10^{-3}} = [2.09]$

∴ The number of bright spots will be two.

7. **(c)** Here $A^2 = a_1^2 + a_2^2 + 2a_1a_2\cos\delta$

$\because a_1 = a_2 = a$

$\therefore A^2 = 2a^2(1+\cos\delta) = 2a^2\left(1 + 2\cos^2\frac{\delta}{2} - 1\right)$

$\Rightarrow A^2 \propto \cos^2\frac{\delta}{2}$

Now, $I \propto A^2 \quad \therefore I \propto A^2 \propto \cos^2\frac{\delta}{2}$

$\therefore I \propto \cos^2\frac{\delta}{2}$.

8. **(b)** $\Delta x_1 = (\mu_1 - 1)t = (1.5-1)t = 0.5t$

and $\Delta x_2 = (\mu_2 - 1)\times 2t = \left(\frac{4}{3} - 1\right)\times 2t = \frac{2}{3}t$.

As $\Delta x_2 > \Delta x_1$, so shift will be along –ve *y*-axis.

9. **(d)** Given: D = 2m; d = 1 mm = 1×10^{-3} m
$\lambda = 600\text{ nm} = 600\times10^{-6}$ m
Width of central bright fringe (= 2β)

$= \frac{2\lambda D}{d} = \frac{2\times600\times10^{-6}\times2}{1\times10^{-3}}\text{ m} = 2.4\text{ mm}$

10. **(d)** Conditions for diffraction minima are
Path diff. $\Delta x = n\lambda$ and Phase diff. $\delta\phi = 2n\pi$
Path diff. $= n\lambda = 2\lambda$
Phase diff. $= 2n\pi = 4\pi \quad (\because n = 2)$

11. **(c)** When the wavelength of light used is comparable with the separation between two points, the image of the object will be a ϕ diffraction pattern whose size will be

$\theta = \frac{1.22\lambda}{D}$

where λ = wavelength of light used
D = diameter of the objective
Two objects whose images are closer than this distance, will not be resolved.

12. **(d)** The waves reflected from the top layer of oil interfere with the wave train reflected from the lower surface of thin oil film producing light and dark coloured pattern.

13. **(d)** Phase difference, $\phi = \frac{2\pi}{\lambda}\times$ Path difference

$\phi = \frac{2\pi}{\lambda}\times\frac{\lambda}{6} = \frac{\pi}{3} = 60°$

As, $I = I_{max}\cos^2\frac{\phi}{2}$

$I = I_0\cos^2\frac{60°}{2} = I_0\times\left(\frac{\sqrt{3}}{2}\right)^2 = \frac{3}{4}I_0 \quad \frac{I}{I_0} = \frac{3}{4}$

14. **(b)**

15. (a) We know that for maxima

$$b\sin\theta = (2n+1)\frac{\lambda}{2}$$

or $\sin\theta = \frac{2n+1}{2}\left(\frac{\lambda}{b}\right)$

So on decreasing the slit width, 'b', keeping λ same, sin θ and hence θ increases.

16. (b) If the angular limit of resolution of human eye is R then

$$R = \frac{1.22\lambda}{a} = \frac{1.22\times5\times10^{-7}}{2\times10^{-3}} \text{ rad}$$

$$= \frac{1.22\times5\times10^{-7}}{2\times10^{-3}}\times\frac{180}{\pi}\times60 \text{ minute} = 1 \text{ minute}$$

17. (c) $\mu = \tan i$

$\Rightarrow i = \tan^{-1}(\mu) = \tan^{-1}(\sqrt{3}) = 60°$.

18. (d) Order of the fringe can be counted on either side of the central maximum. For example, no. 3 is first order bright fringe.

$$\Delta X_C = \lambda,\ \Delta X_A = \frac{\lambda}{2}$$

$$\Delta X_C - \Delta X_A = \frac{\lambda}{2} = 300\text{nm}$$

19. (a) For a circularly polarised light electric field remains constant with time.

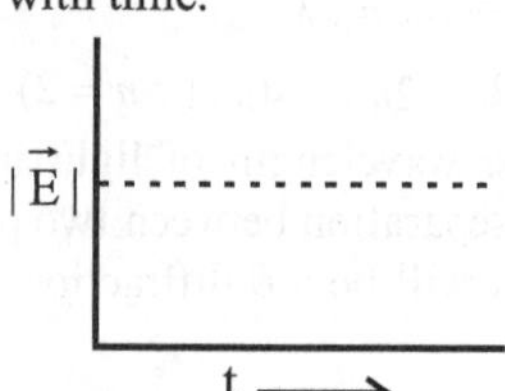

20. (b) $\beta' = \frac{\beta}{\mu} = \frac{0.133}{1.33} = 0.1$ cm

21. (b)

22. (d) Let λ be wavelength of monochromatic light incident on slit S, then angular distance between two consecutive fringes, that is the angular fringe width is

$$\theta = \frac{\lambda}{d}$$

where *d* is distance between coherent sources.

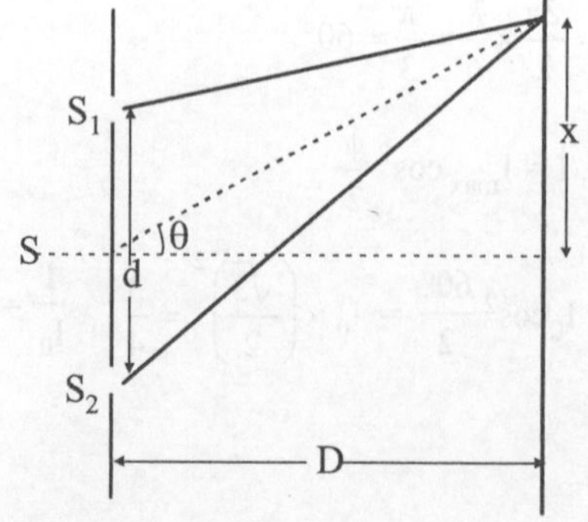

Give, $\frac{\Delta\theta}{\theta} = \frac{10}{100}$

So, from eq. (1),

$$\frac{\Delta\lambda}{\lambda} = \frac{\Delta\theta}{\theta} = \frac{10}{100} = 0.1$$

$\Rightarrow \Delta\lambda = 0.1\lambda = 0.1\times5890\text{Å} = 589\text{Å}$ (increases)

Note : Since, $\theta \propto \lambda$, as θ increases, λ increases.

23. (c) $\sin\theta = \frac{\lambda}{d} = \frac{589\times10^{-9}}{0.589\times10^{-3}} = 10^{-3} = \frac{1}{1000} = 0.001$

24. (c) In Fraunhoffer diffraction, for minimum intensity,

$$\Delta x = m\frac{\lambda}{2}$$

For first minimum, m = 1

$$\therefore\ \Delta x = \frac{\lambda}{2}$$

25. (d) Optical path difference

$\Delta x = (\mu_2 - \mu_1)t$.

26. (b) Separation between slits are (r_1=) 16 cm and (r_2=) 9 cm. Actual distance of separation

$= \sqrt{r_1 r_2} = \sqrt{16\times9} = 12\text{cm}$

27. (b) $\phi = \frac{\pi}{3}$, $a_1 = 4$, $a_2 = 3$

So, $A = \sqrt{a_1^2 + a_2^2 + 2a_1a_2\cos\phi} \approx 6$

28. (c) $\beta = \frac{D\lambda}{d}$, where D is the distance between the slits & screen and d is the separation between the slits.

$$\beta' = \frac{2D\lambda}{d/2} = \frac{4D\lambda}{d} = 4\beta$$

29. (b) For first minima at P

AP – BP = λ

$$AP - MP = \frac{\lambda}{2}$$

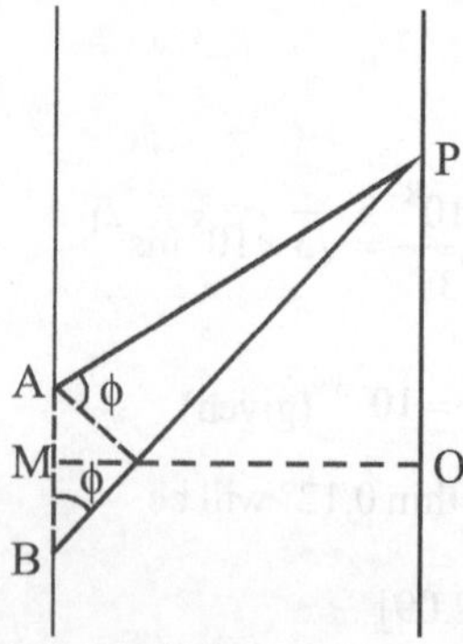

So phase difference, $\phi = \frac{2\pi}{\lambda}\times\frac{\lambda}{2} = \pi$ radian

30. (a) Shift $= \frac{D}{d}(\mu - 1)\,t = \frac{\beta}{\lambda}(\mu - 1)\,t = 4\beta$

$$t = \frac{4\lambda}{\mu - 1} = \frac{4 \times 6000 \times 10^{-10}}{1.5 - 1} = 4.8\ \mu m$$

31. (c) The fringe width is given by, $\beta = \frac{\lambda D}{d}$

The angular width of fringe is given by

$$\frac{d}{D} = \frac{\lambda}{\beta} = \frac{6 \times 10^{-7}}{0.12 \times 10^{-3}} = 5 \times 10^{-3}\ \text{rad.}$$

32. (c) Distance of nth maxima, $x = n\lambda \frac{D}{d} \propto \lambda$

As $\lambda_b < \lambda_g \quad \therefore\ x_{blue} < x_{green}$

33. (a) As $\beta = \frac{\lambda D}{d}$ and $\lambda_b < \lambda_y$,

$\therefore$ fringe width β will decrease

34. (c) At Brewster's angle, only the reflected light is plane polarised, but transmitted light is partially polarised.

35. (b) $\Delta x_{max} = 2\lambda.$

So there are five maxima.

These are for $\Delta x = 0, \pm\lambda, \pm 2\lambda.$

36. (c) The nearest white spot will be at P, the central maxima.

$$\therefore\ y = \frac{2d}{3} - \frac{d}{2} = \frac{d}{6}$$

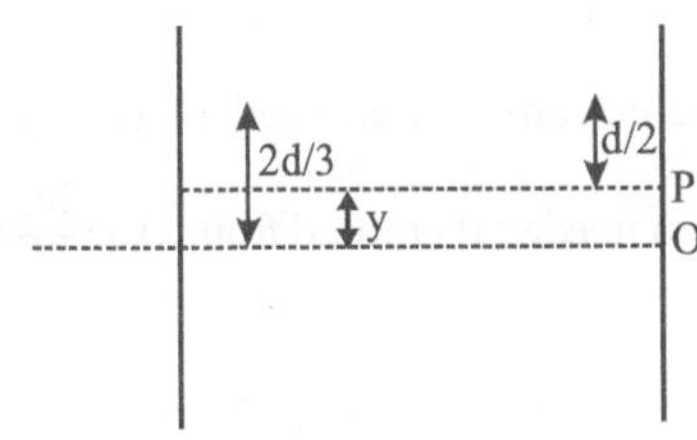

37. (d) : Resultant amplitude,

$$A = \sqrt{(A_1)^2 + (A_2)^2 + 2A_1A_2\cos\theta}$$

Here, $A_1 = A_2 = 1$ cm, $\phi = 3\pi$ rad

$$\therefore\ A = \sqrt{1^2 + 1^2 + 2 \times 1 \times 1 \times \cos 3\pi}$$

$$= \sqrt{2 + 2 \times (-1)} = 0$$

38. (c)

39. (c)

40. (c)

41. (b) (Light bends upwards)

Plane WF

μ increases

Vel decreases

Refracted WF

42. (a) $I = I_0\left(\frac{\sin\phi}{\phi}\right)^2$ and $\phi = \frac{\pi}{\lambda}(b\sin\theta)$

When the slit width is doubled, the amplitude of the wave at the centre of the screen is doubled, so the intensity at the centre is increased by a factor 4.

43. (a)

44. (a) Where n is equivalent number of fringe by which the centre fringe is shifted due to mica sheet

$$\lambda = \frac{(\mu - 1)t}{n} = \frac{(1.5 - 1)6 \times 10^{-6}}{5}$$

$$= 6 \times 10^{-7}\ \text{m} = 6000\ \text{Å}$$

45. (c) Suppose intensity of unpolarised light = 100.

$\therefore$ Intensity of polarised light from first nicol prism

$$= \frac{I_0}{2} = \frac{1}{2} \times 100 = 50$$

According to law of Malus,

$$I = I_0\cos^2\theta = 50\,(\cos 60°)^2 = 50 \times \left(\frac{1}{2}\right)^2 = 12.5$$

Speed Test-25

1. (d) Wavelength of particle $(\lambda_1) = \frac{h}{mv} = \frac{h}{(1\times10^{-3})\times v}$

where v is the velocity of the particle.
Wavelength of electron

$$(\lambda_2) = \frac{h}{(9.1\times10^{-31})\times(3\times10^6)}$$

But $\lambda_1 = \lambda_2$

$$\therefore \frac{h}{(1\times10^{-3})\times v} = \frac{h}{(9.1\times10^{-31})\times(3\times10^6)}$$

$$\Rightarrow v = \frac{9.1\times10^{-31}\times3\times10^6}{10^{-3}}$$
$$= 2.73\times10^{-21}\,ms^{-1}$$

2. (a) For electron De-Broglie wavelength,

$$\lambda_e = \frac{h}{\sqrt{2mE}}$$

For photon $E = pc$

$\Rightarrow$ De-Broglie wavelength, $\lambda_{Ph} = \frac{hc}{E}$

$$\therefore \frac{\lambda_e}{\lambda_{Ph}} = \frac{h}{\sqrt{2mE}}\times\frac{E}{hc} = \left(\frac{E}{2m}\right)^{1/2}\frac{1}{c}$$

3. (d) The electron ejected with maximum speed v_{max} are stopped by electric field $E = 4N/C$ after travelling a distance $d = 1m$

$$\frac{1}{2}mv_{max}^2 = eEd = 4eV$$

The energy of incident photon $= \frac{1240}{200} = 6.2$ eV

From equation of photo electric effect

$$\frac{1}{2}mv_{max}^2 = h\nu - \phi_0$$

$$\therefore \phi_0 = 6.2 - 4 = 2.2\text{ eV}$$

4. (b) $\lambda_{min} = 1$ Å (given)

$$\because \lambda_{min} = \frac{1240}{E}\text{ (eV) (nm)}$$

Thus, $E = \frac{1240(eV)(nm)}{0.01(nm)} = 12400$ eV

E = 12.4 KeV

5. (a) The maximum kinetic energy of an electron accelerated through a potential difference of V volt is $\frac{1}{2}mv^2 = eV$

$\therefore$ maximum velocity $v = \sqrt{\frac{2eV}{m}}$

$$v = \sqrt{\frac{2\times1.6\times10^{-19}\times15000}{9.1\times10^{-31}}}$$

$v = 7.26\times10^7$ m/s

6. (b) Photoelectrons are emitted in A alone. Energy of electron needed if emitted from $A = \frac{h\upsilon}{e}eV$

$$\therefore E_A = \frac{(6.6\times10^{-34})\times(1.8\times10^{14})}{1.6\times10^{-19}} = 0.74\text{ eV}$$

$$E_B = \frac{(6.6\times10^{-34})\times(2.2\times10^{14})}{1.6\times10^{-19}} = 0.91\text{ eV}$$

Incident energy 0.825 eV is greater than E_A (0.74 eV) but less than E_B (0.91 eV).

7. (a) According to relation, $E = \frac{1}{2}mv^2$

$$\sqrt{\frac{2E}{m}} = v$$

$$\lambda = \frac{h}{\sqrt{2mE}}$$

Because $m_1 < m_3 < m_2$

So for same λ, $E_1 > E_3 > E_2$.

8. **(a)** Emission of electron from a substance under the action of light is photoelectric effect. Light must be at a sufficiently high frequency. It may be visible light, U.V, X-rays. So U.V. cause electron emission.

9. **(b)** $\lambda_0 = \frac{c}{v_0} = \frac{3\times10^8}{5\times10^{14}} = 6\times10^{-7}\text{m} = 6000\text{Å}$

10. **(c)** $\lambda = \frac{h}{mv}$, $v = \frac{m_0}{\sqrt{1-\left(\frac{v}{c}\right)^2}}$, $v\to c$, $m\to\infty$

hence, $\lambda \to 0$.

11. **(a)** Give that, only 25% of 200W converter electrical energy into light of yellow colour

$$\left(\frac{hc}{\lambda}\right)\times N = 200\times\frac{25}{100}$$

Where N is the No. of photons emitted per second, h is planck's constant and c is speed of light.

$$N = \frac{200\times25}{100}\times\frac{\lambda}{hc}$$

$$= \frac{200\times25\times0.6\times10^{-6}}{100\times6.2\times10^{-34}\times3\times10^8} = 1.5\times10^{20}$$

12. **(d)** For photon E = hv

$$E = \frac{hc}{\lambda} \Rightarrow \lambda_2 = \frac{hc}{E} \quad \text{...(i)}$$

for proton $E = \frac{1}{2}m_p v_p^2$

$$E = \frac{1}{2}\frac{m_p^2 v_p^2}{m} \Rightarrow p = \sqrt{2mE}$$

From De Broglie Eqn.

$$p = \frac{h}{\lambda_1} \Rightarrow \lambda_1 = \frac{h}{p} = \frac{h}{\sqrt{2mE}} \quad \text{...(ii)}$$

$$\frac{\lambda_2}{\lambda_1} = \frac{hc}{E\times\frac{h}{\sqrt{2mE}}} \propto E^{-1/2}$$

13. **(a)** $h\nu = W_0 + E_k = 3.5 + 1.2 = 4.7$ eV

14. **(a)** $\phi = 6.2\text{ eV} = 6.2\times1.6\times10^{-19}$ J

$V = 5$ volt

$$\frac{hc}{\lambda} - \phi = eV_0$$

$$\Rightarrow \lambda = \frac{hc}{\phi + eV_0}$$

$$= \frac{6.6\times10^{-34}\times3\times10^8}{1.6\times10^{-19}(6.2+5)} \approx 10^{-7}\text{ m}$$

This range lies in ultra violet range.

15. **(c)** Applying Einstein's formula for photo-electricity

$$h\nu = \phi + \frac{1}{2}mv^2; \qquad h\nu = \phi + K$$

$$\phi = h\nu - K$$

If we use 2ν frequency then let the kinetic energy becomes K'

So, $h.2\nu = \phi + K'$

$$2h\nu = h\nu - K + K'$$

$$K' = h\nu + K$$

16. **(a)** $\because \lambda_0 = \frac{hc}{\phi}$

$$\therefore (\lambda_0)_{sodium} = \frac{6.6\times10^{-34}\times3\times10^8}{2\times1.6\times10^{-19}} = 6188\text{ Å}$$

$$\because \lambda_0 \propto \frac{1}{\phi} \Rightarrow \frac{(\lambda_0)_{sodium}}{(\lambda_0)_{copper}} = \frac{(\phi)_{copper}}{(\phi)_{sodium}}$$

$$\Rightarrow (\lambda_0)_{copper} = \frac{2}{4}\times6188 = 3094\text{ Å}$$

To eject photo-electrons from sodium the longest wavelength is 6188 Å and that for copper is 3094 Å.

Hence for light of wavelength 4000 Å, sodium is suitable.

17. **(c)** $\frac{1}{2}mv^2 = \frac{hc}{\lambda} - \phi \Rightarrow v = \sqrt{\frac{2(hc-\lambda\phi)}{\lambda m}}$

18. **(d)** de-Broglie wavelength,

$$\lambda = \frac{h}{p} = \frac{h}{\sqrt{2.m.(K.E)}}$$

$$\therefore \lambda \propto \frac{1}{\sqrt{K.E}}$$

If K.E is doubled, wavelength becomes $\frac{\lambda}{\sqrt{2}}$

19. **(b)** $\frac{1}{2}mv_1^2 = 2W_0 - W_0 = W_0$ and

$$\frac{1}{2}mv_2^2 = 10W_0 - W_0 = 9W_0$$

$$\therefore \frac{v_1}{v_2} = \sqrt{\frac{W_0}{9W_0}} = \frac{1}{3}$$

20. **(a)** The work function has no effect on photoelectric current so long as $h\nu > W_0$. The photoelectric current is proportional to the intensity of incident light. Since there is no change in the intensity of light, hence $I_1 = I_2$.

21. **(c)** $n \to 2-1$

$E = 10.2$ eV

$kE = E - \phi$

$Q = 10.20 - 3.57$

$h\upsilon_0 = 6.63$ eV

$$\upsilon_0 = \frac{6.63\times1.6\times10^{-19}}{6.67\times10^{-34}} = 1.6\times10^{15}\text{ Hz}$$

22. **(d)** $h\nu = W + \frac{1}{2}mv^2$ or $\frac{hc}{\lambda} = W + \frac{1}{2}mv^2$

Here $\lambda = 3000$ Å $= 3000\times10^{-10}$ m

and W = 1 eV $= 1.6\times10^{-19}$ joule

$$\therefore \frac{(6.6\times10^{-34})(3\times10^{8})}{3000\times10^{-10}}$$

$$= (1.6\times10^{-19}) + \frac{1}{2}\times(9.1\times10^{-31})v^2$$

Solving we get, $v \cong 10^6$ m/s

23. **(b)** According to Einstein's photoelectric equation, $h\nu = \phi_0 + K_{max}$

We have

$h\nu = \phi_0 + 0.5$ ...(i)

and $1.2h\nu = \phi_0 + 0.8$ ...(ii)

Therefore, from above two equations $\phi_0 = 1.0$ eV.

24. **(c)** $\lambda_{max.} = \frac{2d\sin\theta}{n_{min.}} = \frac{2\times15\times\sin 90^\circ}{1} = 30$Å

25. **(d)** $W_0 = h\nu_1 - eV_1$

$= h\,\nu_2 - e\,V_2$

$eV_2 = h(\nu_2 - \nu_1) + eV_1$

$$V_2 = \frac{h(n_2 - n_1)}{e} + V_1$$

26. **(b)** $KE_{max} = h\nu - \phi$

$1\text{eV} = h\nu - 1.9\text{eV} \Rightarrow h\nu = 2.9$ eV

Now threshold wavelength (maximum wavelength), $\lambda_0 = \frac{hc}{E}$

$$\Rightarrow \lambda_0 = \frac{6.6\times10^{-34}\times3\times10^{8}}{1.9\times1.6\times10^{-19}} = 6513\text{ Å}$$

And threshold frequency

$$\nu_0 = \frac{c}{\lambda_0} = \frac{3\times10^8}{6513\times10^{-10}} = 4.6\times10^{14}\text{Hz}$$

27. **(b)** $E = W_0 + K_{max}$ ...(i)

$\Rightarrow hf = W_A + K_A$ ...(ii)

and $2hf = W_B + K_B = 2W_A + K_B \left(\because \frac{W_A}{W_B} = \frac{1}{2}\right)$

Dividing equation (i) by (ii)

$$\frac{1}{2} = \frac{W_A + K_A}{2W_A + K_B} \Rightarrow \frac{K_A}{K_B} = \frac{1}{2}$$

28. **(d)** $h\upsilon - h\upsilon_0 = E_K$, according to photoelectric equation, when $\upsilon = \upsilon_0$, $E_K = 0$.

Graph (d) represents $E_K - \upsilon$ relationship.

29. **(d)** $K_{max} = \frac{hc}{\lambda} - W = \frac{hc}{\lambda} - 5.01$

$$= \frac{12375}{\lambda(\text{in Å})} - 5.01$$

$$= \frac{12375}{2000} - 5.01 = 6.1875 - 5.01 = 1.17775$$

$\simeq 1.2$ V

30. **(b)**

31. **(b)** $\lambda \propto \frac{1}{\sqrt{V}}$

$$\Rightarrow \frac{\lambda_1}{\lambda_2} = \sqrt{\frac{V_2}{V_1}} = \sqrt{\frac{100\text{keV}}{25\text{keV}}} = 2$$

$$\Rightarrow \lambda_2 = \frac{\lambda_1}{2}$$

32. **(a)** In the Davisson and Germer experiment, the velocity of electrons emitted from the electron gun can be increased by increasing the potential difference between the anode and filament.

33. **(b)** According to Einsten's photoelectric effect, the K.E. of the radiated electrons

$K.E_{max} = E - W$

$\frac{1}{2}mv_1^2 = (1 - 0.5)$ eV $= 0.5$ eV

$\frac{1}{2}mv_2^2 = (2.5 - 0.5)$ eV $= 2$ eV

$$\frac{v_1}{v_2} = \sqrt{\frac{0.5}{2}} = \frac{1}{\sqrt{4}} = 1/2$$

34. **(b)** By using $h\nu - h\nu_0 = K_{max}$

$\Rightarrow h(\nu_1 - \nu_0) = K_1$ ..... (i)

And $h(\nu_2 - \nu_0) = K_2$ ..... (ii)

$\Rightarrow \frac{\nu_1 - \nu_0}{\nu_2 - \nu_0} = \frac{K_1}{K_2} = \frac{1}{K}$, Hence $\nu_0 = \frac{k\nu_1 - \nu_2}{K - 1}$.

35. **(b)** Cathode rays get deflected in the electric field.

36. **(c)** As we know

$$\lambda \propto \frac{1}{\sqrt{V}}$$

$$\therefore \frac{1}{\sqrt{100}} : \frac{1}{\sqrt{200}} : \frac{1}{\sqrt{300}} = 1 : \frac{1}{\sqrt{2}} : \frac{1}{\sqrt{3}}$$

37. **(d)** Number of emitted electrons N_E

$\propto$ Intensity

$$\propto \frac{1}{(\text{Distance})^2}$$

Therefore, as distance is doubled, N_E decreases by (1/4) times.

38. (d) Photoelectrons are emitted if the frequency of incident light is greater than the threshold frequency.

39. (a) K.E. = $h\nu - h\nu_{th} = eV_0$ (V_0 = cut off voltage)

$$\Rightarrow V_0 = \frac{h}{e}(8.2 \times 10^{14} - 3.3 \times 10^{14})$$

$$= \frac{6.6 \times 10^{-34} \times 4.9 \times 10^{14}}{1.6 \times 10^{-19}} \approx 2V.$$

40. (d) $\frac{hc}{\lambda} - \phi = eV_0$

$$v_0 = \frac{hc}{e\lambda} - \frac{\phi}{e}$$

For metal A For metal B

$\frac{\phi_A}{hc} = \frac{1}{\lambda}$ $\frac{\phi_B}{hc} = \frac{1}{\lambda}$

As the value of $\frac{1}{\lambda}$ (increasing and decreasing) is not specified hence we cannot say that which metal has comparatively greater or lesser work function (ϕ).

41. (c)

42. (d) Potential difference = 100 V

K.E. acquired by electron = e (100)

$$\frac{1}{2}mv^2 = e(100) \Rightarrow v = \sqrt{\frac{2e(100)}{m}}$$

According to de Broglie's concept

$$\lambda = \frac{h}{mv}$$

$$\Rightarrow \lambda = \frac{h}{m\sqrt{\frac{2e(100)}{m}}}$$

$$= \frac{h}{\sqrt{2me(100)}} = 1.2 \times 10^{-10} = 1.2\text{Å}$$

43. (d) Since $p = nh\nu$

$$\Rightarrow n = \frac{p}{h\nu} = \frac{2 \times 10^{-3}}{6.6 \times 10^{-34} \times 6 \times 10^{14}} = 5 \times 10^{15}$$

44. (a) From formula

$$\lambda = \frac{h}{\sqrt{2mKT}}$$

$$= \frac{6.63 \times 10^{-34}}{\sqrt{2 \times 1.67 \times 10^{-27} \times 1.38 \times 10^{-23} T}} m$$

[By placing value of h, m and k)

$$= \frac{30.8}{\sqrt{T}}\text{Å}$$

45. (c) The photoelectric equation

$K_{max} = h\nu - \phi_0$

Explains that the intensity of incident radiation will increase photocurrent only beyond the threshold frequency.

Speed Test-26

1. (b) P.E. $= \frac{-Ze^2}{4\pi\varepsilon_0 r}$. Negative sign indicates that revolving electron is bound to the positive nucleus.
So, it decreases with increase in radii of orbit.

2. (b) $E = Rhc\left[\frac{1}{n_1^2} - \frac{1}{n_2^2}\right]$

E will be maximum for the transition for which $\left[\frac{1}{n_1^2} - \frac{1}{n_2^2}\right]$ is maximum. Here n_2 is the higher energy level.

Clearly, $\left[\frac{1}{n_1^2} - \frac{1}{n_2^2}\right]$ is maximum for the third transition, i.e. $2 \to 1$. I transition represents the absorption of energy.

3. (a) Number of emission spectral lines

$$N = \frac{n(n-1)}{2}$$

$\therefore 3 = \frac{n_1(n_1-1)}{2}$, in first case.

Or $n_1^2 - n_1 - 6 = 0$ or $(n_1 - 3)(n_1 + 2) = 0$
Take positive root.
$\therefore n_1 = 3$

Again, $6 = \frac{n_2(n_2-1)}{2}$, in second case.

Or $n_2^2 - n_2 - 12 = 0$ or $(n_2 - 4)(n_2 + 3) = 0$.
Take positive root, or $n_2 = 4$

Now velocity of electron $\upsilon = \frac{2\pi KZe^2}{nh}$

$\therefore \frac{\upsilon_1}{\upsilon_2} = \frac{n_2}{n_1} = \frac{4}{3}$.

4. (c) $N \propto \frac{1}{\sin^4\theta/2}$; $\frac{N_2}{N_1} = \frac{\sin^4(\theta_1/2)}{\sin^4(\theta_2/2)}$

or $\frac{N_2}{5\times10^6} = \frac{\sin^4(60°/2)}{\sin^4(120°/2)}$

or $\frac{N_2}{5\times10^6} = \frac{\sin^4 30°}{\sin^4 60°}$

or $N_2 = 5\times10^6 \times \left(\frac{1}{2}\right)^4\left(\frac{2}{\sqrt{3}}\right)^4 = \frac{5}{9}\times10^6$

5. (c) Magnetic moment of the hydrogen atom, when the electron is in n^{th} excited state, i.e., $n' = (n+1)$
As magnetic moment $M_n = I_n A = i_n(\pi r_n^2)$

$$i_n = eV_n = \frac{mz^2e^5}{4\varepsilon_0^2 n^3 h^3}$$

$$r_n = \frac{n^2h^2}{4\pi^2 kzme^2}\left(k = \frac{1}{4\pi\epsilon_0}\right)$$

Solving we get magnetic moment of the hydrogen atom for n^{th} excited state

$$M_{n'} = \left(\frac{e}{2m}\right)\frac{nh}{2\pi}$$

6. (a) $E = \frac{hc}{\lambda} \Rightarrow \lambda = \frac{hc}{E} = \frac{6.62\times10^{-34}\times3\times10^8}{12.5\times1.6\times10^{-19}}$
$= 993$ A°

$$\frac{1}{\lambda} = R\left(\frac{1}{n_1^2} - \frac{1}{n_2^2}\right)$$

(where Rydberg constant, $R = 1.097\times10^7$)

or, $\frac{1}{993\times10^{-10}} = 1.097\times10^7\left(\frac{1}{1^2} - \frac{1}{n_2^2}\right)$

Solving we get $n_2 = 3$
Spectral lines
Total number of spectral lines = 3
Two lines in Lyman series for $n_1 = 1, n_2 = 2$ and $n_1 = 1$, $n_2 = 3$ and one in Balmer series for $n_1 = 2, n_2 = 3$

7. (b) $l = \frac{nh}{2\pi}, |E| \propto Z^2/n^2; n = 3$

$\Rightarrow l_H = l_{Li}$ and $|E_H| < |E_{Li}|$

8. (b) $r \propto n^2$

$\therefore \frac{\text{radius of final state}}{\text{radius of initial state}} = n^2$

$\frac{21.2\times10^{-11}}{5.3\times10^{-11}} = n^2$

$\therefore n^2 = 4$ or $n = 2$

9. (a) $R = \frac{R_0 n^2}{Z}$

Radius in ground state $= \frac{R_0}{Z}$

Radius in first excited state $= \frac{R_0\times4}{Z}$ $(\because n = 2)$

Hence, radius of first excited state is four times the radius in ground state.

10. **(a)** Speed of electron in nth orbit

$$V_n = \frac{2\pi KZe^2}{nh}$$

$$V = (2.19 \times 10^6 \text{ m/s}) \frac{Z}{n}$$

$$V = (2.19 \times 10^6) \frac{2}{3} \quad (Z = 2 \;\&\; n = 3)$$

$$V = 1.46 \times 10^6 \text{ m/s}$$

11. **(b)** $KE_{max} = 10\text{eV}$

$\phi = 2.75$ eV

Total incident energy

$E = \phi + KE_{max} = 12.75$ eV

$\therefore$ Energy is released when electron jumps from the excited state n to the ground state.

$\because E_4 - E_1 = \{-0.85 - (-13.6) \text{ ev}\}$

$= 12.75\text{eV}$

$\therefore$ value of n = 4

12. **(a)** As the electron comes nearer to the nucleus the potential energy decreases

$$\left(\because \frac{-k.Ze^2}{r} = \text{P.E. and } r \text{ decreases}\right)$$

The K.E. will increase $\left[\because \text{K.E.} = \frac{1}{2}|\text{P.E.}| = \frac{1}{2}\frac{kZe^2}{r}\right]$

The total energy decreases $\left[\text{T.E.} = -\frac{1}{2}\frac{kZe^2}{r}\right]$

13. **(d)** When one e^- is removed from neutral helium atom, it becomes a one e^- species.

For one e^- species we know

$$E_n = \frac{-13.6Z^2}{n^2} \text{ eV/atom}$$

For helium ion, $Z = 2$ and for first orbit $n = 1$.

$$\therefore \quad E_1 = \frac{-13.6}{(1)^2} \times 2^2 = -54.4 \text{ eV}$$

$\therefore$ Energy required to remove this $e^- = +54.4$ eV

$\therefore$ Total energy required $= 54.4 + 24.6 = 79$ eV

14. **(b)** For 2nd line of Balmer series in hydrogen spectrum

$$\frac{1}{\lambda} = R\,(1)\left(\frac{1}{2^2} - \frac{1}{4^2}\right) = \frac{3}{16}R$$

For Li^{2+} $\left[\frac{1}{\lambda} = R \times 9\left(\frac{1}{x^2} - \frac{1}{12^2}\right) = \frac{3R}{16}\right]$

which is satisfied by $n = 12 \rightarrow n = 6$.

15. **(d)** For an atom following Bohr's model, the radius is given by

$r_m = \dfrac{r_0 m^2}{Z}$ where r_0 = Bohr's radius and m = orbit number.

For *Fm*, $m = 5$ (Fifth orbit in which the outermost electron is present)

$$\therefore \quad r_m = \frac{r_0 5^2}{100} = nr_0 \text{ (given)} \Rightarrow n = \frac{1}{4}$$

16. **(a)** Energy of electron in n^{th} orbit is

$$E_n = -(\text{Rch})\frac{Z^2}{n^2} = -54.4 \text{ eV}$$

For He^+ is ground state

$$E_1 = -(\text{Rch})\frac{(2)^2}{(1)^2} = -54.4 \Rightarrow \text{Rch} = 13.6$$

$\therefore$ For Li^{++} in first excited state (n = 2)

$$E' = -13.6 \times \frac{(3)^2}{(2)^2} = -30.6 \text{ eV}$$

17. **(a)** Angular momentum = mrv = J

$$\therefore \quad v = \frac{J}{mr}$$

$$\text{K. E. of electron} = \frac{1}{2}mv^2 = \frac{1}{2}m\left(\frac{J}{mr}\right)^2$$

$$= \frac{J^2}{2mr^2}$$

18. **(b)** When $F = \frac{k}{r}$ = centripetal force, then $\frac{k}{r} = \frac{mv^2}{r}$

$\Rightarrow mv^2 = \text{constant}$ $\Rightarrow$ kinetic energy is constant

$\Rightarrow$ *T* is independent of *n*.

19. **(b)** $\dfrac{1}{\lambda'} = \dfrac{1}{\lambda}\sqrt{\dfrac{c - v}{c + v}}$

Here, $\lambda' = 706$ nm, $\lambda = 656$ nm

$$\therefore \quad \frac{c - v}{c + v} = \left(\frac{\lambda}{\lambda'}\right)^2 = \left(\frac{656}{706}\right)^2 = 0.86$$

$$\Rightarrow \quad \frac{v}{c} = \frac{0.14}{1.86}$$

$$\Rightarrow \quad v = 0.075 \times 3 \times 10^8 = 2.25 \times 10^7 \text{m/s}$$

20. **(d)** $\because \quad B = \dfrac{\mu_0 I}{2r}$ and $I = \dfrac{e}{T}$

$$B = \frac{\mu_0 e}{2rT} \quad [r \propto n^2, T \propto n^5]; \quad B \propto \frac{1}{n^5}$$

21. **(a)** 53 electrons in iodine atom are distributed as 2, 8, 18, 18, 7

$\therefore n = 5$

$$r_n = (0.53 \times 10^{-10})\frac{n^2}{Z}$$

$$= \frac{0.53 \times 10^{-10} \times 5^2}{53} = 2.5 \times 10^{-11} \text{m}$$

22. **(a)** At closest distance of approach, the kinetic energy of the particle will convert completely into electrostatic potential energy.

Kinetic energy K.E. $= \dfrac{1}{2}mv^2$

Potential energy P.E. $= \frac{KQq}{r}$

$\frac{1}{2}mv^2 = \frac{KQq}{r} \Rightarrow r \propto \frac{1}{m}$

23. (c) $\frac{n(n-1)}{2} = 6$

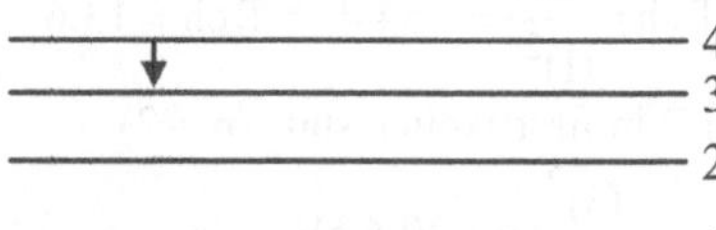

$n^2 - n - 12 = 0$

$(n-4)(n+3) = 0$ or $n = 4$

24. (c) The wavelength of spectrum is given by

$$\frac{1}{\lambda} = Rz^2\left(\frac{1}{n_1^2} - \frac{1}{n_2^2}\right) \quad \text{where } R = \frac{1.097 \times 10^7}{1 + \frac{m}{M}}$$

where m = mass of electron

M = mass of nucleus.

For different M, R is different and therefore λ is different.

25. (a) $\because T \propto n^3$

$Tn_1 = 8\, Tn_2$ (given)

Hence, $n_1 = 2n_2$

26. (d) $\Delta E = h\nu$

$$\nu = \frac{\Delta E}{h} = k\left[\frac{1}{(n-1)^2} - \frac{1}{n^2}\right] = \frac{k(2n-1)}{n^2(n-1)^2}$$

$$\approx \frac{2k}{n^3} \text{ or } \nu \propto \frac{1}{n^3}$$

27. (c) A spectrum is observed, when light coming directly from a source is examined with a spectroscope. Therefore spectrum obtained from a sodium vapour lamp is emission spectrum.

28. (a) Energy of ground state 13.6 eV

Energy of first excited state

$= -\frac{13.6}{4} = -3.4$ eV

Energy of second excited state

$= -\frac{13.6}{9} = -1.5$ eV

Difference between ground state and 2nd excited state $= 13.6 - 1.5 = 12.1$ eV

So, electron can be excited upto 3rd orbit

No. of possible transition

$1 \to 2, 1 \to 3, 2 \to 3$

So, three lines are possible.

29. (b) In Bohr's model, angular momentum is quantised i.e

$$\ell = n\left(\frac{h}{2\pi}\right)$$

30. (b) The smallest frequency and largest wavelength in ultraviolet region will be for transition of electron from orbit 2 to orbit 1.

$$\therefore \frac{1}{\lambda} = R\left(\frac{1}{n_1^2} - \frac{1}{n_2^2}\right)$$

$$\Rightarrow \frac{1}{122 \times 10^{-9} m} = R\left[\frac{1}{1^2} - \frac{1}{2^2}\right] = R\left[1 - \frac{1}{4}\right] = \frac{3R}{4}$$

$$\Rightarrow R = \frac{4}{3 \times 122 \times 10^{-9}} m^{-1}$$

The highest frequency and smallest wavelength for infrared region will be for transition of electron from ∞ to 3rd orbit.

$$\therefore \frac{1}{\lambda} = R\left(\frac{1}{n_1^2} - \frac{1}{n_2^2}\right) \Rightarrow \frac{1}{\lambda} = \frac{4}{3 \times 122 \times 10^{-9}}\left(\frac{1}{3^2} - \frac{1}{\infty}\right)$$

$$\therefore \lambda = \frac{3 \times 122 \times 9 \times 10^{-9}}{4} = 823.5\text{nm}$$

31. (c) $\frac{1}{\lambda} = R\left(\frac{1}{n_1^2} - \frac{1}{n_2^2}\right)$ where R = Rydberg constant

$$\frac{1}{\lambda_{32}} = \left(\frac{1}{4} - \frac{1}{9}\right) = \frac{5}{36}$$

$$\Rightarrow \lambda_{32} = \frac{36}{5}$$

Similarly solving for λ_{31} and λ_{21}

$$\lambda_{31} = \frac{9}{8} \text{ and } \lambda_{21} = \frac{4}{3}$$

$$\therefore \frac{\lambda_{32}}{\lambda_{31}} = 6.4 \text{ and } \frac{\lambda_{21}}{\lambda_{31}} \simeq 1.2$$

32. (d) $b = \frac{Ze^2 \cot\left(\frac{\theta}{2}\right)}{4\pi \epsilon_0 k_i} = 0 \Rightarrow \cot\left(\frac{\theta}{2}\right) = 0$

$$\Rightarrow \frac{\theta}{2} = 90° \text{ or } \theta = 180°$$

33. (a) Speed of electron in nth orbit

$$V_n = \frac{2\pi KZe^2}{nh}$$

$$V = (2.19 \times 10^6 \text{m/s}) \frac{Z}{n}$$

$$V = (2.19 \times 10^6) \frac{2}{3} \quad (Z = 2 \;\&\; n = 3)$$

$V = 1.46 \times 10^6$ m/s

34. (d) $E = E_4 - E_3$

$$= -\frac{13.6}{4^2} - \left(-\frac{13.6}{3^2}\right) = -0.85 + 1.51$$

$= 0.66$ eV

35. (d) $\because$ The frequency of the transition $\nu \propto \frac{1}{n^2}$, when

$n = 1, 2, 3.$

36. (c) According to Bohr's theory, the wave number of the last line of the Balmer series in hydrogen spectrum,

For hydrogen atom z = 1

$$\frac{1}{\lambda} = RZ^2\left(\frac{1}{n_2^2} - \frac{1}{n_1^2}\right)$$

$$= 10^7 \times 1^2\left(\frac{1}{2^2} - \frac{1}{\infty^2}\right)$$

$\Rightarrow$ wave number $\frac{1}{\lambda} = 0.25 \times 10^7\ m^{-1}$

37. (a) Velocity of electron in n^{th} orbit of hydrogen atom is given by :

$$V_n = \frac{2\pi KZe^2}{nh}$$

Substituting the values we get,

$$V_n = \frac{2.2 \times 10^6}{n} m/s \quad \text{or} \quad V_n \propto \frac{1}{n}$$

As principal quantum number increases, velocity decreases.

38. (c) $\frac{1}{\lambda} = R\left[\frac{1}{n_1^2} - \frac{1}{n_2^2}\right]$

$$\Rightarrow \frac{1}{970.6 \times 10^{-10}} = 1.097 \times 10^7\left[\frac{1}{1^2} - \frac{1}{n_2^2}\right] \Rightarrow n_2 = 4$$

$\therefore$ Number of emission line $N = \frac{n(n-1)}{2} = \frac{4 \times 3}{2} = 6$

39. (a) We have $E_n = \frac{-2\pi^2 mK^2 Z^2 e^4}{n^2 h^2}$. For helium Z = 2. Hence requisite answer is $4E_n$

40. (c) As α-particles are doubly ionised helium He^{++} i.e. Positively charged and nucleus is also positively charged and we know that like charges repel each other.

41. (b) $\bar{v} = R\left(\frac{1}{n_1^2} - \frac{1}{n_2^2}\right)$, where $n_1 = 2, n_2 = 4$

$$\bar{v} = R\left(\frac{1}{4} - \frac{1}{16}\right)$$

$$\frac{1}{\lambda} = R\left(\frac{12}{4 \times 16}\right) \Rightarrow \lambda = \frac{16}{3R}$$

42. (a) The kinetic energy of the projectile is given by

$$\frac{1}{2}mv^2 = \frac{Ze(2e)}{4\pi\varepsilon_0 r_0} = \frac{Z_1 Z_2}{4\pi\varepsilon_0 r_0}$$

Thus energy of the projectile is directly proportional to Z_1, Z_2

43. (a) We know that $\frac{1}{\lambda} = RZ^2\left[\frac{1}{n_1^2} - \frac{1}{n_2^2}\right]$

The wave length of first spectral line in the Balmer series of hydrogen atom is 6561Å. Here $n_2 = 3$ and $n_1 = 2$

$$\therefore \frac{1}{6561} = R(1)^2\left(\frac{1}{4} - \frac{1}{9}\right) = \frac{5R}{36} \quad ...(i)$$

For the second spectral line in the Balmer series of singly ionised helium ion $n_2 = 4$ and $n_1 = 2$; Z = 2

$$\therefore \frac{1}{\lambda} = R(2)^2\left[\frac{1}{4} - \frac{1}{16}\right] = \frac{3R}{4} \quad ...(ii)$$

Dividing equation (i) and equation (ii) we get

$$\frac{\lambda}{6561} = \frac{5R}{36} \times \frac{4}{3R} = \frac{5}{27}$$

$\therefore \quad \lambda = 1215$ Å

44. (a) For Lyman series

$$\upsilon = R_C\left[\frac{1}{1^2} - \frac{1}{n^2}\right]$$

where n = 2, 3, 4, ...

For the series limit of Lyman series, $n = \infty$

$$\therefore \quad \upsilon_1 = R_C\left[\frac{1}{1^2} - \frac{1}{\infty^2}\right] = R_C \quad ...(i)$$

For the first line of Lyman series, n = 2

$$\therefore \quad \upsilon_2 = R_C\left[\frac{1}{1^2} - \frac{1}{2^2}\right] = \frac{3}{4}R_C \quad ...(ii)$$

For Balmer series

$$\upsilon = R_C\left[\frac{1}{2^2} - \frac{1}{n^2}\right]$$

where n = 3, 4, 5 .....

For the series limit of Balmer series, $n = \infty$

$$\therefore \quad \upsilon_3 = R_C\left[\frac{1}{2^2} - \frac{1}{\infty^2}\right] = \frac{R_C}{4} \quad ...(iii)$$

From equation (i), (ii) and (iii), we get

$\upsilon_1 = \upsilon_2 + \upsilon_3$ or $\upsilon_1 - \upsilon_2 = \upsilon_3$

45. (d) As $r \propto \frac{1}{m}$ $\quad \therefore r_0' = \frac{1}{2} r_0$

As $E \propto m$ $\quad \therefore E_0' = 2(-13.6) = -27.2$ eV

Speed Test-27

1. **(b)** B.E. $= 0.042 \times 931 \simeq 42$ MeV

Number of nucleons in ${}_{3}^{7}Li$ is 7.

$\therefore$ B.E./ nucleon $= \frac{42}{7} = 6$ MeV $\simeq 5.6$ MeV

2. **(d)** ${}_{Z}^{A}X \longrightarrow {}_{Z+1}^{A}Y : \beta$, ${}_{Z+1}^{A}Y \longrightarrow {}_{Z-1}^{A-4}B^* : \alpha$

${}_{Z-1}^{A-4}B^* \longrightarrow {}_{Z-1}^{A-4}B : \gamma$

(β, α, γ) ($\because \beta = {}_{-1}^{0}e$, $\alpha = {}_{2}^{4}He$, mass number and charge number of a nucleus remains unchanged during γ decay)

3. **(c)** The radius of the nuclears is directly proportional to cube root of atomic number i.e. $R \propto A^{1/3}$

$\Rightarrow$ $R = R_0 A^{1/3}$, where R_0 is a constant of proportionality

$$\frac{R_2}{R_1} = \left(\frac{A_2}{A_1}\right)^{1/3} \left(\frac{64}{27}\right)^{1/3} = \frac{4}{3}$$

where R_1 = the radius of ^{27}Al, and A_1 = Atomic mass number of Al

R_2 = the radius of ^{64}Cu and A_2 = Atomic mass number of C4

$$R_2 = 3.6 \times \frac{4}{3} = 4.8\text{m}$$

4. **(c)** Nuclear forces are short range attractive forces which balance the repulsive forces between the protons inside the nucleus.

5. **(a)** $\lambda = \frac{1}{t}\log_e \frac{A_o}{A} = \frac{1}{5}\log_e \frac{5000}{1250}$

$= \frac{2}{5}\log_e 2 = 0.4 \log_e 2$

6. **(d)** Radioactivity at T_1, $R_1 = \lambda N_1$

Radioactivity at T_2, $R_2 = \lambda N_2$

$\therefore$ Number of atoms decayed in time

$(T_1 - T_2) = (N_1 - N_2)$

$$= \frac{(R_1 - R_2)}{\lambda} = \frac{(R_1 - R_2)T}{0.693} \propto (R_1 - R_2)T$$

7. **(c)** ${}_{1}^{2}H$ and ${}_{1}^{3}H$ requires a and b amount of energies for their nucleons to be separated.

${}_{2}^{4}$He releases c amount of energy in its formation i.e., in assembling the nucleons as nucleus.

Hence, Energy released $= c - (a + b) = c - a - b$

8. **(a)** Mass defect $= ZM_p + (A - Z)M_n - M(A,Z)$

or, $\frac{B.E.}{c^2} = ZM_p + (A-Z)M_n - M(A,Z)$

$\therefore M(A, Z) = ZM_p + (A-Z)M_n - \frac{B.E.}{c^2}$

9. **(d)**

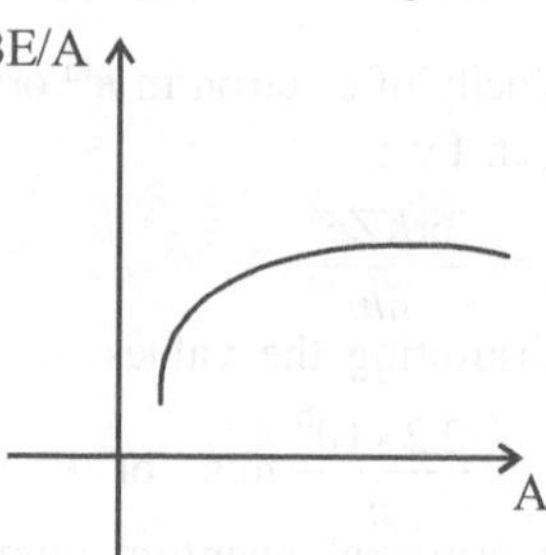

From the graph of BE/A versus mass number A it is clear that, BE/A first increases and then decreases with increase in mass number.

10. **(c)** The range of energy of β-particles is from zero to some maximum value.

11. **(a)** ${}_{72}A^{180} \xrightarrow{\alpha} {}_{70}A_1^{176} \xrightarrow{\beta} {}_{71}A_2^{176}$

$\xrightarrow{\alpha} {}_{69}A_3^{172} \xrightarrow{\gamma} {}_{69}A_4^{172}$

12. **(c)** $\frac{dN}{dt} = KN$

$9750 = KN_0$ .... (1)

$975 = KN$ ..... (2)

Dividing (1) by (2)

$\frac{N}{N_0} = \frac{1}{10}$

$K = \frac{2.303}{t}\log\frac{N_0}{N} = \frac{2.303}{5}\log 10$

$= 0.4606 = 0.461$ per minute

13. **(d)**

14. **(d)** Extremely high temps needed for fusion make K.E. large enough to overcome repulsion between nuclei.

15. **(c)** Binding energy

$= [ZM_P + (A - Z)M_N - M]c^2$

$= [8M_P + (17 - 8)M_N - M]c^2$

$= [8M_P + 9M_N - M]c^2$

$= [8M_P + 9M_N - M_o]c^2$

16. **(c)** In this reaction mass is not conserved.

17. **(a)** $T_{1/2} = \frac{\ln 2}{\lambda} \therefore \lambda = \frac{\ln 2}{T_{1/2}}$

$\Rightarrow \lambda_A = \frac{\ln 2}{T_A}, \lambda_B = \frac{\ln 2}{T_B} \Rightarrow \frac{\lambda_A}{\lambda_B} = \frac{T_B}{T_A}.$

18. (d) $N_1 = N_0 e^{-10\lambda t}$, $N_2 = N_0 e^{-\lambda t}$

$\frac{N_1}{N_2} = e^{-9\lambda t} = e^{-1}$; $9\lambda t = 1 \Rightarrow t = \frac{1}{9\lambda}$

19. (d) Let at time t_1 & t_2, number of particles be N_1 & N_2. So,

$$R_1 = \frac{dN_1}{dt} = -\lambda N_1; \quad R_2 = \frac{dN_2}{dt} = -\lambda N_2$$

$$\frac{R_1}{R_2} = \frac{\lambda N_1}{\lambda N_2} = \frac{N_1}{N_1 e^{-\lambda(t_2 - t_1)}} = e^{\lambda(t_2 - t_1)}$$

$$R_1 = R_2 e^{\lambda(t_2 - t_1)} = R_2 e^{-\lambda(t_1 - t_2)}$$

20. (c) Average life of the nuclei is

$$t_{av} = \frac{1}{\lambda} \quad \text{....(i)}$$

Half life of the nuclei

$$t_{1/2} = \frac{0.693}{\lambda} \quad \text{....(ii)}$$

from (i) and (ii)

$$t_{av} = \frac{t_{1/2}}{0.693}$$

21. (d) Nuclear force is not the same between any two nucleons.

22. (a)

23. (a) $P = n\left(\frac{E}{t}\right) \Rightarrow 1000 = \frac{n \times 200 \times 10^6 \times 1.6 \times 10^{-19}}{t}$

$\Rightarrow \frac{n}{t} = 3.125 \times 10^{13}$.

24. (c) Binding energy per nucleon for fission products is higher relative to Binding energy per nucleon for parent nucleus, i.e., more masses are lost and are obtained as kinetic energy of fission products. So, the given ratio <1.

25. (b) We have $K_\alpha = \frac{m_y}{m_y + m_\alpha}.Q$

$\Rightarrow K_\alpha = \frac{A-4}{A}.Q \Rightarrow 48 = \frac{A-4}{A}.50 \Rightarrow A = 100$

26. (b) Using the relation for mean life.

Given: $t = 2\tau = 2\left(\frac{1}{\lambda}\right) \quad \left(\because \tau = \frac{1}{\lambda}\right)$

Then from $M = M_0 e^{-\lambda t} = 10 e^{-\lambda \times \frac{2}{\lambda}}$

$= 10\left(\frac{1}{e}\right)^2 = 1.35\text{g}$

27. (d) Because radioactivity is a spontaneous phenomenon.

28. (a) α-particle = ${}_2He^4$. It contains 2 p and 2 n. As some mass is converted into B.E., therefore, mass of α particle is slightly less than the sum of the masses of 2 *p* and 2 *n*.

29. (c) $T_{av} = \frac{T_\alpha T_\beta}{T_\alpha + T_\beta}$

If α and *B* are emitted simultaneously.

30. (a) Due to irradiation of α-rays on end A will make it (positive) and irradiation of β-rays on end B will make it (negative) hence current will flow from A to B (or from positive to negative).

31. (b) Momentum

$Mu = \frac{E}{c} = \frac{h\nu}{c}$

Recoil energy

$$\frac{1}{2}Mu^2 = \frac{1}{2}\frac{M^2u^2}{M} = \frac{1}{2M}\left(\frac{h\nu}{c}\right)^2$$

$$= \frac{h^2\nu^2}{2Mc^2}$$

32. (c) No. of nuclide at time t is given by $N = N_0 e^{-\lambda t}$

Where N_0 = initial nuclide

This equation is equivalent to $y = ae^{-kx}$

Thus correct graph is

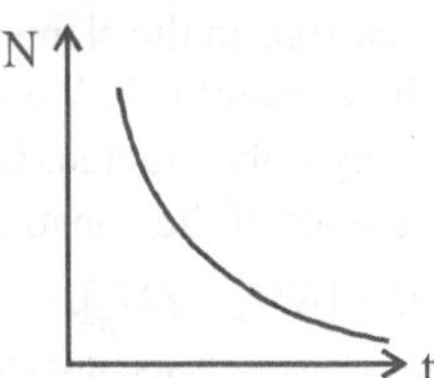

33. (b) By conservation of energy,

$$(M + \Delta m)c^2 = \frac{2M}{2}c^2 + \frac{1}{2}.\frac{2M}{2}v^2,$$

where v is the speed of the daughter nuclei

$$\Rightarrow \Delta mc^2 = \frac{M}{2}v^2 \qquad \therefore v = c\sqrt{\frac{2\Delta m}{M}}$$

34. (a) Suppose that,

The number of ${}^{10}B$ type atoms = x

and the number of ${}^{11}B$ type atoms = y

Weight of ${}^{10}B$ type atoms = $10x$

Weight of ${}^{11}B$ type atoms = $11y$

Total number of atoms = $x + y$

$\therefore$ Atomic weight $= \frac{10x + 11y}{x + y} = 10.81$

$\Rightarrow 10x + 11y = 10.81x + 10.81y$

$\Rightarrow 0.81x = 0.19y \Rightarrow \frac{x}{y} = \frac{19}{81}$

35. (b) Applying law of conservation of momentum,

$m_1 v_1 = m_2 v_2$

$\frac{v_1}{v_2} = \frac{m_2}{m_1}$

As $m = \frac{4}{3}\pi r^3 \rho \Rightarrow m \propto r^3$

Hence, $\frac{m_2}{m_1} = \frac{r_2^3}{r_1^3}$

$\therefore \frac{v_1}{v_2} = \frac{r_2^3}{r_1^3} \Rightarrow \frac{r_2}{r_1} = \left(\frac{1}{2}\right)^{\frac{1}{3}}$

36. **(d)** In an explosion a body breaks up into two pieces of unequal masses both part will have numerically equal momentum and lighter part will have more velocity.

$U \rightarrow Th + He$

$KE_{Th} = \frac{p^2}{2m_{Th}}, KE_{He} = \frac{p^2}{2m_{He}}$

since m_{He} is less so KE_{He} will be more.

37. **(a)** As we know, $R = R_0 (A)^{1/3}$

where A = mass number

$R_{Al} = R_0 (27)^{1/3} = 3R_0$

$R_{Te} = R_0 (125)^{1/3} = 5R_0 = \frac{5}{3} R_{Al}$

38. **(a)** Given : Mass of neutron = M_n

Mass of proton = M_p; Atomic mass of the element = M; Number of neutrons in the element = N and number of protons in the element = Z. We know that the atomic mass (M) of any stable nucleus is always less than the sum of the masses of the constituent particles.

Therefore, $M < [NM_n + ZM_p]$.

X is a neutrino, when β-particle is emitted.

39. **(a)** Activity decreases

5000 dps to 2500 dps in 150 days

$\therefore$ Half life period $T_{1/2} = 150$ days

$\therefore$ 300 days $= 2T_{1/2}$

Therefore, initial activity $= 5000 \times 2T_{1/2} = 5000 \times 2 \times 2 = 20000$ dps

40. **(b)** The order of density of uranium nucleus is 10^{17} kg/m^2.

41. **(b)**

42. **(a)** $B.E_H = \frac{2.22}{2} = 1.11$

$B.E_{He} = \frac{28.3}{4} = 7.08$

$B.E_{Fe} = \frac{492}{56} = 8.78 =$ maximum

$B.E_U = \frac{1786}{235} = 7.6$

${}^{56}_{26}Fe$ is most stable as it has maximum binding energy per nucleon.

43. **(d)** Neutrons can't be deflected by a magnetic field.

44. **(b)** ${}_{-1}e^0$ is known as β-particle & $\overline{\nu}$ is known as antineutrino. Since in this reaction $\overline{\nu}$ is emitted with ${}_{-1}e^0$ (β-particle or electron), so it is known as β-decay.

45. **(a)** Given, $\lambda_A = 8\lambda, \lambda_B = \lambda$

$N_B = \frac{N_A}{e}$

$\Rightarrow N_o e^{-\lambda_B t} = N_o \frac{e^{-\lambda_A t}}{e}$

$e^{-\lambda t} = e^{-8\lambda t} e^{-1}$

$e^{-\lambda t} = e^{-8\lambda t - 1}$

Comparing both side powers

$-\lambda t = -8\lambda t - 1$

$-1 = 7\lambda t$

$t = -\frac{1}{7\lambda}$

The best possible answer is $t = \frac{1}{7\lambda}$

Speed Test-28

1. (d) $\Delta I_E = 8.0\,mA$
$\Delta I_C = 7.9\,mA$
$$\alpha = \frac{\Delta I_C}{\Delta I_E} = \frac{7.9}{8.0} = 0.9875 \simeq 0.99$$
Also, $\beta = \frac{\alpha}{1-\alpha} = \frac{0.9875}{(1-0.9875)} = 79$

2. (d) Here, $n_i = 10^{16}\,m^{-3}$, $n_h = 5 \times 10^{22}\,m^{-3}$
As $n_e n_h = n_i^2$
$$\therefore\ n_e = \frac{n_i^2}{n_h} = \frac{(10^{16}m^{-3})^2}{5\times10^{22}m^{-3}} = 2\times10^9\,m^{-3}$$

3. (d) Energy band gap range is given by,
$$E_g = \frac{hc}{\lambda}$$
For visible region $\lambda = (4 \times 10^{-7} \sim 7 \times 10^{-7})$m
$$E_g = \frac{6.6\times10^{-34}\times3\times10^8}{7\times10^{-7}} = \frac{19.8\times10^{-26}}{7\times10^{-7}} = \frac{2.8\times10^{-19}}{1.6\times10^{-19}}$$
$E_g = 1.75\,eV$

4. (b) Voltage gain = $\beta \times$ Impedance gain
$$50 = \beta \times \frac{200}{100} = 2\beta \Rightarrow \beta = 25$$
and power gain $= \beta^2 \times \frac{200}{100} = 1250.$

5. (b) When either of *A* or *B* is 1 i.e. closed then lamp will glow.
In this case, Truth table

Inputs		Output
A	B	Y
0	0	0
0	1	1
1	0	1
1	1	1

This represents OR gate.

6. (c) In p-region of p-n junction
holes concentration > electrons concentration and in n-region electrons concentration > holes concentration.

7. (c) Peak value of rectified output voltage
= peak value of input voltage – barrier voltage
$= 2 - 0.7 = 1.3$ V.

8. (a) Current gain $(\alpha) = 0.96$
$I_e = 7.2\,mA$
$$\frac{I_c}{I_e} = \alpha = 0.96$$
$$I_c = 0.96 \times 7.2\,mA = 6.91\,mA$$
$I_e = I_c + I_b$
$\Rightarrow I_b = I_e - I_c = 7.2 - 6.91 = 0.29\,mA$

9. (c) No. of electrons reaching the collector,
$$n_C = \frac{96}{100}\times10^{10} = 0.96\times10^{10}$$
Emitter current, $I_E = \frac{n_E \times e}{t}$
Collector current, $I_C = \frac{n_C \times e}{t}$
$\therefore$ Current transfer ratio,
$$\alpha = \frac{I_C}{I_E} = \frac{n_C}{n_E} = \frac{0.96\times10^{10}}{10^{10}} = 0.96$$

10. (c) Here diode is forward biased with voltage $= 2 - 0 = 2$ V.
$V_B = V_{knee} + IR$
$2 = 0.7 + I \times 200$
($\therefore$ Total resistance $= 180 + 20 = 200\Omega$)
$$\therefore\ I = \frac{1.3}{200} = 6.5\,mA$$

11. (b) I $\rightarrow$ ON
II $\rightarrow$ OFF
In IInd state it is used as a amplifier it is active region.

12. (b) In half wave rectifier only half of the wave is rectified.

13. (c) $V' = V + IR = 0.5 + 0.1 \times 20 = 2.5\,V$

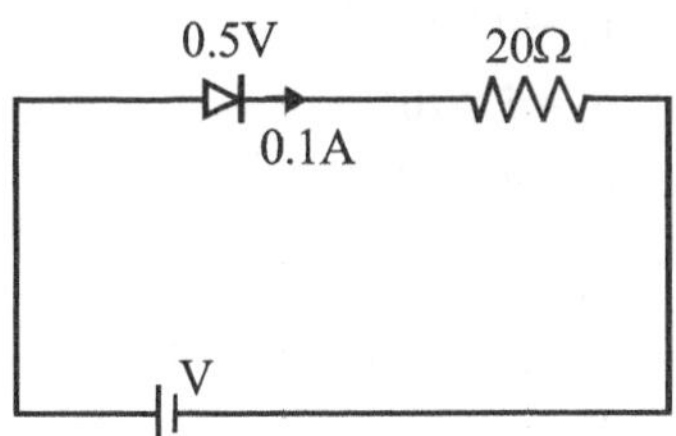

14. (b) $\frac{V_o}{V_{in}} = \frac{R_o}{R_{in}} \times \beta = \frac{5\times10^3\times62}{500} = 10\times62 = 620$
$V_o = 620 \times V_{in} = 620 \times 0.01 = 6.2\,V$
$\therefore V_o = 6.2$ volt.

15. (b) Conductivity $\sigma = n_i e \mu_e = 10^{17} \times (1.6\times10^{-19}) \times 3800$
$= 60.8$ mho/cm

16. (d) Negative feedback is applied to reduce the output voltage of an amplifier. If there is no negative feedback, the value of output voltage could be very high. In the options given, the maximum value of voltage gain is 100. Hence it is the correct option.

17. (a) In the given system all four gate is NOR gate

Truth Table

A	B	$(y' = \overline{A+B})$	$y'' = (\overline{A+y'})$	$y''' = (A+y'')$	$y = \overline{y''+y'''}$
0	0	1	0	0	1
0	1	0	1	0	0
1	0	0	0	1	0
1	1	0	0	0	1

i.e.,

A	B	y
0	0	1
0	1	0
1	0	0
1	1	1

18. (a) Conductivity, $\sigma = \frac{1}{\rho} = e(n_e\mu_e + n_h\mu_h)$

$2.13 = 1.6 \times 10^{-19}(0.38 + 0.18)\,n_i$

(Since in intrinsic semi-conductor, $n_e = n_h = n_i$)

$\therefore$ density of charge carriers, n_i

$$= \frac{2.13}{1.6 \times 10^{-19} \times 0.56} = 2.37 \times 10^{19}\,m^{-3}$$

19. (d) Here $Y = (\overline{\overline{A} + \overline{B}}) = \overline{\overline{A.B}} = A \cdot B$. Thus, it is an AND gate for which truth table is

A	B	Y
0	0	0
0	1	0
1	0	0
1	1	1

20. (d) $n_i^2 = n_e n_h$

$(1.5 \times 10^{16})^2 = n_e(4.5 \times 10^{22})$

$\Rightarrow \quad n_e = 0.5 \times 10^{10}$

or $\quad n_e = 5 \times 10^9$

Given $\quad n_h = 4.5 \times 10^{22}$

$\Rightarrow n_h >> n_e$

$\therefore$ Semiconductor is p-type and

$n_e = 5 \times 10^9\,m^{-3}$.

21. (c) In *n*-type semiconductors, electrons are the majority charge carriers.

22. (d) For semiconductor, $n = AT^{3/2}e^{\frac{E_g}{2KT}}$;

so $n \propto T^{3/2}$

23. (d) When PN junction diode is forward biased both depletion layer width W and barrier height V_0 decrease and current due to molarity carrier increases.

24. (b) D_2 is forward biased whereas D_1 is reversed biased. So effective resistance of the circuit

$R = 4 + 2 = 6\Omega$

$\therefore i = \frac{12}{6} = 2$ A.

25. (d) In common emitter configuration current gain

$$A_i = \frac{-hf_e}{1 + h_{oe}R_L} = \frac{-50}{1 + 25 \times 10^{-6} \times 1 \times 10^3} = -48.78$$

26. (c)

27. (b) It is a *p-n-p* transistor with *R* as base.

28. (c) Here P-N junction diode rectifies half of the ac wave i.e., acts as half wave rectifier. During + ve half cycle Diode $\rightarrow$ forward biased output across will be

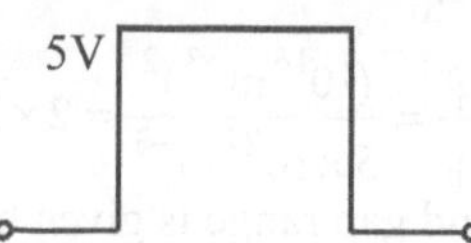

During –ve half cycle Diode $\rightarrow$ reverse biased output will not obtained.

29. (d) Due to heating, when a free electron is produced then simultaneously a hole is also produced.

30. (b) $I = nA\,ev_d$ or $I \propto nv_d$

$$\therefore \frac{I_e}{I_h} = \frac{n_e v_e}{n_h v_h} \text{ or } \frac{n_e}{n_h} = \frac{I_e}{I_h} \times \frac{v_h}{v_e} = \frac{7}{4} \times \frac{4}{5} = \frac{7}{5}$$

31. (c) Electronic configuration of ^6C

$^6C = 1s^2, 2s^2\,2p^2$

The electronic configuration of ^{14}Si

$^{14}Si = 1s^2, 2s^2\,2p^6, 3s^2\,3p^2$

As they are away from Nucleus, so effect of nucleus is low for Si even for Sn and Pb are almost mettalic.

32. (d) V_1 —▷|—/\/\/— V_2

In forward bias, $V_1 > V_2$ i.e., in figure (d) p-type semiconductor is at higher potential w.r.t. n-type semiconductor.

33. (a) A positive feed back from output to input in an amplifier provides oscillations of constant amplitude.

34. (b) The power gain in case of CE amplifier,

Power gain = $\beta^2 \times$ Resistance gain

$= \beta^2 \times \frac{R_o}{R_i}$

$= (10)^2 \times 5 = 500.$

35. (c) **Given :** Voltage gain $A_V = 150$

$V_i = 2\cos\left(15t + \frac{\pi}{3}\right)$; $V_0 = ?$

For CE transistor phase difference between input and output signal is $\pi = 180°$

Using formula, $A_V = \frac{V_0}{V_i}$

$\Rightarrow V_0 = A_V \times V_i$

$= 150 \times 2\cos\left(15t + \frac{\pi}{3}\right)$

or $V_0 = 300\cos\left(15t + \frac{\pi}{3} + \pi\right)$

$$V_0 = 300\cos\left(15t + \frac{4}{3}\pi\right)$$

36. **(a)** To use a transistor as an amplifier the emitter base junction is forward biased while the collector base junction is reverse biased.

37. **(d)** Copper is a conductor, so its resistance decreases on decreasing temperature as thermal agitation decreases; whereas germanium is semiconductor therefore on decreasing temperature resistance increases.

38. **(b)** In forward biasing, the diode conducts. For ideal junction diode, the forward resistance is zero; therefore, entire applied voltage occurs across external resistance R i.e., there occurs no potential drop, so potential across R is V in forward biased.

39. **(a)** Current gain $(\alpha) = 0.96$

$I_e = 7.2\,\text{mA}$

$$\frac{I_c}{I_e} = \alpha = 0.96$$

$$I_c = 0.96 \times 7.2\,\text{mA} = 6.91\text{ mA}$$

$$I_e = I_c + I_b$$

$$\Rightarrow I_b = I_e - I_c = 7.2 - 6.91 = 0.29\,\text{mA}$$

40. **(d)**

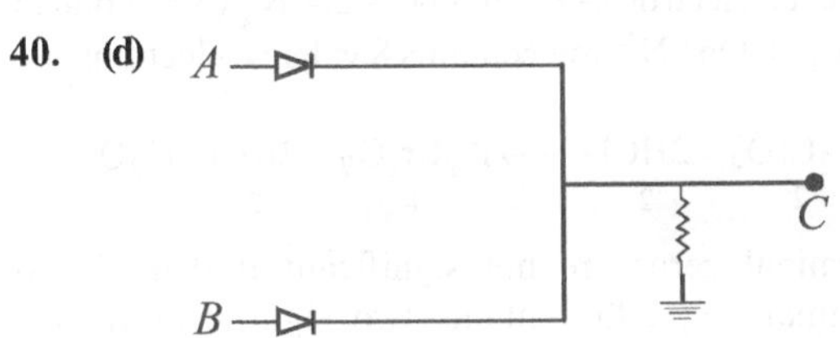

The truth table for the above logic gate is :

A	B	C
1	1	1
1	0	1
0	1	1
0	0	0

This truth table follows the boolean algebra $C = A + B$ which is for OR gate

41. **(b)** $R = \frac{\Delta V}{\Delta I} = \frac{2.1 - 2}{(800 - 400) \times 10^{-3}} = \frac{1}{4} = 0.25\,\Omega$

42. **(c)**

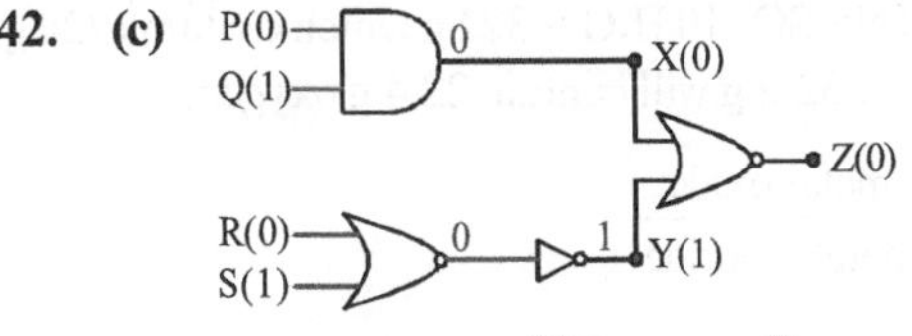

43. **(b)**

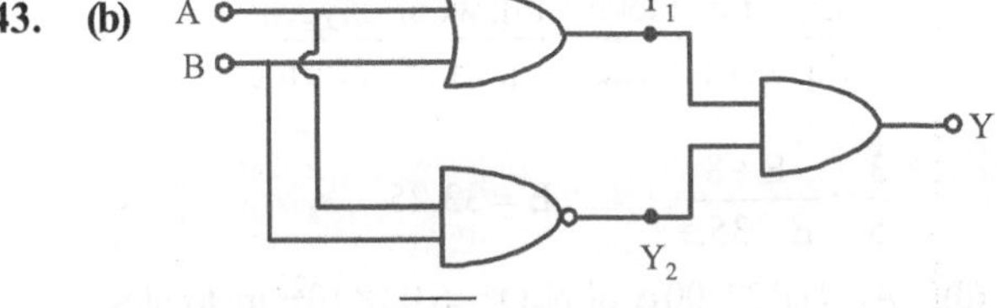

$Y_1 = A + B,\ Y_2 = \overline{A.B}$

$Y = (A + B)\cdot\overline{AB} = A\cdot\overline{A} + A\cdot\overline{B} + B\cdot\overline{A} + B\cdot\overline{B}$

$= 0 + A\cdot\overline{B} + B\cdot\overline{A} + 0 = A\cdot\overline{B} + B\cdot\overline{A}$ (XOR gate)

44. **(b)** $E_g = 2.0\,\text{eV} = 2 \times 1.6 \times 10^{-19}\,\text{J}$

$E_g = h\nu$

$$\therefore\ \nu = \frac{E_g}{h} = \frac{2 \times 1.6 \times 10^{-19}\,\text{J}}{6.62 \times 10^{-34}\,\text{Js}}$$

$= 0.4833 \times 10^{15}\,\text{s}^{-1} = 4.833 \times 10^{14}\,\text{Hz}$

$\simeq 5 \times 10^{14}\,\text{Hz}$

45. **(d)** The average value of output direct current in a full wave rectifier = (average value of current over a cycle)

$$= (2I_0/\pi) = \frac{2I_0}{\pi}$$

HINTS & SOLUTIONS (CHEMISTRY – Chapter-wise Tests)

Speed Test-29

1. (c) Each has three significant figures. When zero is used to locate the decimal point it is not considered as significant figure.

2. (d) Both Y and X are neither precise nor accurate as the two values in each of them are not close. With respect to X & Y, the values of Z are close & agree with the true value. Hence, both precise & accurate.

3. (c) M. Wt of $Na_2SO_4.10\,H_2O$ is 322 g which contains 224 g oxygen. ∴ 32.2 g will contain 22.4 g oxygen.

4. (b) $\frac{\text{Wt. of metal oxide}}{\text{Wt. of metal chloride}}$

$$=\frac{\text{Eq. wt of metal} + \text{Eq. wt of oxygen}}{\text{Eq. wt of metal} + \text{Eq. wt of chlorine}}$$

$$\frac{3}{5}=\frac{E+8}{E+35.5} \qquad \therefore E = 33.25$$

5. (d) At NTP 22400 cc of $N_2O = 6.02\times10^{23}$ molecules

$$\therefore 1\text{ cc } N_2O=\frac{6.02\times10^{23}}{22400}\text{ molecules}$$

$$=\frac{3\times6.02\times10^{23}}{22400}\text{ atoms }=\frac{1.8}{224}\times10^{22}\text{ atoms}$$

No. of electrons in a molecule of $N_2O = 7+7+8=22$

Hence no. of electrons

$$=\frac{6.02\times10^{23}}{22400}\times22\text{ electrons }=\frac{1.32\times10^{23}}{224}$$

6. (c) In law of reciprocal proportions, the two elements combining with the third element, must combine with each other in the same ratio or multiple of that ratio of S and O when combine with C is 2 : 1. Ratio of S and O in SO_2 is 1 : 1

7. (d) Normality of oxalic acid solution

$$=\frac{6.3\times1000}{63\times250}=0.4\text{ N}$$

Now from

$N_1V_1 = N_2V_2$

$0.4 \times 10 = 0.1 \times V_2$

$V_2 = 40$ mL

8. (c) The relation between molarity (M) and molality (m) is

$$d = M\left(\frac{1}{m}+\frac{M_2}{1000}\right),\ M_2 = \text{Mol. mass of solute}$$

On putting value

$$1.252 = 3\left(\frac{1}{m}+\frac{58.5}{1000}\right)$$

on solving m = 2.79 molal.

9. (b) The number of atoms in 0.1 mole of a triatomic gas $= 0.1 \times 3 \times 6.023 \times 10^{23}$.
$= 1.806 \times 10^{23}$

10. (a)

11. (c) 50% of X (Atomic mass 10), 50% of Y (Atomic mass 20).

Relative number of atoms of X $=\frac{50}{10}=5$ and than

$Y=\frac{50}{20}=2.5$

Simple Ratio 2 : 1. Formula X_2Y

12. (c) (a) Weight of H_2 = mole × molecular wt.
$= 0.2 \times 2 = 0.4$ g

(b) $6.023 \times 10^{23} = 1$ mole

Thus $6.023 \times 10^{22} = 0.1$ mole

Weight of $N_2 = 0.1 \times 28 = 2.8$ g

(c) Weight of silver = 0.1 g

(d) Weight of oxygen = 32 × 0.1 = 3.2 g

13. (b) Moles of nitride ion

$$=\frac{4.2}{14}=0.3\text{ mole}=0.3\times N_A\text{ nitride ions.}$$

Valence electrons = 8 × 0.3 N_A = 2.4 N_A (5 + 3 due to charge). One N^{3-} ion contains 8 valence electrons.

14. (a) $\underset{2}{2K_2CrO_4}+\underset{2}{2HCl}\longrightarrow \underset{1}{K_2Cr_2O_7}+\underset{2}{2KCl}+\underset{1}{H_2O}$

15. (b) Terminal zeros are not significant if there is no decimal i.e., 290 contains two significant figures whereas in 29900. there are 5 significant figures; 1.23 × 1.331 = 1.63713 but keeping the mind the 1.23 has only few significant figures i.e., only three significant figures, so result should also be reported in three significant figures only. Thus 1.6373 should be rounded off to 1.64. Value 1.783 is rounded off to 2, so has only one significant figure.

16. (a) No. of molecules in different cases

(a) ∵ 22.4 litre at STP contains
$= 6.023 \times 10^{23}$ molecules of H_2

$$\therefore 15\text{ litre at STP contains}=\frac{15}{22.4}\times6.023\times10^{23}$$
$= 4.03 \times 10^{23}$ molecules of H_2

(b) ∵ 22.4 litre at STP contains
$= 6.023\times10^{23}$ molecules of N_2

$$\because 5\text{ litre at STP contains}=\frac{5}{22.4}\times6.023\times10^{23}$$
$= 1.344 \times 10^{23}$ molecules of N_2

(c) ∵ 2 gm of $H_2 = 6.023\times10^{23}$ molecules of H_2

$\because$ 0.5 gm of $H_2 = \frac{0.5}{2} \times 6.023 \times 10^{23}$

$= 1.505 \times 10^{23}$ molecules of H_2

(d) Similarly 10 g of O_2 gas

$= \frac{10}{32} \times 6.023 \times 10^{23}$ molecules of O_2

$= 1.88 \times 10^{23}$ molecules of O_2

Thus (a) will have maximum number of molecules.

17. **(a)** 21% of 1 litre is 0.21 litre.
22.4 litres = 1 mole at STP

$\therefore$ 0.21 litre $= \frac{0.21}{22.4} = 0.0093$ mole

18. **(a)** $BaCO_3 \longrightarrow BaO + CO_2$

192 g of $BaCO_3$ 1 gives mole of CO_2 = 22.4 L
9.85 g of $BaCO_3$ will give 0.05 mole of CO_2 which is equal to 1.12 litre.

19. **(b)** Moles of Ca^{2+} to be precipitated $= \frac{20 \times 1}{1000} = 0.02$

Moles of Cu^{2+} to be precipitated $= \frac{20 \times 0.5}{1000} = 0.01$

Hence molar amount of H_2S will be in the ratio 2 : 1

$\left(\text{Remember Moles} = \frac{\text{Molarity} \times \text{volume in ml}}{1000}\right)$

20. **(c)** For statement (i) : H, O, C, N = All have different chemical properties.
For statement (ii) : It is true as per Dalton's postulate.
For statement (iii) : N : O = 1 : 1 (NO)
For statement (iv) : Dalton's postulates says, atoms can neither be created nor destroyed.

21. **(d)** No. of moles $= \frac{\text{weight}}{\text{mol. wt.}} = \frac{50}{342} = 0.14$ mole

22. **(b)** For one mole of the oxide
Moles of M = 0.98
Moles of $O^{2-} = 1$
Let moles of $M^{3+} = x$
$\therefore$ Moles of $M^{2+} = 0.98 - x$

on balancing charge

$(0.98 - x) \times 2 + 3x - 2 = 0$
$x = 0.04$

$\therefore$ % of $M^{3+} = \frac{0.04}{0.98} \times 100 = 4.08\%$

23. **(d)** $MgCO_3 \longrightarrow MgO + CO_2$

84 g of $MgCO_3$ form 40 g of MgO

$\therefore$ 20g of $MgCO_3$ form $\frac{40 \times 20}{84}$ g of MgO

= 9.52 g of MgO
Since 8.0 g of MgO is formed

Purity of sample $= \frac{8}{9.52} \times 100 = 84.0\%$

24. **(d)** In, AlF_3 the number of F is 3, for one AlF_3 molecule
$3F^- \equiv 1$ formula unit of AlF_3

$3.0 \times 10^{24}\ F^- \equiv \frac{1}{3} \times 3.0 \times 10^{24}\ AlF_3$ units

25. **(d)** Mass of a substance is the amount of matter present in it while weight is the force exerted by gravity on an object.
Mass is constant while weight may vary from one place to another due to gravity.
SI unit of both mass and weight is kilogram.

26. **(a)** Fe (no. of moles) $= \frac{558.5}{55.85} = 10$ moles $= 10N_A$ atoms.
No. of moles in 60 g of C = 60/12 = 5 moles = $5N_A$ atoms.

27. **(c)** 50 mL of 16.9% solution of $AgNO_3$

$\left(\frac{16.9}{100} \times 50\right) = 8.45$ g of $AgNO_3$

$n_{mole} = \frac{8.45g}{(107.8 + 14 + 16 \times 3)\ g/mol}$

$= \left(\frac{8.45\ g}{169.8 g/mol}\right) = 0.0497$ moles

50 mL of 5.8% solution of NaCl contain

$NaCl = \left(\frac{5.8}{100} \times 50\right) = 2.9$ g

$n_{NaCl} = \frac{2.9g}{(23 + 35.5) g/mol} = 0.0495$ moles

$AgNO_3$ +	NaCl	$\rightarrow AgCl\downarrow + \overset{\oplus}{Na} + \overset{\ominus}{Cl}$
1 mole	1 mole	1 mole
$\therefore$ 0.049 mole	0.049 mole	0.049 mole of AgCl

$n = \frac{w}{M} \Rightarrow w = (n_{AgCl}) \times$ Molecular Mass

$= (0.049) \times (107.8 + 35.5)$
$= 7.02$ g

28. **(d)** $n_C = \frac{26 g}{12 g/mol} = 2.16$

$n_{O_2} = \frac{20 g}{32 g/mol} = 0.625$

O_2 will be a limiting reagent in reaction (i)

$n_{N_2} = \frac{60\,g}{28\,g/mol} = 2.14$

$n_{H_2} = 40$

According to balanced equation,
1 mole of N_2 requires 3 mole of H_2
2.14 mole of N_2 require 6.42 mole of H_2
N_2 will be a limiting reagent in reaction (ii)

$n_{P_4} = \frac{100g}{4 \times 31} = 0.86 \qquad n_{O_2} = 6.25$

According to balanced equation
1 mole of P_4 require 3 mole of O_2
0.86 mole of P_4 require 2.58 mole of O_2
So P_4 is a limiting reagent in reaction (iii)

29. **(a)** Proceed as follows :

Element	%	At. wt.	RNA	Simplest ratio
A	25	12.5	$\frac{25}{12.5} = 2$	1
B	75	37.5	$\frac{75}{37.5} = 2$	1

∴ The simplest formula of compound is AB

30. **(d)** Moles of Iodine present $= \frac{254}{127} = 2$

Moles of oxygen $= \frac{80}{16} = 5$

∴ The molecular formula is $= I_2O_5$

31. **(a)** Change in O.N. of N in HNO_3 is 3, hence one formula weight has 3 equivalents.

$$3Sn + 12HCl + 4H\overset{+5}{N}O_3 \longrightarrow 3SnCl_4 + 4\overset{+2}{N}O + 8H_2O \quad (+3e^-)$$

Since change in O.N. = 3

32. **(c)** Ratio of no. of atoms in the molecule

$= \frac{9}{12} : \frac{1}{1} : \frac{3.5}{14} = 0.75 : 1 : 0.25 = 3 : 4 : 1$

Empirical formula $= C_3H_4N$;
M.F. $= (C_3H_4N)_n$
n × Empirical formula mass = Molecular mass
$n(3 \times 12 + 4 + 14) = 108$
$n \times 54 = 108$
$n = 2$
M.F. $= C_6H_8N_2$

33. **(a)** 2.6 has two significant figures.
0.260 has three significant figures.
0.002600 has four significant figures.
2.6000 has five significant figures.

34. **(d)** Writing the equation for the reaction, we get

$$\underset{\substack{207+16\\=223\text{ g}}}{PbO} + \underset{\substack{2\times 36.5\\=73\text{g}}}{2HCl} \longrightarrow \underset{\substack{207+71\\=278\text{g}}}{PbCl_2} + H_2O$$

No. of moles of PbO $= \frac{6.5}{223} = 0.029$

No. of moles of HCl $= \frac{3.2}{36.5} = 0.0877$

Thus PbO is the limiting reactant 1 mole of PbO produce 1 mole $PbCl_2$.
0.029 mole PbO produces 0.029 mole $PbCl_2$.

35. **(c)** When the weight of different solutes are equal in equal volumes of solutions, the molarity is inversely related to molecular mass of the solute. Mol. mass of NaCl is less than KCl. Hence, molarity of NaCl solution will be more.

36. **(b)** geq of HCl $= \frac{3}{36.5} \times 2.5 = 0.20548 =$ geq of $Al(OH)_3$

Weight of $Al(OH)_3 = \frac{0.20548 \times 78}{3}$

$= 5.342\text{ g} = 5342\text{ mg}$

∴ No of tablets $= \frac{5342}{400} = 13.35 \approx 14$

37. **(a)** Let 100 g of compound be there.

Number of moles of Nitrogen $= \frac{35}{14} = 2.5$

Number of moles of Hydrogen $= \frac{5}{1.008} = 4.9$

Number of moles of Carbon $= \frac{60}{12.01} = 4.9$

Since 2.5 is the smallest value division by it give ratio
N : H : C
1 : 1.96 : 1.96
= 1 : 2 : 2

Empirical formula $= C_2H_2N$
Empirical formula weight = 2 × 12 + 2 + 14 = 40
Molecular mass = 80
Molecular formulae $= n\,(C_2H_2N)$

$\because = 2\,(C_2H_2N)\left(n = \frac{80}{40}\right) = C_4H_4N_2$

38. **(a)** $\underset{a}{C_3H_8} + 5O_2 \rightarrow \underset{3a}{3CO_2} + 4H_2O$

$\underset{(3-a)}{C_4H_{10}} + \frac{13}{2}O_2 \rightarrow \underset{4(3-a)}{4CO_2} + 5H_2O$

But $3a + 4(3 - a) = 10$
∴ a = 2 (Propane) and 3 – 2 = 1 (Butane)

39. **(a)** Mass of 6.023×10^{23} atoms of oxygen = 16 g
Mass of one atom of oxygen

$= \frac{16}{6.023 \times 10^{23}} = 2.66 \times 10^{-23}$ g

Mass of 6.023×10^{23} atoms of nitrogen = 14 g

Mass of one atom of nitrogen

$= \frac{14}{6.023 \times 10^{23}} = 2.32 \times 10^{-23}$ g

Mass of 1×10^{-10} mole of oxygen = 16×10^{-10}

Mass of 1 mole of copper = 63 g

Mass of 1 mole of oxygen = 16 g

Mass of 1×10^{-10} mole of copper = $63 \times 1 \times 10^{-10}$

$= 63 \times 10^{-10}$

So, the order of increasing mass is II < I < III < IV.

40. **(d)** $N_2(g) + 3H_2(g) \longrightarrow 2NH_3(g)$;

N_2 is the limiting reagent in this reaction. 10 L N_2 will react with 30 L H_2 to produce 20 L of NH_3. As the yield of reaction is 50% composition of resultant mixture will be 5 L of N_2, 15 L of H_2 and 10 L of NH_3.

41. **(d)** 1 Mole of $Mg_3(PO_4)_2$ contains 8 mole of oxygen atoms

$\therefore$ 8 mole of oxygen atoms $\equiv$ 1 mole of $Mg_3(PO_4)_2$

0.25 mole of oxygen atom $\equiv \frac{1}{8} \times 0.25$ mole of $Mg_3(PO_4)_2$

$= 3.125 \times 10^{-2}$ mole of $Mg_3(PO_4)_2$

42. **(c)** Let the alcohol be ROH and x its molecular weight

$\underset{x\,g}{ROH} + CH_3MgI \rightarrow \underset{16\,g}{CH_4} + ROMgI$

$\frac{4.12}{1000}$ g of alcohol will produce $\frac{16}{x} \times \frac{4.12}{1000}$ g of methane

Methane actually obtained is $= \frac{16 \times 1.12}{22400}$ g

equal $= \frac{16 \times 4.12}{x \times 1000} = \frac{16 \times 1.12}{22400} \therefore x = 82.4$

43. **(c)** The conditions given are standard conditions

224 mL has mass = 1 g;

22400 mL will have mass = 100 g. This is mol. wt of gas

6.023×10^{23} molecules have $3 \times 6.023 \times 10^{23}$ atoms since gas is triatomic

$\therefore$ weight of one atom

$= \frac{100}{3 \times 6.023 \times 10^{23}} = 5.5 \times 10^{-23}$ g

44. **(b)** Sum of oxidation states must be equal to zero which is given by $A_3(BC_4)_2 = A_3B_2C_8$ $(6 + 10 - 16 = 0)$

45. **(d)**

	SO_2 +	$\frac{1}{2}O_2$ $\rightleftharpoons$	SO_3
Initial	5 mole	5 mole	0 mole
Final	5 – 3 = 2 mole	5 – 1.5 mole = 3.5 mole	3 mole

Total number of moles = 2 + 3.5 + 3.0 = 8.5

Speed Test-30

1. (c) The species CO, NO^+, CN^- and C_2^{2-} contain 14 electrons each.

2. (d) Rutherford used doubly charged helium particle. (α - particle)

3. (d) $E_n^H = -2.18\times10^{-18}\left(\frac{Z^2}{n_H^2}\right)J = \frac{-2.18\times10^{-18}}{n_H^2}J$

$$E_n^{He^+} = -2.18\times10^{-18}\left(\frac{Z^2}{n_{He^+}^2}\right)J = \frac{-2.18\times10^{-18}\times4}{n_{He^+}^2}J$$

$$E_n^H = E_n^{He^+} \Rightarrow \frac{1}{n_H^2} = \frac{4}{n_{He^+}^2} \Rightarrow n_{He^+} = 2\times n_H$$

If $n_H = 1$ Then $n_{He^+} = 2$

If $n_H = 2$ Then $n_{He^+} = 4$

If $n_H = 3$ Then $n_{He^+} = 6$

4. (c) Energy of a photon, $E = \frac{hc}{\lambda}$

$$= \frac{6.626\times10^{-34}(Js)\times3\times10^8(ms^{-1})}{331.3\times10^{-9}(m)} = 6\times10^{-19}J$$

No. of photons emitted per second

$$= \frac{600\ (J)}{6\times10^{-19}(J)} = 10^{21}$$

5. (a) $\Delta E = 2.178\times10^{-18}\left(\frac{1}{1^2}-\frac{1}{2^2}\right) = \frac{hc}{\lambda}$

$$2.17\times10^{-18}\times\frac{3}{4} = \frac{hc}{\lambda} = \frac{6.62\times10^{-34}\times3\times10^8}{\lambda}$$

$$\lambda = \frac{6.62\times10^{-34}\times3\times10^8\times4}{2.17\times10^{-18}\times3} = 1.214\times10^{-7}m$$

6. (d) Energy required to break one mole of Cl – Cl bonds in Cl_2

$$= \frac{242\times10^3}{6.023\times10^{23}} = \frac{hc}{\lambda} = \frac{6.626\times10^{-34}\times3\times10^8}{\lambda}$$

$$\therefore \lambda = \frac{6.626\times10^{-34}\times3\times10^8\times6.023\times10^{23}}{242\times10^3}$$

$= 0.4947\times10^{-6}\ m = 494.7\ nm$

7. (d) For Balmer $n_1 = 2$ and $n_2 = 3$;

$$\bar{v} = R_H\left(\frac{1}{2^2}-\frac{1}{3^2}\right) = \frac{5R_H}{36}\ cm^{-1}$$

8. (c) For 4p electron n = 4, l = 1, m = –1, 0 + 1 and s = $+\frac{1}{2}$ or $-\frac{1}{2}$.

9. (c) Em waves shown in figure A has higher wavelength in comparison to em waves shown in figure B. Thus these waves also differ in frequency and energy. $\nu = \frac{c}{\lambda}$

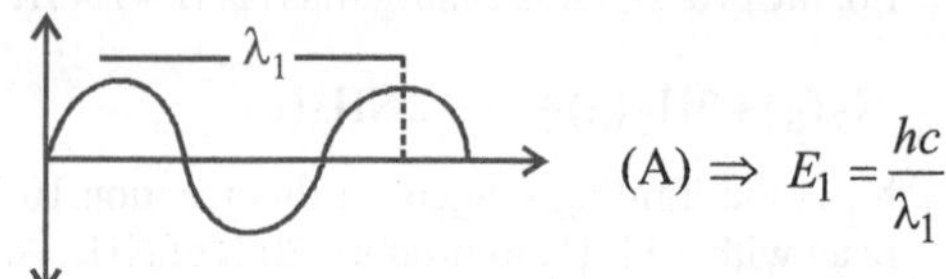

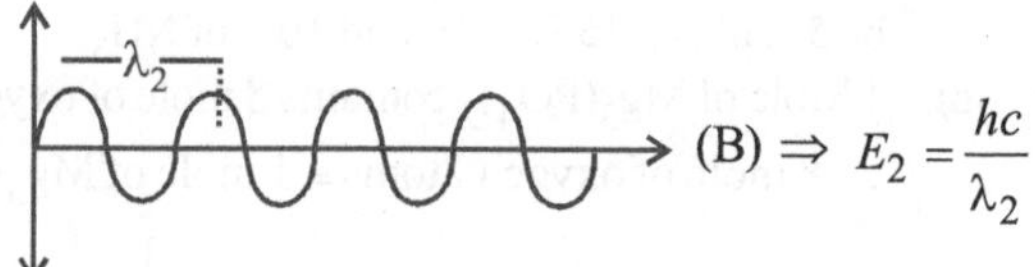

$$\lambda_1 > \lambda_2 \Rightarrow E_1 < E_2$$

10. (a) For *d*-subshell ⇒ Number of orbitals = 5, l = 2
f-subshell ⇒ Number of orbitals = 7, l = 3
s-subshell ⇒ Number of orbitals = 1, l = 0
p-subshell ⇒ Number of orbitals = 3, l = 1

11. (a) For s-electron, l = 0

$\therefore$ Orbital angular momentum $= \sqrt{0(0+1)}\frac{h}{2\pi} = 0$

12. (b) $\Delta E = h\nu = \frac{hc}{\lambda}$;

$$\therefore \lambda = \frac{hc}{\Delta E} = \frac{6.63\times10^{-34}(3\times10^8)}{3.03\times10^{-19}} = 656\ nm$$

13. (a) (n + l) rule the higher the value of (n + l), the higher is the energy. When (n+l) value is the same see value of n.

	I	II	III	IV
(n + l)	(4+1)	(4+0)	(3+2)	(3+1)
	5	4	5	4

$\therefore$ IV < II < III < I

14. (c) (i) Beyond a certain wavelength the line spectrum becomes band spectrum.
(ii) For Balmer series $n_1 = 2$
(iv) For calculation of longest wavelength use nearest value of n_2. Hence for longest wavelength in Balmer series of hydrogen spectrum, $n_1 = 2$ & $n_2 = 3$.

15. (a) $\bar{\nu} = \frac{1}{\lambda} = R_H\left[\frac{1}{n_1^2} - \frac{1}{n_2^2}\right]$

For second line in lyman series

$n_2 = 3$

$\therefore \frac{1}{\lambda} = R_H\left[\frac{1}{1^2} - \frac{1}{3^2}\right] = R_H\left[\frac{1}{1} - \frac{1}{9}\right] = \frac{8R_H}{9}$

16. (c) The kinetic energy of the ejected electron is given by the equation

$$h\nu = h\nu_o + \frac{1}{2}mv^2 \quad \because \nu = \frac{c}{\lambda}$$

or $$\frac{hc}{\lambda} = \frac{hc}{\lambda_o} + \frac{1}{2}mv^2$$

$$\frac{1}{2}mv^2 = \frac{hc}{\lambda} - \frac{hc}{\lambda_o}$$

$$= hc\left(\frac{\lambda_o - \lambda}{\lambda\lambda_o}\right)$$

$\therefore$ $$v^2 = \frac{2hc}{m}\left(\frac{\lambda_o - \lambda}{\lambda\lambda_o}\right)$$

or $$v = \sqrt{\frac{2hc}{m}\left(\frac{\lambda_o - \lambda}{\lambda\lambda_o}\right)}$$

17. (a) $p = \frac{h}{\lambda} = \frac{6.63\times10^{-34}}{2.2\times10^{-11}} = 3\times10^{-23}\text{ kg/s}$

18. (d) Atomic orbitals are 4s, 3s, 3p and 3d. ($n + l$) values being 4, 3, 4 and 5. Hence 3d has highest energy.

19. (a)

20. (b) Since electrons are negatively charged particles they got deflected toward positively charged electrode whereas proton being positively charged will get deflected toward negative electrode. Since neutrons are neutral, so they went straight.

21. (a) The expression for orbital angular momentum is

Angular momentum $= \sqrt{l(l+1)}\left(\frac{h}{2\pi}\right)$

For d orbital, $l = 2$.

Hence, $L = \sqrt{2(2+1)}\left(\frac{h}{2\pi}\right) = \sqrt{6}\left(\frac{h}{2\pi}\right)$

22. (c) $\Delta x \,.\, \Delta p = \frac{h}{4\pi}$ or $\Delta x \,.\, m\Delta v = \frac{h}{4\pi}$;

$$\Delta v = \frac{0.011}{100}\times3\times10^4 = 3.3\text{ cms}^{-1}$$

$$\Delta x = \frac{6.6\times10^{-27}}{4\times3.14\times9.1\times10^{-28}\times3.3} = 0.175\text{ cm}$$

23. (b) $E = h\nu = \frac{hc}{\lambda}$; and $\nu = \frac{c}{\lambda}$

$$8\times10^{15} = \frac{3.0\times10^8}{\lambda}$$

$$\therefore \lambda = \frac{3.0\times10^8}{8\times10^{15}} = 0.37\times10^{-7} = 37.5\times10^{-9}\text{ m} = 4\times10^1\text{ nm}$$

24. (a) According to de-Broglie's equation

$$\lambda = \frac{h}{p} = \frac{h}{mv}$$

Given, $h = 6.6 \times 10^{-34}$ Js, $m = 200 \times 10^{-3}$ kg

$$v = \frac{5}{60\times60}\text{ m/s}$$

$$\lambda = \frac{6.6\times10^{-34}}{200\times10^{-3}\times5/(60\times60)} = 2.38\times10^{-10}\text{ m}$$

25. (b) Average atomic mass of Fe

$$= \frac{(54\times5)+(56\times90)+(57\times5)}{100} = 55.95$$

26. (a) $\Delta E = -2.0\times10^{-18}\times\left(\frac{1}{2^2} - \frac{1}{1^2}\right)$

$$= -2.0\times10^{-18}\times\frac{-3}{4}$$

$$= 1.5\times10^{-18}$$

$$\Delta E = \frac{hc}{\lambda}$$

$$\lambda = \frac{hc}{\Delta E} = \frac{6.6\times10^{-34}\times3\times10^8}{1.5\times10^{-18}} = 1.325\times10^{-7}\text{ m}$$

27. (a) We know $\Delta p.\Delta x \geq \frac{h}{4\pi}$

since $\Delta p = \Delta x$ (given)

$\therefore \Delta p.\Delta p = \frac{h}{4\pi}$

or $m\Delta v.\, m\Delta v. = \frac{h}{4\pi}$ $[\therefore \Delta p = m\Delta v]$

or $(\Delta v)^2 = \frac{h}{4\pi m^2}$

or $\Delta v = \sqrt{\frac{h}{4\pi m^2}} = \frac{1}{2m}\sqrt{\frac{h}{\pi}}$

Thus option (a) is the correct option.

28. (b) The radius of nucleus is of the order of 1.5×10^{-13} to 6.5×10^{-13} cm or 1.5 to 6.5 Fermi (1 Fermi $= 10^{-13}$ cm)

29. (b)

30. (b)

	5p	4f	6s	5d
(n + l)	5+1	4+3	6+0	5+2
	6	7	6	7

Hence the order is 5p < 6s < 4f < 5d

31. (a)

32. (c)

33. (c) Not more than two electrons can be present in same atomic orbital. This is Pauli's exclusion principle.

34. (a)

35. (b)

36. (c)

37. (d) Total energy of a revolving electron is the sum of its kinetic and potential energy.
Total energy = K.E. + P. E.

$$= \frac{e^2}{2r} + \left(-\frac{e^2}{r}\right)$$

$$= -\frac{e^2}{2r}$$

38. (d) From the expression of Bohr's theory, we know that

$$m_e v_1 r_1 = n_1 \frac{h}{2\pi}$$

$$\& \; m_e v_2 r_2 = n_2 \frac{h}{2\pi}$$

$$\frac{m_e v_1 r_1}{m_e v_2 r_2} = \frac{n_1}{n_2} \frac{h}{2\pi} \times \frac{2\pi}{h}$$

Given, $r_1 = 5r_2, n_1 = 5, n_2 = 4$

$$\frac{m_e \times v_1 \times 5r_2}{m_e \times v_2 \times r_2} = \frac{5}{4}$$

$$\Rightarrow \frac{v_1}{v_2} = \frac{5}{4 \times 5} = \frac{1}{4} = 1:4$$

39. (a) The electronic configuration of Rubidium (Rb = 37) is

$1s^2 2s^2 2p^6 3s^2 3p^6 3d^{10} 4s^2 4p^6 5s^1$

Since last electron enters in 5*s* orbital

Hence $n = 5, l = 0, m = 0, s = \pm\frac{1}{2}$

40. (d) Except Al^{3+} all contain one electron and Bohr's model could explain the spectra for one electron system, Bohr's model was not able to explain the spectra of multielectron system.

41. (a)

42. (d) $r_n = 0.529 \frac{n^2}{Z}$ Å

For hydrogen, $n = 1$ and $Z = 1$; $\therefore r_H = 0.529$
For Be^{3+}, $n = 2$ and $Z = 4$;

$$\therefore r_{Be^{3+}} = \frac{0.529 \times 2^2}{4} = 0.529$$

43. (a) Velocity of electron

$$v_n = 2.19 \times 10^6 \frac{Z}{n} ms^{-1}$$

The distance travelled by electron in 10^{-8} s in Second Bohr's Orbit

$$= \frac{2.19 \times 10^6 \times 1 \times 10^{-8}}{2} m$$

$$= 1.095 \times 10^{-2} \text{ m}$$

The circumference of second orbit = $2\pi r_2$

$$= 2\pi \times 0.529 \times 10^{-10} \times 2^2$$

$$= 13.3 \times 10^{-10} \text{ m}$$

$$\therefore \text{ Number of revolutions} = \frac{1.095 \times 10^{-2}}{13.3 \times 10^{-10}} = 8.23 \times 10^6$$

44. (b) de – Broglie wavelength is given by :

$$\lambda = \frac{h}{mv} \quad \text{... (i)}$$

$$K.E. = \frac{1}{2} mv^2$$

$$v^2 = \frac{2KE}{m}$$

$$v = \sqrt{\frac{2KE}{m}}$$

Substituting this in equation (i)

$$\lambda = \frac{h}{m}\sqrt{\frac{m}{2KE}}$$

$$\lambda = h\sqrt{\frac{1}{2m(K.E.)}} \quad \text{...(i)}$$

i.e. $\lambda \propto \frac{1}{\sqrt{KE}}$

$\therefore$ when *KE* become 4 times wavelength become 1/2.

45. (a) $r_n = a_0 \times n^2$

$$r_4 = a_0 \times (4)^2 = 16a_0$$

$$mvr = \frac{nh}{2\pi}; \; mv = \frac{4h}{2\pi \times 16a_0};$$

$$\lambda = \frac{h}{mv} = \frac{h}{h/8\pi a_0} = 8\pi a_0$$

Speed Test-31

1. (d)
2. (d) The additional π-molecular electron in O_2^- is added to the less stable antibonding orbital. Hence, it is easy to remove that electron from O_2^- ion. Thus I.E. (I.P.) of O_2^- is lowest.
3. (a) Continuous increase as no. of shells increases down the group.
4. (b)
5. (b) Closed shell (Ne), half filled (P) and completely filled configuration (Mg) are the cause of higher value of I.E.
6. (d)
7. (b) Cu, Ag and Au are coinage metals. They belong to group IB (*d*-block) of periodic table.
8. (d) In fourth period filling up of 3*d* orbital becomes energetically favourable before the 4*p* orbital is filled.
9. (b) $K^+ \rightarrow K^{2+} + e^-$. Since e^- is to be removed from stable configuration.
10. (a) For isoelectronic species ionic radii decreases as the charge on ion decreases. Further on moving down in a group ionic radii increases. Hence the correct order is

$$O^{2-} < N^{3-} < S^{2-} < P^{3-}$$

11. (c) On moving down a group atomic radii increases.
12. (a) Incoming electrons occupies the smaller n = 2 shell, also negative charge on oxygen (O^-) is another factor due to which incoming electron feel repulsion.
Hence electron repulsion outweigh the stability gained by achieving noble gas configuration.
13. (c)
14. (b) It is electronic configuration of alkali metal. Hence it will form basic oxide.
15. (b) The right sequence of $I.E_1$ of Li < B < Be < C.
16. (c) Al ($3s^2 p^1$) and Mg ($3s^2$). Lower energy is required to remove $3p^1$ electron than $3s^1$ electron (penetrating effect is $s > p > d > f$). Secondly Mg has stable electronic configuration than Al
17. (c) I represents Li, II represents K
III represents Br, IV represents I
V represents He
So, amongst these, II represents most reactive metal and V represents least reactive non-metal.
18. (c)
19. (c) Generally, the ionization enthalpies or energy increases from left to right in a period and decreases from top to bottom in a group. Several factor such as atomic radius, nuclear charge, shielding effect are responsible for change of ionization enthalpies.
Here, Ist ionization enthalpy of *A* and *B* is greater than group I (Li 520 $kJmol^{-1}$ to Cs374 $kJmol^{-1}$), which means element *A* and *B* belong to group –2 and all three given ionization enthalpy values are less for element *B* means *B* will come below *A*.
20. (b) For dissolution, Hydration energy > Lattice energy.
$BaSO_4$ is sparingly soluble in water because its hydration energy is lesser than the lattice energy and thus ions are not separated from each other.
21. (c) The anomalous behaviour of first member of a group in the *s*- and *p*-block element is due to their small size, large charge/radius ratio and high electronegativity.
22. (c) In $3d^6 4s^2$ the differentiating electron enters d sub shell, Hence it represents transition metal, Fe.
23. (b) In the isoelectronic species, all isoelectronic anions belong to the same period and cations to the next period.
24. (b) On passing from left to right in a period acidic character of the normal oxides of the elements increases with increase in electronegativity.
25. (a) The electronic configuration clearly suggests that it is a d-block element (having configuration $(n-1)\,d^{1-10}\,ns^{0-2}$) which starts from III B and goes till II B. Hence with d^3 configuration it would be classified in the group.
26. (b) Correct order of increasing basic strength is
$NH_3 > PH_3 > AsH_3 > SbH_3 > BiH_3$
27. (c) Electron affinity of ^9F is less than that of ^{17}Cl
28. (c) $ns^2\,np^1$ is the electronic configuration of III A period.
Al_2O_3 is amphoteric oxide
29. (d) P^{5+} has more effective nuclear charge and smaller size than P^{3+}.
30. (a) For isoelectronic species, size of anion increases as negative charge increases. Thus the correct order is

$$\underset{(1.71)}{N^{3-}} > \underset{(1.40)}{O^{2-}} > \underset{(1.36)}{F^-}$$

31. (a) Hydrogen bonding increases the boiling point. Hydrogen bonds are formed in compounds having F or O or N with hydrogen. S, Se, Te cannot undergo hydrogen bond formation because of their larger size and lower electronegativity values.

32. (b) A. $Li^+ < Al^{2+} < Mg^{2+} < K^+$
The cation with the greater positive charge will have a smaller radius because of the greater attraction of the electrons to the nucleus. Anion with the greater negative charge will have the larger radius.

$$\text{Positive charge} \propto \frac{1}{\text{ionic radius}}$$

Negative charge $\propto$ ionic radius

B. Greater positive charge, increases effective nuclear charge in case of isoelectronic species. While for same group elements effective nuclear charge decreases down the groups.

C. $Cl > F > Br > I$
electron affinity of Cl is highest in halogen family.

D. $F > Cl > Br > I$
electronegativity of fluorine (F) is higher than Cl, Br and I.

33. (a) Because Al is amphoteric in nature so it dissolve in both acid and base.

34. (b) Pb^{2+} ($5d^{10}\,6s^2$), has the most stable +2 oxidation state because here the *d*-orbital is completely filled and is more stable than Fe^{2+} ($3d^6$). Again Ag^+ ($4d^{10}$) is more stable as here again the *d*-orbital is completely filled and Ag^{2+} is not easily obtained. Pb^{2+} is more stable compared to Sn^{2+} ($4d^{10}\,5s^2$) because of its large size.

35. (b)

36. (a) Iodine with lower atomic weight than that of tellurium (Group VI) was placed in Group VII along with fluorine, chlorine, bromine because of similarities in properties.

37. (c) Covalent radius is radius of an atom in its bound state i.e., in fluorine it is half of distance between two covalently bonded fluorine atoms; van der Waal radii is one-half of the distance between the nuclei of two identical non-bonded isolated atoms. These atoms are attracted toward each other through weak van der Waal's force hence van der Waal radii are very large.

38. (c) According to Dobereneir's triad the atomic mass of Br will be average of the atomic masses of Cl & I

$$= \frac{35.5 + 127}{2} = 81.25$$

39. (b) $\because$ For $Na \longrightarrow Na^+ + e^-$ $\quad IE_1 = 5.1$ eV

$\therefore$ For $Na^+ + e^- \longrightarrow Na$ $\quad EF = -5.1$ eV

(because the reaction is reverse)

40. (b) N has half filled atomic orbital, which is more stable.

41. (d) Number of moles $= \dfrac{1}{35.5}$

Given, 1 eV = 23.06 kcal mol^{-1}

3.7 eV = 3.7 × 23.06 kcal mol^{-1}

i.e. 1 mole realease energy

= 3.7 × 23.06 kcal

$\therefore$ Energy released

$$= \frac{1}{35.5} \times 3.7 \times 23.06 \text{ kcal} = 2.4 \text{ kcal}$$

42. (a)

43. (a) O^- ion exerts a force of repulsion on the incoming electron. The energy is required to overcome it.

44. (d) Oxides of Eka-Aluminium = Ga_2O_3
Oxides of Eka-Silicon = SiO_2
Melting point of Eka-Aluminium = Low (302 K)
Melting point of Eka-Silicon = High (1231 K)

45. (b) In case of halogens covalent radius is considered this bond is formed by overlapping of electron clouds; while noble gases remain monoatomic, in this case only way to obtain radius is through van der Waal radii.

Speed Test-32

1. **(b)** Electronic configuration reveals it is monovalent (in fact Na) hence its oxide will be M_2O.

2. **(c)** CO_3^{2-} Its structure is $\left[\begin{array}{c}\ddot{O}\\ \ \ \backslash\!\backslash C-\ddot{O}: \\ \ddot{O}^{/}\end{array}\right]^{2-}$

3. **(c)** Formation of positive ion involves removal of electron(s) from neutral atom and that of the negative ion involves addition of electron(s) to the neutral atom.

4. **(a)** $$\text{Hybridisation} = \frac{1}{2}\left[\begin{pmatrix}\text{No. of electrons}\\ \text{in valence}\\ \text{shell of atom}\end{pmatrix} + \begin{pmatrix}\text{No.of monovalent}\\ \text{atoms around it}\end{pmatrix} - \begin{pmatrix}\text{charge on}\\ \text{cation}\end{pmatrix} + \begin{pmatrix}\text{charge on}\\ \text{anion}\end{pmatrix}\right]$$

   (a) For AlH_3,

   Hybridisation of Al atom $= \frac{1}{2}[3+3-0+0] = 3 = sp^2$

   For AlH_4^-,

   Hybridisation of Al atom$= \frac{1}{2}[3+4-0+1] = 4 = sp^3$

   (b) For H_2O,

   Hybridisation of O atom $= \frac{1}{2}[6+2-0+0] = 4 = sp^3$

   For H_3O^+, Hybridisation of O atom $= \frac{1}{2}[6+3-1+0]$ $= 4 = sp^3$

   (c) For NH_3

   Hybridisation of N atom $= \frac{1}{2}[5+3-0+0] = 4 = sp^3$

   For NH_4^+, Hybridisation of N atom $= \frac{1}{2}[5+4-1+0]$ $= 4 = sp^3$

   Thus hybridisation changes only in option (a).

5. **(b)** The bond angle decreases on moving down the group due to decrease in bond pair-bond pair repulsion.

NH_3	PH_3	AsH_3	SbH_3	BiH_3
107°	93.5°	91.8°	91.3°	90°

NOTE : This can also be explained by the fact that as the size of central atom increases sp^3 hybrid orbital becomes more distinct with increasing size of central atom i.e. pure p- orbitals are utilized in M–H bonding

6. **(c)** $\left[\begin{array}{c}O\\ |\\ O-P-O\\ \|\\ O\end{array}\right]^{3-} \leftrightarrow \left[\begin{array}{c}O\\ |\\ O-P=O\\ |\\ O\end{array}\right]^{3-} \leftrightarrow \left[\begin{array}{c}O\\ \|\\ O-P-O\\ |\\ O\end{array}\right]^{3-} \leftrightarrow \left[\begin{array}{c}O\\ |\\ O=P-O\\ |\\ O\end{array}\right]^{3-}$

Bond order

$$= \frac{\text{Number of bonds}}{\text{Number of Resonating structures}} = \frac{5}{4} = 1.25$$

Three unit negative charge is being shared by four O atoms. Formal charge = –3/4

7. **(c)** Since F form H-bond $[HF_2]^-$ exists. Therefore KHF_2 gives $K^+ + HF_2^-$

8. **(d)** In alcohol intermolecular H-bonding is possible whereas in ether it is not possible.

9. **(c)** (a) N_2 : bond order 3, paramagnetic
   N_2^- : bond order, 2.5, paramagnetic
   (b) C_2 : bond order 2, diamagnetic
   C_2^+ : bond order 1.5, paramagnetic
   (c) NO : bond order 2.5, paramagnetic
   NO^+ : bond order 3, diamagnetic
   (d) O_2 : bond order 2, paramagnetic
   O_2^+ : bond order 2.5, paramagnetic

10. **(d)**

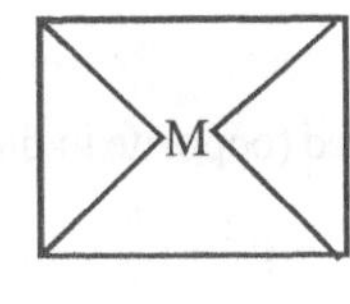

M

dsp^2 hybridisation — sp^3d or dsp^3 hybridisation

Number of 90° angle between bonds = 4 — Number of 90° angle between bonds = 6

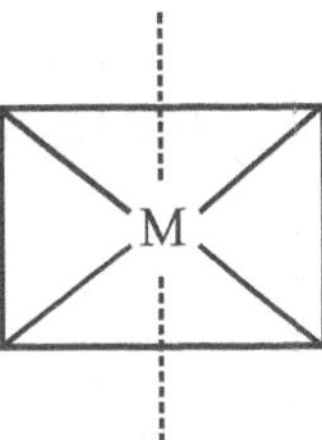

sp^3d^2 hybridisation

Number of 90° angle between bonds = 12

11. **(c)** It is due to H - bonding.

12. **(d)** In XeF_2 Total number of valence electrons of Xe = 8, two electrons shared with 2F atoms, 6 electrons left hence 3 lone pairs, in XeF_4 4 shared with 4 F atoms 4 left hence 2 lone pairs; in XeF_6 6 shared with 6 F atoms 2 left hence 1 lone pair.

13. (b) $NO_2^+ = \frac{1}{2}[5+0+0-1] = 2\ sp$; $NO_2^- = \frac{1}{2}[5+0+1-0]$

$= 3\ sp^2$; $NH_4^+ = \frac{1}{2}[5+4+0-1] = 4\ sp^3$

14. (b) $NH_3 \rightarrow$ 1l.p, 3b.p $\rightarrow$ Trigonal pyramidal
$SO_2 \rightarrow$ 1l.p, 2b.p $\rightarrow$ Bent
$SF_4 \rightarrow$ 1l.p, 4b.p $\rightarrow$ See-saw
$ClF_3 \rightarrow$ 2l.p, 3b.p $\rightarrow$ T-shape

15. (b) Atomic orbitals having same or nearly same energy will not combine if they do not have the same symmetry. $2p_z$ Orbital of one atom cannot combine with $2p_x$ or $2p_y$ orbital of other atom because of their different symmetries.

16. (a) The number of lone pairs of electrons on central atom in various given species are

Species	Number of lone pairs on central atom
IF_7	nil
IF_5	1
ClF_3	2
XeF_2	3

Thus the correct increasing order is
$IF_7 < IF_5 < ClF_3 < XeF_2$
0 1 2 3

17. (c) 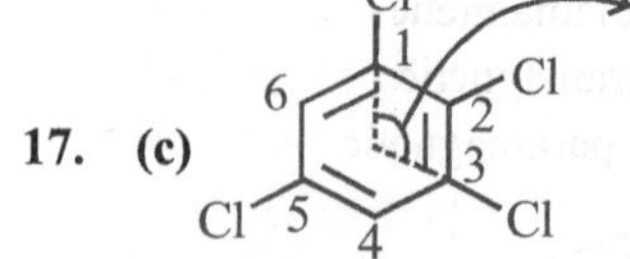

Dipole moments of 2Cl and 5 Cl are vectorically cancelled (opposite in direction).

and now for 1 Cl and 3 Cl, $\mu^2 = \mu_1^2 + \mu_2^2 + 2\mu_1\mu_2\cos\theta$

$= (1.5)^2 + (1.5)^2 + 2 \times 1.5 \times 1.5 \cos 120$

$\therefore\ \mu = 1.5\ D$

18. (b) BCl_3: $Cl-B\langle^{Cl}_{Cl}$; sp^2 - Hybridisation (Trigonal geometry); Bond angle = 120°

In PCl_3 — $\ddot{P}$ (sp^3) with Cl Cl Cl (Pyramidal geometry)
In $AsCl_3$ — $\ddot{As}$ (sp^3) with Cl Cl Cl (Pyramidal geometry)
In $BiCl_3$ — $\ddot{Bi}$ (sp^3) with Cl Cl Cl (Pyramidal geometry)

Bond angle = below 109° 28' and decreases from PCl_3 to $BiCl_3$

In these, order of bond angle : $BCl_3 > PCl_3 > AsCl_3 > BiCl_3$

19. (d) According to Fajan's rule :

Covalent character $\propto \frac{1}{\text{size of cation}}$

$\propto$ size of anion

Among the given species order of size of cations $N^{3+} < O^{2+} < Pb^{2+} < Ba^{2+}$

order of size of anions $O^{2-} < Cl^-$.

Hence the order of covalent character is
$NCl_3 > Cl_2O > PbCl_2 > BaCl_2$
$BaCl_2$ is most ionic in nature.

20. (c) Let amount of compound = 100 g

No. of moles of C $= \frac{92.3}{12} = 7.69 = 7.7$

No. of moles of H $= \frac{7.7}{1} = 7.7$

Empirical formula = CH
Empirical formula mass = 12 + 1 = 13 g/mol
Molecular mass = 52 g/mol

$n = \frac{52}{13} = 4$

$\therefore$ Molecular foumula = Empirical formula × 4
$= C_4H_4$

Possible structures

$H_2C=C=C=CH_2$ (terminal C: sp^2, central C: sp sp), $H-C\equiv C-CH=CH_2$ (sp sp sp^2 sp^2),

cyclobutadiene: $HC=CH$ / $HC=CH$ (all carbons sp^2)

21. (a) NO_3^- and CO_3^{2-} both have same number of electrons (equal to 32) and central atom in each being sp^2 hybridised, are isostructural too.

22. (d) The hybrid state of N in NO_3^- and NO_2^- is the same and it is sp^2 while in NO_2^+ it is sp

23. (d) The molecular orbital configuration of the given molecules is

$H_2 = \sigma 1s^2$ (no electron anti-bonding)

$Li_2 = \sigma 1s^2\, \sigma^* 1s^2\, \sigma 2s^2$ (two anti-bonding electrons)

$B_2 = \sigma 1s^2\, \sigma^* 1s^2\, \sigma 2s^2\, \sigma^* 2s^2 \{\pi 2p_y^1 = \pi 2p_z^1\}$

(4 anti-bonding electrons)

Though the bond order of all the species are same (B.O = 1) but stability is different. This is due to difference in the presence of no. of anti-bonding electron.

Higher the no. of anti-bonding electron lower is the stability hence the correct order is $H_2 > Li_2 > B_2$

24. (b) The formation of a heavy nucleus from those of lighter elements is known as nuclear fusion. The mass of the heavier nucleus is always less than the sum of masses of lighter nuclei which is converted into energy according to Einstein equation $E = mc^2$.

25. (a) A gaseous HCl molecule has hydrogen and chlorine linked by a covalent bond. Here electronegativity of chlorine is greater than that of hydrogen. Due to this the shared pair of electron is more attracted towards chlorine. Thus, chlorine end of molecule has higher electron density and becomes slightly negative and the hydrogen and slightly positive. Hence the covalent bond in HCl has a polar character as shown below

$\overset{\delta^+}{H} \longrightarrow \overset{\delta^-}{Cl}$

26. (c) Hybridisation in NF_3 and H_3O^+ is sp^3 and they have pyramidal shape. Hybridisation in NO_3^- and BF_3 is sp^2 and they have triangular planar shape.

27. (c) $H-C(=\ddot{O}:)(-\ddot{O}:^{\ominus}) \longleftrightarrow H-C(-\ddot{O}:^{\ominus})(=\ddot{O}:)$ $\longleftrightarrow$ or Resonance

hybrid $\left[H-C\begin{smallmatrix}O\\ \vdots\\ O\end{smallmatrix}\right]^-$ due to resonance C – O bond length is the same.

28. (d) Promotion of electron is not an essential condition prior to hybridisation. It is not necessary that only half filled orbitals participate in hybridisation. In some cases, even filled orbitals of valence shell take part in hybridisation.

29. (b) Since XY_2 forms 2σ, 2π bonds and has 1 lone pair of electrons. It must have the structure $Y = \ddot{X} = Y$. Hence Y is divalent. The hybridisation of X is $sp^2\left(\frac{1}{2}(6+0+0-0)=3\right)$. So XY_2 is trigonal planar

(X with Y, Y) (like SO_2).

30. (d) The shape of BF_3 is trigonal planar (${}^{\delta-}F$, ${}^{\delta-}F$ $\rangle B^{\delta+}-F^{\delta-}$) and $\mu = 0$ hence it is non polar. The shape of NF_3 is pyramidal ($\ddot{N}^{\delta+}$ with ${}^{\delta-}F$, $F^{\delta-}$, $F^{\delta-}$) and $\mu \neq 0$ hence it is polar.

31. (b) According to Fajan's rules smaller, highly charged cation has greatest covalent character while large cation with smaller charge has greatest ionic character.

32. (d)

(a) $ONCl = 8+7+17 = 32e^-$, $ONO^- = 8+7+8+1 = 24e^-$ } not isoelectronic

(b) O–Ö–O (1.278Å, 1.278A°, 116.8°) The central atom is sp^2 hybridized with one lone pair.

(c) It is a pale blue gas. At – 249.7°, it forms violet black crystals.

(d) It is diamagnetic in nature due to absence of unpaired electrons.

33. (d) H–O–C₆H₄–O–H   H–S–C₆H₄–S–H

In both the molecules the bond moments are not cancelling with each other and hence the molecules has a resultant dipole and hence the molecule is polar.

34. (b) The delocalised $p\pi - p\pi$ bonding between filled *p*-orbital of F and vacant *p*-orbital of B leads to shortening of B–F bond length which results in higher bond dissociation energy of the B–F bond.

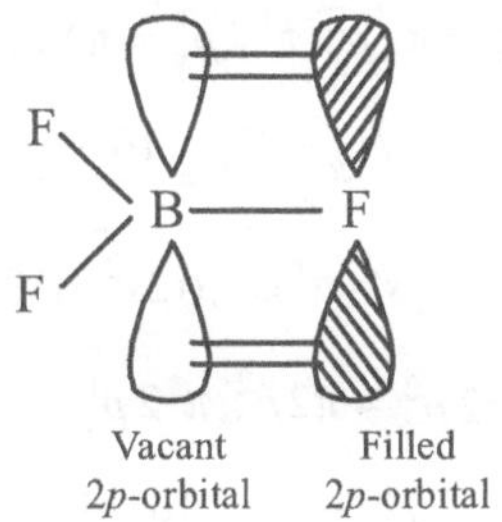

$F_2B=F^+ \longleftrightarrow$ $F^+=BF_2 \longleftrightarrow$ $F^+=BF_2 \equiv$ (B with three F, each $+1/3$)

35. (b) This type of attractive force operates between the polar molecules having permanent dipole and the molecules lacking permanent dipole.

HCl is polar ($\mu \neq 0$) and He is non polar ($r \neq 0$), thus gives dipole-induced dipole interaction.

36. (d) The structure of CaC_2 is $Ca^{2+}[:C\equiv C:]^{2-}$

i.e, one π and two σ bonds

37. (d) Bond lengths are measured by spectroscopic, X-ray diffraction and electron diffraction techniques.

38. (c) In CO (three shared electron pairs between C and O) the bond order is 3. For N_2 bond order is 3 H_2, Cl_2, Br_2 have identical Bond order, Bond order 1.

39. (a) The molecule does not exist for a certain fraction of time in one cannonical form and for other fractions of time in other cannonical forms.

40. **(b)** BF_3 has planar and symmetrical structure thus as a result the resultant of two bond moments, being equal and opposite to the third, cancels out and hence molecule possess zero dipole moment.

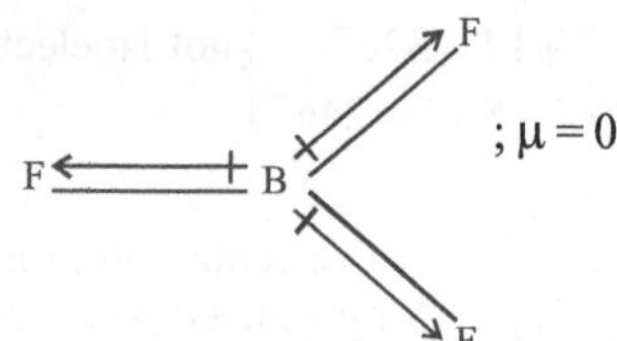

41. **(d)** OSF_2 : $H = \frac{6+2}{2} = 4$. sp^3 hybridization.
It has 1 lone pair and 3-bond pair.

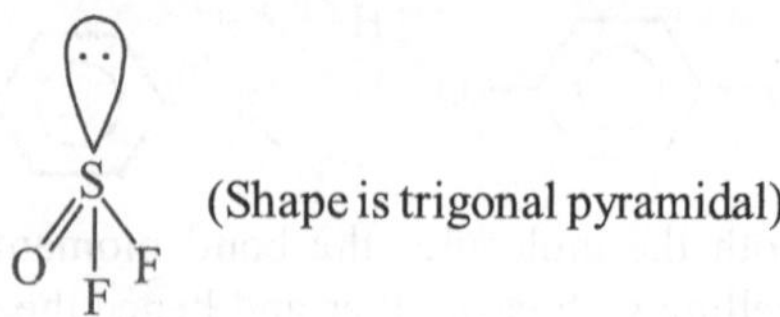

(Shape is trigonal pyramidal)

The shapes of SO_3, BrF_3 and SiO_3^{2-} are triangular planar respectively.

42. **(b)** $(O_2) = \sigma 1s^2, \sigma^* 1s^2, \sigma 2s^2, \sigma^* 2s^2, \sigma 2p_z^2,$

$$\pi 2p_x^2 = \pi 2p_y^2, \pi^* 2p_x^1 = \pi^* 2P_y^1$$

$$\text{Bond order} = \frac{N_b - N_a}{2} = \frac{10-6}{2} = \frac{4}{2} = 2$$

$$\left(O_2^+ \text{ ion}\right) = \sigma 1s^2, \sigma^* 1s^2, \sigma 2s^2, \sigma^* 2s^2, \sigma 2p_z^2,$$

$$\pi 2p_x^2 = \pi 2p_y^2, \pi^* 2p_x^1$$

$$\text{Bond order } \frac{N_b - N_a}{2} = \frac{10-5}{2} = \frac{5}{2} = 2\frac{1}{2}$$

$$\left(O_2^-\right) = \sigma 1s^2, \sigma^* 1s^2, \sigma 2s^2, \sigma^* 2s^2, \sigma 2P_z^2,$$

$$\pi 2p_x^2 = \pi 2p_y^2, \pi^* 2p_x^2 = \pi^* 2p_y^1$$

$$\text{Bond order} = \frac{(N_b - N_a)}{2} = \frac{10-7}{2} = \frac{3}{2} = 1\frac{1}{2}$$

$$\left(O_2^{2-}\right) = \sigma 1s^2, \sigma^* 1s^2, \sigma 2s^2, \sigma^* 2s^2, \sigma 2p_z^2,$$

$$\pi 2p_x^2 = \pi 2p_y^2, \pi^* 2p_x^2 = \pi^* 2p_y^2$$

$$\text{Bond order } \frac{N_b - N_a}{2} = \frac{10-8}{2} = \frac{2}{2} = 1$$

43. **(a)** Nitric oxide is paramagnetic in the gaseous state because of the presence of one unpaired electron in its outermost shell.
The electronic configuration of NO is

$$\sigma_{1s}^2 \, \sigma_{1s}^{*2} \, \sigma_{2s}^2 \sigma_{2s}^{*2} \sigma_{2p_z}^2 \, \pi_{2p_x}^2 = \pi_{2p_y}^2 \, \pi_{2p_x}^{*1}$$

44. **(d)** Smaller the size and higher the charge more will be polarising power of cation. Since the order of the size of cation is $K^+ > Ca^{2+} > Mg^{2+} > Be^{2+}$. So the correct order of polarising power is
$K^+ < Ca^{2+} < Mg^{2+} < Be^{2+}$

45. **(c)** $H_2^{2+} = \sigma 1s^0 \, \sigma^* 1s^0$

$$\text{bond order for } H_2^{2+} = \frac{1}{2}(0-0) = 0$$

$$He_2 = \sigma 1s^2 \sigma^* 1s^2$$

$$\text{bond order for } He_2 = \frac{1}{2}(2-2) = 0$$

so both H_2^{2+} and He_2 do not exist

Speed Test-33

1. (c) Wt. of compound is 96 g. The compound exists as 50% monomer and 50% dimer.

$$\text{Moles of monomer} = \frac{48}{48} = 1,$$

$$\text{Moles of dimer} = \frac{48}{96} = 0.5$$

$$\therefore \quad P = \frac{1.5 \times 0.0821 \times (273 + 273)}{33.6} = 2.00 \text{ atm}$$

2. (d) $u_1 \propto \sqrt{\frac{1}{m_1}}$ and $u_2 \propto \sqrt{\frac{1}{m_2}}$

$$\therefore \frac{u_1^2}{u_2^2} = \frac{m_2}{m_1} \quad \therefore m_1 u_1^2 = m_2 u_2^2$$

3. (c) Gas equation is $PV = \frac{m}{M} RT$ ...(i)

Again $\frac{P}{2} V = \frac{m_1}{M} R . \frac{2}{3} T$ ...(ii)

Divide (i) by (ii)

$2 = \frac{m}{m_1} \times \frac{3}{2} \therefore m_1 = \frac{3}{4} m$. Gas escaped is then $= \frac{1}{4} m$

4. (b) $V_0 = \sqrt{\frac{2RT}{M}} = \sqrt{R(273+t)}$

$$u_{rms} = \sqrt{\frac{3(2t + 273 + 273)R}{1}}$$

$$= \sqrt{6(t+273)R} = \sqrt{6} V_0$$

5. (d) Average velocity $= \sqrt{\frac{8RT}{\pi M}}$

i.e., $v \propto \sqrt{T}$

$$\therefore \frac{v_2}{v_1} = \sqrt{\frac{2T}{T}} = 1.41$$

6. (b) $R = 0.0082$ litre atm K^{-1} mol^{-1}.

7. (d) From the ideal gas equation :

$$PV = nRT$$

$$\text{or } n = \frac{PV}{RT} = \frac{3170 \times 10^{-3}}{8.314 \times 300} = 1.27 \times 10^{-3}$$

8. (c) $\frac{x}{32} + \frac{x}{28} = \frac{60x}{32 \times 28}$,

PV = nRT;

$$P_1 V = \frac{x}{32} RT; \; P_2 V = \frac{x}{28} RT$$

$$\therefore \quad 32 P_{O_2} = 28 P_{N_2}$$

or, $P_{O_2} = 0.875 \, P_{N_2}$

9. (a) Since b = 4 × volume occupied by molecules of 1 mole of a gas

$$b = 4 \, N_A \left(\frac{4}{3} \pi r^3 \right)$$

$$\therefore r = \left(\frac{3b}{16 N_A \pi} \right)^{\frac{1}{3}} = \left[\frac{3 \times 24 cm^3 mol^{-1}}{16 (6.023 \times 10^{23} mol^{-1} \times 3.14)} \right]^{\frac{1}{3}}$$

$$= 1.335 \times 10^{-8} \text{ cm} = 133.5 \text{ pm}$$

Molecular diameter, d = 2r = 267 pm.

10. (d) Let V be the original volume of bubble. The final volume will be 8 V. Let P be the atmospheric pressure and P_1 the pressure at the bottom

$\therefore \quad P \times 8 V = P_1 \times V;$

$8p = P_1$

P_1 = atmospheric pressure + pressure due to water lake

$= P + 7p$

The P = 10 m high, the 7p will be = 70 m high

So the depth = 70 m

11. (a) $d \propto P$, Boyle's law, $\left(d = \frac{MP}{RT} \right)$. At sea level pressure is more, hence density of air is more.

12. (d) $\frac{P}{T}$ = constant (Gay Lussac's law)

$$\Rightarrow \quad \frac{P_1}{T_1} = \frac{P_2}{T_2} \Rightarrow P_1 T_2 = P_2 T_1$$

PV = constant

$P_1 V_1 = P_2 V_2$ [Boyle's law]

13. (a) Given

$P_1 = 1.5$ bar $T_1 = 273 + 15 = 288$ K $V_1 = V$

$P_2 = 1.0$ bar $T_1 = 273 + 25 = 298$ K $V_2 = ?$

$$\frac{P_1 V_1}{T_1} = \frac{P_2 V_2}{T_2}$$

$$\frac{1.5 \times V}{288} = \frac{1 \times V_2}{298}$$

$V_2 = 1.55$ V i.e., volume of bubble will be almost 1.6 time to initial volume of bubble.

14. (a) $r \propto \frac{P}{\sqrt{m}}$

$$\frac{r_A}{r_B} = \frac{P_A}{P_B}\sqrt{\frac{M_B}{M_A}}$$

15. (a) The mean free path, $\lambda = \frac{1}{\sqrt{2}\,\pi a^2 N}$

or $\lambda \propto \frac{1}{a^2}$, where a = molecular diameter

$\therefore$ Smaller the molecular diameter, longer the mean free path. Hence H_2 is the answer.

16. (d) $u_{rms} = \sqrt{\frac{3RT}{M}}$ Using ideal gas equation,

$PV = nRT = \frac{w}{M}RT;\ \frac{RT}{M} = \frac{PV}{w} = \frac{P}{d}$ where d is the density of the gas

$\therefore\ u_{rms} = \sqrt{\frac{3P}{d}}$ at constant pressure, $u_{rms} \propto \frac{1}{\sqrt{d}}$

17. (c) The correct order of viscosity of the given liquids is dimethyl ether < methyl alcohol < water < glycerol.

18. (c) The different type of molecular velocities possessed by gas molecules are

(i) Most probable velocity $(\alpha) = \sqrt{\frac{2RT}{M}}$

(ii) Average velocity $\overline{v} = \sqrt{\frac{8RT}{\pi M}}$

(iii) Root mean square velocity in all three cases

$v = \sqrt{\frac{3RT}{M}}$

In all the above cases

Velocity $\propto \sqrt{T}$

19. (c) $\frac{V_1}{T_1} = \frac{V_2}{T_2}$ at const. pressure

$\Rightarrow \frac{22.4}{273} = \frac{V_2}{373},\ V_2 = 30.6$ litre

20. (a)

21. (c) $u_{rms} = \sqrt{\frac{3RT}{M}} \Rightarrow \sqrt{\frac{3RT_{H_2}}{2}} = \sqrt{7}\sqrt{\frac{3RT_{N_2}}{28}}$;

$\therefore\ T_{N_2} = 2T_{H_2}$ or $T_{N_2} > T_{H_2}$

22. (b) Compressibility factor $(Z) = \frac{PV}{RT}$

(For one mole of real gas)

van der Waals equation

$$\left(P + \frac{a}{V^2}\right)(V - b) = RT$$

At low pressure, volume is very large and hence correction term b can be neglected in comparison to very large volume of V.

i.e. $V - b \approx V$

$$\left(P + \frac{a}{V^2}\right)V = RT$$

$$PV + \frac{a}{V} = RT$$

$$PV = RT - \frac{a}{V}$$

$$\frac{PV}{RT} = 1 - \frac{a}{VRT}$$

Hence, $\boxed{Z = 1 - \frac{a}{VRT}}$

23. (b) For gas A, $a = 0$, $Z = 1 + \frac{Pb}{RT}$ implies Z varies linearly with pressure.

For gas B, $b = 0$, $Z = 1 - \frac{a}{VRT}$. Hence, Z does not vary linearly with pressure.

Given the intersection data for gas C, it is possible to find the values of 'a' and 'b'. All van der Waal gases, like gas C, give positive slope at high pressures.

24. (c) According to Avogadro's law "At same temperature and pressure Volume $\propto$ no. of moles"

$n_{H_2} = \frac{w}{2};\ n_{O_2} = \frac{w}{32};\ n_{CH_4} = \frac{w}{16}$

$\because V_{H_2} : V_{O_2} : V_{CH_4} = n_{H_2} : n_{O_2} : n_{CH_4}$

$= \frac{w}{2} : \frac{w}{32} : \frac{w}{16} = 16 : 1 : 2$

25. (c) As temperature rises the most probable speed increases and the fraction of molecules possessing most probable speed decreases.

26. (a) $\frac{\text{K.E of neon at } 40°C}{\text{K.E of neon at } 20°C} = \frac{\frac{3}{2}K \times 313}{\frac{3}{2}K \times 293} = \frac{313}{293}$

27. (c) The expression of root mean square speed is

$u_{rms} = \sqrt{\frac{3RT}{M}}$

Hence,

$$\frac{u_{rms}(H_2)}{u_{rms}(O_2)} = \left[\frac{3R(50K)/(2\,g\,mol^{-1})}{3R(800K)/(32\,g\,mol^{-1})}\right]^{1/2} = 1$$

28. **(c)** For positive deviation: $PV = nRT + nPb$

$$\Rightarrow \frac{PV}{nRT} = 1 + \frac{Pb}{RT}$$

Thus, the factor nPb is responsible for increasing the PV value, above ideal value. b is actually the effective volume of molecule. So, it is the finite size of molecules that leads to the origin of 'b' and hence positive deviation at high pressure.

29. **(d)** Let the mass of methane and oxygen = m g

Mole fraction of O_2

$$= \frac{\text{Moles of } O_2}{\text{Moles of } O_2 + \text{Moles of } CH_4}$$

$$= \frac{m/32}{m/32 + m/16} = \frac{m/32}{3m/32} = \frac{1}{3}$$

Partial pressure of O_2 = Total pressure × mole fraction of O_2, $P_{O_2} = P \times \frac{1}{3} = \frac{1}{3}P$

30. **(d)** Rate $\propto \sqrt{\frac{1}{M}}$. The smaller the value of M the more is the rate of diffusion

31. **(d)** The given equation is cubic equation in the variable V and, therefore, for a single value of P and T, there should be three values of V, all of which may be real or one real and two imaginary.

At T_c there values of V become identical.

32. **(d)** r.m.s. velocity $v_{rms} = \sqrt{\frac{3RT}{M}}$

i.e., $\frac{v_1}{v_2} = \sqrt{\frac{T_1}{T_2}}$

$$\frac{5 \times 10^4}{10 \times 10^4} = \frac{1}{2} = \sqrt{\frac{T_1}{T_2}}$$

$\therefore\ T_2 = 4T_1$

33. **(b)** $d = \frac{PM}{RT}$

It means density of gas is directly proportional to pressure and inversely proportional to temperature.

Density of neon will be maximum at highest pressure and lowest temperature.

34. **(d)** Above Boyle point, real gases show positive deviation from ideality and Z values are greater than one.

35. **(d)** Induced dipole moment depends upon the dipole moment present in the permanent dipole and the polarisability of the electrically neutral molecule. Molecules of large size can be easily polarized. High polarisability increases the strength of attractive interactions.

36. **(c)** More will be critical temperature easier is the liquification of the gas. Hence correct order will be

$He < H_2 < N_2 < O_2$

37. **(b)** The strength of H-bonding is in the order N....H< O....H <F....H

38. **(b)** Liquid drops assume spherical shape because a sphere has minimum surface area.

39. **(a)** $PV = \frac{1}{3}mnu^2 = \frac{1}{3}Mu^2$

$$= \frac{2}{3}.\frac{1}{2}Mu^2 = \frac{2}{3}E \text{ or } P = \frac{2}{3}E \text{ per unit vol.}$$

40. **(c)** Moles of A, $(n_A) = \frac{p_A v_A}{RT} = \frac{8 \times 12}{RT} = \frac{96}{RT}$

Moles of B, $(n_B) = \frac{p_B v_B}{RT} = \frac{8 \times 5}{RT} = \frac{40}{RT}$

Total pressure × total volume = $(n_A + n_B) \times RT$

$$P \times (12 + 8) = \frac{1}{RT}(96 + 40)RT$$

$P = 6.8$

Partial pressure of A = P × mole fraction of A

$$= 6.8\left(\frac{96}{RT} \Big/ \frac{96+40}{RT}\right)$$

$= 4.8$ atm

Partial pressure of B = 6.8 – 4.8 = 2 atm.

41. **(c)**

42. **(d)** These forces are important only at short distances (~ 500 pm)

43. **(a)** The gas molecules are tiny particles and not rigid in nature rather they are perfect elastic bodies.

44. **(a)** For statement (ii), $p_{real} = p_{ideal} - \frac{an^2}{V^2}$

For statement (iii), value of 'a' is independent of temperature and pressure.

45. **(a)** $P = \frac{n^2 a}{V^2}$; $a = \frac{PV^2}{n^2}$ = atm dm^6 mol^{-2}

Speed Test-34

1. **(b)** In insulated system no heat or matter is exchanged, $q = 0 \therefore \Delta E = W$. The work done on the system increases internal energy.

2. **(c)** $\Delta H = H_2 - H_1 = (E_2 + P_2V_2) - (E_1 + P_1V_1)$
$= (E_2 - E_1) + (P_2V_2 - P_1V_1)$
$= 30 + 4 \times 5 - 2 \times 3 = 44 L$ atm

3. **(d)** Given $\Delta H = 41$ kJ mol^{-1} = 41000 J mol^{-1}
$T = 100°C = 273 + 100 = 373$ K
$n = 1$
$\Delta U = \Delta H - \Delta nRT = 41000 - (1 \times 8.314 \times 373)$
$= 37898.88$ J mol^{-1} $\simeq 37.9$ kJ mol^{-1}

4. **(a)** Process is isothermal reversible expansion, hence $\Delta U = 0$, therefore $q = -W$.
Since $q = +208$ J, $W = -208$ J

5. **(b)** An intensive property is a physical quantity whose value does not depend on the amount of the substance for which it is measured.

6. **(d)** Kirchoff's equation, $\frac{\Delta H_2 - \Delta H_1}{T_2 - T_1} = \Delta C_P$

7. **(a)** Heat capacity at constant volume $(q_v) = \Delta E$
Heat capacity of constant pressure $(q_p) = \Delta H$
$\Delta H = \Delta E + \Delta nRT$ or $\Delta H - \Delta E = \Delta nRT$
Δn = no. of moles of gaseous products – no. of moles of gaseous reactants
$= 12 - 15 = -3$
$\Delta H - \Delta E = -3 \times 8.314 \times 298$ J $= -7.43$ kJ.

8. **(b)** Desired equation is $H_2O(l) \rightarrow H_2O(g)$, $\Delta H = ?$
(Equation II - Equation I)
$\Delta H = -245.5$ kJ $- (-286$ kJ$) = 40.5$ kJ

9. **(a)** $C_2H_5OH(\ell) + 3O_2(g) \longrightarrow 2CO_2(g) + 3H_2O(\ell)$
Bomb calorimeter gives ΔU of the reaction
Given, $\Delta U = -1364.47$ kJ mol^{-1}
$\Delta n_g = -1$
$\Delta H = \Delta U + \Delta n_g RT = -1364.47 - \frac{1 \times 8.314 \times 298}{1000}$
$= -1366.93$ kJ mol^{-1}

10. **(a)** $\Delta S_{(A \to B)} = \Delta S_{(A \to C)} + \Delta S_{(C \to D)} - \Delta S_{(B \to D)}$
$= 50 + 30 - 20 = 60$ e.u.

11. **(a)** $CH_4 + 2O_2 \rightarrow CO_2 + 2H_2O; \Delta H = 20$ kcal........(1)
$C + O_2 \rightarrow CO_2$; $\Delta H = -40$ kcal.....(2)
$2H_2 + O_2 \rightarrow 2H_2O$; $\Delta H = -20$ kcal........(3)
(2) + (3) – (1) we have, $C + 2H_2 \rightarrow CH_4$
or $\Delta H = -20 + (-40) - (-20) = -40$ kcal

12. **(b)** Enthalpy of reaction
$= B.E_{(Reactant)} - B.E_{(Product)}$
$= \left[B.E_{(C=C)} + 4B.E._{(C-H)} + B.E._{(H-H)}\right]$
$- \left[B.E._{(C-C)} + 6B.E._{(C-H)}\right]$
$= [606.1 + (4 \times 410.5) + 431.37)] - [336.49 + (6 \times 410.5)]$
$= -120.0$ kJ mol^{-1}

13. **(a)** $\Delta G = \Delta H - T\Delta S$, ΔH + ve, ΔS is + ve; $T\Delta S > \Delta H$ for spontaneous process. It will make ΔG, –ve

14. **(d)** $\Delta H = \Delta E + \Delta nRT$ For $\Delta H \neq \Delta E, \Delta n \neq 0$
Where Δn = no. of moles of gaseous products – no. of moles of gaseous reactants
(a) $\Delta n = 2 - 2 = 0$
(b) $\Delta n = 0$ ($\because$ they are either in solid or liquid state)
(c) $\Delta n = 1 - 1 = 0$ ($\because$ C is in solid state)
(d) $\Delta n = 2 - 4 = -2$
$\therefore$ (d) is correct answer

15. **(b)** The species in its elemental form has zero standard molar enthalpy of formation at 298 K. At 298K, Cl_2 is gas while Br_2 is liquid.

16. **(b)** High pressure reduces volume, decreases entropy, hence ΔS negative.

17. **(d)** $\Delta S° = 2S°_{HCl} - (S°_{H_2} + S°_{Cl_2})$
$= 2 \times 186.7 - (130.6 + 223.0)$
$= 19.8$ JK^{-1}mol^{-1}

18. **(a)** $\Delta G° = \Delta H° - T\Delta S°$
For a spontaneous reaction $\Delta G° < 0$
or $\Delta H° - T\Delta S° < 0 \Rightarrow T > \frac{\Delta H°}{\Delta S°}$
$\Rightarrow T > \frac{179.1 \times 10^3}{160.2} > 1117.9K \approx 1118K$

19. **(d)** For the reaction, $C_{(s)} + \frac{1}{2}O_{2(g)} \longrightarrow CO$
$\Delta H = \Delta U + \Delta nRT$ or $\Delta H - \Delta U = \Delta nRT$
$\Delta n = 1 - \frac{1}{2} = \frac{1}{2}$; $\Delta H - \Delta U = \frac{1}{2} \times 8.314 \times 298$
$= 1238.78$ J mol^{-1}

20. **(c)** $\Delta G° = \Delta H° - T\Delta S°$; $-RT \ell nK = \Delta H° - T\Delta S°$

$$\ell nK = -\frac{\Delta H° - T\Delta S°}{RT}$$

21. (a) $Fe_2O_3(s) + 3CO(g) \longrightarrow 2Fe(s) + 3CO_2(g)$; $\Delta H = -26.8$ kJ ...(i)

$FeO(s) + CO(g) \longrightarrow Fe(s) + CO_2(g)$; $\Delta H = -16.5$ kJ ...(ii)

eq. (i) – 2 × eq. (ii), we get

$Fe_2O_3(s) + CO(g) \longrightarrow 2FeO(s) + CO_2(g)$

$\Delta H = -26.8 + 33.0 = +6.2$ kJ

22. (b) At equilibrium $\Delta G = 0$

Hence, $\Delta G = \Delta H - T_e\Delta S = 0$

$\therefore \Delta H = T_e\Delta S$ or $T_e = \frac{\Delta H}{\Delta S}$

For a spontaneous reaction

ΔG must be negative which is possible only if

$\Delta H - T\Delta S < 0$

$\therefore \Delta H < T\Delta S$ or $T > \frac{\Delta H}{\Delta S}$; $T_e < T$

23. (b) $N_2 + 3H_2 \longrightarrow 2NH_3$ $\Delta H = 2 \times -46.0$ kJ mol^{-1}

Let x be the bond enthalpy of N – H bond then

[**Note :** Enthalpy of formation or bond formation enthalpy is given which is negative but the given reaction involves bond breaking hence values should be taken as positive.]

$\Delta H = \Sigma$ Bond energies of reactants – Σ Bond energies of products

$2 \times -46 = 712 + 3 \times (436) - 6x$

$-92 = 2020 - 6x$

$6x = 2020 + 92$

$6x = 2112$

$x = +352$ kJ/mol

24. (c) For a reaction to be at equilibrium $\Delta G = 0$. Since $\Delta G = \Delta H - T\Delta S$ so at equilibrium $\Delta H - T\Delta S = 0$ or $\Delta H = T\Delta S$

For the reaction

$\frac{1}{2}X_2 + \frac{3}{2}Y_2 \longrightarrow XY_3$; $\Delta H = -30$kJ (given)

Calculating ΔS for the above reaction, we get

$$\Delta S = 50 - \left[\frac{1}{2} \times 60 + \frac{3}{2} \times 40\right] JK^{-1}$$

$= 50 - (30 + 60)\,JK^{-1} = -40\,JK^{-1}$

At equilibrium, $T\Delta S = \Delta H$ $[\because \Delta G = 0]$

$\therefore T \times (-40) = -30 \times 1000$ $[\because 1kJ = 1000J]$

or $T = \frac{-30 \times 1000}{-40}$ or 750 K

25. (a) According to first law of thermodynamics energy can neither be created nor destroyed although it can be converted from one form to another.

NOTE : Carnot cycle is based upon this principle but during the conversion of heat into work some mechanical energy is always converted to other form of energy hence this data violates 1st law of thermodynamics.

26. (c) The standard enthalpy of the combustion of glucose can be calculated by the eqn.

$C_6H_{12}O_6(s) + 6O_2(g) \rightarrow 6CO_2(g) + 6H_2O(l)$

$\Delta H_C = 6 \times \Delta H_f(CO_2) + 6 \times \Delta H_f(H_2O) - \Delta H_f[C_6H_{12}O_6]$

$\Delta H° = 6(-400) + 6(-300) - (-1300)$

$\Delta H° = -2900$ kJ/mol

For one gram of glucose, enthalpy of combustion

$$\Delta H° = -\frac{2900}{180} = -16.11 \text{kJ/g}$$

27. (d) (i) $2C(s) + H_2(g) \longrightarrow H-C \equiv C-H(g)$ $\Delta H = 225$ kJ mol^{-1}

(ii) $2C(s) \longrightarrow 2C(g)$ $\Delta H = 1410$ kJ mol^{-1}

$C(s) \longrightarrow C(g)$ $\Delta H = \frac{1410}{2} = 705$kJmol^{-1}

(iii) $H_2(g) \longrightarrow 2H(g)$ $\Delta H = 330$ kJ mol^{-1}

From equation (i) :

$225 = [2 \times \Delta H_{C(s) \rightarrow c(g)} + 1 \times BE_{H-H}] - [2 \times BE_{C-H} + 1 \times BE_{C\equiv C}]$

$225 = [1410 + 1 \times 330] - [2 \times 350 + 1 \times BE_{C\equiv C}]$

$225 = [1410 + 330] - [700 + BE_{C\equiv C}]$

$225 = 1740 - 700 - BE_{C\equiv C}$

$BE_{C\equiv C} = 815$ kJ mol^{-1}

28. (b) ΔH_N for strong base and strong acid

$= -13.7$ kcal eq^{-1}

$\Delta H_{ion}(CH_3COOH)$

$= -12.5 - (-13.7) = 1.2$ kcal mol^{-1}

$\Delta H_{ion}(NH_4OH)$

$= -10.5 - (-13.7) - \Delta H_{ion}(CH_3COOH)$

$= 13.7 - 10.5 - 1.2$

$= 2$ kcal mol^{-1}

29. (b) Write the proper chemical equations.

$C(graphite) + O_2(g) \rightarrow CO_2(g)$

$\Delta H = -393$kJ ....(i)

$H_2(g) + \frac{1}{2}O_2(g) \rightarrow H_2O(l)$

$\Delta H = -286$kJ ....(ii)

$C_2H_5OH(l) + 3O_2(g) \rightarrow 2CO_2(g) + 3H_2O(l)$ $\Delta H = -1360$kJ ....(iii)

From $(2 \times I + 3 \times II) - (III)$ we get

$$2C + 3H_2 + \frac{1}{2}O_2 \rightarrow C_2H_5OH$$

$\therefore 2(-393kJ) + 3(-286kJ) - (-1360kJ) = -284kJ$

30. (a) $\Delta H_{hyd.} = \Delta H_{sol.} - \Delta H_{lattice}$

$= 1 - 180 = -179$ kcal mol^{-1}

Then $\Delta H_{hyd.}(Na^+) + \Delta H_{hyd.}(Cl^-) = -179$

or $\Delta H_{hyd.}(Na^+) + \frac{2}{3}\Delta H_{hyd}(Na^+) = -179$

or $\Delta H_{hyd.}(Na^+) = -107.4\ kcal\,mol^{-1}$

31. (a) For non spontaneous reaction

$\Delta G = +ve$

$\Delta G = \Delta H - T\Delta S$ and

$\Delta S = 121\ JK^{-1}$

For $\Delta G = +ve$

ΔH has to be positive. Hence the reaction is endothermic. The minimum value of ΔH can be obtained by putting

$\Delta G = 0$

$\Delta H = T\Delta S = 298 \times 121\ J$
$= 36.06\ kJ$

32. (c) The standard enthalpy of reaction is the enthalpy change for a reaction when all the participating substances are in their standard states. The standard state of a substance at a specified temperature is its pure form at 1 bar. For example, the standard state of liquid ethanol at 298 K is pure liquid ethanol at 1 bar. Standard state of solid iron at 500 K is pure iron at 1 bar.

33. (d)

34. (a) $\Delta C_p = 2 \times 25.1 + 3 \times 75.3 - [103.8 + 3 \times 28.8]$

$= 85.9\ JK^{-1}mol^{-1}$

$\frac{\Delta H_2 - \Delta H_1}{T_2 - T_1} = \Delta C_p$;

$\frac{\Delta H_2 - (-33290)}{358 - 298} = 85.9$

$\Delta H = -28136\ J\,mol^{-1}$

$= -28.136\ kJ\,mol^{-1}$

35. (b) The enthalpy of ionisation of weak acid is given by

$\Delta H_{ion(HA)}$

$= \Delta H_{N(weak\ acid/strong\ base)} - \Delta H_{N(strong\ acid/strong\ base)}$

$= -56.1 - (-57.3) = 1.2\ kJ\,mol^{-1}$

$\Delta H_{(ionisation)} = 1.5\ kJ\,mol^{-1}$

Hence % ionisation in 1 M solution

$= \frac{(1.5 - 1.2)}{1.5} \times 100 = 20$

36. (d) $\frac{1}{2}N_2(g) + \frac{3}{2}F_2(g) \longrightarrow NF_3;\ \Delta H = -113\ kJ$

or $\Delta H_{N\equiv N} + \frac{3}{2}\Delta H_{F-F} - 3\Delta H_{N-F} = -113\ kJ$

Let x $kJ\,mol^{-1}$ be the bond energy of F – F bond then bond energy of N ≡ N bond = 6x

$\therefore\ \frac{1}{2} \times 6x + \frac{3}{2} \times x - 3 \times 273 = -113\ kJ$

On solving,

$x = 156.9\ kJ\,mol^{-1}$ and

N ≡ N bond energy $= 6 \times 156.9 = 941.4\ kJ\,mol^{-1}$

37. (b) Given ΔH

$\frac{1}{2}A \longrightarrow B \quad +150$ ...(1)

$3B \longrightarrow 2C + D \quad -125$ ...(2)

$E + A \longrightarrow 2D \quad +350$ ...(3)

To calculate ΔH operate

$2 \times$ eq. (1) + eq. (2) – eq. (3)

$\Delta H = 300 - 125 - 350 = -175$

38. (a) $q = -W = 2.303nRT\log\frac{V_2}{V_1}$

39. (c)

40. (a) The first reaction is exothermic and the second reaction is endothermic. On passing the mixture of O_2 and H_2O (steam) over coke while keeping the temperature constant ΔH of both the reactions must be same. Moles of O_2 needed to evolve 132 kJ

$= \frac{0.5 \times 132}{110} = 0.6$

Hence steam : O_2 ratio must be 1 : 0.6

41. (a) The greater the (negative value) of heat of neutralisation, the more is the strength of the acid. Hence,

$HCOOH > CH_3COOH > H_2S > HCN$

42. (b) Dissolution of KNO_3 is endothermic, hence heat is absorbed and cooling is observed.

43. (d) The positive sign expresses when work is done on the system. Similarly, negative sign expresses when work is done by the system.

44. (b) This is combustion reaction, which is always exothermic hence

$\Delta H = -ve$

As the no. of gaseous molecules are increasing hence entropy increases so $\Delta S = +ve$.

now $\Delta G = \Delta H - T\Delta S$

For a spontaneous reaction

$\Delta G = -ve$

which is possible in this case as $\Delta H = -ve$ and $\Delta S = +ve$.

45. (c) ΔS has negative value if number of gaseous moles decreases during a reaction, $\Delta n_g = -ve$

For the reaction

$2SO_2 + O_2 \rightarrow 2SO_3$

$\Delta n_g = 2 - 3 = -1$

Speed Test-35

1. (a) $I_2 \rightleftharpoons 2I^-$

$1-x \quad\quad 2x$

$$K_c = \frac{(2x)^2}{(1-x)} = 10^{-6}$$

Soln. shows that $(1-x) > 2x \therefore [I_2(g)] > [I^-(g)]$

2. (c)

	A	+ 2B	$\rightleftharpoons$ 2C
Initial moles in 2 litres	2	3	2
At Equilibrium moles in 2 litres	2.5	4	1
Molar conc. moles in 2 litres	1.25	2	0.5

$$K_c = \frac{(0.5)^2}{(1.25)(2)^2} = 0.05$$

3. (b) $K_p = K_c (RT)^{\Delta n}$ since $\Delta n = 0$, $K_p = K_c$.

4. (a) $\Delta G^o = -2.303\, RT \log K$

$-4.606 \times 10^3 = -2.303 \times 2 \times 500 \log K_c$

$\therefore K_c = 100.$

5. (c) $SO_3(g) \rightleftharpoons SO_2(g) + \frac{1}{2}O_2(g)$

$$K_c = \frac{[SO_2][O_2]^{1/2}}{[SO_3]} = 4.9 \times 10^{-2};$$

On taking the square of the above reaction

$$\frac{[SO_2]^2[O_2]}{[SO_3]^2} = 24.01 \times 10^{-4}$$

now K'_C for $2SO_2(g) + O_2(g) \rightleftharpoons 2SO_3$

$$= \frac{[SO_3]^2}{[SO_2]^2\,[O_2]} = \frac{1}{24.01 \times 10^{-4}} = 416$$

6. (c) The correct order of acidic strength of the given species is

$$\underset{(iv)}{HSO_3F} > \underset{(ii)}{H_3O^+} > \underset{(iii)}{HSO_4^-} > \underset{(i)}{HCO_3^-}$$

or (i) < (iii) < (ii) < (iv)

It corresponds to choice (c) which is correct answer.

7. (d) $N_2O_4 \rightleftharpoons 2NO_2$

$1-\alpha \quad\quad 2\alpha$

Total moles at equ $= 1 - \alpha + 2\alpha = 1 + \alpha$

$$K_c = \frac{p^2_{NO_2}}{p_{N_2O_4}} = \frac{\left(\frac{2\alpha}{1+\alpha}.P\right)^2}{\frac{1-\alpha}{1+\alpha}.P} = \frac{4\alpha^2 P}{1-\alpha^2}$$

8. (b) Let the initial moles of X be 'a' and that of Z be 'b' then for the given reactions, we have

	X	$\rightleftharpoons$ 2Y
Initial a moles		0
At equi (moles)	$a(1-\alpha)$	$2a\alpha$

Total no. of moles $= a(1-\alpha) + 2a\alpha$

$= a - a\alpha + 2a\alpha$

$= a(1+\alpha)$

Now, $$K_{P_1} = \frac{(n_Y)^2}{n_X} \times \left(\frac{P_{T_1}}{\Sigma n}\right)^{\Delta n}$$

$$K_{P_1} = \frac{(2a\alpha)^2.P_{T_1}}{[a(1-\alpha)][a(1+\alpha)]}$$

	Z	$\rightleftharpoons$ P	+ Q
Initial b moles		0	0
At equi (moles)	$b(1-\alpha)$	$b\alpha$	$b\alpha$

Total no . of moles $= b(1-\alpha) + b\alpha + b\alpha$

$= b - b\alpha + b\alpha + b\alpha$

$= b(1+\alpha)$

Now $$K_{P_2} = \frac{n_Q \times n_P}{n_Z} \times \left[\frac{P_{T_2}}{\Sigma_n}\right]^{\Delta_n}$$

or $$K_{P_2} = \frac{(b\alpha)(b\alpha).P_{T_2}}{[b(1-\alpha)][b(1+\alpha)]}$$

or $$\frac{K_{P_1}}{K_{P_2}} = \frac{4\alpha^2.P_{T_1}}{(1-\alpha^2)} \times \frac{(1-\alpha)^2}{P_{T_2}.\alpha^2} = \frac{4P_{T_1}}{P_{T_2}}$$

or $$\frac{P_{T_1}}{P_{T_2}} = \frac{1}{9} \quad \left[\text{given: } \frac{K_{P_1}}{K_{P_2}} = \frac{1}{9}\right]$$

or $$\frac{P_{T_1}}{P_{T_2}} = \frac{1}{36} \text{ or } 1:36$$

i.e., (b) is the correct answer.

9. (b) For the reaction

$$2AB_2(g) \rightleftharpoons 2AB(g) + B_2(g)$$

at equi $\quad 2(1-x) \quad\quad 2x \quad\quad x$

$$K_c = \frac{[AB]^2[B_2]}{[AB_2]^2} \text{ or } K_c = \frac{(2x)^2 \times x}{\{2(1-x)\}^2}$$

$= x^3$ [(1– x) can be neglected in denominator (1– x) $\simeq 1$]

The partial pressure at equilibrium are calculated on the basis of total number of moles at equilibrium.

Total number of moles

$= 2(1-x) + 2x + x = (2 + x)$

$\therefore P_{AB_2} = \frac{2(1-x)}{(2+x)} \times P$, where P is the total pressure.

$$P_{AB} = \frac{2x}{(2+x)} \times P,\ P_{B_2} = \frac{x}{(2+x)} \times P$$

Since x is very small so can be neglected in denominator thus, we get

$P_{AB_2} = (1-x) \times P$ $\qquad$ $P_{AB} = x \times P$

$$P_{B_2} = \frac{x}{2} \times P$$

$$\text{Now, } K_P = \frac{(P_{AB})^2 (P_{B_2})}{(P_{AB_2})^2}$$

$$= \frac{(x)^2 \times P^2 . P \times \frac{x}{2}}{(1-x)^2 \times P^2}$$

$$= \frac{x^3 . P^3}{2 \times 1 \times P^2} \quad [\because 1 - x \simeq 1]$$

$$= \frac{x^3 . P}{2} \text{ or } x^3 = \frac{2 . K_p}{P} \text{ or } x = \left(\frac{2K_p}{P}\right)^{\frac{1}{3}}$$

10. (a) The reaction given is an exothermic reaction thus according to Le Chatelier's principle lowering of temperature, addition of F_2 and Cl_2 favour the forward direction and hence the production of ClF_3.

11. (d)

12. (a)

13. (c) Since reaction is exothermic hence low temperature will favour forward reaction also volume is decreased by applying high pressure.

14. (d) $\Delta G° = 2494.2 J$

$2A \rightleftharpoons B + C.$

$R = 8.314 J/K/mol.$

$e = 2.718$

$$[A] = \frac{1}{2}, [B] = 2, [C] = \frac{1}{2}$$

$$Q = \frac{[B][C]}{[A]^2} = \frac{2 \times 1/2}{\left(\frac{1}{2}\right)^2} = 4$$

$\Delta G° = -2.303\ RT \log K_C$

$2494.2\ J = -2.303 \times (8.314\ J/K/mol) \times (300K) \log K_C$

$$\Rightarrow \log K_C = -\frac{2494.2\ J}{2.303 \times 8.314\ J/K/mol \times 300\ K}$$

$\Rightarrow \log K_C = -0.4341$

$K_C = 0.37$

$Q > K_C$

15. (a) $N_2(g) + O_2(g) \rightleftharpoons 2NO(g)$

$$K = \frac{[NO]^2}{[N_2][O_2]}$$

$$\frac{1}{2}N_2 + \frac{1}{2}O_2 \rightleftharpoons NO$$

$$K' = \frac{[NO]}{[N_2]^{1/2}[O_2]^{1/2}} = K^{1/2}$$

16. (b) $\Delta G°_{NO(g)} = 86.6k\ J/mol = 86600\ J/mol$

$G°_{NO_2(g)} = x\ J/mol$

$T = 298, K_P = 1.6 \times 10^{12}$

$\Delta G° = -RT \ln K_P$

Given equation,

$2NO(g) + O_2(g) \rightleftharpoons 2NO_2(g)$

$\therefore 2\Delta G°_{NO2} - 2\Delta G°_{NO} = -R(298) \ln(1.6 \times 10^{12})$

$2\Delta G°_{NO2} - 2 \times 86600 = -R(298) \ln(1.6 \times 10^{12})$

$2\Delta G°_{NO2} = 2 \times 86600 - R(298) \ln(1.6 \times 10^{12})$

$$\Delta G°_{NO2} = \frac{1}{2}[2 \times 86600 - R(298) \ln(1.6 \times 10^{12}]$$

$= 0.5 [2 \times 86600 - R(298) \ln(1.6 \times 10^{12})]$

17. (d) HNO_2 is a weak acid and $NaNO_2$ is salt of that weak acid and strong base (NaOH).

18. (b) In dibasic acids the loss of second proton occurs much less readily than the first. Usually the K_a values for successive loss of protons from these acids differ by at least a factor of 10^{-3} i.e., $K_{a_1} > K_{a_2}$

$$H_2X \rightleftharpoons H^+ + HX^- (K_{a_1})$$

$$HX^- \rightleftharpoons H^+ + X^{2-} (K_{a_2})$$

19. (b) Van't Hoff reaction isotherm is $\Delta G = \Delta G° + RT \ln Qp$

When the reaction is in a state of equilibrium

$\Delta G = 0$

Then $\Delta G° = -RT \ln Q_p = -RT \ln K_p$

20. (b) At equilibrium the moles of Cl_2 must be $= 0.15 \times 3 = 0.45$

$$PCl_5 \rightleftharpoons PCl_3 + Cl_2$$

$$\frac{x - 0.45}{3} \quad \frac{0.45}{3} \quad \frac{0.45}{3} \quad \text{Eqb. Conc.}$$

$$K_c = \frac{[PCl_3][Cl_2]}{[PCl_5]}$$

$$\therefore 0.04 = \frac{0.15 \times 0.15}{(x-0.45)/3} \qquad \therefore x = 2.1 \text{ moles}$$

21. (a) $A + 3B \rightleftharpoons 2C + D$

$2a \quad a \quad 0 \quad 0$

$2a - x \quad a - 3x \quad 2x \quad x$

$a - 3x = 2x$ (condition given)

$\therefore x = \frac{a}{5}$

The % of B reacted is

$$\frac{3x}{a} \times 100 = \frac{3}{a} \cdot \frac{a}{5} \times 100 = 60\%$$

22. (c) $H_2CO_3 \rightleftharpoons \overset{+}{H} + H\overset{-}{CO_3} \rightleftharpoons \overset{+}{H} + \overset{-}{CO_3}$.

HCO_3^- can donate and accept H^+.

23. (a) (A) $K_P = K_C (RT)^{\Delta n}$

$\frac{K_P}{K_C} = (RT)^{\Delta n}$ as $\Delta n = -ve \Rightarrow K_P < K_C$

(B) $\Delta n > 0$

(C) $\Delta n = 2 - 1 = 1$

(D) As the reaction is not containing any gaseous component therefore K_P is not defined for this.

24. (c) K_w depends upon temperature as it is an equilibrium constant.

25. (b) $[H^+] = \sqrt{C \times K_a} = \sqrt{0.001 \times 1.8 \times 10^{-4}}$ for formic acid

$[H^+] = \sqrt{C_2 \times 1.8 \times 10^{-5}}$ for acetic acid Equating and solving for $C_2 = 0.01$ M.

26. (d) $H_2A \rightleftharpoons H^+ + HA^-$

$$\therefore K_1 = 1.0 \times 10^{-5} = \frac{[H^+][HA^-]}{[H_2A]} \text{ (Given)}$$

$HA^- \longrightarrow H^+ + A^{--}$

$$\therefore K_2 = 5.0 \times 10^{-10} = \frac{[H^+][A^{--}]}{[HA^-]} \text{ (Given)}$$

$$K = \frac{[H^+]^2[A^{2-}]}{[H_2A]} = K_1 \times K_2$$

$$= (1.0 \times 10^{-5}) \times (5 \times 10^{-10}) = 5 \times 10^{-15}$$

27. (b) $[H_3O]^+$ for a solution having pH = 3 is given by

$[H_3O]^+ = 1 \times 10^{-3}$ moles/litre

$[\therefore [H_3O]^+ = 10^{-pH}]$

Similarly for solution having pH = 4,

$[H_3O]^+ = 1 \times 10^{-4}$ moles/ litre and for pH=5

$[H_3O^+] = 1 \times 10^{-5}$ moles/ litre

Let the volume of each solution in mixture be 1L, then total volume of mixture solution $L = (1 + 1 + 1)\,L = 3L$

Total $[H_3O]^+$ ion present in mixture solution $= (10^{-3} + 10^{-4} + 10^{-5})$ moles

Then $[H_3O]^+$ ion concentration of mixture solution

$$= \frac{10^{-3} + 10^{-4} + 10^{-5}}{3} M = \frac{0.00111}{3} M$$

$= 0.00037\,M = 3.7 \times 10^{-4}$ M.

28. (c) Solubility of AgCl

$$[Ag^+] = \frac{K_{sp}}{[Cl^-]} = \frac{4 \times 10^{-10}}{0.08} = 5.0 \times 10^{-9} M$$

[0.08 M is concentration of $[Cl^-]$ from $CaCl_2$]

29. (d) $pOH = -\log K_b + \log \frac{[SALT]}{[BASE]}$

$$= -\log K_b \left(\text{since } \frac{SALT}{BASE} = 1\right)$$

$= -\log 2 \times 10^{-5} = 4.7$

$pH + pOH = 14$

$\therefore pH = 9.3$

30. (c) Let s = solubility

$AgIO_3 \rightleftharpoons Ag^+ + IO_3^-$

$\qquad\qquad s \qquad s$

$K_{sp} = [Ag^+][IO_3^-] = s \times s = s^2$

Given $K_{sp} = 1 \times 10^{-8}$

$\therefore \; s = \sqrt{K_{sp}} = \sqrt{1 \times 10^{-8}}$

$= 1.0 \times 10^{-4}$ mol/lit $= 1.0 \times 10^{-4} \times 283$ g/lit

($\because$ Molecular mass of Ag $IO_3 = 283$)

$$= \frac{1.0 \times 10^{-4} \times 283 \times 100}{1000} \text{ gm/100ml}$$

$= 2.83 \times 10^{-3}$ gm/ 100 ml

31. (d) $pH = pK_a + \log\left[\frac{Salt}{Acid}\right]$

$$\log[H^+] = \log K_a - \log\left[\frac{Salt}{Acid}\right]$$

$$\log[H^+] = \log K_a + \log\left[\frac{Acid}{Salt}\right]$$

$$[H^+] = K_a\left[\frac{Acid}{Salt}\right]$$

$$= 1.8 \times 10^{-5} \times \frac{0.1}{0.2} = 9 \times 10^{-6}$$

32. (b) $Cr(OH)_3(s) \rightleftharpoons Cr^{3+}(aq.) + 3OH^-(aq.)$

$\qquad\qquad s \qquad 3s$

$(s)\,(3s)^3 = K_{sp}$

$27S^4 = K_{sp}$

$$s = \left(\frac{K_{sp}}{27}\right)^{1/4} = \left(\frac{1.6 \times 10^{-30}}{27}\right)^{1/4}$$

33. (c) $K_p = K_c(RT)^{\Delta n}$;

$$\Delta n = 1-\left(1+\frac{1}{2}\right) = 1-\frac{3}{2} = -\frac{1}{2}.\ \therefore\ \frac{K_p}{K_c} = (RT)^{-1/2}$$

34. (d) For the reaction:- $2NO_2(g) \rightleftharpoons 2NO(g) + O_2(g)$

Given $K_c = 1.8 \times 10^{-6}$ at 184 °C

$R = 0.0831$ Kj/mol. K

$K_p = 1.8 \times 10^{-6} \times 0.0831 \times 457 = 6.836 \times 10^{-6}$

[$\because$ 184°C = (273 + 184) = 457 k, $\Delta n = (2+1, -1) = 1$]

Hence it is clear that $K_p > K_c$

35. (b) $HA \longrightarrow H^+ + A^-$

$$K_a = \frac{[H^+][A^-]}{[HA]},\quad \because\ [H^+] = 10^{-pH}$$

$\therefore$ $[H^+] = 10^{-5}$; and at equilibrium $[H^+] = [A^-]$

$$\therefore\ K_a = \frac{10^{-5} \times 10^{-5}}{0.0015} = 2 \times 10^{-8}$$

$$\alpha = \sqrt{\frac{K_a}{C}} = \sqrt{\frac{2\times10^{-8}}{.005}} = \sqrt{4\times10^{-6}} = 2\times10^{-3}$$

Percentage ionization = 0.2

36. (c) Higher the value of K_a lower will be the value of pK_a i.e. higher will be the acidic nature. Further since CN^-, F^- and NO_2^- are conjugate base of the acids HCN, HF and HNO_2 respectively hence the correct order of base strength will be

$F^- < NO_2^- < CN^-$

($\because$ stronger the acid weaker will be its conjugate base)

37. (d) $\because$ pH = 1 ; $H^+ = 10^{-1} = 0.1$ M

pH = 2 ; $H^+ = 10^{-2} = 0.01$ M

$\therefore$ $M_1 = 0.1$ $V_1 = 1$

$M_2 = 0.01$ $V_2 = ?$

From

$M_1V_1 = M_2V_2$

$0.1 \times 1 = 0.01 \times V_2$

$V_2 = 10$ litres

$\therefore$ Volume of water added = 10 – 1 = 9 litres

38. (a) $HCOONH_4$ is a salt of weak acid and weak base ;

$pH = ½\, pK_w + ½\, pK_a - ½\, pK_b$

$$\therefore pH = \frac{1}{2}\times14+\frac{1}{2}\times3.8-\frac{1}{2}\times4.8\ ; pH = 6.5$$

39. (a)

$$\underset{1\times10^{-4}M}{Na_2CO_3} \longrightarrow \underset{1\times10^{-4}M}{2Na^+} + \underset{1\times10^{-4}M}{CO_3^{2-}}$$

$$K_{SP(BaCO_3)} = [Ba^{2+}][CO_3^{2-}]$$

$$[Ba^{2+}] = \frac{5.1\times10^{-9}}{1\times10^{-4}} = 5.1\times10^{-5}M$$

40. (b) $AgBr \rightleftharpoons Ag^+ + Br^-$

$K_{sp} = [Ag^+][Br^-]$

For precipitation to occur

Ionic product > Solubility product

$$[Br^-] = \frac{K_{sp}}{[Ag^+]} = \frac{5\times10^{-13}}{0.05} = 10^{-11}$$

i.e., precipitation just starts when 10^{-11} moles of KBr is added to 1*l* $AgNO_3$ solution

$\therefore$ Number of moles of Br^- needed from KBr = 10^{-11}

$\therefore$ Mass of KBr = $10^{-11} \times 120 = 1.2 \times 10^{-9}$ g

41. (a)

(i) $$\underset{acid_1}{H_3PO_4} + \underset{base_2}{H_2O_4} \longrightarrow \underset{acid_2}{H_3O^+} + \underset{base_1}{H_2PO_4^-}$$

(ii) $$\underset{acid_1}{H_2PO_4^-} + \underset{base_2}{H_2O} \longrightarrow \underset{base_1}{HPO_4^{2-}} + \underset{acid_2}{H_3O^+}$$

(iii) $$\underset{base_1}{H_2PO_4^-} + \underset{acid_2}{OH^-} \longrightarrow \underset{acid_1}{H_3PO_4} + \underset{base_2}{O^{2-}}$$

Hence only in (ii) reaction $H_2PO_4^-$ is acting as an acid.

42. (a) $pOH = -\log[OH^-]$

$pH + pOH = 14$

For 10^{-4} KOH, $[OH^-] = 10^{-4}$

$pOH = -\log[OH^-] = -\log 10^{-4} = 4$

$pH = 14 - pOH = 10$

43. (b) NaCN is a salt of strong base and weak acid ; pH

$$= 7+\frac{1}{2}pK_a+\frac{1}{2}\log C$$

pK_a for HCN = 14–4.70 = 9.30

$$\therefore pH = 7+\frac{1}{2}\times9.30+\frac{1}{2}\log0.5; pH = 11.5$$

44. (c) Reaction (c) can be obtained by adding reactions (a) and (b) therefore $K_3 = K_1 . K_2$

Hence (c) is the correct answer.

45. (a)

	CO_2 +	$C_{(grapnite)}$ ⇌	2CO
$P_{initial}$	0.5atm		0
P_{final}	(0.5 – x)atm		2x atm

Total P at equilibrium = 0.5 – x + 2x = 0.5 + x atm

0.8 = 0.5 + *x*

$\therefore$ x = 0.8 – 0.5 = 0.3 atm

Now $k_p = (P_{CO})^2/P_{CO_2}$

$$= \frac{(2\times0.3)^2}{(0.5-0.3)} = \frac{(0.6)^2}{(0.2)} = 1.8\text{ atm}$$

Speed Test-36

1. **(a)** $[Fe(H_2O)_5NO]SO_4$
Let O.N. of Fe be x then,
$1\times(x)+5\times(0)+1\times(+1)+1\times(-2)=0 \quad \therefore x=+1$

2. **(c)** In $BaO_2 + H_2SO_4 \rightarrow BaSO_4 + H_2O_2$ all atoms are present in the same O.S. in reactants and products.

3. **(a)** $Cr_2O_7^{2-} + 6I^- + 14H^+ \longrightarrow 2Cr^{3+} + 3I_2 + 7H_2O$
+3 oxidation state of Cr.

4. **(d)** O.N. of N in NO_2 and N_2O_4 is +4
$\therefore$ difference is zero.
O.N. of P in P_2O_5 and P_4O_{10} is +5
$\therefore$ difference is zero
O.N. of N in N_2O is +1 and in NO is +2. The difference is 1
O.N. of S in SO_2 is +4 and in SO_3 is +6. The difference is +2.

5. **(d)** Xe = 53.5 % $\therefore$ F = 46.5%
Relative number of atoms Xe

$$=\frac{53.5}{131.2}=0.4 \text{ and } F=\frac{46.5}{19}=2.4$$

Simple ratio Xe = 1 and F = 6
$\therefore$ Molecular formula is XeF_6
O.N. of Xe is +6.

6. **(d)** The element is Ti (At. no. 22). Electronic configuration is $1s^2, 2s^2p^6, 3s^2p^6d^2, 4s^2$, the energy level of 3d and 4s is very close. It can exhibit +4 oxidation state (Ti^{4+}).

7. **(d)** In Ag_2O, O.N. of Ag is +1 and in Ag the O.N. is 0. There is gain of electrons, hence H_2O_2 act as a reducing agent.

8. **(d)** In redox reaction oxidation and reduction take place simultaneoushy. $Cu_2S + 2FeO \rightarrow 2Cu + 2Fe + SO_2$.
O.N. of Cu changes from +1 to 0 (reduction) and O.N. of S changes from –2 to +4 (oxidation).

9. **(d)** Order of decreasing electrode potentials of Mg, K, Ba and Ca is
Mg > Ca > Ba > K
It can be explained by their standard reduction potentials.

$E^\circ_{K^+|K} = -2.925$

$E_{Ba^{2+}|Ba} = -2.90$

$E^\circ_{Ca^{2+}|Ca} = -2.87$

$E^\circ_{Mg^{2+}|Mg} = -2.37$

Highly negative value of E°_{red} shows the least value of electrode potential.

10. **(a)** (i) $Mn^{n+} + ne^- \rightleftharpoons M$, for this reaction, high negative value of E° indicates lower reduction potential, that means M will be a good reducing agent.

Stronger reducing agent ⇒ Easy to oxidise
⇓
Lower reduction potential ⇐ higher oxidation potential

(ii)

Element	F	Cl	Br	I
Reduction potential (E° volt)	+2.87	+1.36	+1.06	+0.54

As reduction potential decreases from fluorine to iodine, oxidising nature also decreases from fluorine to iodine.

(iii) The size of halide ions increases from F^- to I^-. The bigger ion can loose electron easily. Hence the reducing nature increases from HF to HI.

11. **(d)** Negative E° ⇒ Stronger reducing agent or weaker oxidising agent
Positive E° ⇒ Weaker reducing agent or stronger oxidising agent.

12. **(a)** Both Fe(II) and S(IV) in SO_3^{2-} can be oxidised to Fe (III) and $(SO_4)^{2-}$ respectively hence (3/5)×0.5 =0.3 mol /litre.

$$\left[MnO_4^- + 5e^- + 8H^+ \rightarrow Mn^{2+} + 4H_2O\right]\times\frac{3}{5}$$

$$Fe^{2+} \longrightarrow Fe^{3+} + e^-$$

$$SO_3^{2-} \longrightarrow SO_4^{2-} + 2e^-$$

$$\frac{3}{5}MnO_4^- + \frac{24}{5}H^+ + Fe^{2+} + SO_3^{2-} \longrightarrow 3/5\,Mn^{2+} + 12/5\,H_2O + Fe^{3+} + SO_4^{2-}$$

13. **(d)** Reduction potential of Cu(II) is greater than that of Zn(II) and Al(III) thus can be easily replaced by these ions. Moreover solution of copper is blue in color.

14. **(b)** $3SO_2 + O_3 \rightarrow 3SO_3$
O.N. of S changes from +4 to +6. Two electron change
$\therefore$ Eq. Wt = M/2. (molecular wt. = M)

15. **(a)** $2K\overset{+7}{Mn}O_4 + 3H_2SO_4 \rightarrow K_2SO_4 + 2\overset{+2}{Mn}SO_4 + 3H_2O + 5O$

$$2\overset{+2}{Fe}SO_4 + H_2SO_4 + O \rightarrow \overset{+3}{Fe_2}(SO_4)_3 + H_2O$$

O.N. of Mn changes from +7 to +2 (Reduction)

O.N. of Fe changes from +2 to +3 (Oxidation)

16. (c) On balancing the given equations, we get

$$2MnO_4^- + 5C_2O_4^{2-} + 16H^+ \longrightarrow 2Mn^{2+} + 10CO_2 + 8H_2O$$

So, $x = 2, y = 5 \& z = 16$

17. (b) On reaction with hot and concentrated alkali a mixture of chloride and chlorate is formed

$$3Cl_2 + 6\,NaOH(excess) \xrightarrow{Hot} 5Na\overset{-1}{Cl} + Na\overset{+5}{Cl}O_3 + 3H_2O$$

18. (a) $[Co(NH_3)_5Cl.]Cl_2$, $\overset{+1}{H}\overset{+1}{H}\overset{-1}{N}-\overset{-2}{O}-\overset{+1}{H}$, $\left(H_2\overset{-2}{N}-\overset{-2}{N}H_2\right)$, Mg_3N_2

−3, −1, −2, −3

19. (c) The redox couple with maximum reduction potential will be best oxidising agent and with minimum reduction potential will be best reducing agent.

20. (a) $3MnO_4^{2-} + 2H_2O \rightarrow MnO_2 + 2MnO_4^- + 4OH^-$

or $MnO_4^{2-} + \frac{2}{3}H_2O \rightarrow \frac{1}{3}MnO_2 + \frac{2}{3}MnO_4^- + \frac{4}{3}OH^-$

21. (b) In iodometry, $K_2Cr_2O_7$ liberates I_2 from iodides (NaI or KI) which is titrated with $Na_2S_2O_3$ solution.

$$K_2Cr_2O_7 + I^- + H^+ \longrightarrow Cr^{3+} + I_2$$

Here, one mole of $K_2Cr_2O_7$ accepts 6 mole of electrons.

$$\therefore \text{Equivalent weight} = \frac{\text{molecular weight}}{6}$$

22. (d) $\overset{0}{Cl_2} + 2NaOH \rightarrow Na\overset{-1}{Cl} + Na\overset{+1}{Cl}O + H_2O$

$3\overset{+6}{Mn}O_4^{2-} + 2H_2O \rightarrow 2\overset{+7}{Mn}O_4^- + \overset{+4}{Mn}O_2 + 4OH^-$

$2\overset{+4}{N}O_2 + H_2O \rightarrow H\overset{+5}{N}O_3 + H\overset{+3}{N}O_2$

All undergo disproportionation.

23. (c) $\overset{-4\ +4}{N_2H_4} \xrightarrow{\text{loss of } 10e^-} N_2^{+6}(y);$

O.N. of N changes from -2 to +3

24. (b) Phosphorus, sulphur and chlorine disproportionate in the alkaline medium.

25. (c) Oxidation number of oxygen in $OF_2 = +2$ and in $KO_2 = \frac{-1}{2}$.

26. (d) In H_2SO_4, sulphur is in highest oxidation state (+6). Hence H_2SO_4 will be strongest oxidising agent.

27. (c) $K_2Cr_2O_7 + 3SO_2 + 4H_2SO_4 \rightarrow K_2SO_4 + Cr_2(SO_4)_3 + 3SO_3 + 4H_2O$

O.N. of chromium changes from +6 to +3

28. (a) Higher the value of reduction potential higher will be the oxidising power whereas the lower the value of reduction potential higher will be the reducing power.

29. (a) More the reduction potential, more will be the oxidising power.

30. (c) The violent reaction between sodium and water is an example of redox reaction :

$$\underset{0}{2Na} + \underset{+1}{2H_2O} \longrightarrow \underset{+1}{2NaOH} + \underset{0}{H_2}$$

(Oxd. state)

In this reaction, sodium (Na) is oxidised to NaOH while H_2O is reduced to H_2.

31. (a) $FeSO_4$ is oxidised to $Fe_2(SO_4)_3$, change in O.N. of Fe is by 1. Hence equivalent weight of Mohr's salt is M/1 = M.

32. (d) $2K_2CrO_4 + 2HCl \rightarrow K_2Cr_2O_7 + 2KCl + H_2O$

Coefficients are 2, 2, 1, 2, 1

33. (a)

34. (c) In Cannizzaro's reaction

$$2HCHO + KOH \rightarrow CH_3OH + HCOOK$$

formaldehyde is getting reduced as well as oxidised.

35. (a)

36. (d) Zinc gives H_2 gas with dil H_2SO_4/HCl but not with HNO_3 because in HNO_3, NO_3^- ion is reduced and give NH_4NO_3, N_2O, NO and NO_2 (based upon the concentration of HNO_3)

$$[Zn + \underset{\text{(nearly 6\%)}}{2HNO_3} \longrightarrow Zn(NO_3)_2 + 2H] \times 4$$

$$HNO_3 + 8H \longrightarrow NH_3 + 3H_2O$$

$$NH_3 + HNO_3 \longrightarrow NH_4NO_3$$

$$4Zn + 10HNO_3 \longrightarrow 4Zn(NO_3)_2 + NH_4NO_3 + 3H_2O$$

Zn is on the top position of hydrogen in electrochemical series. So Zn displaces H_2 from dilute H_2SO_4 and HCl with liberation of H_2.

$$Zn + H_2SO_4 \rightarrow ZnSO_4 + H_2$$

37. (c)

38. (a) ON of S in $S_8 = 0$

ON of S in $S_2F_2 = +1$

ON of S in $H_2S = -2$

39. (a) More is E°_{RP}, more is the tendency to get itself reduced or more is oxidising power.

40. (a) For statement (iii), $HgCl_2$ is reduced to Hg_2Cl_2

41. (d) More the negative reduction potential, more is the tendency to lose electron. The reducing power increases as the standard reduction potential becomes more and more negative.

Thus, Li is the strongest reducing agent as the standard reduction potential of Li^+/Li is most negative, –3.05 V.

42. (a) $\overset{+5}{ClO_3^-} \longrightarrow \overset{0}{Cl_2}$

$x - 6 = -1 \quad x = 0$

$x = +5 \quad x = 0\,(x = \text{oxidation number})$

$$\text{Equivalent mass} = \frac{\text{Molecular mass}}{\text{Oxidation number}} = \frac{84.45}{5} = 16.89$$

43. (b) In SO_2 the O.N. of S can increase and decrease. Hence can behave as reducing and oxidising agent. Oxidation state of S varies from –2 to 6.

44. (a) –(4/3) is the average oxidation state of C in C_3H_4.

45. (c) The redox reaction involve loss or gain of electron(s) i.e. change in oxidation state. Given reaction is not a redox reaction as this reaction involves no change in oxidation state of reactant or product.

Speed Test-37

1. (c) Hg will not displace hydrogen since it is present below hydrogen in ECS.
2. (c) In metal hydrides the O.S. of hydrogen –1 otherwise it is +1.
3. (c)
4. (c) (i) and (iii) are properties of hydrogen which shows its resemblance with alkali metals whereas (ii), (iv) and (v) shows resemblance with halogens.
5 (b)
6. (c) The unusual properties of water in the condensed phase (liquid an solid states) are due to the presence of extensive hydrogen bonding between the water molecules.
7. (c) Hydrogen bond is weak force of attraction existing between molecules. Its energy is equal to 3-10 k cals.
8. (d) H_2O absorbs neutrons more than D_2O and this decreases the number of neutrons for the fission process.
9. (c)
10. (a) It is due to hydrogen bonding when H_2O forms a cage like structure in solid ice and density is reduced.
11. (a) $CaC_2 + 2D_2O \rightarrow C_2D_2 + Ca(OD)_2$
12. (b) $CO(g) + 2H_2(g) \xrightarrow[\text{catalyst}]{\text{cobalt}} CH_3OH(l)$
13. (b) Due to high dielectric constant, water acts as a good solvent therefore it is also called a universal solvent.
14. (a) ice occupy more volume than liquid water (ice $\rightleftharpoons$ water). Increase of pressure favours forward reaction (Le-Chatelier's principle).
15. (d) On the industrial scale hydrogen is prepared from water gas according to following reaction sequence

$$\underbrace{CO + H_2}_{\text{water gas}} + \underbrace{H_2O}_{\text{(steam)}} \xrightarrow{\text{catalyst}} CO_2 + 2H_2$$

$$\xrightarrow[\text{(alkali)}]{2NaOH} Na_2CO_3 + H_2O$$

From the above reaction it is clear that CO is first oxidised to CO_2 which is then absorbed in NaOH.

16. (a) Normality of 10V of H_2O_2

$$\frac{68\times 10}{22.4} = 17\times N \quad \therefore N = 1.78$$

17. (b) $H^-(aq) + H_2O(l) \rightarrow OH^- + H_2$. Since H^- is a strong base it will abstract H^+ to form H_2.
18. (d) Heavy water is D_2O (1–C); Temporary hard water contains the bi-carbonates of Mg and Ca (2–A); Soft water contains no foreign ions (3–B); Permanent hard water contains the sulphates and chlorides of Mg and Ca (4–D) therefore the answer is D.
19. (a) $\underset{\text{'A'}}{2Na} + 2H_2O \rightarrow \underset{\text{'C'}}{2NaOH} + \underset{\text{'B'}}{H_2} \uparrow$

$\underset{\text{'D'}}{Zn} + \underset{\text{'C'}}{2NaOH} \rightarrow Na_2ZnO_2 + \underset{\text{'B'}}{H_2} \uparrow$

$\underset{\text{'D'}}{Zn} + \text{dil. } H_2SO_4 \rightarrow ZnSO_4 + \underset{\text{'B'}}{H_2} \uparrow$

Na produces golden yellow colour with smokeless flame of Bunsen burner.

20. (b) In the structure of ice each molecule of H_2O is surrounded by three H_2O molecules in hexagonal honey comb manner. On the other in water, each molecule is surrounded by four neighbouring molecules randomly which results an open cage like structure. As a result there are a number of 'hole' or open spaces. In such a structure lesser number of molecules are packed per ml. When ice melts a large no. of hydrogen bonds are broken. The molecules therefore move into the holes or open spaces and come closer to each other than they were in solid state. This result sharp increase in the density. Therefore ice has lower density than water.
21. (c) $BaO_2 + H_2O + CO2 \rightarrow$

$BaCO_3 + H_2O_2$ (Merck process)

22. (c) $Na_2O_2 + 2H_2O \rightarrow 2NaOH + H_2O_2$

$2H_2O_2 \rightarrow 2H_2O + O_2$

23. (c) $2H_2O_2 \rightarrow 2H_2O + O_2$

The reaction is decomposition of H_2O_2.

24. (a) True peroxide contains O – O linkage and O_2^{2-} ion. They give hydrogen peroxide with dil H_2SO_4.

$BaO_2 + H_2SO_4(\text{dil.}) \rightarrow BaSO_4 + H_2O_2$

25. (d) Composition of water gas is 40-50% CO, 44-50% H_2, 3-7% CO_2 and 4-5% N_2
26. (d) H_2 is a highly inflammable gas.
27. (a) $PbO_2 \rightarrow PbO$ (change in O.S. is +4 to +2 hence reduction)
28. (d) SO_2 changes to H_2SO_4 (O.N. changes from +4 to +6 oxidation)

$2KI \rightarrow I_2$ (O.S. changes from –1 to 0 oxidation)

$PbS \rightarrow PbSO_4$ (O.S. changes from –2 to +6 oxidation)

$Ag_2O \rightarrow 2Ag$ (O.S. changes from +1 to 0 reduction)

29. (b) Strength of 10 volume $H_2O_2 = \frac{68 \times 10}{22400} \times 100 = 3.035\%$

30. (a) D_2O actually has higher freezing point (3.8°C) than water H_2O (0°C)

31. (b) Na_2 zeolite + $CaCl_2 \rightarrow$ Ca zeolite + 2NaCl

32. (a) $Na_2O_2 + 2HCl \rightarrow 2NaCl + H_2O_2$

33. (c) Ortho and para forms of hydrogen resemble in their chemical properties.

34. (b) When water is heated from 0°C to 4°C, its density increases and volume decreases. $\left(d = \frac{m}{V}\right)$

35. (a) Polarity of bond depends on difference in electronegativity of the two concerned atoms. H_2O is more polar than H_2S because oxygen (in O–H) is more electronegative than sulphur (in S–H).

36. (b) $LiH + AlCl_3 \longrightarrow (AlH_3)_n \xrightarrow[\text{LiH}]{\text{excess}} LiAlH_4$
Lithuim aluminium hydride is a most useful organic reducing agent. It reduces functional groups but does not attack double bonds.

37. (a) Only elements having reduction potential less than -0.41V liberate hydrogen with cold water.

38. (c) $2H_2O_2 \xrightarrow{\Delta} 2H_2O + O_2$

$2KI + H_2O_2 \rightarrow 2KOH + I_2$

$2KMnO_4 + 3H_2SO_4 + 5H_2O_2 \rightarrow K_2SO_4 + 2MnSO_4 + 8H_2O + 5O_2$

39. (a) PbO_2 is lead dioxide and does not contain O – O bonds and O_2^{2-} ions.

40. (b)

41. (d) d- and f-block elements form metallic hydride. While p-block elements form covalent hydrides, s-block elements except Be and Mg form ionic hydrides. Hydrides of Be, Mg, Cu, Zn, Ca and Hg are intermediate hydrides.

42. (d) Decomposition of H_2O_2 can be accelerated by finely divided metals such as Ag, Au, Pt, Co, Fe etc.

43. (b) $M = \frac{5.1 \times 1000}{34 \times 100} = 1.5$

44. (b) This is an example of exchange of ions.

45. (b) $BaO_2 + H_2SO_4 \rightarrow BaSO_4 + H_2O_2$.
oxygen has common O.S. as –2 and in peroxides as –1.

Speed Test-38

1. (d) Melting point of alkali metals decreases with increase in size.
2. (c)
3. (a) $4KO_2 + 2CO_2 \rightarrow 2K_2CO_3 + 3O_2$.
   KO_2 is used as an oxidising agent. It is used as air purifier in space capsules. Submarines and breathing masks as it produces oxygen and remove carbon dioxide.
4. (d) The stability of alkali metal hydrides decreases from Li to Cs. It is due to the fact that M–H bonds become weaker with increase in size of alkali metals as we move down the group from Li to Cs. Thus the order of stability of hydrides is
   LiH > NaH > KH > RbH > CsH
   i.e. option (d) is correct answer.
5. (c) $Cs + O_2 \rightarrow CsO_2$ (Superoxide)
   $4Li + O_2 \rightarrow 2Li_2O$ (Oxide)
   $2Na + O_2 \rightarrow Na_2O_2$ (Peroxide)
6. (a) $Be(OH)_2$ is amphoteric while $Ca(OH)_2$, $Sr(OH)_2$ and $Ba(OH)_2$ are all basic.
7. (c) $2Al(s) + 2NaOH(aq) + 2H_2O(l) \longrightarrow \underset{\text{sod. meta aluminate}}{2NaAlO_2} + 3H_2$
8. (d) Na_2O_2 is peroxide of sodium not super oxide. The formula of sodium superoxide is NaO_2.
9. (d) Na_2CO_3 does not decompose to form Na_2O.
10. (b)
11. (d) $Na_2S_2O_3 + 2HCl \longrightarrow 2NaCl + H_2O + \underset{\text{colourless}}{SO_2} + S$

    $SO_2 + Br_2 + H_2O \longrightarrow HBr + H_2SO_4$
12. (a)
13. (d) Amongst alkali metal Li ions are highly hydrated.
14. (c) $4S + 6NaOH \rightarrow Na_2S_2O_3 + 2Na_2S + 3H_2O$
15. (c) NaCl (brine), NH_3 and CO_2 are raw materials. $CaCO_3$ is source of CO_2.
16. (b) $\underset{X}{3Mg} + N_2 \xrightarrow{\Delta} \underset{Y}{Mg_3N_2}$;

    $Mg_3N_2 + 6H_2O \longrightarrow 3Mg(OH)_2 + \underset{\text{(colourless)}}{2NH_3 \uparrow}$

    $CuSO_4 + 4NH_3 \longrightarrow \underset{\text{Blue complex}}{[Cu(NH_3)_4]SO_4}$
17. (b) $Na_2S_2O_3 + 2HCl \rightarrow 2NaCl + SO_2 + S + H_2O$
    (Disproportionation)
18. (b) As we move down the group, the lattice energies of fluorides decrease more rapidly than the hydration energy and hence the solubilities of the fluorides increase from top to bottom within a group.
19. (d) When cold calcium hydroxide reacts with chlorine, then bleaching powder is obtained.

    $\underset{\text{slaked lime}}{3Ca(OH)_2} + 2Cl_2 \longrightarrow \underset{\text{Bleaching powder}}{Ca(OCl)_2.Ca(OH)_2.CaCl_2.2H_2O}$
20. (d) $Be(OH)_2$ is amphoteric, but the hydroxides of other alkaline earth metals are basic. The basic strength increases gradually.
21. (a) As the size of the anion increases, the covalent character increases and hence the m.p. decrease.
22. (c) Monovalent sodium and potassium ions and divalent magnesium and calcium ions are found in large proportions in biological fluids.
23. (c) $\underset{\text{temp. hardness}}{Ca(HCO_3)_2} + Ca(OH)_2 \longrightarrow 2CaCO_3 \downarrow + 2H_2O$

    $\underset{A}{Ca(OH)_2} + Na_2CO_3 \longrightarrow \underset{\text{Caustic soda}}{2NaOH} + CaCO_3$

    $\underset{A}{Ca(OH)_2} + CO_2 \longrightarrow \underset{\text{milkiness}}{CaCO_3 \downarrow} + H_2O$
24. (b) During the dissolution of alkali metal hydrides energy is released in large amount, i.e., it is exothermic in nature.
25. (d)
26. (a) The calcium concentration in plasma is regulated at about 100 mgL^{-1}. It is maintained by two hormones: calcitonin and parathyroid hormone.
27. (a) $2CaOCl_2 + dil.H_2SO_4 \rightarrow CaCl_2 + CaSO_4 + 2HClO$

    $HClO \rightarrow HCl + O$
28. (d) $CaO + CO_2 \longrightarrow CaCO_3$

    $CaO + H_2O \longrightarrow Ca(OH)_2$

    hissing sound and $\Delta H = -ve$
29. (c) MgO has high melting point and does not catch fire and hence protects the cooker against fire.
30. (c) The high solubility of $LiClO_4$ is mainly due to high heat of hydration of Li^+ ion.

31. (c)

32. (d) K and Mg are formed at cathode

$K^+ + e^- \longrightarrow K$

$Mg^{2+} + 2e^- \longrightarrow Mg.$

Chlorine is formed at anode $2C\bar{l} - 2\bar{e} \longrightarrow Cl_2.$

33. (b) The $Be(OH)_2$ and $Al(OH)_3$ are amphoteric in nature.

34. (c) $Be(OH)_2$ is insoluble in water value.

35. (d) Nitrites gives NO_2 (brown) with dil. acids. The nitrites and bromides give brown vapours of NO_2 and Br_2 with conc. acids.

36. (c) As Cs^+ ion has larger size than Li^+ and I^- has larger size than F^-, therefore maximum distance between centres of cations and anions is in CsI.

37. (c) The higher the covalent character, the lower the solubility of compound in water.

38. (b)

39. (b) In case of halogens covalent radius is considered this bond is formed by overlapping of electron clouds; while noble gases remain monoatomic, in this case only way to obtain radius is through van der Waal radii.

40. (c) In NO_2^+ odd (unpaired) electron is removed. In peroxides $\left(O_2^{2-}\right)$ no unpaired electrons are persent $\left(AlO_2^-\right)$ containing $Al^{3+}(2s^2p^6)$ configuration and 2 oxides (O^{2-}) ions each of which does not contain unpaired electron. Superoxide O_2^- has one unpaired electron.

41. (b) Magnesium hydroxide is used to prepare an antacid which is used as medicine for stomach acidity. Hence, the metal M is Mg.

42. (c) Na_2O_2 is $Na^{\oplus} O^{\ominus} - O^{\ominus} Na^{\oplus}$; Cr_2O_5 is

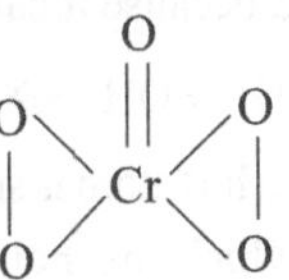

BaO_2 is $Ba^{+2}\left(O^{\ominus} - O^{\ominus}\right)$ while Fe_2O_3 consists of only Fe^{3+} and O^{2-} ions. Thus, Fe_2O_3 does not contain a peroxide $\left(O^{\ominus} - O^{\ominus}\right)$ linkage.

43. (b) The basic character of oxides increases down the group.

44. (a) On moving across a period ionisation energy increases hence the electropositive nature of metals decreases therefore the ease of formation of ion also decreases and hence the basic character decreases. Further basic character of alkali metals oxides increases from Li_2O to Cs_2O. Hence the correct order will be

$Al_2O_3 < MgO < Na_2O < K_2O$

45. (d) All nitrides react with H_2O to give NH_3

$Li_3N + 3H_2O \longrightarrow 3LiOH + NH_3$

$Mg_3N_2 + 6H_2O \longrightarrow 3Mg(OH)_2 + 2NH_3$

$CaNCN + 3H_2O \longrightarrow CaCO_3 + 2NH_3$

Speed Test-39

1. (d) $B(OH)_3$ is acid because it can take OH^- ions.

H_3BO_3 or $B(OH)_3 + OH^- \rightarrow B(OH)_4^-$

2. (b) In Boric acid each B atom is sp^2 hybridized and contains BO_3^{3-} units which are held together by hydrogen bonds.

3. (c) The IE_1 of Ga is more than that of Al because of the small atomic size and greater effective nuclear charge of Ga.

4. (b) In aqueous solution the probable aluminate species is $[Al(H_2O)_2(OH)_4]$ hence Al containing co-ordination number 6.

5. (b) Carbon is non-metal. Germanium and silicon are metalloid. Tin and lead are metals.

6. (c) Due to structural changes, melting point, increases from Ga to Tl and Ga has the lowest melting point.

7. (d) Reluctance of valence shell electrons to participate in bonding is called inert pair effect. The stability of lower oxidation state (+2 for group 14 element) increases on going down the group. So the correct order is $SiX_2 < GeX_2 < SnX_2 < PbX_2$

8. (d) The more the bond energy, the more is the catenation.

9. (d) Borax on heating gives B_2O_3 and $NaBO_2$ which is glassy mass and used for borax-bead test.

10. (a) $Al_2(SO_4)_3 + 6NH_4OH \rightarrow 2Al(OH)_3 + 3(NH_4)_2SO_4$

$Al(OH)_3 + NaOH \rightarrow Na^+[Al(OH)_4]^-$ Soluble complex

it is insoluble in NH_4OH

11. (b) The solution of aluminium chloride in water is acidic due to hydrolysis.

$AlCl_3 + 3H_2O \longrightarrow Al(OH)_3 + 3HCl.$

On heating it till dryness $Al(OH)_3$ is converted into Al_2O_3

$2Al(OH)_3 \xrightarrow{\Delta} Al_2O_3 + 3H_2O$

12. (a) Higher boranes are also spontaneously flammable in air.

13. (a) B_2O_3 is acidic and Al_2O_3 is amphoteric.

14. (b) Aluminium oxide is amphoteric oxide because it shows the properties of the both acidic and basic oxides. It reacts with both acids and bases to form salt and water.

$Al_2O_3.xH_2O + 2NaOH \longrightarrow NaAlO_2 + H_2O$

$Al_2O_3.xH_2O + HCl \longrightarrow AlCl_3 + H_2O$

15. (c) Fused alumina (Al_2O_3) is a bad conductor of electricity. Therefore, cryolite (Na_3AlF_6) and fluorspar (CaF_2) are added to purified alumina which not only make alumina a good conductor of electricity but also reduce the melting point of the mixture to around 1140 K.

16. (c) Due to + I effect of methyl groups the Lewis character of $B(CH_3)_3$ decreases and coordination becomes weaker.

17. (b) The hybridizations of B in H_3BO_3 is sp^2.

18. (a) Lead in +2 oxidation is stable while Sn and C are both stable in +4 oxidation.

19. (b) BCl_3 forms $[B(OH)_4]^-$ in which B is sp^3 hybridized and have +3 oxidation state.

20. (d)

21. (a)

22. (b) Silicon has Si – O – Si – O – Si linkage.

23. (c) CO_2 being more dense covers the igniting material more effectively than N_2.

24. (c) Aluminium chloride in acidified aqueous solution forms octahedral $[Al(H_2O)_6]^{3+}$ ion.

25. (d) H_2CO_3/HCO_3^- buffer system help to maintain pH of blood between 7.26 to 7.42.

26. (b) Grey tin $\rightleftharpoons$ white tin

Grey tin is brittle and crumbles down to powder in very cold climate

The conversion of grey tin to white tin is acompained by increase in volume., This is knwon as tin plaque or tin disease.

27. (c) $SnCl_2 + 2NaOH \rightarrow Sn(OH)_2 + 2NaCl$

$Sn(OH)_2 + 2NaOH \rightarrow Na_2SnO_2 + 2H_2O$

28. (a) The stability of +2 O.S. follows the order

$Pb^{2+} > Sn^{2+} > Ge^{2+}$

Hence reducing power $Ge > Sn > Pb$

29. (d) $2CaF_2 + SiO_2 + H_2SO_4 \longrightarrow$

$SiF_4 + H_2O + CaSO_4 \xrightarrow{\text{hydrolysis}} CaSiF_6$

30. (c) Negative $\Delta_r G^\circ$ value indicates that + 2 oxidation state is more stable for Pb. Also it is supported by inert pair effect that + 2 oxidation state is more stable for Pb and as $\Delta_r G^\circ$ value is positive in second reaction it indicates that + 4 oxidation state is more stable for Sn.

i.e., $Sn^{2+} < Pb^{2+}$, $Sn^{4+} > Pb^{4+}$

31. (a) Metal atom in the lower oxidation state forms the ionic bond and in the higher oxidation state the covalent

bond because higher oxidation state means small size and great polarizing power and hence greater the covalent character. Hence MCl_2 is more ionic than MCl_4.

32. (a) H_3BO_3 is a weak monobasic acid.

33. (d) $Si_2O_7^{6-}$ ion represents pyrosilicate.

34. (d) It is mercury because it exists as liquid at room temperature.

35. (b) F and Cl are more oxidising in nature and can achieve Pb in (IV) O.S. but Br_2 and I_2 can not achieve Pb in (IV) O.S. secondly Pb^{4+} is strong in oxidising nature and in its presence, Br^- and I^- can not exist.

36. (d) Ge(II) tends to acquire Ge (IV) state by loss of electrons. Hence it is reducing in nature. Pb (IV) tends to acquire Pb (II) O.S. by gain of electrons. Hence it is oxidising in nature. This is due to inert pair effect.

37. (d) Hybridisation $=\frac{1}{2}(4+4+0-0)=4$, sp^3 tetrahedral.

38. (b) $8BF_3+6LiH\xrightarrow{\Delta}B_2H_6+6LiBF_4$

39. (d) In artificial respiration a mixture of O_2 with CO_2 or helium is used. Helium is used as it is less soluble in blood.

40. (c) Graphite is composed of flat two-dimensional sheets of carbon atoms. Each sheet is a hexagonal net of C atoms. The 3 e^- of C form σ bond & 4th electron is a π e^- and is delocalized over the whole sheet & is thus mobile. Conduction of electricity is due to these delocalized electrons within each layer. Conduction does not occur from one sheet to another.

41. (c) CO_2 forms carbonic acid H_2CO_3, when dissolved in water, CO is neutral, whereas other two GeO_2 and SnO_2 are solids.

42. (d) Carborundum is SiC.

43. (b) $R_3SiCl+HOH\rightarrow R_3SiOH+HCl$

$$R_3SiOH+HOSiR_3\rightarrow R_3Si-O-SiR_3+H_2O$$

44. (a) Carbon does not contain *d*-orbital hence it cannot expand its octet.

45. (b) Glass being a mixture of sodium and calcium silicates reacts with hydrofluoric acid forming sodium and calcium fluorosilicates respectively.

$$Na_2SiO_3+6HF\rightarrow Na_2SiF_6+3H_2O$$

$$CaSiO_3+6HF\rightarrow CaSiF_6+3H_2O$$

The etching of glass is based on these reactions.

Speed Test-40

1. (a) The correct order of priority for the given functional group is

$$-COOH > -SO_3H > -\overset{O}{\overset{||}{C}}-NH_2 > -\overset{O}{\overset{||}{C}}-H$$

2. (b) When – CHO is treated as side chain, its name is carbaldehyde.

$$\overset{3}{C}H_2 - \overset{2}{C}H - \overset{1}{C}H_2$$

Hence $\underset{CHO}{|}$ $\underset{CHO}{|}$ $\underset{CHO}{|}$ is propane – 1, 2, 3-tri carbaldehyde.

3. (a) Carbinol is methyl alcohol (CH_3OH), hence vinylcarbinol should be $\overset{3}{C}H_2 = \overset{2}{C}H\overset{1}{C}H_2OH$ (prop-2-enol)

4. (a)

5. (a) Cyclohexane (iv) is non-planar and has chair conformation. In this conformation, the bond angle is the normal tetrahedral angle (109°, 28') and thus has no angle strain and hence is most stable. The rest of the molecules are nearly planar and hence their stability depends upon the angle strain in accordance with *Baeyer's strain theory.* Since cyclopropane has higher angle strain $\left(\frac{109°28'-60°}{2} = 24°, 44'\right)$ than cyclopentane $\left(\frac{109°\ 28'-108°}{2} = 0°, 44'\right)$.

Therefore cyclopentane (iii) is more stable than cyclopropane (i). Further, because of the presence of a double bond in a three membered ring, cyclopropene (ii) is the least stable. Thus the order of stability is (iv) > (iii) > (i) > (ii).

6. (b) If there is a small difference (10 or less) in the boiling points of liquids fractional distillation is used e.g. acetone b.p. 333 K and methanol b.p. 338 K.

7. (c) Cl^- is the best leaving group among the given option. As it has high electronegativity thereby generating positive charge on carbonyl carbon atom.

8. (a) $C_6H_5\ddot{O}:^-$ > $C_6H_5\ddot{O}H$

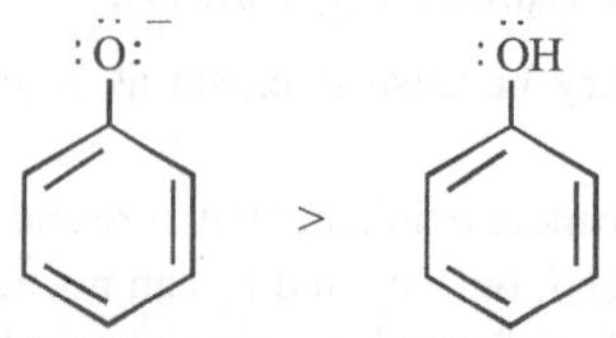

Most electron-releasing due to –ve charge on O; Electron releasing due to –OH group

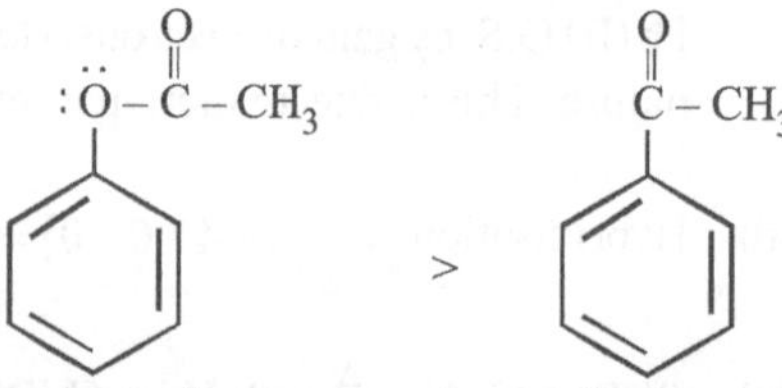

$C_6H_5\ddot{O}-\overset{O}{\overset{||}{C}}-CH_3$ > $C_6H_5-\overset{O}{\overset{||}{C}}-CH_3$

Less electron releasing due to presence of –CO grouping which shows resonance with the electrons on O; Electron-withdrawing group

9. (a) $C_nH_{2n}O_2$ is general formula for carboxylic acid.

10. (a) Since during the reaction, a chiral carbon is created and further since the CN^- ion can attack the planar aldehyde group both from the top and the bottom face of the aldehyde group with equal ease, therefore, a 50:50 mixture of the two enantiomers, i.e. a racemic mixture is obtained.

11. (c) C_5H_{10} has 1° degree of unsaturation since the isomers are acyclic, all of these are alkenes. For writing the isomers, first introduce the double bond at different possible positions, and then consider the possibility of branching in the alkyl group.

$CH_3CH_2CH_2CH=CH_2$ 1-pentene (*i*)

$CH_3CH_2CH=CHCH_3$ 2- pentene, (*cis,- trans*) (*ii*), (*iii*)

$CH_3-\underset{}{\overset{CH_3}{\overset{|}{C}H}}-CH=CH_2$ 3-methyl-1-butene, (*iv*)

$CH_3CH_2\overset{CH_3}{\overset{|}{C}}=CH_2$ 2-methyl-1-butene, (*v*)

$CH_3-\overset{CH_3}{\overset{|}{C}}=CHCH_3$ 2-methyl-2-butene, (*vi*)

12. (d) Since all the six carbon atoms of cyclohexatriene (benzene) are sp^2 hybridized, therefore its stablest structure is planar form.

13. (a) Prussian blue $Fe_4[Fe(CN)_6]_3$ is formed in lassaigne test for nitrogen.

$$3Na_4[Fe(CN)_6] + 2Fe^{3+} \longrightarrow \underset{\text{Prussian blue}}{Fe_4[Fe(CN)_6]_3} + 12Na^+$$

14. (b) Percentage of $P = \frac{62}{222} \times \frac{\text{wt. of } Mg_2P_2O_7}{\text{wt. of compound}} \times 100$

$$= \frac{62}{222} \times \frac{1.332}{2.79} \times 100 = 13.33\%$$

15. (a)

16. (a) It is a bridge compound

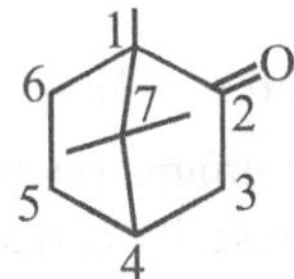

1, 7, 7-trimethyl bicyclo [2. 2. 1] heptan-2-one

17. (c) Convert these Newmann projections into open chain structures.

CH_3 / H—Cl / H—H / CH_3 CH_3 / H—H / H—H / CH_2Cl

Both structures have same molecular formula C_4H_9Cl, thus these are isomers. However, the two have different groups, viz CH_3 and CH_2Cl, so these are neither enantiomers nor diastereomers. Hence these are structural isomers.

18. (b) $(CH)_2(COOH)_2$ is HOOCCH = CHCOOH, hence here geometrical isomerism is possible.

19. (c) $CH_2 = CH - \ddot{C}l\!: \leftrightarrow \bar{C}H_2 - CH = \overset{+}{C}l\!:$ a double bond is formed between C and Cl. Hence it is less reactive due to resonance

20. (b) Among the given compounds naphthelene is volatile but benzoic acid is non-volatile (it forms a dimer). So, the best method for their separation is sublimation, which is applicable to compounds which can be converted directly into the vapour phase from its solid state on heating and back to the solid state on cooling. Hence it is the most appropriate method.

21. (b) $\% \text{ of } S = \frac{32}{233} \times \frac{0.233}{0.32} \times 100 = 10\%$

22. (d) $\overset{6}{C}H_3\overset{5}{C}H_2\overset{4}{C}H = \overset{3}{C}H - \overset{2}{\underset{}{C}}(=O) - \overset{1}{C}H$ (hex – 3 – en – 2 – one)

23. (b)   24. (b)

25. (a) In S_N Ar reactions, a carbanion is formed as an intermediate, so any substituent that increases the stability of carbanion and hence the transition state leading to its formation will enhance the S_NAr reactions. To compare the rates of substitution in chlorobenzene, chlorobenzene having electron-withdrawing group, and chlorobenzene having electron-releasing group, we compare the structures carbanion I (from chlorobenzene), II (from chlorobenzene containing electron-withdrawing group) and III (from chlorobenzene containing electron-releasing group).

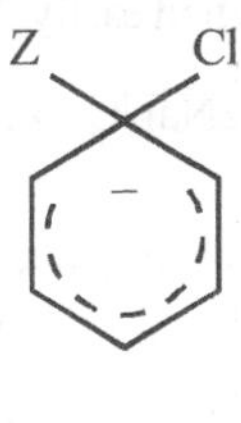

I

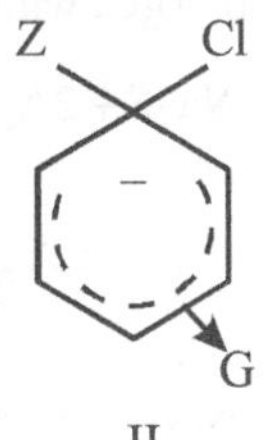

II

G withdraws electrons, neutralises (disperses) –ve charge of the ring, stabilises carbanion, facilitates S_N reaction **(activation effect)**

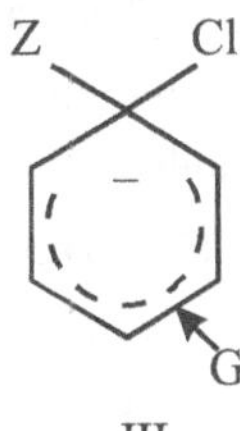

III

G releases electrons, intensifies –ve charge, destabilizes carbanion, retards S_N reaction **(deactivation)**

NO_2 is activating group and CH_3 and OCH_3 are deactivating group towards nucleophilic aromatic substitution reactions.

Hence, the correct order of nucleophilic substitution reactions

Cl / NO_2 > Cl > Cl / CH_3 > Cl / OCH_3

26. (c) As in above question,

$$C = \frac{40}{12} = 3.33;\ H = \frac{13.33}{1} = 13.33;\ N = \frac{46.67}{14} = 3.34$$

Relative No. of atoms,

$$C = \frac{3.33}{3.33} = 1;\ H = \frac{13.33}{3.33} = 4;\ N = \frac{3.34}{3.33} = 1$$

$\therefore$ Empirical formula $= CH_4N$

27. (a) $\overset{5}{C}H_3-\overset{4}{C}H(CH_3)-\overset{3}{C}(=O)-\overset{2}{C}H_2-\overset{1}{C}H_2OH$

1-Hydroxy-4-methyl-3-pentanone

28. (c) Diastereomers have different solubility, m.p. and b.p., hence they can be separated by fractional crystallisation.

29. (b) Na_2S and NaCN, formed during fusion with metallic sodium, must be removed before adding $AgNO_3$, otherwise black ppt. due to Na_2S or white precipitate due to AgCN will be formed and thus white precipitate of AgCl will not be identified easily.

$$Na_2S + 2AgNO_3 \longrightarrow 2NaNO_3 + \underset{\text{Black}}{Ag_2S}\downarrow$$

$$NaCN + AgNO_3 \longrightarrow NaNO_3 + \underset{\text{White}}{AgCN}\downarrow$$

$$NaCl + AgNO_3 \longrightarrow NaNO_3 + \underset{\text{White}}{AgCl}\downarrow$$

$$Na_2S + 2HNO_3 \xrightarrow{\text{boil}} 2NaNO_3 + H_2S\uparrow$$

$$NaCN + HNO_3 \xrightarrow{\text{boil}} NaNO_3 + HCN\uparrow$$

30. (a) Stronger the acid, weaker the conjugate base. Since acidic character follows the order

$$H_2O > NH_3 > HC\equiv CH > CH_3-CH_3$$

the basic character of their conjugate bases decreases in the reverse order, i.e.,

$$CH_3CH_2^- > HC\equiv C^- > NH_2^- > OH^-$$

31. (c) All of these compounds show tautomerism

[Structures: 4,4-dimethylcyclohex-2-enone ⇌ enol form (OH); 6,6-dimethylcyclohex-2-enone ⇌ enol form (OH); 5,5-dimethylcyclohex-2-enone ⇌ enol form (OH)]

H₃C CH₃ / H / O ⇌ H₃C CH₃ / OH

CH₃ CH₃ / H / O ⇌ CH₃ CH₃ / OH

H / CH₃ CH₃ / O ⇌ CH₃ CH₃ / OH

32. (a) 2,4,6-Trinitrophenol (III) $> CH_3COOH$ (II) $>$ Phenol (IV) $>$ Cyclohexanol (I)

Explanation : Presence of three $-NO_2$ groups in *o*–, *p*– positions to phenolic groups (in III) makes phenol strongly acidic because its corresponding conjugate base is highly stabilised due to resonance. Conjugate base of CH_3COOH, II (*i.e.* CH_3COO^-) is resonance hybrid of two equivalent structures. The conjugate base of phenol, IV is stabilized due to resonance (note that here all resonating structures are not equivalent). The conjugate base of cyclohexanol, I does not exhibit resonance, hence not formed.

33. (c) Decreasing order of deactivating effect of the given *m*-directing group is

$$-NO_2 > -CN > -SO_3H > -COOH$$

$-NO_2$ group is most deactivating group due to strong $-E$, $-I$ and $-M$ effects.

34. (a) On moving down a group, the basicity and nucleophilicity are inversely related, i.e. nucleophilicity increases while basicity decreases. i.e RS^- is more nucleophilic but less basic than RO^-. This opposite behaviour is because of the fact that basicity and nucleophilicity depends upon different factors. Basicity is directly related to the strength of the H–element bond, while nucleophilicity is indirectly related to the electronegativity of the atom to which proton is attached.

35. (c) The degree of hydrolysis increases as the magnitude of positive charge on carbonyl group increases. Electron withdrawing group increases the positive charge and electron releasing group decreases the positive charge. Among these NO_2 & CHO are electron withdrawing group from which NO_2 has more –I effect than –CHO. On the other hand CH_3 is a electron releasing group therefore the order of reactivity towards hydrolysis is

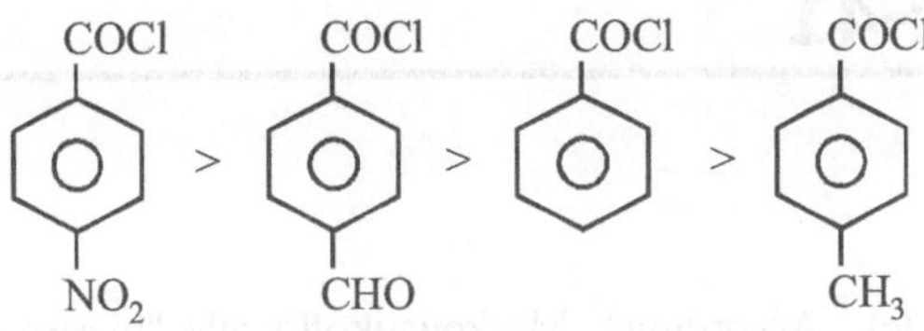

COCl-C_6H_4-NO_2 > COCl-C_6H_4-CHO > COCl-C_6H_5 > COCl-C_6H_4-CH_3

36. **(a)** Enolic form predominates in compounds containing two carbonyl groups separated by a $-CH_2$ group. This is due to following two factors.

(i) Presence of conjugation which increases stability.

(ii) Formation of intramolecular hydrogen bond between enolic hydroxyl group and second carbonyl group which leads to stablisation of the molecule. Hence the correct answer is III > II > I.

37. **(a)**

38. **(b)** – I group destablises carbocation and since inductive effect decreases with increasing length of carbon chain. Therefore (b) is the correct option.

39. **(b)** The octet around N is complete, hence it has no electrophilic character. N has no unshared pair of electrons to act as nucleophile.

40. **(b)** K_2SO_4 raises b.pt. and $CuSO_4$ acts as catalyst.

41. **(b)** Constitutional isomers

Altrose is CHO–C(HO)(H)–$(CHOH)_3$–CH_2OH, Glucose is CHO–C(H)(OH)–C(HO)(H)–$(CHOH)_2$–CH_2OH

$$\text{Altrose is } \begin{array}{c} CHO \\ | \\ HO-C-H \\ | \\ (CHOH)_3 \\ | \\ CH_2OH \end{array}, \quad \text{Glucose is } \begin{array}{c} CHO \\ | \\ H-C-OH \\ | \\ HO-C-H \\ | \\ (CHOH)_2 \\ | \\ CH_2OH \end{array}$$

42. **(c)** It is definition of asymmetric synthesis.

43. **(a)** $$PhCOCOPh \xrightarrow{LiAlH_4} Ph-\overset{OH}{\underset{H}{C^*}}-\overset{OH}{\underset{H}{C^*}}-Ph$$

The product contains two similar asymmetric carbon atoms and two optically active and one optically inactive meso form.

44. **(b)** In carbocations, carbon bearing positive charge is always sp^2-hybridised

45. **(b)** $$\overset{1°}{CH_3}-\underset{3°}{\overset{\overset{1°}{CH_3}}{CH}}-\overset{\overset{1°}{CH_3}}{\underset{Cl}{\overset{4°}{C}}}-\overset{2°}{CH_2}-\overset{1°}{CH_3};$$

Thus all the four types of carbon atoms are present in this compound.

Speed Test-41

1. (c) $$H_3C-\underset{CH_3}{\overset{CH_3}{\underset{|}{\overset{|}{C}}}}-CH_2Br + 2Na + Br-CH_2-\underset{CH_3}{\overset{CH_3}{\underset{|}{\overset{|}{C}}}}-CH_3 \xrightarrow[-2NaBr]{ether}$$

neo-pentyl bromide

$$H_3C-\underset{CH_3}{\overset{CH_3}{\underset{|}{\overset{|}{C}}}}-CH_2-CH_2-\underset{CH_3}{\overset{CH_3}{\underset{|}{\overset{|}{C}}}}-CH_3$$

2,2,5,5-tetramethylhexane

2. (c) $CH_3CHBrCHBrCH_3 \xrightarrow{Zn/alcohol} CH_3CH=CHCH_3$

Since two bromine atoms are lost from different carbon atom, the reaction is known as β-elimination.

3. (a) The intermediate 2° carbocation shows resonance

$$CH_2=CH-CH=CH_2 \xrightarrow{Br^+}$$

$$\left[CH_2Br-\overset{+}{C}H-CH=CH_2 \longleftrightarrow CH_2Br-CH=CH-\overset{+}{C}H_2\right]$$

$$\xrightarrow{Br^-} \underset{\text{1,4-dibromo-2-butene}}{CH_2Br-CH=CH-CH_2Br}$$

4. (d) $$\underset{\text{2,3-dimethyl-2-pentene}}{(CH_3)_2C=C(CH_3)CH_2CH_3} \longrightarrow (CH_3)_2C=O + O=C(CH_3)C_2H_5$$

5. (c) $$CH_3-CH=CH_2+H_2O \xrightarrow{H_2SO_4} CH_3-\underset{OH}{\underset{|}{C}H}-CH_3$$

2° alcohol

$$CH_3-\overset{CH_3}{\overset{|}{C}}=CH_2+H_2O \xrightarrow{H_2SO_4} CH_3-\underset{OH}{\underset{|}{\overset{CH_3}{\overset{|}{C}}}}-CH_3$$

3° alcohol

Addition follows Markownikoff's rule.

6. (b) $$CH_2=CH_2 \xrightarrow{HOCl} \underset{(M)}{\underset{Cl\quad OH}{\underset{|\qquad |}{CH_2-CH_2}}} \xrightarrow{aq.\ NaHCO_3} \underset{\text{Glycol}}{\underset{CH_2OH}{\overset{CH_2OH}{|}}}$$

7. (c) According to Markownikoff's rule, "in case of addition of an unsymmetrical reagent (H–X), the positive part get attached to the C which is least substituted or which bears larger number of hydrogen atoms."

$$\underset{H}{\overset{R}{\ }}\!\!>C=C<\!\!\underset{H}{\overset{H}{\ }} + H-X \longrightarrow R-\underset{X}{\underset{|}{\overset{H}{\overset{|}{C}}}}-\underset{H}{\underset{|}{\overset{H}{\overset{|}{C}}}}-H$$

Markownikoff's rule is based on the stability of carbocations (3° > 2° > 1° > methyl).

8. (a) $$\underset{\text{Ethyne}}{CH\equiv CH}+H_2 \xrightarrow{Pd/C} \underset{\text{Ethene}}{CH_2=CH_2}$$

$$H-\underset{H}{\underset{|}{\overset{H}{\overset{|\beta}{C}}}}-\underset{X}{\underset{|}{\overset{H}{\overset{|\alpha}{C}}}}-H \xrightarrow[\Delta]{alc.KOH} \underset{H}{\overset{H}{\ }}\!\!>C=C<\!\!\underset{H}{\overset{H}{\ }}$$

$(X = Cl, Br, I)$

$$CH_2Br-CH_2Br+Zn \longrightarrow CH_2=CH_2+ZnBr_2$$

$$\underset{\text{Ethanol}}{H-\underset{H}{\underset{|}{\overset{H}{\overset{|\beta}{C}}}}-\underset{OH}{\underset{|}{\overset{H}{\overset{|\alpha}{C}}}}-H} \xrightarrow[\Delta]{Conc.H_2SO_4} CH_2=CH_2+H_2O$$

9. (a) $$CH_2=C=CH-CH_3 \xrightarrow{H^+}$$

$$\left[CH_2=\overset{+}{C}-CH_2CH_3 + CH_2=CH-\overset{+}{C}HCH_3\right]$$

$$\xrightarrow{Cl^-} \underset{\text{2-Chlorobutene}}{CH_2=\underset{Cl}{\underset{|}{C}}-CH_2CH_3} + \underset{\text{3-Chlorobutene}}{CH_2=CH-\underset{Cl}{\underset{|}{C}}HCH_3}$$

10. (c)

11. (d) Writing the reaction we get

$$CH_3MgX+CH_3-C\equiv C-H \longrightarrow CH_3-C\equiv CMgX+CH_4(g)$$

12. (b) –Cl group is o-, p-directing due to +R effect ; however it is deactivating due to strong –I effect of Cl (different from other o-, p-directing groups which are activating). The net result is that chlorobenzene undergoes o-, p-substitution, with difficulty.

13. (b) $CH_3-CH=CH_2+H_2O \xrightarrow[\text{Markonikoff's rule}]{\text{conc. } H_2SO_4}$ $CH_3-\underset{\underset{OH}{|}}{CH}-CH_3$

Isopropyl alcohol

14. (b) Dihydrogen gas adds to alkenes and alkynes in the presence of finely divided catalysts like platinum, palladium or nickel to form alkanes. These metals adsorb dihydrogen gas on their surfaces and activate the hydrogen-hydrogen bond. Platinum and palladium catalyse the reaction at room temperature but relatively higher temperature and pressure are required with nickel catalyst.

15. (a) Electrolysis of a concentrated aqueous solution of either sodium or potassium salts of saturated non-carboxylic acids yields higher alkane at anode.

$$2RCOOK \xrightarrow[\text{Oxidation}]{\text{Electrolytic}} \underset{\text{Anode}}{2RCOO^-} + \underset{\text{Cathode}}{2K^+}$$

At anode : $2RCOO^- \rightarrow 2RCOO + 2e^- \longrightarrow R-R + 2CO_2$

At Cathode : $2K^+ + 2e^- \longrightarrow 2K$
$2K + H_2O \rightarrow 2KOH + H_2\uparrow$

16. (c) Both (a) and (b) are correct. Wet CH_3COOH gives cis addition and dry CH_3COOH gives trans addition products.

17. (a) Oxymercuration leads to hydration according to Markownikoff's rule.

$$CH_3CH_2C\equiv CH \xrightarrow{HgSO_4+H_2SO_4} \left[CH_3CH_2\overset{\overset{OH}{|}}{C}=CH_2\right] \longrightarrow CH_3CH_2COCH_3$$

18. (a)

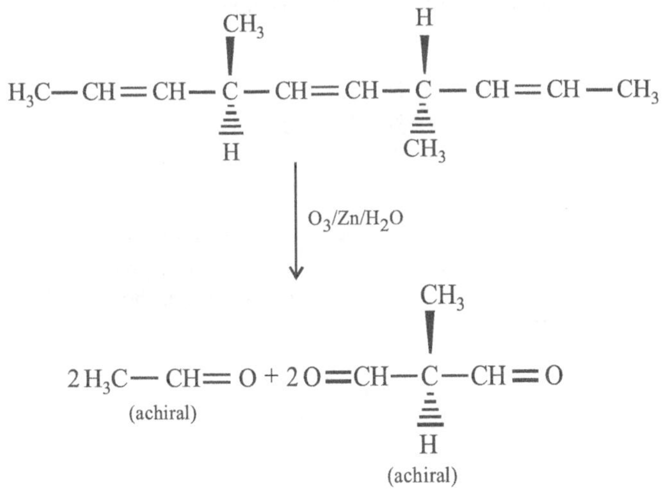

$$H_3C-CH=CH-\underset{H}{\overset{CH_3}{C}}-CH=CH-\underset{CH_3}{\overset{H}{C}}-CH=CH-CH_3$$

$\downarrow O_3/Zn/H_2O$

$$\underset{\text{(achiral)}}{2H_3C-CH=O} + 2O=CH-\underset{H}{\overset{CH_3}{C}}-CH=O$$

(achiral)

19.

$$3CH_3-C\equiv CH \longrightarrow$$ (ring structure: benzene ring with three CH_3 groups at alternate positions)

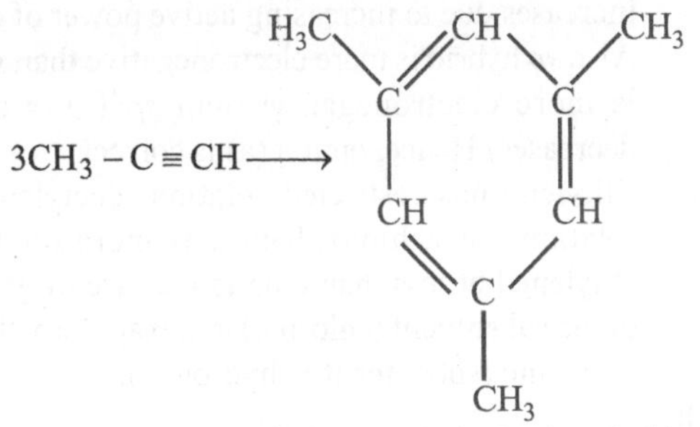

Mesitylene or 1, 3, 5-trimethyl benzene

20. (a) According to experimental evidences, electrophilic substitution reactions are supposed to proceed via the following three steps:
(1) Generation of the electrophile
(2) Formation of carbocation intermediate
(3) Removal of proton from the carbocation intermediate

21. (a) Determine the empirical formula of the two compounds

$$C:H = \left(\frac{12}{13}\times 100\right):\left(\frac{1}{13}\times 100\right) = 92.3:7.7$$

$$= \frac{92.3}{12}:\frac{7.7}{1} = 7.7:7.7 = 1:1$$

∴ The empirical formula of the two compounds is CH. Thus the molecular formula of A and B will be the simple multiple of CH, i.e. C_2H_2, C_3H_3, C_4H_4, C_6H_6, etc.
Thus options (c) and (d) are discarded. Further since A decolourises bromine water and B does not, A and B should be C_2H_2 (acetylene) and C_6H_6 (benzene) respectively.

22. (d) $H_3C-C\equiv C-\boxed{H + CH_3CH_2}MgCl \longrightarrow$

$H_3C-C\equiv C-MgCl + CH_3CH_3$

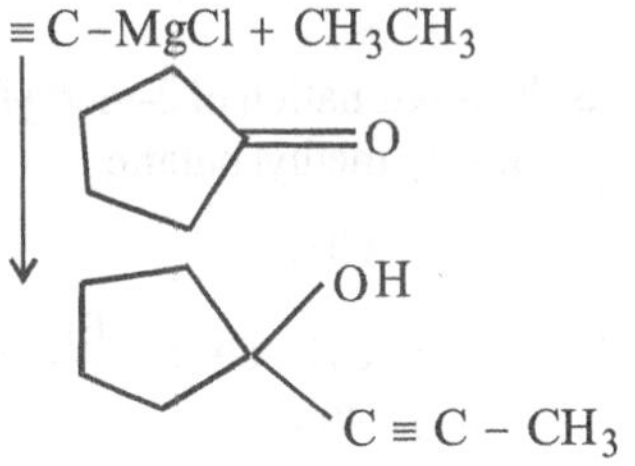

$\downarrow$ (cyclopentanone, C=O)

1-(prop-1-ynyl)cyclopentanol: cyclopentane ring bearing OH and $C\equiv C-CH_3$

23. (b) $(CH_3)_2CH-\underset{\underset{CH_3}{|}}{CH}-CH=CH_2$ contain 7 carbon atoms

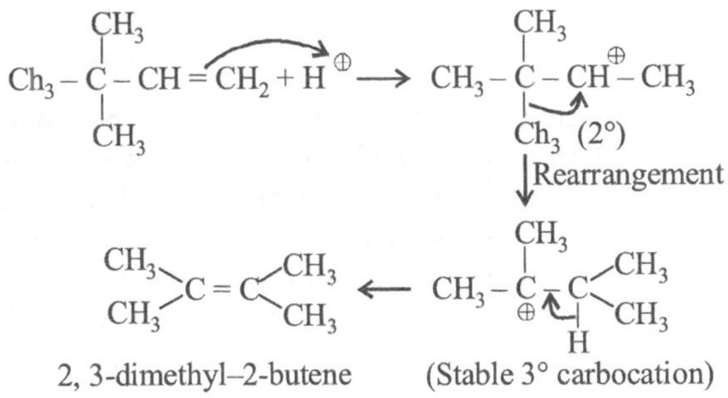

$$Ch_3-\underset{\underset{CH_3}{|}}{\overset{\overset{CH_3}{|}}{C}}-CH=CH_2+H^{\oplus} \longrightarrow CH_3-\underset{\underset{Ch_3\ (2^\circ)}{|}}{\overset{\overset{CH_3}{|}}{C}}-\overset{\oplus}{CH}-CH_3$$

$\downarrow$ Rearrangement

$$\underset{\text{2, 3-dimethyl–2-butene}}{\frac{CH_3}{CH_3}\!\!>C=C<\!\!\frac{CH_3}{CH_3}} \longleftarrow \underset{\text{(Stable 3° carbocation)}}{CH_3-\overset{\overset{CH_3}{|}}{\underset{\oplus}{C}}-\underset{\underset{H}{|}}{C}<\!\!\frac{CH_3}{CH_3}}$$

24. (a) As the number of bonds between carbon atoms increases, electronegativity of that carbon also increases due to increasing active power of electrons. Also *sp* hybrid is more electronegative than sp^2 which is more electronegative than sp^3($\because$ *s* character decreases) Hence, option (a) is correct.

25. (a) Ethylene has restricted rotation, acetylene has no rotation, hexachloroethane has more rotation than ethylene but less than ethane because of greater size of the substituent (chlorine) in hexachloroethane than in ethane (substituent is hydrogen).

26. (d)

27. (a) In $H_2C = C = CH_2$ hybridisation of C atoms is sp^2 and sp. The molecule is monoplanar but H–atoms lie in different planes.

28. (a) $CH \equiv CH \xrightarrow[Hg^{2+}]{CH_3COOH} CH_2 = CHOCOCH_3 \xrightarrow{CH_3COOH} CH_3CH(OCOCH_3)_2$

29. (b) $(CH_3)_2CH - CH_2 - CH(CH_3) - CH_2 - CH_3$ (2,4 dimethyl hexane)

Isopropyl group

It contains isopropyl group.

30. (c) In the given reactions, X is

$CH_3 - CH_2 - CH_2 - \overset{O}{\overset{||}{C}} - CH_3$ and Y is $CH_3CH_2CH_2CH_2CHO$, X will give +ve iodoform test and Y will give +ve silver mirror test.

31. (d) The order of substitution in different alkanes is

$3° > 2° > 1°$

Thus the bromination of 2-methylbutane mainly gives 2-Bromo - 2 - methyl butane

$CH_3 - CH_2 - CH(CH_3) - CH_3 \xrightarrow{Br_2}$
2-methylbutane

$CH_3 - CH_2 - CH(CH_3) - CH_2Br + CH_3 - CH_2 - C(CH_3)(Br) - CH_3$

1-Bromo-2methyl butane (minor)

2-Bromo-2-methyl butane (major)

32. (a) The acidity of acetylene or 1–alkyne can be explained on the basis of molecular orbital concept according to which formation of C—H bond in acetylene involves *sp*-hybridised carbon atom. Now since s electrons are closer to the nucleus than *p* electrons, the electrons present in a bond having more *s* character will be correspondingly more closer to the nucleus.

Thus owing to high *s* character of the C—H bond in alkynes (*s* = 50%), the electrons constituting this bond are more strongly held by the carbon nucleus i.e., the acetylenic carbon atom or the *sp* orbital acts as more electronegative species than the sp^2 and sp^3 with the result the hydrogen present on such a carbon atom (≡C—H) can be easily removed as a proton.

33. (c) Phenol as well as toluene have electron-releasing groups, however –OH group, in phenol, is more electron-releasing (due to +R effect) than the $-CH_3$ group in toluene, so phenol is more easily attacked by an electrophile.

34. (b) The given reaction is Diel's Alder reaction. This reaction involves a cycloaddition between a conjugated diene and a substituted alkene.

35. (a) Reduction of alkynes with Lindar's catalyst ($Pd-BaSO_4$) gives cis-alkenes.

36. (b) $HC \equiv C - CH_2 - CH_2NH_2$ contains three active hydrogen atoms (one attached to sp hybridised carbon atom and two attached to N). Hence, Et.MgBr will give three moles of C_2H_6.

37. (c) Anisole ($:\ddot{O}CH_3$) > Benzene > Nitrobenzene (NO_2)

Electron-releasing group present | No group is present | Electron withdrawing group is present

38. (b) 1-Methylcyclopentene $\xrightarrow{D-Cl}$ carbocation (CH_3, ⊕, D)

Formation of above species is more favourable. The stability order of carbocations is

$-\overset{|}{C}+ < -\overset{|}{\underset{}{C}}+ < -\overset{|}{\underset{|}{C}}+$
1° 2° 3°

Now, carbocation formed is sp^2 hybridised that is triangular planar as shown below

Either the $Cl^{\ominus}$ attack from above or below formation of the plane of the molecule, so there is probability of resultant product as shown below i.e., both product will form.

39. (d) N–bromosuccinimide results into bromination at allylic and benzylic positions

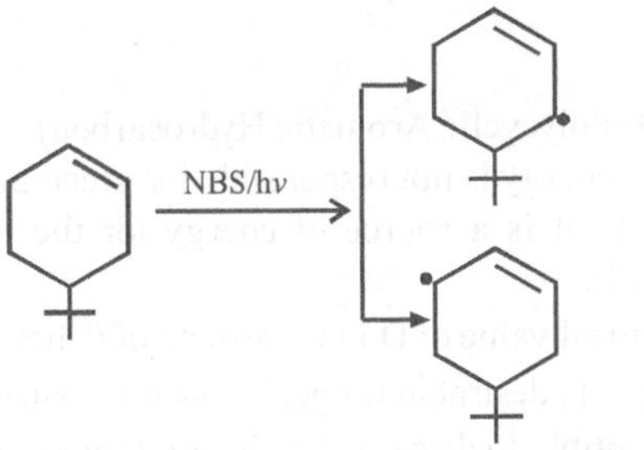

NBS/hν

More stable

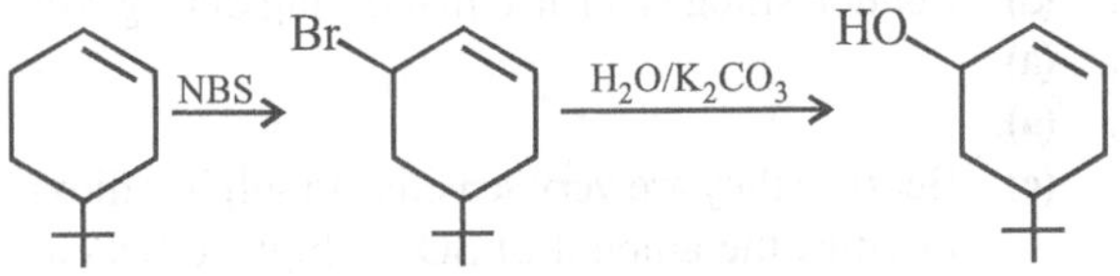

NBS

Br

H_2O/K_2CO_3

HO

40. (c) $CH_3C \equiv CCH_3 \xrightarrow{O_3} CH_3C - CCH_3$ (ozonide, O–O bridge)

$\xrightarrow{H_2O/Zn} CH_3\underset{\underset{O}{\|}}{C} - \underset{\underset{O}{\|}}{C}CH_3 + ZnO$

41. (c) Due to the maximum percentage of *s* character (50%), the *sp* hybridised orbitals of carbon atoms in ethyne molecules have highest electronegativity; hence, these attract the shared electron pair of the C-H bond of ethyne to a greater extent than that of the sp^2 hybridised orbitals of carbon in ethene and the sp^3 hybridised orbital of carbon in ethane. Thus in ethyne, hydrogen atoms can be liberated as protons more easily as compared to ethene and ethane.

42. (a) The heat of hydrogenation of an alkene depends upon its stability. Higher the stability, lower the heat of hydrogenation. Since CH_2=CH_2 has no substituent, it is the least stable alkene and hence has the highest heat of hydrogenation.

43. (c) In neopentane all the H atoms are same (1°).

$$CH_3 - \underset{\underset{CH_3}{|}}{\overset{\overset{CH_3}{|}}{C}} - CH_3$$

44. (a) This is due to acidity of the alkyne hydrogen

$$CH \equiv CH + Cu_2Cl_2 \longrightarrow \underset{\text{Copper acetylide (Red)}}{HC \equiv C^-Cu^+}$$

$AgNO_3$ ↓

$$HC \equiv \overset{\ominus}{C}Ag^+$$

The above reactions forms basis of test to distinguish between terminal and non-terminal alkynes, since non-terminal alkynes ($R - C \equiv C - R'$) do not react with these metal salts.

45. (c) $CH_3CH_2Br \xrightarrow{C_2H_5O^-Na^+} CH_3\overset{\oplus}{C}H_2 + C_2H_5\overset{\ominus}{O}$

Ethoxide ion is a strong base which abstracts proton from carbocation to form alkene.

$$\underset{\underset{H}{|}}{CH_2} - \overset{\oplus}{C}H_2 + C_2H_5\overset{\ominus}{O} \longrightarrow CH_2 = CH_2 + C_2H_5OH$$

Thus, there is a loss of hydrogen and halogen both leading to dehydrohalogenation.

Speed Test-42

1. (b) CO is a primary pollutant.
2. (d) Aerosols use CFC and flying jets release NO. Both causes depletion of ozone layer.
3. (c) CO is converted into CO_2 by microorganism present in soil.
4. (b) Algae
5. (a)
6. (a)
7. (c) For statement (iii), Stratosphere lies above troposphere between 10 and 50 km above sea level cloud formation takes place in troposphere.
For statement (iv), Troposphere is a turbulent, dusty zone containing air, much water vapour and clouds.
For statement (v), Stratosphere contains dinitrogen, dioxygen, ozone and little water vapour.
8. (b) Green chemistry may be defined as the programme of developing new chemical products and chemical processes or making improvements in the already existing compounds and processes so as to make less harmful to human health and environment. This means the same as to reduce the use and production of hazardous chemicals.
9. (c) Chemical pollutants in photochemical smog are nitrogen oxides (NO and NO_2), volatile organic compounds, ozone (O_3) and peroxyacetyl nitrate.
10. (a) PSCs react with chlorine nitrate and HCl to give HOCl and Cl_2.
11. (b)
12. (d) For statement (iii), Methemoglobinemia (blue baby syndrome) is caused due to excess of nitrate in drinking water.
For statement (iv), Excessive sulphate (> 500 ppm) in drinking water causes laxative effect, otherwise at moderate levels it is harmless.
13. (a) Methyl isocyanate, $CH_3-N=C=O$
14. (d) Minamata is caused by Hg poisoning.
15. (a) Eutrophication causes reduction in D.O
16. (d) $3CH_4 + 2O_3 \xrightarrow{\text{Polluted air}}$

$$\underset{\text{Formaldehyde}}{3CH_2=O} + \underset{\text{Acrolein}}{CH_2=CH-CHO} +$$

$$CH_3-\underset{\underset{O}{||}}{C}OONO_2$$

Peroxyacetyl nitrate (PAN)
17. (b) Replacement of earlier used tetra chloroethene as solvent for dry cleaning by liquid CO_2 results in less harm to ground water.
18. (a) Oil slick in sea water decreases D.O value.
19. (a) The average residence time of NO is 4 days.
20. (a) PAH (Polycyclic Aromatic Hydrocarbon)
21. (c) Solar energy is not responsible for green house effect instead it is a source of energy for the plants and animals.
22. (b) The ideal value of D.O for growth of fishes is 8 mg/ℓ. 7mg /ℓ is desirable range, below this value fishes get susceptible to disease. A value of 2 mg/ℓ or below is lethal for fishes.
23. (b) Surface water contains salts + organic matter.
24. (d) London smog is formed in morning during winter.
25. (a)
26. (a)
27. (c) Because they are very sensitive to sulphur dioxide and in cities the amount of SO_2 is high so lichen do not grow in cities.
28. (c) Freons and chlorofluorocarbon find their way to stratosphere through without being destroyed in the troposphere due to their low reactivity. In the stratosphere the Cl and Br atoms are liberated from the parent compounds by the action of ultraviolet light e.g.

$$CF_2Cl_2 + h\nu \longrightarrow CF_2Cl + Cl$$

$$CFCl_3 + h\nu \longrightarrow CFCl_2 + Cl$$

The Cl atoms can destroy ozone molecules through a variety of catalytic cycles.
29. (b) When SO_2 pollution in air is much higher. Sometimes, SO_2 mixes in the air with small particles of metals near the factories and gets oxidised into sulphur trioxide SO_3. These gases are harmful and they react with water to form sulphuric acid (H_2SO_4) or sulphurous acid (H_2SO_3) and come down to earth with rain water, it is called acid rain or acid precipitation.
30. (c) Above 2 ppm concentration of F^- in drinking water cause brown mottling of teeth.
31. (b)
32. (c) The ozone layer, existing between 20 to 35 km above the earth's surface, shield the earth from the harmful U. V. radiations from the sun.
Depletion of ozone is caused by oxides of nitrogen

$$N_2O + h\upsilon \longrightarrow \underset{\text{reactive nitric oxide}}{NO} + N$$

$$NO + O_3 \longrightarrow NO_2 + O_2$$

$$O_3 + h\upsilon \longrightarrow O_2 + O$$

$$NO_2 + O \longrightarrow NO + O_2$$

$$2O_3 + h\upsilon \longrightarrow 3O_2 \text{ (Net reaction)}$$

The presence of oxides of nitrogen increase the decomposition of O_3.

33. (a) BOD is connected with microbes and organic matter
34. (d) The oxidised hydrocarbons and ozone in presence of humidity cause photochemical smong.
Hydrocarbons + O_2, NO_2, NO, O, O_3, Peroxides, formaldehyde, peroxyacetyl-nitrate (PAN), acrodein etc.
Hence chlorofluorocarbons are not common component of photochemical smog.
35. (c) H_2, He and ionic oxygen are present in exosphere.
36. (b) In presence of U.V. rays O_2 is converted into O_3.
37. (c) CO and oxides of nitrogen are poisonous gases present in automobile exhaust gases.
38. (a) Dust
39. (c) Troposphere contains water vapour.
40. (d) Fly ash.
41. (d) Carboxyhaemoglobin is 300 times more stable than oxyhaemoglobin.
42. (a) Normal rain water has pH 5.6. Thunderstorm results in the formation of NO and HNO_3 which lowers the pH.
43. (c) Usually catalytic converters are used in the automobiles, which prevent the release of nitrogen oxide and hydrocarbons to the atmosphere. Certain plants e.g., *Pinus*, *Juniparus*, *Quercus*, *Pyrus* and *Vitis* can metabolise nitrogen oxide and therefore, their plantation could help in this matter.
44. (a) London smog is reducing in nature.
45. (d) Depletion of ozone layer causes skin cancer.

Speed Test-43

1. (c)
2. (b) n-Type, since electron is set free.
3. (a)

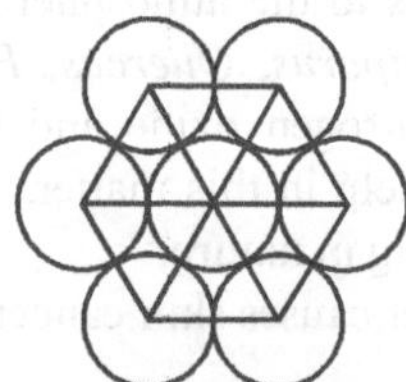

Let radius of the sphere = r

Area occupied by sphere in hexagonal close packing

$$\pi r^2 + 6\times\left(\frac{1}{6}\times\pi r^2\right) = 2\pi r^2$$

$$\text{Area of hexagonal } = 6\times\left[\frac{\sqrt{3}}{4}\times(2r)^2\right]$$

$$= 6\times\frac{\sqrt{3}}{4}\times 4r^2$$

$$= 6\sqrt{3}\times r^2$$

$$\% \text{ occupied by } = \frac{2\pi r^2}{6\times\sqrt{3}\times r^2}\times 100$$

$$= \frac{2\times 3.14}{6\times\sqrt{3}}\times 100 = 60.43\%$$

4. (c) As per formula,

$$\text{radius ratio } = \frac{\text{radius of cation}}{\text{radius of anion}}$$

$$= \frac{94}{146} = 0.643$$

Since the value is between 0.414 – 0.732 hence the coordination no. will be 6 and geometry will be octahedral.

5. (c) As CsCl is body-centred, $d = \sqrt{3}a/2$.
6. (b) It is the property of liquid crystal.
7. (a) $\frac{r+}{r-}$ ratio is $\frac{60}{136} = 0.441$, Hence LiF has NaCl structure with C.N. = 6.
8. (b) Molecular solid is the best description of water in the solid phase. For example ice is hydrogen bonded molecular solid.
9. (c) The hcp arrangement of atoms occupies 74% of the available space and thus has 26% vacant space.
10. (c) The p.f. for body centred cube = 0.68
11. (d) When insulators (non metal atoms) interact to form a solid, their atomic orbitals mix to form two bunch of orbitals, separated by a large band gap. Electrons cannot therefore be promoted to an empty level, where they could move freely.
12. (a) Covalent solids as in case of diamond.
13. (c)
14. (d) For octahedral $r^+/r^- = 0.414 - 0.732$.
15. (c) AgBr exhibits Frenkel defect.
16. (b) $\rho = \frac{zM}{N_A V}$

$$z = \frac{\rho N_A V}{M} = \frac{8.92\times 6.02\times 10^{23}\times(362)^3\times 10^{-30}}{63.55}$$

$$= 4$$

$\therefore$ It has fcc unit cell

17. (a) MnO_2.
18. (c) Amorphous silicon is used as best photovoltaic material available for conversion of sunlight into electricity.
19. (d)
20. (c) $\frac{d_1}{d_2} = \frac{(a_2)^3}{(a_1)^3}\times\frac{z_1}{z_2} = \left(\frac{3}{3.5}\right)^3\times\frac{4}{2} = 1.26$
21. (c) Glass is amorphous solid.
22. (d) $n\lambda = 2d\sin\theta$;

$$2\times 1Å = 2\times d\sin 60 \Rightarrow d = 1.15Å \because \left(\sin 60 = \frac{\sqrt{3}}{2}\right)$$

23. (b)
24. (c) Solid CH_4 is a molecular solid. In this, the constituent molecules are held together by van der Waal's forces.
25. (d) When electrons are trapped in anion vacancies, these are called F-centre.

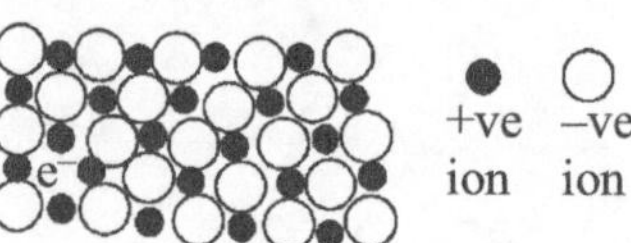

F- centre in crystal

26. (b) Density is given by

$$d = \frac{z\times M}{N_A a^3}\text{; where z = number of formula units}$$

present in unit cell, which is 4 for fcc

a = edge length of unit cell. M = Molecular mass

$$2.72=\frac{4\times M}{6.02\times10^{23}\times\left(404\times10^{-10}\right)^3}$$

$(\because\ 1\text{pm}=10^{-10}\text{cm})$

$$M=\frac{2.72\times6.02\times(404)^3}{4\times10^7}=26.99$$

$=27\text{ g mol}^{-1}$

27. **(a)** It is due to movement of energised electrons (KE $\propto$ T).

28. **(c)** $\frac{M^+}{X^-}$ is highest in CsF

$\therefore$ correct choice : (c)

29. **(d)** The electrical resistance of metals depends upon temperature. Electrical resistance decreases with decrease in temperature and becomes zero near the absolute temperature. Material in this state is said to possess super conductivity.

30. **(c)**

31. **(d)** Number of formulas in cube shaped crystals

$=\frac{1.0}{58.5}\times6.02\times10^{23}$ since in NaCl type of structure

4 formula units form 'a' cell

$\therefore$ units cells $=\frac{1.0\times6.02\times10^{23}}{58.5\times4}=2.57\times10^{21}$ unit cells.

32. **(b)** CsCl has a bcc structure ions touching along body diagonal.

33. **(c)** Rhenium oxide ReO_3 is like metallic copper in conductivity.

34. **(d)**

35. **(b)** Among the given crystals, only silicon exists as a covalent solid. It has diamond like structure.

36. **(d)** The addition of one Sr^{2+} replaces $2Na^+$ and one cationic vacancy is created.

No. of cationic vacancy $=2\times10^{-3}$ mole % of NaCl

$=\frac{2\times10^{-3}}{100}\text{mol}^{-1}$ of NaCl

$=2\times10^{-5}\times6.02\times10^{23}\text{ mol}^{-1}$

$=12.04\times10^{18}\text{ mol}^{-1}$ of NaCl

37. **(d)** In bcc - points are at corners and one in the centre of the unit cell.

Number of atoms per unit cell $=8\times\frac{1}{8}+1=2$.

In fcc - points are at the corners and also centre of the six faces of each cell.

Number of atoms per unit cell $=8\times\frac{1}{8}+6\times\frac{1}{2}=4$.

38. **(b)** For fcc,

$$r=\frac{\sqrt{2}a}{4}=\frac{a}{2\sqrt{2}}=0.3535a$$

given $a=361$ pm

$r=0.3535\times361$

$=128$ pm

39. **(a)**

40. **(a)** Diamond is like ZnS. In diamond cubic unit cell, there are eight corner atoms, six face centered atoms and four more atoms inside the structure.

Number of atoms present in a diamond cubic cell

$=8\times\frac{1}{8}+6\times\frac{1}{2}+4=8$

(corners) (face centered) (inside body)

41. **(b)** Packing fraction is defined as the ratio of the volume of the unit cell that is occupied by the spheres to the total volume of the unit cell.

P.F. for ccp and bcc are 0.74 and 0.68 respectively.

So, the free space in ccp and bcc are 26% and 32% respectively.

42. **(d)** For an Fcc crystal

$$r_{cation}+r_{anion}=\frac{\text{edge length}}{2}$$

$$110+r_{anion}=\frac{508}{2}$$

$r_{anion}=254-110=144$ pm

43. **(b)** CsI_3 dissociates as $CsI_3\rightarrow Cs^++I_3^-$

44. **(b)**

45. **(a)** For bcc lattice body diagonal $=a\sqrt{3}$.

The distance between the two oppositely charged ions

$=\frac{a}{2}\sqrt{3}$

$=\frac{387\times1.732}{2}=335\text{pm}$

Speed Test-44

1. (d) Molarity (M) $= \dfrac{\text{wt} \times 1000}{\text{mol. wt.} \times \text{vol (ml)}}$

$2 = \dfrac{\text{wt.}}{63} \times \dfrac{1000}{250}$

$\text{wt.} = \dfrac{63}{2}$ gm

wt. of 70% acid $= \dfrac{100}{70} \times 31.5 = 45$ gm

2. (b) $p_s = X_A(p_A^o - p_B^o) + p_B^o;$

$p_s = p_A^o \times x_A - p_B^o \times x_A + p_B^o;$

$p_s = p_A^o \times x_A - p_B^o(1 - x_B) + p_B^o$

$\therefore p_s = p_A^o \times x_A + p_B^o \times x_B.$

This is condition for ideal solution.

3. (c) $\Delta T_b = \dfrac{K_b \times w \times 1000}{M \times W};$

$\therefore K_b = \dfrac{\Delta T_b \times 100 \times 100}{10 \times 1000} = \Delta T_b$

4. (d) For $K_4[Fe(CN)_6]$, $i = 5$ hence lowest freezing point.

5. (b) $P_{total} = \overset{o}{P_A} X_A + \overset{o}{P_B} X_B$

$550 = \overset{o}{P_A} \times \dfrac{1}{4} + \overset{o}{P_B} \times \dfrac{3}{4}$

$\overset{o}{P_A} + 3\overset{o}{P_B} = 550 \times 4$ ...(i)

In second case

$P_{total} = \overset{o}{P_A} \times \dfrac{1}{5} + \overset{o}{P_B} \times \dfrac{4}{5}$

$\overset{o}{P_A} + 4\overset{o}{P_B} = 560 \times 5$ ...(ii)

Subtract (i) from (ii)

$\therefore \overset{o}{P_B} = 560 \times 5 - 550 \times 4 = 600$

$\because \overset{o}{P_A} = 400$

6. (b) $M = \dfrac{6.02 \times 10^{20} \times 1000}{6.02 \times 10^{23} \times 100} = 0.01M$

7. (a) $N_1V_1 = N_2V_2$ (H_3PO_3 is dibasic $\therefore M = 2N$)

$20 \times 0.2 = 0.1 \times V$

$\therefore V = 40$ ml

8. (c) There is no change in vapour pressure.

9. (a) In case of osmosis the flow of the solvent, is from lower concentration to higher concentration.

10. (d) According to Henry's law,

$m = k \times p$

given $K_H = 1.4 \times 10^{-3}$

$p_{O_2} = 0.5$ or

$p_{O_2} = K_H \times x_{O_2}$

$\therefore x_{O_2} = \dfrac{0.5}{1.4 \times 10^{-3}}$

No. of moles; $n = \dfrac{m}{M}$

$0.7 \times 10^{-4} = \dfrac{m}{32}$

$m = 22.4 \times 10^{-4}$ g $= 2.24$ mg

11. (b) A mixture of benzene and methanol show positive deviation from Raoult's law

12. (c) Number of moles of urea $= \dfrac{120}{60} = 2$

Total mass of solution $= 1000 + 120 = 1120$ g

Total volume of solution (in L) $= \dfrac{\text{Mass}}{\text{Density}}$

$= \dfrac{1120}{1.15 \times 10^3} = \dfrac{112}{115}$ L

Molarity of the solution $= \dfrac{\text{Number of moles}}{\text{Volume of solution in litre}}$

$= \dfrac{2 \times 115}{112} = 2.05 \text{ mol L}^{-1}$

13. (b) $P_{total} = p_A^o \times x_A + p_B^o \times x_B$

$= 80.0 \times 0.4 + 120.0 \times 0.6 = 104$ mm Hg

The observed P_{total} is 100 mm Hg which is less than 104 mm Hg. Hence the solution shows negative deviation.

14. (d) According to given information

$p_X = 80$ Torr

$p_Y = 60$ Torr

$n_X = 3$ moles

$n_Y = 2$ moles

mole fraction of X$(x_X) = \dfrac{n_X}{n_X + n_Y} = \dfrac{3}{3+2} = \dfrac{3}{5}$

mole fraction of Y$(x_Y) = \dfrac{n_Y}{n_X + n_Y} = \dfrac{2}{3+2} = \dfrac{2}{5}$

Total Pressure, $P = p_X x_X + p_Y x_Y$

$= \dfrac{3}{5} \times 80 + \dfrac{2}{5} \times 60 = 48 + 24 = 72$ Torr.

15. (c)

16. (b) For isotonic solutions

$\pi_1 = \pi_2$

$C_1 = C_2$

$$\frac{5/342}{0.1} = \frac{1/M}{0.1}$$

$$\frac{5}{342} = \frac{1}{M}$$

$$\Rightarrow M = \frac{342}{5} = 68.4 \text{ gm/mol}$$

17. (b) $\Delta T_f = 0.3°C$

$$\Delta T_f = 0.3°C = \frac{K_f \times W_B \times 1000}{M_B \times W_A}$$

$$= \frac{1.86 \times W_B \times 1000}{62 \times 5000}$$

$\therefore W_B = 50$ g

The amount used should be more than 50 g.

18. (b) As $\Delta T_f = K_f \, m$

$\Delta T_b = K_b . m$

Hence, we have $m = \frac{\Delta T_f}{K_f} = \frac{\Delta T_b}{K_b}$

or $\Delta T_f = \Delta T_b \frac{K_f}{K_b}$

$\Rightarrow [\Delta T_b = 100.18 - 100 = 0.18°C]$

$$= 0.18 \times \frac{1.86}{0.512} = 0.654°C$$

As the Freezing Point of pure water is 0°C,

$\Delta T_f = 0 - T_f$

$0.654 = 0 - T_f$

$\therefore T_f = -0.654$

Thus the freezing point of solution will be – 0.654°C.

19. (c) Molar mass of $CHCl_3$ = 119.5 g/mol.

Molar mass of CH_2Cl_2 = 85 g/mol.

Moles of $CHCl_3 = \frac{11.95}{119.5} = 0.1$ mol.

Moles of $CH_2Cl_2 = \frac{8.5}{85} = 0.1$ mol.

Mole fraction of $CHCl_3 = \frac{0.1}{0.2} = 0.5$ mol.

Mole fraction of $CH_2Cl_2 = \frac{0.1}{0.2} = 0.5$ mol.

(Given -

Vapour pressure of $CHCl_3$ = 200 mm Hg = 0.263 atm.

Vapour pressure of CH_2Cl_2 = 415 mm Hg = 0.546 atm.)

(1 atm = 760 mm Hg)

$\therefore P_{\text{(above solution)}}$

= Mole fraction of $CHCl_3$ × (Vapour pressure of $CHCl_3$) + Mole fraction of CH_2Cl_2 × (Vapour pressure of CH_2Cl_2)

$= 0.5 \times 0.263 + 0.5 \times 0.546 = 0.4045$

Mole fraction of $CHCl_3$ in vapour form

$$= \frac{0.1315}{0.4045} = 0.325.$$

20. (c)

	$Na_2SO_4 \longrightarrow$	$2Na^+$ +	SO_4^{2-}
Mol. before dissociation	1	0	0
Mol. after dissociation	$1-\alpha$	2α	1α

$i = 1 - \alpha + 2\alpha + \alpha = 1 + 2\alpha$

21. (c) $M_B = \frac{\Delta T_b \times W_B \times 1000}{K_b \times W_A}$ is wrong. The correct form is $M_B = \frac{K_b \times W_B \times 1000}{\Delta T_b \times W_A}$

22. (c)

23. (b)

24. (d) According to Henry's law the mass of a gas dissolved per unit volume of solvent is proportional to the pressure of the gas at constant temperature m = K p i.e. as the solubility increases, value of Henry's law constant decreases. Since CO_2 is most soluble in water among the given set of gases. Therefore CO_2 has the lowest value of Henry's law constant.

25. (b) For this solution intermolecular interactions between *n*-heptane and ethanol are weaker than *n*-heptane-*n*-heptane & ethanol-ethanol interactions hence the solution of *n*-heptane and ethanol is non-ideal and shows positive deviation from Raoult's law.

26. (a) $K_4[Fe(CN)_6]$ and $Al_2(SO_4)_3$ both dissociates to give 5 ions or $i = 5$

$K_4[Fe(CN)_6] \rightleftharpoons 4K^+ + [Fe(CN)_6]^{4-}$

and $Al_2(SO_4)_3 \rightleftharpoons 2Al^{3+} + 3SO_4^{--}$

27. (b) According to Raoult's law "The partial pressure of a volatile component of a solution is directly proportional to its mole fraction in solution at any temperature".

$p = P^\circ_x$

where, p = Partial pressure of component

P° = Vapour pressure of component in pure form

x = mole fraction of component in solution.

28. (d) To increase the solubility of CO_2 in soft drinks and soda water, the bottle is sealed under high pressure.

29. (d) Gaseous densities of ethanol and dimethyl ether would be same at same temperature and pressure. The heat of vaporisation, V.P. and b.pt. will differ due to H - bonding in ethanol.

30. (c) Molarity (experimental)

$$= \frac{\Delta T_f}{K_f} = \frac{3.82}{1.86} = 2.054 \text{ mol/1000 g solvent}$$

$$\text{Molarity (theartical)} = \frac{\text{mole of solute}}{\text{wt. of solventing(g)}} \times 1000$$

$$= \frac{5 \text{ g}/142 \text{ g/mole}}{x} \times 1000$$

	$Na_2SO_4 \longrightarrow$	$2Na^+$ +	SO_4^{2-}
Moles before dissociation	1	0	0
Moles after dissociation	$1-x$	$2x$	x

$$\text{Von't Hoff Factor } (i) = \frac{\text{Moles after dissociation}}{\text{Moles before dissociation}}$$

$$= \frac{(1-x)+2x+x}{1}$$

Na_2SO_4 is ionised 81.5% means $x = 0.815$

$$= \frac{(1-0.815)+2\times0.815+0.815}{1}$$

$= 2.63.$

$$i = \frac{\text{Observed molarity}}{\text{Calculated molarity}}$$

$$\Rightarrow 2.63 = \frac{2.054}{\frac{0.0352}{x}\times1000} = 45.07 \text{ g.}$$

31. **(d)** Using relation,

$$\frac{p^\circ - p_s}{p_s} = \frac{w_2 M_1}{w_1 M_2}$$

where w_1, M_1 = mass in g and mol. mass of solvent
w_2, M_2 = mass in g and mol. mass of solute
Let $M_2 = x$
$p^\circ = 185$ torr
$p_s = 183$ torr

$$\frac{185-183}{183} = \frac{1.2\times58}{100x} \text{ (Mol. mass of acetone} = 58)$$

$x = 64$

$\therefore$ Molar mass of substance = 64

32. **(b)** $[\Delta H_{mix} < 0]$

33. **(c)** Vant Hoff factor $i = 4$ in case of $(NH_4)_3PO_4$,

$$(NH_4)_3PO_4 \rightleftharpoons 3\overset{+}{N}H_4 + PO_4^{3-}$$

34. **(d)** At 1 atmospheric pressure the boiling point of mixture is 80°C.
At boiling point the vapour pressure of mixture, $P_T = 1$ atmosphere = 760 mm Hg.
Using the relation,

$P_T = P_A^o X_A + P_B^o X_B$, we get

$P_T = 520X_A + 1000(1 - X_A)$

$\{\because P_A^o = 520 \text{mm Hg},$

$P_B^o = 1000 \text{ mm Hg}, X_A + X_B = 1\}$

or $760 = 520X_A + 1000 - 1000X_A$ or $480X_A = 240$

or $X_A = \frac{240}{480} = \frac{1}{2}$ or 50 mol. percent

i.e., The correct answer is (d)

35. **(a)** Given $\pi_{ob} = 10.8$ atm
$\pi_{nor} = CST = 0.10 \times 0.0821 \times 298 = 2.446$
now experimental value of (i)

$$= \frac{\text{Observed osmotic pressure}}{\text{Normal osmotic pressure}} = \frac{10.8}{2.446} = 4.42$$

36. **(d)** Glucose is non electrolyte hence depression in freezing point will be minimum, hence freezing point will be highest.

37. **(b)** Solution always boil at higher temperature
$T_1 - T_2 = \Delta T_b$

38. **(d)** $\Delta T_f = K_f \times m \times i$

$$i = \frac{\Delta T_f}{K_f \times m} = \frac{1.91}{1.86\times1} = 1.02$$

For $HI \rightleftharpoons H^+ + I^-$
$(1-\alpha) \quad \alpha \quad \alpha$
$1 - \alpha + \alpha + \alpha = i = 1.027$
$1 + \alpha = 1.02$
$\alpha = 0.02$ or 2.7%

39. **(b)** $\text{Mol.wt.} = \frac{k_f \times w \times 1000}{\Delta T_f \times W}$

$$= \frac{1.86\times0.85\times1000}{0.23\times125} \approx 55 \text{ gm}$$

Where
$w = 0.85$g
$W = 125$ g
$\Delta T_f = 0°C - (-23°C) = 23°C$

$$\text{Now, } i = \frac{M_{normal}}{M_{observed}} = \frac{136.3}{55} = 2.47$$

$$\underset{1-\alpha}{ZnCl_2} \rightleftharpoons \underset{\alpha}{Zn^{++}} + \underset{2\alpha}{2Cl^-}$$

Van't Hoff factor (i)

$$= \frac{1-\alpha_\eta + \alpha_\eta + 2\alpha_\eta}{1} = 2.47$$

$\therefore \quad \alpha\eta = 0.735 = 73.5\%$

40. **(a)** Liquid solvent and solid solvent are in equilibrium.

41. **(b)** Benzoic acid forms a dimer in benzene.

42. **(d)** $\Delta T_f = K_f m$
where m = molality

$$273 - 268 = 1.86 \times \frac{w}{M \times v}$$

$$5 = 1.86 \times \frac{w}{32\times10}$$

$$w = \frac{5\times32\times10}{1.86}$$

$= 860.2 \approx 868.06$ g

43. **(d)** According to Henry law

$$\frac{P_1}{P_2} = \frac{S_1}{S_2}$$

$$\frac{500}{750} = \frac{0.01}{S_2}$$

$$\therefore S_2 = \frac{750\times0.01}{500} = 0.015 \text{ g/L}$$

44. **(a)**

45. **(d)** Azeotrope of HCl + H_2O contains 20.2% HCl.

Speed Test-45

1. **(a)** The given order of reduction potentials (or tendencies) is Z > Y > X. A spontaneous reaction will have the following characteristics
Z reduced and Y oxidised
Z reduced and X oxidised
Y reduced and X oxidised
Hence, Y will oxidise X and not Z.

2. **(c)** From the given data we find Fe^{3+} is strongest oxidising agent. More the positive value of E°, more is the tendency to get oxidized. Thus correct option is (c).

3. **(b)** $R = 100\,\Omega,\ \kappa = \frac{1}{R}\left(\frac{l}{A}\right)$,

$\frac{l}{A}$ (cell constant) $= 1.29 \times 100\ m^{-1}$
Given, $R = 520\,\Omega, C = 0.2\,M$,
μ (molar conductivity) = ?

$\mu = \kappa \times V$ (κ can be calculated as $\kappa = \frac{1}{R}\left(\frac{l}{A}\right)$

now cell constant is known.)
Hence,

$$\mu = \frac{1}{520} \times 129 \times \frac{1000}{0.2} \times 10^{-6}\ m^3$$

$$= 12.4 \times 10^{-4}\ S\ m^2\ mol^{-1}$$

4. **(b)** For, $M^+ + X^- \longrightarrow M + X$, $E^\circ_{cell} = 0.44 - 0.33 = 0.11V$ is positive, hence reaction is spontaneous.

5. **(b)** RHS : $2H^+ + 2e^- \rightleftharpoons H_2(P_2)$
LHS : $H_2(P_1) \rightleftharpoons 2H^+ + 2e^-$
overall reaction : $H_2(P_1) \rightleftharpoons H_2(P_2)$

$$E = E^\circ - \frac{RT}{nF}\ln\frac{P_2}{P_1} = 0 - \frac{RT}{nF}\ln\frac{P_2}{P_1} = \frac{RT}{nF}\ln\frac{P_1}{P_2}$$

6. **(c)** $\Delta G^\circ = -nFE^\circ;\ E^\circ = \frac{-\Delta G^\circ}{nF}$;

$$E^\circ = \frac{-(-50.61J)}{2 \times 96500 \times 10^{-3}} = 0.26\ V$$

7. **(b)** $Ohm^{-1}\ cm^2\ (g\ eq)^{-1}$

8. **(a)** In case of equivalent conductance of strong electrolyte there is little increase with dilution.

9. **(d)** Here $n = 4$, and $[H^+] = 10^{-3}$ (as pH = 3)
Applying Nernst equation

$$E = E^\circ - \frac{0.059}{n}\log\frac{[Fe^{2+}]^2}{[H^+]^4(p_{O_2})}$$

$$= 1.67 - \frac{0.059}{4}\log\frac{(10^{-3})^2}{(10^{-3})^4 \times 0.1}$$

$$= 1.67 - \frac{0.059}{4}\log 10^7 = 1.67 - 0.103 = 1.567\ V$$

10. **(d)** Cell constant = l/a
Unit $= m/m^2 = m^{-1}$.

11. **(d)** $\Lambda^\circ_{m(NH_4Cl)} = \Lambda^\circ_{m NH_4^+} + \Lambda^\circ_{m Cl^-}$

$$\Lambda^\circ_{m(NaOH)} = \Lambda^\circ_{m Na^+} + \Lambda^\circ_{m OH^-}$$

$$\Lambda^\circ_{m(NaCl)} = \Lambda^\circ_{m Na^+} + \Lambda^\circ_{m Cl^-}$$

$$\therefore\ \Lambda^\circ_{m(NH_4^+)} + \Lambda^\circ_{m(OH^-)}$$

$$= \Lambda^\circ_{m(NH_4^+)} + \Lambda^\circ_{m(Cl^-)} + \Lambda^\circ_{m(Na^+)}$$

$$+ \Lambda^\circ_{m(OH^-)} - \left[\Lambda^\circ_{m(Na^+)} + \Lambda^\circ_{m(Cl^-)}\right]$$

$$\Lambda^\circ_{m(NH_4OH)} = \Lambda^\circ_{m(NH_4Cl)} + \Lambda^\circ_{m(NaOH)} - \Lambda^\circ_{m(NaCl)}$$

12. **(d)**

$$Pb + SO_4^{2-} \longrightarrow PbSO_4 + 2e^-$$

$$PbO_2 + 4H^+ + SO_4^{2-} + 2e^- \longrightarrow PbSO_4 + 2H_2O$$

$$Pb + PbO_2 + 2H_2SO_4 \longrightarrow 2PbSO_4 + 2H_2O$$

The reaction indicates that 2 moles of H_2SO_4 corresponds to 2 × 96500 C and 2 moles $H_2SO_4 \equiv 4$ equiv. of H_2SO_4.

2 × 96500 C consumed 4 equiv. of H_2SO_4

and $100 \times 10^{-3} \times 9.65 \times 10^5$ C consumed

$$= \frac{4 \times 100 \times 10^{-3} \times 9.65 \times 10^5}{2 \times 96500} = 2 \text{ equiv. } H_2SO_4$$

$$\therefore \text{ Decrease in normality} = \frac{2}{5} = 0.40$$

13. **(b)** For $Zn^{2+} \rightarrow Zn$

$$E_{Zn^{2+}/Zn} = E^\circ_{Zn^{2+}/Zn} - \frac{2.303RT}{nF}\log\frac{[Zn]}{[Zn^{2+}]}$$

$$= -0.76 - \frac{0.06}{2}\log\frac{1}{[0.1]} = -0.76 - 0.03$$

$$E_{Zn^{2+}/Zn} = -0.79V$$

14. (c) Reduction half reaction :

$$Cr_2O_7^{2-} + 6e^- + 14H^+ \longrightarrow 2Cr^{3+} + 7H_2O$$

Oxidation half reaction :

$$Cr \longrightarrow Cr^{3+} + 3e^-$$

Overall reaction :

$$Cr_2O_7^{2-} + Cr + 14H^+ + 3e^- \longrightarrow 3Cr^{3+} + 7H_2O$$

3F of electricity = 3 moles of Cr^{3+}

1F of electricity = $\frac{3}{3}$ moles of Cr^{3+}

15. (a) $2Cr^{3+} + 7H_2O \rightarrow Cr_2O_7^{2-} + 14H^+$

O.S. of Cr changes from +3 to +6 by loss of electrons. At anode oxidation takes place.

16. (b) In $H_2 - O_2$ fuel cell, the combustion of H_2 occurs to create potential difference between the two electrodes.

17. (b) $E^o_{cell} = \frac{0.059}{2} \log K_C$ or $\frac{1.10 \times 2}{0.059} = \log K_C$

$\therefore K_C = 1.9 \times 10^{37}$

18. (a) The value of $E^o_{M^{2+}/M}$ for given metal ions are

$E^o_{Mn^{2+}/Mn} = -1.18$ V,

$E^o_{Cr^{2+}/Cr} = -0.9$ V,

$E^o_{Fe^{2+}/Fe} = -0.44$ V and $E^o_{Co^{2+}/Co} = -0.28$ V.

The correct order of $E^o_{M^{2+}/M}$ values without considering negative sign would be

$$Mn^{2+} > Cr^{2+} > Fe^{2+} > Co^{2+}.$$

19. (d) For spontaneous reaction ΔG should be negative. Equilibrium constant should be more than one ($\Delta G = -2.303\,RT \log K_c$, If $K_c = 1$ then $\Delta G = 0$; If $K_c < 1$ then $\Delta G = +ve$). Again $\Delta G = -nFE^o_{cell}$.

E^o_{cell} must be +ve to have ΔG –ve.

20. (d) Standard Gibbs free energy is given as $\Delta G^o = -nE^oF$

If $E^o_{cell} < 0$ i.e., – ve

$\Delta G^o > 0$

Further $\Delta G^o = -RT \ln K_{eq}$

$\therefore \Delta G^o > 0$ and $K_{eq} < 0$

21. (c) Conductivity of an electrolyte depends on the mobility of ions and concentration of ions. The motion of an ionic species in an electric field is retarded by the oppositely charged ions due to their interionic attraction. On dilution, concentration of electrolyte decreases and the retarding influence of oppositely charged ions decreases. Therefore mobility of ions increases.

22. (d) Higher the value of standard reduction potential, stronger is the oxidising agent, hence MnO_4^- is the strongest oxidising agent.

23. (c) As the value of reduction potential decreases the reducing power increases i.e.

C < B < D < A

(0.85). (0.6). (–0.76) (–1.2)

24. (b) Specific conductance decreases with dilution.

25. (a) $\Lambda^\infty_m = 57 + 73 = 130\ S cm^2 mol^{-1}$

26. (d) $E_{cell} = 0$; when cell is completely discharged.

$$E_{cell} = E^o_{cell} - \frac{0.059}{2} \log\left(\frac{[Zn^{2+}]}{[Cu^{2+}]}\right)$$

$$\text{or } 0 = 1.1 - \frac{0.059}{2} \log\left(\frac{[Zn^{2+}]}{[Cu^{2+}]}\right)$$

$$\log\left(\frac{[Zn^{2+}]}{[Cu^{2+}]}\right) = \frac{2 \times 1.1}{0.059} = 37.3$$

$$\therefore \left(\frac{[Zn^{2+}]}{[Cu^{2+}]}\right) = 10^{37.3}$$

27. (c) Reduction potential of Cu is more than H_2.

28. (d) Reducing character decreases down the series. Hence the correct order is

$$Al < Fe^{2+} < Br^-$$

29. (c) Writing the equation for pentane-oxygen fuel cell at respective electrodes and overall reaction, we get

At Anode:

$$\underset{\text{(pentane)}}{C_5H_{12}} + 10H_2O \rightarrow 5CO_2 + 32H^+ + 32e^-$$

At Cathode:

$$8O_2 + 32H^+ + 32e^- \rightarrow 16H_2O$$

$$\text{Overall}: C_5H_{12} + 8O_2 \rightarrow 5CO_2 + 6H_2O$$

Calculation of ΔG^o for the above reaction

$\Delta G^o = [5\times(-394.4) + 6\times(-237.2)] - [-8.2]$

$= -1972.0 - 1423.2 + 8.2 = -3387.0$ kJ

$= -3387000$ Joules.

From the equation we find n = 32

Using the relation, $\Delta G^o = -nFE^o_{cell}$ and substituting various values, we get

$-3387000 = -32 \times 96500 \times E^o_{cell}$ (F = 96500C)

$$\text{or } E^o_{cell} = \frac{3387000}{32 \times 96500}$$

$= \frac{3387000}{3088000}$ or $\frac{3387}{3088}$ V = 1.0968 V

Thus option (c) is correct answer.

30. (d) From the given representation of the cell, E_{cell} can be found as follows.

$$E_{cell} = \left(E^o_{Fe^{2+}/Fe} - E^o_{Cr^{3+}/Cr}\right) - \frac{0.059}{6}\log\frac{[Cr^{3+}]^2}{[Fe^{2+}]^3}$$

[Nernst -Equ.]

$$= -0.42 - (-0.72) - \frac{0.059}{6}\log\frac{(0.1)^2}{(0.01)^3}$$

$$= -0.42 + 0.72 - \frac{0.059}{6}\log\frac{0.1\times0.1}{0.01\times0.01\times0.01}$$

$$= 0.3 - \frac{0.059}{6}\log\frac{10^{-2}}{10^{-6}} = 0.3 - \frac{0.059}{6}\times 4$$

$= 0.30 - 0.0393 = 0.26$ V

Hence option (d) is correct answer.

31. (b) $H_2O \rightleftharpoons H^+ + OH^-$

$H^+ + e^- \longrightarrow \frac{1}{2}H_2$

$\therefore$ 0.5 mole of H_2 is liberated by 1 F = 96500 C

0.01 mole of H_2 will be liberated by

$= \frac{96500}{0.5}\times 0.01 \quad = 1930$ C

$Q = I \times t$

$$t = \frac{Q}{I} = \frac{1930\ C}{10\times10^{-3}\ A} = 19.3\times10^4 \text{ sec}$$

32. (d)

33. (b) Conductivity (X) = conductance (c) × cell constant

$\therefore$ Cell constant $= \frac{X}{Y}$

Conductivity of NaOH $= \frac{X}{Y}.Z$

$$\Delta m\,(NaOH) = \frac{X}{Y}.Z\times\frac{1000}{0.1} = \frac{XZ}{Y}10^4$$

34. (b) Total of 6 electrons are required to form 2 moles of Cr^{3+} therefore to form 1 mole of Cr^{3+} 3F of charge is required.

35. (a) When platinum electrodes are dipped in dilute solution H_2SO_4 than H_2 is evolved at cathode.

36. (a) Specific conductance = Conductance × Cell constant

$$k = \frac{1}{2.5\times10^3}\times1.15;$$

$$\Lambda_{eq} = \frac{1.15}{2.5\times10^3}\times\frac{1000}{0.1} = 4.6$$

37. (a) Thus difluoro acetic acid being strongest acid will furnish maximum number of ions showing highest electrical conductivity. The decreasing acidic strength of the carboxylic acides given is difluoro acetic acid > fluoro acetic acid > chloro acetic acid > acetic acid.

38. (a) No. of moles of silver $= \frac{9650}{96500} = \frac{1}{10}$ moles

$\therefore$ Mass of silver deposited $= \frac{1}{10}\times108 = 10.8$ g

39. (c) $H^+ + e^- \longrightarrow \frac{1}{2}H_2$

$$E = E^o - \frac{0.059}{1}\log\frac{[P(H_2)]^{1/2}}{[H^+]}$$

Now if $p_{H_2} = 2$ atm and $[H^+] = 1M$

then $E = 0 - \frac{0.059}{1}\log\frac{2^{1/2}}{1} = \frac{-0.059}{2}\log 2$

40. (a) 112 mL of H_2 at STP $= \frac{2\times112g}{22400}$

(Since 22400 mL at STP = M.wt)

Amount deposiled $= \frac{Eq.wt\times i\times t}{96500}$

$\therefore \frac{2\times112}{22400} = \frac{1\times965\times i}{96500};$

i = 1 amp

41. (d) $\frac{W_A}{E_A} = \frac{W_B}{E_B}; \ \frac{1.6}{8} = \frac{\text{Wt. of Ag}}{108}$

$\therefore$ Wt. of Ag = 21.6 g

42. (d) Correct matching for pair (iii) will be [G (conductance) – siemens or ohm^{-1}(S).]

43. (a) The charge carried by 1 mole of electrons is one faraday. Thus for a reaction

$M^{n+} + ne^- \longrightarrow M$

nF = 1 mole of M

$Al^{3+} + 3e^- \longrightarrow Al$
3F — 1 mole
1F — 1/3 mole

$Cu^{2+} + 2e^- \longrightarrow Cu$
2F — 1 mole
1F — 1/2 mole

$Na^+ + e^- \longrightarrow Na$
1F — 1 mole

The mole ratio of Al, Cu and Na deposited at the respective cathode is $\frac{1}{3}:\frac{1}{2}:1$ or 2 : 3 : 6.

44. (a) Reciprocal of resistance is conductance. We can add the conductance and not resistance.

Hence $\frac{1}{r} = \frac{1}{\rho} + \frac{1}{\rho} + ...$

45. (c) The correct relation is $\Delta G^\circ = -nFE^\circ$

Speed Test-46

1. (d) $k = \frac{2.303}{t}\log\frac{a}{a-x} = \frac{2.303}{24}\log\frac{1}{\frac{1}{8}} = \frac{2.303}{24}\log 8$

2. (b) Since doubling the concentration of B does not change half life, the reaction is of 1st order w.r.t. B.
Order of reaction with respect to $A = 1$ because rate of reaction doubles when concentration of A is doubled keeping concentration of B constant.
$\therefore$ Order of reaction = 1 + 1 = 2 and units of second order reaction are L mol^{-1} sec^{-1}.

3. (d) The molecularity of a reaction is the number of reactant molecules taking part in a single step of the reaction. Thus the reaction involving two different reactant can never be unimolecular.

4. (a) Let the rate law be $r = k[A]^x[B]^y$

Divide (3) by (1) $\frac{0.10}{0.10} = \frac{[0.024]^x[0.035]^y}{[0.012]^x[0.035]^y}$

$\therefore 1 = [2]^x, x = 0$

Divide (2) by (3) $\frac{0.80}{0.10} = \frac{[0.024]^x[0.070]^y}{[0.024]^x[0.035]^y}$

$\therefore 8 = (2)^y, y = 3$

Hence rate equation, $R = k[A]^0[B]^3 = k[B]^3$

5. (a) If we write rate of reaction in terms of concentration of NH_3 and H_2, then

Rate of reaction $= \frac{1}{2}\frac{d[NH_3]}{dt} = -\frac{1}{3}\frac{d[H_2]}{dt}$

So, $\frac{d[NH_3]}{dt} = -\frac{2}{3}\frac{d[H_2]}{dt}$

6. (a) As doubling the initial conc. doubles the rate of reaction, order = 1

7. (b) Rate law has to be determined experimentally as Cl_2 is raised to power $\frac{1}{2}$ in rate law whereas its stichiometric coefficient in balanced chemical equation is 1.

8. (a)

9. (c) $\frac{(t_{1/2})_1}{(t_{1/2})_2} = \left(\frac{a_2}{a_1}\right)^{n-1}$; $\frac{120}{240} = \left(\frac{4\times10^{-2}}{8\times10^{-2}}\right)^{n-1}$; $n = 2$

10. (b)

11. (b)

12. (c) Activation energy is lowered in presence of +ve catalyst.

13. (d) Overall order = sum of orders w.r.t each reactant.
Let the order be x and y for G and H respectively

Exp.No.	[G]mole $litre^{-1}$	[H]mole $litre^{-1}$	rate(mole $litre^{-}time^{-1}$)
1	a	b	r
2	$2a$	$2b$	$8r$
3	$2a$	b	$2r$

$\because$ For (1) and (3), the rate is doubled when conc. of G is doubled keeping that of H constant i.e., rate $\propto [G]$ $\therefore x = 1$

From (2) and (3), $y = 2$

$\therefore$ Overall order is 3.

14. (b) For a first order reaction

$k = \frac{2.303}{t}\log\frac{a}{a-x} = \frac{2.303}{40}\log\frac{0.1}{0.025}$

$= \frac{2.303}{40}\log 4 = \frac{2.303\times0.6020}{40}$

$= 3.47\times10^{-2}\ min^{-1}$

Rate $= k[A] = 3.47\times10^{-2}\times0.01$

$= 3.47\times10^{-4}$ M/min

15. (c) Third order

16. (c) For a first order reaction

$k = \frac{2.303}{t}\log_{10}\frac{a}{a-x}$

when $t = t_{½}$

$k = \frac{2.303}{t_{½}}\log_{10}\frac{a}{a-a/2}$

or $t_{½} = \frac{2.303}{k}\log_{10}2 = \frac{\ln 2}{k}$

17. (d) The integrated rate equations are different for the reactions of different reaction orders. We shall determine these equations only for zero and first order chemical reactions.

18. (b) $T_2 = T$(say), $T_1 = 25°C = 298K$,
$E_a = 104.4\ kJ\ mol^{-1} = 104.4\times10^3\ J\ mol^{-1}$
$k_1 = 3\times10^{-4}$, $k_2 = ?$,

$\log\frac{k_2}{k_1} = \frac{E_a}{2.303R}\left[\frac{1}{T_1} - \frac{1}{T_2}\right]$

$\log\frac{k_2}{3\times10^{-4}} = \frac{104.4\times10^3\ J\ mol^{-1}}{2.303\times(8.314\ J\ K^{-1}mol^{-1})}\left[\frac{1}{298} - \frac{1}{T}\right]$

As $T\to\infty, \frac{1}{T}\to 0$

$$\therefore \log\frac{k_2}{3\times10^{-4}}=\frac{104.4\times10^3\ \text{J mol}^{-1}}{2.303\times8.314\times298}$$

$$\log\frac{k_2}{3\times10^{-4}}=18.297, \frac{k_2}{3\times10^{-4}}=1.98\times10^{18}$$

$$k_2=(1.98\times10^{18})\times(3\times10^{-4})=6\times10^{14}\text{s}^{-1}$$

19. **(c)** Adsorption lowers the activation energy.

20. **(a)** For the change $2A+3B\rightarrow$ products

$$-\frac{1}{2}\frac{d[A]}{dt}=-\frac{1}{3}\frac{d[B]}{dt}, \frac{1}{2}r_1=\frac{1}{3}r_2;\quad 3r_1=2r_2$$

21. **(c)** The $t_{1/2}$ is 15 minutes. To fall the concentration from 0.1 to 0.025 we need two half lives i.e., 30 minutes.

22. **(b)** According to Arrhenius equation

$$\ln\frac{k_2}{k_1}=\frac{E_a}{R}\left(\frac{1}{T_1}-\frac{1}{T_2}\right)$$

$$=-\frac{E_a}{R}\left(\frac{1}{T_2}-\frac{1}{T_1}\right)$$

$$\ln\frac{k_1}{k_2}=-\frac{E_a}{R}\left(\frac{1}{T_1}-\frac{1}{T_2}\right)$$

23. **(c)** $t_{1/4}=\frac{2.303}{k}\log\frac{1}{3/4}=\frac{2.303}{k}\log\frac{4}{3}$

$$=\frac{2.303}{k}(\log 4-\log 3)=\frac{2.303}{k}(2\log 2-\log 3)$$

$$=\frac{2.303}{k}(2\times0.301-0.4771)=\frac{0.29}{k}$$

24. **(d)** For a zero order reaction,

$t_{1/2}\propto a_0$ (initial concentration or initial pressure)

$(t_{1/2})_1\propto P_1$

$(t_{1/2})_2\propto P_2$

$$\frac{(t_{1/2})_2}{(t_{1/2})_1}=\frac{P_2}{P_1}, \frac{(t_{1/2})_2}{45}=\frac{16}{4}$$

$$(t_{1/2})_2=\frac{16}{4}\times45=180\text{ min}$$

25. **(b)**

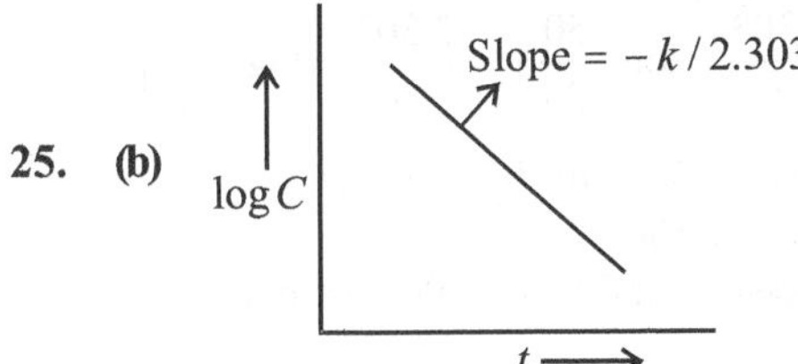

26. **(b)** Plot given is for zero order reaction.

27. **(c)** Since for every 10°C rise in temperature rate doubles for 50°C rise in temperature increase in reaction rate $=2^5=32$ times

28. **(a)** $k=\frac{2.303}{1386}\log\frac{100}{100-75}$ On solving we get . $k=10^{-3}$

29. **(a)**

30. **(a)** Presence of catalyst does not affect enthalpy change of reaction $\Delta H_R=E_f-E_b=180-200=-20$ kJ/mol

31. **(c)** Given $t_{1/2}=15$ minutes

Total time $(T)=1$ hr $=60$ min

From $T=n\times t_{1/2}$

$$n=\frac{60}{15}=4$$

Now from the formula $\frac{N}{N_0}=\left(\frac{1}{2}\right)^n$

$$=\left(\frac{1}{2}\right)^4=\frac{1}{16}$$

Where N_0 = initial amount

N = amount left after time t

hence the amount of substance left after 1 hour will be $\frac{1}{16}$

32. **(d)** $\text{Rate}_1=k[A]^n[B]^m$

$$\text{Rate}_2=k[2A]^n\left[\frac{1}{2}B\right]^m$$

$$\therefore \frac{\text{Rate}_2}{\text{Rate}_1}=\frac{k[2A]^n\left[\frac{1}{2}B\right]^m}{k[A]^n[B]^m}=(2)^n\left(\frac{1}{2}\right)^m$$

$$=2^n\cdot(2)^{-m}=2^{n-m}$$

33. **(a)** On adding eq. (i) and eq. (ii) we get

$$O_3(g)+O(g)\longrightarrow 2O_2(g)$$

Hence overall rate constant $=K_i\times K_{ii}$

$=5.2\times10^9\times2.6\times10^{10}\approx1.4\times10^{20}\text{ mol}^{-1}\text{ L s}^{-1}$

$$O_3(g)+Cl^\bullet(g)\longrightarrow O_2(g)+ClO^\bullet(g),\ K_i$$

$$ClO^\bullet(g)+O^\bullet(g)\longrightarrow O_2(g)+Cl^\bullet(g),\ K_{ii}$$

$$O_3(g)+O^\bullet(g)\longrightarrow 2O_2(g),\ K_{Rate}=K_i\times K_{ii}$$

34. **(b)** $k=Ae^{-E_a/RT}$ $\log k=\log A-\frac{E_a}{2.303R}\cdot\frac{1}{T}$

Plot of log k Vs. $\frac{1}{T}$

Straight line Slope $=\frac{-E_a}{2.303R}$

35. **(b)** $r=k[O_2][NO]^2$. When the volume is reduced to 1/2, the conc. will double

$\therefore$ New rate $=k[2O_2][2NO]^2=8k[O^2][NO]^2$

The new rate increases to eight times of its initial.

36. **(d)** From rate law

$$-\frac{1}{2}\frac{dSO_2}{dt} = -\frac{dO_2}{dt} = \frac{1}{2}\frac{dSO_3}{dt}$$

$$\therefore -\frac{dSO_2}{dt} = -2\times\frac{dO_2}{dt}$$

$= -2 \times 2.5 \times 10^{-4}$

$= -5 \times 10^{-4}\ \text{mol L}^{-1}\ \text{s}^{-1}$

37. **(c)** $k_1 = A_1 e^{-E_{a_1}/RT}$ ....(i)

$k_2 = A_2 e^{-E_{a_2}/RT}$ ....(ii)

On dividing eqn (i) from eqn. (ii)

$\frac{k_1}{k_2} = \frac{A_1}{A_2}(E_{a_2} - E_{a_1})/RT$ ....(iii)

Given $E_{a_2} = 2E_{a_1}$

On substituting this value in eqn. (iii)

$k_1 = k_2 A \times e^{E_{a_1}/RT}$

38. **(d)** Enthalpy of reaction $(\Delta H) = E_{a\,(f)} - E_{a\,(b)}$ for an endothermic reaction ΔH = +ve hence for ΔH to be positive

$E_{a\,(b)} < E_{a\,(f)}$

39. **(d)**

40. **(a)** $\ln\frac{K_1}{K_2} = \frac{E_a}{R}\left(\frac{1}{T_1}, -\frac{1}{T_2}\right)$

$$\ln 4 = \frac{E_a}{8.314}\left(\frac{310-300}{310\times300}\right)$$

$$2\ln 2 = \frac{E_a}{8.314}\left(\frac{310-300}{310\times300}\right)$$

$$E_a = \frac{0.693\times2\times8.314\times300\times310}{10} = 107.2\ \text{kJ/mol}$$

41. **(d)** Since the slow step is the rate determining step hence if we consider option (A) we find

Rate $= k[Cl_2][H_2S]$

Now if we consider option (B) we find

Rate $= k[Cl_2][HS^-]$ ...(i)

For equation,

$H_2S \rightleftharpoons H^+ + HS^-$

$$K = \frac{[H^+][HS^-]}{H_2S}$$

$$\text{or } [HS^-] = \frac{K[H_2S]}{H^+}$$

Substituting this value in equation (i) we find

$$\text{Rate} = k[Cl_2]K\frac{[H_2S]}{H^+} = k'\frac{[Cl_2][H_2S]}{[H^+]}$$

Thus slow step should involve 1 molecule of Cl_2 and 1 molecule of H_2S.

hence only, mechanism (A) is consistent with the given rate equation.

42. **(a)** Arrhenius equation is given by

$k = Ae^{-E_a/(2.303RT)}$

Taking log on both sides, we get

$$\log k = \log A - \frac{E_a}{2.303RT}$$

Arrhenius plot a graph between log k and $\frac{1}{T}$ whose slope is $\frac{-E_a}{2.303R}$.

43. **(d)** The graph show that reaction is exothermic.

$$\log k = \frac{-\Delta H}{RT} + 1$$

For exothermic reaction $\Delta H < 0$

$\therefore$ log k Vs $\frac{1}{T}$ would be negative straight line with positive slope.

44. **(a)** As per Arrhenius equation $(k = Ae^{-E_a/RT})$, the rate constant increases exponentially with temperature.

45. **(a)** Rate law for first order reaction $= k[N_2O_5]$

	$2N_2O_5(g) \longrightarrow$	$4NO_2(g) +$	$O_2(g)$
t = 0 min (Pressure in mm Hg)	50	0	0
t = 30 min (Pressure in mm Hg)	$50 - 2p$	$4p$	p

Total pressure $50 - 2p + 4p + p = 50 + 3p$

$= 87.5$ mm Hg

$\therefore$ P = 12.5 mm Hg

$\therefore P_0 = 50$ & P (t = 30 min)

= 25 for N_2O_5 reactant

$$\therefore\ k = \frac{2.303}{30\,\text{min}}\times\log\left(\frac{50}{25}\right) = \frac{2.303}{60\,\text{min}}\times\log\left(\frac{50}{x}\right)$$

On solving x = 12.5 mm Hg = $50 - 2p$

$\therefore$ P = 18.75 mm Hg

$\therefore$ Total pressure = 50 + 3P = 106.25 mm Hg

Speed Test-47

1. (d)
2. (d)
3. (b) When oppositely charged sols are mixed their charges are neutralised. Both sols may be partially or completely precipitated.
4. (a) Brownian movement is the random motion of particles suspended in a fluid (a liquid or gas) resulting from their collision with the fast moving atom or molecules in the liquid or gaseous state of the matter. That means smaller particles are responsible for the Brownian movement than for bigger particles.
5. (b)
6. (a) Chemical adsorption involves formation of monolayer.
7. (d) Adsorption is accompanied by evolution of heat as the residual forces acting along the surface of adsorbent decrease i.e., adsorption is accompanied by decrease in enthalpy.
8. (c)
9. (b)
10. (c) Hydrolysis of urea can be represented as follows

$$H_2N-\underset{\underset{O}{\|}}{C}-NH_2 + H_2O \xrightarrow[\text{(enzyme)}]{\text{Urease}} 2NH_3 + CO_2$$

Since it involves biological catalyst (enzyme) so it is an example of biochemical catalysis.

11. (c) Alum coagulates mud particles and helps in purifying water.
12. (d) Efficiency of catalysing property of a catalyst is inversely proportional to activation energy.
13. (a) Tyndall effect is shown by sols.
14. (c) It is due to impact of molecules of dispersion medium on the colloidal particles.
15. (c)
16. (c) Adsorption theory is applied to heterogeneous catalysis.
17. (d) Electrolytic (Ionic) impurities can be most easily removed on application of electric field.
18. (d) All are irreversible colloidal systems.
19. (d)
20. (a) Gold number $\propto \frac{1}{\text{Protective power}}$

i.e., The smaller the value of gold number of lyophilic sol, the greater is the protective action. Hence, gelatin will be better protective colloid.

21. (c) Colloidal gold is prepared by Bredig's arc method.
22. (b) According to Freundlich equation,

$$\frac{x}{m} \propto p^{1/n} \text{ or } \frac{x}{m} = Kp^{1/n}$$

$$\text{or } \log\frac{x}{m} = \log Kp^{1/n} \text{ or } \log\frac{x}{m} = \log K + \frac{1}{n}\log p$$

23. (c) V_2O_5 is used as catalyst in contact process of manufacturing H_2SO_4.
24. (d) Linseed oil, lanolin and glycogen attract water hence contain a hydrophilic structure but rubber does not attract water and thus does not contain a hydrophobic structure.
25. (c) For physiosorption the ΔH value is 10 - 40 kJ/mol.
26. (a) As adsorption is an exothermic process.

∴ Rise in temperature will decrease adsorption.

27. (d) Greater the surface area, greater the van der waal forces of attraction and therefore at lesser concentration micelle formation will take place. In case of $CH_3(CH_2)_{15}\overset{\oplus}{N}(CH_3)_3Br\overset{\ominus}{}$ due to greater chain length, greater will be van der waal forces.
28. (d) In first case the given compounds have same anion but different cations having different charge hence they will precipitate negatively charged sol i.e. 'A'.

In second case the given compounds have similar cation but different anion with different charge. Hence they will precipitate positively charged sol. i.e. 'B'.

29. (d) Volume of gold present in solution

$$= \frac{\text{Mass of gold}}{\text{Density of gold}} = \frac{1.9\times10^{-4}\,g}{19 g/cm^3}$$

$$= 0.1 \times 10^{-4}\,cm^3.$$

For spherical particles of gold with radius equal to 10 nm

The volume of each particle

$$= \frac{4}{3}\pi r^3 = \frac{4}{3}\times\frac{22}{7}\times(10\times10^{-7}\,cm)^3$$

$$= \frac{88}{21}\times10^{-18}\,cm^3$$

Number of gold particles present

$$= \frac{\text{Volume of gold in solution}}{\text{Volume of each particle}}$$

$$= \frac{0.1\times10^{-4}\,cm^3}{\frac{88}{21}\times10^{-18}\,cm^3}$$

$$= \frac{21}{88}\times10^{13} \text{ particles}$$

$$= 2.4 \times 10^{12} \text{ particles}$$

2.4×10^{12} particles of gold are present in 1000 cm^3 (1 litre).

$\therefore$ Number of particles present per mm^3

$$= \frac{2.4 \times 10^{12}}{10^6} \; [1\,L = 10^6\,mm^3]$$

$$= 2.4 \times 10^6$$

30. (d) The stability of lyophilic colloids is due to layer of dispersion medium around sol particles.

31. (d)

32. (a) On shaking with the dispersion medium, colloids directly form the colloidal sol. Hence they are called intrinsic colloids. i.e., glue.

33. (d) The characteristics given suggests that this should be physical adsorption.

Physical adsorption usually takes place at low temperature and decreases with increase in temperature. The force of attraction holding the adsorbate are van der Waal's forces. Heat of adsorption is low. It is reversible and forms multimolecular layer. It does not acquire any activation energy.

34. (b) ZSM-5 is a shape selective catalyst. Zeolites are good shape selective catalysts because of the honey comb like structure.

35. (d)

36. (a) According to Langmuir's model of adsorption of a gas on a soild surface the mass of gas adsorbed(x)per gram of the adsorbent (m) is directly proportional to the pressure of the gas (p) at constant temperature i.e.

$$\frac{x}{m} \propto p$$

37. (a) Smaller the charge on anion, lesser will be its coagulating power.

$\therefore$ KBr have Br^- with least charge of – 1 on Br thus KBr is least effective in coagulating $Fe(OH)_3$.

38. (a)

39. (c) Protein is an emulsifying agent for O/W emulsion.

40. (b)

41. (c) At low pressure the extent of adsorption is directly proportional to pressure which follows first order kinetics.

42. (c) Adsorption is a phenomena of attracting and retaining the molecules of a substance on the surface of a liquid or a solid resulting into a higher concentration of the molecules on the surface.

After adsorption there is a decrease in the residual forces due to bond formation ΔG, ΔH & ΔS all are negative in the case of adsorption.

43. (b) Peptisation is disintegration of colloidal aggregate.

44. (b) At isoelectric point there is no migration of dispersed phase in an electric field.

45. (c) Let the amount of iodine in water be a gm., $C_1 = 5g$ in x ml of CS_2, $C_2 = 5 - a$ g in x ml of H_2O. Then

$$\frac{5-a}{a} = 420, \quad \therefore = 0.0118$$

Speed Test-48

1. (b)
2. (d) Zincite is ZnO.
3. (c) The reduction of metal sulphides by carbon reduction process is not spontaneous because ΔG for such a process is positive. The reduction of metal oxide by carbon reduction process is spontaneous as ΔG for such a process is negative. From this we find that on thermodynamic considerations CO_2 is more stable than CS_2 and the metal sulphides are more stable than corresponding oxides.
In view of above the factor listed in choice (c) is incorrect and so is of no significance.
4. (b) When reduction by carbon is not satisfactory in case of metals having high m.pt., aluminothermic process is used.
5. (c)
6. (d)
7. (c) $\text{Nacl} \rightleftharpoons Na^+ + Cl^-$

$$H_2O \rightleftharpoons H^+ + OH^-$$
$$\downarrow e^-$$
$$\frac{1}{2}H_2 \leftarrow H; \quad Cl^- \rightarrow Cl \rightarrow \frac{1}{2}Cl_2 + e^-$$
(At cathode) (At anode)

Reduction potential of H is more than Na.
8. (b) Pig iron or cast iron contains 3 – 5% carbon and varying amounts of Mn, Si, P and S which makes the iron hard and brittle.
9. (c)
10. (a)
11. (b) PbO and $PbSO_4$ get reduced by PbS itself which is already present in mixture so because the reduction took place by itself, hence is known as self reduction.

$$2PbO + PbS \xrightarrow{\Delta} 3Pb + SO_2 \uparrow$$

$$PbSO_4 + PbS \xrightarrow{\Delta} 2Pb + 2SO_2 \uparrow$$

12. (c)
13. (c) Fused alumina (Al_2O_3) is a bad conductor of electricity. Therefore, cryolite (Na_3AlF_6) and fluorspar (CaF_2) are added to purified alumina which not only make alumina a good conductor of electricity but also reduce the melting point of the mixture to around 1140 K.
14. (b) For a spontaneous reaction , ΔG^o must be negative and it can be possible only in this case when $x < y$
15. (d) Most electropositive metals are obtained by electrolysis of their fused ionic salts.
16. (b) Zr and Ti are purified by van Arkel method.

$$Zr(s) + 2I_2(g) \xrightarrow{870K} ZrI_4(g)$$

$$ZrI_4(g) \xrightarrow[\text{Tugsten filament}]{2075K} Zr(s) + 2I_2(g)$$

$$Ti(s) + 2I_2(s) \xrightarrow{523K} TiI_4(g)$$
$$\downarrow 1700K$$
$$Ti(s) + 2I_2(g)$$
Pure titanium

17. (b) Cyanide process is for gold (A-IV); floatation process - pine oil (B-II); Electrolytic reduction - Al (C-III); Zone refining -Ge (D-I).
18. (d) Blister-Copper contains 1 – 2 % impurities. It is obtained after Bessemerisation of crude copper.
19. (c) Because Na is very reactive and cannot be extracted by means of the reduction by C, CO etc. So it is extracted by electrolysis.
20. (d) Leaching is the selective dissolution of the desired mineral leaving behind the impurities in a suitable dissolving agent, e.g. Argentitie or Silver glance, Ag_2S is an ore of silver. Silver is extracted from argentite by the mac-Arthur and Forest process (leaching process).

$$Ag_2S + 4NaCN \rightarrow 2Na[Ag(CN)_2] + Na_2S$$

$$4Au + 8KCN + 2H_2O + O_2 \rightarrow 4K[Au(CN)_2] + 4KOH$$

21. (d) Decomposition of carbonates and hydrated oxides.
22. (d)
23. (b) Highly electropositive elements are obtained by electrolytic reduction.
24. (a) Ag is leached by cyanide process.
25. (c)
26. (a) Calcination is heating ore in absence of air to remove moisture and volatile impurities. Carbonate ores decomposed to corresponding oxides as a result of calcination.
27. (b) Zinc dust is used as a reducing agent in the manufacture of dye-stuffs, paints etc.
28. (b) Silver containing lead is purified by cupellation.
29. (c) Ca and K are strong reducing agents, hence their oxides cannot be reduced with carbon.
30. (d)
31. (a)

32. (a) Cuprous oxide formed during roasting of cuprous sulphide is mixed with few amount of cuprous sulphide and heated in a reverberatory furnace to get metallic copper.

$$2Cu_2O + Cu_2S \rightarrow 6Cu + SO_2$$

33. (d) Na reacts vigorously with water (exothermic process)

34. (b) In the graph of $\Delta_r G°$ vs T for formation of oxides, the Cu_2O line is almost at the top. So, it is quite easy to reduce oxide ores of copper directly to the metal by heating with coke both the lines of C, CO and C, CO_2 are at much lower temperature (500 - 600 K).

$$Cu_2O + C \longrightarrow 2Cu + CO$$

35. (c) Hematite is Fe_2O_3. Thus it is the ore of iron (Fe).

36. (a) Chalcopyrite : $CuFeS_2$
Fool's gold : FeS_2
Carnalite : $KMgCl_3.6H_2O$
Bauxite : $Al_2O_3.2H_2O$

37. (a) To remove moisture and non-metallic impurities like S, P and As are oxidised and are removed as volatile substances.

$$S_8 + 8O_2 \rightarrow 8SO_2 \uparrow ; \ P_4 + 5O_2 \rightarrow P_4O_{10} \uparrow$$

$$4As + 3O_2 \rightarrow 2As_2O_3 \uparrow$$

38. (d) Si obtained by reduction of $SiCl_4$ with H_2 is further purified by zone refining method to get Si of very high purity. Silicon is purified by zone-refining process because the impurities present in it are more soluble in the liquid phase than in the solid phase.

39. (d) $2CuO + CuS \rightarrow 3Cu + SO_2$ (Self - reduction)

40. (d) Cast iron is different from pig iron and is made by melting pig iron with scrap iron and coke using hot air blast. It has slightly lower carbon content (about 3%) and is extremely hard and brittle.

41. (c) In blast furnace at about 1270 K, calcium carbonate is almost completely decomposed to give CaO which acts as a flux and combines with SiO_2 present as impurity (gangue) in the ore to form calcium silicate (fusible slag)

$$CaO(s) \text{ (basic flux)} + SiO_2(s) \text{ (acidic flux)} \longrightarrow CaSiO_3(s) \text{ (slag)}$$

42. (a) FeO is capable forming slag with SiO_2

$$SiO_2 + FeO \rightarrow FeSiO_3$$

43. (b) Since silica is acidic impurity the flux must be basic.

$$CaO + SiO_2 \rightarrow CaSiO_3$$

44. (b) This process is also called autoreduction process or air reduction process. The sulphide ores of less electropositive metals are heated in air to convert part of the ore into oxide or sulphate which then react with the remaining sulphide ore to give the metal and sulphur dioxide.

$$2Cu_2S + 3O_2 \longrightarrow 2Cu_2O + 2SO_2$$

$$Cu_2S + 2Cu_2O \longrightarrow 6Cu + SO_2$$

45. (d) Pure metal always deposits at cathode.

Speed Test-49

1. (c) $[Fe(H_2O)_5NO]^{2+}$ ion is formed.
2. (c)

Compound	O.S. of N
N_2O	+1
NO	+2
NO_2	+4
NO_3^-	+5
NH_4^+	−3

Therefore increasing order of oxidation state of N is:

$NH_4^+ < N_2O < NO < NO_2 < NO_3^-$.

3. (d) Among the hydrides of group 16 elements, boiling point of H_2O is higher than H_2S (difference in boiling points of H_2O and H_2S is around 200°C) because of strong intermolecular hydrogen bonding. After the decrease in boiling point from H_2O to H_2S, from H_2S to H_2Te, it increases due to increase in size of the atoms from S to Te which increases the magnitude of van der Waal's forces among the molecules. So, the correct order of boiling points is

$$H_2O > H_2Te > H_2Se > H_2S$$

4. (d) (i) The geometry of phosphorus is tetrahedral in all the three.

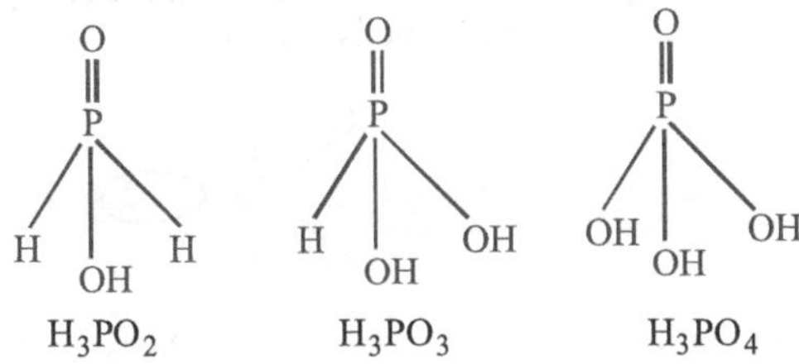

(ii) The acidity increases with increase in oxidation number of central atom

$$\overset{+1}{H_3PO_2} < \overset{+3}{H_3PO_3} < \overset{+5}{H_3PO_4}$$

(iii) H_3PO_4 is not reducing.

(iv) H_3PO_3 is diabasic, while H_3PO_2 is monobasic.

5. (b) HO– P(=O)(OH) –H it can form two series of salts by replacement of H attached to oxygen

6. (d) $N{\equiv}N{\rightarrow}O$ (i) $O{=}N{-}N{\overset{\nearrow O}{\searrow O}}$ (ii) $O{=}N{-}N(\rightarrow O){=}O$ with $O \swarrow$ (iii) $O{=}N{-}O{-}N(\rightarrow O){=}O$ with $O \swarrow$ (iv)

7. (b) Hybridisation is sp^3 and shape pyramidal

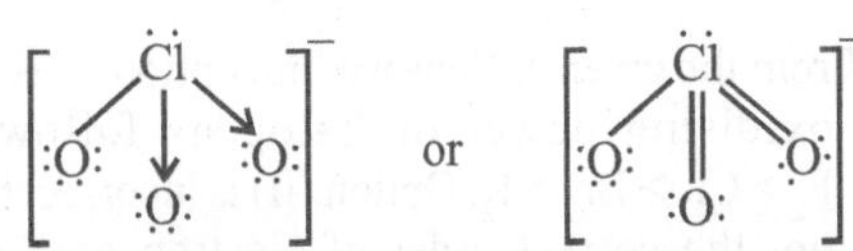

8. (c) Air is liquified by making use of the joule-Thomson effect (cooling by expansion of the gas). Water vapour and CO_2 are removed by solidification. The remaining constituents of liquid air i.e., liquid oxygen and liquid nitrogen are separated by means of fractional distillation (b.p. of O_2 = –183°C : b. P. of N_2 = – 195.8°C).
9. (b) More the oxidation state of the central atom (metal) more is its acidity. Hence SeO_2 (O. S. of Se = +4) is acidic. Further for a given O.S., the basic character of the oxides increases with the increasing size of the central atom. Thus Al_2O_3 and Sb_2O_3 are amphoteric and Bi_2O_3 is basic.
10. (d)
11. (a) Hypophosphorous acid is H_3PO_2 in which O.S. of P is +1.
12. (b) [H—P(=O)(—O—H)—H] Hypophosphorous acid (H_3PO_2) is a monobasic acid. i.e., it has only one ionisable hydrogen atom or one OH is present.
13. (d) The products of the concerned reaction react each other forming back the reactants.

$$XeF_6 + 3H_2O \longrightarrow XeO_3 + 6HF.$$

14. (a) Due to large enthalpy of vaporisation SO_2 can be used as refrigerant.
15. (d) $2Ag_2O\,(s) \rightarrow 4Ag\,(s) + O_2\,(g)$
$2Pb_3O_4\,(s) \rightarrow 6PbO\,(s) + O_2\,(g)$
$2PbO_2\,(s) \rightarrow 2PbO\,(s) + O_2\,(g)$
16. (a) Phosphorus occurs in minerals of the apatite family, $Ca_9(PO_4)_6$, CaX_2 (X = F, Cl or OH) which are main components of phosphate rocks whereas arsenic and antimony are found as sulphide minerals. The increase in covalent radii from N to P is greater in comparison to increase from As to Bi.
17. (d) (i) The first ionization energy of xenon (1, 170 kJ mol^{-1}) is quite close to that of dioxygen (1,180 kJ mol^{-1}).

(ii) The molecular diameters of xenon and dioxygen are almost identical.

Based on the above similarities Barlett (who prepared $O_2^+[PtF_6]^-$ compound) suggested that since oxygen combines with PtF_6, so xenon should also form similar compound with PtF_6.

18. (a) $2S_2O_3^{2-} + I_2 \rightarrow \underset{\text{Tetrathionate}}{S_4O_6^{2-}} + 2I^-$

19. (a) ICl_7. The hybridisation is $\frac{1}{2}(7+7+0-0) = 7\ (sp^3d^3)$

20. (b)

21. (c) From the given options we find option (i) is correct. The oxidising power of halogens follow the order $F_2 > Cl_2 > Br_2 > I_2$. Option (ii) is incorrect because it in not the correct order of electron gain enthalpy of halogens.
The correct order is $Cl_2 > F_2 > Br_2 > I_2$. The low value of F_2 than Cl_2 is due to its small size.
Option (iii) is incorrect. The correct order of bond dissociation energies of halogens is
$Cl_2 > Br_2 > F_2 > I_2$.
Option (iv) is correct. It is the correct order of electronegativity values of halogens. Thus option (ii) and (iii) are incorrect.

22. (c) Oxides which are more ionic in nature (salt - like) are known as saline oxides e.g. oxides of alkali metals.

23. (b) $XeOF_4$ square pyramidal.

24. (b) ClO_2 contains 7 + 12 i.e. 19 electrons (valence) which is an odd number, i.e. there is (are) free electron(s). Hence it is paramagnetic in nature.

25. (c) All the members form volatile halides of the type AX_3. All halides are pyramidal in shape. The bond angle decreases on moving down the group due to decrease in bond pair-bond pair repulsion.

NCl_3	PCl_3	$AsCl_3$	$SbCl_3$
107°	109.5°	98°	97.2°

26. (d) $\underset{+1}{HOCl} < \underset{+3}{HOClO} < \underset{+5}{HOClO_2} < \underset{+7}{HOClO_3}$
In case of oxyacids of similar element as the oxidation number of the central atom increases, strength of acid also increases.

27. (a) As size increases, van der Waal's forces of attraction between noble gas atoms also increases. Consequently, ease of their liquefaction increases.

28. (b) KI reacts with $CuSO_4$ solution to produce cuprous iodide (white precipitate) and I_2 (which gives brown colour). Iodine reacts with hypo ($Na_2S_2O_3.5H_2O$) solution. Decolourisaiton of solution shows the appearance of white precipitate.

$$2CuSO_4 + 4KI \rightarrow 2K_2SO_4 + \underset{\substack{\text{Cuprous iodide} \\ \text{(White ppt.)}}}{2CuI} + \underset{\substack{\text{(Brown colour} \\ \text{in solution)}}}{I_2}$$

$$2Na_2S_2O_3 + I_2 \longrightarrow \underset{\substack{\text{Sod. tetra} \\ \text{thionate} \\ \text{(colourless)}}}{Na_2S_4O_6} + 2NaI$$

29. (b) $RCOO^-$ is not pseudo halide.

30. (d)

31. (a) (Bonus)
$CaC_2 + N_2 \rightarrow Ca(CN)_2 + C$

32. (d) Electron gain enthalpy for noble gases is positive and it becomes less positive with increase in size of atom. Value of electron gain enthalpy
He – 48 kJ mol^{-1}, Ne – 116 kJ mol^{-1}
Ar, Kr – 96 kJ mol^{-1}, Xe – 77 kJ mol^{-1}
Hence, Ne has highest negative electron gain enthalpy.

33. (d) In gaseous state the HCl is covalent in nature while in aqueous solution it ionises to give H^+ and Cl^- ions.

34. (a) Air contains about 1% inert gases, mainly Ar (At.wt = 40). The atomic wt. of N_2 is 28.

35. (a) Non-metallic oxides are acidic and acidic character decreases with decreasing non-metallic character.

36. (b) $Fe_2(SO_4)_3 \xrightarrow{\Delta} Fe_2O_3 + SO_3$

37. (c) The correct order of increasing bond angle is
$Cl_2O < ClO_2^- < ClO_2$

Cl_2O (110°) ClO_2^- ClO_2 (118°)

* In ClO_2^- there are 2 lone pairs of electrons present on the central chlorine atom. Therefore the bond angle in ClO_2^- is less than 118° which is the bond angle in ClO_2 which has less number of electrons on central chlorine atom.

38. (c) Pure ClO_2 is obtained by passing dry Cl_2 over $AgClO_3$ at 90°C.

$$2AgClO_3 + Cl_2(\text{dry}) \xrightarrow{90°C} 2AgCl + 2ClO_2 + O_2$$

39. (d) XeO_2F_2 has trigonal bipyramidal geometry, but due to presence of lone pair of electrons on equitorial position, its actual shape is *see-saw*.

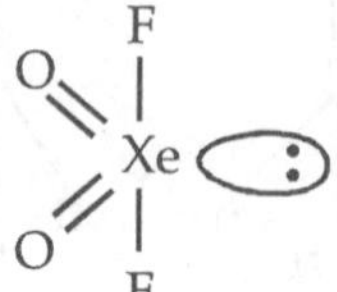

40. (a)

	XeF_2	XeF_4	XeF_6
Valence electrons of Xe	8	8	8
Electrons involved in bond formation	2	4	6
Lone pairs left	3	2	1

41. (a) $XX' \rightarrow$ Linear (e.g. ClF, BrF)
$XX_3' \rightarrow$ T-Shape (e.g. ClF_3, BrF_3)
$XX_5' \rightarrow$ Square pyramidal (e.g. BrF_5 IF_5)
$XX_7' \rightarrow$ Pentagonal bipyramidal (e.g. IF_7)

42. (c) $FeSO_4.7H_2O \rightarrow FeSO_4 + 7H_2O$

$$2FeSO_4 \xrightarrow{\Delta} Fe_2O_3 + SO_2 + SO_3$$

43. (b) $2F_2 + 4KOH \rightarrow 4KF + O_2 + 2H_2O$ for 1 mole of F_2 the molar ratio.

F_2	KOH	KF	O_2	H_2O
1	2	2	$\frac{1}{2}$	1

44. (b) $3Cl_2 + 6KOH \rightarrow KClO_3 + 5KCl + 3H_2O$
$KClO_3$ is used in fire works and safety matches and Cl_2 is greenish yellow gas.

45. (c) Yellow ammonium sulphide is $(NH_4)_2S_x$.

Speed Test-50

1. (b) Mn - $3d^5 4s^2$ | 1 | 1 | 1 | 1 | 1 | | 1l |

The no. of various oxidation states possible are +2, +3, +4, +5, +6 and +7.

2. (b)

3. (c) The number of unpaired electrons in $Ni^{2+}(aq) = 2$

Water is weak ligand hence no pairing will take place spin magnetic moment

$= \sqrt{n(n+2)} = \sqrt{2(2+2)} = \sqrt{8} = 2.82$

4. (b)

5. (d) $(n-1)d^5ns^2$ attains the maximum O.S. of +7.

6. (c)

7. (a) $Mn^{2+} = 3d^5$ i.e. no. of unpaired $e^- = 5$

$Cu^{2+} = 3d^9$ i.e. no. of unpaired $e^- = 1$

$Fe^{2+} = 3d^6$ i.e. no. of unpaired $e^- = 4$

$Zn^{2+} = 3d^{10}$ i.e. no. of unpaired $e^- = 0$

$Ni^{2+} = 3d^8$ i.e. no. of unpaired $e^- = 3$

Higher the number of unpaired electrons higher will be the magnetic moment. Hence Mn^{2+} having maximum unpaired electrons will have the maximum magnetic moment.

8. (a) Given magnetic moment of transition metal

$= \sqrt{n(n+2)} = 5.92$

i.e., n = 5

Number of unpaired electrons in $Mn^{2+} = 5$

Number of unpaired electrons in $Ti^{3+} = 1$

Number of unpaired electrons in $Cr^{3+} = 3$

Number of unpaired electrons in $Cu^{2+} = 1$

Number of unpaired electrons in $Co^{2+} = 3$

Thus Mn^{2+} have magnetic moment = 5.92 BM

9. (a) Zn, Cd and Hg due to presence of completely filled *d*-orbitals in ground state as well as in their common oxidation states are not regarded as a transition metals but they are studied along with the transition metals.

10. (d) Super conductors are derived from compounds of transition metals.

11. (a) Electronic configuration of Mn is $[Ar]3d^5 4s^2$. Being transition metal it has 7 valence electrons and all are involved in bond formation in MnO_4^-. Hence it has no unpaired electron

12. (d) Mischmetall consists of a lanthanoid metal (~95%) and iron (~ 5%) and traces of S,C,Ca and Al.

13. (a) $Tb^{4+} = 4f^7$ — 3 unpaired e^-

$Lu^{3+} = 4f^{14}$ — 0 unpaired e^-

$Ce^{4+} = 4f^0$ — 0 unpaired e^-

$La^{3+} = 4f^0$ — 0 unpaired e^-

14. (b) In neutral or faintly alkaline medium thiosulphate is quantitatively oxidized by $KMnO_4$ to SO_4^{2-}

$$8KMnO_4 + 3Na_2S_2O_3 + H_2O \longrightarrow 3K_2SO_4 + 8MnO_2 + 3Na_2SO_4 + 2KOH$$

15. (a) They contain different percentage of carbon.

16. (b) In vertice columns of transition elements, there is an increase in size from first member to second member as expected but from second member to third member, there is very small change in size and some times sizes are same. This is due to lanthanide contraction. This is the reason for Zr and Hf to have same radius.

17. (b) HCl and SO_2 are reducing agents and can reduce MnO_4^-. CO_2 which is neither oxidising and nor reducing will provide only acidic medium. It can shift reaction in forward direction and reaction can go to completion.

18. (b) Mn^{2+} (d^5) is more stable than Mn^{3+} (d^4), thus

$E^\circ_{Mn^{3+}/Mn^{2+}} = +ve$

19. (a) Green vitrol is $FeSO_4.7H_2O$.

20. (a) $Cr_2O_7^{2-} + 6e^- + 14H^+ \rightarrow 2Cr^{3+} + 7H_2O$

$Sn^{2+} \rightarrow Sn^{4+} + 2e^-$

one mole of Sn^{2+} provide 2 mole of e^- which will reduce $1/3\,Cr_2O_7^{2-}$.

21. (c) $E^o_{Cu^{+2}/Cu} = 0.34\,V$

other has – ve $E^o_{R.P.}$

$E^o_{Co^{2+}/Co} = -0.28\,V$

$E^o_{Ni^{2+}/Ni} = -0.25V$

$E^o_{Fe^{2+}/Fe} = -0.44V$

22. (b) In lanthanides, there is poorer shielding of 5*d* electrons by 4*f* electrons resulting in greater attraction of the nucleus over 5*d* electrons and contraction of the atomic radii.

23. (c) $AgCl(s) + 2NH_4OH(aq) \rightarrow [Ag(NH_3)_2]Cl(aq) + 2H_2O(l)$

24. (d) (i) Haematite is Fe_2O_3 in which Fe is present in III oxidation state.

(ii) Magnetite (Fe_3O_4) is an equimolar mixture of FeO and Fe_2O_3.

Oxidation state of Fe in FeO is II.

Oxidation state of Fe in Fe_2O_3 is III.

25. (b) $1M\ KMnO_4 \equiv 5\ N\ KMnO_4 \equiv 5\ N\ FeSO_4$

$\therefore\ 10 \times 1M \equiv 10 \times 5N \equiv 10 \times 5N$

$KMnO_4$ $KMnO_4$ $FeSO_4$

26. (b) Eu^{2+} has electronic configuration $[Xe]4f^7$ hence stable due to half filled atomic orbitals.

27. (b) $H_2Cr_2O_7 + 4O \rightarrow \underset{\text{Blue peroxide of chromium}}{2CrO_5} + H_2O$

28. (c) Both MnO_2 and $KMnO_4$ used for the preparation of chlorine by the action of conc. HCl

$MnO_2 + 4HCl \rightarrow MnCl_2 + 2H_2O + Cl_2$

$2KMnO_4 + 16HCl \rightarrow 2KCl + 2MnCl_2 + 8H_2O + 5Cl_2$

Chlorine is not obtained by dil HCl

29. (a) $2KMnO_4 + H_2SO_4\,(conc.) \rightarrow K_2SO_4 + \underset{\text{Explosive}}{Mn_2O_7} + H_2O$

30. (b) In any row the melting points of transition metals rise to a maximum at d^5 except for anomalous values of Mn and Tc and falls regularly as the atomic number increases.

31. (c) In laboratory, manganese (II) ion salt is oxidised to permagnate ion in aqueous solution by peroxodisulphate.

$2Mn^{2+} + \underset{\text{peroxodisulphate ion}}{S_2O_8^{2-}} + 8H_2O \rightarrow 2MnO_4^- + 10SO_4^{2-} + 16H^+$

32. (a) In interstitial compounds small atoms like H, B and C enter into the void sites between the packed atoms of crystalline metal. They retain metallic conductivity and are chemically inert.

33. (d)

Eu	La	Gd	Am
O.S = +2, +3	+3	+3	+4, +5, +6

34. (b) $2MnO_2 + 4KOH + O_2 \longrightarrow \underset{\text{dark green}}{2K_2MnO_4} + 2H_2O$

35. (b) $Ag_2S + 4NaCN + 2O_2 \longrightarrow 2Na[Ag(CN)_2] + Na_2SO_4$

36. (b) Ferrous ferricyanide is known as Turbull's blue.

37. (b) Oxidation of water takes place in presence of Mn in biological process.

38. (b) As a result of lanthanide contraction Zr^{4+} and Hf^{4+} possess almost the same ionic radii. Ce^{4+} is an oxidising agent. Ce^{4+} gains electron to acquire more stable Ce^{3+}state. $La(OH)_3$ is the most basic among lanthanide hydroxides.

39. (a) When $AgNO_3$ reacts with PH_3, then Ag is obtained.

$\underset{\text{silver nitrate}}{6AgNO_3} + \underset{\text{phosphene}}{2PH_3} \longrightarrow 6Ag + \underset{\text{phosphorous acid}}{2H_3PO_3} + 6NO_2$

40. (c) I^- is converted to IO_3^- by neutral or faintly alkaline MnO_4^- as shown below.

$2MnO_4^- + H_2O + I^- \longrightarrow 2MnO_2 + 2OH^- + IO_3^-$

41. (c) The transition metals and their compounds are used as catalysts. Because of the variable oxidation states they may form intermediate compound with one of the readtants. These intermediate provides a new path with lowe activation energy. $V_2O_5 + SO_2 \rightarrow V_2O_4 + SO_3$

$2V_2O_4 + O_2 \rightarrow 2V_2O_5$

42. (b)

43. (a) The basic character of the transition metal monoxide is TiO > VO > CrO > FeO because basic character of oxides decrease with increase in atomic number. Oxides of transitional metals in low oxidation state i.e., + 2 and + 3 are generally basic except Cr_2O_3.

44. (b) After crystal field spliting, the five d-orbitals. get separated as three t_{2g} and two orbitals. For Mn^{2+}, last shell has 5 e^-s i.e., $3d^5\,4s^0$. So according to Hund's rule of maximum multiplicity the excited state configuration will be $t_{2g}^3 e_g^2$.

45. (a) $2K_2CrO_4 + 2HNO_3 \rightarrow K_2Cr_2O_7 + 2KNO_3 + H_2O$

$\Rightarrow 2CrO_4^{2-} \overset{H^{\oplus}}{\rightleftharpoons} Cr_2O_7^{2-} + H_2O$

Speed Test-51

1. (c) $[PtCl_2(NH_3)_4]Br_2$ and $[PtBr_2(NH_3)_4]Cl_2$ are ionisation isomers
2. (b)
3. (a) In octahedral complex the magnitude of Δ_o will be highest in a complex having strongest ligand. Out of the given ligands CN^- is strongest. So, Δ_o will be highest for $[Co(CN)_6]^{3-}$. Thus option (a) is correct.
4. (a) As + ve charge on the central metal atom increases, the less readily the metal can donate electron density into the π^* orbitals of CO ligand to weaken the C – O bond. Hence, the C – O bond would be strongest in $Mn(CO)_6^+$.
5. (b)
6. (b) The chemical formula of Pentamminenitrochromium (III) chloride is

   $\left[Cr(NH_3)_5NO_2\right]Cl_2$

   It can exist in following two structures

   $\left[Cr(NH_3)_5NO_2\right]Cl_2$ and

   $\left[Cr(NH_3)_5ONO\right]Cl_2$

   Therefore the type of isomerism found in this compound is linkage isomerism as nitro group is linked through N as $-NO_2$ or through O as – ONO.
7. (d) In silver plating $K[Ag(CN)_2]$ is used which provides constant and required supply of Ag^+ ions as $Ag(CN)_2^-$ is very stable. But if $AgNO_3$ is used concentration of $[Ag^+]$ in solution will be very large. In that case Ag will be deposited at faster rate without any uniformity.
8. (a) Chromium in $Cr(CO)_6$ is in zero oxidation state and has $[Ar]^{18}\,3d^5 4s^1$ as the electronic configuration. However, CO is a strong ligand, hence pairing up of electrons takes place leading to following configuration in $Cr(CO)_6$.

3d					4s	4p		
↑↓	↑↓	↑↓	××	××	××	××	××	××

   d^2sp^3 Hybridisation

   Since the complex has no unpaired electron, its magnetic moment is zero.
9. (b) $d^6 - t_{2g}^{\;2,2,2}\; eg^{\;0,0}$ (in low spin)

   $$CFSE = -0.4 \times 6\Delta_0 + 3P$$

   $$= -\frac{12}{5}\Delta_0 + 3P$$
10. (d) $K_2SO_4 \cdot Al_2(SO_4)_3 \cdot 24H_2O$
11. (b) Ionisation isomer of $[Cr(H_2O)_4Cl(NO_2)]Cl$ is $[Cr(H_2O)_4Cl_2]NO_2$.
12. (a) The given compound may have linkage isomerism due to presence of NO_2 group which may be in the form $-NO_2$ or $-ONO$.

    It may have ionisation isomerism due to presence of two ionisable group $-NO_2$ & $-Cl$. It may have geometrical isomerism in the form of *cis-trans* form as follows :

    $[Co(NH_3)_4Cl(NO_2)]NO_2$ and $[Co(NH_3)(NO_2)_2]Cl$ — ionisation isomers.

    $[Co(NH_3)_5(NO_2)_2]Cl$ and $[Co(NH_3)_5(ONO)_2Cl$ — Linkage isomers

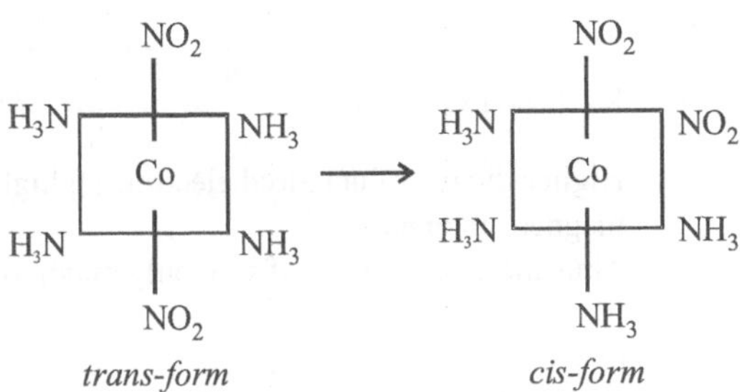

    Geometrical isomers
13. (b) IUPAC name of $K_3[Ir(C_2O_4)_3]$ is potassium trioxalato iridate (III)
14. (a) $[Co(NH_3)_5CO_3]ClO_4$. Six monodentate ligands are attached to Co hence C. N. of Co = 6;

    O. N. = x + 5 × (0) + 1 × (–2) + 1× (–1) = 0 ∴ x = + 3 ; electronic configuration of $Co^{3+}[Ar]\ 3d^6 4s^0$ hence number of d electrons is 6. All d-electrons are paired due to strong ligand hence unpaired electron is zero.
15. (b)
16. (a) Since the precipitate of AgCl shows two ionisable chloride ion the complex must have the structure.

    $$[Co(NH_3)_5Cl]Cl_2 + 2AgNO_3 \rightarrow [Co(NH_3)_5Cl](NO_3)_2 + 2AgCl$$

    Hence two chlorine atoms satisfy the primary valency and one secondary valency.
17. (d) d_5 —— strong ligand field

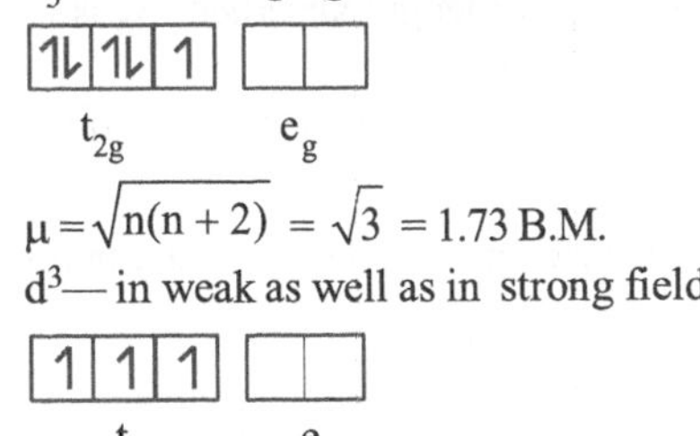

    $\mu = \sqrt{n(n+2)} = \sqrt{3} = 1.73$ B.M.

    d^3— in weak as well as in strong field

    $\mu = \sqrt{3(5)} = \sqrt{15} = 3.87$ B.M.

    d^4– in weak ligand field

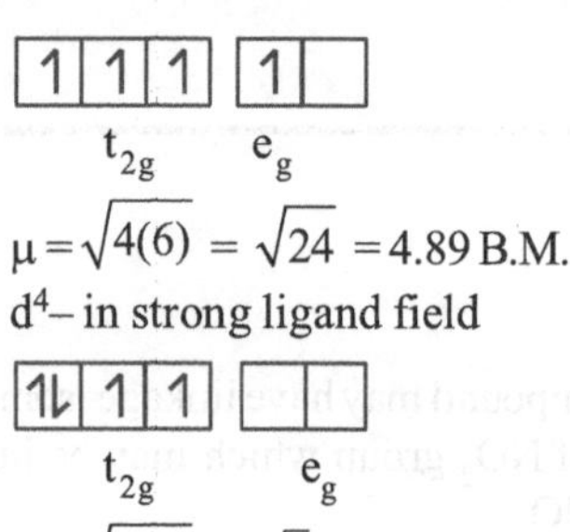

$\mu = \sqrt{4(6)} = \sqrt{24} = 4.89$ B.M.

d^4– in strong ligand field

$\mu = \sqrt{2(4)} = \sqrt{8} = 2.82$ B.M.

18. **(b)** The electronic configuration of central metal ion in complex ions P, Q and R are

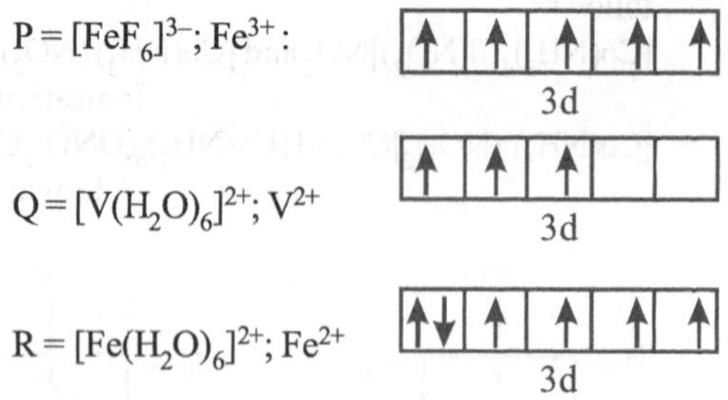

$P = [FeF_6]^{3-}$; Fe^{3+}: 3d

$Q = [V(H_2O)_6]^{2+}$; V^{2+} 3d

$R = [Fe(H_2O)_6]^{2+}$; Fe^{2+} 3d

Higher the no. of unpaired electron(s), higher will be magnetic moment.

Thus the correct order of spin only magnetic moment is

Q < R < P

19. **(a)** $Ti(C_2H_4)_4$ is an organometallic compound due to Ti directly attached to C- atom

20. **(b)**

Atom/Ion Complex	Configuration (3d, 4s, 4p)	No. of unpaired electrons	Magnetic nature
Ni^{2+} (d^8)	3d: ↑↓ ↑↓ ↑↓ ↑ ↑; 4s: ☐; 4p: ☐ ☐ ☐	2	Paramagnetic
$[NiCl_4]^{2-}$	3d: ↑↓ ↑↓ ↑↓ ↑ ↑; 4s: :; 4p: : : : (sp^3)	2	Paramagnetic
$[Ni(CN)_4]^{2-}$	3d: ↑↓ ↑↓ ↑↓ ↑↓ :; 4s: :; 4p: : : ☐ (Rearrangement, dsp^2)	0	Diamagnetic
Ni (d^8s^2)	3d: ↑↓ ↑↓ ↑↓ ↑ ↑; 4s: ↑↓; 4p: ☐ ☐ ☐	2	Paramagnetic
$[Ni(CO)_4]$	3d: ↑↓ ↑↓ ↑↓ ↑↓ ↑↓; 4s: :; 4p: : : : (Rearrangement, sp^3)	0	Diamagnetic

21. **(a)** For any metal cation, the magnitude of Δ_0 depends upon the nature of ligand. Higher the value of Δ_0, lower will be the wave length absorbed. Δ_0 is crystal field stabilisation energy.

The value of Δ_0 for legands varies as follows

$H_2O < NH_3 < NO_2^-$

So, the wavelength absorbed will vary in reverse order

$NO_2^- < NH_3 < H_2O$

22. **(c)** In Na_2CdCl_4, Cd has oxidation state +2.

So, its electronic configuration is $4d^{10}4s^0$.

All the 4d orbitals are fully filled.

Hence, there will not be d-d transition resulting in colour.

So, it is colourless.

23. **(d)** Tetraethyl lead $Pb(C_2H_5)_4$ is not π bonded complex. It is σ bonded organometallic compound.

24. **(c)** $[Mn(CN)_6]^{3-}$ and $[Fe(CN)_6]^{3-}$ are inner orbital complexes and paramagnetic while $[Co(C_2O_4)_3]^{3-}$ is diamagnetic in nature.

25. **(c)** Naming should be done alphabetically. Hence 'carbonyl' is followed by 'chloro' and then 'phosphine'. bis used to denote two same groups and trans denotes the position. 'CO', and 'PH_3,' are neutral ligands. Only Cl^- is charged. Hence oxidation state of Ir is (+ I) only. Thus correct IUPAC name of given complex is carbonylchlorobistransphosphineiridium (I).

26. **(d)** The optical isomers are pair of molecules which are non super imposable mirror images of each other

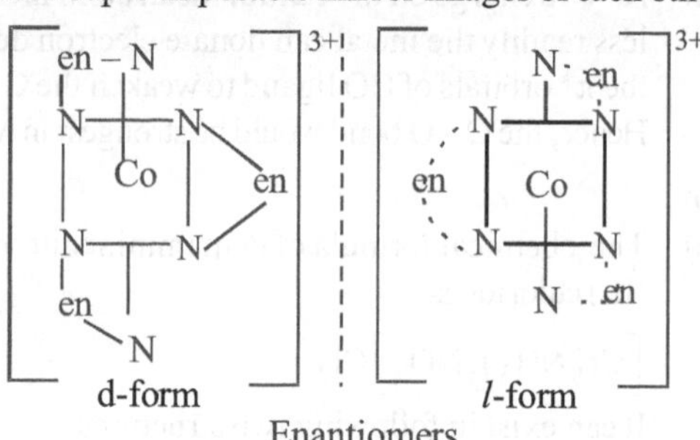

Enantiomers

The two optically active isomers are collectivity called enantiomers.

27. **(d)** $[Cr(H_2O)_4Cl_2]Cl + AgNO_3 \longrightarrow AgCl + [Cr(H_2O)_4Cl_2]NO_3$

$$\text{Molarity} = \frac{\text{wt}}{\text{mol. mass}} \times \frac{1000}{\text{vol.}}$$

$$\frac{\text{wt}}{\text{mol. mass}} = \text{molarity} \times \frac{\text{vol.}}{1000} = \frac{0.01 \times 100}{1000}$$

$$= 0.001$$

28. **(d)** $K_2[Ni(EDTA)]$. Since EDTA is hexadentate and chelating and coordinates from six sides forming more stable complex

29. **(d)** isomers

$[Ru(NH_3)_4Cl_2]^+$, $[Co(NH_3)_5Cl]^{2+}$,
cis and trans — none

$[Ir(PR_3)_2H(CO)]^{2+}$, $[Co(en)_2Cl_2]^+$
cis and trans — cis and trans and optical isomers

30. **(d)** CN^- is a strong field ligand and form low spin complexes thus $\Delta_o > P$.

31. **(b)** $\beta = K_1K_2K_3K_4$

$\log\beta = \log(K_1K_2K_3K_4)$

$\log\beta = \log K_1 + \log K_2 + \log K_3 + \log K_4$

$\log K_3 = 11.9 - (3.20 + 2.0 + 4.0)$

$\log K_3 = 2.7$

32. **(a)** Triethoxyaluminium has no Al – C linkage

$$Al\begin{cases} O-CH_2CH_3 \\ O-CH_2CH_3 \\ O-CH_2CH_3 \end{cases}$$

33. (d) Due to some backbonding by sidewise overlapping between d-orbitals of metal and p-orbital of carbon, the Fe – C bond has σ and π character.

34. (c)

	$Ni(CO)_4$	$Ni(PPh_3)_2Cl_2$
O.S.	Ni^0	Ni^{2+}
E.C.	$[Ar]3d^84s^2$	$[Ar]3d^84s^0$
	Pairing of e^-	No pairing of e^-
Hybridization	sp^3 (tetrahedral)	sp^3 (tetrahedral)

35. (b) The crystal field splitting in tetrahedral complexes is lower than that in octahedral complexes, and $\Delta_t = -\frac{4}{9}\Delta_0$.

36. (a) $[NiCl_4]^{2-}$ is sp^3 hybridised and paramagnetic in nature $[Ni(CN)_4]^{2-}$ is square planar and diamagnetic. Chlorophyll contains Mg^{2+}, Ziegler – Natta catalyst contains Ti^{4+}, Deoxyhaemoglobin is nonplanar and oxyhaemoglobin planar.

37. (d) Magnetic moment can be calculated by using the relation $\sqrt{n(n+2)}$B.M. Where n = number of electrons and B.M. is Bohr magneton.

$\therefore\ 5.9 = \sqrt{n(n+2)}$

$\therefore\ n = 5$

38. (c) The correct structure of EDTA is

$$\begin{matrix} HOOC-H_2C \\ HOOC-H_2C \end{matrix} \!\!> N-CH_2-CH_2-N <\!\! \begin{matrix} CH_2-COOH \\ CH_2-COOH \end{matrix}$$

39. (a) The complex chlorodiaquatriamminecobalt (III) chloride can have the structure $[CoCl(NH_3)_3(H_2O)_2]Cl_2$

40. (b) According to spectrochemical series $C_2O_4^{2-} > F^-$.

41. (a)

42. (a) Structure of $[Co_2(CO)_8]$

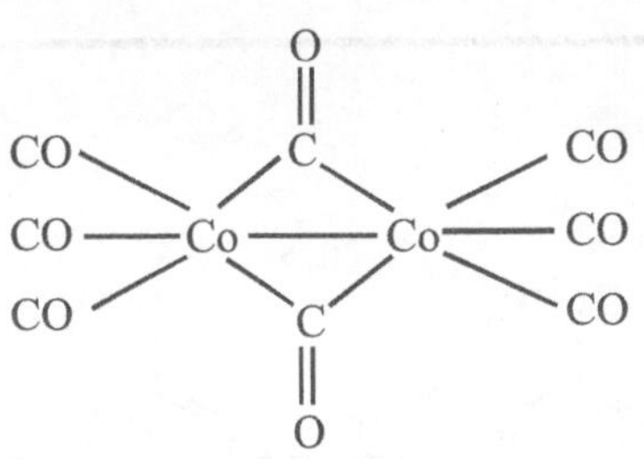

Total M – C bonds = 10, Total M – M bonds = 1

43. (b) $\left[Pt(NH_3)_6\right]Cl_4 \rightleftharpoons \left[Pt(NH_3)_6\right]^{4+} + 4Cl^-$;

$Ag^+ + Cl^- \rightarrow AgCl$ (ppt)

44. (c) In both states (paramagnetic and diamagnetic) of the given complex, Ni exists as Ni^{2+} whose electronic configuration is $[Ar]\,3d^84s^0$.

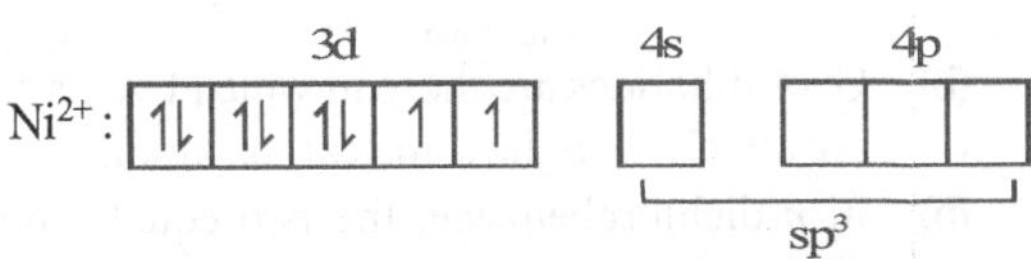

In the above paramagnetic state the geometry of the complex is sp^3 giving tetrahedral geometry.

The diamagnetic state is achieved by pairing of electrons in $3d$ orbital.

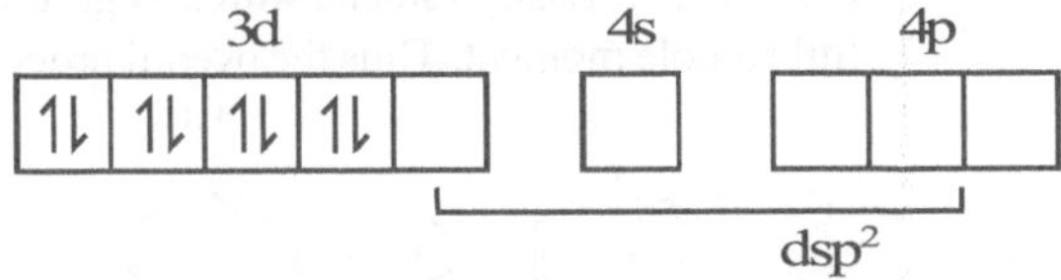

Thus the geometry of the complex will be dsp^2 giving square planar geometry.

45. (d)

Speed Test-52

1. (d) [Anisole with Br at ortho] $\xrightarrow[(-HBr)]{NaNH_2}$ [Benzyne intermediate] $\xrightarrow{NH_2^-}$ [OCH_3, NH_2 carbanion] + [OCH_3, carbanion, NH_2 at meta] $\xrightarrow[(-NH_2^-)]{NH_3}$ [OCH_3 with NH_2 at meta]

Benzyne intermediate

More stable — *m*-Methoxyaniline

2. (b) Gem-dihalides are those in which two halogen atoms are attached on the same carbon atom.

3. (b) In *p*-dichlorobenzene, the two equal dipoles are in opposite direction, hence the molecule has zero dipole moment. In *o*- and *m*- dichlorobenzenes, the two dipoles are at 60° and 120° apart respectively, and thus according to parallelogram law of forces, the dipole moment of *o*-dichlorobenzene is much higher than that of *m*-isomer. Lastly, toluene with a +I group possesses little dipole moment. Thus the overall order is

p-dichlorobenzene (IV) < toluene (CH_3) (I) < m-dichlorobenzene (II) < o-dichlorobenzene (III)

4. (b) DDT is prepared by heating chlorbenzene and chloral with concentrated sulphuric acid

$CCl_3CHO + 2\ H-C_6H_4-Cl \xrightarrow[-H_2O]{H_2SO_4} CCl_3CH(C_6H_4Cl)_2$

1,1,1-trichloro–2,2 bis (p-chlorophenyl) ethane
or
DDT

5. (a) 1° Alkyl halides (having least steric hindrance at the α-carbon atom) are most reactive towards S_N2 reaction.

6. (c) $C_6H_5NH_2 \xrightarrow[\text{(Diazotization)}]{HNO_2,\ HCl} C_6H_5\overset{+}{N}\equiv NCl^- \xrightarrow[\text{Sandmeyer's reaction}]{Cu_2Cl_2} C_6H_5Cl$

7. (d) –Cl is *o, p*–directing.

8. (d) [o-CH_2Br, CH_3 benzene] A $\xrightarrow[AgNO_3]{\text{Alcholic}}$ $AgBr\downarrow$

A $\xrightarrow{\text{Oxidation}}$ [o-$C_6H_4(COOH)_2$] $\xrightarrow{\Delta}$ [$C_6H_4(CO)_2O$]

Acid (B) — Phthalic Anhydride

9. (a)

10. (b) $R-X + NaI \xrightarrow{\text{acetone}} R-I + NaX\downarrow$

Soluble in (CH_3OH, Me_2CO) — Insoluble in (CH_3OH, Me_2CO)

(where X = Cl or Br)

11. (a) Due to steric hindrance tertiary alkyl halide do not react by S_N2 mechanism they react by S_N1 mechanism. S_N2 mechanism is followed in case of primary and secondary alkyl halides of

$CH_3-X > CH_3-CH_2X > (CH_3)_2-CH.X > (CH_3)_3-C-X$

12. (c) S_N1 reactions involve the formation of carbocations, order of stability of carbocation is 3° > 2° > 1° hence higher the stability of carbocation, more will be the reactivity of the parent alkyl halide. Moreover the tertiary carbocation formed from (c) is stabilized by two phenyl groups.

13. (d) $CH_3-\underset{Br}{CH}-CH_2-\underset{Br}{CH}-CH_2-CH_3 \xrightarrow[E2]{KOH,\ CH_3OH\ \Delta} CH_3-CH=CH-CH=CH_2-CH_3$

(Saytzeff product)

14. (a) Only 1° alkyl halides (i.e. CH_3Br) undergo S_N2 reaction.

15. (d) It is an example of intramolecular Wurtz reaction.

$\square$(Br, Cl) $\xrightarrow[\text{ether}]{Na}$ $\xrightarrow{Na}$ bicyclobutane + NaCl

Br^- is a better leaving group than chloride. In this reaction alkali metal (Na) is electron donor.

16. (d) $C_6H_5CH_3 \xrightarrow[\text{heat}]{3Cl_2,\,h\nu} C_6H_5CCl_3 \xrightarrow{\text{aq. NaOH}} [C_6H_5C(OH)_3] \xrightarrow{-H_2O} C_6H_5COOH$

17. (c) CH_3OH does not undergo iodoform reaction, all others do so.

18. (d) Mechanism of Hunsdiecker's reaction is

$$R-CO\bar{O}\,\overset{+}{Ag} \xrightarrow[-Ag\,Br]{Br_2} RCOOBr \longrightarrow RCO\dot{O} + \dot{B}r$$

$$\longrightarrow R^{\bullet} + CO_2\,;$$

$$R^{\bullet} + RCOO\,Br \longrightarrow R-Br + RCO\dot{O}$$

19. (b) $C_2H_5\overset{\ominus}{O}$ abstracts the more acidic H:

$C_6H_5-CH(H)-C(CH_3)(Br)-CH(H)-CH_3$

(–I effect) (+I effect)

$\xrightarrow[C_2H_5OH]{C_2H_5ONa}$ $C_6H_5-CH=C(CH_3)-CH_2-CH_3$

20. (c) Alkyl halides can be prepared by treating alcohol with $SOCl_2$.

$$CH_3CH_2OH + SOCl_2 \longrightarrow CH_3CH_2Cl + SO_2 + HCl$$

This reaction is known as Darzen's procedure.

Note : $SOBr_2$ and SOI_2 are not used in this reaction because $SOBr_2$ is less stable and SOI_2 does not exist.

21. (b)

22. (d) $H_3C-CCl_2-CH_3$ $(C_3H_6Cl_2)$ (I) $\xrightarrow[\text{(aq.)}]{KOH}$ $CH_3-C(OH)_2-CH_3$ Unstable

$\xrightarrow{-H_2O} CH_3-\overset{O}{\overset{\|}{C}}-CH_3$ (II) $\xrightarrow[\text{(II) } H_2O/H^{\oplus}]{\text{(I) } CH_3MgBr}$

$CH_3-C(CH_3)(OH)-CH_3 \xrightarrow{ZnCl_2+HCl}$ given turbidity immediately

23. (a) Although all the three compounds can be used for preparing Grignard reagents, diethyl ether is considered as the best because it provides electron pairs to Mg of the reagent fully for coordination, in case of $C_6H_5OCH_3$ and $C_6H_5N(CH_3)_2$ electron pair on O and N are partialy delocalised over the benzene and hence are less available for coordination with Mg.

R, X–Mg ← $O(C_2H_5)_2$, ← $O(C_2H_5)_2$

24. (d) $CH_2=CH-Cl$ (Vinyl Chloride)

The halogen atom in vinyl chloride is not reactive as in other alkyl halides. The non-reactivity of chlorine atom is due to resonance stabilisation. The $\ell.p.$ on Cl-atom can participate in delocalisation (Resonance) to give two canonical structure.

$$CH_2=CH-\ddot{C}l: \longrightarrow \overset{\ominus}{C}H_2-CH=\overset{+}{C}l:$$

25. (d) Chlorination of n-butane taken place via free radical formation i.e., $Cl_2 \xrightarrow{h\nu} Cl^{\bullet} + Cl^{\bullet}$

$CH_3-CH_2-CH_2-CH_3 \xrightarrow{Cl_2/h\nu}$ $H-C(CH_3)(C_2H_5)-Cl$ (d) + $Cl-C(CH_3)(C_2H_5)-H$ (*l*)

Racemic mixture

50% d form + 50% *l* form

$Cl^{\bullet}$ may attack on either side and give a racemic mixture of 2 chloro butane which contain 50% d form and 50% *l*-form.

26. (c)

$$C_6H_5CH_3 \xrightarrow[FeCl_3]{Cl_2} o\text{-}ClC_6H_4CH_3 + p\text{-}ClC_6H_4CH_3$$

$$C_6H_5CH_3 \xrightarrow{Cl_2,hv} C_6H_5CH_2Cl \xrightarrow{Cl_2,hv} C_6H_5CHCl_2 \xrightarrow{Cl_2,hv} C_6H_5CCl_3$$

27. (b)

28. (c) $\underset{(A)}{Me_2C.Cl} \xrightarrow{KOH} \underset{\text{tert. alcohol}}{Me_3COH} \xrightarrow{Cu/300°}$

$$CH_3-\underset{CH_3}{\underset{|}{C}}=CH_2+H_2O \text{ or } \underset{(C)}{Me_2C=CH_2}$$

29. (c) The acid character follows the order :
$CH_3COOH > C_6H_5OH > H_2O > CH_3OH$
The basic character will follow the order
$CH_3COO^- < C_6H_5O^- < \bar{O}H < CH_3O^-$
The stronger the acid, the weaker the conjugate base formed.

30. (b) The compound has two similar assymmetric C-atoms. It has plane of symmetry and exist in meso form.

CH₃ / H–C–Cl / - - - - Plane of symmetry / H–C–Cl / CH₃

Meso - 2, 3 dichlorobutane

31. (d) $Cl_3C-CH_2CH_3+KOH \xrightarrow{heat} (OH)_3C-CH_2CH_3+3KCl$

$$\downarrow$$

$$CH_3CH_2\overset{O}{\overset{||}{C}}-OH$$

32. (b) Elimination reaction is highly favoured if
(a) Bulkier base is used
(b) Higher temperature is used
Hence in given reaction biomolecular elimination reaction provides major product.

$$C_6H_5CHBr-CH_2C_6H_5 \xrightarrow[\text{1, 2 elimination}]{\text{t-BuOK}} C_6H_5CH=CHC_6H_5 + \text{t-BuOH} + Br$$

33. (c) The major component of Borsch reagent is 2,4-dinitrophenyl hydrazine which can be obtained by reaction of 2,4-dinitrochloro benzene and hydrazine

$$O_2N-C_6H_3(NO_2)-Cl + H.NH-NH_2 \longrightarrow O_2N-C_6H_3(NO_2)-NH-NH_2$$

2,4 -dinitrophenyl hydrazine

34. (d) $C_6H_5I \xrightarrow{NaOH} C_6H_5ONa \xrightarrow{HNO_3/H^+}$

$C_6H_5OH \xrightarrow{AgNO_3}$ No yellow ppt.

$C_6H_5CH_2I \xrightarrow{NaOH} C_6H_5CH_2ONa$

$\xrightarrow{HNO_3/H^+} C_6H_5CH_2OH$

$\xrightarrow{AgNO_3}$ yellow ppt.

Since benzyl iodide gives yellow ppt. hence this is compound B and A was phenyl iodide (C_6H_5I).

35. (a)

$$C_6H_5N{=}NCl \xrightarrow{HBF_4} C_6H_5F + N_2 + BF_3 + NaCl$$

(Balz-Schiemann's reaction)

36. (b) $BrCH_2-CH_2Br \xrightarrow[-HBr]{Alc.KOH} CH_2=CHBr$

$\xrightarrow[-HBr]{NaNH_2} CH \equiv CH$

Elimination of HBr from $CH_2=CHBr$ requires a stronger base because here, Br acquires partial double bond character due to resonance.

37. (a) $CH_3-\underset{CH_3}{\overset{CH_3}{C}}-Cl + 2Na + Cl-\underset{CH_3}{\overset{CH_3}{C}}-CH_3$

t-Butyl chloride

$\xrightarrow{\text{Wurtz Rxn}}$ $CH_3-\underset{CH_3}{\overset{CH_3}{C}}-\underset{CH_3}{\overset{CH_3}{C}}-CH_3 \xrightarrow{\text{Mono Chlorination}} CH_3-\underset{CH_3}{\overset{CH_3}{C}}-\underset{CH_3}{\overset{CH_3}{C}}-CH_2Cl$

38. (d) The boiling points of isomeric haloalkanes decrease with increase in branching. For example, 2-bromo-2-methylpropane has the lowest boiling point among the three isomers.

	$CH_3CH_2CH_2CH_2Br$	$CH_3CH_2\underset{Br}{CH}CH_3$	$H_3C-\underset{Br}{\overset{CH_3}{C}}-CH_3$
b.p./K	375	364	346

Boiling points of isomeric dihalobenzenes are very nearly the same. However, the para-isomers are high melting as compared to their ortho and meta-isomers. It is due to symmetry of para-isomers that fits in crystal lattice better as compared to ortho- and meta-isomers.

	o-dichlorobenzene	m-dichlorobenzene	p-dichlorobenzene
b.p/K	453	446	448
m.p/K	256	249	323

39. (a) $\underset{\text{Ethanol}}{CH_3CH_2OH} + Cl_2 \xrightarrow{\text{oxidation}} \underset{\text{Ethanal}}{CH_3CHO} + 2HCl$

$\underset{\text{Ethanal}}{CH_3CHO} + 3Cl_2 \longrightarrow \underset{\text{Chloral}}{CCl_3CHO} + 3HCl$

$2CCl_3CHO + Ca(OH)_2 \longrightarrow \underset{\text{Chloroform}}{2CHCl_3} + \underset{\text{Cal. formate}}{(HCOO)_2Ca}$

$\underset{\text{Acetone}}{CH_3COCH_3} + 3Cl_2 \longrightarrow \underset{\text{Trichloroacetone}}{CCl_3COCH_3} + 3HCl$

$2CCl_3CO.CH_3 + Ca(OH)_2 \longrightarrow 2CHCl_3 + (CH_3COO)_2Ca$

40. (d) $C_6H_5COOAg + Br_2 \xrightarrow{\text{Hunsdiecker reaction}} C_6H_5Br + CO_2 + AgBr$

41. (d) $C_6H_6 + CH_3CH_2CH_2Cl \xrightarrow[AlCl_3]{\text{Anhyd.}} \underset{\text{Isopropyl benzene}}{C_6H_5-\overset{CH_3}{CH}-CH_3}$

42. (a) Alkyl iodides are often prepared by the reaction of alkyl chlorides/bromides with NaI in dry acetone. This reaction is known as Finkelstein reaction.

$R-X + NaI \longrightarrow R-I + NaX$

X = Cl, Br

NaCl or NaBr thus formed is precipitated in dry acetone. It facilitates the forword reaction according to le chatelier's principle. The synthesis of alkyl fluorides is best accomplished by heating an alkyl chloride/bromide in the presence of a metallic fluoride such as AgF, Hg_2F_2, CoF_2 or SbF_3. The reaction is termed as Swarts reaction.

$H_3C-Br + AgF \longrightarrow H_3C-F + AgBr$

43. (d) In case of optically active alkyl halides, the product formed as a result of S_N2 mechanism has the inverted configuration as compared to the reactant. This is because the nucleophile attaches itself on the side opposite to the one where the halogen atom is present. In case of optically active alkyl halides, S_N1 reactions are accompanied by racemisation. The carbocation formed in the slow step being sp^2 hybridised is planar (achiral).

44. (c) Inversion in configuration occurs in S_N2 reactions.

45. (a)

Speed Test-53

1. (c) Boron trifluoride being a lewis acid forms adduct with diethyl ether which is a lewis base.

2. (c) Primary alcohol on oxidation give aldehyde which on further oxidation give carboxylic acid whereas secondary alcohols give ketone.

$$\underset{\text{n-propyl alcohal}}{CH_3CH_2CH_2OH} \xrightarrow{[O]}$$

$$CH_3CH_2CHO \xrightarrow{[O]} CH_3CH_2COOH$$

$$\underset{\text{isopropyl alcohal}}{(H_3C)_2CH-OH} \xrightarrow{[O]} \underset{\text{Ketone}}{(H_3C)_2C=O}$$

3. (d) Phenol has active (acidic) hydrogen so it reacts with CH_3MgI to give CH_4, and not anisole

$$C_6H_5OH + CH_3MgI \longrightarrow CH_4 + C_6H_5OMgI$$

4. (d) Hydrogen bonding is formed in compounds in which H is attached to highly electronegative element like F, O and N.

(i) In $H-\overset{\overset{O}{||}}{C}-H$, O is not having H atom so it shows very little H-bonding.

(ii) N is less electronegative than O, so H— bond formed by amines will be weak than that by alcohols.

(iii) C_6H_5OH forms weak H-bonding due to steric hinderance due to bulky phenyl group.

5. (a) Methyl alcohol (CH_3OH) is also known as carbinol. Hence vinyl carbinol is $CH_2=CH-CH_2OH$

6. (a) Lucas reagent is conc. HCl + anhyd. $ZnCl_2$.

7. (c) The order of reactivity depends upon the stability of the carbocations formed.

From (I) 2° carbocation

From (II) 2°

From (III) 2°

From (IV). 1°, Most stable benzyl carbocation

Remember that presence of electron-withdrawing group intensifies i.e., destabilises the carbocation thus (i) and (ii) are less stable than (iii). Further (i) is less stable than (ii) because –I effect is more pronounced in (i) due to less distance between F and + charge. Thus the stability order of the four carbocations and reactivity of their parent alcohols will be

IV > III > II > I

8. (b) $p\text{-}BrC_6H_4CH_3 \xrightarrow[\text{CCl}_4\text{ heat allylic bromination}]{\text{NBS, benzoyl peroxide}} p\text{-}BrC_6H_4CH_2Br \xrightarrow[CH_3CH_2OH]{CH_3CH_2ONa} p\text{-}BrC_6H_4CH_2OCH_2CH_3$

9. (c) $\underset{1}{CH_2}-\underset{2}{CH}\underset{3}{CH_2}Cl$ (epoxide O bridging C1 and C2) – 3-chloro -1, 2-epoxy propane

10. (c)

11. (c) If a tertiary alkyl halide is used, an alkene is the only reaction product and no ether is formed. For example, the reaction of CH_3ONa with $(CH_3)_3C–Br$ gives exclusively 2-methylpropene.

$$(CH_3)_3C-Br + \overset{+}{Na}\overset{-}{\ddot{O}}-CH_3 \longrightarrow$$

$$\underset{\text{2-Methylpropene}}{CH_3-\underset{CH_3}{C}=CH_2} + NaBr + CH_3OH$$

It is because alkoxides are not only nucleophiles but strong bases as well. They react with alkyl halides leading to elimination reactions.

12. (b) The commercial alcohol is made unfit for drinking by mixing in it some copper sulphate (to give it colour) and pyridine (a foul smelling liquid). It is known as denaturation of alcohol.

13. (d) 2-Phenylethanol, $\overset{1}{C}H_2OH\overset{2}{C}H_2C_6H_5$, is a 1° alcohol which can be prepared from C_6H_5MgBr by treating with ethylene oxide (note that HCHO will introduce only one carbon atom, i.e. it will give $C_6H_5CH_2OH$ and not $C_6H_5CH_2CH_2OH$).

$$C_6H_5MgBr + \text{(ethylene oxide)} \longrightarrow C_6H_5CH_2CH_2OH;$$

$$C_6H_5MgBr + HCHO \longrightarrow C_6H_5CH_2OH$$

14. (d) o-cresol, Salicylic acid, Phenol

Electron releasing groups ($-CH_3$, $-OCH_3$, $-NCH_3$ etc) intensify the negative charge of phenoxide ion, i.e., destablises it hence decrease ionization of parent phenol. Therefore decreases acidity while electron with drawing groups ($-NO_2$, $-COOH$, $-CHO$ etc.) increases acidity.

15. (a) Here also, carbocation is formed as an intermediate, hence the species capable of forming most stable carbocation will be most reactive.

$C_6H_5\overset{+}{C}HCH_2CH_3$ > $C_6H_5CH_2\overset{+}{C}HCH_3$ > $C_6H_5CH_2CH_2\overset{+}{C}H_2$

Benzyl carbocation 2° carbocation 1° carbocation

16. (c) $C_6H_5OH + H_2O \rightleftharpoons C_6H_5O^- + H_3O^+$

Phenoxide ion

The phenoxide ion is stable due to resonance.

The negative charge is delocalized in the benzene ring which is a stabilizing factor in the phenoxide ion and because of this reason ionization constant of phenol is higher whereas no resonance is possible in alkoxide ions (RO^-) derived from alcohol. The negative charge is localized on oxygen atom in case of alcohols.

17. (d)

18. (c) Hydration of alkenes

$$CH_2 = CH_2 + \overset{+}{H}\overset{-}{HSO_4} \rightarrow CH_3 - CH_2 - HSO_4$$

$$CH_3 - CH_2HSO_4 \xrightarrow[\text{Boil}]{H_2O} CH_3 - CH_2 - OH + H_2SO_4$$

Fermentation of sugar :

$$\underset{}{C_{12}H_{22}O_{11}} + H_2O \xrightarrow{\text{Invertase}} \underset{\text{Glucose}}{C_6H_{12}O_6} + \underset{\text{Fructose}}{C_6H_{12}O_6}$$

$$\underset{\text{Glucose or Fructose}}{C_6H_{12}O_6} \xrightarrow{\text{Zymase}} 2C_2H_5OH + 2CO_2$$

19. (c) The mechanism of the reaction involves the following three steps:

Step 1: Protonation of alkene to form carbocation by electrophilic attack of H_3O^+

$H_2O + H^+ \rightarrow H_3O^+$

$$>C=C< + H-\overset{H}{\underset{..}{O^+}}-H \rightarrow -\underset{H}{\overset{|}{C}}-\overset{+}{C}< + H_2O$$

Step 2: Nucleophilic attack of water on carbocation.

$$-\underset{H}{\overset{|}{C}}-\overset{+}{C}< + H_2O \longrightarrow -\underset{H}{\overset{|}{C}}-\overset{|}{\underset{|}{C}}-\overset{H}{O^+}-H$$

Step 3: Deprotonation to form an alcohol.

$$-\underset{H}{\overset{|}{C}}-\overset{|}{\underset{|}{C}}-\overset{H}{O^+}-H + H_2\ddot{O} \rightarrow -\underset{H}{\overset{|}{C}}-\overset{:\ddot{O}H}{\underset{|}{C}}- + H_3O^+$$

20. (c)

21. (d) $(C_2H_5O)_2Mg + H_2O \xrightarrow{\text{distill}}$

$$\underset{\text{(distillate)}}{2C_2H_5OH} + \underset{\text{(residue)}}{Mg(OH)_2}$$

22. (c) p-cresol (CH_3, OH) $\xrightarrow[\text{Reimer Tiemman reaction}]{CHCl_3 + NaOH}$ (aldehyde with CH_3, OH, $-\underset{H}{C}=O$) $\xrightarrow{HCN}$

(Cyanohydrin, with substituents CH_3, OH and $-\underset{H}{C}(OH)(CN)$ on the ring) $\xrightarrow{HOH}$ (ring with CH_3, OH and $-CH(OH)\,COOH$)

Cyanohydrin

23. (a) In case of m–nitrophenol operational effect of nitrogroup is electron withdrawing inductive effect while in case of b and c, both –R and –I effect are operational.

24. (d) Diethyl ether, being a Lewis base, is not attacked by nucleophiles, while all others contain electrophilic carbon, hence attacked by nucleophiles like OH^- ions.

$$CH_3-\overset{O\delta-}{\underset{\delta+}{C}}-OCH_3 \qquad \overset{\delta+}{CH_3-C}\equiv\overset{\delta-}{N}$$

$$CH_3-\overset{O\delta-}{\underset{\delta+}{\overset{||}{C}}}-NH_2 \qquad C_2H_5-\ddot{\underset{..}{O}}-C_2H_5$$

25. (b) Number of active hydrogen in a compound corresponds to the number of moles of CH_4 evolved per mole of the compound.

$$-NH_2, -SH, -OH \text{ or } -C\equiv CH \xrightarrow{CH_3MgI} ClCH_4\uparrow (2CH_4 \text{ from } -NH_2)$$

26. (b) $\underset{\text{Sod. ethoxide}}{C_2H_5Br + C_2H_5ONa} \xrightarrow[-NaBr]{} \underset{\text{diethyl ether}}{C_2H_5-O-C_2H_5}$

27. (a) A methanol poisoned patient is treated by giving intravenous injection of ethanol.

28. (d) $CH_3CH_2OH \xrightarrow{P+I_2} \underset{A}{CH_3CH_2I} \xrightarrow[\text{Ether}]{Mg}$

$$\underset{(B)}{CH_3CH_2MgI} \xrightarrow{HCHO} \underset{(C)}{H-\overset{CH_2CH_3}{\underset{H}{C}}-OMgI}$$

$$\xrightarrow{H_2O} \underset{\text{n-propyl alcohol}}{\underset{(D)}{H-\overset{CH_2CH_3}{\underset{H}{C}}-OH}}$$

29. (b)

30. (d) $CH_3-CH_2-\underset{OH}{CH}-\underset{OH}{CH}-CH_2-CH_3 \xrightarrow{HIO_4} 2CH_3-CH_2-CHO$

31. (b) (dihydropyran) $\xrightarrow{H^+}$ (oxocarbenium ion) $\longrightarrow$ (cyclic cation) +

$\xrightarrow{RCH_2OH}$ (tetrahydropyranyl–$\overset{+}{O}(H)CH_2R$) $\xrightarrow{-H^+}$ (tetrahydropyranyl–OCH_2R)

an acetal

32. (c) 1, 2 – Diols, when treated with an aqueous solution of periodic acid give aldehyde

$$\underset{CH_2OH}{\overset{CH_2OH}{|}} \xrightarrow{HIO_4} CH_2O + CH_2O$$

Note that a 1° alcohol gives CH_2O. Since in glycol both the OH groups, are primary hence give 2 molecules of CH_2O as by product.

33. (a)

34. (a) $CH_2\overset{O}{\diagup\diagdown}\underset{CH_3}{C}-CH_3 \xrightarrow[H_2SO_4]{CH_3OH} H_2\overset{OH}{C}-\overset{OCH_3}{\underset{CH_3}{C}}-CH_3$

35. (b) $CH_3-CH\langle{}^{OLi}_{CH_2.CH(CH_3)_2} + CH_3CHO$

$$\longrightarrow CH_3-\overset{OH}{CH}-CH_2-\overset{CH_3}{CH}-CH_3$$

36. (d) 2-methyl-2-propanol is $CH_3-\overset{OH}{\underset{CH_3}{C}}-CH_3$. It cannot be obtained by reduction of an aldehyde or ketone with $NaBH_4$.

37. (b)

38. (b) Reaction of sodium ethoxide with ethyl iodide to produce diethyl ether is known as Williamson synthesis. It is a nucleophilic substitution reaction and proceeds via S_N2 mechanism.

39. (b) $\overset{5}{CH_3}-\overset{4}{\underset{OH}{CH}}-\overset{3}{CH_2}-\overset{2}{\underset{OH}{\overset{CH_3}{C}}}-\overset{1}{CH_3}$

2-methyl- 2, 4-pentanediol.

40. (c)

41. (b)

42. (c) $(CH_3CH_2)_2O + (CH_3CO)_2O$ (Ether) (Acid anhydride) $\xrightarrow{\text{anhy. } AlCl_3} CH_3COOCH_2CH_3$ (Ester)

43. (b) $CH_3CH_2CH_2CH_2OH \xrightarrow{\text{Oxidation}} CH_3CH_2.CH_2CHO$

44. (c)

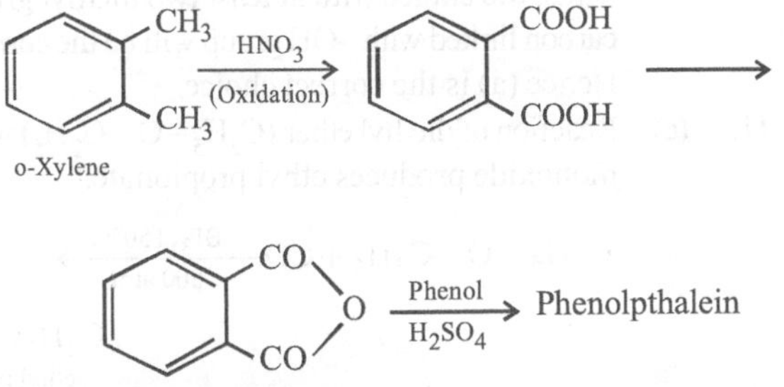

o-Xylene $\xrightarrow[\text{(Oxidation)}]{HNO_3}$ (phthalic acid, COOH / COOH) $\longrightarrow$

Phthalic anhydride, X $\xrightarrow[H_2SO_4]{\text{Phenol}}$ Phenolpthalein (Y)

45. (a)

(a) $\xrightarrow{\text{tert-BuONa}}$ O-tBu (fails to decolorise the colour of bromine) due to unsaturation

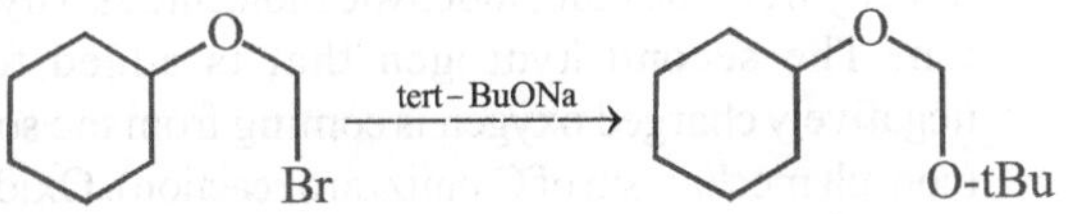

(b) Br, C_6H_5 $\xrightarrow{\text{tert-BuONa}}$ C_6H_5 (it decolorises bromine solution)

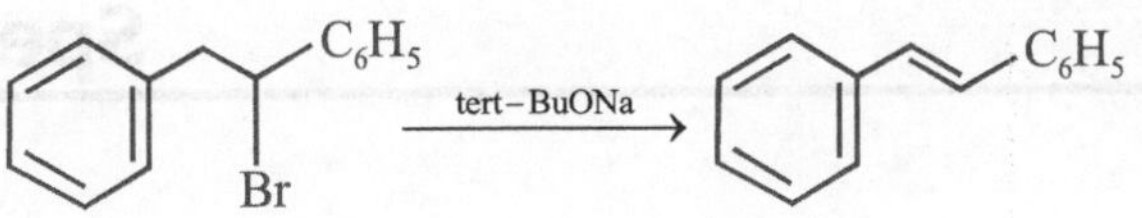

(c) O, Br $\xrightarrow{\text{tert-BuONa}}$ O (it decolorises bromine solution)

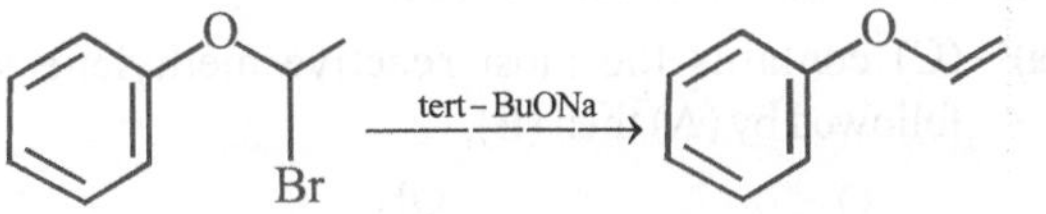

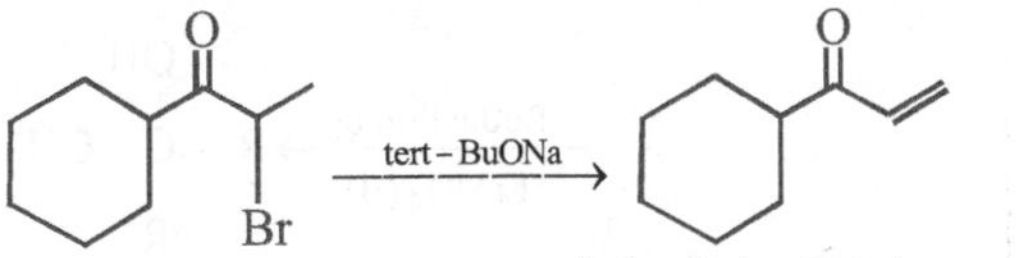

(d) O, Br $\xrightarrow{\text{tert-BuONa}}$ O (it decolorises bromine solution)

Products formed in option (2), (3) & (4) decolorises bromine solution due to presence of double bond.

Speed Test-54

1. (a) (B) followed by (A) then (C).
2. (a) (C) contains the most reactive methylene group followed by (A) then (B).
3. (a) $R-\overset{O}{\overset{\|}{C}}-R' \xrightarrow[KCN]{HCN} \underset{(A)}{R-\overset{OH}{\overset{|}{\underset{R'}{\underset{|}{C}}}}-CN} \xrightarrow[LiAlH_4 (B)]{\text{Reduction by}} R-\overset{OH}{\overset{|}{\underset{R'}{\underset{|}{C}}}}-CH_2NH_2$
4. (b) Acetaldehyde reacts only with nucleophiles. Since the mobile p electrons of carbon–oxygen double bond are strongly pulled towards oxygen, carbonyl carbon is electron-deficient and carbonyl oxygen is electron-rich. The electron deficient (acidic) carbonyl carbon is most susceptible to attack by electron rich nucleophilic reagents, that is, by base. Hence the typical reaction of aldehydes and ketones is nucleophilic addition.
5. (b) $NaBH_4$ selectively reduces the aldehyde group to alcohol without affecting double bond in a organic compound. So, X is $NaBH_4$.
6. (a)
7. (c) $\underset{(\beta\text{ - keto acid})}{PhCOCH_2^*COOH} \xrightarrow[-CO_2]{Heat} \underset{(E)}{PhCO\overset{*}{C}H_3} \xrightarrow{I_2/NaOH} \underset{(F)}{PhCO\overset{-}{O}\overset{+}{Na}} + \underset{(G)}{\overset{*}{C}HI_3}$
8. (c) By oxidation of tertiary alcohol with stronger oxidising agents, ketones may be formed along with carboxylic acid.

$$(CH_3)_3COH \xrightarrow{4[O]} CH_3COCH_3 + CO_2 + 2H_2O$$

$$(CH_3)_3COH \xrightarrow{8[O]} CH_3COOH + 2CO_2 + 3H_2O$$

9. (d)
10. (a) Recall that, esters react with excess of Grignard reagents to form 3° alcohols having at least two identical alkyl groups corresponding to Grignard reagent.

$$R-\overset{O}{\overset{\|}{C}}-OR' + R''MgX \longrightarrow R-\overset{OH}{\overset{|}{\underset{R''}{\underset{|}{C}}}}-R''$$

Since here Grignard reagent is CH_3MgBr, the 3° alcohol should have at least two methyl groups

Thus, the choice with at least two methyl groups at the carbon linked with –OH group will be the correct choice. Hence (a) is the correct choice.

11. (c) Reaction of diethyl ether ($C_2H_5-O-C_2H_5$) with carbon monoxide produces ethyl propionate.

$$C_2H_5-O-C_2H_5 + CO \xrightarrow[500\text{ atm}]{BF_3, 150°C} \underset{\text{ethyl propionate}}{C_2H_5COOC_2H_5}$$

12. (b) 13. (b)
14. (b) The hydrogen atom that is added to the carbonyl carbon of the aldehyde in the reduction is derived directly from the other aldehyde molecule as a hydride ion. The second hydrogen that is added to the negatively charged oxygen is coming from the solvent (consult mechanism of Cannizzaro reaction). Oxidation of one molecule of the compound at the expense of other molecule of the same compound is known as disproportionation.
15. (d) Use of $SOCl_2$ and ClCOCOCl forms gaseous by-products which can be easily removed, giving better yield of RCOCl. Further, oxalyl chloride is particularly easy to use becasue any excess of it can be easily evaporated due to its low b.p. (62°C)

$$R-\overset{O}{\overset{\|}{C}}-OH + Cl-\overset{O}{\overset{\|}{C}}-\overset{O}{\overset{\|}{C}}-Cl \longrightarrow R-\overset{O}{\overset{\|}{C}}-Cl + HCl\uparrow + CO\uparrow + CO_2\uparrow$$

16. (a) More the magnitude of positive charge on the carbonyl carbon, higher will be its reactivity toward nucleophilic attack.

$CH_3-\overset{O}{\overset{\|}{C}}-Cl$ $\quad CH_3-\overset{O}{\overset{\|}{C}}-H$

$CH_3-\overset{O}{\overset{\|}{C}}-OCH_3$ $\quad CH_3-\overset{O}{\overset{\|}{C}}-OCOCH_3$

Chlorine being more electron-withdrawing than oxygen develops more positive charge on carbonyl carbon.

17. (b)

18. (b) Pinacolone is oxidation product of pinacol.

$$CH_3-\overset{OH}{\underset{CH_3}{C}}-\overset{OH}{\underset{CH_3}{C}}-CH_3 \xrightarrow[\text{rearrangement}]{\text{oxidation with}} CH_3-\overset{CH_3}{\underset{CH_3}{C}}-\overset{O}{\overset{||}{C}}-CH_3$$

Pinacol → Pinacolone (3, 3-dimethyl-2-butanone)

19. (a) 4-formylcyclohexanone (CHO) $\xrightarrow[\text{Tollens reagent}]{[Ag(NH_3)_2]OH}$ 4-oxocyclohexanecarboxylic acid (CO_2H) $\xrightarrow[\text{(esterification)}]{H^+/CH_3OH}$ methyl ester ($O=C-OCH_3$) $\xrightarrow{CH_3MgBr}$ product with ring carbon bearing CH_3 and $H_3C-\underset{OH}{C}-CH_3$

20. (b) When benzaldehyde is refluxed with aqueous alcoholic potassium cyanide, two molecules of benzaldehyde condense together to form benzoin

$$C_6H_5-\overset{H}{\underset{O}{C}} + \overset{O}{\underset{H}{C}}-C_6H_5 \xrightarrow[\Delta]{\text{KCN (alc)}} C_6H_5-\overset{H}{\underset{OH}{C}}-\overset{O}{\overset{||}{C}}-C_6H_5$$

Benzoin

21. (b)

$$\underset{\text{acetaldehyde}}{CH_3-\overset{O}{\overset{||}{C}}-H} \xrightarrow{HCN} CH_3-\overset{OH}{\underset{CN}{C}}-H \xrightarrow{\text{Hydrolysis}} \underset{\text{Lactic acid}}{CH_3-\overset{OH}{\underset{COOH}{C}}-H}$$

22. (c) Catalytic reduction, Na/C_2H_5OH and $LiAlH_4$ reduce $>C=O$ group to $>CHOH$ and not $>CH_2$.

23. (c) $RX \xrightarrow{CN^-} \underset{(A)}{RCN} \xrightarrow[H_2O]{NaOH} \underset{(B)}{RCOO^-Na^+}$

The conversion of an alkyl halide into nitrile followed by hydrolysis (alkaline or acidic), provides a method for preparing carboxylic acid containing one carbon atom more than the starting alkyl halide.

24. (b) $C_6H_5-\overset{O}{\overset{||}{C}}-CH_3 \xrightarrow{\text{Zn-Hg/HCl}} C_6H_5-CH_2-CH_3$

Phenyl methyl ketone → Ethyl benzene

This reaction is known as Clemmensen's reduction.

25. (c) Aldehydes having α-H atom, when treated with aluminium ethoxide (in place of NaOH or KOH), undergo Cannizzaro type of reaction with a difference that the product isolated is an ester rather than salt of acid or alcohol. Such reaction in called Tischenko reaction.

$$\underset{\text{Acetaldehyde}}{2CH_3CHO} \xrightarrow{Al(OC_2H_5)_3}$$

$$[CH_3COOH + CH_3CH_2OH] \rightarrow \underset{\text{Ethyl acetate}}{CH_3COOC_2H_5}$$

26. (c)

27. (d) $A \xrightarrow[(I)]{NH_3} B \xrightarrow[II]{\Delta} C \xrightarrow[KOH,(III)]{Br_2} CH_3CH_2NH_2$

Reaction (III) is a Hoffmann bromamide reaction. Now formation of $CH_3CH_2NH_2$ is possible only from a compound $CH_3CH_2CONH_2$(C) which can be obtained from the compound $CH_3CH_2COO^-NH_4^+$(B).

Thus (A) should be CH_3CH_2COOH

$$\underset{(A)}{CH_3CH_2-\overset{O}{\overset{||}{C}}-OH} \xrightarrow{NH_3} \underset{(B)}{CH_3CH_2COO^-NH_4^+}$$

$$\xrightarrow{\Delta} \underset{(C)}{CH_3CH_2CONH_2} \xrightarrow{KOH\,|\,Br_2} CH_3CH_2NH_2$$

28. (a) Carbonyl compounds (aldehydes and ketones) are obtained by the oxidation of 1° and 2° alcohols respectively. Among the given options, only (a) is 2° alcohol hence it can be oxidized to ketone.

$$\underset{\text{2-hydroxypropane}}{H_3C\overset{OH}{\overset{|}{C}}HCH_3} \xrightarrow{\text{oxidation}} \underset{\text{Acetone}}{H_3C\overset{O}{\overset{||}{C}}CH_3}$$

29. (d) I_2 and Na_2CO_3 react with acetophenone ($C_6H_5COCH_3$) to give yellow ppt. of CHI_3 but benzophenone ($C_6H_5COC_6H_5$) does not and hence can be used to distinguish between them.

30. (a) $RCH_2CH_2OH \xrightarrow{PBr_2} RCH_2CH_2Br$

$\xrightarrow{KCN} RCH_2CH_2CN \xrightarrow{H^+} RCH_2CH_2COOH$

31. (d) $\underset{'x'}{Na_2C_2O_4} + \underset{\text{(conc.)}}{H_2SO_4} \rightarrow Na_2SO_4 + CO\uparrow + CO_2\uparrow + H_2O$

$\underset{'x'}{Na_2C_2O_4} + CaCl_2 \rightarrow \underset{\text{(white ppt.)}}{CaC_2O_4\downarrow} + 2NaCl$

$5CaC_2O_4\downarrow + \underset{\text{(purple)}}{2KMnO_4} + 8H_2SO_4 \rightarrow$

$K_2SO_4 + 5CaSO_4 + \underset{\text{(colourless)}}{2MnSO_4} + 10CO_2 + 8H_2O$

32. (a) $CH_3COOH + PCl_5 \rightarrow \underset{[A]}{CH_3COCl}$ $\xrightarrow[\text{Anhyd}AlCl_3]{C_6H_6}$ $C_6H_5COCH_3$ (Friedel Craft reaction)

$$\underset{(C)}{C_2H_5-\overset{OH}{\overset{|}{C}}(C_6H_5)-CH_3} \xleftarrow[\text{ether hydrolysis}]{H^+} C_2H_5-\overset{OMgBr}{\overset{|}{C}}(C_6H_5)-CH_3 \xleftarrow{MgBrC_2H_5}$$

33. (a) Compound (a) undergoes dehydration easily as the product obtained is conjugated and thus more stable.

34. (d) Vanillin -vanilla beans
Salicylaldehyde - meadow sweet
Cinnamaldehyde -from cinnamon.

35. (a)

36. (b) In structure II, presence of positive charge on oxygen causes the displacement of π electrons toward oxygen, making carbon more electron deficient than that in unprotonated carbonyl group.

37. (a) The optically active acid will react with *d* and *l* forms of alcohol present in the racemic mixture at different rates to form two diastereomers in unequal amounts leading to optical activity of the product.

38. (d) *m*-Chlorobenzaldehyde does not contains α-H atom. It is an example of Cannizzaro reaction

$$m\text{-}ClC_6H_4CHO \xrightarrow{\text{conc. KOH}} m\text{-}ClC_6H_4COOK + m\text{-}ClC_6H_4CH_2OH$$

39. (c)

40. (a) The correct order of increasing acid strength
$CF_3COOH > MeOCH_2COOH > CH_3COOH > (Me)_2CH.COOH$
Electron withdrawing groups increase the acid strength and electron donating groups decrease the acid strength.

41. (a) Addition of HCN to carbonyl compounds is nucleophilic addition reaction. The order of reactivity of carbonyl compounds is
Aldehydes (smaller to higher), ketones (smaller to higher), Then
$HCHO > CH_3COCH_3 > Ph.COCH_3 > PhCOPh$
The lower reactivity of ketones is due to presence of two alkyl group which shows +I effect. The reactivity of ketones decreases as the size of alkyl group increases.

42. (d) 2,4,6-$(O_2N)_3C_6H_2OH$ (Picric acid); (Barbituric acid); (Ascorbic acid); $o\text{-}HOOC\text{-}C_6H_4\text{-}O\text{-}\overset{O}{\overset{||}{C}}\text{-}CH_3$ (Aspirin)

43. (a) $CH_3-CH_2-\overset{H}{\overset{|}{C}}=\underset{CH_3}{\underset{|}{\overset{CH_3}{\overset{|}{C}}}} \xrightarrow{O_3}$ ozonide $\xrightarrow{(-H_2O)} CH_3-\overset{O}{\overset{||}{C}}-CH_3 + CH_3-CH_2-CHO$

44. (d) It is Clemmensen's reduction

$$\underset{\text{Butan-2-one}}{CH_3-\overset{O}{\overset{||}{C}}-CH_2-CH_3} \xrightarrow[\text{Conc. HCl}]{Zn-Hg} CH_3CH_2-CH_2CH_3$$

45. (a)

Speed Test-55

1. (d) Reduction with iron scrap and hydrochloric acid is preferred because $FeCl_2$ formed gets hydrolysed to release hydrochloric acid during the reaction. Thus, only a small amount of hydrochloric acid is required to initiate the reaction.

2. (b) *o*-Nitrophenol shows intramolecular H-bonding and forms chelate. Compounds involved in chelation become non-polar. Consequently such compounds are soluble in non-polar solvents like ether, benzene etc. and are only sparingly soluble in water whereas meta and para isomers are more soluble in water & less soluble in non-polar solvents.

O intra-molecular H-bonding

3. (d) The reaction can be completed as follows:

'A' (Aniline) $\xrightarrow[\text{(diazotisation)}]{NaNO_2/HCl}$ $C_6H_5N_2Cl$ 'B' Benzene diazonium chloride + $C_6H_5N(CH_3)_2$ N,N-dimethylaniline $\xrightarrow{\text{cold}}$ $C_6H_5-N=N-C_6H_4-N(CH_3)_2$

'C'

p-dimethylaminoazobenzene

4. (c) 1° amines have $-NH_2$ group in their structure. 4 primary amines are possible by $C_4H_{11}N$.

$CH_3-CH_2-CH_2-CH_2NH_2$ (i)

$CH_3-CH_2-CH(NH_2)-CH_3$ (ii)

$CH_3-CH(CH_3)-CH_2-NH_2$ (iii)

$CH_3-C(CH_3)(NH_2)-CH_3$ (iv)

5. (c) CH_3NC (methyl isocyanide) on reduction with $LiAlH_4$ gives secondary amine.

6. (b) Wurtz reaction is for the preparation of hydrocarbons from alkyl halide

$$RX + 2Na + XR \longrightarrow R-R + 2NaX$$

7. (d) Benzylamine ($C_6H_5CH_2NH_2$) is most basic. In others the basic character is suppressed due to resonance.

8. (d) Nitrous acid reacts differently with aliphatic and aromatic amines in cold.

$$\underset{1^\circ\text{ Amine}}{C_2H_5NH_2} + HONO \longrightarrow \underset{\text{Alcohol}}{C_2H_5OH} + N_2$$

$$C_6H_5NH_2 + \underset{(NaNO_2 + HCl)}{HONO} \xrightarrow{\text{Cold}} [C_6H_5\overset{\oplus}{N}\equiv N]\overset{\ominus}{Cl}$$

Benzene diazonium chloride

9. (c) Aliphatic amines are more basic than aromatic amines thus methylamine is most basic. Electron donating groups increase the basicity whereas electron withdrawing groups decrease the basicity of the aromatic amines. Thus *p*-methoxyaniline is more basic then aniline which is further more basic then *p*-nitroaniline.

$$p\text{-}NO_2C_6H_4NH_2 < C_6H_5NH_2 < p\text{-}CH_3OC_6H_4NH_2 < CH_3-NH_2$$

10. (d)

11. (d) $CH_3CH_2N \equiv C + H_2O \xrightarrow{H^+} CH_3CH_2NH_2 + HCOOH$

12. (d) Aromatic amines are less basic than aliphatic amines. Among aliphatic amines the order of basicity is 2° > 1° > 3°. The electron density is decreased in

3° amine due to crowding of alkyl group over N atom which makes the approach and bonding by a proton relatively difficult. Therefore the basicity decreases. Further Phenyl group show – I effect, thus decreases the electron density on nitrogen atom and hence the basicity.

∴ dimethylamine (2° aliphatic amine) is strongest base among given choices.

∴ The correct order of basic strength is

Dimethylamine > Methyl amine > Trimethyl amine > Aniline.

13. (d) Nitro compounds having α-hydrogen show tautomerism

$$RCH_2-\overset{+}{N}(=O)O^- \rightleftharpoons RCH=\overset{+}{N}(OH)O^-$$

14. (c) Only primary aromatic amines undergo diazotisation followed by coupling.

15. (c)

16. (a) This is carbylamine reaction.

$$CH_3CH_2NH_2 + CHCl_3 + 3KOH \longrightarrow C_2H_5NC + 3KCl + 3H_2O$$

17. (b) Explosives invariably contain two or more $-NO_2$ groups, hence *o*-aminotoluene (not having any $-NO_2$ group) is not an explosive. All other three compounds have three $-NO_2$ groups per molecule.

18. (c) The first compound will give azo dye

$H_3C-C_6H_4-N=N-$(naphthyl with OH)

19. (a) Secondary amines are more basic than tertiary amines due to stabilisation of 2° amine by hydrogen bonding with solvent molecule.

20. (b)

21. (b) Benzene $\xrightarrow[333\,K]{HNO_3,\,H_2SO_4}$ Nitrobenzene (NO_2) $\xrightarrow{Cl_2/Fe}$ m-Chloronitrobenzene (NO_2, Cl) $\xrightarrow{\text{reduction}}$ m-Chloroaniline (NH_2, Cl)

(i) In case chlorination is done earlier than nitration, chlorobenzene formed at first step would introduce $-NO_2$ group in ortho-position, not in m-position

(ii) Again if $-NO_2$ group is reduced earlier than the chlorination step, $-NH_2$ group formed on reduction will again introduce –Cl in o-position

22. (d) Proceed backward ; tribromobenzene is produced by boiling compound Z with C_2H_5OH ; Z in turn is obtained by diazotisation of Y, so Y and Z should have $-NH_2$ and $-N_2Cl$ groups respectively, in addition to three Br atoms. Hence X should be $C_6H_5NH_2$

Aniline (X) $\xrightarrow{\text{bromination}}$ 2,4,6-Tribromoaniline (Y) $\xrightarrow[HCl]{NaNO_2}$ 2,4,6-Tribromobenzenediazonium chloride (N_2Cl) (Z) $\xrightarrow[\text{boil}]{C_2H_5OH}$ 1,3,5-Tribromobenzene

23. (a) Acylation occurs in one step only because lone pair of nitrogen is delocalized with acyl group.

$$R-\ddot{N}H-\overset{O}{\overset{\|}{C}}-CH_3 \longleftrightarrow R-\overset{\oplus}{N}H=\overset{O^-}{\overset{|}{C}}-CH_3$$

24. (d) **Hofmann's rule :** When theoretically more than one type of alkenes are possible, the alkene containing least alkylated double bond is formed. Hence

(cyclohexyl with Me, n-Bu, $\overset{+}{N}$(Me)(Et)) $\overset{-}{O}H \xrightarrow{\Delta}$ (cyclohexyl with Me, $\ddot{N}$(Me)(n-Bu)) $+ CH_2=CH_2 + H_2O$

25. (b) The hydrogen attached to nitrogen in sulphonamide is strongly acidic due to the presence of strong electron withdrawing sulphonyl group. Hence, it is soluble in alkali.

26. (b)

27. (a) 1° amines (aliphatic and aromatic) react with $CHCl_3/KOH$ to yield isocyanide (foul smelling). This is known as carbylamine test which is not given by 2° and 3° amines.

28. (b)

29. (c) (a) $C_6H_5-\ddot{N}H_2$ + R effect

the lone pair of electron is less easily available for protonation.

(b) 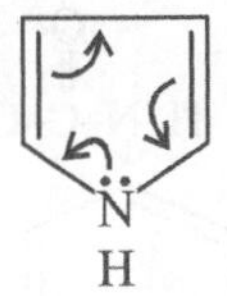 [Pyrrole structure with curved arrows] + R effect

the lone pair of electron is not available for proton.

(c) 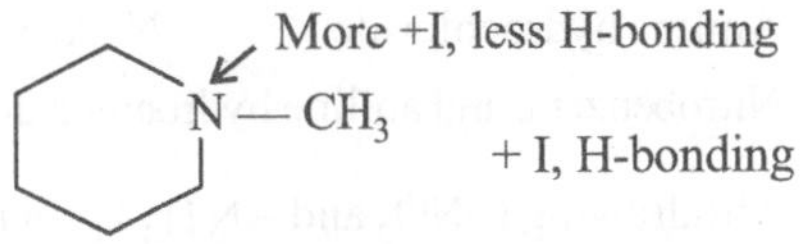 [N-methylpiperidine] N— CH_3: More +I, less H-bonding; + I, H-bonding

+I more preferred than H-bonding, is due to steric hindrance to H-bonding in 1° amine.

(d) 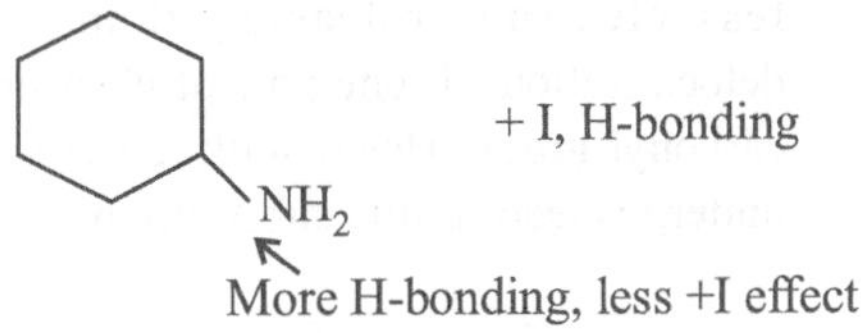 [Cyclohexylamine] NH_2: + I, H-bonding; More H-bonding, less +I effect

Unstable Thus, the correct order is
(II) < (I) < (IV) < (III).

30. **(c)** Aliphatic amines are more basic than aromatic amines. Resonance decreases the basic character due to delocalisation of shared pair of electrons on nitrogen within benzene nucleus.

31. **(d)**

32. **(b)** $\underbrace{R-NH_2}_{\text{Mol.Mass}=16} + CH_3-\overset{\overset{O}{\|}}{C}-Cl \xrightarrow[-HCl]{} \underbrace{R-NH-\overset{\overset{O}{\|}}{C}-CH_3}_{\text{Mol.mass}=58}$

Now since the molecular mass increases by 42 unit as a result of the reaction of one mole of CH_3COCl with one-NH_2 group and the given increase in mass is 210. Hence the number of –NH_2 groups is = 210/42 = 5.

33. **(c)** 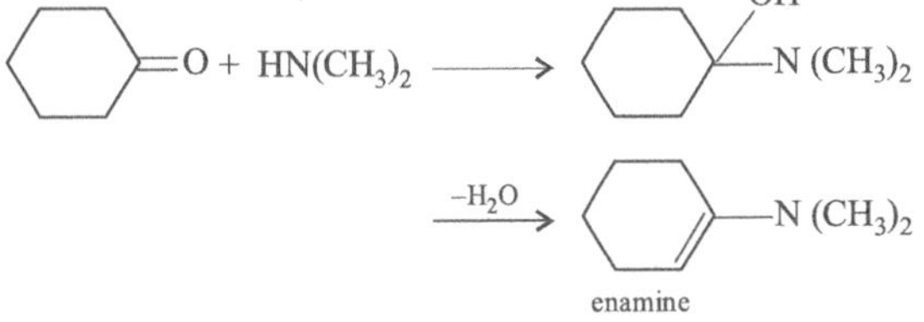 [Cyclohexanone]=O + HN$(CH_3)_2$ ⟶ [Cyclohexane with OH and N$(CH_3)_2$] $\xrightarrow{-H_2O}$ [Cyclohexene]–N$(CH_3)_2$
enamine

34. **(a)** Acetamide is basic due to the presence of lone pair of electrons of N; it is also acidic because its conjugte base shows resonance.

$CH_3-\overset{\overset{O}{\|}}{C}-NH_2 \xrightarrow{\text{base}}$

$CH_3-\overset{\overset{O}{\|}}{C}-\bar{N}H \longleftrightarrow CH_3-\overset{\overset{O^-}{|}}{C}=NH$

(more stable due to –ve charge on O)

∴ Acetamide is neutral. Benzonitrile ($C_6H_5C{\equiv}N$) acts as an electrophile (Lewis acid) due to electron deficiency of C of CN as well as nucleophile (Lewis base) in nature due to presence of lone pair electrons on N; hence it is neutral. Triethyl amine and phenol are basic and acidic in nature respectively.

35. **(c)** Since the organic amino compound on reaction with nitrous acid at low temperature produces an oily nitrosoamine so the organic amino compound is a secondary aliphatic amines.

36. **(a)** $R_2NNO + H_2O \rightarrow R_2NH + HNO_2$

37. **(c)**

38. **(d)** $CH_3C \equiv CH + AgNO_3 \xrightarrow{C_2H_5OH} CH_3C \equiv CAg \downarrow + HNO_3$

$CH_3CHO + 2Cu(OH)_2 \rightarrow CH_3COOH + Cu_2O + 2H_2O$

$\underset{\substack{\text{Insoluble in } H_2O \\ \text{due to no H-bond}}}{C_6H_5COOC_2H_5} + NaOH \xrightarrow{\text{heat}} \underset{\text{(soluble)}}{C_6H_5COONa} + \underset{\text{(soluble)}}{C_2H_5OH}$

$C_6H_5NH_2 + HCl \rightarrow$
$\underset{\text{(soluble)}}{C_6H_5N^+H_3Cl^-} \xrightarrow{NaOH} \underset{\text{(Insoluble)}}{C_6H_5NH_2 \downarrow}$

39. **(d)**

40. **(c)**

41. **(d)** For the preparation of Me_3CNH_2, the required alkyl halide is Me_3CX which will react with potassium phthalimide, a strong base, to form alkene rather than substituted product. For preparing $C_6H_5NH_2$, C_6H_5Cl will be the starting halide in which Cl is non-reactive.

42. **(b)** 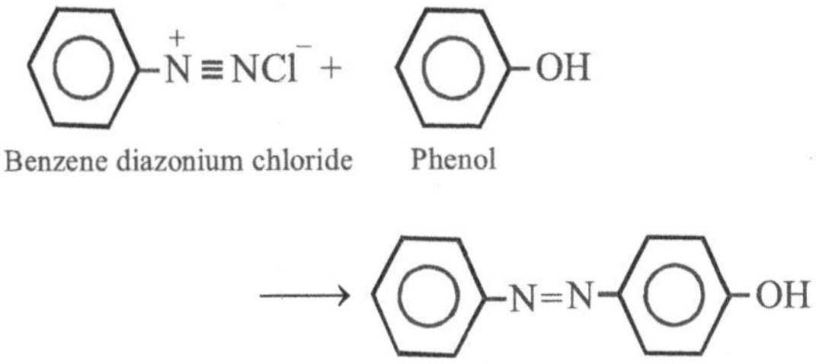 [Benzene]–$\overset{+}{N} \equiv N\overset{-}{Cl}$ + [Benzene]–OH
Benzene diazonium chloride; Phenol

⟶ [Benzene]–N=N–[Benzene]–OH
p-Hydroxyazobenzene (orange dye)

43. (d)

44. (a) $CH_3CH_2Cl \xrightarrow{NaCN} \underset{X}{CH_3CH_2CN} \xrightarrow{Ni/H_2}$

$\underset{Y}{CH_3CH_2CH_2NH_2} \xrightarrow{(CH_3CO)_2O} \underset{Z}{CH_3CH_2CH_2NHCOCH_3}$

45. (b)

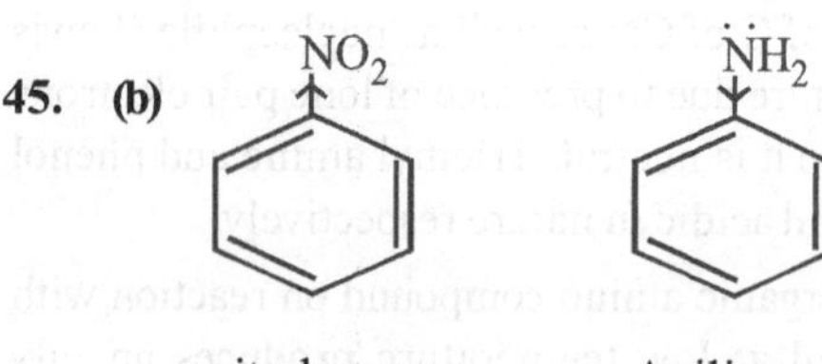

nitrobenzene Aniline

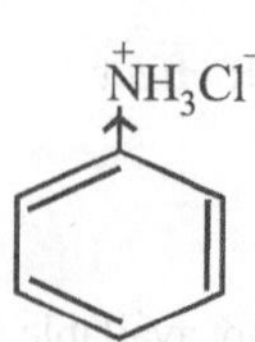

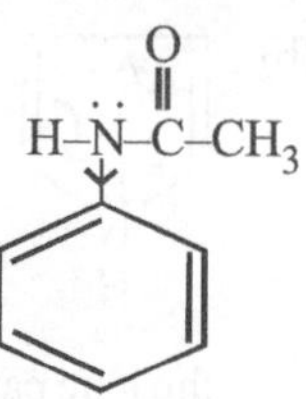

Aniline hydrochloride N- Acetylaniline

Nitrobenzene and aniline hydrochloride have electron-withdrawing ($-NO_2$ and $-\overset{+}{N}H_3$) groups, hence these will undergo electrophilic substitution with difficulty. Aniline and N– acetylaniline (acetanilide) have electron– releasing groups, however $-NHCOCH_3$ is less electron- releasing than $-NH_2$ due to delocalisation of lone pair of electron on N toward carbonyl group. Hence aniline (having $-NH_2$) will undergo electrophilic substitution most easily.

Speed Test-56

1. (c) Chemically amylose is a long unbranched chain with 200-1000 α-D-(+ -glucose units held by C1-C4 glycosidic linkage.
2. (a)
3. (c)
4. (c) Amylose is water soluble component which constitutes about 15-20% of strach. Amylopectin is insoluble in and constitutes about 80-85% of starch.
5. (d) Histidine is an acidic amino acid whereas rest are neutral amino acids.
6. (a) On the basis of structure of guanine and complementary bases present in them, we can say that if the sequence of bases in one strand of DNA is I, then the sequence in the second strand should be II

   A:T:G:C:T:T :G :A I

   T:A:C:G:A:A:C:T II
7. (b) Glucogen is produced by pancreas.
8. (a)
9. (d) The correct structure of thymine is

   Thymine (T)
10. (c) Due to resonance, $-\overset{O}{\overset{\|}{C}}-\ddot{N}H- \longleftrightarrow -\overset{O^-}{\overset{|}{C}}=\overset{+}{N}H-$,

    C – N bond in proteins acquires some double bond character, hence shorter in length.
11. (b) RNA has D (–) – Ribose and the DNA has 2–Deoxy D (–) – ribose as the carbohydrate unit.

    ribose 2-deoxy ribose

    From the structures it is clear that 2nd carbon in DNA do not have OH group.
12. (b) **Molisch's Test :** This is a general test for carbohydrates. One or two drops of alcoholic solution of α-naphthol is added to 2 ml glucose solution. 1 ml of conc. H_2SO_4 solution is added carefully along the sides of the test-tube. The formation of a violet ring at the junction of two liquids confirms the presence of a carbohydrate or sugar.
13. (b) Night blindness is caused by deficiency of vitamin A.
14. (d)

    Deoxyribose-Adenine ... Thymine -Deoxyribose

    Deoxyribose-Guanine ... Cytosine -Deoxyribose

    Deoxyribose-Guanine ... Cytosine -Deoxyribose

    Deoxyribose-Adenine ... Thymine -Deoxyribose

    The hydrogen bonds are formed between the base (shown by dotted lines). Because of size and geometrics of the bases, the only possible pairing in DNA and between G(Guanine) and C(Cytosine) through three H-bonds and between A (Adenine) and T (Thymine) through two H-bonds.
15. (a) Isoelectric point (pH)

    $$= \frac{pK_{a_1} + pK_{a_2}}{2} = \frac{2.34 + 9.60}{2} = 5.97$$
16. (b) The secondary structure of a protein refers to the shape in which a long peptide chain can exist. There are two different conformations of the peptide linkage present in protein, these are α-helix and β-conformation. The α-helix always has a right handed arrangement. In β-conformation all peptide chains are stretched out to nearly maximum extension and then laid side by side and held together by intermolecular hydrogen bonds. The structure resembles the pleated folds of drapery and therefore is known as β-pleated sheet.
17. (c) DNA fingerprinting is same for every cell and cannot be altered by any known treatment.
18. (d) Alitame is an artificial sweetner that is 2,000 times as sweet as sugar.
19. (b) Since sucrose is dextrorotatory while hydrolysis product of sucrose, having equimolar mixture of glucose and fructose, is leovorotatory. Hence the hydrolysed product of sucrose is known as inversion.
20. (a)

    $\xrightarrow[-CH_3COOK]{Aq.KOH}$ Hemiketal $\rightleftharpoons$ (Ring opening)

    ⊕ve silver mirror test $\xleftarrow{\text{Tollen's Reagent}}$

    (a Reducing sugar) α-hydroxy ketone

21. (b)

22. (c) It is found in liver, egg, milk, meat, and fish. Minute amounts are probably present in all animal cells. Peculiarly, unlike other vitamins, B_{12} is found in significant amounts in green plants.

23. (b) 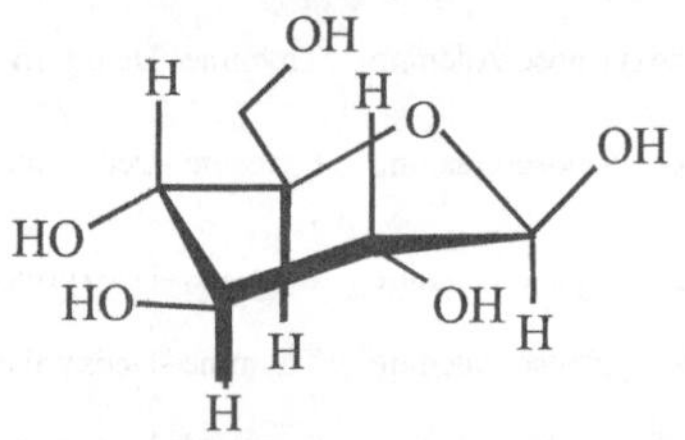 [Structure: β-D-glucopyranose]

It is a β-pyranose hence it is an aldohexose.

24. (c) Glucose is considered as a typical carbohydrate which contains –CHO and –OH group.

25. (c) Vitamin E (Tocopherol) is a fat or oil soluble vitamin . It is present in ghee milk and egg yolk. Deficiency of vitamin E causes loss of sexual power of reproduction and degeneration of muscle fibres in animals.

26. (d) Quaternary structure refers to the overall structure of a multiprotein complex where as primary, secondary and tertiary structure refer to the different structural levels of a single protein.

27. (b) Cyclisation of the open chain structure of D-(+)-glucose has created a new stereocenter at C_1 which explains the existence of two cyclic forms of D-(+)-glucose, namely α– and β–. These two cyclic forms are *diasteromers, such diastereomers which differ only in the configuration of chiral carbon developed on hemiacetal formation* (it is C_1 in glucose and C_2 in fructose) *are called* **anomers** and the hemiacetal carbon (C_1 or C_2) is called the **anomeric carbon.**

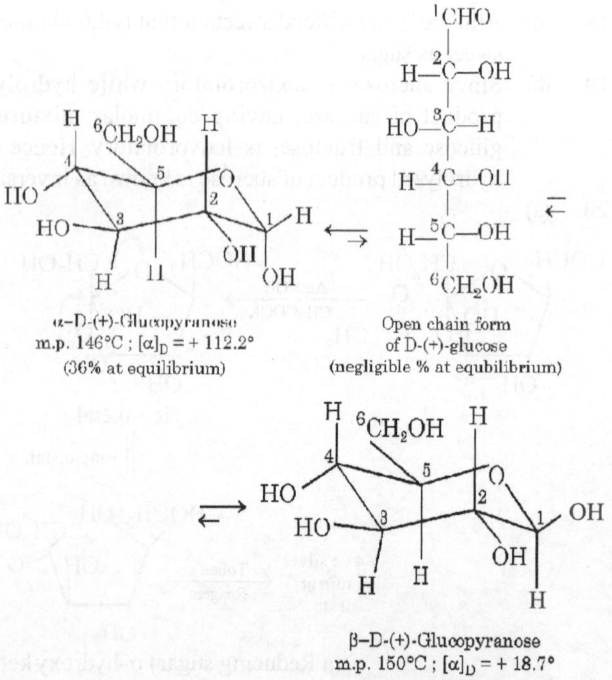

α-D-(+)-Glucopyranose m.p. 146°C ; $[\alpha]_D = +112.2°$ (36% at equilibrium) ⇌ Open chain form of D-(+)-glucose (negligible % at equbilibrium) ⇌ β-D-(+)-Glucopyranose m.p. 150°C ; $[\alpha]_D = +18.7°$ (64% at equilibrium)

28. (b) In DNA and RNA heterocyclic base and phosphate ester are at C_1' and C_5' respectively of the sugar molecule. Each corners is shared by 8 cubes and each face is shared by 2 faces

29. (b) Adrenaline is amine hormone.

30. (d) Zwitter ion contains both +ve and –ve charge. Proton of –COOH group is transferred to the $-NH_2$ group.—NH_3^+ group is acidic since it can donate a proton and $-COO^-$ group is basic since it can accept a proton.

31. (d)

32. (a)

33. (a) Glucose contains an aldehyde group. It is oxidised into acidic group by bromine water and gluconic acid is formed

$$CH_2OH-(CHOH)_4-CHO \xrightarrow{(O)} CH_2OH-(CHOH)_4-COOH$$

$$Br_2 + H_2O \longrightarrow 2HBr + O$$

34. (c) Deficiency of vitamin D causes rickets.

35. (a)

36. (a) CHO–CHOH–$(CHOH)_3$–CH_2OH $\xrightarrow{3PhNHNH_2}$ CH=N.NHPh–CH=N.NHPh–$(CHOH)_3$–CH_2OH + $PhNH_2$ + NH_3

37. (b)

38. (d)

39. (d) Glucose being an aldose responds to Tollen's test while fructose, although a ketose, undergoes rearrangement in presence of basic medium (provided by Tollen's reagent) to form glucose, which then responds to Tollen's test.

40. (b)

41. (b) Hydrogen bonding

42. (c) When the proteins are subjected to the action of heat, mineral acids or alkali, the water soluble form of globular protein changes to water insoluble fibrous protein. This is called denaturation of proteins. During denaturation secondary and tertiary structures of protein destroyed but primary structures remains intact.

43. (a) When antigens enter in to the body cells and destroy them, then antibodies being proteins are synthesised in the body and combine with antigens and destroy these antigens by forming inactive complexes. Therefore antibodies protein destroy antigens.

44. (d) Glucose is aldohexose. Glucose is a monosaccharide, i.e. it can not be hydrolysed further to simple sugars. Oligosaccharides on hydrolysis give 2-10 molecules of monosaccharides.

45. (d) Since sucrose is dextrorotatory while hydrolysis product of sucrose, having equimolar mixture of glucose and fructose, is laevorotatory. Hence the hydrolysed product of sucrose is known as invert sugar and the hydrolysis of sucrose is known as inversion.

Speed Test-57

1. (b) High density polythene is formed when addition polymerisation of ethene takes place in a hydrocarbon solvent in presence of catalyst such as Ziegler-Natta catalyst.
2. (d) Nylon and cellulose, both have intermolecular hydrogen bonding, polyvinyl chloride has dipole-dipole interactions, while natural rubber has van der Waal forces which are weakest.
3. (b) Vinyl alcohol, $CH_2=CHOH$, monomer of polyvinyl alcohol exists mainly as CH_3CHO; hence polyvinyl alcohol is best prepared by the alkaline hydrolysis of polyvinyl acetate which in turn is prepared by the polymerisation of vinyl acetate
4. (d) Silk is protein fibre. Dacron is polyester fibre and Nylon-6, 6 is polyamide fibre.
5. (d) Nylon–6 can be manufactured from

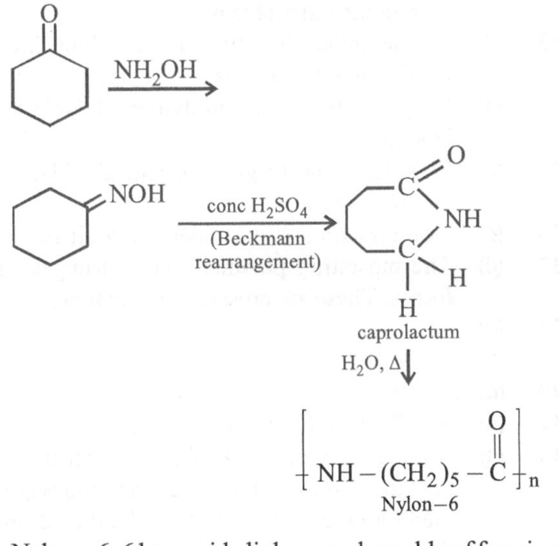

Cyclohexanone $\xrightarrow{NH_2OH}$ Cyclohexanone oxime (=NOH) $\xrightarrow[\text{(Beckmann rearrangement)}]{\text{conc } H_2SO_4}$ caprolactum $\xrightarrow{H_2O,\ \Delta}$ $\left[NH-(CH_2)_5-\overset{O}{\overset{||}{C}} \right]_n$

Nylon–6

6. (b) Nylon – 6, 6 has amide linkage and capable of forming hydrogen bonding.
7. (d) Copolymer of adipic acid and hexamethylene diamine.

$$\underset{\text{Adipic acid}}{n\,HOOC(CH_2)_4COOH} + \underset{\text{Hexamethylene diamine}}{nH_2N(CH_2)_6NH_2} \rightarrow \underset{\text{Nylon 6, 6}}{\left(\overset{O}{\overset{||}{C}}-(CH_2)_4-\overset{O}{\overset{||}{C}}-NH-(CH_2)_6-NH \right)_n}$$

8. (b) Thermosetting plastics consist of chain molecules which are chemically bonded, or cross-linked, with each other when heated. When thermosetting plastics cross-link, the molecules create a permanent, 3-D network that can be considered one giant molecule.
9. (b) Elastomers are the polymers having very weak intermolecular forces of attraction between the polymer chain. The weak forces permit the polymer to be stretched.
10. (b) $\underset{\text{adipic acid}}{nHOOC(CH_2)_4COOH} + \underset{\text{Hexamethylene diamine}}{nH_2N(CH_2)_6NH_2}$

$$\xrightarrow[\text{Polymerisation}]{525K} \underset{\text{Nylon 6, 6}}{[-\overset{O}{\overset{||}{C}}-(CH_2)_4-\overset{O}{\overset{||}{C}}-NH-(CH_2)_6-NH-]_n}$$

11. (b) Buna – N is a copolymer of butadiene ($CH_2=CH-CH=CH_2$) and acrylonitrile ($CH_2=CHCN$).
12. (b) Nylon-6, 6 is a polyamide having –CONH–; oxygen of CO of amide linkage is linked to H of NH of the other –CONH– linkage
13. (a) Formula of the monomer indicated in bracket, $(CH_3)_2C=CH_2$, corresponds to 2-methylpropene
14. (b) Nylon-6,6 is a polyamide, hence it has only –CONH– linkage and no –COO– linkage
15. (c)
16. (d)
17. (d) Phenol and formaldehyde undergo condensation polymerisation under two different conditions to give a cross linked polymer called bakelite.

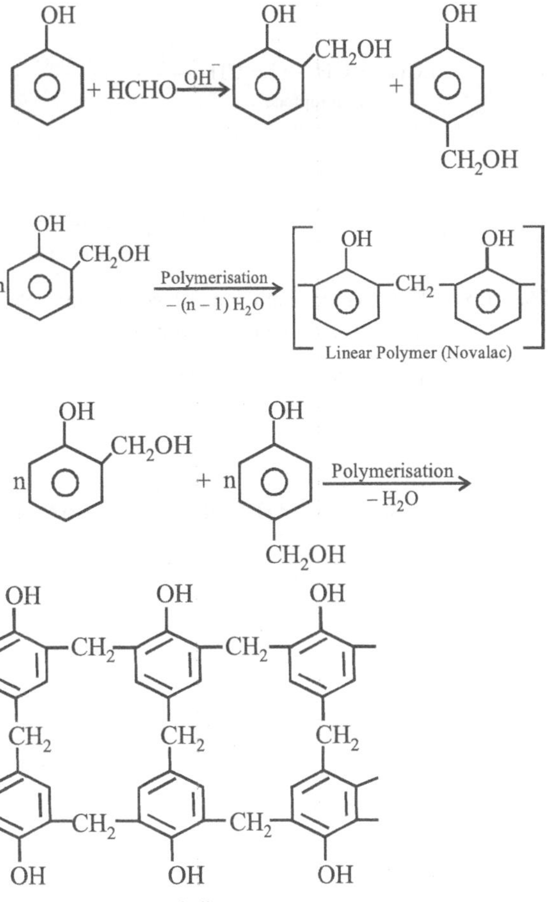

Phenol + HCHO $\xrightarrow{OH^-}$ o-hydroxybenzyl alcohol (CH_2OH) + p-hydroxybenzyl alcohol (CH_2OH)

n o-hydroxybenzyl alcohol $\xrightarrow[-(n-1)H_2O]{\text{Polymerisation}}$ [phenol–CH_2–phenol] Linear Polymer (Novalac)

n o-hydroxybenzyl alcohol + n p-hydroxybenzyl alcohol $\xrightarrow[-H_2O]{\text{Polymerisation}}$ cross-linked network of phenol rings (OH) joined by CH_2 bridges

Bakelite

18. (a) Polymerisation starts either by condensation or addition reactions between monomers. Condensation polymers are formed by the combination of monomers with the elimination of simple molecules. Where as the addition polymers are formed by the addition together of the molecules of the monomer or monomers to form a large molecule without elimination of any thing.

19. (a) Melamine plastic crockery is a copolymer of HCHO and melamine.

20. (c) Nylon-6, 6 is a general name for all synthetic fibres forming polyamides.

21. (d)

22. (a) Addition of monomers follows isoprene rule

$$(CH_3)_2C=CH_2 + (CH_3)_2C=CH_2 \rightarrow$$

H T H T

$$\overset{\oplus}{C}(CH_3)_2-CH_2-C(CH_3)_2-CH_2$$

23. (d) 24. (c)

25. (d) Neoprene is an addition polymer of isoprene.

$$\underset{\text{Chloroprene}}{nCH_2=CH-\overset{Cl}{\overset{|}{C}}=CH_2} \xrightarrow{O_2 \text{ or peroxides}} \underset{\text{Neoprene}}{\left(CH_2-\overset{Cl}{\overset{|}{C}}=CH-CH_2\right)_n}$$

26. (a) The polymer of ethylene glycol and tere-phthalic acid is known as **terylene** or **dacron**.

$$\underset{\text{Ethylene glycol}}{n(HO-CH_2-CH_2-OH)} + \underset{\text{Terephthalic acid}}{n\left(HOOC-C_6H_4-COOH\right)} \longrightarrow$$

$$\underset{\text{Terylene or Dacron}}{\left(OCH_2CH_2-O-\overset{O}{\overset{\|}{C}}-C_6H_4-\overset{O}{\overset{\|}{C}}\right)_n} + nH_2O$$

It is a **condensation polymer.**

[**Note:** Now a days dimethyl terepthalate is used instead of terephthalic acid. This is due to the fact that terephthalic acid is non-volatile and very slightly soluble in most of the solvents. Dimethyl terepthalate on the other hand, can be purified by distillation very easily]. Thus, option (a) is correct.

27. (c) Neoprene is a homopolymer of chloroprene.

28. (c)

29. (a) Dacron is a polyester and is the condensation polymer of ethylene glycol and terephthalic acid. It is a crease resistant.

30. (a) Molecules of a polymer, being large in size, scatter light.

31. (c) Polythene is a linear polymer

32. (c) Biodegradable polymers are manufactured because conventional polymers are quite resistant to the environmental degradation which leads to accumulation of polymeric solid waste materials causing acute environmental problems.

33. (d) As the amide density along the chain increases the melting point increases.

34. (a) Butyl rubber is a copolymer of isobutylene and isoprene.

35. (c) Ebonite is a hard highly vulcanized rubber, containing 20-30%, rubber

36. (d) Orlon is a trade name of polyacrylonitrile

37. (d) Thermosetting polymers have strongest molecular forces. These are crosslinked polymers.

38. (d)

39. (b) A – V; B – I; C – III; D – II

40. (d)

41. (a) A – III; B – I; C – II; D – V; E – IV

42. (d) Number of hydrogen bonds is greater in polymer (1) than in (2) as the density of amide bond is greater in (1) therefore the chain links to each other strongly in (1) than in (2) hence (1) melts at higher temperature.

43. (a) Bakelite is used for making phonograph records.

44. (c)

45. (b)

Speed Test-58

1. (a) These drugs induce sleep and are habit forming common example of hypnotic drugs are Luminal and Saconal.
2. (b) p-chloro-m-xylenol is phenolic antibacterial deodorants.
3. (b) Aluminium salts present in deodorants act as antibacterial agents.
4. (b)
5. (a) Bactericidal are the drugs that kills bacteria. Ofloxacin works by stopping the growth of bacteria. This antibiotic treats only bacterial infections.
6. (b) It is acetyl salicylic acid i.e., aspirin, analgesic and antipyretic.
7. (d) Sucrose is natural sweetner.
8. (d)
9. (a) Phenelzine is an antidepressant, while others are antacids.
10. (c) Any oils which are good for eating or cooking, can be used in making soap. One of the best is said to be coconut oil. Groundnut, Shea butter, Cocoa butter, Sun flower and many other vegetable oils are also used.
11. (d) Cetyltrimethyl ammonium bromide possess germicidal properties. Thus it is used as a cationic detergent in hair conditioners.
12. (d)
13. (a) [structure: HO, Cl, O, HO, OH, Cl, O, OH, Cl, O] is sucralose.
14. (c) Diphenhydramine is used as antihistamine.
15. (d) The mixture of chloroxylenol and terpenol is dettol which is used as antiseptic.
16. (a) Whiteware possesses good strength, translucency, and low porosity.
17. (a) Antiseptic drugs cause destruction of micro-organism that produce septic disease e.g. Dettol, Savlon, Boric acid, Phenol, Iodoform, $KMnO_4$ and some dye such as methylene blue, genation violet.
18. (b) Bithional is a well known antiseptic, added in soaps to reduce odours produced by bacterial decomposition of organic matter of skin.

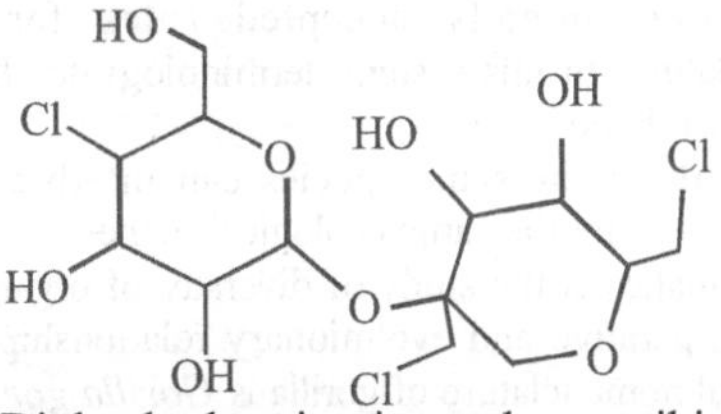

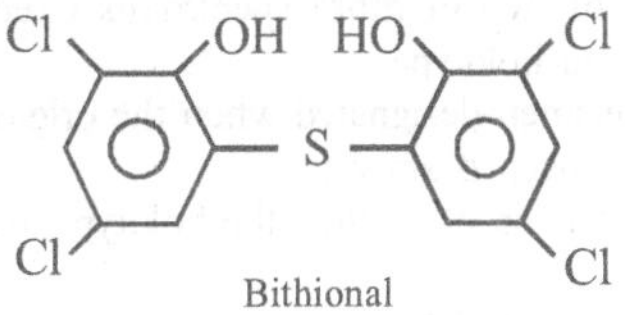

   [structure: Cl, OH, HO, Cl, S, Cl, Cl]

   Bithional
19. (b) It is the known structure of Penicillin G
20. (a) Pheromones are the chemical substances used by insects for communication.
21. (a) The aminoglycosides are among the oldest antibiotics.
22. (c) Non- ionic detergent is formed when stearic acid reacts with polyethylene glycol.
23. (b) For statement (ii), drug which brings major change in the treatment of hyperacidity was histamine. For statement (iv), antidepressant drugs like iproniazid and phenelzine inhibit the enzymes which catalyse the degradation of noradrenaline when the enzyme is inhibited, this important neurotransmitter is slowly metabolised and can activate its receptor for longer periods of time, thus counteracting the effect of depression.
24. (b)
25. (d) Aspirin is an non-narcotics analgesic.
26. (a)
27. (d) Neither any of the substances among given options possess nutritive value.
28. (c) The antifertility drugs are those chemical compounds which prevent pregnancy in woman. These, drugs controls the menstrual cycle and ovulation and so used as birth control drug or contraceptives.
29. (c) The most widely used domestic detergent is the sodium dodecyl benzene sulphonate (SDS).

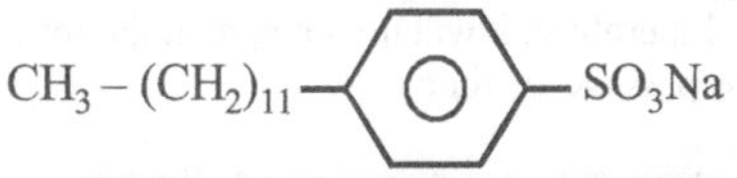

   $CH_3 - (CH_2)_{11} - C_6H_4 - SO_3Na$

   (Sodium dodecyl benzene sulphonate)
30. (c) Sulphonamides act as antimicrobials.
31. (a) Butylated hydroxy anisole (BHA) is an antioxidant.
32. (c) For statement (ii), 2–3% solution of iodine in alcohol water mixture is known as tincture of iodine. For statement (iii), SO_2 in very low concentrations are used as disinfectants.
33. (d)
34. (c) Aspartame is stable under cold conditions.
35. (b) Zinc salts in deodorants act as astringents and antiseptics.
36. (c) Structural features of soaps and detergents are almost same except that the polar end in detergents is $-OSO_3^-Na^+$ while in soaps polar end is $-COO^-Na^+$. Detergents have an advantage over soaps that its polar end sulphate and sulphonate retain their efficiency in hard water, since the corresponding Ca and Mg salts are soluble. Being salts of strong acids, they yield neutral solution, in contrast, to the soaps, which being salts of weak acids yield slightly alkaline solutions.
37. (c) Broad spectrum antibiotics act on different antigens.
38. (a) Novalgin is most widely used as analgesic. Analgesics are pain releiving
39. (c) An antipyretic is a drug which is responsible for lowering the temperature of the feverish organism to normal but has no effect on normal temperature states.
40. (b) Dilute solutions of boric acid and hydrogen peroxide are weak antiseptics.
41. (c)
42. (c)

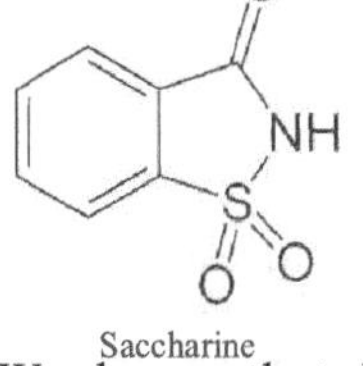

   [structure: O, NH, S, O, O]

   Saccharine
43. (c) We know that N-acetyl-para-aminophenol (or paracetamol) is an antipyretic which can also be used as an analgesic to relieve pain.
44. (b) 45. (c)

HINTS & SOLUTIONS (BIOLOGY – Chapter-wise Tests)

Speed Test-59

1. **(b)** There are several factors and processes which differentiate living beings with non-living beings like reproduction, respiration, growth, etc. But among them reproduction is the only characteristic which differentiates without any exception, living being from non-living beings.
2. **(a)** *Panthera tigris* is the scientific name of tiger.
3. **(a)** 4. **(b)** 5. **(c)**
6. (a) The common characteristics between brinjal and wheat can be observed maximum at the level of their division.
7. **(c)** Cytotaxonomy is the study of chromosome number, size and behaviour.
8. **(b)** The original scientific names were taken from Latin and Greek languages. New names are now derived either from Latin language or are latinised. This is because Latin language is dead and therefore, it will not change in the form or spellings with the passage of time.
9. **(d)**
10. **(b)** The number of similar characters of categories decreases from lowest rank to highest rank in a taxonomic hierarchy. Out of the given categories i.e., family, class, genus and species, the class being the highest category possesses the least similar characters.
11. **(c)** Hierarchy of categories is the classification of organisms in a definite sequence of categories (taxonomic categories) in a descending order starting from kingdom and reaching upto species or an ascending order from species to kingdom. The number of similar characters of categories decreases from lowest rank (species) to highest rank (kingdom). The taxonomic hierarchy includes seven obligate categories-kingdom, division or phylum, class, order, family, genus and species. Some subcategories like tribe, subfamily, subspecies are also used whenever required.

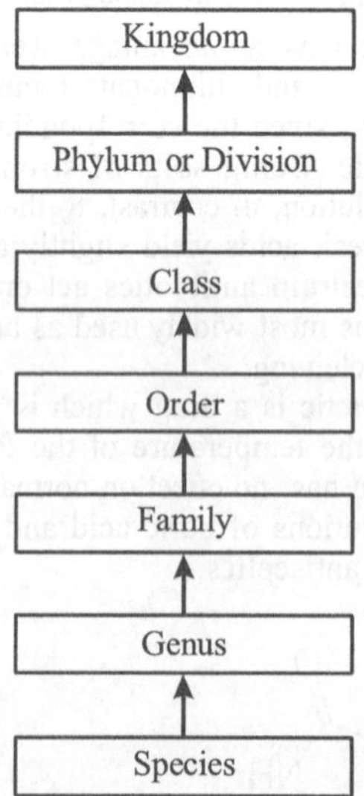

Fig: Taxonomical hierarchy showing arrangement in ascending order

12. **(c)** Teleology is the unscientific explanation of phenomena, while study of vestigeal organs is known as dysteleology.
13. **(d)** International code for Zoological Nomenclature is responsible for setting rules for naming of animals and resolution of nomenclature problems.
14. **(b)** When external temperature is warm, the superficial blood vessels dilate to lose the body heat.
15. **(c)** The biological species concept was formulated by Theodosium Dobzhansky and Ernst Mayr. According to this concept "A species is a reproductive community of populations whose members can interbreed with each other but not with the members of other species.
16. **(b)** Carolus Von Linnaeus in his book Genera Plantanum made use of the artificial system of classification. He distinguished between the natural and artificial systems. He used the binomial nomenclature system and classified organisms into genius and species.
17. **(a)** Species is the lowest taxonomic category. Class is a category made of one or more related orders possessing similar correlated characters, Family is composed of one to many related genera. Division comprises of several related classes.
18. **(d)** Taxon is a grouping of organisms of any level in hierarchy of classification based on some common characteristic.
19. **(c)** Species is the lowest or basic taxonomic category comprising of one or more natural population of individuals that interbreed freely.
20. **(b)** Carolus Linnaeus system of classification is artificial.
21. **(a)** Carolus Von Linnaeus wrote the book systema Naturae.
22. **(d)** Benthem and Hooker system was published well before there were internationally accepted rules for botanical nomenclature. In this system, terminology for families was not so as it is now.
23. **(c)** Individuals of the same species can interbreed. No two individuals share the same ecological niche.
24. **(d)** Biosystematics is the study of diversity of organism and all their comparative and evolutionary relationships.
25. **(b)** Trinomial nomenclature of gorilla is *Gorilla gorilla gorilla.*
26. **(a)** Isotype refers to the duplicate of holotype. When the original material is missing, the new nomenclatural type is termed as neotype. When there is no holotype, any of two or more specimens cited by the author is named as syntype.
27. **(c)** Carnivora and Insectivora are two orders of mammals. Mastigophora is a class of Protozoa. Any plant-eating animal can be termed as a herbivore.
28. **(c)** Many related families can be grouped under an order.
29. **(d)** NBRI is a research institute situated in Lucknow that is engaged in the field of taxonomy and Modern biology.
30. **(c)** Holotype- a specimen on which the original description of the species is based.
Syntype- any of two or more specimens cited by author when there is no holotype.
Neotype- a specimen designated when the original types are known to have been destroyed.
Paratype- a specimen other than the holotype available with the author.
Isotype- a duplicate of the type.
31. **(a)** Chemotaxonomy is the method of biological classifi cation based on similarities in the structure of certain compounds among the organisms being classified.
32. **(b)** Tautonym is the name in which both genus and species epithet are identical
33. **(c)** Lectotype is a specimen later selected to serve as the single type specimen for species originally described from a set of syntypes.

34. (d) Neotype is a type specimen that is selected subsequent to the description of a species to replace a pre-existing type that has been cost or destroyed.
35. (a) Dried specimens are poisoned not by DDT but by others like formaldehyds.
36. (a) Reproduction is a characteristic feature of all living organisms.
37. (b) Animals in lower hierarchy possess more characters in common.
38. (c) Phylum, class and family are classificatory units.
39. (c) Homonym is a name for a taxon that is identical in spelling to another such name, that belongs to a different taxon.
40. (a) Autonyms are automatically created names as regulated by the International code of Nomenclature for algae, fungi, and plants.
41. (d) A binomial name in which the specific name repeats the generic.
42. (b) The most important process for formation of new species is reproductive isolation as this prevents interbreeding in between members of a population, thus giving rise to new species.
43. (c) Two or more species which are reproductively isolated from each other but are morphologically quite similar are known as sibling species. Sympatric species are developed due to reproductive isolation and occur in over lapping or same area of geographical distribution. Parapatric species are developed in adjacent geographical areas meeting in very narrow regions of overlap.
44. (b) Members of same species form population and members of different species form community.
45. (d) Exobiology is the study of possible extra-terrestrial life.

Speed Test-60

1. (b) 2. (d)
3. (c) Cyanobacteria, chlorophyll a, PS I and II.
4. (d)
5. (c) Vegetative phase-animal-like and reproductive phase- plant-like.
6. (c) Desmids i.e golden algae belongs to group chrysophytes. These are found in freshwater as well as marine environment.
7. (a)
8. (c) T_2 phage consists of linear ds DNA.
9. (b) Cell wall is absent in Mycoplasma.
10. (d) Non-motile spores, saprophytic protists.
11. (c) Eubacteria can be differentiated from archaebacteria and bacteria on the basis of cell wall. Eubacteria possess true cell wall, made up of NAM and NAG i.e. N-acetyl muramic acid and N-acetyl glucoseamine. Cell wall of archaebacteria is made up of N-acetyl talosaminuric acid.
12. (d) Pathogen of cholera is *Vibrio cholerae* bacterium. Cholera is transmitted by contaminated water. Typhoid or enteric fever spreads through contaminated water in which bacterium *Salmonella typhi* is present. Citrus canker and crown gall are bacterial disease of plants caused by *Xanthomonas citri* and *Agrobacterium tumefaciens* respectively.
13. (a) Cyanobacteria or blue-green algae are Gram + photosynthetic prokaryotes which perform oxygenic photosynthesis. Photosynthetic pigments include chlorophyll *a*, carotenoids and phycobilins. Cyanobacteria are classified under kingdom Monera. Cyanobacterial cell structure is typically prokaryotic – one envelope organisation with peptidogolycan wall, naked DNA, 70S ribosomes and absence of membrane bound structure like endoplasmic reticulum, mitochondria, golgi bodies, plastids, lysosomes, sap vacuoles. The outer part of the protoplast, called chromoplasm, contains a number of photosynthetic thylakoids.
14. (d) Saprophytic bacteria are free living bacteria which obtain their food from organic remains, plant and animal origin. Aerobic breakdown of organic compounds is known as decay. In nature saprophytic bacteria alongwith saprotrophic fungi are the decomposers of organic remains.
15. (a) Diatoms are very important photosynthesizers. About half of all the organic matter synthesized in the world is believed to be produced by them. Diatoms are probably the most numerous of all plants like protists. Because of this abundance, they are one of the most important primary producers of the sea. There are about 5,500 species of diatoms, mainly marine. The diatoms constitute an important phytoplankton component of the oceans.
16. (c) Fungi is a large kingdom of over 100,000 species. They are achlorophyllous, heterotrophic, spore-forming, non-vascular, eukaryotic organisms which often contain chitin or fungal cellulose in their walls and possess glycogen as food reserve. They are cosmopolitan in occurrence being present in air, water, soil, over and inside animals and plants.
17. (d) Virus is an obligate parasite and is inert outside the host cell. An inert virus outside host is called virion.
18. (d) Monera is the kingdom of all prokaryotes and includes bacteria, blue green algae (cyanobacteria) and archae- bacteria- a group of ancient bacteria kingdom. Protista includes slime unicellular and colonial eukaryotes. The important members are diatoms, dinoflagellates, euglenoids, alone moulds and protozoans. Fungi the kingdom of multicellular or multinucleate heterophyllous and spore producing eukaryotic organisms like *Rhizopus* mildews, mushroom etc. Kingdom plantae includes all coloured multicellular photosynthetic organisms (plants).
19. (c) Viruses that get integrated with the bacterial host genome are called Lysogenic. Lysozymes are present in the saliva and are antibacterial agents. Lipolytic enzymes are the enzymes which catalyse breakdown (lysis) of fats (Lipids).
20. (a) Phenetic classification is purely based on appearances. Phylogenetic classifiaction is based on ancestral lineage. Karyotaxonomy is based on DNA characteristics. Morphotaxonomy involves morphological characters.
21. (d) Biological classification is the scientific arrangement of organisms in a hierarchical series of groups and subgroups on the basis of similarities and differences in their traits. It helps in building evolutionary pathways and in identifying new organisms.
22. (c) Artificial system of classification is based on comparison of on or a few characters. Phylogenetic system of classification indicates the evolutionary or phylogenetic relationship of organisms.
23. (b) The five kingdom classification is a mode of classification based on the following criteria.
   - Complexity of cell structure
   - Complexity of body structure
   - Modes of nutrition
   - Ecological life styles
   - Phylogenetic relationship
24. (c) Phylogenetic system of classification is a system indicating the evolutionary or phylogenetic relationship of organisms.
25. (a) Bacteria are prokaryotes which are grouped under Monera. Protista is a kingdom of unicellular eukaryotes. Fungi is a kingdom of multicellular spore-producing eukaryotes. Plantae are photosynthetic eukaryotes.
26. (a) Retroviruses have RNA as the genetic material and hence they exhibit reverse transcription whereby DNA is synthesized on RNA template. They have reverse transcriptase as the enzyme.

27. (b) Four criteria are : (i) complexity of cell, (ii) complexity of organism, (iii) mode of nutrition and (iv) major ecological role
28. (b) First phylogenetic classification was given by Eichler but that was partially phylogenetic and first true phylogenetic classification was given by Engler and Prantl.
29. (a) *Taenia*, commonly known as tapewom is not a protist, it belongs to phylum Platyhelminthes (Kingdom Animalia)
30. (c)
31. (b) Physiological characters
32. (c) During the origin of life, the first organisms evolved were chemoheterotrophs. They obtained the organic material from outside which they utilized in energy production and synthesis of their own organic material.
33. (d) Bacteria posses various forms and shapes and are of 4 different types - coccus (round), bacillus (rod shaped), vibrio (comma shaped) and spirillum (spiral like cork screw).
34. (c) Slime moulds in the division of myxomycota have spores that develop into flagellated gametes.
35. (b) While working at the Rockefeller Institute, Brown reported isolation of a PPLO from human arthritic joint tissue in 1938. In discussing the significance of this observation, Brown reported successful treatment of arthritic patients in 1949 with a new antibiotic called aureomycin.
36. (c)
37. (c) *Saccharomyces cervisiae* is a yeast used in making bread (Baker's yeast) and commercial production of ethanol. *Paramecium* & *Plasmodium* are of animal kingdom while *Pencillium* is a fungi. Lichen is composite organism formed from the symbiotic association of an algae and a fungus. *Nostoc* & *Anabaena* are examples of kingdom monera.
38. (a) 39. (a) 40. (b) 41. (b) 42. (a)
43. (a)
44. (b) The correct labeling in the figures of bacterial cell and *Nostoc* are - A- cell wall, B - cell membranes, C - DNA, D- heterocysts, E - mucilaginous sheath.
45. (a) A - Cocci (spherical), B - Bacilli (rod shaped), C - Spirilla (spiral), D - Vibrio (comma shaped). These are all the shapes of the bacteria.

Speed Test-61

1. (b) Reserve food in red algae (Rhodophyceae) is floridean starch. In green algae (Chlorophyceae), reserve food is starch. In brown algae Phaeophyceae, reserve food is laminarin and mannitol. In Cyanophyceae, reserve food is cyanophycean starch.
2. (a) Peat moss is another name for *Sphagnum*. It is also known as famine food in China.
3. (b) Well developed vascular system is present in the members of pteridophytes but absent in mosses as the plant body is sporophyte which is distinguished into true root, stem and leaves.
4. (c) The leaves appear green because of the pigment chlorophyll which does not absorb green light rather reflects it back.
5. (b) In chlorophyceae, sexual reproduction takes place by all the three processes :
Isogamy – fusion of morphologically and physiologically similar gametes. Anisogamy – morphologically similar but physiologically dissimilar gametes. Oogamy – fusing gametes are dissimilar in all respect.
6. (d) *Azolla* has been used as a green manure crop in Vietnam and China for centuries. The ability of *Azolla* to shade out weeds in wetland rice and taro has been noted by farmers and researchers since the early 20th century.
7. (a) *Rafflesia* or Corpse flower is a total root parasite. It obtains the total nourishment from the root of the host plant. Its flowers only come out of the host plant and they have a diameter of 1 m and weight around 10 kg.
8. (a)
9. (b) *Laminaria* (kelp) and *Fucus* (rock weed) are marine algae. They are the members of class- phaeophyceae (brown) algae.
10. (b) Algae *Spirulina* is one of the richest sources of protein, containing 40–50 percent crude protein on dry weight basis which under favourable condition may reach upto 70 percent. So, the people recovering from long illness are advised to take it in the diet.
11. (b) The membrane surrounding a lysosome allows the digestive enzymes to work at the 4.5 pH they require. They are created by the addition of hydrolytic enzymes to early endosomes from the Golgi apparatus.
12. (d) 13. (a) 14. (c)
15. (a) Statement (i) and (ii) are correct.
Riccia is liverwort in which simplest sporophyte consists of capsule only while *Polytrichum* is moss in which sporophyte consists of foot, seta & capsule. *Volvox* is a fresh water green colonial alga. Reproduction is both sexual and asexual. Sexual reproduction is oogamous. Slime moulds are consumer decomposer protists. They possess characters of plants (cellulosic cell wall), animals (phagotrophic nutrition) and fungi (spores).
16. (d)
17. (d)
(a) Gametophyte of bryophytes bears protonemal & leafy stage.
(b) In gymnosperm female gametophyte is not free living.
(c) They are present in *Marchantia* or which is a bryophyte.
(d) Origin of seed habit started in pteridophyte *Selaginaella.*
18. (d) 19. (b) 20. (a) 21. (a) 22. (d)
23. (a) 24. (b) 25. (d) 26. (b)
27. (a) Prothallus of pteridophytes is free-living, mostly photosynthetic small but multicellular and inconspicuous.
28. (d)
- Psilopsida – *Psilotum* – rootless
- Sphenopsida – *Equisetum* – Strobilus
- Lycopsida – *Lycopodium* – Homosporous
- Lycopsida – *Selaginella* – Heterosporous

29. (a) Angiosperms are highly evolved and well adapted land plants. They have both vessels and tracheids in xylem for better conduction of water. Roots are modified into tap roots, adventitious roots, pneumatophores etc. to suit the desired climate.
Sex organs are highly developed, sporophylls are organised into flowers and the flowers are highly coloured or modified to attract pollinators ar different times and places. Insect pollination is more prevalent because it is more efficient and leads to less wastage of pollen grains as compared to wind pollination. So the flowers are made attractive to attract a variety of insects. Seed are more protected as they are enclosed inside a fruit.
All these adaptations have made angiosperms more adaptative in diverse habitats.
30. (d) Tracheophyta are those plants which possess conducting or vascular tissue, xylem and phloem. Xylem transports water and minerals while phloem conducts organic food. Tracheophytes include pteridophytes, gymnosperms and angiosperms.

31. (c) Nearly 50% of total carbon dioxide fixation of photosynthesis of world is carried out by algae.
Photosynthesis by algae releases oxygen in the immediate aquatic environment. It is essential for respiration of aquatic life. Algae are primary producers of food in large bodies of fresh, brackish and sea water.

32. (d) In bryophytes, the zygote develops into a multicellular, undifferentiated structure called embryo. The embryo, within venter of archegonium, by further segmentation and differentiation finally develops into a full fledged sporophyte called sporogonium.

33. (d)

34. (d) The gymnosperms are comparatively more ancient than the angiosperms in evolutionary terms. Most of the gymnosperms have now become extinct and the group is presently represented by only 900 living species. The living gymnosperms are widely distributed in the cold climates where snow is the source of water. *Cycas* and *Ginkgo* are referred to as living fossils.

35. (d) In gymnosperms, pteridophytes and angiosperms, the sporophytic phase is dominant and the gametophytic phase is dependent on sporophyte.

36. (b) In diplontic life cycle, the dominant free living phase is the diploid (2n). Sporophyte is photosynthetic. The gametophytic phase is represented by single to few-celled haploid gametophyte e.g., all seed-bearing plants i.e., gymnosperms and angiosperms.

37. (d) Algae and fungi are grouped under thallophyta. Bryophytes are non vascular embryophytes having an independent gametophyte and parasitic sporophyte.

38. (a) Angiosperms have adapted themeslves to all kinds of habitat-terrestial, aquatic, tropical, deciduous and alpine. Self pollination is seen in very few angiosperms. Production of large number of seeds ensure that at least some will germinate. Not all plants have been domesticated by man.

39. (d) Blue-green algae which grow in hot water springs (at about 70°C) are *Oscillatoria terebriformis*, *Oscillatoria brevis* etc. These blue-green algae are also called thermophytes. The temperature tolerance of these algae is due to the presence of homopolar bonds in their proteins.

40. (b) *Cladophora* is an autotrophic and filamentous algae which occurs in fresh as well as in marine water.

41. (a) The pyrenoids are small spherical protein bodies surrounded by starch deposition. They are found singly or in numbers embedded in the chloroplast of many algae and bryophytes.

42. (c) Phycocyanin pigment is found in blue-green algae (myxophycean algae). The reserve food material is in the form of cyanophycean starch.

43. (c) *Cephaleuros virescens* grows as a parasite on the leaves of tea and causes red rust of tea. It is the common intercellular parasitic algae of chlorophyceae.

44. (b)

45. (b)

Speed Test-62

1. (b) The terms Porifera was given by Grant, the phylum includes animals with pores in their body. Its classification based on skeleton or spicules.

2. (c) Chordates are featured by the presence of the following characters : Notochord (cephalic or head region), Pharyngeal gill silts, Postanal tail.

3. (b) Lampreys and hagfishes are unusual, jawless fish that comprise the order Cyclostomata, so named because of the circular shape of the mouth.

4. (d)

5. (a) Aschelminthes is bilaterally symmetrical and triploblastic. These are mostly aquatic, free living or parasitic. Their body is three layered which is ectoderm, mesoderm and endoderm.

6. (c)

7. (c) Characteristic of phylum-Annelida is pseudocoelomate. Pseudocoelomate is any invertebrate animal whose body cavity is a pseudocoel, a cavity between the gut and the outer body wall derived from a persistent blastocoel, rather than a true coelom. Pseudocoelomate animals include the Rotifera and Nematoda.

8. (c) Mammals have 12 pairs of cranial nerves.

9. (b)

10. (d) Poison glands of snake are modified parotid salivary gland.

11. (c)

12. (a) All sponges are marine and have collared cells without any exception. Sponges are animals of the phylum Porifera. They are multicellular organisms which have bodies full of pores and channels allowing water to circulate through them, consisting of jelly-like substance sandwiched between two thin layers of cells.

13. (b) 14. (b) 15. (c) 16. (c) 17. (a)

18. (c)

19. (d) Annelids are first to evolve true metameric segmentation. They are present in embryo as well as in adults. They are present both in ectoderm as well as in mesoderm and are repetitive.

20. (c) Presence of coelom posses a problem for circulation of oxygen and nutrients.

21. (c) Birds belong to class Aves. Bats belong to class Mammalia. Both are warm blooded, endothermic and maintain a constant body temperature. Non-vascular air sacs connected to lungs to supplement respiration are present only in birds not bats.

22. (d) In the molluscs mantle is a loose fold of skin, not concerned with locomotion.

23. (a) In birds syrinx is the sound box.

24. (c) *Tubifex* is blood worm, it is an annelid.

25. (c) In all chordates notochord is present at some stage of embryonic development. Hemichordates do not possess notochord; instead of this they possess stomochord, ectodermal in origin.

26. (d) Birds have internal fertilization.

27. (b) *Adamsia* – Sea anemone (coelenterate)

28. (a) In whales, *Balaenoptera* external ear pinna is absent.

29. (a) A body cavity can mean any internal space, or a series of spaces present inside body, whereas coelom or true body cavity generally refers to a large fluid-filled space (cavity) lying between the outer body wall and the inner digestive tube. In acoelomates, no body cavity or coelom is present. Embryonic mesoderm remains as a solid layer, space between endoderm (gut wall) and ectoderm (body wall) is filled with mesenchyme and muscle fibres. In pseudocoelomates, body space is a pseudocoelom or false coelom. In coelomates or eucoelomates, body space is a true coelom, enclosed by mesoderm on both sides. Aschelminthes are pseudocoelomates. Molluscs and insects are coelomates while flatworms are acoelomates.

30. (b) Mollusca is normally oviparous and its development may be direct or indirect. If development is indirect then it occurs through trochophore or veliger larva. Echinoderms show bilateral symmetry in larvae but pentamerous radial symmetry adult. Fertilization is external. In arthopods, body is divided into head, thorax and abdomen. Respiratory organs consists of book gills, book lungs and tracheae. Notochord is present in chordates at some stage of their lives. Urinary and anal openings, may or may not be separate.

31. (b) In reptiles, fertilization is internal and development is direct.

32. (d) The body cavity of coelomates develops from the mesoderm and contains a peritoneum. The acoelomates lack a body cavity.

33. (b) Because they are not structurally robust, heavy wave action would destroy large, upright sponges.

34. (c) The Ctenophora have evolved a complete gut with a mouth and two anal pores.

35. (c) There are no eyes but photoreceptors do occur on prostomium and dorsal epidermis. They have been, of course, called "ocelli of earthworm".

36. (b) The phylum Rotifera are pseudocoelomates and have a pseudocoel.

37. (a) The segmentation of the annelids allows for more complex coordinated movement.

38. (c) Similar body halves could be obtained with either radial or biradial symmetry. Spherical symmetry has no main body axis along which to cut, and bilateral symmetry produces mirror-image halves.

39. (d) Bilateral animals tend to move through the environment. cephalization is important in the control and coordination of this locomotion.

40. (b) Olfactory chemoreceptors means olfactoreceptors.

41. (d) Corals and sea anemones are members of the cnidarian class Anthozoa.

42. (d) Nematocysts, the stinging cells found in cnidocytes, are the only item in this list that the cnidarians possess exclusively.

43. (d) Flatworms are bilaterally symmetrical and triploblastic animals.

44. (d) A garden snail possesses all of these structures.

45. (a) Medusa and polyp are two types of body shapes of Cnidaria, which includes jellyfish, sea anemones, corals and hydrozoans. Medusa has an umbrella shape. Polyp is umbrella in shape also but inverted. Both medusae and polyps have gastrovascular cavities, tentacles and a mouth. Spongin is a protein found in the inside layer of a sponge. it helps in its structural support.

Speed Test-63

1. (d) The fruit is a mature or ripened ovary. When a fruit develops exclusively from the ovary, it is said to be true fruit. When in addition to the ovary, some other floral part also participates in the formation of fruits, then it is known as false fruit. Apple, pear, cashewnut, mulberry etc. are all false fruits.

2. (a)

3. (a) Single cotyledon of embryo in cereal grain is represented by scutellum. Coleoptile represents the covering of stem. Coleorrhiza represents the covering of root.

4. (d) Desert plants have well developed root system so that they can absorb water from the deeper layers of soil. They have sunken stomata and reduced leaves which reduce the rate of water loss through transpiration.

5. (a)

6. (d) Insectivorous plants grown in nitrogen deficient soil. Therefore, these plants capture insects and have the ability to digest them (their protein). Since proteins are made up of amino acids, having nitrogen in their structure (amino group), these plants overcome the deficiency of nitrogen which is essential for their growth.

7. (b) 8. (b) 9. (d) 10. (d) 11. (d)

12. (c) 13. (a)

14. (c) In *Cocos nucifera* (coconut) milky endosperm is found in which many nuclei, vitamins and growth hormone e.g., cytokinins, auxin and induced cytokinin is found.

15. (a) 16. (d) 17. (c) 18. (a)

19. (a) Epigynous flower ⇒ $\overline{G}$ e.g. Cucumber
Perigynous flower ⇒ G – e.g. Rose and plum
Hypogynous flower ⇒ $\underline{G}$ e.g. Brinjal

20. (c)

21. (b) Caryopsis is a small, indehiscent, one seeded fruit developing from a monocarpellary ovary in which the pericarp is fused with the seed coat. The seed completely fills the chamber, e.g., wheat, maize.

22. (c) Polyarch condition

23. (a)

24. (c) Opuntia has phylloclade for food synthesis.

25. (a) Sub-aerial stem

26. (c) Inferior ovary

27. (c) Drupe is the fruit type in mango & coconut.

28. (c) When stamens are attached to the perianth, they are known as epiphyllous, e.g., Asparagus, lily.

29. (b) In perigynous condition of a flower, the gynoecium is situated in the centre and other floral parts are located on the rim of the thalamus almost at the same level. Ovary is said to be half-inferior, e.g., *Rosa* (Flask-shaped thalamus), *Prunus* (Cup-shaped thalamus).

30. (a) The given floral diagram is of family Solanaceae (potato family). Its flower is bisexual and actinomorphic, abracteate or bracteate, pentamerous, cyclic. Calyx 5, gamosepalous, persistent. Corolla 5, gamopetalous, often plicate in bud. Androecium 5, polyandrous and epipetalous. Gynoecium bicarpellary and syncarpous. Ovary superior, placed obliquely, placentation axile with swollen-placenta. Fruit is berry or capsule.

31. (c) Liliaceae (Lily family) and Poaceae (= Gramineae, gross family) are the two monocot families.

32. (b) In *Nepenthes*, the pitchers are meant for catching and digesting insects. The lamina is modified into pitcher. The leaf apex gives rise to a coloured lid for attracting the insects.

33. (a) In Dahlia, roots do not originate from radicles and are therefore, adventitious. These roots are fleshy having no definite shape, i.e. tuberous in nature. The tuberous roots occur in group or fascicle and are also called fasciculated. Roots of radish, carrot and beet that originate from radicle are the examples of modified tap root.

34. (d) The main function of root-cap is to protect the growing apex from soil particles. Plant growing in water (hydrophytes) or on another plant (epiphytes) or in another plant (parasites) are devoid of root-cap.

35. (d) The coralloid root of *Cycas* and pneumatophores of mangroves (like *Rhizophora*) become negatively geotropic i.e., come above the soil surface, due to bacterial infection and for aeration, respectively.

36. (b) *Santalum album* (Sandal wood plant) is a small tree, but at the young stage remains as a parasite on the roots of other plants.

37. (b) For storage, tap roots are modified into four ways i. e., napiform, fusiform, conical and tuberous. In the latter form there is no definite shape, as found in *Mirabilis*. A point to note that tuberous root may develop either from tap root or from adventitious root.
38. (c)
39. (b) In many monocots, the stem is represented by underground modifications. However, the flowers are developed on a axis called scape or pseudostem. Such type of development is found in onion, aroids, banana etc.
40. (a) Sweet potato represents the adventitious modified root of *Ipomoea* plant.
41. (c) Epiphyllous bud is a type of adventitious bud, i.e, not originating from stem apex or axil of a leaf. Usually it develops from margin (or leaf surface) of leaf as in *Bryophytlum, Kalanchoe etc.* It serves the function of vegetative propagation.
42. (d) Tuber is a modified stem. A stem can not be developed on root. In potato plant, tubers develop on a special branch of the stem called stolon.
43. (b) 44. (b)
45. (b) Like phylloclade, cladode is also a modification of stem. But here the branch or axillary bud is only modified into a flat, tree like structure with only one internode.

Speed Test-64

1. (b)
2. (d) Function of companion cell is to load sugar and amino acids into sieve elements. These cells use transmembrane proteins to take up by active transport.
3. (c) Phellem, phellogen and phelloderm are collectively called periderm.
4. (d) Submerged hydrophytes do not have stomata (a protective mechanism in aquatic plants against water logging of internal cells and tissues).
5. (d) Tracheids are chief water conducting elements of xylem in gymnosperms. They are devoid of protoplasm and hence dead. The wall constituting the tracheids is hard, thick and lignified. These are elongated cells with tapering ends.
6. (d)
7. (b) Vascular cambium is produced by two types of meristems, fascicular and interfascicular cambium.
8. (d) Vessels are elongated, multicellular water conducting channels with wide lumen formed by end to end fusion of a large number of vessel elements. Tracheids are elongated dead cells with tapering ends having lignified walls with large or wide lumen. Their main function is conduction of water and minerals from root to leaf.
9. (c) The concept of quiescent centre was proposed by Clowes in 1961. On the basis of autoradiographic studies of DNA synthesis in the root tip of *Zea*, he found a reservoir of cells having low DNA, RNA and protein concentration. They may or may not divide. It is resistant to damages.
10. (d) 11. (b)
12. (b) The common bottle cork is the product of phellogen. Phellogen produces cork or phellem on the outer side. It consists of dead and compactly arranged rectangular cells that possess suberised cells walls. The cork cells contain tannins. Hence, they appear brown or dark brown in colour. The cork cells of some plants are filled with air *e.g.*, *Quercus suber* (Cork Oak or Bottle Cork).
13. (b)
14. (d) In submerged hydrophytes, whole plant body remains under water. *e.g. Ceratophyllum* and *Utricularia*. In these plants, stomata is absent and gaseous exchange takes place through general body surface.
15. (d) In collenchyma cell walls show localized thickenings due to presence of approximately 45% pectin, 35% hemicellulose and 20% cellulose.
16. (c) Being a xerophytic plant, *Nerium* bears multiple epidermis to cut the rate of transpiration.
17. (a)
18. (a) Secondary wall situated near the plasma membrane after the formation of primary wall.
19. (d) 20. (a) 21. (d) 22. (d)
23. (a) Based on position of protoxylem in relation to metaxylem, the xylem may be exach/centripetal, endarch/centrifugal, mesarch and centerarch. In endarch condition, protoxylem lies on the inner side of metaxylem e.g., dicot and monocot stems.
24. (a) A monocot stem lacks secondary growth. The vascular bundles are oval or rounded in outline. They contain both phloem and xylem. Phloem lies towards the outside and the xylem on the inner side. Cambium is absent as the whole procambium is consumed in the formation of vascular tissues. Xylem is in the form of the letter Y. It is endarch, i.e., protoxylem lies towards the centre of the stem. Xylem is made up of vessels, tracheids, xylem parenchyma and a few xylem fibres. Metaxylem generally consists of two large oval of rounded vessels lying at the upper two angles of xylem. Protoxylem cavity is present at the end of protoxylem vessels.
25. (d) Heart wood (duramen) is the central wood of an old stem. It is dark coloured. Living cells are absent. Heart wood is the part of secondary xylem. The tracheary elements are plugged by tyloses. Tracheary elements have deposition of tannins, resins, gums, etc. Heart wood is heavier. It is more durable due to its little susceptibility to the attack of pathogens and insects. Heart wood is mechanical in function. The outer or peripheral portion of the trunk is lighter in colour and soft which performs the functions of conduction of water and minerals and it is known as sap wood or alburnum.
26. (d) Intercalated between mature tissues, it helps in regeneration.
27. (d) Spring wood or earlywood
28. (a) Shoot apical meristem
29. (c) Companion cells control activities of sieve tube.
30. (c)
31. (d) Internal (physiological) and external (environmental) factors.
32. (d)
33. (d) Meristematic zone
34. (b) Thickening of wall is due to deposition of cellulose, hemicellulose and pectin.
35. (b) Endodermis with casparian strips is found in dicot stem.
36. (d)
37. (d) The electron microscope revealed al the structural details of the cell.
38. (c)
39. (d) Important functions of veins are : (i) Conduction of water through xylem; (ii) Providing channels for translocation of organic nutrients; (iii) Conduction of minerals; (iv) By their large number, the veins and veinlets provide skeletal support to the lamina so that it can remain stretched for its optimum functioning; (v) Veins and veinlets reduce the effect of wilting.
40. (b) *Cuscuta* is a total parasite so it absorbs the prepared food from the phloem of the host, hence haustoria reaches upto phloem of host.
41. (c) Tylose is a balloon-like outgrowth of paratracheal parenchyma into a pit in the wall of a vessel or tracheid and a xylem parenchyma cell lying next to it. This xylem parenchyma occurs at the edge of annual ring around the vessels.

42. (c) Epidermis is generally uniseriate. i.e., compsoed of single layer of epidermal cells.
In some cases, it is multilayered also. e.g., *Ficus*, *Nerium*, *Peperomia*, etc.
43. (a) In the cortex of monocot root, we observe a few layers of cell below the epidermis which have thick walls due to the deposition of a chemical suberin. These layers of suberized cells are called exodermis.
There are also number alternating zones of xylem present in root. The number of xylem patches far exceeds to ten. That is why, they are called polyarch. In monocot root, there is a large sized pith made up of parenchyma tissues.
44. (c) Phellem is a suberized cell formed outside the region of stem followed by endodermis, inside the phloem.
Pericycle lies immediately inside the endodermis of the dicotyledonous stem phloem. Phloem in characterized by the presence of sieve tubes.
45. (c) Tunica corpus theory was proposed by Schmidt. According to this theory, two tissue zones occur at the apex.

Speed Test-65

1. (d) Squamous epithelium is formed of thin discoidal and polygonal cells that fit like tiles in a floor, so is also called pavement epithelium. It is found in the walls of blood vessels, in the alveoli of lungs for exchange of gas, and in Bowman's capsule of nephron for ultra filtration.
2. (b) The cell junctions called tight, adhering and gap junctions are found in epithelial tissue. Epithelial tissue covers the whole surface of the body. It is made up of cells closely packed and arranged in one or more layers.
3. (b) 4. (d)
5. (d) Myoglobin is a single-chain globular protein of 153 amino acids, containing a heme (iron-containing porphyrin) prosthetic group in the center around which the remaining apoprotein folds. It has a molecular weight of 16,700 daltons, and is the primary oxygen-carrying pigment of muscle tissues. Unlike the blood-borne hemoglobin, to which it is structurally related, this protein does not exhibit cooperative binding of oxygen, since positive cooperativity is a property of multimeric/oligomeric proteins only.
6. (a)
7. (c) Silver fish (Insecta), scorpion (Arachnida); crab (Crustacea) and honey bee (Insecta) all belong to phylum Arthropoda which is characterized by the presence of jointed appendages. Poison glands occur only in scorpion. Compound eyes and metamorphosis are the characteristic of insects.
8. (c)
9. (a) Lymph differs from blood in that it contains less protein and no red blood cells. Lymph contains white blood cells.
10. (b)
11. (c) Dolphin is an aquatic mammal and breathes through lungs.
12. (c) 13. (b) 14. (a) 15. (a) 16. (c)
17. (a) Sexual dimorphism is found in cockroach. A pair of anal style are present in male cockroach only. Female has broader abdomenal segments.
18. (a) Presence of air passages in the bones (pneumatic bones) is a characteristic of birds.
19. (a) 20. (c)
21. (b) Nephridia in earthworm, malpighian tubules in cockroach and urinary tubules in the rat are excretory in function.
22. (c) 23. (a) 24. (c) 25. (b) 26. (d)
27. (d) 28. (b) 29. (c) 30. (c)
31. (c) Spiracles are 20 in number
32. (c)
33. (d) Propelling mucus is the function of simple epithelium.
34. (c) Imitability is a property only shown by cardiac muscles
35. (b) 36. (b) 37. (c)
38. (c) Myocardium is the muscular part. Pericardium and endocardium are the linings of epithelium.
39. (c) This cartilage is found in intervertebral discs.
40. (d) These granules are composed of RNA and protein.
41. (b) The GI tract is lined with simple columnar epithelium, which allows a maximum number of cells to contact food particles.
42. (a) Most epithelia have a basement membrane between the epithelial cells and the underlying connective tissue.
43. (a)
44. (b) Bone is surrounded by dense, white fibrous sheath called periosteum.
45. (b) A - Ocellus; B - Compound eye; C - Mandible;
D - Maxilla; E - Labrum; F - Labium.

Speed Test-66

1. (c) Glycosylation is the process or result of addition of saccharides to proteins and lipids. The process is one of the four principal co-translational and post-translational modification steps in the synthesis of membrane and secreted proteins and the majority of proteins synthesized in the rough ER undergo glycosylation.
2. (b) Vacuoles are present mainly in the plant cells. Each vacuole is surrounded by cytoplasmic membrane called as tonoplast which is similar to plasma membrane.
3. (b) The membrane surrounding a lysosome allows the digestive enzymes to work at the 4.5 pH they require. They are created by the addition of hydrolytic enzymes to early endosomes from the Golgi apparatus.
4. (c)
5. (c) Nucleolus was discovered by Fontana (1781) and given name by Bowman (1840). It does not have membrane and is attached to chromatin at nucleolar organiser region (NOR). Nucleolus is the site for elaboration of r-RNA and synthesis of ribsomes, hence called ribosomal factory.
6. (b)
7. (a) The fluidity of membranes in a plant in cold weather may be maintained by increasing the number of phospholipids with unsaturated hydrocarbon tails.
8. (c) 9. (a) 10. (b)
11. (b) Fimbriae are hair like structures present in large number in bacteria. They help in attaching bacteria to solid surfaces or host tissues.
12. (d) Proteins have very specific shapes which make them ideal as receptor molecules for chemical signalling between cells. Branching side chain glycolipids on the outer surface of cell membranes are also involved in cell-cell recognition.
13. (a) The SER provides surface for the synthesis of lipids, including phospholipids, cholesterol, steroid hormones (sex hormones, adrenal corticoid hormones), ascorbic acid and visual pigments.
14. (a)
15. (b) Phospholipids in the lipid bilayer limit the permeability of the membrane.
16. (c) Vacuole is a non - living reservoir, bounded by a selectively permeable membrane, the tonoplast. It is not a air filled cavity but it is filled with a highly concentrated solution called vascular sap or cell sap. pH of vacuolar cell sap is acidic and hypertonic.
17. (c) Plastids are double membranous, semi-autonomous organelles which store and synthesise various types of organic compounds. They develop from colourless precursor proplastids. Proplastids have the ability to divide and differentiate into various types of plastids.
18. (c) Only statements B and E are incorrect as plastids have circular DNA and are found to be present in higher plants.

19. (b) 20. (a)
21. (d) Prokaryotes possess gas vacuole.
22. (d) Membrane-less organelles.
23. (b)
24. (d) All of these
25. (b) 2n = 34
26. (d) 27. (a) 28. (b) 29. (d) 30. (b)
31. (d) 32. (c)
33. (b) In 1935, Danielli and Davson proposed that cell membrane is made of a double layer of phospolipid molecules sandwiched between two single layers of proteins. The three layers are held together by electrostatic forces while phospholipid layers are kept adhered by vander Waal's forces.
34. (a)
35. (d) The cell membrane is asymmetric and has different properties, and functions of the cytoplasmic side versus the extracellular side. These properties arise from differences in the constituents of the membrane.
36. (b) Both glycolipids and glycoproteins serve as recognition signals.
37. (a) The charged or polar lining of the channel proteins allows passage of polar and charged molecules.
38. (d) All cells have a plasma membrane. The other structures listed are organelles and therefore are present only in eukaryotes.
39. (d)
40. (c) The cytoskeleton supports the cell and allows for movement of the entire cell and listed are part of the cytoskeleton.
41. (d) 42. (c) 43. (b)
44. (c) Plants are autotrophs and synthesize their food in the process of photosynthesis with the help of chloroplast (plastid).
45. (d) Peroxisomes contain glycolic acid and oxidase, which oxidises glycolic acid (a product of photosynthesis) to glyoxylic acid.

Speed Test-67

1. (c) The nucleic acid (DNA and RNA) are repeating units of nucleotides i.e. polynucleotides. Each nucleotide comprises of nitrogenous heterocyclic bases viz. purines or pyrimidines, pentose sugar and phosphoric acid.
2. (b) Glycogen is an animal starch, stored in the liver and is polysaccharide of α – Glucose. About 30,000 glucose molecules joined by 1-4 α -glycosidic bonds and its branches by 1-6 glycosidic bonds. It gives red colour with iodine solution.
   - Galactose is a monosaccharide from milk.
   - Fructose is a monosaccharide from fruit.
   - Sucrose is a disaccharide (Glucose + Fructose).
3. (b) Cellulose is the most abundant organic compound, most abundant polysaccharide and most abundant biopolymer found on earth.
4. (c) In the cytoplasm, protein synthesis is restricted to the ribosomes. Mitochondria being a semiautonomous organelle, has its own genetic machinery to synthesize its proteins.
5. (d) RNA is a single chain of ribonucleotides. Each ribonucleotide consists of nitrogenous bases (adenine, guanine, cytosine and uracil), ribose sugar and phosphoric acid.
6. (a) Reducing sugar is any sugar that has an aldehyde group or is capable of forming one in solution through isomerisation. Reducing monosaccharides include glucose, fructose, glyceraldehyde and galactose. Many disaccharides, like lactose and maltose also have a reducing form, as one of the two units may have an open- chain form with an aldehyde group.
However, sucrose and trihalose in which the anomeric carbons of the two units are linked together, are non reducing disaccharides since neither of the rings is capable of opening.
7. (d) α-amylase enzyme stimulates the germination of barley seed.
8. (a) Massive ions like Na^+ facilitate the absorption of substances like amino acid and glucose through cotransport.
9. (d) Enzymes accelerate chemical reaction by lowering the activation energy.
10. (c) Competitive inhibition is the reversible inhibition of enzyme activity due to presence of substrate analogues. Non competitive inhibition is the reduction of enzyme activity by a factor that has no real structural similarity with the substrate. Allosteric inhibition is reversible non-competitive inhibition occurring in case of allosteric enzymes . Herein, the inhibitors are the products or intermediates of reactions catalyzed by the enzymes. Hence, it is also called end product inhibition or feedback inhibition.
11. (c) There are only 20 amino acids . These can be arranged in different order in the polypeptide chain to form a diverse array of proteins.
12. (a) Length of one turn of DNA helix is 34Å.
$1Å = 10^{-1}$ nm
13. (c) K_m (Michealis Menten constant) is defined as that substrate concentration at which under optimum conditions the rate of an enzyme catalysed reaction reaches half the maximum rate. K_m is inversely proportional to affinity of enzyme for its substrate.
14. (b) 15. (a) 16. (d) 17. (a) 18. (a)
19. (d) 20. (b) 21. (d) 22. (c) 23. (b)
24. (c) 25. (b)
26. (b) Phospholipids are triglyceride lipids, in which one fatty acid is replaced by phosphoric acid residue often linked to additional nitrogenous groups like choline (in lecithin), ethanolamine (in cephalin) etc.

$$\begin{array}{l} CH_2-O-CO-R_1 \\ | \\ CH-O-CO-R_2 \\ | \qquad\qquad O \\ | \qquad\qquad \| \\ CH_2-O-\underset{\underset{O}{\|}}{P}-(CH_2)_2-\overset{+}{N}(CH_3)_3 \end{array}$$

Phosphate; Choline

Fig. : Structure of lecithin.

27. (b) Polysaccharides, monosaccharides are linked together by glycosidic bond (C–O–C). Water has hydrogen bonding. Proteins and polymers of different amino acids, which are linked by peptide (CONH) bond formed by dehydration (polymerisation) between COOH group of one amino acid and NH_2 group of next amino acid with the removal of H_2O. The three hydroxyl groups of a glycerol molecule join with the the carboxyl groups of three fatty acid molecules to form a fat or triglyceride molecule. The chemical linkage between the glycerol and fatty acids is called the ester bond.
28. (a) Chitin is the second most abundant polysaccharide (after cellulose). Chitin is not a storage polysaccharide rather it is a structural homopolysaccharide, formed of N-acetylglucosamine (NAG) monomers joined together by β-1, 4 linkages. Also, it forms the structural component of fungal walls and exoskeleton of arthropods.

29. (b)

Some Secondary Metabolites	
Pigments	Carotenoids, anthocyanins, etc.
Alkaloids	Morphine, Codeine, etc.
Terpenoids	Monoterpenes, Diterpenes, etc.
Essential oils	Lemon grass oil, etc.
Toxins	Abrin, Ricin
Lectins	Concanavalin A
Drugs	Vinblastin, Curcumin, etc.
Polymeric substances	Rubber, Gums, Cellulose.

Vinblastin is used as an anticancer drug, whereas curcumin is a component of turmeric and also used as drug.

30. (b) Lyases enzyme catalyze the breakage of specific covalent bonds and removal of groups without hydrolysis producing double bonds or removal of double bonds by adding groups e.g., histidine decarboxylase that splits C–C bond of histidine, forming CO_2 and histamine.

$$\underset{\mid}{\overset{X}{C}}-\underset{\mid}{\overset{Y}{C}} \xrightarrow{\text{lyase}} X-Y+C=C$$

Fructose-1, 6 diphosphate $\xrightarrow{\text{Aldolase}}$ Dihydroxyacetone-3-phosphate + Glyceraldehyde-3-phosphate.

31. (c) Successive glucose units are linked together by $\alpha\ 1 \rightarrow 4$ linkage and at branchings $\alpha\ 1 \rightarrow 6$ linkage is present.

32. (c) 33. (c)

34. (b) Tertiary structure of proteius is devoid of phosphodiester bonds. There bonds are present in nudeic acids.

35. (b)

36. (a) A high k_m indicates low affinity of an enzyme for its substrate.

37. (d) The multiple molecular forms of an enzyme occuring in the same organisms and having a similar substrate activity are called isoenzymes or isozymes. They have similar properties but different molecular weights and location. Over 100 enzymes are known to have isoenzymes. α-amylase of wheat endosperm has 16 isozymes, lactate dehydrogenase has 5 isozymes.

38. (d) Essential amino acids are the amino acids which cannot be synthesized by organisms in the body and are obtained from plants e.g., valine, leucine, isoleucine, phenylalanine, threonin, lysine, tryptophan, methionine.

Non-essential amino acids can be synthesized by the organism and may not be the requisite components of diet e.g., serine, tryosine, aspartate, cysteine, glutamate, proline, glycrine, alanine, asparagine, glutamine and tyrosine.

39. (a) Acidic amino acids have an extra carboxylic group (mono-amino dicarboxylic), e.g., glutamate (glutamic acid, Glu), asparate (aspartic acid, Asp).

Basic amino acids have an additional amino group without forming amides (diamino monocarboxylic), e.g., arginine (Arg), lysine (Lys).

Neutral amino acids have one amino group and one carboxylic group (mono-amino mnocarboxylic) with noncyclic hydrocarbon chain, e.g., glycine (Gly), alanine (Ala), valine (Val), Leucine (Leu), isoleucine (lle). Essential amino acids are the amino acids which cannot be synthesized by organisms in the body and are obtained from plants e.g., valine, leucine, isoleucine, phenylalanine, threonin, lysine, tryptophan, methionine.

Non-essential amino acids can be synthesized by the organism and may not be the requisite components of diet e.g., serine, tryosine, aspartate, cysteine, glutamate, proline, glycrine, alanine, asparagine, glutamine and tyrosine.

40. (d)

41. (b) Trehalose is a non-reducing sugar. It is made up to 2 molecules of glucose

42. (c) 43. (a) 44. (d)

45. (a) Palmitic acid is one of the most common saturated fatty acids found in animals and plants. It has 16 carbons including the carboxyl carbon.

Speed Test-68

1. (d) G_1 phase, also called Gap I phase is characterized by increase in cell size. In the S phase or synthetic phase DNA molecules replicate. G_2 is the second growth phase or Gap II where in there is intensive formation of RNAs and proteins. In the mitotic metaphase, the chromosomes are arranged at the equatorial plate.

2. (b) Kinetochore is the proteinaceous covering of centriole, to which spindle fibers attach.

3. (b) Mitosis is the process in which eukaryotic cell separates the chromosomes in its cell nucleus, into two identical sets in two daughter nuclei. It is generally followed immediately by cytokinesis, which divides the nuclei, cytoplasm, organelles and cell membrane into two daughter cells containing roughly equal shares of these cellular components. Mitosis and cytokinesis together define the mitotic (M) phase of the cell cycle - the division of the mother cell into two daughter cells, genetically identical to each other and to their parent cell.

4. (d) In bivalent formation of chromosomes during meiosis, the homologous chromosomes are arranged in pairs. The phenomenon is called synapsis and it occurs during zygotene stage. DNA replication occurs during S phase or synthetic phase which is the second phase of interphase.

5. (a) 6. (b) 7. (b) 8. (b) 9. (b)

10. (c) 11. (b)

12. (d) During telophase, the individual chromosomes are no longer seen and chromatin material tends to collect in a mass at the two poles. Chromosomes cluster at opposite spindle poles and their identity is lost as discrete elements. Nuclear envelope assembles around the chromosome clusters. Nucleolus, Golgi complex and ER reform.

13. (a) 14. (c)

15. (a) Condensation initiates in prophase.

16. (c) Interkinesis is the stage that occurs in between meiosis-I and meosis-II

17. (a) During anaphase, centromeres split resulting in the separation of sister chromatids towards opposite poles.

18. (c) 19. (d) 20. (a)

21. (d) A = Diplotene B = Dissolution
C = Pachytene D = Anaphase - II

22. (d) The lampbrush chromosomes occuring in prophase of meiosis II are highly elongated special kind of synapsed mid-prophase or diplotene chromosome bivalents which have already undergone crossing over. Lampbrush chromosomes occur in pairs. Each chromosome of a pair has a double main axis due to presence of two elongated chromatids. Both the adjacent chromatids bear rows of large number of chromomeres. Two adjacent chromomeres are separated by interchromomeric stretches. Many of the chromomeres give out lateral projections or loops. The lateral loops provide a test tube or lampbrush-like appearance to the chromosome pair. Lateral loops take part in rapid transcription of DNA to mRNA meant for synthesis of yolk and other substances required for growth and development of meiocytes.

23. (a) The mitotic spindle forms and the nuclear membrane disperses during prophase.
24. (b) If at G_1 cells are given the signal to divide, they are unlikely to be stopped at subsequent checkpoints.
25. (a) Sister chromatids are the two identical strands of a duplicated chromosome.
26. (d) Meiosis reduces the chromosome count from diploid to haploid and halves the amount of genetic material.
27. (d) Kinetochores are assembled at the centromere of each chromosome and are the sites where microtubules attach to segregate the chromosomes. In meiosis there is only one fused kinetochore per chromosome; in mitosis there are two kinetochores per chromosome.
28. (d) Chromosomes are attached tot he microtubules at their kinetochores. There are molecular motors at the kinetochores which help move the chromosomes to the poles by the shortening of the kinetochore microtubules.
29. (c) Programmed cell death occurs during the development of many organisms (for instance, tadpoles lose their tails to become adult frogs). One of the stimuli for programmed cell death. Necrosis (cell death that is not programmed) occurs when cells have been deprived of cell cycle, in which cells reproduce, and is not a step in programmed cell death.
30. (b) After fertilization, the DNA content in the cell increases because of the fusion of genetic material of the parents. Mitosis then occurs and is followed by cytokinesis at x, which is the division of the cytoplasm into 2 compartments, i.e. 2 cells.
31. (a) Although no centrioles are visible, there is spindle formation and the chromosomes do exhibit equatorial arrangement. Spindle formation is probably by another organelle, unknown as yet.
32. (c) At prophase I, DNA replication has already occurred, and the original amount of DNA has been doubled to x. At anaphase I, the amount of DNA in the cell remains the same because no cytokinesis has occurred yet to separate the cytoplasm.
33. (d) G_0 represents a stage in G_1 in which cells are supposed to be withdrawn from division.
34. (c) Restriction point represents a stage in G_1 phase If the cell has passed restriction point, it would divide.
35. (c) Pairing can be procentric proterminal pairing or intermediate condition (also called as random synapsis which may occur simultaneously at all chromomeres).
36. (b) Stock is the one that receives the graft which has 2n = 48. This would produce the root which will have 2n = 48. Scion has 2n = 24, would produce microspore (n = 2)
37. (c) The number of chromosome will be same (50), but each chromosome will have 2 chromatids.
38. (a) No. of required meiosis $= n + \frac{n}{4} = \frac{5n}{4}$

where n = no. of seeds.

$$= \frac{5 \times 10}{4} = \frac{50}{4} = 12.5 = 13$$

10 Megaspore + 10 Microspore = 10 seeds

To produce 10 Megaspores, 10 meiotic division would be needed

13 – 10 = 3 meiosis will produce 12 microspore

So, wastage of pollen grain = 2
39. (d) The correct order of mitotic events which occur during meiosis is: Formation of synaptonemal complex, recombination, separation of homologous chromosomes, separation of sister chromatids.
40. (b)
41. (c) Any agent that stimulates cell division is called mitogen e.g., temperature, cytokinin, auxin, gibberellin, insulin and steroids.
42. (c)
43. (d) During the S-period, the centrioles separate and undergo duplication which produces two pairs of centrioles still contained within the radiating masses of microtubules.
44. (a)
45. (c) The given figure shows anaphase I of meiosis. In anaphase I, the homologous chromosomes break apart while sister chromatids remains associated at their centromere. At the end of anaphase I, two groups of chromosomes are produced at two poles, having half the number of parental chromosomes.

Speed Test-69

1. (d)
2. (c) Osmosis is the movement of solvent particles from a region of low solute concentration to a region of high solute concentration through a selectively permeable membrane.
3. (b) 4. (c)
5. (d) The factors which affect the rate of transpiration are light – stomatal opening, temperature – increases rate of transpiration, humidity – low humidity increases the rate of transpiration whereas high humidity exerts an opposite effect *i.e.* decreases the rate, wind – high wind causes stomatal closure, thereby, reducing the rate of transpiration in plants.
6. (a) Osmotic potential is the potential of a solution to cause water movement into it across a semi- permeable membrane. Water potential is the tendency of water to leave a system.
7. (d) Turgor pressure is the pressure that develops in a cell due to osmotic diffusion of water inside it and is responsible for pushing the membrane against cell wall. Stomata open under conditions of increased turgor pressure of guard cells and stomata gets closed under conditions of decreased turgor pressure of guard cells. When turgid, they swell and bend outward. As a result, the stomatal aperture opens. When they are flaccid, the tension from the wall is released and stomatal aperture closes.
8. (b) Active transport involves movement of ions against concentration gradient involves the expenditure of energy. Diffusion involves the movement of solute particles from region of higher concentration to a region of lower concentration. Pinocytosis is cell drinking. Brownian movement is the random to and fro movement of atoms and molecules.
9. (c)
10. (d) A solution having more solutes as compared to solution having less number of solutes : former is known as hypertonic and latter hypotonic. Hence, solution outside the cytoplasm has more solutes (higher concentration) and are hypertonic. If two solutions have same solute concentration then they are isotonic.
11. (b)
12. (a) During sodium-potassium pump, the concentration of sodium ions will be about 14 times more in extra cellular fluid (outside) and concentration of potassium ions will be about 28-30 times more in axoplasm (inside). Thus, $3Na^+$ and $2K^+$ are transported during the process.
13. (a) In rainy season, door gets swelled due to the phenomenon of imbibition. It is the process of absorption of water without forming a solution.
14. (c) Cell placed in a hypotonic solution becomes turgid due to endosmosis. Water exerts a pressure on the walls of the cell called turgor pressure. Cell wall being a rigid and hard structure also exerts a pressure on Cytoplasm in response to Turgor pressure when TP = WP, DPD = 0 (No net exchange of water).

15. (a) The pure water, at atmospheric pressure has zero water potential. The addition of any solute particles reduces the free energy of water. Thus, the water potential will be negative.
16. (b)
17. (b) Water logging of soil makes it physiologically dry because this condition does not allow oxygen to enter the soil.
18. (c) 19. (b) 20. (b)
21. (b) The absorption of water still occurs when concentration of outer soil water is more than root hair cell sap.
22. (d)
23. (b) With increasing humidity, the rate of transpiration decreases linearly, because the high saturation of water vapour in the atmosphere prevents the evaporation of more water from the leaf interior to the exterior.
24. (b) 25. (b)
26. (d) If we cut a small soft-stemmed plant on a day, when there is plenty of atmospheric moisture, early in the morning we will soon see drops of solution ooze out of the cut stem; this comes out due to the positive root pressure. If we fix a rubber tube to the cut stem as a sleeve we can actually collect and measure the rate of exudation, and also determine the composition of the exudates. Root pressure is a positive pressure that develops in the xylem sap of the root of some plants. It is a manifestation of active water absorption. Root pressure is observed in certain seasons which favours optimum metabolic activity and reduce transpiration. It is more during rainy season in the tropical countries and during spring in temperate habitats.
27. (c) Cohesion tension theory (Cohesion-tension and transpiration pull theory) explains the ascent of sap best. It was put forward by Dixon and Jolly in 1894. It was further improved by Dixon in 1914. Therefore, the theory is also named after him as Dixon's theory of ascent of sap. Today most of the workers believe in this theory.
28. (a) Sap will flow from high to low pressure areas in the plant. Adding sugars to the sap causes water to enter the phloem, thus increasing pressure. Removing sugars causes water to leave the phloem, thereby reducing pressure.
29. (c) The water potential is the sum of the osmotic potential (usually negative) and the pressure potential (usually positive), so WP = –0.24 + 0.16 = –0.08 mPa.
30. (a) Guttation is caused by root pressure. It is only important to the movement of water in quite small plants.
31. (d) As leaf cells lose water, they release abscisic acid, which causes potassium ions to leave guard cells, decreasing their pressure potential and closing stomata.
32. (b) As carbon dioxide is fixed into organic acids at night the pH decreases; metabolism of these acids during the day (with the carbon dioxide going into the citric acid cycle) causes the pH to increase.
33. (a) Choices b, c, and d are true for phloem transport only.
34. (c) Sugar molecules diffuse through the symplast of mesophyll cells, are pumped into the apoplast near a vein, re-enter the symplast of a companion cell, and then move into a sieve tube element.
35. (a) The intercellular spaces and cell walls of the plant constitute the apoplast.
36. (a) Transpiration causes tension.
37. (d) Abscisic acid, light, and carbon dioxide levels all regulate stomatal opening and closing.
38. (a) Stomatal regulators work by activating and deactivating the proton pump in guard cells.
39. (d) 40. (c) 41. (c) 42. (a)
43. (b) The tension created by the evaporation of water from leaf surfaces generates a pull on the water column that moves water and nutrients up the xylem from the roots to the leaves.
44. (c) 45. (d)

Speed Test-70

1. (b) 2. (c)
3. (a) Molybdenum is a component of nitrogenase and nitrate reductase involved during N_2 fixation. Copper is essential for photosynthesis and respiration. Zinc is involved in synthesis of auxin. Manganese is activator of enzymes involved in nitrogen metabolism.
4. (b) The root nodules of leguminous plants contain a symbiotic nitrogen fixing bacteria *Rhizobium*. Root nodules are small irregular outgrowth of the roots which are pinkish internally due to presence of a pigment called leghaemoglobin. It is related to blood pigment haemoglobin. The cells of root nodules are tetraploid and contain polyhedral bacteria called bacteroids. Leghaemoglobin is an oxygen scavenger and protects the nitrogen fixing enzyme nitrogenase of bacteroids.
5. (c) 'Whip-tail' disease in cauliflower is noted due to deficiency of molybdenum. Cauliflower is the most sensitive of crops to molybdenum (Mb) deficiency. Light sandy soils with pH levels close to or below pH 6 under conditions of high fertility can show severe Mb deficiency. Molybdenum is the only plant essential micronutrient that becomes less available as the soil acidifies–the opposite of copper, zinc and iron.
6. (b) The essential elements are divided into macroelements and microelements based on the quantity in which they are required by the plants. Mn, Fe, Cu, Mo, Zn, B, and Cl are the micronutrients needed in very small quantities by the plants. C, H, O, N, P, S, K, Ca, Mg, Fe are the macronutrients required in more quantity.
7. (d) Heterotrophic plants are less dependent on nitrogen obtained from nitrification since they receive some nitrite and nitrate through their parasitic or carnivorous nutritional modes.
8. (d) 9. (b)
10. (d) Root hairs absorb water, minerals and oxygen but they do not absorb CO_2. CO_2 intake takes place in leaves.
11. (c) The ash that is left after burning any dry part of the plant contains only mineral elements and is called plant ash.
12. (b) The atmospheric nitrogen is fixed in the soil in the form of nitrate. Nitrate and ammonium can be taken up by plants or used by other soil organisms. Any nitrate or ammonium that is not used for growth is added to the pool of inorganic nitrogen in the soil.
13. (c) Cultivation of plants by placing the roots in the nutrient solution without any soil is called hydroponics. It is also known as soilless culture/ water culture/ solution culture. It is used to determine which elements are essential for plant growth and what symptoms are produced by the absence or deficiency of essential elements.
14. (c) 15. (c)
16. (a) Cobalt stimulates growth of legumes such as beans, clover and alfalfa. This stimulation of growth by cobalt is due to its use, not by the plant itself, but by nitrogen-fixing bacteria that live in roots of plants.
17. (b) 18. (a) 19. (a) 20. (b) 21. (b)
22. (d)
23. (b) Magnesium activates the enzymes of respiration, photosynthesis and is involved in the synthesis of DNA and RNA. Manganese activates many enzymes which are involved in photosynthesis, respiration and nitrogen metabolism.
24. (a) NO_3^-, is negatively charged and not tightly bound to soil particles.
25. (d) Legume roots have swellings called nodules that contain nitrogen-fixing bacteria of the genus Rhizobium.

26. (b) The main difference between micronutrients and macronutrients is in how much of them a plant needs to survive.
27. (c) Symptoms caused by deficiency of essential mineral elements on plants are called Hunger signs.
28. (a) The deficiency of calcium results in death of leaf, stem and root apices.
29. (c) Hydrogen sulphide has little to do with ion exchange.
30. (b) Due to immobile property of sulphur, chlorosis occurs first in young leaves.
31. (c) All other statements are false.
32. (a) The characteristic symptom of iron deficiency is the interveinal chlorosis. The symptom may be general or localised to a single leaf or a single branch because of the limited mobility of iron in the tissues. The deficiency symptom first appears in young leaves.
33. (d) An iron deficiency is suspected in a plant. If the older leaves are yellow, a nitrogen deficiency would be suspected because nitrogen is easily relocated in the plant while iron is not.
34. (d) 35. (d)
36. (d) The bulk of the organic material of a plant is derived from carbon dioxide assimilated from the atmosphere.
37. (b) For chlorophyll formation, a plant needs Fe, Mg & light
38. (c) 39. (a) 40. (b) 41. (c) 42. (a)
43. (b) "Reclamation" and "Little leaf" disease is caused by deficiency of Cu and Zn.
44. (a) 45. (a)

Speed Test-71

1. (a)
2. (c) The C_4 pathway allows photosynthesis to occur at very low concentrations of carbon dioxide as PEP carboxylase has an extremely high affinity for carbon dioxide. This pathway also works well at high temperatures and light intensity, enabling efficient photosynthesis in tropical plants.
3. (a) Photorespiratory loss of CO_2 occurs when RuBisCo starts functioning as an oxygenase instead of carboxylase under conditions of high O_2 and low CO_2. It involves three organelles chloroplast, mitochondria and peroxisomes. Half of the photosynthetically fixed carbon (in the form of RuBP) may be lost into the atmosphere through this process and no ATP formation occurs.
4. (d) 5. (a)
6. (c) The process of photorespiration requires 3 cell organelles- mitochondria, chloroplasts and peroxisomes. In chloroplasts glycolate is formed from ribulose biphosphate which passes into peroxisomes to be changed into glyoxylate. In this reaction H_2O_2 is evolved. Glyoxylate is changed to glycine which now enters mitochondria. Two molecules of glycine combine to form one molecule of serine with the evolution of CO_2.
7. (b) Grana are present inside the chloroplasts. Each granum may contain 10 – 100 thylakoids. Thylakoids or baggy trousers are membrane lined flattened sacs. Thylokoids (or granna) contain chloroplast proteins, photosynthetic pigments and other factors required for photosynthesis.
8. (b) Photosynthesis takes place only in the visible part (400 - 700 nm wavelength) of electromagnetic radiations. Hence, this component comprises the photo-synthetically active radiation.
9. (a) 10. (a) 11. (a)
12. (b) RuBisCo is the enzyme involved in Calvin cycle. Nitrogenase catalyses nitrogenation. Invertase catalyses breaking of sucrose to glucose and fructose.
13. (a) The primary acceptor of CO_2 in C_4 plants is phosphoenol pyruvate or PEP. PEP in mesophyll cells combine with CO_2 and is converted into 4 carbon compound oxaloacetic acid by PEP carboxylase. In C_3 plant, Ribulose 1, 5–diphosphate is primary acceptor of CO_2.
14. (a) Photolysis is catalysed by the protein-bound inorganic complex containing manganese ions (oxygen evolving complex) of photosystem II.
15. (c) 16. (c) 17. (d) 18. (d) 19. (d) 20. (a)
21. (b) 22. (c) 23. (c) 24. (a) 25. (d) 26. (b)
27. (c) 28. (c) 29. (d)
30. (a) Oxygen is a product of photosynthesis. A small quantity of O_2 is essential for photosynthesis to take place. But as O_2 concentration rises, rate of photosynthesis decreases. It may be because (i) Oxygen takes part in oxidation of photosynthetic pigments, intermediates and enzymes in the presnce of strong light (photo-oxidation), (ii) Oxygen is a strong quencher of excited state of chlorophyll. Oxygen competes with CO_2 for reducing power. It converts RuBP-carboxylase to RuBP-oxygenase. At very high oxygen concentration, the rate of photosynthesis begins to decline in all plants. This phenomenon is referred to as Warburg effect.
31. (c) PS I is involved in both cyclic and non-cyclic photophosphorylation. PS II is involved only in non-cyclic photophosphorylation. PS II is present in the appressed (linner) part of grana thylakoids. PS I is located in the non-appresed (outer) part of grana thylakoids as well as stroma thylakoids.
32. (d) In cyclic photophosphorylation, only PS–I is involved.
33. (a) In Calvin cycle, three molecules of CO_2 will require 3 x 3 = 9 ATP and 2 x 3 = 6 $NADPH_2$.
34. (c) In photosynthesis, light energy trapped by chlorophyll is used to excite electrons in the chlorophyll. (An electron extracted from water by photolysis fills the electron hole.) The excited electrons are then transferred through the electron transport chain in the thylakoid membrane to $NADP^+$, forming NADPH in the stroma.
35. (b) The key compound of C-3 cycle or Calvin cycle is 3-PGAL as it is starting point for many other metabolic pathways in the plant.
36. (d) Photosynthesis is the process by which plants manufacture food. This occurs when CO_2 combines with ribulose 1,5-bisphosphate (RuBP) to form the products of photosynthesis.
37. (d) 38. (d) 39. (c) 40. (b) 41. (b)
42. (a) 43. (c) 44. (a) 45. (a)

Speed Test-72

1. (b) During aerobic respiration, oxygen is consumed and CO_2 is released. R.Q is defined as ratio of volume of CO_2 released and O_2 consumed by the respiratory substrate.

$$R.Q. = \frac{\text{Volume of } CO_2}{\text{Volume of } O_2}$$

2. (b) As a result of glycolysis, one molecule of glucose is broken down to two molecules of pyruvate. During glycolysis, 4 molecules of ATP are produced but 2 molecules of ATP are consumed in the activation of glucose molecule. Therefore, there is a net gain of 2 molecules of ATP.
3. (d) The end product of glycolysis is pyruvate. It enters mitochondria and is oxidatively decarboxylated to acetyl CoA before entering into Krebs cycle.

4. (c) Mesosomes are the invaginations of the plasma membrane that can form into vesicles. They are found to be present in both gram-positive and gram-negative bacteria. Mesosomes may play a role in cell wall formation during cell division and/or chromosome replication and distribution and/or electron transfer systems of respiration.
5. (d) Terminal cytochorome is cyt a_3. cyt a_3 posseses two copper centers. It helps in transfer of electrons to oxygen.
6. (c)
7. (d) Glycolysis is a reductive process in which glucose is broken down in the absence of oxygen within the cytoplasm of the cell. It forms 2 pyruvate molecules, 2 net ATP molecules, 2 $NADH_2$ molecules.
8. (d) In Kreb's cycle, the FAD participates as electron acceptor during the conversion of succinic acid to fumaric acid.
9. (d) 10. (a) 11. (a) 12. (a) 13. (d)
14. (d) 15. (d) 16. (b) 17. (c) 18. (b)
19. (b) 20. (a) 21. (b) 22. (b) 23. (d)
24. (c) Muscle fatigue is the reduction in force of contraction of a muscle after prolonged stimulation. In the absence of oxygen, skeletal muscle of human beings can contract for a short time, but it gets fatigued soon. This is due to the fact that in the absence of oxygen, products of glycolysis mainly lactic acid is not disposed off and accumulates in the muscles. This leads to muscle fatigue and pain in the muscles. A muscle gets fatigued sooner after a strenuous exercise than after a mild exercise. Faster breathing for sometime after a strenuous exercise supplies extra oxygen, disposes off excess lactic acid and muscle fatigue disappears.
25. (b)

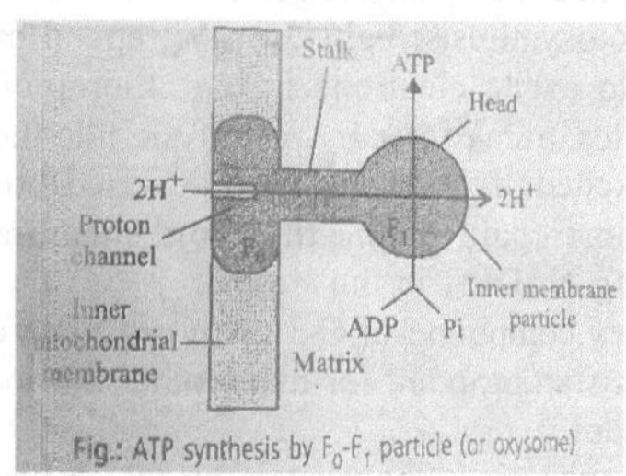

Fig.: ATP synthesis by F_0-F_1 particle (or oxysome)

26. (a) Under normal circumstances, the cell must have sodium pumps (Na^+/K^+ ATPase) which actively transport ATP into the cell. When KCN is added, the carriers are destroyed, thus ATP can enter freely.
27. (c) Since oxygen will not participate, the Pasteur effect will not take place.
28. (d) During Krebs cycle fumarate is formed from succinate and hence, synthesis of fumarate is blocked.
29. (a) Substrate-level-phosphorylation means synthesis of ATP by utilizing energy released directly by the substrates. In glycolysis, there are two steps in which ATP is synthesized. In Krebs cycle, there is only one step where GTP is synthesized when succinyl CoA is converted to succinic acid.
30. (c) Mitochondria oxidize not only carbohy drates but also the products of fats i.e. fatty-acids through acetyl CoA and glycerol through phosphoglyceraldehyde.
31. (b) Yeast causes alcoholic fermentation without using oxygen and hence depletion of oxygen has no effect on the metabolism or growth of yeast cells.
32. (c) When oxygen is available $NADH_2$ produced in EMP-Krebs cycle pathway is released in the form of NAD. When there is shortage of oxygen NAD is not available and NADP takes up its place.
33. (d)
34. (d) ATP molecules from ADP are generated maximum in electron transport chain.
35. (b) 12 kcal of energy present in one molecule of ATP & on oxidation of one mole of glucose into CO_2 and H_2O energy released in 686 kcal. So no. of ATP which can store this energy would be = 57.1 = 57 ATPs.
36. (c) Succinate:ubiquinone oxidoreductase, also known in mitochondria as Complex II, provides a link between the citric acid cycle and the membrane-bound electron-transport system. The membrane extrinsic, water-soluble domain, known as succinate dehydrogenase (SDH), contains the fumarate/succinate active site with a covalently bound FAD group and three iron-sulfur clusters: $[2Fe\text{-}2S]^2$ +/1+, $[4Fe\text{-}4S]^2$+/1+, and $[3Fe\text{-}4S]^1$ +/0. The enzyme catalyzes the interconversion of fumarate and succinate, and is closely related to fumarate reductase.
37. (d) Glycolysis takes place in all body cells and is of two types-
   (a) Anaerobic glycolysis-From glycogen or glucose to lactic acid in muscles.
   (b) Aerobic glycolysis- From glycogen or glucose to pyruvic acid (all cells of body).
38. (d)
39. (b) One of the functions of the electron transport chain and the conversion of pyruvate to lactate is the regeneration of NAD from reduced NAD. NAD is needed in glycolysis.
40. (d) ATP formation occurs both at 2, where glyceraldehyde-3-phosphate is converted to pyruvate; and at 5, where the six-carbon compound, citrate, releases water and CO_2 in the Krebs cycle.
41. (a) $FADH_2$ is produced during the formation of fumaric acid from succinic acid in the kreb's cycle of aerobic respiration.
42. (d) The oxygen obtained from cellular respiration combines with the hydrogen obtained from the oxidation of organic molecules to form water.
43. (d) Fats make more electrons available to the electron transport system and more hydrogen ions available for chemiosmosis.
44. (c)
45. (c) Primary respiratory substrate is carbohydrate and secondary respiratory substrate is fat.

Speed Test-73

1. (d) Long day plants undergo flowering after receiving light above a critical day length. *e.g.* spinach, sugarbeet. Short day plants flower only when they receive light below a critical day length, *e.g. Glycine max,* tobacco.
2. (d) The hormone, which controls cell division and cell differentiation, is cytokinin. Both the auxin and gibberellins cause elongation of cell and plants.
3. (d) Long-day plants usually flower in the spring or early summer; they flower only if the light periods are longer than a critical length, which is usually 9-16 hours. For example, wheat plants flower only when light periods exceed fourteen hours.
4. (c)
5. (c) Abscisic acid (ABA), also known as abscisin II and dormin, is a plant hormone. It functions as many plant developmental processes, including bud dormancy. Abscisic acid is a derivative of carotenoids. It was called "abscisin II" originally because it was thought to play a major role in abscission of fruits. At about the same time another group was calling it "dormin" because they thought it had a major role in bud dormancy. The name abscisic acid (ABA) was coined by a compromise between the two groups.
6. (c) Differentiation of root is controlled by high auxin concentration. in tissue culture auxin concentration is made high to promote rooting.

7. (c) 8. (c) 9. (b) 10. (a) 11. (c)
12. (b)
13. (d) Parthenocarpy refers the development of fruits without fertilization. Such fruits are seedless but otherwise normal in appearance, e.g. banana, pineapple etc. The auxins (IAA, IBA, 2, 4-D) are applied in low concentration in a lanolin paste to the stigma of flower to induce parthenocarpy.
14. (c) 15. (a)
16. (b) Cytokinin are usually amino purine so they resemble nucleic acids in structural aspects.
17. (a) Natural auxin are naturally occurring auxin plant hormones which are called phytohormones. Eg. IAA and IBB. These are synthesized in shoot apices, leaf primordial and developing seeds from tryptophan. Some of the important synthetic auxins are 2, 4-D; 2, 4, 5-T (2, 4, 5- trichlorophenoxy acetic acid).
18. (c) 2, 4-Dichlorophenoxy acetic acid is used for causing defoliation of forest trees.
2, 4-D or 2, 4 dichlorophenoxy acetic acid is an auxin hormone. It stimulates the growth activities of the cells of the root due to which roots get destroyed and thus plants finally destroys. 2, 4-D is used as a defoliant for broad leaved dicots.
19. (d) 20. (a) 21. (c) 22. (d) 23. (b)
24. (c) Geometric growth is quite common in unicellular organisms when growth is nutrient rich medium. Here, every cell divides. The daughter cells grow and divide, the grand daughter cells repeat the process and so on. Number of cells in initially small so that initial growth is slow. Later on, there is rapid growth at exponential rate (log or exponential growth).
Sigmoid Growth Curve : Geometric growth cannot be sustained for long. Limited nutrient availability slows down the growth. It leads to stationary phase. Plotting the growth against time gives a typical sigmoid or S-curve.
The exponential growth can be expressed as
$W1 = W_0 e^{rt}$
where W_1 = final size (weight, height, number etc.)
W_0 = initial size at the beginning of the period
r = growth rate
t = time of growth
e = base of natural logarithms

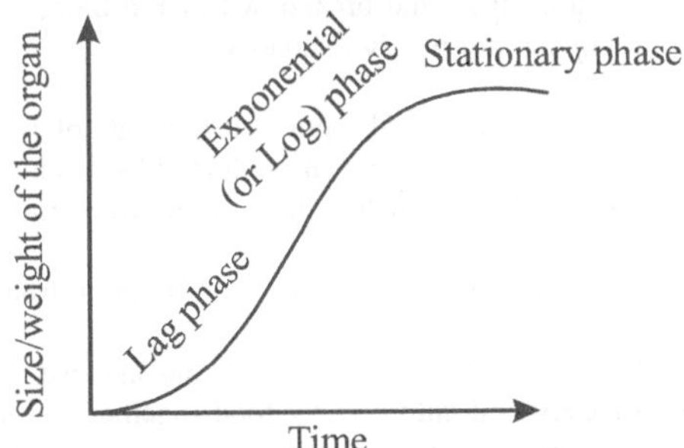

25. (a) Low temperature required for vernalization is usually 0—5°C. In nature, the plants requiring vernalization are commonly biennials (e.g., cabbage, sugarbeet, carrot), which complete their life cycle in two years. They germinate and grow vegetatively in the first year and produce flowers in the second year of growth. These plants fulfill their cold requirement during winters. However, such biennial plants can be made to flower in one growing season by providing low temperature treatment (i.e., 0—5°C temperature) to young plants or moistened seeds.
26. (c) The pulse of red light converts P_r to P_{fr}. Subsequent pulses of far-red light stimulate changes that lead to chlorophyll synthesis.
27. (d) Mechanical abrasion, leaching of inhibitors by water, and exposure to fire may all trigger germination, but actual germination cannot begin until the seed imbibes water.
28. (b) Ethylene gas promotes senescence and is one of the by products of burning your gas grill. You should move your grill or your camellia bush.
29. (b) Less of chlorophyll and degeneration of proteins are the two important symptoms of senescence. Cytokinins delay these processes and, thus the senescence is also delayed. This effect of cytokinin is known as Richmond-Lang effect.
30. (d) Receptors receive environmental cues and trigger hormone release or a signal transduction pathway that involves hormones. The signal alters gene expression by altering genes which are transcribed and translated. Cellular response depends on expression of those genes.
31. (b) The ratios of cytokinins to auxins control cell differentiation in plant tissue culture. When both are present in relatively equal quantities, cells divide but do not differentiate. If there is more of cytokinin than auxin, shoot buds develop from a callus. If there is relatively more auxin than cytokinins, roots develop. Thus proportion of these two hormones control organ formation in callus tissues. Abscissic acid (ABA) is a naturally occurring growth inhibitor.
32. (c) Cryptochromes respond to blue and ultraviolet light.
33. (d) The curvature induced in plant organs in response to the unidirectional light is called photoropism.
34. (a) The first naturally occuring auxin was isolated by Kogl and Haagen-Smit (1931) from human urine. It was identified as auxin-a (auxentriolic acid). Later, in 1934 Kogl, Haagen-Smit and Erxleben obtained another auxin called auxin-b (auxenolonic acid) from corn germ oil (extracted from germinating corn seeds).
35. (b) Altering the plasticity allows for permanent changes in cell wall shape. The cell wall must increase in size in order for cell growth to occur.
36. (b) Dwarf strains were genetically unable to produce gibberellin, so additional fertilizers would have no effect.
37. (a) Paratonic movements are induced by external stimuli.
38. (d) 39. (a) 40. (d) 41. (c) 42. (a)
43. (c) Prunning of plants promotes branching, because the axillary buds get sensitized to cytokinin.
44. (c) 45. (d)

Speed Test-74

1. (b) Spleen (also known as blood bank and graveyard of RBCs) is a dark, purple gland present in the left side of abdomen against the stomach. It is internally made up of white pulp and red pulp. Its main functions are storage of blood and break down of old and senescent RBCs.
2. (a) Vitamins are accessory food factors required in small amount for growth and metabolism. Vitamins are either water soluble → B. complex and vit.C or fat soluble → vit. A, D and K.
3. (c) 4. (d)
5. (b) Premolar and molar are lophodont teeths. Lophodont teeth with the cusps elongated to form narrow ridges. The molars in elephants and horses have cusps fused by means of intermediate masses of dentine to form ridges or lophs.
6. (d)

7. (c) Continued consumption of fat rich diet causes hypercholesterolemia. Hypercholesterolemia is the presence of high levels of cholesterol in the blood. High cholesterol raises risk for heart disease, heart attack, and stroke. Kidney stones are solid mass made up of tiny crystals. There are different types of kidney stones. The exact cause depends on the type of stone like, calcium stones, uric acid stone *etc.* Vitamin A toxicity or hypervitaminosis A is having too much of vitamin A in the body. Ketonuria is condition in which ketone bodies are present in urine. Body productes excess ketone bodies as an alternate source of energy during starvation or diabetes mellitus (type 1).

8. (a) Fat is mainly digested by pancreatic lipase while protein is digested by enzymes in pancreatic juice, intestinal juice and stomach.

9. (c) Beri-beri is a deficiency disease caused by the lack of vitamin B_1 (Thiamine) in the diet. The deficiency of riboflavin (Vit.B_2) causes ariboflavinosis. Scurvy is the result of lack of vitamin C in the diet. Deficiency of calciferol (vitamin D) in the diet causes rickets in children and osteomalacia in adults.

10. (a) Oxyntic cells or Parietal cells, are the stomach epithelium cells that secrete gastric acid and intrinsic factor. These cells secrete hydrochloric acid (HCl) which makes the gastric juice acidic (pH = 2.0-3.0).
Alpha cells of islets of Langerhans secretes glucagon hormone which increase the glucose level in the blood by converting glycogen to glucose in liver cells. Kupffer's cells are specialized cells in the liver that destroy bacteria, foreign proteins, and worn-out blood cells. Sebaceous glands and microscopic glands in the skin that secrete an oily/waxy matter (called sebum) to lubricate the skin and hair of mammals.

11. (c) Kwashiorkor and Beri-Beri are deficiency diseases which occur mostly in children. Kwashiorkar occurs due to deficiency of protein and Beri-Beri due to deficiency of vit-B_1 (Thiamine).

12. (d) Colostrum (also known as beesting or first milk) is a form of milk produced by the mammary glands in late pregnancy and the few days after giving birth. Human and bovine colostrums are thick, sticky and yellowish. In humans, it has high concentrations of nutrients and antibodies, but it is small in quantity.
Colostrum is high in carbohydrates, high in protein, high in antibodies, and low in fat (as human new borns may find fat difficult to digest). Newborns have very small digestive systems, and colostrum delivers its nutrients in a very concentrated low-volume form. It has a mild laxative effect, encouraging the passing of the baby's first stool, which is called meconium. This clears excess bilirubin, a waste product of dead red blood cells which is produced in large quantities at birth due to blood volume reduction, from the infant's body and helps to prevent jaundice.

13. (b) Long term intake of alcohol causes damage to liver which is known as cirrhosis of liver with continued alcohol intake, there is destruction of hepatocytes and fibroblasts (cell which form fibres) and stimulates of collagen protein formation.

14. (d) 15. (d) 16. (b) 17. (b) 18. (d) 19. (a)
20. (d) 21. (b)

22. (a) The chylomicrons are formed inside enterocytes and are absorbed in lacteals.

23. (a) The caecum is a pouch-like portion of the large intestine which hosts some symbiotic micro-organism. The caecum absorbs water and salts from undigested foods before they continue on to the large intestine.

24. (b) 25. (a)

26. (d) In the small intestine, pancreatic juice containing an enzyme, α-amylase acts on starch and converts it into dissacharide, maltose and isomaltose and 'limit' dextrins.

$$\text{Starch} \xrightarrow[\alpha-\text{aMylase}]{\text{Pancreatic}} \text{Maltose} + \text{Isomaltose} + \text{'Limit' dextrins}$$

27. (a) Fructose is generally absorbed by facilitated transport. The digestive wastes, solidified into coherent faeces in the rectum initiate a neural reflex causing an urge or desire for its removal.

28. (c) Many of the water-soluble vitamins play a vital role in enzyme function.

29. (d) The pancreas produces a mumber of important digestive enzymes, without which digestion and nutrient absorption are greatly hampered.

30. (c) A gastrovascular cavity has a single opening.

31. (d) Enzymes that digest proteins, lipids, and carbohydrates all function in the small intestine.

32. (c) Essential amino acids must be acquired through diet because an animal cannot directly synthesize all of the amino acids needed for protein

33. (d) The stomach is protected from digestive enzymes and low pH by the neutralizing, buffering, and coating mucus secreted over its inner surface.

34. (a) The small intestines are the site for the majority of digestion in humans.

35. (c) The large intestine is the site of water and ion absorption. The large population of bacteria in the large intestine contributes vitamins that are useful to the host.

36. (b) The membranes of the digestive tract are, from the inside to the outside: mucosa, submucosa, circular and longitudinal muscles, serosa.

37. (c) the stomach stores food (and performs some digestion too) before passing it on to the intestines. The small intestine (midgut) finishes tint digestion and carries out most of the nutrient absorption, while the large intestine (hindgut) reabsorbs water and ions.

38. (d) Insulin increases the rate of glucose uptake from the blood into the muscle cells by increasing the number of glucose transporters in the plasma membrane.

39. (a) The liver produces bile salts and add to the bile pigments bilirubin from the breakdown of red blood cells. The bile pigments are purely excretory.

40. (c)

41. (d) Generally, fatty acids upto a chain length of 10 carbon atoms are primarily absorbed through the blood caillaries, but those with higher chain length through lymphatic route (lymph vessels).

42. (c) Mammals may drink water and also get it from oxidation of glucose.

43. (b) Because saliva converts starch into maltose.

44. (a) Anxiety and eating spicy food together in normal healthy man can lead to indigestion which is difficulty in digestion.

45. (a) Young infant may be feeding entirely on mother's milk which is white in colour but the stools which the infant passes out is quite yellowish because bile pigments passed through bile juice. Bile pigments are any of several coloured compounds derived from porphyrin that are found in bile; principally bilirubin and biliverdin. Bile pigment is produced regularly when old red blood cells are broken down, mainly by the spleen. In some blood-disorders where the red cells are destroyed, more bile pigment is produced.

Speed Test-75

1. (a) 70% to 75% CO_2 is transported as primary buffer of the blood bicarbonate ion (HCO_3) in blood plasma. When CO_2 diffuses from tissues into blood then it is acted upon by the enzyme carbonic anhydrase.
2. (a) A large portion of oxygen is left unused in the human blood even after its uptake by the body tissues. This O_2 acts as a reserve during muscular exercise.
3. (a) It is the relationship between the percentage saturation of haemoglobin (by volume) in the blood and the oxygen tension (in partial tension) pO_2 of the blood.
   It is usually a sigmoid plot. Haemoglobin molecules can bind up to four oxygen molecules in a reversible way. The shape of the curve results from the interaction of bound oxygen molecules with incoming molecules. The binding of the first molecule is difficult. However, this facilitates the binding of the second and third molecules, and it is only when the fourth molecule is to be bound that the difficulty increases, partly as a result of crowding of the haemoglobin molecule, partly as a natural tendency of oxygen to dissociate.
4. (d) Brain is the most vital organ. It stops functioning in the absence of O_2.
5. (d) When the CO_2 concentration in blood increases, breathing becomes faster and deeper. As CO_2 levels increase, patients exhibit a reduction in overall level of consciousness as well as respiratory effort. Severe increase in CO_2 levels can lead to respiratory arrest.
6. (c) CO_2 enters RBC and reacts with water to form carbonic acid. Carbonic acid dissociates to form bicarbonate and hydrogen ions. Some bicarbonate ions are transported in erythrocytes while some diffuse into the blood plasma. Exit of bicarbonate ions change the ionic balance between the plasma and erythrocytes. To restore this balance chloride ions diffuse from plasma into erythrocytes. Due to this, the pH of blood is maintained.
7. (a)
8. (c) The maximum volume of air a person can breath in after a forced expiration or the maximum volume of air a person can breathe out after a forced inspiration is called vital capacity (VC). This includes tidal volume, inspiratory reserve volume and expiratory reserve volume.
   (TV + IRV + ERV). VC varies from 3400 ml – 4800 mL, depending upon age, sex and height of the individual.
9. (b) 10. (d)
11. (c) Emphysema is lung condition that causes shortness of breath due to damage of air sacs in the lungs (alvcoli). The main cause of emphysema is a long-term exposure to air-borne irritants including tobacco smoke, air pollution, dust.
12. (b) 13. (d) 14. (b) 15. (d) 16. (d)
17. (a) 18. (a)
19. (c) When the external intercostal muscles and diaphragm relax, the ribs move downward and inward and diaphragm becomes convex (dome shaped), thus decreasing the volume of thoracic cavity and increasing the pressure inside as compared to the atmospheric pressure outside. This will cause the air to move out (expiration).
20. (d) Pulmonary, CO_2 is found to be lower than cutaneous O_2 at all temperatures. Statement A is a wrong answer. This is because at 5°C, pulmonary O_2 is lower than cutaneous O_2, although as the temperature increases, the reverse becomes true.
21. (c) Myoglobin has an affinity for oxygen. It is present in the muscles. As oxygen levels reduce, myoglobin would release the stored oxygen to keep the muscles working.
22. (a) This decreases the size of the thoracic cavity, which increases the pressure within the thoracic cavity, forcing air out of the lungs.
23. (d) Debris normally gets trapped in mucus lining the respiratory passage ways. This mucus is then swept up and away from the lungs by the action of cilia.
24. (d) Myoglobin has the greatest affinity for oxygen and does not unload the oxygen until very low partial pressures of oxygen (below 20 mmHg). Foetal haemoglobin has a higher affinity for oxygen than adult haemoglobin, thus facilitating the transfer of oxygen from maternal haemoglobin to fetal, haemoglobin at the placenta. When respiration is occurring a fast rate, more oxygen is needed. High levels of respiration are associated with high levels of carbon dioxide, hence the affinity of haemoglobin for oxygen decreases at higher carbon dioxide partial pressures so that oxygen can be released to respiring tissues.
25. (a) Inspiration in the mammalian lung occurs by means of negative pressure produced by contraction of the diaphragm. Thus, the pressure in the lungs falls below atmospheric pressure.
26. (d) The Bohr effect describes the action of pH on the oxygen-binding curve. Decreases in pH result in a net right shift of the entire oxygen equilibrium curve.
27. (d) Movement of O_2 and CO_2 from the blood to the tissues always occurs by diffusion of O_2 and CO_2 down their partial pressure gradients.
28. (d) This mechanism serves a very important cleansing role for the mammalian respiratory system.
29. (d) A left shift in the oxygen-binding curve means that the pigment operates at lower PO_2 values.
30. (d) Actively respiring tissues require more oxygen. They are also associated with high partial pressures of carbon dioxide since it is a product of respiration. The curves show that oxygen would be more readily released at higher partial pressures of carbon dioxide, i.e. at active tissues.
31. (c) When the chest expands, stretch receptors in the lungs reflexly excite the expiratory center in the medulla which tends to produce expiration. Partial exhalation lessens the intensity of this reflex, allowing breath to be held for a longer time. Exhalation does not change the blood CO_2 concentration unless fresh air (low in CO_2) is brought into the lungs, allowing more CO_2 to diffuse out of the blood.
32. (b) Thin layer of water on the inner surface of alveoli serves to contract the alveoli and makes them behave like unfilled balloons that resist inflation. This would mean tremendous effort to inhale and expand the alveoli and therefore to overcome this, cells of the alveoli secrete pulmonary surfactant to decrease the surface tension of water lining the alveoli.
33. (d) Gas is brought into the lungs when the negative pressure exists between the lungs and the rest of the chest. This negative intrapleural pressure is aided to occur by all the choices mentioned.
34. (c) 35. (d)
36. (c) Changes in pH due to the accumulation of acidic metabolites resulting from increased cell activity are the basis of the Bohr effect.
37. (d)
38. (d) The hyoid is a bone of the skeletal system that supports the larynx and tongue.
39. (c) The alveoli do not contain "air" with 20.9% O_2 because incoming air is mixed with air left in the "dead space" of the trachea and bronchi that has had some of the O_2 removed by the lungs.

40. (c) Water breathing is more difficult than air breathing because the higher density of water makes it more expensive to move across the respiratory surfaces than air, it has less oxygen than air, and the oxygen content is very dependent on the temperature of the water. CO_2 however, dissolves easily into water and is easy to get rid of.

41. (d) All of the listed choices have larger volume than the resting tidal volume.

42. (a) Myoglobin has only one haem group and there can be no co-operative binding, hence the shape of the dissociation curve is hyperbolic rather than sigmoidal. Also, myoglobin has a very high affinity for oxygen and does not release oxygen until a very low oxygen tension.

43. (b)

44. (a) During the transport of CO_2 through the blood, bicarbonate ions diffuse out of RBCs while chloride ions from plasma enter the RBCs to maintain ionic equilibrium. This is called chloride shift.

45. (b) The total volume of air that can be expelled from the lungs after maximum inspiration and then expiring to the maximum is known as the vital capacity. The volume of air that remains inside lungs at the end of maximum forceful expiration is the residual volume. Expiratory reserve volume is the maximum extra volume of air that can be expired by forceful expiration after a normal tidal expiration. Total lung capacity is the maximum volume of air that can be contained in the lungs after maximum inspiration.

Speed Test-76

1. (a)
2. (c)
3. (a) Lubb sound is caused partly by the closure of the bicuspid and tricuspid valves and partly by the contraction of the muscles in the ventricles. Lubb is the first heart sound.
4. (b) Rh factor was discovered by Karl Landsteiner. A child of Rh^+ man will be Rh^+ whether the mother is Rh^+ or Rh^-. If the mother is Rh^+ then there will be no problem but if mother is Rh^- so when the blood of Rh^+ child (in womb) mixes with the blood of Rh^- mother then some antibodies in mother's blood are formed against Rh^+ factor which coagulate the womb blood causing death. If birth takes place then there is a possibility of child death in early years. This in known as erythroblastosis foetalis. In most cases the Ist pregnancy may succeed but after that it fails.
5. (c)
6. (c) Peak P-causes diastolic phase in ventricle while R-Peak causes systole in ventricle means diastolic and systolic phases represented by P & R.
7. (c) Sino-Auricular node (SA node) present in the walls of right auricle has a myogenic initiation of heartbeat in a regular fashion and controls the pace of heartbeat called pacemaker.
8. (c)
9. (d) Haemoglobin has 250 times more affinity for CO as compared to oxygen. Hb readily combines with CO, forming carboxyhaemoglobin (COHb), COHb interferes with the transport of oxygen.
10. (c) An adult healthy human has average systolic and diastolic blood pressure as given below :

$$\text{B.P.} = \frac{\text{Systolic}}{\text{Diastolic}} = \frac{120 \text{ mm Hg}}{80 \text{ mm Hg}}$$

11. (b) Blood group A – Antigen-A & Antibody 'b' or Anti A or a.
Blood group B – Antigen-B & antibody a or Anti B or b.
Blood group AB – Antigen-A & B and no antibody.
Blood group O – No antigen & Antibodies a & b both.
12. (d) The number of blood platelets per cubic mm in human blood is 3 lacs while WBCs are 5000/cubic mm of blood. Veins are as complex as the arteries. Veins and arteries both are types of blood vessels. Arteries carry blood from heart to different organs while vein carries blood from different organs to heart. At any given time in a healthy human, the blood amount is same in both, as the circulation of blood never stops.
Blood consists of two parts:
The **plasma** (water, proteins, inorganic salts and other elements) constitutes 55-60% of blood while **cellular** part constitutes 40-45% of total blood. WBC are produced in red bone marrow, lymph nodes and sometimes even in liver and spleen.
13. (a) High proportion of cholesterol in blood leads to deposition of cholesterol on the walls of blood vessels. This causes the arteries to lose their elasticity and get stiffened. This is called arteriosclerosis or hardening of arteries.
14. (d)
15. (b) 'Bundle of His' are a typical cardiac muscle fibres, connecting the atria with ventricle.
16. (d) 17. (d) 18. (a) 19. (c) 20. (d)
21. (d) 22. (c) 23. (a) 24. (a) 25. (a)
26. (d) 27. (b) 28. (a)
29. (a) The degree of oxygenation of blood markedly affects the amount of CO_2 transported in blood. The lower the pO_2 and the haemoglobin saturation with O_2, the more the CO_2 that can be carried in the blood. This phenomenon, is called the Haldane effect. It depicts the greater ability of reduced haemoglobin to form carbaminohaemoglobin and to buffer H^+ by combining with it. In the pulmonary circulation, uptake of O_2 facilitates the release of CO_2. As haemoglobin becomes saturated with O_2, the hydrogen ions released combine with HCO_3^-, helping to unload CO_2 from the pulmonary blood. The Haldane effect is quantitatively more important in promoting O_2 transport than the Bohr effect in promoting O_2 transport. It results from the simple fact that combination of O_2 with haemoglobin causes the haemoglobin (oxyhaemoglobin) to become a stronger acid. This in turn displaces CO_2 from the blood.
30. (d) Christmas factor (factor IX) is a plasma thromboplastin component i.e. a thromboplastin activator present in blood plasma. Its deficiency causes congenital disease called hemophilia B (also called Christmas disease).
31. (c) Veins bring blood from different body parts to the heart. The flow of blood in veins is not so fast because the blood in veins is under low pressure. Veins possess valves which prevent backward flow of blood.
32. (d) Cardiac output = Stroke volume × heart beats per minute

$$\therefore \text{ Stroke volume} = \frac{\text{Cardiac output}}{\text{Heart beats per minute}}$$

$$= \frac{5250}{75} = 70 \text{ ml}$$

33. (a) Heart valves only permit unidirectional flow of blood.
34. (b)
35. (c) The left ventricle pumps blood into the aorta.
36. (a) Contraction of the ventricle produces pressure in the human circulatory system. Blood leaves the ventricles and then immediately enters the arteries moving away from the heart. Blood pressure will have its highest recording in these arteries.

37. (c) The small diameter of capillaries offers great resistance to blood flow. This slows the blood to a speed at which nutrient and gas exchange with neighboring cells is more efficient.
38. (b) The atrium has thinner walls and generates lower pressures than the ventricles.
39. (a)
40. (c) The left ventricle generates a greater pressure in the blood flowing to the systemic circuit than the right ventricle with blood flowing to the pulmonary circuit.
41. (c) The AV node delays the ventricular depolarization relative to atrial depolarization, so atrial contraction occurs before ventricular contraction. The Purkinje fibers transmit the cardiac impulse to very small localized groups of ventricular fibers.
42. (d)
43. (a) Presence of calcium will remove heparin - blood anticoagulant and will promote blood clotting. Sodium oxalate and heparin containing test tubes will not allow the blood to clot.
44. (a) Blood serum is liquid minus clotting elements of pale yellow colour. It does not have fibrinogen and other clotting materials. It does not take part in blood clotting.
45. (a) Folic Acid (Cyanocobalamine vit. B_{12}) works in the formation and maturation of RBCs. In the deficiency of this RBCs formation decreases and the formed RBCs will not mature i.e. they will not loose the nucleus and hence remain nucleated and lack haemoglobin. Such RBCs cannot carry oxygen & person suffers from anaemia. Supplementing his diet with folic acid and cobalamine will lead to the increased formation and proper maturation of enucleated RBCs with haemoglobin and eliminate anaemia.

Speed Test-77

1. (c) Liver is the primary site of detoxification and elimination of body wastes and poisons. Liver detoxifies endotoxins, *e.g.* toxic NH_3 combined with CO_2 to form less toxic urea. It also detoxifies alcohol and convert them to acetaldehyde and then harmless acetyl CoA.
2. (d) Renin (also called rennet or chymosin) is an coagulating enzyme produced from stomach of human body. It catalyzes the coagulation of milk by converting milk with soluble protein caesin into insoluble semi fluid calcium paracaesinate. This is called curdling of milk. Rennin produced in the infants immediately after birth. As the child grows, rennin production goes down and is replaced by pepsin digestive enzymes.
Renin is an enzyme which acts as hormone secreted by juxtaglomerular cells. It converts angiotensinogen into angiotensin.
3. (b) Nephron is the excretory unit of human excretory system. Each nephron has a Bowman's Capsule, a Proximal Convoluted Tubule (PCT), Loop of Henle (Descending & Ascending limbs) and Distal Convoluted Tubule (DCT) which then enter into collecting duct.
4. (d)
5. (b) Thermoregulation is the ability of an organism to keep its body temperature within certain boundaries, even when temperature surrounding is very different. In humans, sweating is primarily a means of thermoregulation.
6. (c) Due to a long hunger strike and survival on water, a person will have less urea in his urine because urea comes to kidney as a waste product from liver which is formed after the breakdown of protein fat, carbohydrate during hunger. It is not synthesised but the synthesised ones are catabolised.
7. (c)
8. (b) It is named after its discoverer, F. G. J. Henle. In the kidney, the loop of Henle is the portion of the nephron that leads from the proximal convoluted tubule to the distal convoluted tubule. The loop has a hairpin bend in the renal medulla. The main function of this structure is to reabsorb water and ions from the urine. To do this, it uses a countercurrent multiplier mechanism in the medulla.
9. (a) 10. (d) 11. (c) 12. (b) 13. (d)
14. (a) Glomerular podocytes are highly specialized cells with a complex cytoarchitecture plays a major role in establishing the selective permeability of glomerular filtration barrier.
15. (c) Haematuria is the presence of blood cells in urine.
16. (c) 17. (c)
18. (a) ANF stimulates the loss of sodium in urine while aldosterone absorbs sodium from glomerular filtrate.
19. (b) 20. (d) 21 (d) 22. (b)
23 (a) Kangaroo rat lives in desert, therefore, it needs to conserve water in the body. In kangaroo rat, loop of Henle is significantly longer as it descends further into the medulla and produces a higher concentration gradient in the surrounding tissue so as to produce urine which is 18 times concentrated than that of their blood. This gradient allows more water to diffuse into the surrounding tissues to be reabsorbed.
24. (b) Dialysis is of two types : haemodialysis and peritoneal dialysis. Peritoneal dialysis uses a natural filter inside the body i.e. peritoneal membrane to remove wastes and extra fluid from the body. The dialysis fluid fills the belly and pulls out wastes and extra fluid from the body. Blood is not removed from the body as in the case of haemodialysis.
25. (b) If the walls of the collecting duct are water-permeable, water leaves the ducts to pass into the hyperosmotic surrounding and concentrated urine is produced. Thus, when there is insufficient ADH, less water is reabsorbed and more dilute urine is produced in copious amounts.
26. (c) Ectotherms on poikilothermic animals are cold-blooded animals whose body temperature is dependent upon their environment.
27. (c) A and B involve ultrafiltration.
In the proximal convoluted tubules, the mitochondria provide energy for active transport. The cells here are adapted for reabsorption. The amino acids diffuse into the cells and are actively transported to the intercellular spaces, where they diffuse into the surrounding capillaries.
28. (a) The removal of urea and excess ions occurs by diffusion from the blood in the abdominal capillaries to the dialysis fluid, down a concentration gradient.
29. (d) This is the correct flow of urine after it leaves the kidney.
30. (b) About 1 percent of the filtrate is excreted as urine, so about 1.5 litres of the original 150 litres would be urinated.
31. (c) Antidiuretic hormone acts on the collecting ducts by increasing the permeability to water. Antidiuretic hormone secretion is stimulated by a decrease in blood pressure.
32. (b) Reabsorption returns substances to the blood, secretion moves substances from blood into the kidney tubules.
33. (a) The route of water and solutes through the nephron from the glomerulus, to Bowman's capsule, to proximal tubule, to loop of Henle, to distal tubule, to collecting ducts.
34. (d) Glucose and amino acids found in the filtrate are reabsorbed.
35. (a) The proximal tubule is the site of active transport of Na^+ out of the tubule. Na^+ also moves out of the tubule at the ascending limb of the loop of Henle, but this is a passive transport with Cl^- being actively transported out.
36. (a) Red blood cells are too large to be filtered out of the blood at the glomerulus and thus will not be found in the filtrate.

37. (b) Glucose is 100% reabsorbed and thus a healthy person will excrete no glucose in the urine. Sodium and water are usually over 99% reabsorbed. Urea is the main excretory product formed as a result of protein breakdown.
38. (b) The sole mechanism for water reabsorption in the renal tubules is by osmosis.
39. (d) A – Adrenal gland – located at the anterior part of kidney, secrete Catecholamines which stimulate glycogen breakdown.
40. (d)
41. (c) Salamander (Amphibia; Caudata) excrete urea by help of kidneys.
42. (c) Normally albumin can't pass out through the filtering pores due to their large size but in some pathological conditions viz. anoxia or heart failure, the filtration membrane becomes damaged and filtering pores enlarge in size, so that serum albumin passes out in the largest amount and appears in the urine.
43. (b) 44. (b) 45. (c)

Speed Test-78

1. (c) Movement of Ca^{2+} out in sarcoplasmic reticulum controls the making and breaking of actin and myosin complex actomyosin due to which muscle contraction and relaxation takes place. Albert Szent Gyorgyi worked out biochemical events of muscle contraction.
2. (a) Elbow joint is an example of hinge joint. The elbow is a hinge joint; it can open and close like a door. Hinge joint is a form of diarthrosis (freely movable joint) that allows angular movement in one plane only, increasing or decreasing the angle between the bones e.g. elbow joint, knee joint etc.
3. (b) MRI machine does not show face image of bone and calcium, *e.g.* scapula, canine. It is also not suitable for patients with cardiac pacemakers.
4. (b) Hyoid is a horse shoe shaped bone present in neck between lower law and sound box (larynx). It is not articulated to any bone, but is simply suspended, from temporal bones by means of ligaments. Hyoid provides surface for the attachment of tongue muscles.
5. (b)
6. (d) Ball and socket joint is a type of synovial joint in which two bones are articulated. Shoulder joint is an example of ball and socket joint in which humerus is joined with pectoral girdle.
7. (a) Actin and tropomyosin are part of thin filaments of skeletal muscle. Tubulin is presents in microtubules. Myosin is muscle protein.
8. (d)
9. (a) The pelvic girdle is formed by two innominate bones consists of three separate bones ilium, ischium and the pubis.
10. (d) The last two pairs *i.e.* 11th and 12th pairs ribs remain free anteriorly, hence, they are called as floating ribs.
11. (d)
12. (d) The sensation of fatigue in the muscles after prolonged strenuous physical work is caused by the accumulation of lactic acid.
13. (d) 14. (c) 15. (c) 16. (c) 17. (a)
18. (c) Troponin is a protein which is found on actin filament and myosin protein is found in myosin filament. Both actin and myosin are complex proteins in striated muscles. Thymosin is a hormone secreted by the thymus that stimulates development of T-cells. Prolactin is a hormone released by the pituitary gland that stimulates breast development and milk production in women. Rhodopsin, also known as visual purple, is not a hormone. It is a biological pigment in photoreceptor cells of the retina that is responsible for the first events in the perception of light.
19. (a) 20. (d) 21. (a) 22. (a) 23. (a)
24. (a) Smooth muscles are non-straited, unbranched and spindle shaped. Skeletal muscles are unbranched. Cardiac muscles fibres are uni-nucleated.
25. (d) Tarsals, femur, metatarsals and tibia are boned of the legs which are involved in running during chasing the ball by cricket player.
26. (b) Bone is made up of 60&70% inorganic matter and 30&40% organic matter.
27. (a) Hyaline cartilage is most abundant cartilage in body.
28. (b) The ER releases calcium ions only if stimulated by an action potential, which requires acetylcholine to diffuse across the neuromuscular junction.
29. (c) Fine motor control is accomplished by the presence of smaller, more numerous motor units. Each motor unit requires an individual motor neuron.
30. (c) Smooth muscle is found mainly in the walls of hollow organs, such as digestive tract organs and blood vessels. Smooth muscles propel substances through the hollow organ by alternately contracting and relaxing.
31. (b) A hydrostatic skeleton consists of fluid held under pressure in a closed body compartment.
32. (a) Mandible is a large bone constituting the lower jaw.
33. (b) Stapes is one of the three ear ossicles in the middle ear resembling a tiny stirrup. It transmits sound vibrations from the incus to the internal ear.
34. (b) ATP provides energy that is used to detach myosin from actin.
35. (b) Endoskeletons (such as those of mammals) are found inside the body, and exoskeletons (such as those of insects) are found outside the body.
36. (c) In gout, there occurs a defect in uric acid metabolism resulting into its elevated level in blood (hyperuricemia). This is followed by precipitation of excessive uric acid which gets deposited in the joint spaces. These deposited crystals of uric acid causes pain in different bony joints.
37. (b) 38. (c) 39. (d)
40. (a) Glenoid cavity is a shallow concavity on the lateral side of pectoral girdle in which the head of humerus fits making the shoulder joint.
41. (c) 42. (c) 43. (b) 44. (b) 45. (a)

Speed Test-79

1. (b) Afferent nerve fibres – sensory nerve fibres which carry senses from receptors to brain or spinal cord (CNS). Efferent nerve fibres – motor nerve fibres that carry orders or responses from CNS to effectors (muscles and glands).
2. (a) Hypothalamus contains important nerve centres that controls the body temperature, thirst, hunger, eating, water balance and sexual function.
3. (c) The rods and cones are exceptionally specialized bipolar neurons which have developed some structural features to carry out the transduction of light energy into neuronal signals.
4. (c) The transmission of nerve impulse through synapse requires a chemical neuro transmitter. The most common neurotransmitter is acetylcholine.
5. (b) Alzheimer disease in humans is associated with the deficiency of acetylcholine. Acetylcholine is the neurotransmitter produced by neurons (referred to as cholinergic neurons). Acetylcholine plays a role in skeletal muscle movement, as well as in the regulation of smooth muscle and cardiac muscle. Acetylcholine is synthesized from choline and acetyl coenzyme-A through the action of the enzyme choline acetyltransferase and becomes packaged into membrane-bound vesicles.

6. (c) Conditioned reflexes are acquired reflexes and are dependent on past experiences, training and learning. I.R. Pavlov demonstrated conditioned reflexes in a hungry dog. He called food and salivation in response to it as unconditioned stimulus and sound of bell and salivation in response to bell as conditioned reflexes.
7. (a) The inner layer of the posterior two-thirds of the eyeball consists of a light sensitive layer, called retina that possesses two types of photoreceptors called the rods and the cone cells. Retina reduces the internal reflection, so any damage to it leads to greater internal reflection of light often causing an increase in light sensitivity.
8. (c) Epinephrine or adrenaline, norepinephrine or noradrenaline and acetylchloline are the neurotransmitters. These are released by the nerve fibres to transmit the impulse to the next neurone. Cortisone is not a neurotransmitter.
9. (d) Total sum of physio-electrochemical changes that takes place along the length of nerve fibre is known as nerve impulse. Change in potential due to stimulation of nerve fibre is called action potential. During propagation of nerve impulse, Na^+ enters inside so (+ve) change is formed inside the membrane. K^+ ions come out.
10. (c) 11. (c) 12. (b)
13. (c) The intensity of movement of basilar fibres regulates the loudness or amplitude of sound.
14. (d) 15. (a) 16. (b)
17. (a) Epinephrine and norepinephrine are secreted by adrenalmedulla in response to stress of any kind and during emergency situations and are called emergency hormones or hormones of flight, or fight.
18. (c) 19. (a) 20. (d) 21. (d) 22. (b)
23. (a)
24. (a) During stress condition, stimulation of the sympathetic nerves to adrenal medulla causes large quantities of adrena-line to be released into the blood circulation and then this hormone is carried to the specific tissues of the body where it produces its effect e.g., increase in heart beat.
25. (b) Tectorial membrane is a gelatinous membrane covering the sensory hair cells in the scala media of cochlea.
26. (b) Once differentiated, nerve cells do not divide as they lack mitotic activity. Lack of mitotic activity indicates that they do not have centrosome.
27. (d) Reflex arcs allow for rapid processing and response.
28. (d) These drugs alter perception of stimuli and work mainly at the axon or the synapse
29. (b) An action potential is a localized electrical event—a membrane depolarization at a specific point of stimulation.
30. (d) An influx of sodium depolarizes the membrane and opens more sodium channels, causing still more depolarization, an example of positive feedback.
31. (c) The embryonic forebrain gives rise to the telencephalon and the diencephalon. The thalamus and the hypothalamus develop from the diencephalon; the cerebral cortex develops from the telencephalon.
32. (c) Since the action potential started in the middle of the axon, rather than at the axon hillock as typically occurs, there is no previous patch of membrane currently undergoing a refractory period. The action potential is thus free to propagate in both directions.
33. (b) Hyperpolarizing neuron B by 15 mV would make its membrane potential –65mV, actually taking it further away from the threshold voltage needed to fire an action potential.
34. (d) The medulla oblongata contains centers that control several visceral functions, such as breathing, heart and blood vessel activity, swallowing, vomiting, and digestion.
35. (d) For an action potential to occur in an axon, the membrane must be depolarized above a certain level. This level is known as the threshold.
36. (d) Electrical synapses join two cells with protein tunnels known as connexons. The junctions that are formed provide for very fast transmission between cells.
37. (c) Atropine is a substance that blocks the inhibitory effects of muscarinic receptors in muscle tissue, especially the heart.
38. (b)
39. (c) Arbor vitae is composed of white matter.
40. (a)
41. (c) The white matter in the CNS consists of tracts that convey sensations from one structure or region to another.
42. (c)
43. (c) The olfactory epithelium lining the superior border of the nasal cavity is innervated by the olfactory (first cranial) nerve.
44. (a) These are called the limits of audibility. Actual value is 20 to 20000 cycles/sec.
45. (c)

Speed Test-80

1. (a) Cortisol is secreted by the middle region of adrenal cortex. It increases the blood glucose level (which is anti-insulin effect) by converting proteins & fats into glucose.
2. (b) Pancreas is a gland which is both exocrine and endocrine. Cells of acini are exocrine which secrete enzymes and islet of Langerhans part is endocrine which secretes hormones like insulin, glucagon, *etc.*
3. (b) Hormones are chemical messengers formed by endocrine cells. Chemically hormones are of the following types: Amines–composed of amino group e.g., Melatonin.
Amino acids – eg. thyroxine
Peptides –eg. insulin
Steroids –eg. aldosterone
4. (a) Parathamone is a peptide hormone secreted by the parathyroid gland in response to low levels of calcium in the blood. It acts to maintain normal blood levels of calcium by increasing the number of osteoclasts, which break down the bone matrix and release calcium into the blood. It also increases the reabsorption of calcium and magnesium ions in the kidney tubules, so that their concentration is maintained in the blood.
5. (d) Electroencephalogram is the recording of electric potentials originating from different parts of the brain in the form of waves. Fractionation is the technique of rupturing cells and separating their components especially cell organelles for studying their chemistry and functions. Electrophoresis is the technique of separation of charged solutes on the basis of their differential migration in an applied electric field.
6. (b)
7. (a) Luteinizing hormone (LH) stimulates ovulation. Deficiency of insulin causes diabetes mellitus. Deficiency of ADH or vasopressin causes diabetes insipidus. Deficiency of parathormone causes tetany. Deficiency of thyroxine causes cretinism in infants and myxoedema in adults.
8. (b) In heart cells AMP acts as secondary messenger which is made in the response of adrenaline and it stimulates Ca^{2+} ions to come out from the sarcoplasmic reticulum of muscle fibres which causes muscle contraction.
cGMP (Cyclic Guanosine Monophosphate) which acts as secondary messenger works on the action of acetylcholine, increase in flow of Ca^{2+} into muscle fibres & hence causes muscle relaxation. There is no role of sodium in hormonal action.

9. (c) Pancreas is a heterocrine gland comprising both endocrine and exocrine parts. Its endocrine part consists of small masses of hormone secreting cells called islets of Langerhans. The α-cells of latter secrete glucagons and its β-cells secrete insulin. These two hormones have antagonistic effects on the glucose level in the blood which means that insulin decreases the blood glucose level while glucagon increases blood glucose level.
10. (a) Neurons regulate endocrine activity, but not *vice-versa*.Neurons in the hypothalamus secrete thyroid releasing hormone (TRH), which stimulates cells in the anterior pituitary to secrete thyroid-stimulating hormone (TSH).
11. (b) Posterior pituitary releases vasopressin which stimulates reabsorption of water in the distal tubules in nephron.
12. (d) Osmotic pressure of body fluids is mainly maintained by the plasma proteins (albumins, globulins) and electrolyte ions (Na^+, K^+ etc). Phosphorus has nothing to do with the osmotic pressure of body fluids.
13. (c) Sertoli cells are found in the walls of seminiferous tubules of the testes. They anchor and provide nutrition to the developing germ cells especially the spermatids.
14. (b) In menstrual cycle, menstrual phase lasts for 4 days, proliferating/ovulating phase for about 10 days and secretory phase for 14 days.
15. (c) 16.(a) 17. (a) 18. (b) 19. (b)
20. (c) 21.(d) 22. (a) 23. (b) 24. (d)
25. (c) Calcium plays an important role in blood clotting. Parathormone, a hormone released by parathyroid glands, increases calcium level in the blood. Therefore, deficiency of this hormone will decrease Ca^{2+} level in the blood, thus leading to delay in blood clotting and increase in bleeding time.
26. (d) Estrogen and testosterone being steroid hormones are soluble in lipids, therefore they can cross the plasma membrane and bind to the cytoplasmic receptors to trigger their action.
27. (b)
28. (d) Hydrophobic molecules, such as steroid based hormones, can move easily through the plasma membrane.
29. (d) Insulin acts to lower blood sugar levels.
30. (d) Receptors on target cells react specifically to chemical messengers. The way they react will determine the cellular response.
31. (d) The adrenal glands secrete hormones in response to stress.
32. (b) Hormones typically act on a receptor in or on target cells to stimulate the production of proteins.
33. (d) The internal transport system may be the cardiovascular system in animals or the xylem and phloem in plants.
34. (c) Oxytocin stimulates muscle contractions during childbirth and milk letdown.
35. (c) In diabetics, the rise in blood glucose above the normal level of 80–90 mg/100ml fails to stimulate the production of insulin from the pancreatic β-cells of the islets of Langerhans. As a result, the glucose is not removed from the blood to be stored in muscle cells as glycogen, resulting in a high blood glucose level for a long period of time.
36. (c) Paracrine hormones act on local cells that are hormones act on the very same cells that secrete them.
37. (a) "Upregulation" of hormone receptors on a cell is the production of more receptors when the hormone is present over time in the blood or other fluids surrounding the cell.
38. (b) Thymic hormones stimulate T cell development.
39. (c) In many cases, hormones trigger cyclic AMP when they bind with the target cells. Cyclic AMP then carries out the action of the hormone within the cell as a second messenger.
40. (d) The pituitary gland is considered the master gland because it produces hormones that control endocrine glands throughout the body.
41. (c) Inhibited release of a releasing hormone will lead to a reduction in the secretion of a specific anterior pituitary hormone.
42. (d) 43. (c) 44. (b)
45. (d) Iodine is essential for the normal rate of hormone synthesis in the thyroid. Deficiency of iodine in our diet results in **hypothyroidism** and enlargement of the thyroid gland, commonly called **goitre.**
Hypothyroidism during pregnancy causes defective development and maturation of the growing baby leading to stunted growth (cretinism), mental retardation, low intelligence quotient, abnormal skin, deaf-mutism, etc.

Speed Test-81

1. (c)
2. (b) Cloning is a technique by which genetically same individuals can be produced without including any sexual reproduction eg. Dolly sheep.
3. (d) 4. (d)
5. (b) The parents that have survived to reproduce asexually are able to survive in the current stable environment. Therefore, the offspring should be preadapted for this stable environment.
6. (a) Species that exhibit parthenogenesis develop from unfertilized eggs produced by the mother. Therefore, the genetic make-up should be 100 percent the same as the mother.
7. (a) Since external fertilization can only take place in an aquatic habitat, there are no terrestrial animals that use it.
8. (a) Many animals reproduce both by asexual and sexual means.
9. (b) All these animals can reproduce sexually. However, only the chicken lays an external egg.
10. (b) All of these statements concerning asexual reproduction are correct, except that asexual reproduction is best in favorable, stable environments, ones that don't change rapidly. The reason for this is that asexual reproduction, in contrast to its sexual counterpart, results in the formation of identical offspring. Although asexual organisms can often produce many more offspring in a single reproductive event than sexual organisms, these asexually produced young do not usually have the genetic variation caused by meiosis and crossing-over to be able to survive a rapidly changing environment or times of environmental stress.
11. (a) Buds in 'eyes' form new plants.
12. (b) Bud giving rise to new plant is present towards base.
13. (b) New plants in cane-sugar are formed from nodes which are absent.
14. (b) Water absorption & gaseous exchange stop due to presence of wax
15. (c) Parthenocarpy is the development of a fruit without the formation of seeds as a result of lack of pollination, lack of fertilization and lack of development. This condition can be artificially induced by application of hormones.
16. (a) 17. (a) 18. (a) 19. (d)
20. (c) Most of banana varieties are triploid and triploidy is associated with seedlessness.
21. (d) 22. (b) 23. (b) 24. (a) 25. (d)
26. (a) Homothallic and monoecious are terms used to denote bisexual condition. The example indudes fungi and plants. Heterothallic and dioecious are terms used to denote unisexual condition.
27. (b) Morphallaxis is a mechanism of regeneration involving reorganization of body cells. In epimorphosis, new cells proliferate from the surface of the wound to form the missing structure. In accretionary growth some specialized cells retain the ability to divide and produce new cells to replace the worn-out.

28. (a) Cells become variable in shape, size & getting their specialization for the formation of particular tissue or organ in future foetus. They place themselves at some specific regions in embryo for further organogeny.

29. (d) Earthworm, sponges, tapeworms are bisexual animals and hermaphrodites as they prossess both male and female reproductive organs.

30. (c)

31. (c) Sowing is related with sexual reproduction.

32. (c) Vegetative propagation in mint occurs through sucker. Vegetative reproduction is a type of asexual reproduction for plants, and is also called vegetative propagation, vegetative multiplication, or vegetative cloning. It is a process by which new plant "individuals" arise or are obtained without production of seeds or spores. It is a natural process in many plant species (as well as non-plant organisms such as bacteria and fungi) and used or encouraged by horticulturists to obtain quantities of economically valuable plants. A related technique used in cultivation is tissue culture, which involves vegetative reproduction under sterile conditions.

33. (d) Vegetative reproduction and apomixis, both are asexual methods of reproduction, which gives the progeny genetically similar to parent.

34. (c) 35. (c) 36. (b) 37. (d) 38. (d)

39. (c) 40. (d)

41. (b) In oomycetes female gamete is large and non motile while male gamete is small & motile.

42. (c) Male sex organ is called antheridium or globule while female sex organ is called oogonium. They develop on the same branchlet in the same plant in *chara.*

43. (c)

44. (c) In most aquatic organisms, such as a majority of algae and fishes as well as amphibians, syngamy occurs in the external medium (water), *i.e.*, outside the body of the organism. This type of gametic fusion is called external fertilisation.

45. (d)

Speed Test-82

1. (c) In porogamy the tip of pollen tube enters the micropyle, pushes through the nucellar tissue & finally pierces the egg-apparatus end of the embryo sac. If pollen tube enters through the chalazal side it is called chalazogamy & if it enters laterally it is called mesogamy.

2. (b) Dry indehiscent single-seeded fruit formed from bicarpellary syncarpous inferior ovary is cypsela. Cypsela is also called inferior, false or pseudocarpic achene, the thin fruit wall (developed from pericarp and thalamus)is attached to the seed at one point but the fruits develops from an inferior, unilocular and uniovuled ovary, *e.g.*, sunflower, marigold. Some cypsela develop pappus for dispersal *e.g. Sonchus*, *Taraxacum.*

3. (d) Each pollen has two layered wall. The outer layer is thick, tough, cuticularised called exine which is composed of a material called "sporopollenin". It is highly resistant to biological and physical decomposition, due to which pollens are preserved for a long time in fossils.

4. (b) 5. (d)

6. (c) Embryo sac is 7-celled structure. There is a large central cell with two polar nuclei, egg apparatus with egg cell and 2 synergids present at micropylar end and its chalazal end, 3 antipodal cells are present.

7. (b) Nucellus - 2n, antipodal cells - n
Antipodal cells - n, egg cell - n
Antipodal cells - n, megaspore mother cell - 2n
Nucellus - 2n primary endosperm nucleus - 3n
Antipodal and egg cell are the product of meiotic division and rest are not.

8. (a) Polyembryony refers to the formation of more than one embryo within a seed of a flowering plant. *e.g.* Citrus.

9. (c)

10. (b) In oogamy male and female gametes are morphologically as well as physiologically different. Female gametes are large and non-motile. Male gametes are small but motile.

11. (d) Cotyledons and testa respectively are edible parts in groundnut and pomegranate. A cotyledon is a significant part of the embryo within the seed of a plant. Upon germination, the cotyledon may become the embryonic first leaves of a seedling. Testa is often thick or hard outer coat of a seed.

12. (a) 13. (c)

14. (a) Some fleshy fruits such as mango, plum etc. usually have a single hard stone that encloses a seed, called drupe.

15. (a) Herkogamy – when there is some physical barrier present between the stamens and carpels avoiding any chance of self pollination.
Cleistogamy – when the flowers remain closed, self-pollination is the rule.
Dichogamy – when the two sexes mature at different times.

16. (b)

17. (a) Unisexuality of flowers prevents autogamy, but not geitonogamy. In self fertilisation , the male and female gametes are derived from the same individual. Among plants, self fertilization also called autogamy is common in many cultivated species, *eg*., wheat and oats. However, self fertilization is a form of inbreeding and does not allow for the mixing of genetic material; if it occurs over a number of generations it will result in offspring being less vigorous and productive than those resulting from cross fertilization.

18. (a) Amphitropous : Both body of ovule and embryo sac are curved. The embryo sac assumes horse-shoe shape. *e.g. Papaveraceae.*

19. (d) The male gamete will be haploid (n). 2 polar nuclei will be diploid (2n). Endosperm formed by fusion of male gamete with two polar nuclei will be pentaploid.

$$\text{Male gamete} + 2\text{ polar nuclei} \rightarrow \text{Endosperm}$$
$$(n) \qquad (2n)+(2n) \qquad (5n)$$

20. (a) Monocarpic plants are the plants in which flowers and fruits are formed only once after vegetative growth of several years e.g., some bamboos, *Agave*, etc.

21. (c) In angiosperms, microsporangium is equivalent to pollen sac, megasporangium is equivalent to nucellus and embryo sac is equivalent to female gametophyte. Pollen grain or microspore represents immature male gametophyte.

22. (a) Ovule is an integumented megasporagium found in spermatophytes which develops into seed after fertilization. An angiospermic ovule is typically an ovoid and whitish structure. It occurs inside ovary where it is attached to a parenchymatous cushion called placenta either singly or in a cluster. The ovule is stalked. The stalk is called funiculus or funicle. The point of attachment of the body of the ovule with the funiculus is known as hilum.

23. (d) Autogamy (Gk. autos-self, gamos-marriage) is a type of self pollination in which an intersexual or perfect flower is pollinated by its own pollen.
Geitonogamy (Gk. geiton-neighbour, gamos-marriage) is a type of pollination in which pollen grains of one flower are transferred to the stigma of another flower belonging to either the same plant or genetically similar plant. In geitonogamy, the flowers often show modifications similar to ones found in xenogamy or cross pollunation.
Xenogamy (Gk. xenos-strange, gamos-marriage) or cross pollination is the transfer of pollen grains from anther of one flower to the stigma of a genetically different flower.

24. (d) *Cannabis* is wind pollinated plant.
25. (b) The typical and the most common type of embryo sac, found in 80% flowering plants is called *Polygonum* type of embryosac. It contains 8 nuclei but 7 cells – 3 micropylar, 3 chalazal and one central. It is formed by one meiosis and three mitosis.
26. (a) The pollen tube eats its way through the solid part of the stigma and style by secreting pectinases and hydrolytic enzymes. Pollen tube travels intercellularly and chemotropically along the concentration gradient of calcium – boron -inositol sugar complex.
27. (a) Stigma is the terminal receptive part of the pistil which functions as landing platform for the pollen grains. It also determines the compatibility of the pollen grains.
28. (c) The tapetal layer is of great physiological significance as all the food material entering into the sporogenous tissue diffuses through this layer. Ultimately, the cells of tapetal layer disorganise. Thus, tapetum makes a nutritive layer for the developing microspores.
29. (b) The typical and the most common type of embryo sac, found in 80% flowering plants is called *Polygonum* type of embryosac. It contains 8 nuclei but 7 cells – 3 micropylar, 3 chalazal and one central. It is formed by one meiosis and three mitosis.
30. (b) Outer layer (exine) of pollen grain is made of a highly resistant substance called sporopollenin (Zelisch, 1932). Sporopollenin is not degraded by any enzyme. It is not affected by high temperature, strong acid or strong alkali. Because of sporopollenin, pollen grains are well preserved as fossils.
31. (c) One or more thin areas present in the exine of pollen grain are known as germ pores. The germ pores are apertures in the exine layer of the pollen grain where the sporopollenin is absent. The germ pore helps in the formation of the pollen tube and the release of the male gametes during fertilization. There are usually three germ pores in dicots (tricolpate) and one in monocots (monocolpate).
32. (a) Megaspore mother cell (MMC) is the sporogenous cell that divides to give 4 haploid megaspores. Out of these 4 megaspores, only one is functional and other three degenerate. Hence 100 meiotic divisions are required for the formation of 100 functional megaspores.
33. (c)
34. (c) Autogamy is possible only when anther and stigma are close together and there is synchrony in pollen release and stigma receptivity. As in case of cleistogamous flowers, the flowers remain closed so that anthers and stigmas are never exposed. The flowers undergo only self pollination. No external pollinating agency is required.
35. (b) Apogamy is the reproduction without the fusion of gametes, and usually without meiosis. The term may include any form of vegetative reproduction. The production of a diploid gametophyte from the sporophyte due to the absence of meiosis is known as apospory. Parthenogenesis is the development of an unfertilized egg into a complete individual without fertilization. Production and development of seedless fruits is called parthenocarpy.
36. (a) Endosperm represents the food storing tissue of a seed. It is produced as a result of double fertilization in angiosperms. In most monocots and some dicot seeds, the food reserve remains in the endosperm. They are called endospermic or albuminous seeds, e.g., cereals, castor, coconut, rubber. However, in the majority of dicot seeds (e.g., pea, gram, bean, mustard, groundnut) and some monocot seeds (e.g., orchids, *Sagittaria*), the endosperm is consumed during seed development and the food is stored in cotyledons and other regions. They are called nonendospermic or exalbuminous seeds.
37. (b) Part of embryo axis between the plumule and cotyledonary node is epicotyl (above the level of cotyledons) while the part between radicle and cotyledonary node is called hypocotyl (below the level of cotyledons).
38. (b) Pollination will not occur
39. (b) There will not be insect pollination
40. (a) Germination of pollens will not occur in ovule.
41. (d)
42. (c) Embryo can not grow without food stored in cotyledons.
43. (b) Pollens are formed by meiosis.
44. (b)
45. (c) Obligate symbiotic relationship is present between *Yucca* flowers and moth, *Tageticula*.

Speed Test-83

1. (c) During breast feeding, prolactin hormone (required for the release of milk) present in the blood inhibits the release of LH from pituitary. This will counter the effect of LH on the ovarian follicles and therefore no ovulation will occur. Hence, no pregnancy occurs during this period.
2. (a) 3. (d)
4. (b) The corpus luteum is essential for establishing and maintaining pregnancy in females. In the ovary, the corpus luteum secretes estrogens and progesterone, which are steroid hormones responsible for the thickening of the endometrium and its development and maintenance, respectively.
5. (b)
6. (b) Foetal ejection reflex in human female is induced by fully developed foetus and placenta. When a woman is in a lithotomy or semi-sitting position, the foetal ejection reflex is impaired and the increased pain caused by the sacrum's inability to move as the baby descends can be intolerable.
7. (b) Acrosome a small pointed structure at the tip of nucleus. It breaks down just before fertilization, releasing hydrolytic enzymes that assist penetration between follicle cells that surrounds the ovum, thus facilitating fertilization.
8. (c) Sertoli cells are found in the walls of seminiferous tubules of the testes. They anchor and provide nutrition to the developing germ cells especially the spermatids.
9. (b) In menstrual cycle, menstrual phase lasts for 4 days, proliferating/ovulating phase for about 10 days and secretory phase for 14 days.
10. (a) Menopause is the period when ovulation and menstrual cycle stop in human females. The period of menopause is between 45-55 years.
11. (d)
12. (c) The gland corresponding to this in female is Bertholin.
13. (a) 14. (a) 15. (b) 16. (b)
17. (b) The part of fallopian tube closest to the ovary is infundibulum. Infundibulum possess finger-like projections called fimbriae that help in collection of ovum after ovulation. It leads to wider part of oviduct called ampulla. The last part of oviduct is isthmus that has a narrow lumen and joins the uterus.
18. (c) 19. (b) 20. (b)
21. (a) Vasa efferentia are fine ciliated ductules that arise from the seminiferous tubules of testis (where sperms are formed) and open into epididymis which is a mass of long, narrow, closely coiled tubule lying along the inner side of testis. Epididymis stores the sperms. Thus, if vasa efferentia get blocked, sperms will not be transported from testes to epididymis.
22. (c) Wall of each seminiferous tubule is formed of a single layered germinal epithelium. Majority of cells in this epithelium are male germ cells and at certain places, there are present tall Sertoli cells. These cells act as nurse cells providing nutrition to the developing sperms.

23. (d) Secretion of seminal vesicle, prostrate gland and bulbourethral gland constitute seminal plasma which is rich in fructose, calcium and certain enzymes.
24. (c) The prostate gland is a single large gland that surrounds the urethra. It produces a slightly alkaline, milky secretion which forms 25% of the volume of semen. It possesses citric acid, enzymes (acid phosphatase, amylase, pepsinogen) and prostaglandins. Secretion of the prostate gland nourishes and activates the spermatozoa to swim.
25. (c) The epididymis is a mass of long narrow closely coiled tubule which lies along the inner side of each testis. Coiling forms three parts - upper caput epididymis or head, middle corpus epididymis or body and lower cauda epididymis or tail.
26. (d) Release of ovum from the ovary is called ovulation. The graafian follicle rises to the surface, sends out a protuberance or stigma and everts to release the ovum into peritoneal cavity. The empty Graafian follicle contains a blood clot which is called corpus haemorrhagic. Its granulosa cells continue to proliferate, develop yellow carotene pigment or lutein and get converted into lutein cells. This converts the ruptured a temporary endocrine gland secreting progesterone with small quantity of estrogen.
27. (c) The female external genitalia include mons pubis, labia majora, labia minora, hymen and clitoris.
28. (a) Secondary spermatocyte contains half the number of chromosomes i.e., 8 Each chromosome has 2 chromatids, therefore, 8 chromosomes will have 16 chromatids in all.
29. (d) During spermatogenesis, at the end of first maturation division (reductional division or meiosis), the primary spermatocyte divides into two haploid daughter cells called secondary spermatocytes.
30. (c) In the head of the epididymis, the sperms undergo physiological maturation, acquiring increased motility and fertilizing capacity.
31. (d) Oogenesis is the process of formation of functional haploid ova from the diploid germinal cells in the ovary. Oogenesis begins during embryonic development but is completed only after fertilization of the secondary oocyte with the sperm.
32. (b) The middle piece of sperm contains mitochondria coiled around the axial filament. They provide energy for the movement of the sperm.
33. (a) Release of ovum from the ovary is called ovulation. The Graafian follicle rises to the surface, sends out a protuberance or stigma and everts to release the ovum into peritoneal cavity. The empty Graafian follicle contains a blood clot which is called corpus haemorrhagic. Its granulosa cells continue to proliferate, develop yellow carotene pigment or lutein and get converted into lutein cells. This converts the ruptured a temporary endocrine gland secreting progesterone with small quantity of estrogen.
34. (a) FSH acts on the Sertoli cells and stimulate secretion of some factors which help in the process of spermiogenesis.
35. (a)
36. (d) TSH or thyroid stimulating hormone has no role in menstruation.
37. (c) On the 14th day of menstrual cycle, ovulation occurs, so chances of conception are optimum.
38. (c) Estrogen secreted from ovarian follicles under the influence of FSH, causes proliferation of the endometrium of the uterine wall.
39. (a)
40. (a)
41. (d) Acrosome, a cap like structure present at the tip of the sperm, is a lysosome like organelle derived from golgi apparatus.
42. (b) Prolactin is secreted by the anterior lobe of pituitary gland. After parturition, secretion and storage of milk in mammary glands is under the influence of this hormone.
43. (c) After birth, the first milk released by mammary glands is called colostrum. It is released for 2-3 days. It is thin, yellowish fluid containing cells from the alveoli of glandular tissue of mammary glands and is rich in protein, antibodies, but low in fat.
44. (a) Fusion of male and female gamete produces a zygote. Repeated division of the zygote is called cleavage forming a solid morula. After further division and rearrangement a fluid filled cavity surrounded by blastomeres - blastula is formed. The appearance of germ layers mark the gastrula.
45. (b) The type of reproduction shown in the given figure of yeast is budding. In budding, a daughter individual is formed from a small projection, the bud, arising from the parent body. In yeast, the division is unequal and a small bud is produced that remains attached initially to the parent body. Later on the bud gets separated and matures into a new yeast organism.

Speed Test-84

1. (c) Statements (i) and (iii) are correct.
- Medical Termination of Pregnancy (MTP) during first trimester is generally safe.
- Intrauterine device like copper-T are effective contraceptives.
2. (b) Amniocentesis is the most widely used method for prenatal detection of many genetic disorders. It is also a technique used for determining the sex of the foetus.
3. (d)
4. (a) Copper T is an intrauterine device which prevents the fertilized egg becoming implanted in the wall of the womb.
5. (b) 6. (a)
7. (a) Gamete intrafallopian transfer (GIFT) is recommended for those females who cannot produce an ovum. In this process, the eggs of the donor woman are removed and in a form of mixture with sperm, transferred into fallopian tube of another woman who cannot produce ovum, but can provide suitable environment for fertilization. Thus in GIFT, site of fertilization is fallopian tube, not laboratory.
8. (a)
9. (b) Condoms are barriers made of thin rubber/latex sheath that are used to cover the penis in the male or vagina and cervix in the female, just before coitus so that the ejaculated semen would not enter into the female reproductive tract. This can prevent conception.
10. (c) 11. (a) 12. (d) 13. (a) 14. (b) 15. (b)
16. (c) 17. (c) 18. (b) 19. (d)
20. (b) The birth control pill interferes with the maturation of the follicles and the ova, inhibiting release of an egg.
21. (d) Sterilization techniques can be considered as the safest birth control measures. It provides a permanent and sure birth control. It is called vasectomy in male and tubectomy in female.
22. (c)
23. (a) Copper 'T' is an intrauterine device which prevents the fertilized egg from becoming implanted in the wall of the womb.
24. (c) Cu ions released by copper releasing intra uterine devices suppresses sperm motility.
Intra-uterine devices are inserted by doctors in the uterus through vagina. They are available as the non-medicated IUDs, copper releasing IUDs and hormonereleasing IUDs.
25. (d) Intra uterine device (IUD) is a method of contraception in India. The IUD is inserted in the woman's uterus through the cervix.

26. (d) Test-tube baby programme employs zygote intrafallopion transfer (ZIFT) technique. In this technique fusion of ovum and sperm is done outside the body of woman to form zygote which is allowed to divide forming 8 blastomeres, then it is transfered the fallopion tube of the woman.

27. (d)

28. (c) Jaundice cannot be detected in a developing foetus by amniocentesis. It is a foetal sex determination test based on chromosomal pattern in the amniotic fluid surrounding the developing embryo. It is now legally ban in India.

29. (d) Medical termination of pregnancy (MTP) or induced abortion became legal in India from 1971 with some strict conditions to avoid its misuse. Such restrictions are important to check indiscriminate and illegal female foeticides which are reported to be high in India. All the other options are of natural methods of contraception.

30. (c) Oxytocin is birth hormone and acts on the smooth muscles of our body and stimulates their contraction. Vasopressin acts mainly at the kidney and stimulates resorption of water and electrolytes and reduces loss of water through urine. Hence, it is also called as anti-diuretic hormone (ADH).

31. (a) STDs are more common in 15-24 years age group. Gonorrhoea, syphilis, genital herpes, chlamydiasis, genital warts, trichomoniasis, hepatitis-B and AIDS are some of the common STDs. Haemophilia is sex-linked recessive disease, which show its transmission from unaffected carrier female to some of male progeny. Sickle cell anaemia is an autoimmune linked recessive trait in which both the partners are carriers for the gene.

32. (d) In Intra-Uterine Transfer (IUT), embryo with more than 8-blastomeres stage (morula) is used for transfer into the uterus.

33. (c) Reproductive health in society can be improved by creating awareness among people about various reproduction related aspects and providing facilities and support for building up a reproductively healthy society.

34. (b) 35. (b) 36. (b) 37. (a)

38. (d) Amniocentesis involves prenatal diagnosis of metabolic error and other genetic abnormalities.

39. (a) The programmes called 'family planning' for reproductive health awareness were initiated in 1951.

40. (d) Reproduction-related areas are currently in operation in India come under the popular name 'Reproductive and Child Health Care (RCH) programmes.

41. (b) 'Saheli'–an oral contraceptive for the females was developed at Central Drug Research Institute (CDRI) in Lucknow, India.

42. (b) In artificial insemination (AI) technique, the semen collected either from the husband or a healthy donor is artificially introduced either into the vagina or into the uterus (IUI – intrauterine insemination) of the female.

43. (c) An ideal contraceptive should be user-friendly, easily available, effective and reversible with no or least side-effects.

44. (c) Reproductive health is a crucial part of general health and a central feature of human development. It is a reflection of health during childhood, and crucial during adolescence and adulthood, Reproductively healthy societies have normal sex related emotional and behavioural interactions.

45. (a) To get rid of unwanted pregnancies and to prevent the fatality or harmfulness to the mother or to foetus or both due to the continuation of pregnancy are the reasons on the basis of which pregnancy can be terminated

Speed Test-85

1. (a) AaBB × aaBB on crossing gives 50% individuals having genotype AaBB and 50% individuals having genotype aaBB.

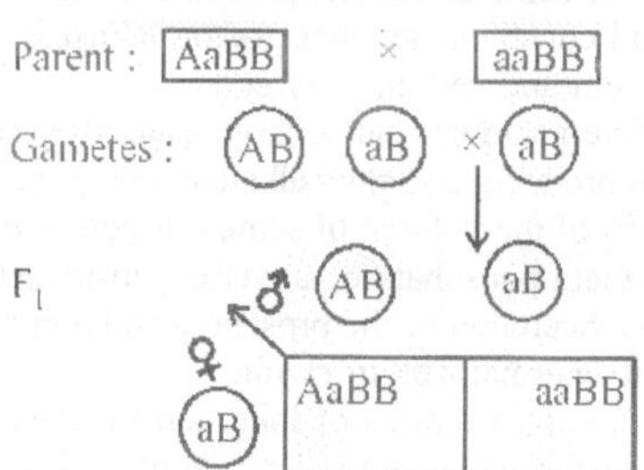

2. (b) Incomplete dominance is the phenomenon where none of the alleles are dominant, with the effect that the hybrid produced by crossing two pure individuals is a mixture between the parents.

3. (d) When a pair of contrasting characters are studied during hybridization, it is called dihybrid cross. In F_2-generation, its ratio is 9 : 3 : 3 : 1.
It means when parents having –
Yellow, round Crossed with green wrinkled
seeds seeds
(IIRR) × (iirr)
will give 9 – Yellow round seeds.
3 – Yellow wrinkled seed.
3 – Green round seeds.
1 – Green wrinkled seeds

4. (b) Genetic mapping help in studying the architecture of the chromosomes and of entire genome.

5. (a) Epistasis is the phenomenon of masking or suppressing the phenotypic impression of a gene pair by a non allelic gene pair which impresses its own effect.

6. (b) Independent assortment of genes takes place only when they are located on separate non-homologus chromosomes. Where two or more than two genes are located on same chromosome, independent assortment will not be possible.

7. (b) In eukaryotic cells, two cytoplasmic organelles, mitochondria and chloroplast of green plants, contain their own genetic materials.

8. (b) A cross of F_1 hybrid with its recessive homozygous parent is called the test cross. It is done to determine the genotype of a given plant. If the given plant has homozygous dominant traits then on test cross it gives all dominant trait plants but if it is heterozygous dominant than it gives dominant and recessive phenotypes in 1 : 1 ratio.

9. (b) Pleiotropy is the condition in which a single gene influences more than one trait.
Polyploidy is a condition in which individuals have more than two complete sets of chromosomes.
Apomixis is a reproductive process in plants that superficially resembles normal sexual reproduction but there is no fusion of gametes.

10. (c) A gene may have more than two alternative forms occupying the same locus on a chromosome, such alleles are known as multiple alleles and the phenomenon is turned as multiple allelism. ABO blood group has 3 alleles. I^O, I^A or A, I^B or B.

11. (b) Aneuploidy is the numerical change in the chromosome number of the genome. Euploidy is the phenomenon of having multiple or more than twice the number of genome.

12. (d) Haemophilia is a sex linked recessive trait carried by X chromosome (also known as bleeder's disease).

13. (d) Sickle cell anaemia (in which nucleotide triplet CTC is changed to CAC) affects the β-globin chain of haemoglobin. Since these changes occur at a particular locus or point of a chromosome where specific gene is located, they are called as point mutation.

14. (b) Down's syndrome is due to trisomy of 21st chromosome and is an autosomal abnormality.
15. (d) A barr body is one of the X-chromosomes in somatic cells of females. If there are more X-chromosomes, then there will be more barr bodies.
16. (b) Down's syndrome develops due to trisomy of chromosome number 21. In Turner's syndrome, the effect appears due to fusion of a gamete without sex chromosome and a gamete with one X-chromosome (44 + X). Klinefelter individuals are phenotypically males. The defect appears due to fusion of egg having unreduced sex complement (A + X X) with a gamete carrying Y chromosome (44 + XXY). Gynandromorphism occurs among *Drosophila*. In such individuals one half of the body shows male characters and the other half shows female characters.
17. (c) Sex in *Drosophila* is a function of the ratio of the number of X chromosomes to the number of autosomal sets. Therefore a *Drosophila* with a X/A =1.0 will be a female whereas the one with a X/A ratio = 0.5 will be male. However, in humans the presence or absence of the Y chromosome determines sex.
18. (c) The lack of independent assortment in sweet pea and *Drosophila* is due to linkage.
19. (c) Baldness is a sex influenced trait. The dominance of alleles may differ in heterozygotes of the two sexes.
20. (a) Cri-du-chat/cat cry syndrome is due to the deletion of a large part of the small or one of the 5th chromosome.
21. (d) Biometric genetics is the mathematical or statistical study of genetic phenomenon. In this branch, data of various genetic traits are analysed by applying the principles of statistics. It helps in the investigation of various genetic principles and checks their correctness and probability.
22. (b) In grasshopper the males lack a Y-sex chromosome and have only an X-chromosome. They produce sperm cells that contain either an X chromosome or no sex chromosome, which is designated as O.
23. (d) Linkage is the inheritance of genes of same chromosome together and capacity of these genes to retain their parental combination in subsequent generation. The strength of linkage between two genes is inversely proportional to the distance between the two. This means, two linked genes show higher frequency of recombination if the distance between them is higher and lower frequency if the distance is smaller.
24. (a)
25. (c) Genotype is the genetic make up of an individual irrespective of the mendelian characters or genes impressing.

Parent : AABB × aabb

Gametes : (AB) ↓ (ab)

F_1 : AaBb

	AB	Ab	aB	ab
AB	AABB	AABb	AaBB	AaBb
Ab	AABb	AAbb	AaBb	Aabb
aB	AaBB	AaBb	aaBB	aaBb
ab	AaBb	Aabb	aaBb	aabb

26. (d)
27. (c)
28. (d) Phenylketonuria is a human genetic disorder in which the body does not contain the enzyme phenylalanine hydroxylase, necessary to metabolize phenylalanine to tyrosine, and converts phenylalanine instead to phenylpyruvic acid. As PKU is an autosomal recessive genetic disorder each parent must have at least one defective allele of the gene for PAH, and the child must inherit a defective allele from each parent. As such, it is possible for a parent with a PKU phenotype to have a child without PKU if the other parent possesses at least one functional allele of the gene for PAH. A child of two parents with the PKU phenotype will always receive two defective alleles so will always have PKU. The gene for PAH is located on chromosome 12.
29. (a) Chromosomes occur in homologous pairs. Somatic cells have diploid number of chromosomes. Humans have 23 pairs *i.e.* 46 chromosomes. 22 pairs of autosomes and 1 pair of sex chromosomes i.e. XX in females and XY in males.
30. (a)
31. (d) Given that recombinant percentage is 7% and 5% therefore, total recombinants would be 7 + 5 = 12%. It is known that one map unit is the distance that yields 1% recombinant chromosomes. Hence distance between two non-allelic genes = 12 map units.
32. (b) In the given cross, passing of disease is from carrier female to male progeny (criss-cross inheritance). Any trait that shows criss-cross inheritance is located on the sex chromosome. Presence of a single recessive gene i.e. X^c in carrier individuals (XX^c) does not cause the disease, thus the trait is recessive.
33. (b)
34. (b) A cross between heterozygous long-winged flies and (homozygous) vestigial winged flies represents an example of test cross, in which the exact Mendelian ratio of 1 : 1 is obtained. i.e., 96 long-winged flies and 96 vestigial winged flies.
35. (b) Incomplete dominance is the phenomenon of neither of the two alleles being dominant so that expression in the hybrid is intermediate between the expressions of the two alleles in homozygous state. F_2 phenotypic ratio is 1 : 2 : 1, similar to genotypic ratio.
36. (a) To determine the genotype of a tall plant of F_2 generation, Mendel crossed the tall plant from F_2 generation with a dwarf plant. He called this a test cross. In a typical test cross an organism (pea plants) showing a dominant phenotype whose genotype is to be determined is crossed with the recessive parent instead of self-crossing. The progenies of such a cross can easily be analysed to predict the genotype of the test organism. Normal test cross ratio for a monohybrid cross is 1 : 1 and for a dihybrid cross is 1 : 1 : 1 : 1.
37. (a) Quantitative inheritance (polygenic inheritance) is a type of inheritance controlled by one or more genes in which the dominant alleles have cumulative effect with each dominant allele expressing a part or unit of the trait, the full trait being shown only when all the dominant alleles are present. e.g., kernel colour in wheat, skin colour in human beings, human intelligence, height in human beings and several plants, etc.

The ability of a gene to have multiple phenotypic effects because it influences a number of characters simultaneously is known as pleitropy. The genes involved are called pleiotropic genes. It is not essential that all the traits are equally influenced. Sometimes the effect of a pleiotropic gene is more evident in case of one trait (major effect) and less evident in case of others (secondary effect). An example of this in humans is the disease phenylketonuria, which also produces abnormal phenotypic traits such as mental retardation, widely placed incisors, pigmented patches on the skin and excessive sweating for multiple alleles.

38. (b) Chromosomal theory of inheritance believes that chromosomes are vehicles of hereditary information which possess Mendelian factors or genes and it is the chromosomes which segregate and assort independently during transmission from one generation to the next. Chromosomal theory of inheritance was proposed by Walter Sutton and Theodore Boveri independently in 1902. But it was later modified and expanded by Morgan, Sturtevant and Bridges.

39. (c) Linked genes are those genes which do not show independent assortment but remain together because they are present on the same chromosome. In linkage, there is a tendency to maintain the parental gene combination except for occasional crossovers.

40. (b) In ZW-ZZ type of sex determination, the male has two homomorphic sex chromosomes (ZZ) and is homogametic, and the female has two heteromorphic sex chromosomes (ZW) and is heterogametic. There are, thus, two types of eggs: Z and W, and only one type of sperms, i.e., each with Z. Fertilization of an egg with Z chromosome by a sperm with Z chromosome gives a zygote with ZZ chromosomes (male). Fertilization of an egg with W chromosome by a sperm with Z chromosome yields a zygote with ZW chromosomes (female). This mechanism operates in some vertebrates (fishes, reptiles and birds).

41. (c) Since colourblindness is a sex-linked recessive trait and males just have one X chromosome, they can never be the carriers. Males will always express the disease/phenotype.

42. (d) In a stable population, for a gene with two alleles, 'A' (dominant) and 'a' (recessive), if the frequency of 'A' is p and the frequency of 'a' is q, then the frequencies of the three possible genotypes (AA, Aa and aa) can be expressed by the Hardy-Weinberg equation:
$p^2 + 2pq + q^2 = 1$
where p^2 = Frequency of AA (homozygous dominant) individuals q^2 = Frequency of aa (homozygous recessive) individuals
$2pq$ = Frequency of Aa (heterozygous) individuals
so, $p = 0.6$ and $q = 0.4$ (given)
$\therefore$ 2pq (frequency of heterozygote) $= 2 \times 0.6 \times 0.4 = 0.48$.

43. (b) The distance between genes is measured by map unit. 1% crossing over between two linked genes is known as 1 map unit or centi Morgan (cM). 100% crossing over is termed as Morgan (M) and 10% crossing over as deci Morgan (dm).

44. (d) Dominant autosomal traits are caused by dominance autosomal genes. Some of the dominantly autosomal inherited disorder in human beings are : Polydactyly– presence of extra fingers and toes , Huntington's disease or Huntington's chorea — a disorder in which muscle and mental deterioration occurs and there is gradual loss of motor control resulting in uncontrollable shaking and dance like movement (chorea), phenylthiocarbamide (PTC) tasting, etc.

45. (a) Most of the gene mutations involve a change in only a single nucleotide or nitrogen base of the cistron. These gene mutations are called point mutations. e.g. sickle cell anaemia in which polypeptide chain coding for hemoglobin contains valine, instead of glutanic acid due to substitution of T by A in second position of triplet codon.

Speed Test-86

1. (d) rRNA occurs inside ribosomes. m RNA brings information from DNA to polypeptides. hnRNA are heterogenous nuclear RNA.

2. (d) (a) **Helicase** also known as unwindase, these enzymes separate the two strands of DNA.
(b) **Topoisomerases :** Tension produced by unwinding of DNA strands is reduced by these enzymes.
(c) **RNA Primase :** This is an RNA polymerase, which helps in the synthesis of a small fragment of RNA called primer.

3. (a) DNA ligase is the enzyme which helps in joining two fragments of DNA. The enzyme is used in DNA replication as it joints the Okazaki segments (also in proof reading). It also finds its use in genetic engineering as it can join two or more desired nucleotide sequences of DNA.

4. (a) In 1953 Wilkins obtained very fine X-ray crystallographic pictures of DNA from which Watson and Crick developed the double helix model of DNA.

5. (c) Okazaki fragments in DNA are linked up by the enzyme DNA *ligase*. Replication always occurs in 5' - 3' direction. Okazaki fragments synthesized on 3' - 5' DNA template, join to form lagging strand which grows in 3' - 5' direction.

6. (d) The phenomenon of making DNA over RNA genome through enzyme reverse transcriptase is called reverse transcription or teminism.

7. (c) Telomerase is a ribonucleoprotein which synthesize the rich strand of telomers in DNA. **Telomerase** is an enzyme that adds specific DNA sequence repeats ("TTAGGG" in all vertebrates) to the 3' ("three prime") end of DNA strands in the telomere regions, which are found at the ends of eukaryotic chromosomes. The telomeres contain condensed DNA material, giving stability to the chromosomes. The enzyme is a reverse transcriptase that carries its own RNA molecule, which is used as a template when it elongates telomeres, which are shortened after each replication cycle. Telomerase was discovered by Carol W. Greider in 1984.

8. (b) During transcription, from the DNA template, complementary mRNA is formed and thymine is replaced by uracil.

9. (d) Replication begins at the *Ori* - origin of replication and proceeds on both sides from the Ori. Unidirectional replication is rare. RNA primers are involved in both prokaryotes and eukaryotes.

10. (c) During the process of replication the enzyme that helps to cut one strand of DNA duplex to release the tension of coiling of two strands is topoisomerase.

11. (c)

12. (d) It was given by Geneticists George W. Beadle and E. L. Tatum which states that each gene in an organism controls the production of a specific enzyme. It is these enzymes that catalyze the reactions that lead to the phenotype of the organism.

13. (b) The transforming chemical discovered by Griffith in his experiments with *Pneumococcus*, was confirmed as DNA by Avery, McLeod and McCarty.

14. (a)

15. (a) Statement (i) and (iv) are / is correct
Regulation of *lac* operon by repressor is referred to as negative regulation. In negative regulation, a repressor molecule binds to the operator of an operon and terminates transcription. In positive regulation, an activator interacts with the RNA polymerase in the promoter region to initiate transcription. Human genome contains some 20,000-25,000 billion genes bases.

16. (a) In negative (repressible) operon, the repressor co-repressor complex binds with the operator. The free repressor cannot bind to the operator.
17. (b)
18. (a)
19. (c) In eukaryotes, DNA organization is complex. There is a set of positively charged, basic proteins called histones. Histones are rich in the basic amino acid residues lysine and arginine. There are five types of histone proteins – H_1, H_2A, H_2B, H_3 and H_4. Four of them (H_2A, H_2B, H_3 and H_4) produce histone octamer called nu body or core of nucleosome. The negatively charged DNA is wrapped around the positively charged histone octamer to form nucleosome. DNA connecting two adjacent nucleosomes is called linker DNA which bears H_1 histone proteins.
20. (c) Transformation is a phenomenon by which DNA isolated from one type of cell when introduced into another type is able to give some of its properties to the latter. In 1944, Avery, McCarty and MacLeod discovered that protein-digesting enzymes (proteases) and RNA-digesting enzymes (RNase) did not affect transformation, so the transforming substance was not a protien or RNA. Digestion with DNase did inhibit transformation, suggestion that the DNA caused did inhibit transformation, suggesting that the DNA caused the transformation. They concluded that DNA is the hereditary material.
21. (d) Synthesis in DNA by DNA polymerases occurs only in 5' $\rightarrow$ 3' direction. One strand called leading strand, is copied in the same direction as the unwinding helix. The other strand is known as the lagging strand. Replication of lagging strand is in a discontinuous way, synthesizing short segments of DNA which are always in the 5' $\rightarrow$ 3' direction. These short segments are called Okazaki fragments joined together by the action of DNA ligase.
22. (b) In tRNA, there is a TΨC loop which contains pseudouridine and ribothymidine. The loop is the site for attaching to ribosomes. Another loop, DHU loop contains dihydrouridine. It is binding site for aminoacyl synthetase enzyme. tRNA molecules have unpaired (single stranded) CCA–OH sequence at the 3' end. This is called amino acid attachment site, because the amino acid becomes covalently attached to adenylic acid or A of CCA sequence during polypeptide synthesis. Anticodon loop is made up of three nitrogen bases for recongnising and attaching to the codon of mRNA.
23. (d) According to Chargaff's rules (1950), purine and pyrimidine base pairs are present in equal amounts in a DNA molecule. i.e., [A + G] = [T + C]

$$\text{or } \frac{[A+G]}{[T+C]} = 1.$$

24. (c) 2'–OH group present in ribose sugar of every nucleotide of RNA is a reactive group. Uracil present in RNA is less stable as compared to thymine (= methyl uracil) of DNA. Being unstable, RNA mutates at a much faster rate and there is no repairing system. That is why RNA viruses have shorter life span. They mutate and evolve very fast.
25. (c) The segment of DNA that takes part in transcription is called transcription unit. It has three components (i) a promoter, (ii) the structural gene and (iii) a terminator. Besides a promoter, eukaryotes also require an enhancer. Promoter is located upstream of structural gene. It is called 5' end of the coding strand which is 3' end of template strand. Terminator region is present downstream of structural gene at the 3' end of coding strand which if actually 5' end of the template strand. Promoter has different parts for attachment to various transcription factors. In many cases, the promoter has an AT rich region called TATA box. The area has a groove to which specific protein components can combine. TATA containing region is also called Pribnow box.
26. (b) Eukaryotes have three RNA polymerases. RNA polymerase I is located in the nucleolus and transcribes for rRNAs (28s, 18s and 5.8S), RNA polymerase II is localized in the nucleoplasm and used for hnRNA, mRNA and RNA polymerase III is localized in the nucleus, possibly the nucleolar-nucleoplasm interface and transcribes for tRNA, 5s tRNA and snRNAs.
27. (a) UAA is a nonsense codon. It signals for polypeptide chain termination. Hence, only 24 amino acids chain will be formed.
28. (d) Regulation of gene expression can be exerted at four levels:
(i) Transcriptional level during formation of primary transcript.
(ii) Processing like splicing, terminal additions or modifications
(iii) Transport of RNAs from nucleus to cytoplasm and
(iv) Translational level
29. (c) A typical nucleosome contains 200 bp of DNA helix. Nucleosomes constitute the repeating unitof a structure in nucleus called chromatin. Chromatin is held over a scaffold of non histone chromosomal (or NHC) proteins. At some places chromatin is densely packed to form darkly stainned heterochromatin. At other places chromatin is loosely packed. It is called euchromatin. It is transcriptionally active chromatin whereas heterochromatin is transcriptionally inactive and late replicating or heteropycnotic.
30. (d) Process of DNA synthesis where by a parent DNA molecule is faithfully copied, giving rise to two identical daughter molecules is called DNA replication. In DNA synthesis, DNA polymerase plays important role having the capability to elongate an existing DNA strand but cannot initiate the synthesis. So, the synthesis is initiated with the help of RNA primer formed by RNA primase. RNA primase synthesizes the short primer RNA of about 10 nucleotides that is elongated by DNA polymerase to form an okazaki fragment of DNA during DNA replication. Helicase unzips the two strands of DNA and topoisomerase reduces the coiling tension developed due to the unwinding of the two strands.
31. (b) Lactose operon in *E.coli* is a catabolic pathway in which the structural genes remain switched off unless the inducer (Lactose) is present in the medium.
32. (d)
33. (a) DNA fingerprinting is the technique of determining nucleotide sequences of certain areas of DNA which are unique to each individual. DNA contains non cistronic hypervariable repeat sequences called VNTR. DNA fingerprinting involves the identification of these VNTRs.
34. (a) In negative (repressible) operon, the repressor co-repressor complex binds with the operator. The free repressor cannot bind to the operator.
35. (a) Operator gene allows the functioning of the operon.
36. (c) If the *lac* repressor is non functional, it cannot bind the operator site and transcription of the *lac* operon will occur at all times, whether or not lactose is present.
37. (d) Option *a* refers to the *lac* and *trp* repressors, option *b* to the CRP protein, and option *c* refers to promoter that have different transcriptional efficiencies.
38. (a) **39.** (b) **40.** (b) **41.** (a)
42. (b) The presence or absence of tryptophan determines whether the genes that code the necessary enzymes in tryptophan synthesis will even be transcribed.
43. (c) Option (a) describes transcription in eukaryotic cells; Option (b) describes translation.

44. (c) DNA replication is an energy-consuming process that must have an input of energy to proceed. Energy is provided in the breaking of the triphosphate tails of each nucleotide.
45. (a) AUG is initiating codon. UCG codes for serine, UUU codes for phenylalanine, UGU codes for cysteine.

Speed Test-87

1. (a) Genetic drift can operate only on smaller populations where its fluctuation can be observed in the proportion of allele distribution in the presence of external disturbances. Genetic drift is the random change in allele number and frequency in a gene pool.
2. (a)
3. (d) Flipper of seal and wing of birds are modified forelimbs, thus, have same fundamental structure but have different functions. Flippers are meant for swimming and wings are meant for flying. Therefore, these organs are homologous organs.
4. (c) Prevalence of pesticide resistant insects supports natural selection theory e.g., DDT was thought to be an effective insecticide against household pests (like mosquitoes houseflies, body lice) in 1945. But, within 2 to 3 years of its introduction, new DDT resistant mosquitoes appeared in the population. These mutant strains, soon became well established in the population by natural selection and thus replaced the original DDT-sensitive mosquitoes.
5. (b) Paleozoic era is the era of ancient life. The correct arrangement of periods of this era is Cambrian → Ordovician (age of invertebrates) → Silurian → Devonian (age of fishes) → Carboniferous (age of Amphibians) → Permian.
6. (b) *Homo erectus* appeared about 1.7 million years ago in middle pleistocene. Its brain capacity was about 900 cc. He was about 1.5-1.8 m tall having erect posture.
7. (b) Stabilizing selection favours average sized individuals while eliminates small sized individuals. It reduces variation and thus, does not promote evolutionary change. But it maintains the mean value from generation to generation. In directional selection, the population changes towards one particular direction. It favours small or large sized individuals and more individuals of that type will be present in next generation. The mean size of the population changes. Disruptive selection favours both small-sized and large-sized individuals, It eliminates most of members with mean expression, so produces two peaks in the distribution of the trait that may lead to development of two different individuals. It is important in bringing about evolutionary change.
8. (b) It is presumed that the first living organisms were chemoheterotrophs that obtained energy by the fermentation of complex organic substances available to them from the sea broth. They were anaerobes.
9. (d) The cranial capacity of Neanderthal man was 1400 cc, of Peking man was 850 - 1100 cc, of java ape man was 800 - 1000 cc and of African man was 500 cc.
10. (b) Hardy-Weinberg principle describes a theoretical situation in which a population is undergoing no evolutionary change. It states that allele frequencies in a population are stable and constant from generation to generation. There are five factors that affect Hardy-Weinberg Principle. These are - mutation, gene flow, genetic drift, genetic recombination and natural selection pressure.
11. (c) In allopatric speciation, a part of the population becomes geographically isolated from the main population. The population becomes entirely separated and finally constitutes a new species in Galapagos Islands is an example of allopatric speciation.
12. (d) In a stable population, for a gene with two alleles, 'A' (dominant) and 'a' (recessive), if the frequency of 'A' is p and the frequency of 'a' is q, then the frequencies of the three possible genotypes (AA, Aa and aa) can be expressed by the Hardy-Weinberg equation:

$p^2 + 2pq + q^2 = 1$

where p^2 = Frequency of AA (homozygous dominant) individuals

q^2 = Frequency of aa (homozygous recessive) individuals

$2pq$ = Frequency of Aa (heterozygous) individuals

so, $p = 0.6$ and $q = 0.4$ (given)

$\therefore$ $2pq$ (frequency of heterozygote) $= 2 \times 0.6 \times 0.4 = 0.48$.
13. (d)
14. (b) According to Lamarckism (proposed by Lamarck), whatever characters an individual acquires in its life time due to internal vital force, effect of environment, new needs, use/disuse of organs, they are inherited to next generations. This process continues and after several generations, the variations are accumulated upto such an extent that they give rise to new species. Melanization in peppered moth favours Drawin's theory of natural selection.
15. (c)
16. (a) In 1953, Stanley Miller and Harold Urey created, in the laboratory, conditions comparable to those of early Earth, with water vapour, hydrogen, methane, and ammonia. The Miller-Urey apparatus produced a variety of amino acids and other organic compounds found in living organisms today.
17. (b) This is the definition of fitness.
18. (b)
19. (d) Fitness is a measure of an organism's genetic contribution to the next generation.
20. (b) 21. (b)
22. (b) The analogous organs show convergent evolution due to similar adaptation. They do not support organic evolution. Whale, seal and shark shows convergent evolution due to similar habitats.
23. (b) Speciation takes place via reproductive isolation which is the most important consequence of geographical isolation.
24. (d) Scales on their hind limbs and eggs with calcareous shell, indicates in birds about their reptilian ancestry.
25. (d) Jurassic period of meoszoic era was about 19-20 crore years ago & lasted for about 5.5-6 crore years. The climate was hot and damp. It is called the age of dinosaurs. Ist primitive bird *Archaeopteryx* evolved from reptiles. I[st] angiosperm appeared as a dicotyledon but gymnosperms were dominant.
26. (a) The theory of the continuity of the germplasm was published by August Weismann (1834-1914) in 1886. It proposes that the contents of the reproductive cells (sperms and ova) are passed on unchanged from one generation to the next, unaffected by any changes undergone by the rest of the body. It thus, rules out any possibility of the inheritance of acquired characteristics, and has become fundamental to Neo-Darwinian theory.
27. (b) The eye of octopus and eye of cat show different patterns of structure, yet they perform similar functions. This is an example of analogous organs.

Analogous organs have evolved due to convergent evolution . Analogous organs have developed in the evolutionary process through adaptation of quite different organisms to similar mode of life.
28. (a) Genetic drift is variation in gene frequencies within populations that can occur by chance rather than by natural selection. Sometimes the change in allele frequency is so different in the new sample of population that they become a different species. The original drifted population becomes founder and the effect is called founder effect.

29. (b) Darwin observed an amazing diversity of creatures on Galapagos islands. He realised that there were many varieties of finches in the same island like seed-eating, with altered beaks insectivorous and vegetarian finches. Carrion are dead bodies. No finches feed on carrion.

30. (b) The term Evolution was given by Herbert Spencer that is "Descent with modifications". Evolution helps us to understand the history of life.
Evolution is a process in which something changes into a different and usually more complete or better form over time and in response to environment. This results in descendents becoming different from ancestors.

31. (c) Organs that are similar in fundamental structure but different in functions are "Homologous organs", Richard Owen, introduced the term homologous. Pectoral fins of fish and fore limbs of horse similar in structure but different in functions are homologous organs.
Rest of the organs compared in the question are analogous organs.

32. (b) One of the first attempts to explain the mechanism of evolution was made by Jean Baptiste de Lamarck. His theory was Inheritance of Acquired Characters. The theory states that the characters acquired during life time are passed on to the progeny and then to subsequent generations and new species are produced.

33. (b) Progressive evolution is development of organisms with more elaborate and specialized structures from those having less elaborate features e.g. amphibians from reptiles .Retrogressive or degenerative evolution is development of simpler forms from more complex ones. Such evolution has occurred in case of vestigial organs, parasitic forms, and in reduction of overspecialized structures such as wings in flightless birds. Parallel evolution is formation of similar traits in related groups of organisms independently due to similar requirement e.g. running of two toed deer and one toed Horse. Evolution of wings in insects and birds serve as example of convergent evolution.

34. (b) In the embryos of all vertebrates, the presence of gill slits supports the theory of recapitulation (repeating the early stages of embryogenesis in earlier evolved animals).

35. (a) The change in the colour of peppered moth is due to the mutation of single mendelian gene for the survival in the smoke-laden industrial environment. It is called Industrial melanism.

36. (c) Chimpanzees and gorillas are our closest relatives among the living primates.

37. (c) Electron Spin Resonance method is the most accurate method for dating of fossils.

38. (a) Adaptive radiation refers to evolution of different species from a common ancestor. The mammals are adapted for different mode of life i.e. they show adaptive radiation. They can be aerial (bat), aquatic (whale and dolphins), burrowing or fossorial (rat), cursorial (horse), scantorial (squirrel) or arboreal (monkey). The adaptive radiation, the term by Osborn, is also known as Divergent evolution.

39. (d) The most significant trend in evolution of modern man (*Homo sapiens*) from his ancestors is development of brain capacity.

40. (b) According to Oparin, the atmosphere of primitive earth was reducing because its atoms were most numerous and most reactive. Free oxygen was not present in significant amount. Large quantities of H_2, N_2, water vapour, CO_2, CH_4 and NH_3 were present.

41. (b) There is no life on moon due to absence of water. There are many other reasons for being no life on moon, like insufficient oxygen, unsuitable temperature etc.

42. (b) *Cro-Magnon* fossils have been found in Europe. Neanderthal man is a transitional stage. *Australopithecus* appeared in early Pleistocene.

43. (c) The primitive atmosphere was reducing due to lack of free molecular oxygen. The early atmosphere contained ammonia (NH_3), water vapour (H_2O), hydrogen (H_2), methane (CH_4).

44. (a) Marsupials in Australia and placental mammals in North America show convergent evolution. These two subclasses of mammal have adapted in similar ways to a particular food supply, locomotor skill or climate.

45. (b) *Australopithecus* is one of the longest-lived and best-known early human species whose remains were found between 3.85 and 2.95 million years ago in Eastern Africa (Ethiopia, Kenya, and Tanzania). Evidences shows that they hunted with stone weapons but essentially ate fruits.

Speed Test-88

1. (c) A special defence system works specially against viral infection. It has no effect on micro-organism. Cells invaded by a virus produce an antiviral protein called interferon (IFN). The latter is released from the infected cell and on reaching the nearby non-infected cells it makes them resistant to the virus infection.

2. (c) Syphilis is caused by bacteria *Treponema pallidum*.

3. (c) The lymphocytes which differentiate in the thymus are known as the T - lymphocytes. T-lymphocytes are responsible for the cellular immune response.

4. (b) The major obstacle in transplantation of organs is that the recipient body does not accept the donor's organ. The body defence mechanism rejects & treats the transplanted organ as a foreign particle and reacts actively.

5. (b) Tranquilizers bring about depression of brain activity and feeling of calmness. Stimulants stimulate the nervous system, and increase alertness and activity. Hallucinogens (*Cannabis* products) alters thoughts, perceptions and feelings.

6. (b) *Rauwolfia serpentina* belong to the family *Apocynaceae*, its roots yield a chemical useful for high blood pressure.

7. (d) Tetanus and typhoid are caused by bacteria. Whooping cough is caused by bacteria. Sleeping sickness is caused by parasitic flees. Syphilis is caused by bacteria while AIDS is the final stage of HIV viral disease. Measles and Rabies are caused by virus.

8. (a) Allergy means all kinds of untoward reactions manifested in the body due to hypersensitivity of substances called allergens. Allergy reactions occur due to liberation of histamine by tissue cells.

9. (c) Carcinomas are malignant growths of the epithelial tissue that cover or line the body organs.

10. (c) HIV is a spherical, enveloped virus of about 90-120 nm diameter. Its nucleocapsid is icosahedral and its genome consists of a single-stranded RNA filament segmented into two identical filaments and associated with a "reverse transcriptase enzyme".

11. (c)

12. (d) AIDS is caused by HIV virus and Gonorrhoea is caused by *Neisseria gonorrhoea*. Urethritis is inflammation of the urethra by bacteria. Syphilis is caused by *Treponema pallidum*.

13. (c) The saliva in the mouth and the tears from the eyes belong to physiological barriers.

14. (d) Widal test is used for the diagnosis of typhoid. It is an agglutination test for the presence of antibodies against the *Salmonella* organisms, which cause typhoid fever.

15. (b) Amphetamines bring about increased alertness and sleeplessness. Hashish is a hallucinogen. Valium is a tranquilizer. Valium depresses brain activity and produces feeling of calmness, relaxation and drowsiness. Morphine is an opiate narcotic.

16. (c) Whenver our body gets attacked by some foreign invadors, our body's immune system produces some chemicals to kill or to react against the invader. These chemicals are actually made up of carbohydrates & proteins *i.e.* glycoproteins called antibodies.

17. (a) B and T-lymphocytes produce antibodies against pathogen in the body, if due to some reason B and T-lymphocytes are damaged the body will not produce antibodies against a pathogen. Each B cell and T cell is specific for a particular antigen.

18. (b) Pollen–grains of many species are responsible for some of the severe allergies and bronchial affliction in some people often lead to chronic respiratory disorders - asthma, bronchitis.

19. (c) Tetanus toxoid is a vaccine consisting of growth products of *Clostridium tetani* treated with formaldehyde serving as an active immunising agent. Hence it is weakened germs. The first tetanus toxoid (inactivated toxin) was produced in 1924 and was used successfully to prevent tetanus in the armed services during World War II. In the mid-1940s, tetanus vaccine was combined with diphtheria toxoid and inactivated pertussis vaccine to make the combination DTP vaccine for routine childhood immunization.

20. (d) AIDS (Acquired Immune Deficiency Syndrome) is caused by HIV retrovirus. The virus destroys the helper T lymphocytes thus reducing their numbers.

21. (d) 22. (a) 23. (a) 24. (b)

25. (a) Preformed antibodies need to be injected to treat the bite by a viper snake. It is also a type of immunization which is called as passive immunization.
Antibodies, produced by B-cells, are typically made of basic structural units—each with two large heavy chains and two small light chains. B cells differentiate into plasma cells that secrete antibodies. Antibodies are proteins that bind to specific antigens and mark them for destruction by, for example, making them more recognizable to phagocytic cells. Rejection of a kidney graft is not a function of B lymphocyte.

26. (b) Infectious diseases are those diseases that can spread from one person to another e.g., AIDS. Non-infectious diseases are those diseases that cannot spread from one person to another e.g., cancer.

27. (a) Common cold is caused by some 100 types of Rhino viruses. Symptoms of common cold are irritation of nasal tract, nasal congestion, flow of mucus, sore throat, sneezing, cough, headache and slight fever.

28. (c) Elephantiasis or filariasis is caused by a number of worms. However, in India only two types of worms are responsible for this disease, *Wuchereria bancrofti* and *W. malayi*. This disease is transmitted by female *Culex* mosquitoes. Elephantiasis affects lymphatic vessels of the lower limbs.

29. (d)

30. (d) Hepatitis B is a viral disease, transmitted through both blood and sexual intercourse.

31. (d) Plague is a bacterial disease caused by *Yersinia pestis*. Symptoms of this disease are high fever and a bubo in the groin or armpit. It is primarily a disease of rodents but accidently affects man. The vector of this disease is rat fleas that carries germs of plague from rat to rat. When the rats dies of plague, the fleas leave the dead rat and if any man is nearby, they bite him and inject some plague germs into his blood. Shigellosis or bacillary dysentery, is a diarrheal illness resulting from an acute inflammatory reaction caused by *Shigella*.

32. (a) Skin amd mucous membrane are the physical barriers that provide the first line of defence or the external defence. These barriers prevent the enrty of micro-organisms into the body. Outer tough layer of the skin, the stratum corneum prevents the enrty of bacteria and viruses. Mucus secreted by mucous membrane traps the microorganisms and immobilises them.

33. (a) The substances to which an exaggerated response of the immune system occurs are called allergens. The antibodies produced to these are of lgE type.

34. (d) If the immune system fails to recognize 'self' from 'non-self' and starts destroying the body's own cells, this leads to some malfunctions, which are termed as autoimmune diseases. Both rheumatoid arthritus and myasthenia gravis are autoimmune diseases. In rheumatoid arthritis, inflammation of the synovial membrane in synovial joints occurs. When this membrane, which is the source of synovial fluid, becomes inflamed, it produces too much fluid. Thus, the joints swell and become extremely painful. Myashtenia gravis is a chronic disease marked by abnormal fatigability and weakness of selected muscles. The degree of fatigue is so extreme that these muscles are temporarily paralysed. In this disease, antibodies bind to cholinergic receptors on muscle cells, which impairs the ability of the neurotransmitter acetylcholine to induce muscle contraction.

35. (b) 'A'-lymph nodes, 'B'-Thymus, 'C'-spleen, 'D'-Bone marrow. Thymus and bone marrow are the primary lymphoid organs where maturation of T-cells and B-cells take place respectively. Lymph nodes and spleen are the secondary lymphoid organs where T-cells and B-cells undergo proliferation and differentiation.

36. (c) When a host is exposed to antigens, which may be in the form of living or dead microbes or other proteins, antibodies are produced in the host body. This type of immunity is called active immunity. Infecting the microbes deliberately during immunization/vaccination induces active immunity e.g., polio vaccine.

37. (c) 38. (d)

39. (d) The given figure is of cannabinoid molecule. Cannabinoids are hallucinogenic chemicals obtained from leaves, resin and inflorescence of hemp plant, Cannabis sativa. Marijuana, hashish and ganja and cannabinoids.

40. (c) Cannabinoids bring about euphoria, excitement, sometimes uncontrolled laughter and dilation of pupil of eyes. These days cannabinoids are taken by some sports persons.

41. (d) Rabies, Influenza and AIDS are viral diseases, Amoebiasis, Ascariasis and Trypanosomiasis are caused by Protozoa; Taeniasis, Ascariasis and Elephantasis are the diseases caused by Helminths but Cancer, Tuberculosis and Tetanus are not related diseases. Tuberculosis and Tetanus are bacterial diseases while cancer is not.

42. (c) Lipoproteins are conjugated proteins having polypeptides in association with lipids. Immunoglobulins are the constituent of antibodies. Interferons (INFs) are a group of three vertebrate glycoproteins.
Interferon induces among adjacent cells, as antiviral state by inducing synthesis of the enzymes which inhibit the viral production cycle.

43. (d) 44. (b) 45. (a)

Speed Test-89

1. (a) Parthenocarpy is the development of fruits without prior fertilization which results in the formation of seedless fruits. In some plant species, parthenocarpic fruits are produced naturally or they may be induced by treatment of the unpollinated flowers with auxin.

Removal of androecium before pollen release is called emasculation which is helpful in preventing unwanted pollination. Vernalized seeds are the chilled treated seeds for breaking dormancy. Phenyl Mercuric Acetate is an antitranspirant.
Gibberellins and Auxins are known to induce parthenocarpy in plants. If a tomato plant is treated with a low concentration of auxin and gibberellic acid it wll produce fruits without fertilization i.e. parthenocarpic fruits.

2. (a)
3. (b) Breeding of crops with high levels of minerals, vitamin and minerals is called biofortification. This is most practical aspect to improve the health of people.
4. (b) Jaya and Ratna are two rice varieties developed for green revolution in India.
- The scientific name of Jaya is IET-723. This paddy variety takes about 130 days to grow and the grain is long, bold and white. Its yield is 50-60 quintals per hectare.
- The scientific name of 'Ratna' is IET-1411. It takes about 130-135 days to grow. The grain is long, slender and white. Its yield is 45-50 quintal/hectare.

5. (a) DDT was subsequently banned for agricultural use worldwide under the Stockholm Convention, but its limited use in disease vector control continues to these days in certain parts of the world and remains controversial. Along with the passage of the endangered Species Act, the US ban on DDT is cited by scientists as a major factor in the comeback of the bald eagle in the contiguous US.
6. (c) *Catla catla* and *Labeo rohita* are the two Indian major carps whereas *Heteropneustes* is a catfish. *Cyprinus* is the exotic breed.
7. (a) Food chain is the transfer of energy from green plants (primary producers), through a sequence of organisms in a food chain occupying different trophic level. Therefore, statements (ii) and (iii) are correct.
8. (a) Azadirachtin is a chemical compound belonging to the limonoids. It is a secondary metabolite present in the Neem tree seeds. The molecular formula is $C_{35}H_{44}O_{16}$. Azadirachtin is a highly oxidised tetranortriterpenoid which boosts a plethora of oxygen functionality, comprising an enol ether, acetal, hemiacetal, and tetra-substituted oxirane as well as a variety of carboxylic esters. It is classified among the plant secondary metabolites.
9. (c) 10. (d) 11. (c) 12. (d)
13. (d) In superovulation, a high milk yielding cow is induced to shed 4–6 eggs (instead of one) every 6–8 weeks (instead of 20–21 days). The superovulated donor is artificially inseminated with semen from a quality bull. The embryos developing from the eggs so fertilised are flushed out. These good quality embryos are now transferred to surrogate mother for delivery.
14. (d) Karl Von Frisch, carried out many experiments and determined that when a foraging bee returns to the hive, it performs a waggle dance. Honey is predominantly glucose and fructose. *Dorsata* is a bigger bee than *Apis indica* (a medium sized bee). Bees wax is secreted by special wax glands to make compartments.
15. (a) 16. (a) 17. (a) 18. (b) 19. (b) 20. (a)
21. (a) White leghorn is a mediterranean breed.
22. (a)
23. (c) Golden rice is vitamin A rich variety developed by rDNA technology and used in the treatment of vitamin A deficiency.
24. (d) Golden rice is a transgenic crop of the future with high Vit. A content. Millions of people suffer from Vit. A deficiency which leads to vision impairment. Transgenic rice has been developed which is capable of synthesizing beta carotene, the precursor of Vitamin A. The rice variety is now being crossed into adapted varieties with field tests possible in an year or two.
25. (a)
26. (d) Main objective of production/use of herbicide resistant GM crops is to reduce herbicide accumulation in food articles for health safety. GM plants has been useful in many ways. Genetic modifications has made crops more tolerant to abiotic stresses, reduced reliance on chemical pesticides, enhanced nutritional value of food.
27. (d) In order to obtain virus-free plants through tissue culture, the best method is meristem culture. Meristem tip culture is used successfully to remove viruses, bacteria, in order to produce the greatest number of plants. Meristem culture is used to produce healthy propagation stock for crops and ornamentals.
28. (c) Gene library contains DNA fragments representing the entire genome of an organism. So collection of alleles of the genes of a crop is called gene library.
29. (b) Vector DNA are the DNA molecules that can carry a foreign DNA segment and replicate inside the host cells. Vector DNA may be plasmids, a bacteriophage, cosmids, yeast artificial chromosomes.
30. (c)
31. (a) Three crops that contribute maximum to global food grain production are Wheat, rice and maize, which belong to the family *Poaceae* (*Graminae*).
32. (d) 'Himgiri' developed by hybridisation and selection for disease resistance against rust pathogens is a variety of wheat. It is resistant to leaf/stripe rust and hill bunt.
33. (b)
34. (b) Controlled breeding experiments are carried out using artificial insemination. The semen is collected from the male and is injected either deep into the cervix or at the beginning of the body of the uterus of the selected female by the breeder. The semen may be used immediately or can be frozen and used later. It can also be transported in a frozen form.
35. (b) Breed is a group of animals related by descent and similar in most characters like general appearance, features, size, configuration, etc.
36. (b) Inbreeding strategies allow the desirable qualities of more closely related individuals to be continued within the same breed for 4-6 generations. It increases homozygosity and thus, is necessary for evolving a pure line. Continued inbreeding, especially close inbreeding usually leads to reduces fertility and even productivity. This is called inbreeding depression.
37. (b) Products of honey bee are honey, bee wax, bee venom and royal jelly. Medicinal importance includes its uses as laxative, antiseptic, sedative, etc. It is also used against digestive disorders. Bee venom is used to cure gout and arthritis. Bee was is used is producing cosmetics, paints polishes, etc. It is not a labour intensive process and is source of additional income to the farmers.
38. (c) Germplasm is the sum total of all the alleles of the genes present in a crop and its related species. The germplasm of any crop species consists of the following types of materials: cultivated improved varieties, improved varieties that are no more in cultivation, old local or 'desi' varieties, pure lines produced by plant breeders, and wild species related to the crop species.
39. (d) Tobacco mosaic is caused by Tobacco Mosaic Virus. The infection causes characteristic patterns, such as "mosaic"-like mottling and discolouration on the leaves. Turnip Mosaic Virus causes turnip mosaic. Chlorotic lesions, mosaic and mottling are the common symptoms of this disease.

40. (d) The cell from micro-organisms such as bacteria, fungi, filamentous algae, treated in various ways and used as food, are called single cell protein (SCP). The biomass is not only obtained from unicellular microorganisms but also from multicellular microorganisms.
41. (d) Meristem is a localized group of cells, which are actively dividing and undifferentiated but ultimately give rise to permanent tissue. Cultivation of axillary or apical shoot meristems is called meristem culture. Meristem culture is carried out in potato, banana, cardamom, orchids (protocorm stage), sugarcane, strawberry, sweet potato, etc.
42. (b) The plant cell without cell wall are called protoplasts.
43. (b) The above figures of maize, wheat and garden pea are some Indian hybrid crops. The term "hybrid" refers to a plant variety which is developed through the interbreeding of two or more varieties, genera or species. Though hybrids contain the best properties of the parent plants, they usually do not breed true and often revert to one of the parent plants. Hybrids are favoured for greater disease resistance, more vigorous growth, earlier maturity, higher quality of vegetables, better uniformity and improved flavour.
44. (b)
45. (c) Because iron promotes the formation of chlorophyll and magnesium is an integral part of chlorophyll molecule so in the absence of these nutrients plants show chlorosis & leaves get yellowing. Application of iron and magnesium to promote the synthesis of chlorophyll can cure the disease.

Speed Test-90

1. (d) Activated sludge is a process for treating sewage and industrial wastewaters using air and a biological floc composed of bacteria and protozoans. During the process, the primary effluent is taken to aeration tank that contain large number of aerobic heterotrophic microbes. They form flocs that digest a lot of organic matter. As the biological oxygen demand of waste water is reduced, it is passed into settling tank to undergo sedimentation. The sediment of the settling tank is called activated sludge that is a rich source of aerobic bacteria. Hence, the statement (d) is correct.
Biogas is produced by anaerobic breakdown of biomass with the help of methanogenic bacteria. It is made up of methane, carbon dioxide with traces of nitrogen, hydrogen sulphide and hydrogen.
Methanobacterium is an anaerobic bacterium that is found in rumen of cattle and is helpful in the breakdown of cellulose.
2. (c) 'Each antibiotic is effective only against one particular kind of germ' is not correct.
3. (d) *Monascus purpureus* is a yeast used in the production of statins which are used in lowering blood cholestrol.
4. (d) A common biocontrol agent for control of plant diseases is *Trichoderma*. *Trichoderma* is a tree living fungus that exerts biocontrol over several plant pathogens for the control of plant diseases. It is the natural method of pest and pathogen control.
5. (c) A fed batch is a biotechnological batch process which is based on feeding of a growth limiting nutrient substrate to culture. It is done for purifying enzymes.
6. (a) 2100 antibiotics have been reported so far from actinomycetes alone. Of these maximum antibiotics have been reported from streptomyces alone. Waksman isolated streptomycin from *Streptomyces griseus*.
7. (c) 8. (a)
9. (c) *Aspergillus niger* is used for production of citric acid in industries.
10. (d)
11. (a) Human insulin is being commercially produced from a transgenic species of *Escherichia coli*. *E. coli* is a bacterium that is commonly found in the lower intestine of warm blooded animals. The bacteria can also be grown easily and its genetics are comparatively simple and easily manipulated, making it one of the best studied prokaryotic model organisms, and an important species in biotechnology.
12. (d) Organic farming involves use of organic wastes and other biological material along with beneficial microbes to release nutrients to crop to increase the soil fertility in an ecofriendly, and pollution free environment. *Glomus*, earthworm and *Oscillatoria* can be used in organic farming while snail cannot.
13. (d)
14. (c) *Clostridium butylicum* industrially produces butyric acid.
15. (b) 16. (b) 17. (c) 18. (c)
19. (b) 20. (a) 21. (c)
22. (a) Farmers have reported over 50% higher yields of rice by using the biofertilizer *Azolla pinnata*.
23. (d) Microbes are omnipresent, found in soil, water, air, ice, iside bodies of human beings, animals and plants. Some are found in hot springs (upto 80°–100°C) and even in geysers (thermal vents).
24. (b) Prions are highly resistant glycoportein particles which function as infectious agents. Prions can also act as catalyst converting nomal protein into prion state. Prions are not affected by proteases, nucleases, temperature upto 800°C, UV radiations and formaldehyde.
25. (c) Probiotics are live microgranisms (bacteria in most cases) that are similar to beheficial micriorganisms found in the human gut. They are also called "friendly bacteria" or " good bacteria". Probiotic microorganisms consist mostly of strains of *Lactobacillius, Bifidobcterium* and *Streptococcus*. Probiotics are taken as food supplement and energy drinks (e.g. Yakult).
26. (c)
27. (b) Flocs are masses of bacteria held together by slime and fungal filaments to form mesh like structures.
28. (a) Secondary treatment of sewage (or biological treatment) depletes 90-95% of the BOD and many pathogens are removed. Reduction of BOD by 90% is achieved through mineralization of small fraction of organic matter and conversion of large proportion to removable solids.
29. (d) Methanogens are microorganisms that produce methane as a metabolic byproduct in anoxic condition. They include *Methanobcterium, Methanobrevibacter* and *Methanococcus*.
30. (d) 31. (b)
32. (b) Organic farming includes serval methods to enhance soil fertility. In such farming, methods of biological origin are used e.g., biopesticides biofertilizers, IPM (Integrated Pest Management) green manure, bioherbicides etc. Chemical fertilizers are not used in organic farming.
33. (b)
34. (c) *Oscillatoria* and *Nostoc* are nitrogen fixing cyanobacteria. They add orgnaic matter as well as extra nitrogen to the soil. Cyanobacteria are very important and low-cost biofertilizers.
35. (d) Commercial ethanol or ethyl alcohol is produced by yeast *Saccharomyces cerevisiae*.
36. (d) Lactic acid bacteria help in souring milk. Ripening of cheese is done by bacteria (*Propionibacterium shermanii*) or moulds (*Penicillium roqueforti*).
37. (a) Brewer's yeast lack sufficient diastase and amylase therefore if complex carbohydrates have to be acted upon by them, 1% malt or inoculation with fungus like *Rhizopus* is done to degrade sugars.

38. (b) Baggasse is crushed sugarcane from which sugar has been extracted. It is used for fuel in sugar refineries and in making of fibre board.
39. (b) The bacteria *Clostridium acetobutylicum* is used to produce butanol and acetone from starch. This bacteria was first used by Chaim Weizmann in 1920.
40. (a) 41. (d)
42. (c) *Aspergillus niger* is related with production of gallic acid.
43. (b) The label A represents sludge, label B represents methane and carbon dioxide, and the label C represents dung and water.
44. (a)
45. (a) BOD is the method of determining the amount of oxygen required by microorganisms to decompose the waste present in the water supply. It is a measure of organic matter present in the water. If the quantity of organic wastes in the water supply is high then the number of decomposing bacteria present in the water will also be high. As a result, BOD value will increase.

Speed Test-91

1. (a) The linking of antibiotic resistance gene with the plasmid vector became possible with DNA ligase. DNA ligase is an enzyme that is able to join together two portions of DNA and therefore plays an important role in DNA repair. DNA ligase is also used in recombinant DNA technology as it ensures that the foreign DNA is bound to the plasmid into which it is incorporated.
2. (b) DNA or RNA segment tagged with a radioactive molecule is called probe. They are used to detect the presence of complementary sequences in nucleic acid samples. Probes are used for identification and isolation of DNA and RNA.
3. (a) Restriction endonucleases are enzymes that makes cuts at specific positions within the DNA molecule. They acts as molecular scissors. They recognise specific base sequence at palindromic sites in DNA duplex and cut its strands.
4. (d) In gel electrophoresis, agarose extracted from sea weed used as gel agarose, made of 0.7% gel show good resolution of large DNA and 2% gel will show good resolution of small fragments.
5. (d)
6. (b) Cloning is the production of an organism with exactly similar genetic make up as in the mother individual. Cloning is done to preserve genotype of an individual. This is achieved by cell culture, tissue culture or genetic engineering.
7. (d) Retrovirus has the ability to transform normal cells into cancerous cells. Hence, it can used as a vector for cloning desirable genes into animal cells.
8. (d) In pBR 322;
-ori-represents site of origin of replication
-rop-represents those proteins that take part in replication of plasmid.
-*Hind* III, *Eco*RI- Recoginition sites of Restriction endonucleases
-amp^R and tet^R - They are antibiotic resistant gene part.
9. (c) Electroporation is the method of making cell membrane permeable for the entry of recombinant DNA into the bacteria.
10. (c) The Southern blot is used to detect and identify certain DNA sequences in a sample of bodily fluid. It uses single-stranded DNA to search out their complementary strands. When a Southern blot is performed on DNA, the first step is digestion of DNA with restriction enzymes. Restriction enzymes cut DNA at known sequences, and produces DNA fragments of a certain length. Once the DNA is cut into pieces, scientists conduct electrophoresis to separate them by size.
11. (a) PCR is now a common and often indispensable technique, developed in 1984 by Kary Mullis, used in medical and biological research labs for a variety of applications. These include DNA cloning for sequencing, DNA-based phylogeny, or functional analysis of genes; the diagnosis of hereditary diseases; the identification of genetic fingerprints (used in forensic sciences and paternity testing); and the detection and diagnosis of infectious diseases. In 1993, Mullis won the Nobel Prize in Chemistry for his work on PCR.
12. (d) For gene transfer into the host cell without using vector microparticles made of tungsten and gold coated with foreign DNA are bombarded into target cells at a very high velocity.
13. (b) The first fecombinant DNA was constructed by Stanley Cohen and Herbert Boyer in 1972. They cut the piece of DNA from a plasmid carryign antibotic-resistance gene in the bacterium *Salmonella typhimurium* and linked it to the plasmid of *Escherichia coli*. The vector transfers the piece of DNA attached to it.
14. (a) Genetic engineering is the artificial synthesis, isolation, modification, combination, addition and repair of the genetic material (DNA) to alter the phenotype of the host organims to suit human needs. It is the manipulation of genes by man in vitro. Restriction endonucleases play major role in genetic engineering as they can cut DNA at specific sites.
15. (c) Electrophoresis is a technique of separation of molecules such as DNA, RNA or protein, under the influence of an electrical field, so that they migrate in the direction of electrode bearing the opposite charge, viz, positively charged molecule move towards cathode (–ve electrode) and negatively charged molecues travel towards anode (+ve electrode) under an electric filed through a matrix of agarose gel. The DNA fragments separate according to their size through the agarose gel, with smaller fragments moving farther away as compared to larger ones. The DNA fragments can be visualized by staining them with ethidium bromide followed by exposure to UV radiations. Bright orange coloured bands of DNA can be observed. The separated DNA bands are then cut out from the agarose gel and extracted from the gel piece. This step is known as elution. The DNA fragments purified in this manner are used in constructing recombinant DNA by joining them with cloning vectors.
16. (c) The DNA used as a carrier for transferring a fragment of foreign DNA into a suitable hosts is called vehicle DNA of cloning vector or gene carrier. When desired gene is introduced into a vector, recombinant DNA is formed. Vectors may be plasmids, bacteriophages, cosmids, phagemids, Yeast Artificial Chromosomes (YACs) Bacterial Artificial Chromosomes (BACs), transposons, viruses, etc.
17. (d) 18. (b)
19. (d) *Escherichia coli* is a bacterium found in human colon. On this bacterium scientists have made extensive genetic experiments to make some vital chemicals like insulin. Another bacterium is *Agrobacterium tumefaciens* which causes crown gall in plants is extensively used for genetic experiments.
20. (c) PCR is a technique for enzymatically replicating DNA without using a living organism such as *E. coli* or yeast. It is commonly used in medical and biological research labs for a variety of tasks like detection of hereditary diseases, identification of genetic fingerprints etc.
The correct steps shown in the given figure are:
A – Denaturation at a temperature of about 94° to 98°C. During the denaturation, the double strand melts open to single stranded DNA, and all enzymatic reactions stop.

B – Annealing (binding of DNA primer to the separated strands. Occurs at 50° to 65°Celsius, which is lower than the optimal temperature of the DNA polymerases)

C – Extension or elongation of the strands using the DNA primer with heat-stable DNA polymerases, most frequently Taq (*Thermus aquaticus*) at 72°C.

21. (d) 22. (c) 23. (a) 24. (b)

25. (c) Transformation is a process by which a cell takes up naked DNA fragment from the environment, incorporates it into its own chromosomal DNA and finally expresses the trait controlled by the incoming DNA. Since DNA is a hydrophilic molecule, it can not pass through membranes, so that bacterial cells must be made competent to take up DNA. This is done by treating them with a specific concentration of a divalent cation, such as calcium (Ca^{2+}) which increases the efficiency with which DNA enters the bacterium through pores in its cell wall. Recombination DNA (rDNA) can then be forced into such cells by incubating them briefly at 42° C (heat shock), and then putting them back on ice. This enables the bacteria to take up the recombination DNA.

26. (c) Polymerase chain reaction is a technique used to replicate a fragment of DNA so as to produce many copies of a particular DNA sequence. A single PCR amplification cycle involves three basic steps: denaturation, annealing and extension (polymerisation).

27. (a) Eukaryotic genes do not function properly when transferred into bacterial cell because introns are present in eukaryotic cells but are absent in prokaryotic cells. Hence, when bacterial cell is transformed with recombinant DNA generated using human gene, it could not process it. As a result desired protein will not be produced.

28. (b) 29. (b) 30. (a) 31. (c)

32. (d) Direct gene transfer is the transfer of naked. DNA into plant cells but the presence of rigid plant cell wall acts as a barrier to uptake. Therefore, protoplasts are the favoured target for direct gene transfer. Polyethylene glycol mediated DNA uptake is a direct gene transfer method that utilizes the interaction between polyethylene glycol, naked DNA, salts and the protoplast membrane to effect transport of the DNA into the cytoplasm.

33. (d) 34. (c)

35. (d) The fact that DNA is structured the same way in all known organisms means that similar methods can be used to study the hereditary material.

36. (a) pBR 322 is an artificially constructed vector plasmid. It is widely used in gene cloning experiments.

37. (d) *EcoR*I is an endonuclease enzyme isolated from strains of *E.coli* and a part of restriction modified system. So, .co part stands for *coli*.

38. (a) Restriction endonuclease-*Hind* II, always cuts DNA molecules at a particular point by recognizing a specific sequence of six base pairs. This specific base sequence is known as the recognition sequence for *Hind* II.

39. (c) Chitinase is an enzyme that cleaves the glycosidic bonds in chitin, thereby breaking down the structural polysaccharide component of the hard outer covering of many animals and of the cell wall of fungi.

40. (d)

41. (c) Palindromic sequences in DNA molecule are group of bases that forms the same sequence when read in both forward and backward direction. In the given question, only option (c) represents a palindromic sequence.

42. (d) During heat shock to the bacterium, the temperature used for giving thermal shock is 42° C. This enables the bacteria to take up the recombinant DNA.

43. (d) A stirred-tank bioreactors is usually cylindrical or with a curved base to facilitate the mixing of the reaction contents. The stirrer facilitates even mixing and oxygen availability throughout the bioreactor. Alternatively air can be bubbled through the reactor.

44. (b) Downstream processing refers to the recovery and purification of biosynthetic products, particularly pharmaceuticals. It is an essential step in the manufacture of pharmaceuticals such as antibiotics, hormones (e.g. insulin and human growth hormone), antibodies and vaccines; antibodies and enzymes used in diagnostics; industrial enzymes; and natural fragrance and flavour compounds.

45. (d) Polymerase chain reaction (PCR) is a technique of synthesizing multiple copies of the desired gene (or DNA) *in vitro*.
At the start of PCR, the DNA from which a segment is to be amplified, an excess of the two primer molecules, the four deoxynucleoside triphosphates and the DNA polymerase are mixed together in reaction mixture that has appropriate quantities of Mg^{2+}. The PCR operation is followed in a sequence where denaturation, primer extention occurs.

Speed Test-92

1. (b) In this technique nematode specific genes are introduced in the host plant in such a way that it produces both sense and antisense RNA. The two RNA's being complementary to each other form a double stranded RNA (dsRNA) which is also called interfering RNA responsible for initiating RNA interference (RNA i). This (dsRNA) bind to and prevent translation of specific mRNA of nematode (gene silencing). Thus transgenic plants based on RNAi technology are resistant to nematode.

2. (a)

3. (a) RNA interference technique, sense & antisense RNA fused to form dsRNA that silent the expression of m- RNA of nematode. RNA interference is a novel strategy adopted to prevent infestation of nematode *Meloidegyne incognitia* in roots of tobacco plants. .

4. (a) Recombinant DNA technology is the process joining together two DNA molecules from two different species that are inserted into a host organism to produce new genetic combination.

5. (d) Transgenic Rosie is actually cow. Restriction enzymes cut the DNA at specific sites.

6. (b)

7. (c) Common activities in bioinformatics include mapping and analysing DNA and protein sequences, aligning different DNA *etc.* are the part of human genome project.

8. (a) Dolly sheep was obtained by cloning the udder cell (somatic cell) fused with enucleated oocyte.

9. (a)

10. (a)

11. (b) Biowar or biological war or bioterrorism is the development of biological weapons against people, their crops and animals.

12. (d) The transgenic food, containing enzyme produced by antibiotic resistance gene, can cause allergies because it is a foregin protein. The bacteria present in alimentary cancal can take up antibiotic resistance gene and become resistant to that antibiotic. Transgenes can endanger native species if Bt toxin is expressed in pollens which are transported by pollinator honey bees. GM crop prodution causes changes in natural environment which may be harmful for all organisms.

13. (c) Two cry genes, cry IAc and cry IIAb have been incorporated in cotton. The genetically modified crop is called Bt cotton as it contains Bt toxin genes. The genes cry I Ac and cry II Ab control cotton bollworms.

14. (c) Hirudin is a protein that stops blood clotting. The gene encoding hirudin was chemically synthesized. This gene was then transferred ito *Brassica napus*, where hirudin accumulaes in seeds. The hirudin is purified and used as medicine.

15. (d) Using conventional methods of diagnosis (serum and urine analysis, etc.) early detection is not possible. Recombinant DNA technology, Polymerase Chain Reaction (PCR) and Enzyme Linked Immunosorbent Assay (ELISA) are some of the techniques that serve the purpose of early diagnosis.

16. (b) Gene therapy is a collection of methods that allows correction of gene defect that has been diagonsed in a child/embryo. Correcting of a genetic defect involves delivery of a normal gene into the individual or embryo to take over the function of and compensate for the non-functional gene.

17. (a) Bioethics may be viewed as the set of standards that may be used to regulate various activites based on their effects on the biological world. This is because biotehncology has aroused social as well as political concerns, which have ranged from biotechnology being unnatural to detrimental to biodiversity.

18. (c) 19. (d) 20. (b) 21. (b) 22. (a)
23. (b) 24. (d) 25. (d) 26. (b) 27. (c)
28. (c) 29. (a)

30. (d) The first commercial example of enzyme modification of a protein for human use is the conversion of pig insulin to human insulin called "humulin".

31. (a)

32. (b) These are all good examples of the end products of various r-DNA technologies.

33. (c) The use of BGH does not appear to have serious health or environmental drawbacks, but it could offer such a competitive edge to corporate farming operations that smaller, more traditional family farms might be forced out of business. This scenario is a good example of how genetic engineering can have unintended social consequences.

34. (d) DNA vaccines are used as injection of pure DNA or RNA into skeleton muscles leading to expression of DNA in the muscle cell.

35. (c) 36. (c)

37. (d) Golden rice is a transgenic food crop which may help in solving the problem of night blindness in developing countries. Golden rice or miracle rice is rich in vitamin A or β-carotene and iron and decaffeinated coffee are also valuable achievements of gene transfer technology.

38. (d) Bt toxin genes were isolated from *Bacillus thuringiensis* and incorporated into cotton plant to form a genetically modified crop called Bt cotton. Bt cotton has high yield and resistance to bollworms.

39. (c) Only mammalian cells can correctly attach these sugars to proteins.

40. (b) *Agrobacterium tumefaciens* is the causal agent of crown gall disease (the formation of tumours) in over 140 species of dicot. This disease caused by a DNA plasmid (T_i plasmid) carried by bacterium and transferred to the plant cells. T_i plasmid has been widely used in plant engineering as a vector in order to inject gene in host plant to form transgenic plant.

41. (d) 42. (b) 43. (b) 44. (b) 45. (a)

Speed Test-93

1. (d) Tropical rain forests occur in equatorial and subequatorial regions. The forests receive all the external inputs for optimum plant growth. Due to abundant plant growth, a large number of animals live in tropical rain forests. In grasslands fire occur periodically which prevent tree growth. In savannahs, periods of drought are common. In deciduous forests broad leaved hard wood deciduous trees are found predominantly.

2. (b) Competition is most severe between the members of a population belonging to same habitat.

3. (a) Symbiosis or mutualism is a mutually beneficial association necessary for the survival of both the partners.

4. (c) Praying mantis is a good example of camouflage. Camouflage is the natural colouring of an animal which enables it to blend in with its surroundings.
A praying mantis, or praying mantid, is the common name for an insect of the order Mantodea. Often mistakenly spelled **preying mantis** (a tempting mistake, as they are notoriously predatory) they are in fact named for the typical "prayer-like" stance. The word *mantis* derives from the Greek word mantis for prophet or fortune teller.

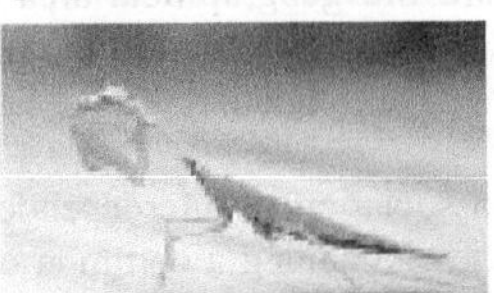

A praying mantis from **India**

5. (a) Population is an aggregation or grouping of individuals of the same species at the same time in a particular area. Species is a grouping of individuals of one or more populations resembling each other in important morphological, anatomical and biochemical characters and can potentially interbreed. Biotic community is an assemblage of interdependent, and ecosystem is a self sufficient and self regulating segment of nature comprising of a biotic community and its physical environment, both interacting and exchanging materials. The basic level of ecological organisation starts with the individual, the next more complex levels are populations, species, community and then ecosystem.

6. (d) The keystone species in an ecosystem are those who are the main contributors to the ecosystem.

7. (b) Niche indicate the habitat of a particular species and the interaction of that species with the resources present in the habitat. Niche overlap means that two or more species sharing the resources present in a particular niche.

8. (a) **Stenohaline :** Steno meaning narrow and haline meaning salt. A fish cannot handle a wide fluctuation of salt content in water. Many fresh water fish tend to be stenohaline and die in environments of high salinity such as the ocean. Fish living in coastal estuaries and tide pools are often euryhaline (tolerant to changes in salinity) as are many species which have life cycle requiring tolerance to both fresh water and sea water environments such as *Salmon*.

9. (d) Human population growth in India can be regulated by following the national programme of family planning.

10. (b) Some species make permanent burrows deep into the soil to escape high temperature or sunlight and some cold blooded animals often like to bask in the sun to warm up their body.

11. (b) 12. (b) 13. (c)

14. (c) This age pyramid represents the declining population of any organism. Population decline is the reduction over time in region's census. It can be caused for several reasons that includes heavy immigration disease, famine or sub-replacement fertility.

15. (b) The logistic population growth is expressed by the equation
$$\frac{dN}{dt} = rN\left[\frac{(K-N)}{K}\right]$$ where N is population density at time t, r is the Malthusian parameter (rate of maximum population growth) and K is the so called carrying capacity (*i.e.* maximum sustainable population). It is a type of population growth when resources are limiting.

16. (b) The best pH of soil for cultivation of plants is 6.5 – 7.5.

17. (d) A self regulatory mechanism of maintaining favourable internal conditions for uninterrupted chemical reactions in the living system despite changes in the external environment is homeostasis. Total energy stored within system is enthalpy.
18. (b) Gause's hypothesis states that two different competing species cannot coexist together for a long in the same niche, one has to get eliminated by the other competing species, if they do coexist, then they do so as a result of niche differentiation, i.e. differentiation of then realized niches.
19. (b) Speciation takes place via reproductive isolation which is the most important consequence of geographical isolation.
20. (d) Hotspots are the geographical area where biodiversity is maximum. Two hotspots in India are Western ghats and North eastern himalayan region.
21. (b) 22. (c)
23. (d) A natural association of interdependent populations of different species inhabiting a common environment or habitat as a visible, self-contained unit is called a biotic community or biocoenosis.
24. (b) A biome is a large regional unit characterized by a major vegetation type and associated fauna found in a specific climatic zone some examples of terrestrial biomes are desert, temperate deciduous forest, tropical rain forest, etc.
25. (d) Protoplasm is the material comprising the living content of a cell. It consists of 90% water alongwith the minerals, sugars, amino acids, proteins, enzymes, etc. The translocation of nutrients inside the body occurs via blood which also majorly consists of water. In an environment with excessive heat, water loss in the form of sweating and transpiration keeps the body cool. Thus, water maintains the body temperature.
26. (a) The red colour of red algae is due to abundant formationof phycoerythrin which is able to absorb blue green wavelengths of light. Being shorter, these wavelengths are able to reach the maximum depth in water. Therefore, red algae can be found in deepest ocean waters.
27. (c) The seasonal movement of complete populations of animals to a more favourable environment is called migration. It is usually in response to uneven precipitation and lower temperatures resulting in a reduced food supply and is often triggered by a change in day length. Migration is common in mammals (e.g. porpoises), fish (e.g. eels and salmon) and some insects but is most marked in birds.
28. (d) Competition is defined as the active demand by two or more individuals of the same species or members of two or more species at same trophic levels for a common resource. Intraspecific competition is competition amongst members of the same species for a common resource such as for food, space and mate. Interspecific competition amongst members of different species for a common resource such as for food, space and mate. Interspecific competition is rivalry amongst members of different species. The severity of competition depends upon similarity in the requirement of food and shelter.
29. (b) Population density is the number of individuals present per unit area of volume at a given time. If the total number of individuals is represented by letter N and the number of units of space (area for land organisms and volume for water organisms) by letter S, then the population density D can be represented as D = N/S. For instance, number of animals per square kilometer, number of trees per acre in a forest etc.
30. (a) $$\text{Date rate} = \frac{\text{Number of deaths}}{\text{Initial number of individuals}}$$

$$= \frac{200}{800} = \frac{1}{4} = 0.25$$

31. (d) Tropical rain forest shows the maximum diversity and also the maximum productivity. More solar energy and resources are available in tropics which promotes higher productivity. On land the maximum primary production rate is found in tropical rain forests, followed by tropical deciduous forests, temperate forests, savannah, temperate grasslands and desert shrubs.
32. (c) 33. (a) 34. (c) 35. (c) 36. (c) 37. (a)
38. (c) Permafrost, a permanently frozen subsoil, is a distinctive characteristic of the tundra.
39. (a) Grasslands are typically maintained by grazing herbivores and by periodic fires. Overgrazing, such as may occur if agricultural livestock are introduced, which can lead to destruction of the grassland.
40. (c) Deserts have less than 25 centimeters of rainfall per year.
41. (c) Aestivation is the cessation or slowing of metabolic activity during the summer period to avoid problems of heat and desiccation etc.
42. (d) Blubber is the fatty layer present between the skin and muscle of whales and other cetaceans. It acts as an insulator and protects the animal from heat loss and serves as a food reserve.
43. (a) Predation is a relation between two organisms in which one organism captures and feeds on other. Commensalism is a relation between two organisms in which one benefits and the other neither derives benefit nor harms. Parasitism is a relation between organisms in which one lives as a parasite on another and harms the host. Competition is process in which the fitness and survival ability of one species is significantly lower in the presence of another species.
44. (a) Population density varies due to changes in the following basic process - A: Natality + Immigration; B: Mortality + Emigration

    Natality is the proportion of births to the total population in a place in a given time. Immigration is the number of individuals of the same species that have come into the habitat from elsewhere during the time period under consideration. Mortality is the number of deaths in the population during a given period of time. Emigration is the number of individuals of the population who left the habitat and have gone elsewhere during a given period of time.
45. (c)

Speed Test-94

1. (c) 2. (b)
3. (a) A blanket of air surrounding the earth is called as atmosphere and it is divided into different strata (zone). The zone of atmosphere that lies near the ground is troposphere.
4. (b) Detritus food chain begins with dead organic matter of dead plant parts, animals and their excretory product which is being acted upon by decomposers such as saprophytes to obtain energy needed for their survival.
5. (b) Biogeochemical cycles : Two types :
   (i) Gaseous : Biogenetic materials involved in circulation are gases *e.g.* N_2, O_2, CO_2 *etc.*
   (ii) Sedimentary : Biogenetic materials involved in circulation are non-gaseous *eg.* P, Ca, S etc. form rocks.
6. (a) A standing crop is the quantity or total weight or energy content of the organism, which are in a particular location at a particular time.
7. (c) The decomposers act on the dead organic matter and break them down into simpler compounds and minerals.

8. (d) In soil science, humus refers to any organic matter which has reached a point of stability where it will break down no further and might, if conditions do not change, remain essentially as it is for centuries, if not millennia. In agriculture, humus is sometimes also used to describe mature compost, or natural compost extracted from a forest or other spontaneous source for use to amend soil. It is also used to describe a topsoil horizon that contains organic matter (humus type, humus form, humus profile).

9. (b) The rate at which organic molecules are formed in a green plant is called gross productivity.

10. (a) An ecosystem having low stability can be easily damaged. An ecosystem having high resilience will take less time to recover.

11. (a) Hydrarch succession takes place in wetter areas and xerarch succession respectively, which takes place in dry areas. So, both hydrarch and xerarch successions leads to medium water conditions.

12. (c) Coral reefs are often called "rainforest of the sea". It forms some of the most diverse ecosystem on earth. Coral reef ecosystem have the highest gross primary productivity in the sea.

13. (c) Polar ice caps & glaciers have the largest amount of pure and fresh water without any dissolved salt or impurity.

14. (d) Four important functional aspects of the ecocystem are (i) Productivity (ii) Decomposition, (iii) Energy flow and (iv) Nutrient cycling.

15. (a) 16. (a) 17. (a)

18. (b) The rate at which food energy is assimilated at the trophic level of consumers is called secondary productivity. In other words, the rate of synthesis of organic matter by consumers is called as secondary productivity. The primary producers have produced the food for consumers, and secondary productivity reflects only the utilization of this food for the production of consumer biomass.

19. (d) Humus constitutes the organic component of soil and is rich in lignin and cellulose. Humus is formed from organic remains through the activity of decomposer microorganisms. Process of formation of humus from raw organic remains is called humification. Humus is quite resistant to microbial action.

20. (c) Less than 50% of the solar energy incident over earth is present in PAR (photosynthetically active radiation).

21. (a) A single species may occupy more than one trophic level. Sparrow can be a primary consumer if it feeds on seeds, fruits and peas or a secondary consumer if it feeds on insects and worms.

22. (b) Secondary sucession (= subsere) is the biotic succession that occurs in an area which become secondarily bare due to the destruction of community previously present there. Secondary succession starts from previously built up substrata with already existing living matter. The action of any external force, such as sudden change in climatic factors, biotic intervention, fire, etc. had resulted in the destruction of previous community. Thus, area become devoid of living matter but its substratum, instead of primitive, is built up. It has organic matter so is biologically fertile and thus the successions are comparatively more rapid.

23. The cycling pool of carbon consists of 6×10^{14} kg (29%) of free CO_2 in the atmosphere, 1.45×10^{15} kg (71%) of dissolved CO_2 occurs in the oceans. Oceans also regulate the amount of CO_2 in the atmosphere.

24. (d) 25. (b) 26. (a) 27. (d) 28. (c)

29. (c) 30. (a) 31. (b) 32. (b) 33. (b)

34. (b) Phosphorus is mostly used as phosphate. Its reservoir pool is phosphate rocks while cycling pool is soil for terrestrial ecosystems and water for aquatic ecosystems.

35. (b) Only 10% of the mass is flown from one trophic level to another in the form of energy.

36. (c) Lichens are the early settlers on a barren area because they can tolerate desiccation, heating during summer noon or excessive cooling during winter nights. They secrete lichen acids and carbonic acid. The acids slowly corrode rock surface and release minerals required for proper growth of lichens.

37. (a) The first biotic community which develops in a bare area is called pioneer community. It has very little diversity. This stage takes the longest time to change the environment for invasion of the next community.

38. (d) Climax community is the stable, self perpetuating and final biotic community that develops at the end of biotic succession and is in perfect harmony with the physical environment.

39. (c) Identification and enumeration of plants and animal species of an ecosystem gives its species composition.

40. (d) Communities is an assemblage of interacting populations occupying a given area. Climate, species interaction, feeding relationship among organisms and succession are the factors which influence communities.

41. (d) Grassland can support greater grazing rates by herbivores than forests because grassland produces less woody plant tissue.

42. (a)

43. (c) Arrow III is incorrect.

44. (d) A : Presence of 3 - 4 storeys of plant grown in a forest is called stratification.

B : A biome having grasses with scattered trees is called savannah.

C : Man made ecosystem is dam. Man - made ecosystem are the artificial ecosystems which rely on the human efforts to sustain.

D : Pioneer in hydrosere is blue green algae.

45. (d) Decomposition involves breakdown of complex organic matter by decomposer to inorganic raw materials like CO_2, water & various nutrients. It consists of the following processes:

Fragmentation : It is the formation of smaller pieces of dead organic matter or detritus by detritivores.

Catabolism : Chemical conversion of detritus into simpler inorganic substances with the help of bacterial and fungal enzymes is called catabolism.

Leaching : Water soluble substances (formed as a result of decomposition) are leached to deeper layers of soil.

Humification : If decomposition leads to the formation of colloidal organic matter (humus), the process is called humification.

Mineralization : Formation of simpler inorganic substances (like CO_2, water and minerals) is termed mineralization.

Speed Test-95

1. (a) In situ means keeping endangered species of animals or plants into natural environment and not in the environment that looks like natural but is man made, like zoological & botanical gardens. *In situ* includes, national parks, sanctuaries and biosphere reserve.

2. (d) Biodiversity Act of India was passed by the parliament in the year 2002.

3. (b) Biodiversity is the number of variety of organism found within a specified geographic region.

4. (d) The 'Cheetah' has become extinct from India. The endangered subspecies *Acinonyx jubatus venaticus* lives in Asia (Iran). In 1990, there were reports in the Times of India of a cheetah sighting in eastern India. There is a chance some cheetahs remain in India, though it is doubtful. There have also been reports of Asiatic cheetahs in the Balochistan Province of Pakistan, though these continue to be unverified. The cheetah prefers to live in an open biotope, such as semi-desert, prairie, and thick bushes.

5. (d) Hot spots are those areas which were rich in biodiversity but now are under threat due to direct or indirect interference of human activites. These regions are on the edge to get some of their species extinct due to humans. Western Ghats in India are under threat due to continuous developmental activities and Doon valley is under threat due to continuous mining activities.

6. (b)

7. (d) *Podophyllum* is one of the endangered species of Indian medicinal plants. It is used to remove benign (not cancer) growths, such as certain kinds of warts. It works by destroying the tissue

8. (a) Kaziranga National Park in Assam is famous as a protection environmental park for rhinoceros.

9. (c) 10. (b)

11. (c) Lesser inter-specific competition is not observed in biodiversity hotspots.

12. (b) In India maximum genetic diversity is seen in rice. Total of 23 variety of irrigated ecology and 8 varieties of rainfed ecology has been invented in India.

13. (d) The statements (i) and (ii) are correct. The statement (iii) is incorrect because predators cannot lead to the extinction of prey species. Predator and prey evolve together. The statement (iv) is incorrect because chemical such as nicotine and strychnine produced by the plants are not metabolic disorders but are metabolic wastes.

14. (b) Diversity is due to the long term evolutionary changes. Adaptability to continuous changes in environmental conditions is important for natural selection of variants and variations generation after generation leading to emergence of diverse descendants.

15. (d) Higher diversity in tropical areas is because (i) Speciation is a function of time. Temperate areas have undergone frequent glaciation in the past. It killed most of the species. No such disturbances occured in tropics where species continuted to flourish and evolve undisturbed for millions of years (ii) There are no unfavouable seasons in tropics. Continued favourable environment has helped tropical organisms to gain more niche specialisation and increased diversity. (iii) More solar energy is available in tropics. This promotes higher productivity and increased biodivesity. (iv) Resoruce availability is higher in tropics (v) There is reduced competition in tropics due to favourable environment. (vi) Rate of extinction is low in tropics.

16. (b) *Lantana*, *Eichhornia* and Arican catfish are exotic species. Non-native or exotic species are often introduced inadvertently for their economic and other uses. They often become invasive and drive away the local species. These species are considered to be second major cause of extinction of species. Exotic species have proved harmful to both aquatic and terrestrial ecosystems.

17. (d) A stable community is self-prepetuating and final biotic community that is in perfect harmony with the physical environment. It does not show much of changes and is usually resilient to natural or man made disturbances, it is also resistant to evasion by alien species.

18. (b) The number of species of aves, reptiles, amphibians and mammals are 1232, 456, 209 and 300 respectively.

19. (a) IUCN is International Union of Conservation of Nature and Natural Resources, which is now called World Conservation Union (WCU).It has its headquarters at Morges, Switzerland. It maintains a red data book or red list which is a catalogue of taxa facing risk of extinction.

20. (a) The relationship between species richness and area is rectangular hyperbola for a wide variety of taxa whether they are birds, bats, fresh water fishes or flowering plants and the equation can be given as $S = CA^Z$. On a logarithimic scale, it is straight line described by the eqution log S = log C + z log A. Where S is species richness, Z is slope of line or regression coefficient, C is Y-intercept while A is area.

21. (b) Genetic diversity is the diverty in the numbers and types of genes as well as chromosomes present in different species and the variations in the genes and their allels in the same species. Genetic variation in *Rauwolfia vomitoria* indicates genetic diversity. Another example is the presence of more than 50,000 genetically different strains of rice,and 1000 varieties of mango in India.

22. (d) Keystone species are those species which have significant and disproportinonaely large influence on the community structure and characteristics. It often has considerably low abundance and biomass as compared to dominant species. Removal of such species causes serious disruption in structure and function of community.

23. (b) National park is a reserved area used for conservation purposes. It is maintained by the government. Cultivation grazing, forestry and habitat manipulation are not allowed. Protection is provided to the entire ecosystem.

24. (d) Bishnois of Rajasthan protect *Prosopis cineraria* and Black buck religiously.

25. (b) Exotic species tend to cause a the reat to biodivesity. They are not found in hot spots which are regions of high biodiversity. In India, 3 hotspots ae found, i.e., Western Ghats and Sri Lanka, Indo-Burma (NE India) and Himalays.

26. (c) Ex situ (off site) conservation is conservation of selected rare plans/animals in places outside their natural homes. Ex situ conservation includes offsite collections, gene banks in vitro fertilization, cryopreservation techniques and tissue culture.

27. (a) Jim Corbett National Park (district Nainita Uttrakhand) is the first national park of Inida, established in 1936.

28. (b) Earth Summiti at Rio de Janeiro (1992), Brazil, promoted Convention on Biological Diversity (CBD) which was signed by 152 nations, Its recommendations came into effect on 29th Dec, 1993. India became a party to this Convention on Biological Diversity in May, 1994.

29. (a)

30. (a) Alpha diversity is present within community.

31. (d) 32. (b) 33. (c) 34. (d)

35. (b) Those species whose populations have been seriously depleted and whose ultimate security is not assured are known as Endangered species.

36. (b) 37. (c)

38. (d) Chiru is Himalayan Ibex, also called Tibetan Antelope. Shahtoosh is obtained from its neck hair. It is banned under the law.

39. (c)

40. (d) Nature selects those set of characters that are best adapted to the environment. This has resulted in the great diversity seen in the population of finches.

41. (d) 42. (b) 43. (b) 44. (d) 45. (b)

Speed Test-96

1. (a) NO_2 and SO_2 after reacting with water in atmosphere produce HNO_3 & H_2SO_4 which fall down as acid rain.

2. (d) DDT residues are rapidly passed through food chain causing biomagnification because DDT is liposoluble. Biomagnification, also known as bioamplification or biological magnification, is the increase in concentration of a substance, such as the pesticide DDT, that occurs in a food chain as a consequence of:
-Persistence (slow to be broken down by environmental processes)
-Food chain energetics
-Low (or non-existent) rate of internal degradation/excretion of the substance
(often due to water-insolubility).

3. (d) Silicosis is caused by exposure to dust containing silica.

4. (d) In secondary treatment mainly settled sewage flows to an aerobic biological treatment stage where it comes into contact with micro-organisms which remove and oxidise most of the remaining organic pollutants.

5. (c) Biochemical Oxygen Demand (BOD) in river water increases when sewage gets mixed with river water. Biochemical oxygen demand or biological oxygen demand (BOD) is a chemical procedure for determining how fast biological organisms use up oxygen in a body of water. It is used in water quality management and assessment, ecology and environmental science. BOD is considered as an indication of the quality of a water source.

6. (d) 7. (a) 8. (a)

9. (b) Ozone layer is present in the stratosphere in the atmosphere of the earth. It protects the earth from UV rays (less than 300 nm). Hole in the ozone layer means thining of ozone layer that allows harmful UV rays to reach earth which cause skin diseases.

10. (a) Lots of urea and phosphate fertilizer were used in the crops in the vicinity and the lake water turned green and stinky. Due to this, lake near a village suffered heavy mortality of fishes within a few days.

11. (c) If natural habitat is destroyed, wild life is affected worstly.

12. (c)

13. (d) The correct acronym is IUCN, International Union for Conservation of Nature and Natural resources.

14. (b) Photochemical smog is made by the deposition of dust & carbon particles on the pollutant gases and water vapours. The gases found in photochemical smog are NO_2, PAN, O_3 etc.

15. (a) Due to dumping of huge amount of sewage, the oxygen levels are depleted, which are reflected in terms of BOD values of water. The number of microbes also increases tremendously and these also consume most of the oxygen. Thus BOD of the river water will increase.

16. (c) Primary pollutants perist in the form they are released in the environment. Secondary pollutants are formed by reaction amongst the primary pollutants. Secondary pollutants are more toxic than primary pollutants. So, DDT is a primary pollutant.

17. (c) Bhopal gas tragedy, the world's worst industrial catastrophes was not due to radioactive fallout, but it was because of leakage of phosgene and methyl isocyanate gas.

18. (b) Lichens are indicators of air polution, especially of the concentration of sulphur dioxide in the atmosphere. Air pollutants dissovled in rain water, mainly sulphur dioxide can damage lichens and prevent them from growing. So, lichens are natural indicators of air pollution.

19. (b) Noise pollution causes anxiety, stress and irritability. Adernaline hormone is released when body is under stress. So noise pollution leads to secretion of adernaline hormone, which provides added energy to the body to deal the stressful situation.

20. (b)

21. (a) In the given pie diagram, greenhouse gases are shown. 'A' is CO_2 which is produced due to deforestation and large scale combustion of fossil fules. 'B' is CH_4 which is produced by incomplete biogas combustion and is the major constituent of biogas. 'C' is water vapour.

22. (b) Ultraviolet radiations are of three types - UV - C (100) - 280 nm), UV - B (280 - 320 nm) and UB - A (320 - 390 nm). UV radiation of wavelengths shorter than UV-B, are almost completely absorbed by earth's atmosphere, given that the ozone layer is intact. But, UV-B damages DNA and mutation may occur. It causes aging of skin, damage to skin cells and various types of skin cancers.

23. (b) In Jhum cultivation crops are cultivated for 2-3 years without manuring. It results in nutrient depletion, reduced moisture retention of soil and increased soil erosion.

24. (b) 25. (c) 26. (d) 27. (b)

28. (c) Yellowing and blackening of Taj Mahal at Agra is due to SO_2 and other pollutants released by Mathura refinery.

29. (b) 30. (b) 31. (c) 32. (a) 33. (d) 34. (a)

35. (a) The 'Jhum cultivation' is also known as 'Slash and burn agriculture'.

36. (c)

37. (a) Unlike domestic sewage, waste water from industries like petroleum, paper manufacturing, metal extraction and processing, chemical manufacturing, etc. often contain toxic substances, notably heavy metals (defined as elements with density > $5 g/cm^3$); such as mercury, cadmium, copper, lead etc.) and a variety of organic compounds.

38. (b) DDT causes egg shell thinning in birds because it inhibits calcium ATPase.

39. (b) Friends of the Arcata Marsh (FOAM) is a non-profit organization which for the last twenty years has advanced knowledge and educated the public about treatment and reuse of wastewater. The purpose of the FOAM is to stimulate understanding of the Arcata Marsh and Wildlife Sanctuary, its relationship with Arcata's integrated wastewater treatment system, the surrounding watersheds and bay, and their link with the earth's water cycle.

40. (d) The green house effect is a naturally occuring phenomenon that is responsible for heating of Earth's surface and atmosphere. Without a green house effect, the average temperature at earth's surface would have been around –18°C, rather than the present average of +15°C.

41. (a) The presence of a large amount of nutrients in water causes excessive growth of planktons or free-floating algae to produce algal bloom. Such algal blooms deteriorate the quality of water, cause the mortality of fishes and impart distinct colour to water bodies.

42. (b) A : Catalytic converter is a device incorporated in the exhaust system of a motor vehicle, containing a catalyst for converting pollutant gases into less harmful ones. As the exhaust passes through the converter, unburnt hydrocarbons are converted into carbon dioxide, water, carbon monoxide and nitric oxide are changed to carbon dioxide and nitrogen gas respectively.
B : Electrostatic precipitator is a device that removes suspended dust particles from a gas or exhaust by applying a high-voltage electrostatic charge and collect the particles on charged plates.
C : Earmuffs is a pair of soft fabric coverings, connected by a band across the top of the head, that are worn over the ears to protect them from cold or high noise level.
D : Land - fill is a site for the disposal of solid waste in which refuse is buried between layers of dirt so as to fill in or reclaim low-lying ground.

43. (a) Electrostatic precipitator is a device that removes suspended dust particles from a gas or exhaust by applying a high-voltage electrostatic charge and collecting the particles on charged plates. In the given diagram of electrostatic precipitator, the parts marked as A, B and C are respectively discharge corona, negatively charged ions, and collection plate grounded.

44. (d)

45. (a) An algal bloom is a rapid increase in the population of phytoplankton algae in an aquatic system. Typically only one or a few species are involved and the bloom is recognized by discoloration of the water resulting from the high density of pigmented cells.

HINTS & SOLUTIONS (PHYSICS – Subject-wise Test)

Speed Test-97

1. (a) $[A]=[E][x^3]; [B]=\dfrac{[E]}{[y]}; [C]=\dfrac{[E]}{[z^2]}$

2. (c) For *a–t* curve, area under the graph gives change in velocity at $t = 10$ sec, $v = 40$ m/s.

For 10 – 30 sec, $\Delta v = -80$, $v_{30sec} - 40 = -80$.

Speed at 30 sec = – 40 m/s

3. (d) $W = W_1 - W_2 = mgh - mgh' = mg\,(h - h')$

$= 5 \times 10\ (20 - 0.2) = 5 \times 10 \times 19.8$

$= 5 \times 198 = 990$ joule

This energy is converted into heat when the ball strikes the earth. Heat produced is

$$Q = \frac{990}{4.2}\ \text{calorie}$$

$$\Delta T = \frac{Q}{mc} = \frac{99 \times 100}{42 \times 5000 \times 0.09} = \frac{11}{32}\ {}^\circ C$$

4. (c) $T_1 = 77^\circ C = 350\,K$

$V_1 = V$ and $V_2 = \dfrac{125V}{343}$

Ratio of specific heats for monoatomic gas, $\gamma = \dfrac{5}{3}$

In an adiabatic process,

$T_1 V_1^{\gamma-1} = T_2 V_2^{\gamma-1}$

or $T_2 = \left(\dfrac{V_1}{V_2}\right)^{\gamma-1} \times T$,

$$T_2 = 350 \times \left(\frac{1}{125/343}\right)^{(5/3)-1}$$

$= 686\,K$

Hence, rise in temperature

$= T_2 - T_1 = 686 - 350 = 336\,K$

5. (b)

6. (d) For nuclear disintegration

$$\lambda = \frac{2.303}{t} \log \frac{N_o}{N_o - N}$$

$$= \frac{2.303}{24 \times 60 \times 60} \log \frac{100}{82} = 2.1 \times 10^{-6} \text{sec}^{-1}$$

7. (a) The mean value of refractive index,

$$\mu = \frac{1.34 + 1.38 + 1.32 + 1.36}{4} = 1.35$$

and

$$\Delta\mu = \frac{|(1.35-1.34)| + |(1.35-1.38)| + |(1.35-1.32)| + |(1.35-1.36)|}{4}$$

$= 0.02$

Thus $\dfrac{\Delta\mu}{\mu} \times 100 = \dfrac{0.02}{1.35} \times 100 = 1.48$

8. (a) The magnetic dipole moment of diamagnetic material is zero as each of its pair of electrons have opposite spins, i.e., $\mu_d = 0$.

Paramagnetic substances have dipole moment > 0, i.e. $\mu_p \neq 0$, because of excess of electrons in its molecules spinning in the same direction.

Ferro-magnetic substances are very strong magnets and they also have permanent magnetic moment, i.e. $\mu_f \neq 0$.

9. (a) Distance covered in one circular loop $= 2\pi r$

$= 2 \times 3.14 \times 100 = 628$ m

Speed $= \dfrac{628}{62.8} = 10$ m/sec

Displacement in one circular loop = 0

Velocity $= \dfrac{0}{\text{time}} = 0$

10. (a) Let velocity at $A = v_A$ and velocity at $B = v_B$

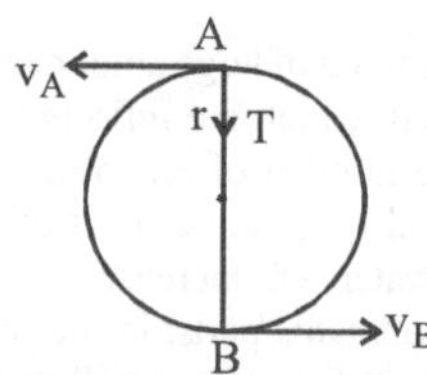

Applying conservation of energy at A & B

$$\frac{1}{2} m v_A^2 + 2gmr = \frac{1}{2} m v_B^2$$

$v_B^2 = v_A^2 + 4gr$.........(i)

Now as it is moving in circular path it has centripetal force.

At point $A \Rightarrow T + mg = \dfrac{mv_A^2}{r}$

for minimum velocity $T \geq 0$

or $\dfrac{mv_A^2}{r} \geq mg \Rightarrow v_A^2 \geq gr \Rightarrow v_A \geq \sqrt{gr}$

11. (c) Power $= V \cdot I = I^2 R$

$$i_2 = \sqrt{\frac{\text{Power}}{R}} = \sqrt{\frac{2}{8}} = \sqrt{\frac{1}{4}} = \frac{1}{2}\ \text{A}$$

Potential over $8\Omega = Ri_2 = 8 \times \dfrac{1}{2} = 4V$

This is the potential over parallel branch. So,

$i_1 = \dfrac{4}{4} = 1\,A$

Power of $3\Omega = i_1^2 R = 1 \times 1 \times 3 = 3W$

12. (c) For n^{th} orbit, energy, $E_n = \frac{2\pi^2 em^4 z^2}{n^2 h^2}$

$$\frac{E_5}{E_7} = \frac{7^2}{5^5}$$

$$\Rightarrow \frac{25}{49} E = E_7$$

13. (c) Conserving Linear Momentum

$2Mv_c = 5Mv - 2Mv \Rightarrow v_c = 3v/2.$

14. (c) $\frac{R_s}{R_\alpha} = \left(\frac{A_s}{A_\alpha}\right)^{1/3} = \left(\frac{32}{4}\right)^{1/3} = 2$

15. (d) $\frac{dH}{dt} \propto (\theta_2 - \theta_1) = (\Delta\theta)^n \Rightarrow n = 1$

16. (d) Use $a = \mu g$ and $v^2 = u^2 + 2as$

17. (c) When the arrangement is dipped in water;

$$\beta' = \beta/\mu = \frac{x}{4/3} = \frac{3}{4} x = 0.75x$$

18. (d) The charge q, which is kept at the centre of metallic spherical shell transfered to the outer surface of shell & inside the shell the electric field is zero & hence force is also zero.

19. (c) $F_n = q(\vec{v} \times \vec{B})$

$= qvB \sin\theta = 0$ (because $\theta = 0°$)

20. (b) The time of cooling increases as the difference between the temperature of body & surrounding is reduced. So $T_1 < T_2 < T_3$ (according to Newton's law of cooling).

21. (a) In uniform circular motion speed is constant. So, no tangential acceleration.

It has only radial acceleration

$a_R = \frac{v^2}{R}$ [directed towards center]

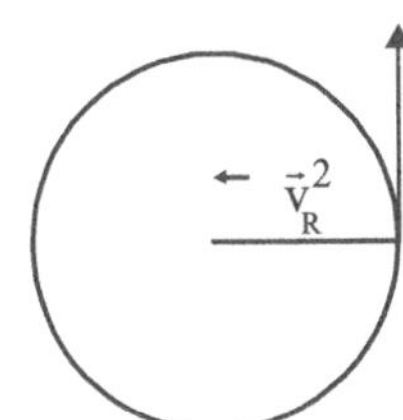

and its velocity is always in tangential direction. So these two are perpendicular to each other.

22. (a) $e = \frac{LdI}{dt} = \frac{40 \times 10^{-3}(11-1)}{4 \times 10^{-3}} = 100V$

23. (c) $C_s = \frac{C_1 C_2}{C_1 + C_2} = 3$

$C_p = C_1 + C_2 = 16 \therefore C_1 C_2 = 48$

$$C_1 - C_2 = \sqrt{(C_1 + C_2)^2 - 4C_1 C_2}$$

$$= \sqrt{16^2 - 4 \times 48} = \sqrt{64} = 8$$

$\therefore C_1 = 12\mu F$ and $C_2 = 4\mu F$

24. (d) At the centre of the earth gravity is zero.

25. (b) Frequency does not depend upon the medium, so, it will remain same in the material of the tuning fork and in air.

26. (a) The highest energy level occupied by an electron in the energy band at zero kelvin is called Fermi level and the energy associated is known as Fermi energy. So, it is independent of T.

27. (b) The intersection of medians is the centre of mass of the triangle. Since distances of centre of mass from the sides are related as : $x_{BC} < x_{AB} < x_{AC}$ therefore $I_{BC} > I_{AB} > I_{AC}$ or $I_{BC} > I_{AB}$.

28. (c) If $\vec{F}$ force acts for short interval Δt, then

$\vec{F}\,\Delta T = m\Delta\vec{v}$.

29. (b) For electromagnetic wave,

$F_E = F_M \Rightarrow eE = BeC \Rightarrow E = B.C$

$= 2 \times 10^{-7} \times 3 \times 10^8 = 60\ V/m$

30. (a) According to Biot Savart's law

$$dB = \frac{\mu_0}{4\pi} \cdot \frac{Id\ell \sin\theta}{r^2}$$

$$dB \propto \frac{1}{r^2}$$

So, graph (a) is correct.

31. (b) According to Stefan' law heat emitted per second per unit area $\alpha(T_1^4 - T_2^4)$ where T_1 is the temperature of body & T_2 is the temperature of surrounding (T_1 & T_2 are on Kelvin scale).

32. (a) $\frac{1}{f_\omega} = \left({}^{\omega}\mu_g - 1\right)\left(\frac{1}{r_1} - \frac{1}{r_2}\right)$

[f_ω is focal length of lens in water]

$\frac{1}{f} = ({}^{a}\mu_g - 1)\left(\frac{1}{r_1} - \frac{1}{r_2}\right)$ [f is focal length of lens in air]

Dividing,

$$\frac{f}{f_\omega} = \frac{({}^{\omega}\mu_g - 1)}{({}^{a}\mu_g - 1)}; {}^{\omega}\mu_g = \frac{{}^{a}\mu_g}{{}^{a}\mu_w} = \frac{3/2}{4/3} = \frac{3}{2} \times \frac{3}{4} = \frac{9}{8}$$

$$\frac{f}{f_w} = \frac{9/8 - 1}{\frac{3}{2} - 1} = \frac{1/8}{1/2} = \frac{1}{4}$$

$f_w = 4 \times f = 4 \times 10 = 40$ cm.

33. (b) If current passes through a spring, it shrinks as in two adjacent wire, current is flowing in the same direction. Even if direction of current is reversed still the spring will shrink. As AC current is a periodically changing current, the process of shrinking will also be periodic in nature.

34. (a)

35. (c) $Y = \frac{F/A}{\Delta\ell/\ell} = \frac{\frac{250\times10}{50\times10^{-6}}}{\frac{0.5\times10^{-3}}{2}} = \frac{250\times9.8}{50\times10^{-6}}\times\frac{2}{0.5\times10^{-3}}$

$\Rightarrow 19.6\times10^{10}\,N/m^2$

36. (c) Max. force = mass × max. acceleration
$= m\,4\pi^2 v^2 a = 1\times4\times\pi^2\times(60)^2\times0.02 = 288\,\pi^2$

37. (b) Changing electric field gives rise to displacement current which creates magnetic field around it.

38. (d)

39. (c)

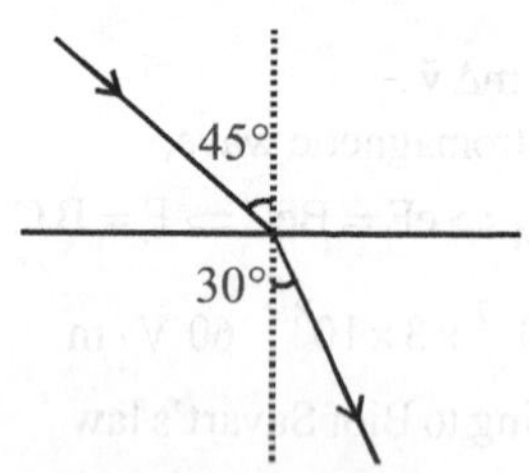

Refractive index, $\mu = \frac{\sin 45^\circ}{\sin 30^\circ}$

$\mu = \frac{1}{\sqrt{2}}\times2 = \sqrt{2}$

Now, $\mu = \frac{\text{Velocity of light in air}}{\text{Velocity of light in medium}} = \sqrt{2}$

Velocity of light in medium

$= 3\times10^8\times\frac{1}{\sqrt{2}} = 2.12\times10^8\,m/sec$

40. (c) Rain drops are in spherical shape due to surface tension.

41. (d) $\delta_1 = 40^\circ, \delta_2 = 30^\circ, \delta = ?$

$\cot\delta = \sqrt{\cot^2\delta_1 + \cot^2\delta_2} = \sqrt{\cot^2 40^\circ + \cot^2 30^\circ}$

$\cot\delta = \sqrt{1.19^2 + 3} = 2.1$

$\therefore\ \delta = 25^\circ$ i.e. $\delta < 40^\circ$.

42. (a) $\mu = \frac{1}{\sin C} = \frac{1}{\sin 30^\circ} = \frac{1}{1/2} = 2$

Velocity of light in the medium

$= \frac{3\times10^8}{2} = 1.5\times10^8\,m/sec$

43. (a)

44. (d) $P_T = P_C\left(1+\frac{m_a{}^2}{2}\right)$

$\therefore\ 600 = 400\left(1+\frac{m_a{}^2}{2}\right) \Rightarrow \frac{3}{2} = 1+\frac{m_a{}^2}{2}$

or $\frac{m_a{}^2}{2} = \frac{1}{2} \Rightarrow m_a = 1$

45. (a)

HINTS & SOLUTIONS (CHEMISTRY – Subject-wise Test)

Speed Test-98

1. (a) Given

$$A \xrightarrow{Cl_2} B \xrightarrow{alc./KOH} \underset{\text{Hydrocarbon}}{C} \xrightarrow{O_3/H_2O} CH_2O$$

Since hydrocarbon C give only CH_2O, on ozonolysis, C should be $CH_2 = CH_2$ hence on going backward, A should be ethane. Thus the reactions are

$$\underset{(A)}{CH_3CH_3} \xrightarrow{Cl_2/hv} \underset{(B)}{CH_3CH_2Cl} \xrightarrow{alc. KOH}$$

$$\underset{(C)}{CH_2{=}CH_2} \xrightarrow[\Delta]{O_3/H_2O} HCHO$$

2. (c) The cyclic portion contains more C-atoms than acyclic portion. Hence it is derivative of cyclopentane.

3. (d) In $\left[Ni(NH_3)_2 Cl_2\right]$, Ni^{2+} is in sp^3 hybridisation, thus tetrahedral in shape. Hence the four ligands are not different to exhibit optical isomerism.

4. (a) Addition of HCN to carbonyl compounds is nucleophilic addition reaction. The order of reactivity of carbonyl compounds is :

$$HCHO > CH_3COCH_3 > PhCOCH_3 > PhCOPh$$

The lower reactivity of Ketones is due to the presence of two alkyl group which shows + I effect. The reactivity of Ketones decreases as the size of alkyl group increases.

5. (c) $\underset{1-x}{PCl_5(g)} \rightleftharpoons \underset{x}{PCl_3(g)} + \underset{x}{Cl_2(g)}$

Total moles after dissociation

$1-x+x+x=1+x$

p_{PCl_3} = mole fraction of PCl_3 ×

Total pressure $= \left(\dfrac{x}{1+x}\right)P$

6. (c) $(H_3C)(H_3C)C=CH-CH_2-CH_3$

Due to the presence of two similar methyl group at same carbon atom, above compound doesn't show geometrical isomerism.

7. (c) Liquid - liquid system is known as emulsion.

8. (d) $P=P_AX_A+P_BX_B$

$= P_AX_A+P_B(1-X_A)$

$\Rightarrow P_AX_A+P_B-P_BX_A$

$\Rightarrow P_B+X_A(P_A-P_B)$

9. (c) For $SbCl_5^{2-}$, $H = \dfrac{5+5+2}{2} = 6$ means sp^3d^2 hybridization I_3^-, SF_4, and PCl_5; all have sp^3d hybridization.

10. (d) Hemiacetal → presence of alcohol and ether on same carbon.

11. (b) During disproportionation same compound undergo simultaneous oxidation and reduction.

Oxidation

$$3H\overset{-}{O}\overset{+}{Cl} \longrightarrow 2H\overset{-1}{Cl} + H\overset{+5}{Cl}O_3$$

reduction

12. (c)

13. (d) Chloramphenicol is

$$O_2N-C_6H_4-\underset{OH}{CH}-\underset{CH_2OH}{CH}-NH-\overset{O}{\overset{\|}{C}}-CHCl_2$$

14. (b) Number of A ions in the unit cell. $= \dfrac{1}{8} \times 8 = 1$

Number of B ions in the unit cell $= \dfrac{1}{2} \times 6 = 3$

Hence empirical formula of the compound $= AB_3$

15. (c) Since rate of reaction becomes four times on doubling concentration of reactant, it is second order reaction.

16. (a)

17. (d) $K_2Cr_2O_7 + \text{conc.}HCl \rightarrow Cl_2\uparrow$

18. (d) Pressure exerted by the gas, $P = \dfrac{1}{3}\dfrac{mnu^2}{V}$ ...(i)

Here, u = root mean square velocity

m = mass of a molecule, n = No. of molecules of the gas

Hence (a) & (b) are clearly wrong.

Again $u^2 = \dfrac{3RT}{M}$ [explained from (i)]

Here, M = Molecular wt. of the gas;

Hence (c) is wrong

Further, Average K.E. $= \dfrac{3}{2}$ KT; Hence (d) is true.

19. (b) The main reason for exhibiting larger number of oxidation states by actinoids as compared to lanthanoids is lesser energy difference between $5f$ and $6d$ orbitals as compared to that between $4f$ and $5d$ orbitals.

In case of actinoids we can remove electrons from $5f$ as well as from $6d$ and due to this actinoids exhibit larger number of oxidation state than lanthanoids.

20. (b and c) From the various given option we find option (a) correct. The oxidising power of halogen follow the order $F_2 > Cl_2 > Br_2 > I_2$. Option (b) incorrect because it in not the correct order of electron gain enthalpy of halogens.

The correct order is $Cl_2 > F_2 > Br_2 > I_2$. The low value of F_2 than Cl_2 is due to its small size.
Option (c) incorrect. The correct order of bond dissociation energies of halogens is $Cl_2 > Br_2 > F_2 > I_2$.
Option (d) correct. It is the correct order of electronegativity values of halogens. Thus option (b) and (c) are incorrect.

21. **(d)** $Al_2O_3.2H_2O \rightarrow Al_2O_3 + 2H_2O$ is calcination.

22. **(c)** According to Arrhenius equation, the rate constant of reaction is given by,

$$k = Ae^{-Ea/RT}$$

where A is pre-exponential factor, E_a is activation energy and T is absolute temperature.

when $T \rightarrow \infty$, $\frac{E_a}{RT} \rightarrow 0$

then $k = Ae^0$

or $k = A$

23. **(a)** Co^{3+} : [⇅|↑|↑|↑|↑] 3d-orbital

$[Co(CN)_6]^{3-}$: [⇅|⇅|⇅| |] 3d-orbital

CN^- is a strong field ligand and it causes pairing of electrons, as a result number of unpaired electrons in Co^{3+} becomes zero and hence it has lowest value of paramagnetic behaviour.

24. **(a)** Given, for reaction

(i) $H_2O(l) \longrightarrow H^+(aq.) + OH^-(aq.)$; $\Delta H_r = 57.32$ kJ

(ii) $H_2(g) + \frac{1}{2}O_2(g) \longrightarrow H_2O(l)$; $\Delta H_r = -286.20$ kJ

For reaction (i)

$$\Delta H_r = \Delta H°_f(H^+aq) + \Delta H°_f(OH^-aq) - \Delta H°_f(H_2O, l)$$

$$57.32 = 0 + \Delta H°_f(OH^-, aq) - \Delta H°_f(H_2O, l) \quad ...(iii)$$

For reaction (ii)

$$\Delta H_r = \Delta H°_f(H_2O, l) - \Delta H°_f(H_2, g) - \frac{1}{2}\Delta H°_f(O_2, g)$$

$$-286.20 = \Delta H°_f(H_2O, l)$$

On replacing this value in equ. (iii) we have

$$57.32 = \Delta H°_f(OH^-, aq) - (-286.20)$$

$$\Delta H°_f = -286.20 + 57.32 = -228.88 \text{ kJ}$$

25. **(c)** Applying VSEPR theory, both NF_3 and H_2O are sp^3 hybridized.

26. **(a)** $C_6H_5Cl + (CH_3)_2NLi \xrightarrow{(CH_3)_2NH} C_6H_5N(CH_3)_2 + LiCl$

27. **(b)** Tertiary alcohols react fastest with conc. HCl and anhydrous $ZnCl_2$ (lucas reagent) as its mechanism proceeds through the formation of stable tertiary carbocation.

Mechanism

Step 1: $CH_3-C(CH_3)_2-OH + H-Cl \rightleftharpoons (CH_3)_3C-\overset{+}{O}H_2 + Cl^-$

2-Methylpropan-2-ol

Step 2: $(CH_3)_3C-\overset{+}{O}H_2 \rightleftharpoons (CH_3)_3C^+ + H_2O$

3° Carbocation

Step 3: $(CH_3)_3C^+ + Cl^- \rightleftharpoons (CH_3)_3C-Cl$

t-Butyl chloride

28. **(a)**

$$2KMnO_4 + 3H_2SO_4 \longrightarrow K_2SO_4 + 2MnSO_4 + 3H_2O + 5(O)] \times 3$$

$$2\,(COO)_2Fe + 3(O) \longrightarrow Fe_2O_3 + 2CO_2 \quad] \times 5$$

$$6KMnO_4 + 9H_2SO_4 + 10\,(COO)_2Fe \longrightarrow 3K_2SO_4 + 6MnSO_4 + 9H_2O + 5Fe_2O_3 + 10CO_2$$

(6 moles) (10 moles)

From above equation 6 moles MnO_4^- required to oxidise 10 moles of oxalate.
Thus number of moles of MnO_4^- required to oxidise one mole of oxalate $= \frac{6}{10} = 0.6$ moles

29. **(d)**

30. **(b)** C_6H_5–CH_2–$CH(OH)$–$CH(CH_3)_2$ $\xrightarrow{H^+}$ carbocation $\xrightarrow{\text{rearranges}}$ carbocation

Benzyl carbocation is more stable

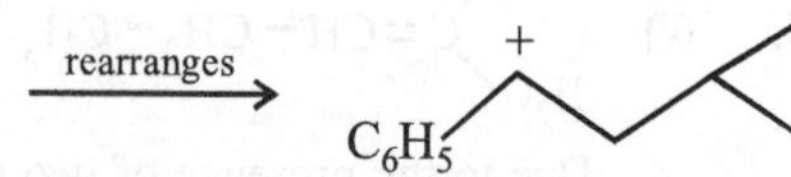

trans–(more stable due to steric relief)   *cis*– (less stable due to bulky gps. lying on same side)

31. **(a)** Eq. wt. of $H_2O_2 = 17$

$$N = \frac{30.36}{17} = 1.78 \text{ N}$$

Volume strength $= 5.6 \times$ normality $= 5.6 \times 1.78 = 10$ V

32. **(d)** The metal placed below in electrochemical series does not react with that metal salt solution whose metal is placed above in electrochemical series.

33. **(b)**

34. **(b)** More will be the electronegativity of X, lesser will be the bond length of X-O bond.

35. **(a)** $C_6H_5CH_2Cl \xrightarrow{NaCN} C_6H_5CH_2CN \xrightarrow{H_2/Ni} C_6H_5CH_2CH_2NH_2$

Benzyl chloride; β–Phenylethylamine

36. **(b)** (4) $Ph-\overset{O}{\overset{\|}{C}}-NH_2$ is weak base due to resonance.

(3) One to –M effect of NO_2 and ortho effect it is weak base.

(2) Strong base because lone pair is not involved in resonance.

37. **(b)** Protonation at β–N leads to imidazolium ion, which is stabilized by two equivalent resonating structures.

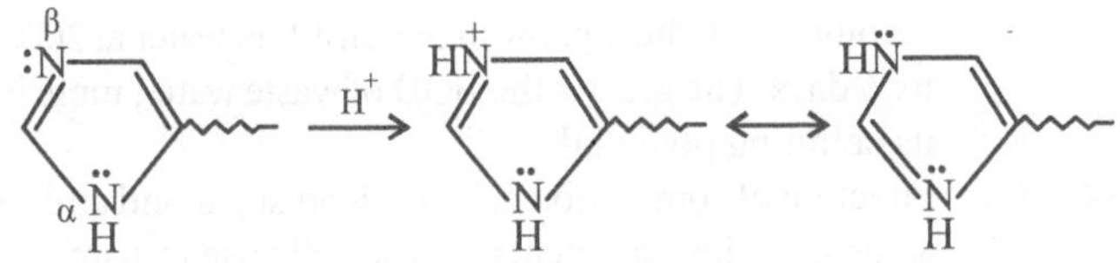

Equivalent resonating structures

38. **(d)** Boron nitride (BN) is known as inorganic graphite. The most stable form is hexagonal one. It has layered structure similar to graphite.

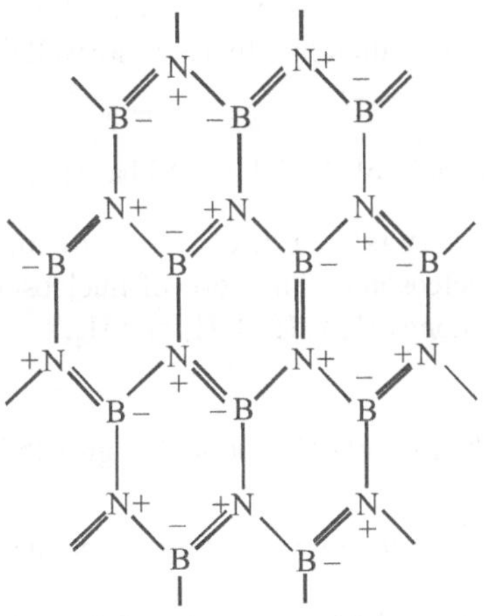

39. **(c)** The correct order of acidic strength of the given species in

$$\underset{(iv)}{HSO_3F} > \underset{(ii)}{H_3O^+} > \underset{(iii)}{HSO_4^-} > \underset{(i)}{HCO_3^-}$$

(i) < (iii) < (ii) < (iv)

It corresponds to choice (c) which is correct answer.

40. **(b)** Stability depends on number of hyperconjugative structures.

41. **(d)** $A \xrightarrow[(I)]{NH_3} B \xrightarrow[II]{\Delta} C \xrightarrow[KOH,(III)]{Br_2} CH_3CH_2NH_2$

Reaction (III) is a Hofmann bromamide reaction. Now formation of $CH_3CH_2NH_2$ is possible only from a compound $CH_3CH_2CONH_2$(C) which can be obtained from the compound $CH_3CH_2COO^-NH_4^+$(B).

Thus (A) should be CH_3CH_2COOH

$$\underset{(A)}{CH_3CH_2-\overset{O}{\overset{\|}{C}}-OH} \xrightarrow{NH_3} \underset{(B)}{CH_3CH_2COO^-NH_4^+} \xrightarrow{\Delta} \underset{(C)}{CH_3CH_2CONH_2} \xrightarrow{KOH/Br_2} CH_3CH_2NH_2$$

42. **(c)**

43. **(a)** As the nuclear charge increases, the force of attraction between the nucleus and the incoming electron increases and hence the elecron gain enthalpy becomes more negative, hence the correct order is Ca < Al < C < O < F

44. **(a)** Addition of monomers follows isoprene rule

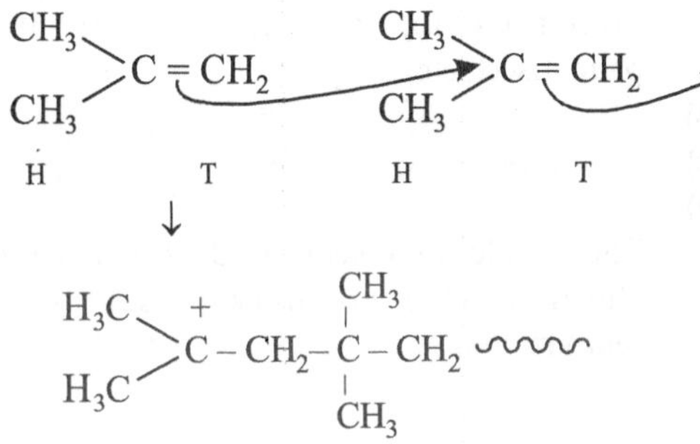

$(CH_3)_2C{=}CH_2$ (H T) + $(CH_3)_2C{=}CH_2$ (H T) →

$(H_3C)_2\overset{+}{C}-CH_2-C(CH_3)_2-CH_2$ ~~~

45. **(d)** Rate $\propto \sqrt{\dfrac{1}{M}}$. The smaller the value of M the more is the rate of diffusion.

HINTS & SOLUTIONS (BIOLOGY – Subject-wise Test)

Speed Test-99

1. (a)
2. (b) Modern day classification is new systematics or biosystematics which includes all the characteristics of organisms gathered from the study of different sections like physiology, ecology, anatomy, biochemistry, cytology.
3. (b)
4. (a)
5. (b)
6. (a)
7. (b)
8. (d)
9. (b)
10. (d) The members of division basidiomycota (class basidiomycetes) are commonly called club fungi because the basidia are club shaped.
11. (c)
12. (d)
13. (c)
14. (b) A leaf having a single or undivided lamina is called simple leaf. The lamina can have different types of incisions, which may reach upto half (-fid), more than half (-partite) or near the base or midrib (-sect). Depending upon the pinnate or palmate venation, the incisions are known as pinnatifid palmatifid, pinnatipartite, palmatipartite, pinnatisect and palmatisect, etc.
15. (b)
16. (b)
17. (a)
18. (d) The complex of protein and DNA is called chromatin. Chromosomes are only present during cell reproduction.
19. (a)
20. (a) $C_6H_{12}O_6 + 6O_2 \longrightarrow 6CO_2 + 6H_2O$

$$R.Q. = \frac{\text{Vol. of } CO_2 \text{ evolved}}{\text{Vol. of } O_2 \text{ absorbed}} = \frac{6}{6} = 1$$

21. (a)
22. (b)
23. (d)
24. (c)
25. (c)
26. (d)
27. (c)
28. (a) The genetically modified brinjal in India has been developed for insect resistance. *Bt* brinjal is a transgenic brinjal that is developed by inserting a crystal gene from the *Bacillus thuringiensis* into the brinjal's genome. This process of insertion is accomplished using *Agrobacterium* mediated recombination.
29. (a)
30. (c) It would make only two types of gametes, these are ABC & AbC.
31. (a) The main precursors of acid rain are SO_2 and NO_2 in atmosphere which form H_2SO_4 (Sulphuric acid) and HNO_3 (nitric acid) with H_2O and these come down with rain. Such rains are called acid rains.
32. (d) Hot spots are those areas which were rich in biodiversity but now under threat due to direct or indirect interference of human activites. These regions are on the edge to get some of their species extinct due to humans. Western Ghats in India are under threat due to continuous developmental activities and Doon valley is under threat due to continuous mining activities.
33. (a) BOD is a measure of organic matter present in water. It refers to amount of O_2 consumed by microbes to decompose all the organic matter in 1 L of water at 20°C for 5 days. The greater the BOD of waste water, more is its polluting potential.
34. (d) Function of companion cell is to load sugar and amino acids into sieve elements. These cells use transmembrane proteins to take up by active transport.
35. (d) They are found in the equatorial regions rainfall exceeds 140 cm. The warm humid climate supports broad leaved evergreen plants. Productivity is very high (12000 k. cal/m^2/ year). The vegetation show stratification into two or more well defined layers.
36. (b)
37. (a) A chain of DNA has 140 base pairs, make $1\frac{3}{4}$ turns and twist around a histone octamer forming nucleosome. The core of nucleosome consists of 4 histones H_2A, H_2B, H_3 and H_4.
38. (b)
39. (c) The formula of exponential growth is $\frac{dN}{dt} = rN$ where $\frac{dN}{dt}$ is the rate of change in population size, r is the biotic potential and N is the population size.
40. (b)
41. (d) '*Himgiri*' developed by hybridisation and selection for disease resistance against rust pathogens is a variety of wheat. It is resistant to leaf/stripe rust and hill bunt.
42. (a)
43. (a)
44. (b)
45. (b) In case of vegetatively propagated crops, pure line selection is not required. Pure-line selection is useful only for sexually reproducing plants. Hybrid vigour is most profitably used in vegetatively propagated crops because they do not involve sexual reproduction and hence loss of hybrid superiority.

46. (d) Biological classification is the scientific arrangement of organisms in a hierarchial series of groups and subgroups on the basis of similarities and differences in their traits. It helps in building evolutionary pathways and in identifying new organisms.
47. (a) Tiger and *tigris* both are from same genus with particular taxonomic category.
48. (b) Glucagon is secreted by α (alpha) cells of islets of langerhans.
49. (a)
50. (d)
51. (c)
52. (a)
53. (b) Acrosome is a small pointed structure at the tip of nucleus. It breaks down just before fertilization, releasing hydrolytic enzymes that assist penetration between follicle cells that surrounds the ovum, thus facilitating fertilization.
54. (b) Sponges belong to Porifera and they have characteristic canal system.
55. (b)
56. (d)
57. (d)
58. (a) Glenoid cavity is a shallow concavity on the lateral side of pectoral girdle in which the head of humerus fits making the shoulder joint.
59. (c) *Clostridium butylicum* industrially produces butyric acid.
60. (b)
61. (b) Morphine is potent opioid analgesic that is often given to persons (who have undergone surgery) as a pain killer. It is mainly used to relieve severe and persistent pain. It is administrated by mouth, injection or suppositories.
62. (c)
63. (a) Common cold, AIDS is a pair of viral diseases. Viruses are a very common type of infectious disease. Viruses are the smallest life-form existing, since they are not even a single cell. It is almost like they are not alive at all. They are small strands of DNA-like cell material. A virus consists mostly of RNA and cannot survive without host cells.
64. (c)
65. (d) We are told that the allele frequency for D = 0.8; therefore, the frequency of d = 0.2. These values are the p and q that we need to calculate the genotype frequencies in the next generation. Using the **Hardy-Weinberg** equation, p^2 (DD) = 0.64, 2pq (Dd) = 0.32, and q^2 (dd) = 0.04.
66. (d)
67. (a) Aschelminthes is bilaterally symmetrical and triploblastic. These are mostly aquatic, free living or parasitic. Their body is three layered which is ectoderm, mesoderm and endoderm.
68. (c) This disease is due to an X-linked recessive mutation. Males suffer this disorder since they have only one X chromosome and hence express any trait on this chromosome.
69. (d)
70. (c)
71. (b)
72. (d)
73. (b)
74. (a)
75. (c) The pathway of inhaled air is - Nostrils - pharynx (common passage for food & air) - larynx (voice box) - trachea (the wind pipe) - bronchi (2 for each side lungs) - bronchioles (give arise to alveolar ducts) - alveoli (the exchange site for gases in the form of small sacs or pouches).
76. (b)
77. (b)
78. (a)
79. (d) A combination of a nitrogen base with a pentose sugar is known as **nucleoside**. The nitrogen base combines with the sugar molecule at its carbon atom 1′ in a glycosidic bond (C – N – C) by one of its nitrogen atoms (usually 1 in pyrimidines and 9 in purines). Depending upon the type of pentose sugar, nucleosides are differentiated into **ribonucleosides** and **deoxyribonucleosides**.
80. (d)
81. (c) In a standard ECG, the P-wave is a small upward wave that indicates the depolarisation of the atria. This is caused by the activation of SA node.
82. (a)
83. (a)
84. (a) Gamete intrafallopian transfer (GIFT) is recommended for those females who cannot produce an ovum. In this process, the eggs of the donor woman are removed and in a form of mixture with sperm transferred into fallopian tube of another woman who cannot produce ovum, but can provide suitable environment for fertilization. Thus in GIFT, site of fertilization is fallopian tube, not laboratory.
85. (d)
86. (c)
87. (d)
88. (c) The point of attachment between homologous chromosomes after the partial dissolution of nucleoprotein complex are called chiasmata. It occurs during diplotene substage of prophase I.
89. (d) The fact that DNA is structured the same way in all known organisms means that similar methods can be used to study the hereditary material.
90. (a)

HINTS & SOLUTIONS (FULL TESTS)

Speed Test-100

PHYSICS

1. **(d)** Speed, $u = 60 \times \frac{5}{18}$ m/s $= \frac{50}{3}$ m/s

$d = 20\text{m},\ u' = 120 \times \frac{5}{18} = \frac{100}{3}$ m/s

Let declaration be a then $(0)^2 - u^2 = -2ad$

or $u^2 = 2ad$ ...(i)

and $(0)^2 - u'^2 = -2ad'$

or $u'^2 = 2ad'$ ...(ii)

(ii) divided by (i) gives,

$4 = \frac{d'}{d} \Rightarrow d' = 4 \times 20 = 80\text{m}$

2. **(d)** For angular momentum, the dimensional formula is $[ML^2T^{-1}]$. For other three, it is $[ML^{-1}T^{-2}]$.

3. **(a)**

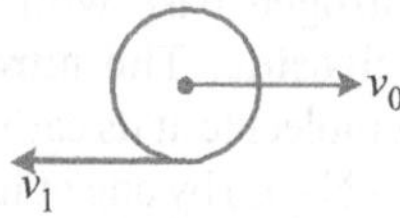

With respect to ground it has only rotation, so

$$v_1 = \omega r$$

Now using conservation of angular momentum about a fixed point at the level of bottom of the sphere,

$$mv_0 r = I\omega$$

$$= \frac{2}{5}mr^2 \times \frac{v_1}{r}$$

$$\therefore \quad v_0 = \frac{2}{5}v_1.$$

4. **(d)** c = a + b.

$$V_A = \frac{\sigma a}{\varepsilon_0} - \frac{\sigma b}{\varepsilon_0} + \frac{\sigma c}{\varepsilon_0} = \frac{\sigma}{\varepsilon_0}[c - (b - a)]$$

$$V_B = \frac{-\sigma b}{\varepsilon_0} + \frac{1}{4\pi\varepsilon_0} \cdot \frac{\sigma \times 4\pi a^2}{b} + \frac{\sigma c}{\varepsilon_0}$$

$$= \frac{\sigma}{\varepsilon_0}\left[c - \frac{(b^2 - a^2)}{b}\right]$$

$$V_C = \frac{\sigma c}{\varepsilon_0} - \frac{1}{4\pi\varepsilon_0} \cdot \frac{\sigma \times 4\pi b^2}{c} + \frac{1}{4\pi\varepsilon_0} \cdot \frac{\sigma \times 4\pi a^2}{c}$$

$$= \frac{\sigma}{\varepsilon_0}\left[c - \frac{(b^2 - a^2)}{c}\right] = \frac{\sigma}{\varepsilon_0}[c - (b - a)]$$

$V_C = V_A \neq V_B$

5. **(c)** Maximum force by surface when friction works

$$F = \sqrt{f^2 + R^2} = \sqrt{(\mu R)^2 + R^2} = R\sqrt{\mu^2 + 1}$$

Minimum force = R when there is no friction

Hence ranging from R to $R\sqrt{\mu^2 + 1}$

[where, R = Mg]

6. **(a)** Acceleration due to gravity at a height h above the earth's surface is

$$g_h = g\left(1 - \frac{2h}{R}\right)$$

Acceleration due to gravity at a depth d below the earth's surface is

$$g_d = g\left(1 - \frac{d}{R}\right)$$

Now, $\frac{g_h}{g_d} = \frac{\left(1 - \frac{2h}{R}\right)}{\left(1 - \frac{d}{R}\right)} = \frac{(R - 2h)}{(R - d)}$

As h = 1 km, d = 1 km

$\therefore \frac{g_h}{g_d} = \frac{R - 2}{R - 1}$

7. **(b)** $I = 1.2\ \text{kg m}^2, E_r = 1500\ \text{J}$,

$\alpha = 25\ \text{rad/sec}^2, \omega_1 = 0, t = ?$

As E_r

$$= \frac{1}{2}I\omega^2,\ \omega = \sqrt{\frac{2E_r}{I}} = \sqrt{\frac{2 \times 1500}{1.2}} = 50\ \text{rad/sec}$$

From $\omega_2 = \omega_1 + \alpha t$

$50 = 0 + 25t, \quad \therefore t = 2$ seconds

8. **(c)** Applying conservation of momentum,

$m_1 v_1 = (m_1 + m_2)v$

$$v = \frac{m_1 v_1}{(m_1 + m_2)}$$

Here, $v_1 = 36$ km/hr = 10 m/s

$m_1 = 2$ kg, $m_2 = 3$ kg

$$v = \frac{10 \times 2}{5} = 4\ \text{m/s}$$

$$\text{K.E. (initial)} = \frac{1}{2} \times 2 \times (10)^2 = 100\ \text{J}$$

$$\text{K.E. (Final)} = \frac{1}{2} \times (3 + 2) \times (4)^2 = 40\ \text{J}$$

Loss in K.E. = 100 – 40 = 60 J

9. **(d)** The total volume remains the same before and after stretching.

Therefore $A \times \ell = A' \times \ell'$

Here $\ell' = 2\ell$

$$\therefore A' = \frac{A \times \ell}{\ell'} = \frac{A \times \ell}{2\ell} = \frac{A}{2}$$

Percentage change in resistance

$$=\frac{R_f - R_i}{R_i}\times 100 = \frac{\rho\left(\frac{\ell'}{A'}-\frac{\ell}{A}\right)}{\rho\frac{\ell}{A}}\times 100$$

$$=\left[\left(\frac{\ell'}{A'}\times\frac{A}{\ell}\right)-1\right]\times 100 = \left[\left(\frac{2\ell}{A/2}\times\frac{A}{\ell}\right)-1\right]\times 100$$

$=300\%$

10. (b) When a ball is dropped on a floor,

$$y=\frac{1}{2}gt^2 \qquad \text{..... (i)}$$

So the graph between y and t is a parabola. Here as time increases, y decreases.
When the ball bounces back, then

$$y = ut+\frac{1}{2}gt^2 \qquad \text{..... (ii)}$$

The graph between y and t will be a parabola. But here as time increases, y also increases. So (b) represents the graph.

11. (a) By conservation of linear momentum, we have

$$mv - mv = (m+m+m)v_{cm}$$

or $v_{cm} = 0$

Now using conservation of angular momentum, we get

$$mv\ell = I\omega$$

$$=\left[\frac{m\ell^2}{12}+2m(\ell/2)^2\right]\omega$$

$$\therefore \quad \omega = \frac{12v}{7\ell}$$

12. (d) Given, $F=m\omega^2 r$ ...(i)

and $F+60=m(3\omega)^2 r$

$= 9(m\omega^2 r)$ ...(ii)

From above equations, we get

$F+60=9F$

or $F=7.5$ N

Initial acceleration $=\omega^2 r$

$=F/m$

$=\frac{7.5}{3}=2.5\ \text{m/s}^2$

Final acceleration $=(3\omega)^2 r$

$=9\times\omega^2 r$

$=9\times 2.5=22.5\ \text{m/s}^2$

13. (d) The velocity to escape earth's gravitational field, $v_e=\sqrt{2gR}$, it is independent of mass of rocket.

14. (b) Magnetic flux linked with the loop is $\phi=B\pi r^2$

$$|e|=\frac{d\phi}{dt}=B\pi\cdot 2r\frac{dr}{dt}$$

When $r=2$ cm, $\frac{dr}{dt}=1\ \text{mm s}^{-1}$

$e=0.025\times\pi\times 2\times 2\times 10^{-2}\times 10^{-3}$
$=0.100\times\pi\times 10^{-5}=\pi\times 10^{-6}\ \text{V}=\pi\mu\text{V}$

15. (b) Along ab, $Q=0+5=5$. $\Delta U_{ab}=0$

Along bc, $0=\Delta U_{bc}+4$, $\therefore\ \Delta U_{bc}=-4$J

In cyclic process $abca$,

$\Delta U_{ab}+\Delta U_{bc}+\Delta U_{ca}=0$

or, $0-4+\Delta U_{ca}=0$

$\therefore\ \Delta U_{ca}=+4$J

Thus, $\Delta U_{ac}=-4$ J

16. (a) In figure, (2, 3, 4) the potential difference across diode is greater than zero (V > 0) and so these are in forward bias.

17. (b) At CD solid will completely convert into liquid.

18. (b) Air medium is non-dispersive in nature.

19. (c) From Newtwon's law of cooling

$$\frac{dQ}{dt}=-KA\frac{dT}{dx}$$

Area of cross-section A and thickness dx is the same.

Also $dQ=mCd\theta$

Thus in first case

$$\frac{m\times C\times(61°-59°)}{4}=\frac{-KA}{dx}\left[\left(\frac{61°+51°}{2}\right)-30°\right] \quad \text{(i)}$$

In second case,

$$\frac{m\times C\times(51°-49°)}{t}=\frac{-KA}{dx}\left[\left(\frac{51°+49°}{2}\right)-30°\right] \quad \text{(ii)}$$

Dividing equation (i) by equation (ii)

$$\frac{t}{4}=\frac{30}{20}$$

or $t=6$ minutes.

20. (b) $\Delta I_b=+50\mu A$, $\Delta I_c=5\times 10^{-3} A$

$$\beta=\frac{\Delta I_c}{\Delta I_b}=\frac{5\times 10^{-3}}{50\times 10^{-6}}=\frac{5\times 1000}{50}=100$$

21. (c) Intensity $I=I_0.e^{-\mu d}$,

Applying logarithm on both sides,

$$-\mu d=\log\left(\frac{I}{I_0}\right)$$

$$-\mu\times 36=\log\left(\frac{I/8}{I}\right) \quad \text{.........(i)}$$

$$-\mu\times d=\log\left(\frac{I/2}{I}\right) \quad \text{..........(ii)}$$

Dividing (i) by (ii),

$$\frac{36}{d}=\frac{\log\left(\frac{1}{8}\right)}{\log\left(\frac{1}{2}\right)}=\frac{3\log\left(\frac{1}{2}\right)}{\log\left(\frac{1}{2}\right)}=3 \text{ or } d=\frac{36}{3}=12\text{ mm}$$

22. **(c)** We have, $U+K=E$
where, U = Potential energy, K = Kinetic energy, E = Total energy.
Also, we know that, in S.H.M., when potential energy is maximum, K.E. is zero and vice-versa.

$\therefore U_{max}+0=E \Rightarrow U_{max}=E$

Further,

$$K.E.=\frac{1}{2}m\omega^2a^2\cos^2\omega t$$

But by question, $K.E.=K_0\cos^2\omega t$

$$\therefore K_0=\frac{1}{2}m\omega^2a^2$$

Hence, total energy, $E=\frac{1}{2}m\omega^2a^2=K_0$

$\therefore U_{max}=K_0$ & $E=K_0$.

23. **(d)** Load supported by sonometer wire = 4 kg
Tension in sonometer wire = 4 g
If μ = mass per unit length

then frequency $\upsilon=\frac{1}{2l}\sqrt{\frac{T}{\mu}}$

$$\Rightarrow 416=\frac{1}{2l}\sqrt{\frac{4g}{\mu}}$$

When length is doubled, i.e., $l'=2l$
Let new load = L
As, $\upsilon'=\upsilon$

$$\therefore \frac{1}{2l'}\sqrt{\frac{Lg}{\mu}}=\frac{1}{2l}\sqrt{\frac{4g}{\mu}}$$

$$\Rightarrow \frac{1}{4l}\sqrt{\frac{Lg}{\mu}}=\frac{1}{2l}\sqrt{\frac{4g}{\mu}}$$

$$\Rightarrow \sqrt{L}=2\times2 \Rightarrow L=16\,kg$$

24. **(b)** $\cos\phi=\frac{R}{Z}$, where Z is the impedance &

$Z=\sqrt{R^2+(X_L-X_C)^2}$, if there is only resistance then $Z=R \Rightarrow \cos\phi=1$

25. **(c)** No current flows through 6 Ω resistor as a capacitor offers infinite resistance to a D.C.
The equivalent circuit is thus as shown below in which 2Ω and 3Ω are in parallel

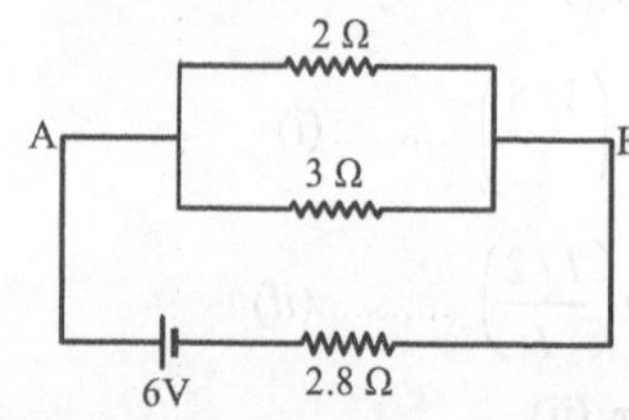

$$\therefore \frac{1}{2}+\frac{1}{3}=\frac{1}{R'} \text{ or } R'=\frac{6}{5}\Omega=1.2\Omega$$

Current drawn from the battery

$$I=\frac{E}{R}=\frac{6}{4}=1.5 \text{ Ampere } [R=1.2+2.8=4\Omega]$$

Potential difference between A and B

$$V=IR'=1.5\times1.2=1.8V$$

$\therefore$ Current through 2Ω resistor

$$=\frac{V}{2}=\frac{1.8}{2}=0.9\,A$$

26. **(a)** When tension in the cable is equal to the weight of cable, the system is in equilibrium. It means the system is at rest or moving with uniform velocity.

27. **(c)** At the two points of the trajectory during projection, the horizontal component of the velocity is the same.

$\Rightarrow$ u cos 60° = v cos 45°

$$\Rightarrow 147\times\frac{1}{2}=v\times\frac{1}{\sqrt{2}} \Rightarrow \frac{147}{\sqrt{2}}\,m/s$$

Vertical component of u = u sin 60°

$$=\frac{147\sqrt{3}}{2}\,m$$

Vertical component of v = v sin 45°

$$=\frac{147}{\sqrt{2}}\times\frac{1}{\sqrt{2}}=\frac{147}{2}\,m$$

but $v_y=u_y+a_yt \Rightarrow \frac{147}{2}=\frac{147\sqrt{3}}{2}-9.8t$

$$\Rightarrow 9.8t=\frac{147}{2}(\sqrt{3}-1) \Rightarrow t=5.49s$$

28. **(b)** **Given :** $M_1=1.20\,Am^2$

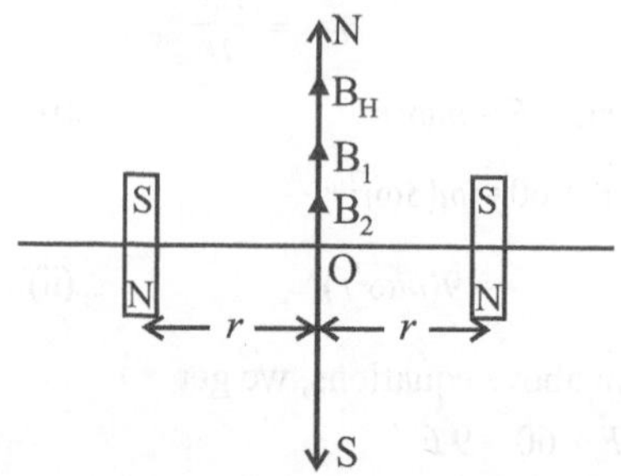

$M_2=1.00\,Am^2$

$$r=\frac{20}{2}cm=0.1m$$

$$B_{net}=B_1+B_2+B_H$$

$$B_{net}=\frac{\mu_0}{4\pi}\frac{(M_1+M_2)}{r^3}+B_H$$

$$=\frac{10^{-7}(1.2+1)}{(0.1)^3}+3.6\times10^{-5}=2.56\times10^{-4}\text{ wb/m}^2$$

29. (d)

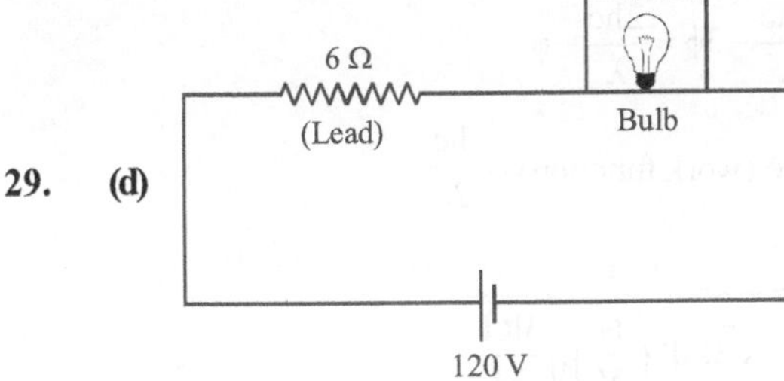

Power of bulb = 60 W (given)

Resistance of bulb $= \frac{120\times120}{60} = 240\Omega$

$$\left[\because P = \frac{V^2}{R}\right]$$

Power of heater = 240W (given)

Resistance of heater $= \frac{120\times120}{240} = 60\Omega$

Voltage across bulb before heater is switched on,

$V_1 = \frac{240}{246}\times120 = 117.73$ volt

Voltage across bulb after heater is switched on,

$V_2 = \frac{48}{54}\times120 = 106.66$ volt

Hence decrease in voltage

$V_1 - V_2 = 117.073 - 106.66 = 10.04$ Volt (approximately)

30. (d) Current in the ring due to rotation,

$$I = \frac{q}{T} = \frac{q\omega}{2\pi} = \frac{q\cdot2\pi f}{2\pi}$$

Therefore, magnetic field at the centre of the ring is

$$B = \frac{\mu_0 I}{2R} = \frac{\mu_0}{2R}\frac{q\,2\pi f}{2\pi} = \frac{\mu_0 q f}{2R}$$

31. (c) Let initial velocity of the bullet be v.

By linear momentum conservation

$$\frac{m}{2}v = \left(\frac{m}{2}+m\right)v_1$$

(v_1 = combined velocity)

$$v_1 = \frac{v}{3} \quad \text{.......... (a)}$$

retardation = μg

$$0 = \left(\frac{v}{3}\right)^2 - 2\mu g d \Rightarrow v = 3\sqrt{2\mu g d}$$

32. (a) Given, $B = 4\times10^{-5}$ T

$R_E = 6.4\times10^6$ m

Dipole moment of the earth M = ?

$$B = \frac{\mu_0}{4\pi}\frac{M}{d^3}$$

$$4\times10^{-5} = \frac{4\pi\times10^{-7}\times M}{4\pi\times\left(6.4\times10^6\right)^3}$$

$\therefore \quad M \cong 10^{23}\ \text{Am}^2$

33. (d) Total internal resistance = (50+2950) Ω = 3000 Ω

Emf of the cell, ε = 3V

$\therefore$ Current $= \frac{\varepsilon}{R} = \frac{3}{3000} = 1\times10^{-3}\,A = 1.0\,mA$

∴ Current for full scale deflection of 30 divisions is 1.0 mA.

∴ Current for a deflection of 20 divisions,

$$I = \left(\frac{20}{30}\times1\right)mA \text{ or } I = \frac{2}{3}mA$$

Let the resistance be x Ω. Then

$$x = \frac{\varepsilon}{I} = \frac{3V}{\left(\frac{2}{3}\times10^{-3}A\right)} = \frac{3\times3\times10^3}{2}\Omega$$

$= 4500\ \Omega$

But the resistance of the galvanometer is 50Ω.

∴ Resistance to be added

$= (4500 - 50)\ \Omega = 4450\ \Omega$

34. (c) Growth in current in LR_2 branch when switch is closed is given by

$$i = \frac{E}{R_2}[1 - e^{-R_2t/L}]$$

$$\Rightarrow \frac{di}{dt} = \frac{E}{R_2}.\frac{R_2}{L}.e^{-R_2t/L} = \frac{E}{L}e^{-\frac{R_2t}{L}}$$

Hence, potential drop across

$$L = \left(\frac{E}{L}e^{-R_2t/L}\right)L = Ee^{-R_2t/L}$$

$$= 12e^{-\frac{2t}{400\times10^{-3}}} = 12e^{-5t}V$$

35. (a) The magnetic field at O due to current in DA is

$$B_1 = \frac{\mu_o}{4\pi}\frac{I}{a}\times\frac{\pi}{6} \quad \text{(directed vertically upwards)}$$

The magnetic field at O due to current in BC is

$$B_2 = \frac{\mu_o}{4\pi}\frac{I}{b}\times\frac{\pi}{6} \quad \text{(directed vertically downwards)}$$

The magnetic field due to current AB and CD at O is zero.

Therefore the net magnetic field is

$B = B_1 - B_2$ (directed vertically upwards)

$$= \frac{\mu_o}{4\pi}\frac{I}{a}\frac{\pi}{6} - \frac{\mu_o}{4\pi}\frac{I}{b}\times\frac{\pi}{6}$$

$$= \frac{\mu_o I}{24}\left(\frac{1}{a}-\frac{1}{b}\right) = \frac{\mu_o I}{24ab}(b-a)$$

36. (a) According to Kirchhoff law, good absorbers are good emitters. Since black spot is good absorber so it is also a good emitter & will be brighter than plate.

37. (a) The angular dispersion θ i.e., the angle between the extreme rays of light,
$\theta = (\delta_V - \delta_R)$ where $\delta_V = (\mu_V - 1)A$, $\delta_R = (\mu_V - 1)A$ & A is angle of prism.
So if refractive index increases, then δ increases & hence θ increases.

38. (c) Heat gain = heat lost

$$C_A(16-12) = C_B(19-16) \Rightarrow \frac{C_A}{C_B} = \frac{3}{4}$$

and $C_B(23-19) = C_c(28-23) \Rightarrow \frac{C_B}{C_C} = \frac{5}{4}$

$$\Rightarrow \frac{C_A}{C_C} = \frac{15}{16} \quad ...(i)$$

If θ is the temperature when A and C are mixed then,

$$C_A(\theta-12) = C_C(28-\theta) \Rightarrow \frac{C_A}{C_C} = \frac{28-\theta}{\theta-12} \quad ...(ii)$$

On solving equations (i) and (ii) θ = 20.2°C

39. (b) Let nth fringe of 2500 Å coincide with (n – 2)th fringe of 3500Å.
∴ 3500 (n – 2) = 2500 × n
1000 n = 7000, n = 7
∴ 7th order fringe of 1st source will coincide with 5th order fringe of 2nd source.

40. (b) In the first process W is + ve as ΔV is positive, in the second process W is – ve as ΔV is – ve and area under the curve of second process is more
∴ Net Work < 0 and also $P_3 > P_1$.

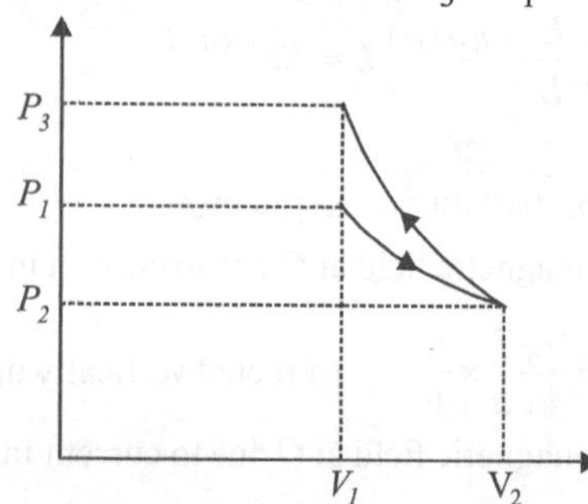

41. (d) Photoelectric equations

$$Ek_{1max} = \frac{hc}{\lambda} - \phi \quad ...(i)$$

and $Ek_{2max} = \frac{hc}{\lambda/2} - \phi$

$$EK_{2max} = \frac{2hc}{\lambda} - \phi \quad ...(ii)$$

From question, $Ek_{2max} = 3Ek_{1max}$
Multiplying equation (i) by 3

$$3Ek_{1max} = 3\left(\frac{hc}{\lambda} - \phi\right) \quad ...(iii)$$

From equation (ii) and (iii)

$$\frac{3hc}{\lambda} - 3\phi = \frac{2hc}{\lambda} - \phi$$

$$\therefore \phi \text{ (work function)} = \frac{hc}{2\lambda}$$

42. (a) $\tau = \dfrac{1}{\sqrt{2}\pi d^2 \left(\frac{N}{V}\right)\sqrt{\frac{3RT}{M}}}$

$$\tau \propto \frac{V}{\sqrt{T}}$$

As, $TV^{\gamma-1} = K$
So, $\tau \propto V^{\gamma + 1/2}$

Therefore, $q = \dfrac{\gamma+1}{2}$

43. (c)

A	B	$\bar{A}$	$\bar{B}$	$\bar{Y} = \bar{A} + \bar{B}$	Y
0	0	1	1	1	0
0	1	1	0	1	0
1	0	0	1	1	0
1	1	0	0	0	1

This table is of AND gate.

44. (c) Let r be the radius of each small drop.
Volume of big drop = 64 × Volume of each small drop

$$\frac{4}{3}\pi R^3 = 64 \times \frac{4}{3}\pi r^3$$

∴ R = 4r
Surface area of big drop = $4\pi R^2$
Surface area of 64 small droplets = $64 \times 4\pi r^2$
∴ Increase in surface area = $64 \times 4\pi r^2 - 4\pi R^2$
$= 4\pi[64r^2 - R^2]$

$$= 4\pi\left[64\left(\frac{R}{4}\right)^2 - R^2\right]$$

$= 4\pi[4R^2 - R^2] = 12\pi R^2$
Energy needed = Surface tension × Increase in surface area
$= T \times 12\pi R^2 = 12\pi R^2 T$

45. (c) Magnetic moment of the hydrogen atom, when the electron is in n^{th} excited state, i.e., $n' = (n + 1)$
As magnetic moment $M_n = I_n A = i_n(\pi r_n^2)$

$$i_n = eV_n = \frac{mz^2e^5}{4\varepsilon_0^2 n^3 h^3}$$

$$r_n = \frac{n^2h^2}{4\pi^2 kzme^2}\left(k = \frac{1}{4\pi\epsilon_0}\right)$$

Solving we get magnetic moment of the hydrogen atom for n^{th} excited state

$$M_{n'} = \left(\frac{e}{2m}\right)\frac{nh}{2\pi}$$

CHEMISTRY

46. (a) Given $A \xrightarrow{Cl_2} B \xrightarrow{alc./KOH} \underset{\text{Hydrocarbon}}{C} \xrightarrow{O_3/H_2O} CH_2O$

Since hydrocarbon C give only CH_2O, on ozonolysis, C should be $CH_2 = CH_2$ hence on going backward, A should be ethane. Thus the reactions are

$$\underset{(A)}{CH_3CH_3} \xrightarrow{Cl_2/hv} \underset{(B)}{CH_3CH_2Cl} \xrightarrow{alc.\ KOH}$$

$$\underset{(C)}{CH_2{=}CH_2} \xrightarrow[\Delta]{O_3/H_2O} HCHO$$

47. (a)

48. (d) In $\left[Ni(NH_3)_2Cl_2\right]$, Ni^{2+} is in sp^3 hybridisation, thus tetrahedral in shape. Hence the four ligands are not different to exhibit optical isomerism.

49. (a) Addition of HCN to carbonyl compounds is nucleophilic addition reaction. The order of reactivity of carbonyl compounds is :

$HCHO > CH_3COCH_3 > PhCOCH_3 > PhCOPh$

The lower reactivity of Ketones is due to the presence of two alkyl group which shows +I effect. The reactivity of Ketones decreases as the size of alkyl group increases.

50. (c) $\underset{1-x}{PCl_5(g)} \rightleftharpoons \underset{x}{PCl_3(g)} + \underset{x}{Cl_2(g)}$

Total moles after dissociation

$1-x+x+x=1+x$

p_{PCl_3} = mole fraction of PCl_3 ×

Total pressure $= \left(\frac{x}{1+x}\right)P$

51. (c) $(H_3C)_2C{=}CH-CH_2-CH_3$

Due to the presence of two similar methyl group at same carbon atom, above compound doesn't show geometrical isomerism.

52. (c) Liquid - liquid system is known as emulsion.

53. (d) $P = P_AX_A + P_BX_B$

$= P_AX_A + P_B(1-X_A)$

$\Rightarrow P_AX_A + P_B - P_BX_A$

$\Rightarrow P_B + X_A(P_A - P_B)$

54. (c) For $SbCl_5^{2-}$, $H = \frac{5+5+2}{2} = 6$ means sp^3d^2 hybridization I_3^-, SF_4, and PCl_5 ; all have sp^3d hybridization.

55. (c) A strong base can abstract an α-hydrogen from a ketone.

56. (b) During disproportionation same compound undergo simultaneous oxidation and reduction.

$$3H\overset{-}{O}\overset{+}{Cl} \longrightarrow 2H\overset{-1}{Cl} + H\overset{+5}{Cl}O_3$$

(Oxidation; reduction)

57. (c) $Cu + HCl \rightarrow$ No reaction as copper is less reactive than hydrogen while others will give H_2.

58. (d) Chloramphenicol is

$O_2N-C_6H_4-CH(OH)-CH(CH_2OH)-NH-C(=O)-CHCl_2$

59. (b) Number of A ions in the unit cell. $= \frac{1}{8} \times 8 = 1$

Number of B ions in the unit cell $= \frac{1}{2} \times 6 = 3$

Hence empirical formula of the compound $= AB_3$

60. (c) Since rate of reaction becomes four times on doubling concentration of reactant, it is second order reaction.

61. (a)

62. (d) $K_2Cr_2O_7 + conc.HCl \rightarrow Cl_2\uparrow$

63. (d) Pressure exerted by the gas, $P = \frac{1}{3}\frac{mnu^2}{V}$ ...(a)

Here, u = root mean square velocity

m = mass of a molecule, n = No. of molecules of the gas

Hence (a) & (b) are clearly wrong.

Again $u^2 = \frac{3RT}{M}$ [explained from (a)]

Here, M = Molecular wt. of the gas;

Hence (c) is wrong

Further, Average K.E. $= \frac{3}{2}$ KT; Hence (d) is true.

64. (b) The main reason for exhibiting larger number of oxidation states by actinoids as compared to lanthanoids is lesser energy difference between $5f$ and $6d$ orbitals as compared to that between $4f$ and $5d$ orbitals.

In case of actinoids we can remove electrons from $5f$ as well as from $6d$ and due to this actinoids exhibit larger number of oxidation state than lanthanoids.

65. **(2 and 3)** From the various given option we find option (a) correct. The oxidising power of halogen follow the order $F_2 > Cl_2 > Br_2 > I_2$. Option (b) incorrect because it in not the correct order of electron gain enthalpy of halogens.

The correct order is $Cl_2 > F_2 > Br_2 > I_2$. The low value of F_2 than Cl_2 is due to its small size.

Option (c) incorrect. The correct order of bond dissociation energies of halogens is

$Cl_2 > Br_2 > F_2 > I_2$.

Option (d) correct. It is the correct order of electronegativity values of halogens. Thus option (b) and (c) are incorrect.

66. (d) $Al_2O_3.2H_2O \rightarrow Al_2O_3 + 2H_2O$ is calcination.

67. (c) According to Arrhenius equation, the rate constant of reaction is given by,

$k = Ae^{-Ea/RT}$

where A is pre-exponential factor, E_a is activation energy and T is absolute temperature.

when $T \to \infty$, $\frac{E_a}{RT} \to 0$

then $k = Ae^0$

or $k = A$

68. (a) Co^{3+} : ⥮ 1 1 1 1 3*d*-orbital

$[Co(CN)_6]^{3-}$: ⥮ ⥮ ⥮ 3*d*-orbital

CN^- is a strong field ligand and it causes pairing of electrons, as a result number of unpaired electrons in Co^{3+} becomes zero and hence it has lowest value of paramagnetic behaviour.

69. (a) Given, for reaction

(i) $H_2O(l) \longrightarrow H^+(aq.) + OH^-(aq.)$; $\Delta H_r = 57.32$ kJ

(ii) $H_2(g) + \frac{1}{2}O_2(g) \longrightarrow H_2O(l)$; $\Delta H_r = -286.20$ kJ

For reaction (i)

$\Delta H_r = \Delta H°_f(H^+aq) + \Delta H°_f(OH^-aq) - \Delta H°_f(H_2O, l)$

$57.32 = 0 + \Delta H°_f(OH^-, aq) - \Delta H°_f(H_2O, l)$ ...(iii)

For reaction (ii)

$\Delta H_r = \Delta H°_f(H_2O, l) - \Delta H°_f(H_2, g) - \frac{1}{2}\Delta H°_f(O_2, g)$

$-286.20 = \Delta H°_f(H_2O, l)$

On replacing this value in equ. (iii) we have

$57.32 = \Delta H°_f(OH^-, aq) - (-286.20)$

$\Delta H°_f = -286.20 + 57.32$

$= -228.88$ kJ

70. (c) Applying VSEPR theory, both NF_3 and H_2O are sp^3 hybridized.

71. (a) $C_6H_5Cl + (CH_3)_2NLi \xrightarrow{(CH_3)_2NH} C_6H_5N(CH_3)_2 + LiCl$

72. (b) Tertiary alcohols react fastest with conc. HCl and anhydrous $ZnCl_2$ (lucas reagent) as its mechanism proceeds through the formation of stable tertiary carbocation.

Mechanism

Step 1 : $(CH_3)_3C-OH + H-Cl \rightleftharpoons (CH_3)_3C-\overset{+}{O}H_2 + Cl^-$

(2-Methylpropan-2-ol)

Step 2 : $(CH_3)_3C-\overset{+}{O}H_2 \rightleftharpoons (CH_3)_3C^+ + H_2O$ (3° Carbocation)

Step 3 : $(CH_3)_3C^+ + Cl^- \rightleftharpoons (CH_3)_3C-Cl$ (t–Butyl chloride)

73. (a)

$[2KMnO_4 + 3H_2SO_4 \longrightarrow K_2SO_4 + 2MnSO_4 + 3H_2O + 5(O)] \times 3$

$[2\,(COO)_2Fe + 3(O) \longrightarrow Fe_2O_3 + 2CO_2] \times 5$

$6KMnO_4 + 9H_2SO_4 + 10\,(COO)_2Fe \longrightarrow 3K_2SO_4 + 6MnSO_4 + 9H_2O + 5Fe_2O_3 + 10CO_2$

(6 moles) (10 moles)

From above equation 6 moles MnO_4^- required to oxidise 10 moles of oxalate.

Thus number of moles of MnO_4^- required to oxidise one mole of oxalate $= \frac{6}{10} = 0.6$ moles

74. (d)

75. (a) Sodium Phenoxide $(C_6H_5ONa) + CO_2 \longrightarrow$ o-$HOC_6H_4COONa \xrightarrow{H_2SO_4}$ o-HOC_6H_4COOH (Salicylic acid) $\xrightarrow{(CH_3CO)_2O}$ o-$CH_3COOC_6H_4COOH$ + CH_3COOH

Aspirin (Acetyl Salicylate)

76. (a) Eq. wt. of $H_2O_2 = 17$

$N = \frac{30.36}{17} = 1.78$ N

Volume strength $= 5.6 \times$ normality $= 5.6 \times 1.78 = 10$ V

77. (d) The metal placed below in electrochemical series does not react with that metal salt solution whose metal is placed above in electrochemical series.

78. (b)

79. (d) According to Fajan's rule :

Covalent character $\propto \frac{1}{\text{size of cation}}$

$\propto$ size of anion

Among the given species order of size of cations $N^{3+} < O^{2+} < Pb^{2+} < Ba^{2+}$

Order of size of anions $O^{2-} > Cl^-$.

Hence the order of covalent character is

$NCl_3 > Cl_2O > PbCl_2 > BaCl_2$

$BaCl_2$ is most ionic in nature.

80. (a) $C_6H_5CH_2Cl \xrightarrow{NaCN} C_6H_5CH_2CN \xrightarrow{H_2/Ni} C_6H_5CH_2CH_2NH_2$

Benzyl chloride ... β–Phenylethy lamine

81. (a) $F-C_6H_4-NO_2 \xrightarrow[DMF, \Delta]{(CH_3)_2\ddot{N}H} (CH_3)_2N-C_6H_4-NO_2 \xrightarrow{Reduction} (CH_3)_2N-C_6H_4-\ddot{N}H_2$

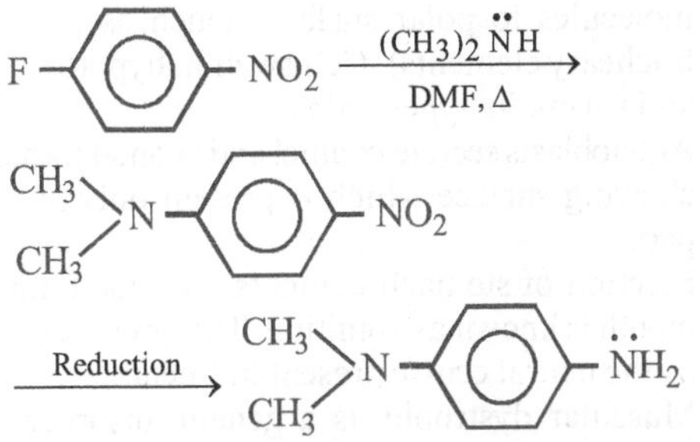

82. (c) With the exception of glycine all the 19 other common amino acids have a uniquely different functional group on the central tetrahedral alpha carbon.

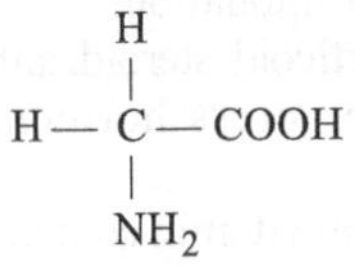

$H-CH(NH_2)-COOH$

glycine

83. (d) Boron nitride (BN) is known as inorganic graphite. The most stable form is hexagonal one. It has layered structure similar to graphite.

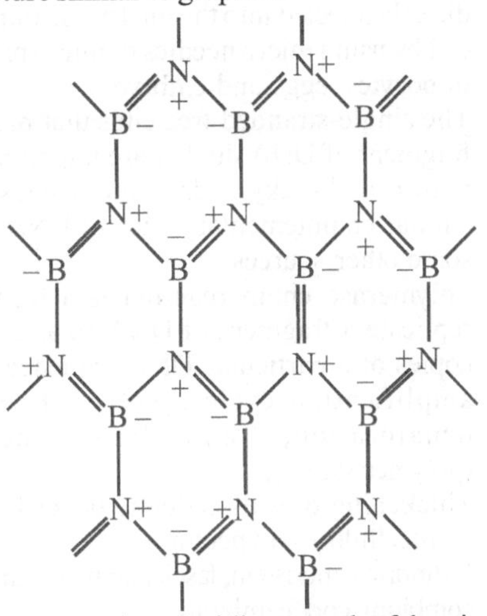

84. (c) The correct order of acidic strength of the given species in

$HSO_3F > H_3O^+ > HSO_4^- > HCO_3^-$

(iv) (ii) (iii) (i)

(i) < (iii) < (ii) < (iv)

It corresponds to choice (c) which is correct answer.

85. (b) Stability depends on number of hyperconjugative structures.

86. (d) $A \xrightarrow[(I)]{NH_3} B \xrightarrow[II]{\Delta} C \xrightarrow[KOH,(III)]{Br_2} CH_3CH_2NH_2$

Reaction (III) is a Hofmann bromamide reaction. Now formation of $CH_3CH_2NH_2$ is possible only from a compound $CH_3CH_2CONH_2$(C) which can be obtained from the compound $CH_3CH_2COO^-NH_4^+$ (B).

Thus (A) should be CH_3CH_2COOH

$$\underset{(A)}{CH_3CH_2-\overset{O}{\overset{\|}{C}}-OH} \xrightarrow{NH_3} \underset{(B)}{CH_3CH_2COO^-NH_4^+} \xrightarrow{\Delta} \underset{(C)}{CH_3CH_2CONH_2} \xrightarrow{KOH \mid Br_2} CH_3CH_2NH_2$$

87. (d) Ionisation energy $= E_\infty - E_1$

For $H = 0-(-13.6)$. For $Be^{3+} = 0-(-13.6 \times 4^2)$.

Therefore Ratio is 1 : 16.

88. (a)

89. (b) Due to the presence of strong C–F bonds, teflon has high thermal stability and chemical inertness.

90. (d) Rate $\propto \sqrt{\frac{1}{M}}$. The smaller the value of M the more is the rate of diffusion

BIOLOGY

91. (b) Phosphorus cycle is an example of sedimentary cycle. Pyramid of biomass of aquatic ecosystem is inverted. If decomposition leads to the formation of colloidal organic matter (humus), the process is called humification. Simple food chains are very rare in nature. This is because each organism may obtain food from more than one trophic level.

92. (b) The proteins encoded by the genes cry I Ac and cry II Ab control the cotton bollworms, that of cry I Ab controls corn borer.

93. (d) The anthers following meiosis produces pollen grains. In an embryosac, the primary endosperm nucleus (PEN) is triploid.

94. (d) Curcumin and vinblastine are secondary metabolites that belong to drugs. Morphine and codeine belong to alkaloids and abrin belongs to toxins.

95. (b) FAD is an electron acceptor in TCA cycle during oxidation of succinic acid to malic acid.

96. (c)

97. (b) Experimental evidences of DNA replication is carried in *E.coli*.

98. (a) The RNA polymerase II transcribes precursor of mRNA, the heterogenous nuclear RNA (hnRNA).

99. (c) Epiglottis is a cartilaginous flap of glottis.

100. (a)

101. (d) *Albugo* is the parasitic fungi which is found on mustard. It is the member of phycomycetes that are found in aquatic habitats and on decaying wood in moist and damp places.

102. (d) The fertile region of microsporophyll bears a number of microsporangia or pollen sacs arranged in sori. The pollen chamber represents microsporangium in which pollen grains develop.
103. (a) Iodine is extracted from brown algae, *laminaria* which is also known as Kelps.
104. (c) The body cavity which is lined by mesoderm is called coelom. Animals possessing coelom are called coelomates, e.g., annelids, molluscs, arthropods, echinoderms, hemichordates and chordates.
105. (c) In class Aves, endoskeleton is almost completely ossified. Bones are spongy or pneumatic. Long bones are hollow with air cavities.
106. (c) Monosaccharides are simple sugars that have 3-7 carbon atoms. Pentose sugar ribose is found in RNA. Most important sugar occuring in animals is glucose.
107. (b) A = Diplotene
B = Dissolution
C = Pachytene
D = Anaphase-II
108. (d) A–II ; B–IV ; C–I; D–III
109. (a) (A) Pulled
(B) Guttation
(C) Root hair
110. (d) Cyanide inhibits terminal electron transfer to O_2 complex IV
111. (c) UTRs are found at both 3' and 5' ends.
112. (c) Interferons are released as cytokine barriers under non-specific immunity.
113. (d) Selection and testing of superior recombinants require scientific evaluation of the progeny.
114. (a) Ganga Action plan was initiated by ministry of Environment and forests.
115. (c)
116. (b) Mixotrophy is the mode of nutrition which includes both phototrophy and heterotrophy.
117. (d) Gymnosperms and angiosperms are seed producing plants.
118. (c) Internal organs are formed for the first time in platyhelminthes. They have blind sac type of body plan with two way digestion.
119. (b)
120. (d) The vascular bundles are present in veins.
121. (5) The ascending limb of Henle's loop is non-permeable to water.
122. (a) Multinucleated animal cells are known as syncytium.
123. (d) Crista ampullaris possess hair cells.
124. (d) Somatostatin from the hypothalamus inhibits the release of growth hormone from the pituitary.
125. (c) NADPH + H^+ never formed in cyclic reaction.
126. (b) A keel is a structure of the papilionaceous type of flower, made up of two petals loosely united along their edges.
127. (d) Initiation of lateral roots during secondary growth takes place in the pericycle.
128. (d) Collagen and elastin are structural proteins present in white collagen fibres and yellow elastic fibres respectively, which are connective tissue fibres. Collagen fibres are present in white fibrous connective tissue. Yellow elastic fibres are present in yellow elastic connective tissue.
Neuroglia cells are specialized cells found in the brain and spinal cord supporting the neurons and their fibres. The muscles of biceps are voluntary and striated.
129. (d) Amyloplasts store carbohydrates (starch), e.g., potato whereas proteins are stored by aleuroplasts. chlorophyll pigments are presents in the thylakoid.
130. (a)
131. (c) Cohesion is the mutual attraction between water molecules whereas adhesion is the attraction of water molecules to polar surfaces (such as the surface of tracheary elements). Cell swell in hypotonic solutions and shrink in hypertonic ones.
132. (a) Ameloblasts secrete enamel and enamel forms the hard chewing surface which is present only in the crown part.
133. (d) Ejection of stomach contents, i.e., food, through the mouth is known as vomiting. This process is controlled by the neural centre present in 'medulla'.
134. (d) Muscular dystrophy is a genetic disorder in which there is continuous weakness and breakdown of skeletal muscles.
135. (a) Ciliary body muscle, lens and suspensory ligament are associated with accommodation.
136. (b) Cortisol is a gluco-corticoid, steroid, anti-inflammatory, immunosuppressive, stress hormone produced by adrenal gland.
137. (c) During biofortification vitamin content is the objective undertaken for improvement.
138. (c) Southern blotting
139. (d) Micro-injection method is the direct or vectorless method of gene transfer, in which foreign DNA is directly injected into the nucleus of animal cell or plant cell by using micro needles or micro pipettes. It is used in oocytes, eggs and embryo.
140. (c) The single-stranded free ends that project from each fragment of DNA duplex are unpaired bases and are known as "sticky ends". Sticky ends can join with similar complementary ends of DNA fragment from some other sources.
141. (d) Polymerase chain reaction is a technique used to replicate a fragment of DNA so as to produce many copies of a particular DNA sequence. A single PCR amplification cycle involves three basic steps: denaturation, annealing and extension (polymerisation).
142. (d) Thickening of wall is due to deposition of cellulose, hemicellulose and pectin.
143. (b) Cylindrical meristem, fascicular meristem, interfascicular combium, cork cambium.
144. (d)
145. (d) The ozone hole over Antarctica develops each year between late August and early October.
146. (c)
147. (b) *Salvinia* and *Selaginella* are heterosporous pteridophytes.
148. (a)
149. (d) Diaphragm is present below lung and separates thoracic cavity from abdominal cavity. Its up and down movement helps in expiration and inspiration during breathing.

150. (d) Hormones of adrenal medulla include noradrenaline and adrenaline. Nor-adrenaline regulates blood pressure and cardiac output under normal conditions.

151. (b) IVF is *in vitro* fertilization which is a method of assisted reproduction for infertile couples.

152. (a)

153. (c)

154. (c) XX-XO type of sex determination is found in roundworms and some insects like tree bugs, grasshoppers etc. Here, the females have two sex chromosome XX, while the males have only one sex chromosome X. There is no second sex chromosome. Females show homogamety and produce all X containing eggs while males show heterogamety and produce both X containing sperms and sperms without sex chromosomes.

155. (b) Pancreatic juice is secreted from aciner cells of exocrine part of pancreas. Its secretion is stimulated by secretin and cholecystokinin (CCK) hormones. Secretin increases the amount of bicarbonates (fluid) in pancreatic juice.

156. (d) Myelinated nerve fibres are found in spinal and cranial nerves. Retina has bipolar neurons with one axon and one dendrite. Electrical synapses are rarely present in human. In a resting neuron, the axonal membrane is high permeable to K^+ ions as compare to Na^+ ions. As a result, it contains low concentration of Na^+.

157. (b) Insulin lowers blood sugar levels, while Glucagon raises blood sugar levels.

158. (b) Synergid cell is haploid (n). If angiosperm plant is 2n = 14, then n = 7.

159. (a)

160. (c) The germ layer mesoderm forms in the embryos of animals more complex than cnidarians, making them triploblastic. Mesoderm forms during gastrulation when some of the cells migrating inward to the endoderm form an additional layer between the endoderm and the ectoderm. This key innovation evolved hundreds of millions of years ago and led to the evolution of nearly all large, complex animals. The formation of a mesoderm led to the formation of a coelom. Organs formed inside a coelom (body cavity) can freely move, grow, and develop independently of the body wall while fluid cushions and protects them from shocks.

161. (d)

Hypothalamus	–	GnRH
Acrosome	–	Sperm lysins
Graafian follicle	–	Estrogen
Leydig cells	–	Testosterone
Parturition	–	Relaxin

162. (a) Osmoconformers are the organisms that change the osmotic concentration of their body with the change in ambient conditions. Their body fluids are in osmotic balance with the environment. For many marine invertebrates, the osmolarity and ionic concentrations of their body fluids are similar to those of the sea-water in which they live.

163. (c)

164. (b) Different age groups have different reproduction capabilities. Pre-reproductive individuals are the young individuals which will enter the reproductive age after some time. They are the potential source of increase in population. Reproductive individuals are the ones which are actually adding new members to the population. Post-reproductive individuals are older individuals which no longer take part in reproduction.

165. (c) (a) - Partial regulators
(b) - Regulators
(c) - Conformers

Conformers :
Majority of the animals (up to 99%) and nearly all plants, cannot maintain a constant internal environment. Their body temperature and osmotic concentration changes according to the surrounding conditions . Such animal and plants are called conformers.

Regulators :
Some animals maintain their homeostasis by physiological or behavioural means. All birds and mammals (homeothermic or warm blooded) and a few lower vertebrates and invertebrates can maintain constant body temperature and constant osmotic concentration regardless of the surrounding conditions. Such organisms are called regulators.

Partial regulators :
If the stressful conditions are localized, the animals can '*escape in place*' and migrate to nearby region, having better environmental conditions. If the unfavourable conditions are for a shorter duration then the animals can '*escape in time*' and avoid those conditions suspending their activities. Such organisms are partial regulators.

166. (a) LNG - 20 and progestasert are the hormone producing intra uterine Devices (IUDs).

167. (d)

168. (d) Cytokine barrier is interferon. Virus infected cells secrete proteins called interferons which protect non-infected cells from further viral infection.

169. (a) The adult echinoderms are radially symmetrical but larvae are bilaterally symmetrical. They are triploblastic and coelomate animals. Fertilization is usually external and indirect development is observed.

170. (c) 171. (b)

172. (c) It is mode of fertilization of seed plant, that involves passage of pollen tube into ovule by the micropyle.

173. (a) AIH is artificial insemination by husband.

174. (a) The level of progestrone and estrogen is essential during pregnancy. Progesterone is essential for the establishment and maintenance of foetus and estrogen promotes parturition by inducing labor and delivery.

175. (a) A– IV ; B – I; C– II; D – III

176. (d) GAG is replaced by GTG

177. (b)

178. (d) Topoisomerse releases the tension in the DNA during replication.

179. (c) F.Griffith performed transformation experiment on *Streptococcus pneumoniae.* Avery, Macleod and Mac Carty used protease, RNAse and DNAse. DNAase inhibits transformation.

180. (c) A– IV ; B – III; C– II; D – I

Speed Test-101

PHYSICS

1. **(c)** Previously, if V_1 and V_2 are the potentials of inner and outer shells due to own charge respectively, then

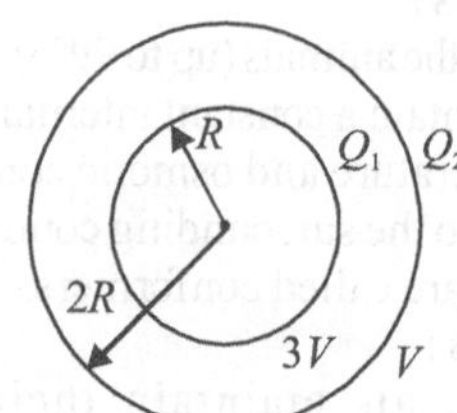

$V_1 + V_2 = 3V$

$\therefore V_1 + V = 3V$ or $V_1 = 2V$

When outer shell is earthed, its potential becomes zero, and so potential of inner shell becomes

$V_1' = 2V + 0 = 2V$

2. **(b)** $W_{ABD} = W_{AB} + W_{BD}$

$= 0 + 6 \times 10^4 \times 4 \times 10^{-3}$

$= 240$ J.

Now, $Q = \Delta U + W$

or $500 + 150 = \Delta U + 240$

$\therefore \Delta U = 410$ J.

3. **(b)** In CGS system,

$d = 4\dfrac{g}{cm^3}$

The unit of mass is 100g and unit of length is 10 cm, so

$$\text{density} = \frac{4\left(\frac{100g}{100}\right)}{\left(\frac{10}{10}cm\right)^3} = \frac{\left(\frac{4}{100}\right)}{\left(\frac{1}{10}\right)^3}\frac{(100g)}{(10cm)^3}$$

$$= \frac{4}{100} \times (10)^3 \frac{100g}{(10cm)^3} = 40 \text{ unit}$$

4. **(d)** $g = \dfrac{GM}{R}$ and $g' = \dfrac{GM}{(R+h)^2} \Rightarrow \dfrac{g'}{g} = \left(\dfrac{R}{R+h}\right)^2$

$\therefore g' = g\left(\dfrac{R}{R+h}\right)^2$

$\Rightarrow \dfrac{g}{2} = g\left(\dfrac{R}{R+h}\right)^2 \Rightarrow \dfrac{1}{\sqrt{2}} = \dfrac{R}{R+h}$

$\Rightarrow R + h = \sqrt{2}R$ or $h = (\sqrt{2} - 1)R$

5. **(a)** Given, h = 60m, g = 10 ms^{-2},

Rate of flow of water = 15 kg/s

$\therefore$ Power of the falling water

$= 15 \text{ kgs}^{-1} \times 10 \text{ ms}^{-2} \times 60 \text{ m} = 900$ watt.

Loss in energy due to friction

$= 9000 \times \dfrac{10}{100} = 900$ watt.

$\therefore$ Power generated by the turbine

$= (9000 - 900)$ watt $= 8100$ watt $= 8.1$ kW

6. **(a)** $N_1 = 25 \sin\theta$,

$\therefore \quad f_1 = \mu N_1 = \dfrac{2}{5} \times 25 \times \dfrac{3}{5} = 6N.$

$f_2 = \mu N_2 = \dfrac{2}{5} mg = \dfrac{2}{5} \times 1 \times 10$

$= 4N.$

Now from Newton's second law

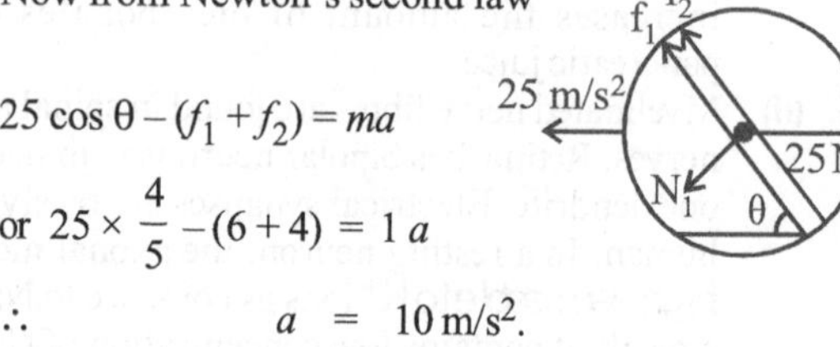

$25\cos\theta - (f_1 + f_2) = ma$

or $25 \times \dfrac{4}{5} - (6 + 4) = 1\,a$

$\therefore \quad a = 10 \text{ m/s}^2.$

7. **(d)** $\dfrac{1}{2}mv^2 = \dfrac{hc}{\lambda} - W_0$ or $\dfrac{hc}{\lambda} = \dfrac{1}{2}mv^2 + W_0$ and

$\dfrac{1}{2}mv_1^2 = \dfrac{hc}{(3\lambda/4)} - W_0 = \dfrac{4}{3}\left(\dfrac{1}{2}mv^2 + W_0\right) - W_0$

So, v_1 is greater than $v\left(\dfrac{4}{3}\right)^{1/2}$.

8. **(a)** Current through each bulb is same because these are connected in series.

since $\left(R = \dfrac{V^2}{P}\right)$, resistance of 40 W bulb is more, hence greater heat is produced in the 40 W bulb, it glows brightest

$H = I^2 R t$

9. **(a)** M.I. of disc about tangent in a plane $= \dfrac{5}{4}mR^2 = I$

$\therefore mR^2 = \dfrac{4}{5}I$ ...(i)

M.I. of disc about tangent ⊥ to plane $I' = \dfrac{3}{2}mR^2$

Substituting the value of mR^2 from equation (i) we get

$I' = \dfrac{3}{2}\left(\dfrac{4}{5}I\right) = \dfrac{6}{5}I$

10. (a) Process AB is isobasic and BC is isothermal, CD isochoric and DA isothermic compression.

11. (c) Electric field lines at each point of the ball must crosses normally.

12. (a) $E = \frac{hc}{\lambda} \Rightarrow \lambda = \frac{hc}{E} = \frac{6.62 \times 10^{-34} \times 3 \times 10^{8}}{12.5 \times 1.6 \times 10^{-19}}$

$= 993\,\text{A}^{\circ}$

$$\frac{1}{\lambda} = R\left(\frac{1}{n_1^2} - \frac{1}{n_2^2}\right)$$

(where Rydberg constant, $R = 1.097 \times 10^{7}$)

or, $\frac{1}{993 \times 10^{-10}} = 1.097 \times 10^{7}\left(\frac{1}{1^2} - \frac{1}{n_2^2}\right)$

Solving we get $n_2 = 3$

Spectral lines

Total number of spectral lines = 3

Two lines in Lyman series for $n_1 = 1, n_2 = 2$ and $n_1 = 1, n_2 = 3$ and one in Balmer series for $n_1 = 2, n_2 = 3$

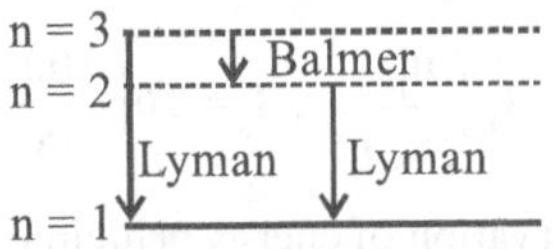

n = 3
Balmer
n = 2
Lyman Lyman
n = 1

13. (b) Boat covers distance of 16km in a still water in 2 hours.

i.e. $v_B = \frac{16}{2}$ km/hr

Now velocity of water $\Rightarrow v_w = 4$ km/hr

Time taken for going upstream

$$t_1 = \frac{8}{v_B - v_w} = \frac{8}{8-4} = 2\text{hr}$$

(As water current oppose the motion of boat)

Time taken for going down stream

$$t_2 = \frac{8}{v_B + v_w} = \frac{8}{8+4} = \frac{8}{12}\text{hr}$$

(As water current helps the motion of boat)

$\therefore$ Total time $= t_1 + t_2 = \left(2 + \frac{8}{12}\right)$hr or 2 hr 40 min.

14. (c) Current in circuit $= \frac{(3-1)V}{200\Omega} = \frac{2}{200} = 0.01$ A.

15. (c) Given $t = d^{a/2}, r^{b/2}, s^{c/2}$. Substituting dimensions, we have

$(T) = (ML^{-3})^{a/2}(L)^{b/2}(MT^{-2})^{c/2}$
$= M^{(a+c)/2}.L^{(-3a/2\,+\,b/2)}\,T^{-c}$

Equating powers of L, we have,

$-\frac{3}{2}a + \frac{b}{2} = 0.$ Given a = 1.

$\therefore -\frac{3}{2} + \frac{b}{2} = 0$ or $b = 3$

16. (b) Distance covered by lift is given by

$y = t^2$

$\therefore$ Acceleration of lift upwards

$$= \frac{d^2y}{dt^2} = \frac{d}{dt}(2t) = 2\ \text{m/s}^2 = \frac{g}{5}$$

Now, $T = 2\pi\sqrt{\frac{\ell}{g}}$

$$T' = 2\pi\sqrt{\frac{\ell}{g + \frac{g}{5}}} = 2\pi\sqrt{\frac{\ell}{\frac{6}{5}g}} = \sqrt{\frac{5}{6}}T.$$

17. (c) Angular limit of resolution of eye, $\theta = \frac{\lambda}{d}$, where, d is diameter of eye lens.

Also, if y is the minimum separation between two objects at distance D from eye then

$$\theta = \frac{y}{D}$$

$$\Rightarrow \frac{y}{D} = \frac{\lambda}{d} \Rightarrow y = \frac{\lambda D}{d} \quad ...(a)$$

Here, wavelength $\lambda = 5000\text{Å} = 5 \times 10^{-7}$ m

$D = 50$ m

Diameter of eye lens = 2 mm = 2×10^{-3} m

From eq. (a), minimum separation is

$$y = \frac{5 \times 10^{-7} \times 50}{2 \times 10^{-3}} = 12.5 \times 10^{-3}\ \text{m}$$

18. (d) The equivalent circuit is as shown in figure.

The resistance of arm AOD (= R + R) is in parallel to the resistance R of arm AD.

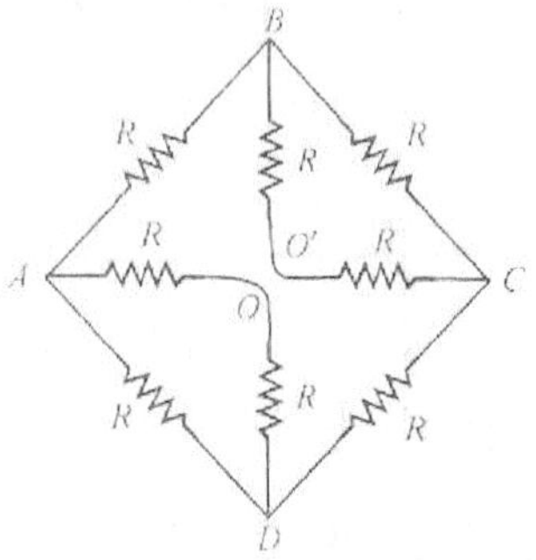

Their effective resistance $R_1 = \frac{2R \times R}{2R \times R} = \frac{2}{3}R$

The resistance of arms AB, BC and CD is

$$R_2 = R + \frac{2}{3}R + R = \frac{8}{3}R$$

The resistance R_1 and R_2 are in parallel. The effective resistance between A and D is

$$R_3 = \frac{R_1 \times R_2}{R_1 + R_2} = \frac{\frac{2}{3}R \times \frac{8}{3}R}{\frac{2}{3}R + \frac{8}{3}R} = \frac{8}{15}R.$$

19. (b) Both the charges are identical and placed symmetrically about $ABCD$. The flux crossing $ABCD$ due to each charge is $\frac{1}{6}\left[\frac{q}{\epsilon_0}\right]$ but in opposite directions. Therefore the resultant is zero.

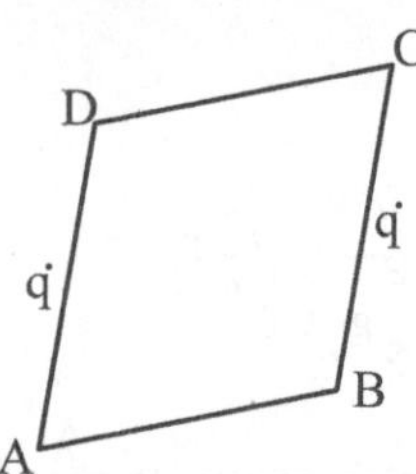

20. (d) C_v for hydrogen $= \frac{5}{2}R$

C_v for helium $= \frac{3R}{2}$

C_v for water vapour $= \frac{6R}{2} = 3R$

$$\therefore (C_v)_{mix} = \frac{4\times\frac{5}{2}R + 2\times\frac{3}{2}R + 1\times 3R}{4+2+1} = \frac{16}{7}R$$

$\therefore C_p = C_v + R$

$C_p = \frac{16}{7}R + R$ or $C_p = \frac{23}{7}R$

21. (b) The effective circuit is shown in the figure

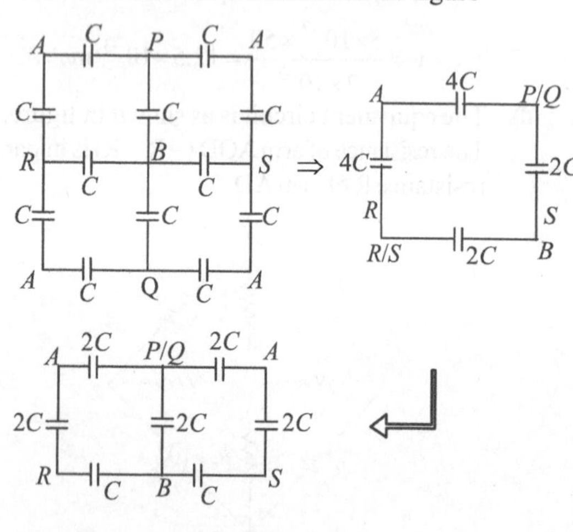

Now $C_{AB} = 2\times\frac{4C\times 2C}{4C+2C} = \frac{8C}{3}$.

22. (d) Work done by tension + Work done by force (applied) + Work done by gravitational force = change in kinetic energy

Work done by tension is zero

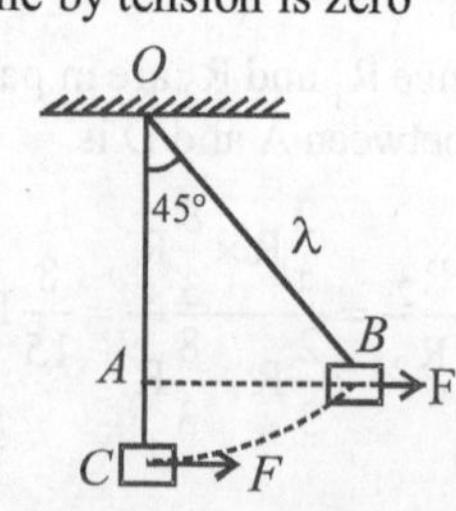

$\Rightarrow 0 + F\times AB - Mg\times AC = 0$

$$\Rightarrow F = Mg\left(\frac{AC}{AB}\right) = Mg\left[\frac{1-\frac{1}{\sqrt{2}}}{\frac{1}{\sqrt{2}}}\right]$$

[$\because AB = \ell\sin 45° = \frac{\ell}{\sqrt{2}}$ and

$AC = OC - OA = \ell - \ell\cos 45° = \ell\left(1-\frac{1}{\sqrt{2}}\right)$

where ℓ = length of the string.]

$\Rightarrow F = Mg(\sqrt{2}-1)$

23. (a) $\frac{E_s}{E_p} = \frac{n_s}{n_p}$ or $E_s = E_p\times\left(\frac{n_s}{n_p}\right)$

$\therefore E_s = 120\times\left(\frac{200}{100}\right) = 240\,V$

$\frac{I_p}{I_s} = \frac{n_s}{n_p}$ or $I_s = I_p\left(\frac{n_p}{n_s}\right)$ $\therefore I_s = 10\left(\frac{100}{200}\right) = 5$ amp

24. (c) Applying conservation of energy principle, we get

$$\frac{1}{2}mk^2v_e^2 - \frac{GMm}{R} = -\frac{GMm}{r}$$

$$\Rightarrow \frac{1}{2}mk^2\frac{2GM}{R} - \frac{GMm}{R} = -\frac{GMm}{r}$$

$$\Rightarrow \frac{k^2}{R} - \frac{1}{R} = -\frac{1}{r} \Rightarrow \frac{1}{r} = \frac{1}{R} - \frac{k^2}{R}$$

$$\Rightarrow \frac{1}{r} = \frac{1}{R}(1-k^2) \Rightarrow r = \frac{R}{1-k^2}$$

25. (a) Water rises upto the top of capillary tube and stays there without overflowing.

26. (c)

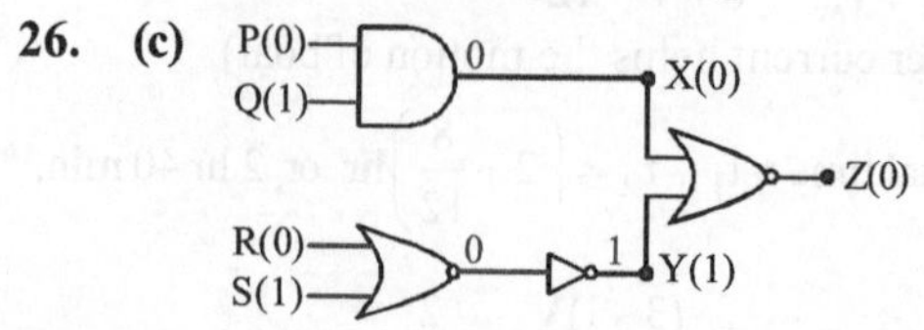

27. (d) The self inductance of a long solenoid is given by

$L = \mu_r\mu_0 n^2 Al$

Self inductance of a long solenoid is independent of the current flowing through it.

28. (b) It means that car which is moving on a horizontal road & the necessary centripetal force, which is provided by friction (between car & road) is not sufficient.

If μ is friction between car and road, then max speed of safely turn on horizontal road is determined from figure.

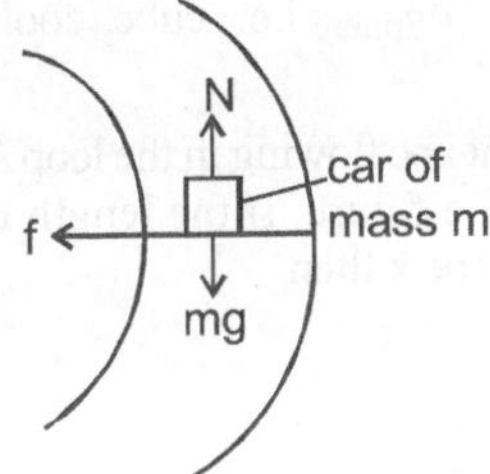

$N = mg$ ...(i)

$f = \frac{mv^2}{r}$ ...(ii)

Where f is frictional force between road & car, N is the normal reaction exerted by road on the car. We know that

$f = \mu_s N = \mu_s mg$ ......(iii)

where μ_s is static friction

so from eq (ii) & (iii) we have

$\frac{mv^2}{r} \le \mu_s mg \Rightarrow v^2 \le \mu_s rg$ or $v \le \sqrt{\mu_s rg}$

& $v_{max} = \sqrt{\mu_s rg}$

If the speed of car is greater than v_{max} at that road, then it will be thrown out from road i.e., skidding.

29. **(a)** Time period of simple pendulam is given by :

$T = 2\pi\sqrt{\frac{\ell}{g_{eff}}}$ or, $T = \frac{k}{\sqrt{g_{eff}}}$

Now, $T_1 = \frac{k}{\sqrt{g}}$ and $T_2 = \frac{k}{\sqrt{g\left(1-\frac{d}{R}\right)}}$

So, $\frac{T_1}{T_2} = \sqrt{1-\frac{d}{R}} = \left(\frac{T_1}{T_2}\right)^2 = 1-\frac{d}{R}$

$d = \left[1-\left(\frac{T_1}{T_2}\right)^2\right]R$

30. **(a)** Black board paint is quite approximately equal to black bodies.

31. **(a)** Here, $r = 6$ cm $= 6 \times 10^{-2}$ m, $N = 20$, $\omega = 40$ rads^{-1}

$B = 2 \times 10^{-2}$ T, $R = 8\Omega$

Maximum emf induced, $\varepsilon = NAB\omega$

$= N(\pi r^2)B\omega$

$= 20 \times \pi \times (6 \times 10^{-2})\ 2 \times 10^{-2} \times 40 = 0.18$ V

Average value of emf induced over a full cycle

$\varepsilon_{av} = 0$

Maximum value of current in the coil.

$I = \frac{\varepsilon I}{R} = \frac{0.18}{8} = 0.023$ A

Average power dissipated,

$P = \frac{\varepsilon I}{2} = \frac{0.18 \times 0.023}{2} = 2.07 \times 10^{-3}$ W

32. **(c)** Angle of prism A = 60°

By prism formula

$\mu = \frac{\sin\left(\frac{A+\delta_m}{2}\right)}{\sin\left(\frac{A}{2}\right)}$ or $\sqrt{3} = \frac{\sin\left(\frac{60^\circ+\delta_m}{2}\right)}{\sin\left(\frac{60^\circ}{2}\right)}$

$\frac{\sqrt{3}}{2} = \sin\left(\frac{60^\circ+\delta_m}{2}\right)$; $\sin 60^\circ = \sin\left(\frac{60^\circ+\delta m}{2}\right)$

$60^\circ = \frac{60^\circ+\delta_m}{2} \Rightarrow \delta_m = 60^\circ$

As we know,

$\delta_m = 2\theta - A$

$\theta = \frac{\delta_m + A}{2} = \frac{60^\circ+60^\circ}{2} = 60^\circ$

33. **(d)** Torque on the solenoid is given by

$\tau = MB\sin\theta$

where θ is the angle between the magnetic field and the axis of solenoid.

$M = niA$

$\therefore\ \tau = niA\,B\sin 30^\circ$

$= 2000 \times 2 \times 1.5 \times 10^{-4} \times 5 \times 10^{-2} \times \frac{1}{2}$

$= 1.5 \times 10^{-2}\ N-m$

34. **(a)** $mg = 72$ N (body weight on the surface)

$g = \frac{GM}{R^2}$

At a height $H = \frac{R}{2}$, $g' = \frac{GM}{\left(R+\frac{R}{2}\right)^2} = \frac{4\ GM}{9\ R^2}$

Body weight at height $H = \frac{R}{2}$,

$mg' = m \times \frac{4\ GM}{9\ R^2}$

$= m \times \frac{4}{9} \times g = \frac{4}{9}mg = \frac{4}{9} \times 72 = 32$ N

35. **(c)** If ℓ is the original length of wire, then change in length of first wire, $\Delta\ell_1 = (\ell_1 - \ell)$

change in length of second wire, $\Delta\ell_2 = (\ell_2 - \ell)$

Now, $Y = \frac{T_1}{A} \times \frac{\ell}{\Delta\ell_1} = \frac{T_2}{A} \times \frac{\ell}{\Delta\ell_2}$

or $\frac{T_1}{\Delta\ell_1} = \frac{T_2}{\Delta\ell_2}$ or $\frac{T_1}{\ell_1 - \ell} = \frac{T_2}{\ell_2 - \ell}$

or $T_1\ell_2 - T_1\ell = T_2\ell_1 - \ell T_2$ or $\ell = \frac{T_2\ell_1 - T_1\ell_2}{T_2 - T_1}$

36. (b) $Q_a = \Delta U + 0 = \Delta U$

and $Q_b = \Delta U + P\Delta V$

As $Q_b > Q_a$, $\therefore$ Change in entropy is greater in case(b).

37. (b) According to the principal of circular motion in a magnetic field

$$F_c = F_m \Rightarrow \frac{mv^2}{R} = qVB$$

$$\Rightarrow R = \frac{mv}{qB} = \frac{P}{qB} = \frac{\sqrt{2m.k}}{qB}$$

$$R_\alpha = \frac{\sqrt{2(4m)K'}}{2qB}$$

$$\frac{R}{R_\alpha} = \sqrt{\frac{K}{K'}}$$

but $R = R_\alpha$ (given)

Thus $K = K' = 1$ MeV

38. (b) Rate of flow of liquid $V = \frac{P}{R}$

where liquid resistance $R = \frac{8\eta l}{\pi r^4}$

For another tube liquid resistance;

$$R' = \frac{8\eta l}{\pi\left(\frac{r}{2}\right)^4}.16 = 16R$$

For the series combination

$$V_{New} = \frac{P}{R+R'} = \frac{P}{R+16R} = \frac{P}{17R} = \frac{V}{17}$$

39. (c) The distance of object from mirror

$$= 15 + \frac{33.25}{4} \times 3 = 39.93 \text{ cm}$$

Distance of image from mirror

$$= 15 + \frac{25 \times 3}{4} = 33.75 \text{ cm}$$

Using mirror formula,

$$\frac{1}{v} + \frac{1}{u} = \frac{1}{f}$$

$$\text{or } \frac{1}{-33.93} + \frac{1}{-33.75} = \frac{1}{f}$$

$$\therefore \quad f = -18.3 \text{ cm}$$

40. (b) Rate of cooling of a body $R = \frac{\Delta\theta}{t} = \frac{A\varepsilon\sigma(T^4 - T_0^4)}{mc}$

$$\Rightarrow R \propto \frac{A}{m} \propto \frac{\text{Area}}{\text{Volume}} \quad [m = \rho \times V]$$

$\Rightarrow$ For the same surface area. $R \propto \frac{1}{\text{Volume}}$

$\because$ Volume of cube < Volume of sphere

$\Rightarrow R_{cube} > R_{Sphere}$ i.e., cube, cools down with faster rate.

41. (b) Let a current i be flowing in the loop ABC in the direction shown in the figure. If the length of each of the sides AB and BC be x then

$|\vec{F}| = i x B$

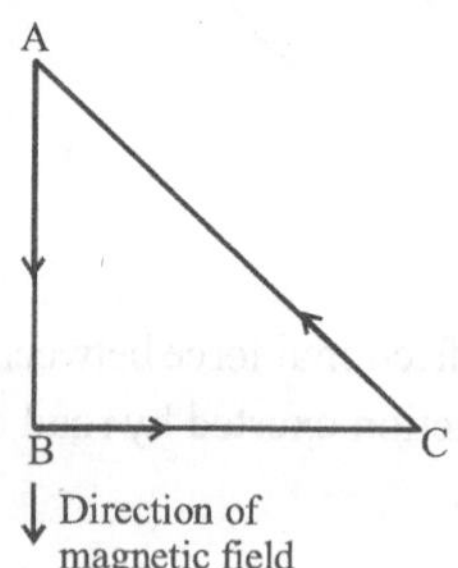

where B is the magnitude of the magnetic force.

The direction of $\vec{F}$ will be in the direction perpendicular to the plane of the paper and going into it.

By Pythagorus theorem,

$$AC = \sqrt{x^2 + x^2} = \sqrt{2}x$$

$\therefore$ Magnitude of force on AC

$$= i\sqrt{2} \text{ x B} \sin 45° = i\sqrt{2} \text{ x B} \times \frac{1}{\sqrt{2}} = ixB = |\vec{F}|$$

The direction of the force on AC is perpendicular to the plane of the paper and going out of it. Hence, force on $AC = -\vec{F}$

42. (b) A nucleus is denoted by ${}_ZX^A$

An isotope should have same Z.

α–particle $= {}_2He^4$; β–particle $= {}_{-1}\beta^0$

The emission of one α particle and the emission of two β particles maintain the Z same.

Hence, for isotope formation 2β particles and one α particle are emitted.

43. (b) Fundamental frequency of closed organ pipe

$$V_c = \frac{V}{4l_c}$$

Fundamental frequency of open organ pipe

$$V_0 = \frac{V}{2l_0}$$

Second overtone frequency of open organ pipe $= \frac{3V}{2l_0}$

From question,

$$\frac{V}{4l_c} = \frac{3V}{2l_0}$$

$$\Rightarrow \quad l_0 = 6l_c = 6 \times 20 = 120 \text{ cm}$$

44. (b) If a body slides down, then the force of friction acts upwards along the plane weight(mg) act vertically downwards.

45. (b) Forward bias opposes the potential barrier and if the applied voltage is more than knee voltage it cancels the potential barrier.

CHEMISTRY

46. (c) This is Avogadro's hypothesis.

According to this, equal volume of all gases contain equal no. of molecules under similar condition of temperature and pressure.

47. (d) $Q = m \times L$

where, L = latent heat of vapourisation of water

$= 2260$ kJ/kg

$= 2260 \times 10^3$ J/kg

$Q = 70 \times 10^{-3} \times 2260 \times 10^3 = 1,58,200$ Joule

48. (d)

49. (d) Oxidation state of Ti in the given compounds. as follows:

TiO – +2

TiO_2 – +4

K_2TiF_6 – +4

K_2TiO_4 – +6

The oxidation states exhibited by Ti is +2, +3, +4. So K_2TiO_4 does not exist.

50. (a)

$$\underset{\text{Isobutylene}}{(CH_3)_2C=CH_2} \xrightarrow{HBr} \underset{\text{Isobutyl bromide}}{(CH_3)_2CHCH_2Br}$$

Note that, here HBr is added in anti-Markownikoff's manner, so reaction should take place in presence of peroxide. Hydroquinone and diphenylamine are not free-radical producing substances but scavangers.

51. (a) The sequence of bases in mRNA are read in a serial order in groups of three at a time. Each triplet of nucleotides (having a specific sequence of bases) is known as codon. Each codon specifies one amino acid. Further since, there are four bases, therefore, $4^3 = 64$ triplets or codons are possible.

52. (d) In FeS_2, Fe^{2+} is converting into Fe^{3+} and sulphur is changing from –1 oxidation state to +4 oxidation state.

There are two S^- and one Fe^{2+} in FeS_2. Thus total no. of electrons lost in the given reaction are 11.

53. (b) $2Al + \frac{3}{2}O_2 \rightarrow Al_2O_3,\ \Delta H = -1596$ kJ .....(i)

$2Cr + \frac{3}{2}O_2 \rightarrow Cr_2O_3,\ \Delta H = -1134$ kJ ....(ii)

By (i) –(ii)

$2Al + Cr_2O_3 \rightarrow 2Cr + Al_2O_3,\ \Delta H = -462$ kJ.

54. (b) It is an example of concentration cell, E_{cell} cannot be zero since $[H^+]$ are different (HCl is strong and CH_3COOH weak acid).

55. (a) CaO is basic as it form strong base $Ca(OH)_2$ on reaction with water.

$$CaO + H_2O \longrightarrow Ca(OH)_2$$

CO_2 is acidic as it dissolve in water forming unstable carbonic acid.

$$H_2O + CO_2 \longrightarrow H_2CO_3$$

Silica (SiO_2) is insoluble in water and acts as a very weak acid.

SnO_2 is amphoteric as it reacts with both acid and base.

$$SnO_2 + 2H_2SO_4 \longrightarrow Sn(SO_4)_2 + 2H_2O$$

$$SnO_2 + 2KOH \longrightarrow K_2SnO_3 + H_2O$$

56. (a)

(A) Sulphuric acid (iv) Contact process

(B) Steel (ii) Bessemer's process

(C) Sodium hydroxide (iii) Leblanc process

(D) Ammonia (i) Haber's process

57. (d) When both double and triple bonds are present, then double bond is considered as the principal group.

58. (c) Butter of tin is $SnCl_4.5H_2O$.

59. (b) Forward reaction is favoured by removal of products.

60. (c) Reaction rate $= k[A]^2[B]$

Now increase conc. of A by three times and conc. of B by two times. Then new rate

$R_2 = k[3A]^2[2B]$

$$\frac{R_1}{R_2} = \frac{k[A]^2[B]}{k[3A]^2[2B]} = \frac{1}{3^2} \times \frac{1}{2} = \frac{1}{18}$$

$R_2 = 18 \times R_1$

Hence rate increases by 18 times.

61. (b) Since the leaving group breaks away as a base, it is easier to displace weaker bases as compared to stronger bases. Thus less basic the substituent, the more easily it is displaced.

Since the basic strength of the given groups is in order.

$I^- < Br^- < Cl^-$

Thus the order of halogen leaving groups is

$I^- > Br^- > Cl^-$

62. (d)

63. (c) Electrolytic reduction of nitrobenzene in weakly acidic medium gives aniline, whereas in strongly acidic medium it gives *p*-hydroxyaniline

64. (d) $2CaOCl_2 \xrightarrow{CoCl_2} 2CaCl_2 + O_2$

65. (a) $\overset{\ominus}{\ddot{C}}H_2 - \underset{\underset{O}{\|}}{C} - CH_3 \leftrightarrow CH_2 = \underset{\underset{\ddot{O}:^{\ominus}}{|}}{C} - CH_3$

I II

66. (b) After every 30 minutes the amount is reduced to $\frac{1}{2}$ therefore $t_{1/2}$ is 30 minutes. In 90 minutes the amount is reduced to $\frac{1}{8}$ i.e. $\frac{1}{2^n}$. Here n = 3. True for 1st order reaction.

67. (d) $H \overset{\sigma}{-} C \overset{\sigma}{\underset{\pi}{=}} C \overset{\sigma}{-} H$ (each C bonded to H by σ bond: $\sigma|$ H, $|\sigma$ H)

68. (c) $(4n+2)\pi$ electrons and planar structure are the essential conditions for aromaticity.

69. (a) Normally $NaBH_4$ as well as $LiAlH_4$ reduce only –CHO group without effecting carbon-carbon double bond, however when it is present in conjugation with benzene ring and aldehydic group it is also reduced along with the reduction of –CHO group.

$$C_6H_5CH = CHCHO \xrightarrow{NaBH_4} C_6H_5CH_2CH_2CH_2OH$$

70. (b)
71. (a) It is due to movement of energised electrons (KE $\propto$ T).
72. (b)
73. (d)
74. (d) He_2 Bond order $= \frac{1}{2}(2-2) = 0$ Hence cannot be formed.
75. (d) Interstitial compounds of transition metal exhibit metallic conductivity.
76. (d) The drugs which act on the central nervous system and help in reducing anxiety are called tranquilizers.
77. (d) Colligative properties depends upon the no. of particles. Since methanol is non electrolyte hence cannot be considered.
78. (c)
79. (b) Aryl halides are less reactive towards nucleophilic substitution because of the partial double bond character of carbon-halogen bonds. It is also partly due to repulsion between the electron cloud of the benzene ring and the nucleophile.
80. (d) Pressure exerted by the gas, $P = \frac{1}{3}\frac{mnu^2}{V}$ ...(a)

Here, u = root mean square velocity
m = mass of a molecule, n = No. of molecules of the gas
Hence (a) & (b) are clearly wrong.

Again $u^2 = \frac{3RT}{M}$ [explained from (a)]
Here, M = Molecular wt. of the gas;
Hence (c) is wrong

Further, Average K.E. $= \frac{3}{2}$ KT; Hence (d) is true.

81. (c) As MgO is a weak base hence some energy got consumed to break MgO (s). Hence enthalpy is less than $-57.33\ kJ\ mol^{-1}$.
82. (a) Smaller the charge on anion, lesser will be its coagulating power.
$\therefore$ KBr have Br^- with least charge of -1 on Br thus KBr is least effective in coagulating $Fe(OH)_3$.
83. (a) Calcium and magnesium form complexes with EDTA.
84. (d) Since Sc^{3+} does not contain any unpaired electron it is colourless in water.
85. (a) ABS is acrylonitrile-butadiene-styrene rubber which is obtained by copolymerisation of acrylonitrile, 1, 3-butadiene and styrene.

$$\underset{\text{Acrylonitrile}}{\underset{|\atop CN}{CH_2 = CH}} + \underset{\text{1,3–Butadiene}}{\underset{|\atop CH=CH_2}{CH_2 = CH}} + \underset{\text{Styrene}}{CH_2 = CHC_6H_5} \longrightarrow$$

$$\underset{\text{ABS rubber}}{\left[CH_2 - \underset{|\atop CN}{CH} - CH_2CH = CHCH_2 - CH_2 - \underset{|\atop C_6H_5}{CH} \right]_n}$$

86. (a) Cl_2 is obtained by electrolysis of (aqueous) NaCl.
87. (b) Stability of an alkene depends upon the heat of hydrogenation of an alkene. The lower the heat of hydrogenation of an alkene higher will be stability.

Order of stability	Heat of hydrogenation (kJ/mol)
trans-2-butene	115.5
cis-2-butene	119.6 and
1-butene	126.8

88. (c)
89. (d) We can distinguish between formic acid and acetic acid by their action on Fehling's solution. Formic acid gives a red ppt of cuprous oxide but acetic acid does not give red ppt.
90. (c) In presence of non-protic solvent such as $CHCl_3$ or CCl_4, concentration of electrophile (Br^+) is less, hence reaction stops at the monobromo stage

BIOLOGY

91. (d) Early blight of potato is caused by a fungus called *Alternaria solani*. Late blight of potato (which claimed more than one million lives in 1845 in Ireland) is caused by another fungus called *Phytopthora infestens*.
92. (d) *Chlorella* is a unicellular green alga, rich in proteins and is used as food supplement even by space travellers.
93. (d) Within the sporangia spore mother cell undergoes meiosis to form spores. If all the spores are of the same size the plant is said to be homosporous (*Lycopodium Psilotum, Adiantum, Equisetum* and *Dryopteris*), and if they are of two different sizes, the plant is called heterosporous (*Selaginella, Isoetes, Marsilea, Azolla* and *Salvinia*).
94. (d) *Asterias* (Star fish) belongs to phylum Echinodermata in which an excretory system is absent.
95. (c) *Struthio* (Ostrich) is the largest living flightless bird.
96. (d) R.Q. value for fatty acid is lees than one. When tripalmitin (a fatty acid) is used as respiratory substrate, the R.Q. is 0.7 as shown below.

$$2\,(C_{51}H_{98}O_6) + 145\,O_2 \rightarrow 102\,CO_2 + 98\,H_2O \text{ (fat tripalmitin)}$$

$$R.Q. = \frac{102\ CO_2}{145\ O_2} = 0.7$$

97. (d) Apical dominance is regulated by auxins. Auxin like 2, 4-D are widely used as herbicides. ABA stimulates the closure of stomata in the epidermis and increases the tolerance of plants to various kinds of stresses.
98. (c) Larynx is a cartilaginous box which helps in sound production and hence called the sound box. Much developed larynx of human male is called Adam's apple.
99. (d) A single layer of **odontoblast cells** line the pulp cavity. These cells secrete enamel, which is a bluishwhite shiny translucent and the hardest substance of the body and helps in the mastication of food.
100. (b) Dead space is the air that is inhaled by the body in breathing but does not take part in gas exchange. In man, it is 150 ml. E.g; the amount of air present in trachea, bronchi and bronchioles, which is not used in respiration.
101. (d) Placenta functions as a gland, secreting human chorionic gonadotrophin, progesterone, and oestrogens, which regulate the maintenance of pregnancy. Its primary function is to provide the embryo with nourishment, eliminate its wastes, and exchange respiratory gases.

102. (b) Copper-T is copper releasing intra uterine devices (IUD). It increases phagocytosis of sperms within the uterus and suppress sperm motility and fertilising capacity of sperms.

103. (a) Use of contraceptive pills is a widespread form of birth control. Contraceptive pills contain oestrogen and progesterone. The production of the pituitary hormones FSH and LH in the normal sexual cycle of a female is shut down by these hormones. In the absence of FSH, the ovarian follicles do not ripen and ovulation does not occur in the absence of LH.

104. (c) Haemophilia and colour blindness both are recessive X-linked traits. They express in males when present in single copy (heterozygous) but in females, they express only when present in homozygous condition.

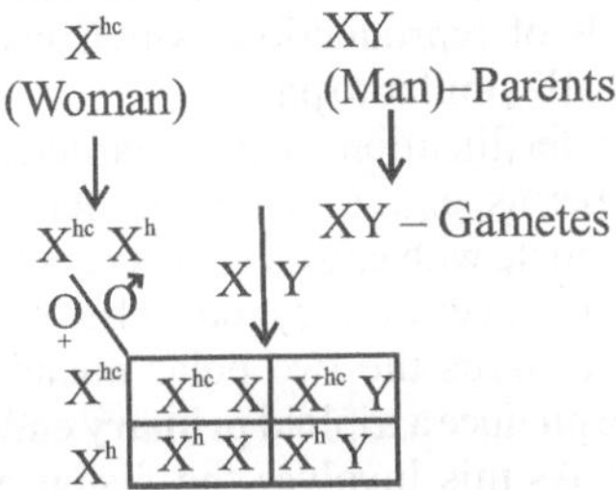

Results

(a) 50% sons are colorblind and haemophilic.

(b) 50% sons are haemophilic only.

(c) 50% daughters are carrier for colour blindness and haemophilia.

(d) 50% daughters are carrier for haemophilia only.

105. (a) X-linked recessive trait shows transmission from carrier female to male progeny. It is also celled criss-cross inheritance in which sex-linked characters are inherited from male parent to male grand children through females.

106. (c) Few pteridophytes are heterosporous i.e., with two types of spores, microspores and megaspores, e.g., *Selaginella*, Salvinia, Marsilea.
Plants of *Cycas* are also heterosporous and invariably dioecious, i.e. male and female reproductive organs occur on separate individuals.

107. (b) Circulatory system in arthropods is of open type. i.e. blood flows in irregular spaces called lacunae. It does not flow in definite blood vessels.

108. (c) Reptiles usually possess 3-chambered heart but crocodiles are an exception with 4-chambered heart. Not all chordates have a mouth with upper and lower jaw. Egg laying mammals include duck-billed platypus. Chondrichthyes (cartilaginous fishes) are the fishes that have cartilaginous endoskeleton. There is no exception to this.

109. (b) Xylem is a complex permanent tissue, which consists of tracheids, vessels, xylem parenchyma and xylem fibres. It functions as a conducting tissue for water and minerals from roots to the stem and leaves. Tracheids are elongated or tube like cells with thick and lignified walls and tapering ends. These are dead and are without protoplasm. Vessel is a long cylindrical tube-like structure made up of many cells called vessel members, each with lignified walls and a large central cavity. Vessel members are interconnected through perforations in their common walls. Xylem fibres have highly thickened walls and obliterated central lumens. These may either be septate or aseptate. Xylem parenchyma cells are living and thin-walled, and their cell walls are made up of cellulose.

110. (d) Epidermal tissue system forms outer covering of plant, which is in direct contact with external environment. The tissue system consists of the epidermis derived from protoderm and its associated structers; epidermal outgrowths. The cells perform different functions like protection, absorption, excretion, gaseous exchange, secretion and control of transpiration, etc.
The tissue present between epidermis and vascular tissue system constitutes ground tissue system. It forms the major part of a plant's body.
Vascular tissue system is composed of a number of vascular bundles, present in the central cylinder or column of the axis of root and stem which is known as stele. The vascular bundle is composed of primary xylem, primary phloem and cambium.

111. (c) AIDS is caused by HIV. When HIV enters into helper T-cells, it replicates and produces other viruses that kill the helper T-cells. Thus, the number of helper T-cells decreases in the body of the infected person and the person starts suffering from various infections.

112. (a) Holstein-Friesian from Holland, Brown Swiss from Switzerland and Jersey from Island of Jersey in English channel are exotic breeds of cattle.

113. (d) The cell from micro-organisms such as bacteria, fungi, filamentous algae, treated in various ways and used as food, are called single cell protein (SCP). The biomass is not only obtained from unicellular microorganisms but also from multicellular microorganisms.

114. (a) Yoghurt (yogurt) is produced by curdling milk with the help of *Streptococcus thermophilus* and *Lactobacillus bulgaricus*. The temperature is maintained at about 45°C (40° – 46°C) for four hours. It has a flavour of lactic acid and acetaldehyde.

115. (c) Sacred forests (= sacred groves) are forest patches around places of worship which are held in high esteem by tribal communities. They are the most undisturbed forest patches (island of pristine forests) which are often surrounded by highly degraded landscapes. They are found in several parts of India, e.g., Karnataka, Maharashtra, Rajasthan, etc. Many endemic species which are rare or have become extinct elsewhere can be seen to flourish here.

116. (c) The Government of India has instituted Amrita Devi Bishnoi Wildlife Protection Award for individuals or communities from rural areas that have shown extraordinary courage and dedication in protecting wildlife.

117. (b) Couplet, Lead, Analytical are the features associated with keys

118. (d) Hartig net, mantle and extracellular sheath are ectomycorrhizal while arbuscule is endouycorrhizal

119. (c) Roundworms are pseudocoelomate animals. The coelom is not completely lined by mesoderm, there are scattered patches or pouches of mesoderm inbetween ectoderm and endoderm.

120. (c) Ephyra is the second larval stage in the life cycle of *Aurelia* or Jelly fish. Planula larva forms Scyphistoma. Budding in Scyphistoma forms Ephyra. The process of Ephyra formation is called strobilation. One scyphistoma forms several Ephyra larva.

121. (b) Aril is the edible

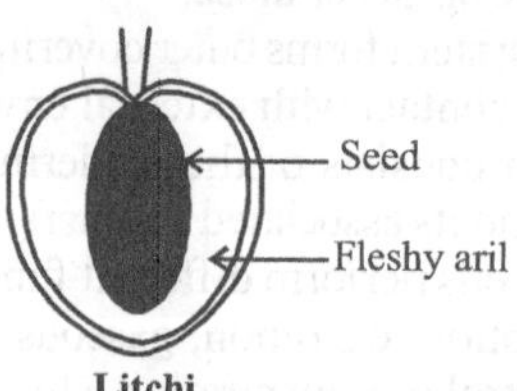

Litchi

part of litchi fruit (*Litchi sinensis*). Its a simple fruit (nut). The fruit has one seed and its covering is hard and woody. The fleshy and juicy aril is edible.

122. (a) *Pisum sativum* (Sweet Pea) belongs to the family Fabaceae which possess ten stamens, diadelphous and dithecous anther.

123. (b) The wood of the older stems gets differentiated into two zones, the outer light coloured and functional sapwood or alburnum which is involved in the conduction of water and minerals from root to leaf and the inner darker and nonfunctional heartwood or duramen. The heartwood is stronger and more durable than the sapwood and provide resistant to the attacks of micro-organisms and insects.

124. (a) Companion cells are part of phloem which in turn are a part of vascular tissue system and not epidermal tissue system.

125. (d) Except the first, the last and clitellar segment in each segment bears a ring of tiny curved, chitinous structure known as setae. Setae helps in locomotion and copulation.

126. (d) In peroxidase and catalase which catalyse the break down of hydrogen peroxide to water and oxygen, heme is a prosthetic group.

127. (b) Colchicine is an alkaloid obtained from the plant *Colchicum autumnale*. During mitosis it does not interfere with the replication of chromosome but prevents the formation of spindle fibres. During metaphase it inhibits the assemblage of microtubules hence spindle formation does not occur. Colchicine is used to induce polyploidy in plant breeding.

128. (b) pH of the guard cells rises due to active H^+ concentration. A rise pH causes hydrolysis of starch to form malic acid. Malic acid dissociates into H^+ and malate. H^+ ions pass out of the guard cells in exchange for K^+ ions. This lowers the osmotic potential of guard cells. As a result movement of water begins from neighbouring cells into guard cells which leads to opening of stomata.

129. (b) A herbicide DCMU (also known as diuron) blocks electron flow at the quinone acceptors of photosystem II, by competing for the binding site of plastoquinone.

130. (a) Birds are uricotelic animals which excrete nitrogenous waste materials in the form of uric acid.

131. (a) Axis vertebra possesses a peg-like structure called the odontoid process which projects forward from the centrum. It fits into the cavity of the atlas below the ligament so that it is separated from the neural canal. Such an arrangement gives a pivot joint which allows head to shake (rotate from one side to the other).

132. (c) Fenestra ovalis is membrane covered opening leading from tympanic cavity into the vestibule of the internal ear.

133. (c) Autonomic nervous system (ANS) automatically regulates the activities of smooth muscles, cardiac muscles and glands. This coordination is involuntary.

134. (c) The inner layer of eye is the retina and it contains three layer of cells—from inside to outside-ganglion cells, bipolar cells and photoreceptor cells.

135. (c) *Cholecystokinin* is a peptide hormone of mucosa of small intestine. It causes pancreas to release pancreatic enzymes and gall bladder to eject bile juice.

136. (d)

137. (d) Vegetative reproduction and apomixis both are asexual methods of reproduction, which gives the progeny genetically similar to parent.

138. (d) Double fertilization is the characteristic feature of angiosperms, e.g., *Capsella*. It includes fusion of one male gamete with egg cell. This result in the formation of a diploid cell, the zygote. The other male gamete moves towards the two polar nuclei and fuses with them to produce a triploid **primary endosperm nucleus** (PEN). As this involves the fusion of three haploid nuclei it is termed **triple fusion**. Since two types of fusions, syngamy and triple fusion take place in an embryo sac the phenomenon is termed double fertillisation.

139. (c) Cleistogmous flowers do not open or bloom at all. Thus, they cannot receive foreign pollens and invariably show autogamy, *i.e.*, self pollination. *E.g., Commellina, Viola* and *Oxalis*. These plants possess both cleistogamous and chasmogamous (flowers which bloom) flowers.

140. (c) Estrogen produced by ovary have wide range of actions such as stimulation of growth and activities of female secondary sex organs, development of growing ovarian follicles, appearance of female secondary sex characters. It also regulates female sexual behavior.

141. (b) Morgan identified linkage in fruitfly hence the percentage of white eyed and miniature winged recombinants are fewer than the expected ratio.

142. (c) Yellow round heterozygous pea plant may be represented by genotype RrYy. On selfing such plants following results will be obtained.

Parents: ♂ RrYy (Round Yellow) (X) ♀ RrYy (Round Yellow)

Gametes: (RY) (Ry) (rY) (ry) (RY) (Ry) (rY) (ry)

Offsprings:

♀ \ ♂	(RY)	(Ry)	(rY)	(ry)
(RY)	RRYY	RRYy	RrYY	RrYy
(Ry)	RRYy	RRyy	RrYy	Rryy
(rY)	RrYY	RrYy	rrYY	rrYy
(ry)	RrYy	Rryy	rrYy	rryy

Hence, total 26 genotypes will be obtained in the next generation, out of which the frequency of occurrence of RrYY genotype is 2, as illustrated in the table above.

143. (a) In a DNA molecule the amount of purine is equal to the amount of pyrimidine. Purine are adenine and guanine, Pyrimidine are cytosine and thymine. The number of adenine is equal to the number of thymine always. The number of cytosine is always equal to that of guanine.

$A = T$

$C = G$

If $C = 18\%$, then $G = 18\%$

$C + G = 36\%$

So, $A + T = 100 - 36 = 64\%$

$A = 32\%$, $T = 32\%$

So, adenine is 32%.

144. (a) There are three nonsense codons – UAA, UAG and UGA. These codons are not recognised by any of the tRNAs. Therefore, no more aminoacyl tRNA is formed and reaches A-site on ribosome.

145. (d) During Meselson and Stahl's experiments, heavy DNA was distinguished from normal DNA by centrifugation in CsCl gradient. When DNA is mixed with caesium chloride it will settle down at a particular height in centrifugation, heavier one higher up.

146. (d) The *lac* operon consists of one regulatory gene (the i gene) and three structural genes (*z*, *y*, and *a*). The i gene codes for the repressor of the *lac* operon. The *z* gene codes for beta-galactosidase (β-gal), which is primarily responsible for the hydrolysis of the disaccharide, lactose into its monomeric units, galactose and glucose. The *y* gene codes for permease, which increases permeability of the cell to β-galactosides. The *a* gene encodes a transacetylase. Hence, all the three gene products in *lac* operon are required for metabolism of lactose.

147. (a) Atavism is the phenomenon of sudden appearance of ancestral characters, not parental, in young ones, e.g., tail in newly born babies, dense and long hairs on body.

148. (c) Plague is a disease of the rats caused by a rod-shaped, non-motile bacillus, *Yersinia pestis*. The rat fleas leave the rats that die of plague, and bite human beings, thus infecting them with the disease.

149. (b) Morphine is the principle opium alkaloid. It is a strong analgesic. Opium is dried latex of unripe capsular fruits of poppy plant, *Papaver somniferum*. It is eaten or smoked. Morphine depresses respiratory centre, contributes to the fall in BP and cause bradycardia. It causes addiction.

150. (a) *Azolla* and BGA are biofertilizer which increases the fertility of soil.

151. (c) Alkaline phosphatase has become a useful tool in molecular biology laboratories, since DNA normally possesses phosphate groups on the 5' end. Removing these phosphates prevents the DNA from ligating thereby keeping DNA molecules linear until the next step of the process for which they are being prepared; also, removal of the phosphate groups allows radiolabeling in order to measure the presence of the labeled DNA through further steps in the process or experiment. For these purposes, the alkaline phosphatase from shrimp is the most useful, as it is the easiest to inactivate once it has done its job. Another important use of alkaline phosphatase is as a label for enzyme immunoassays.

152. (a) Restriction endonuclease-Hind II, always cut DNA molecules at a particular point by recognising a specific sequence of six base pairs. This specific base sequence is known as the recognition sequence for Hind II.

153. (c) The formula of exponential growth is $\frac{dN}{dt} = rN$ where $\frac{dN}{dt}$ is the rate of change in population size, r is the biotic potential and N is the population size.

154. (b) The body parts like ears, tail, limbs of animals living in colder climates become small to reduce the loss of heat from the body and thereby conserving energy. Such animals have to conserve body heat which is necessary to survive in colder climatic conditions. This is called Allen's Rule. Its an important law related with evolution.

155. (d) An ecosystem comprises of various biotic and abiotic components. In biotic components living beings (plants, animals and microbes) are included. These living beings may be various species. Those species which have important impact on ecosystem or which the characteristics of the ecosystem are called keystone species.

156. (c) Every enzyme possesses an optimum pH value, where it is most effective. Most enzymes show maximum activity in a pH range of about 6.0 to 7.5, i.e., near neutral pH. Some digestive enzymes have their optimum pH in the acidic or activity alkaline range. e.g., pepsin of gastric juice has its optimum at pH 2 (acidic), and trypsin of pancreatic juice shows maximum activity at pH 8.8 (alkaline). A rise and fall in pH reduces enzyme activity by changing the degree of ionisation of its side chain.

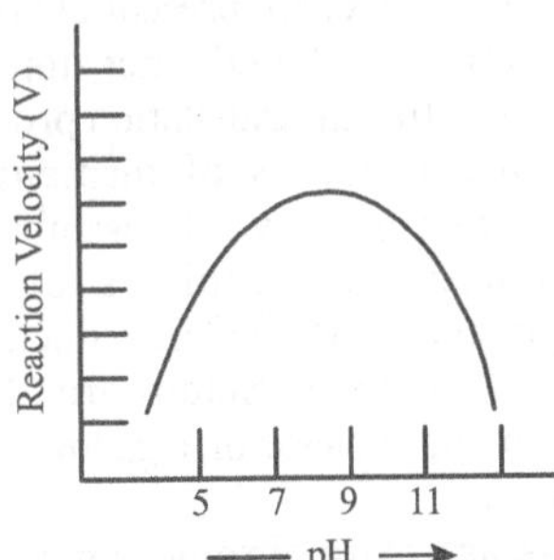

Fig. Effect of pH on the velocity of enzyme action

157. (c) The diameter of afferent arteriole is larger than the efferent arteriole. This increases the volume of blood in glomerulus and increases the filtration rate. This causes the effective filtration pressure thus, promoting filtration.

158. (c) In a mature pollen grain, the generative cell is smaller and the tube (or vegetative) cell is larger. In the later stages of development of pollen grain, callose dissolves and the naked generative cell comes to lie freely in the cytoplasm of the tube cell. The tube cell has a cytoplasm which is rich in the food reserve (starch, protein, fat with mostly unsaturated fatty acids).

159. (d) Given figure represents castor seed. It is oblong mottled brown endospermic and dicotyledonous seed. A thick hard but brittle testa covers the seed. A thin perisperm lies below it and around the kernel. A white oily endosperm lies below the perisperm. It stores food reserve as oil drops and proteins. Endosperm is source of castor oil. Embryo lies in the centre of seed. It consists of a short embryo axis bearing two thin semi-transparent oval cotyledons, a small indistinct plumule and a knob-shaped radicle.

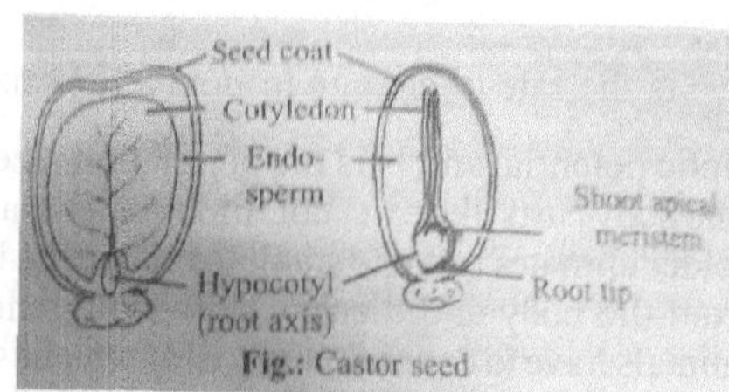

Fig.: Castor seed

160. (d) Third stage of parturition (placental stage) is the time after the delivery until the placenta or after birth is expelled by powerful uterine contractions. Umbilical cord is cut close to the baby's navel. It lasts for 10-15 minutes after the birth of child.

161. (c) P —(4 m.u.)— Q —(7 m.u.)— R; P to R = 11 m.u.

162. (d) Repeated or repetitive sequences make up a large portion of human genome. Repetitive sequences are nucleotide sequences that are repeated many times, sometimes hundred to thousand times. They have no direct coding function but provide information as to chromosome structure, dynamics and evolution. They represent junk DNA.

163. (c) mRNA has some additional sequences that are not translated and are referred as untranslated regions (UTRs). The UTRs are present at both 5'-end (before start codon) and at 3'-end (after stop codon). They are required for efficient translation process.

164. (d) Statins are products of fermentation by yeast *Monascus purpureus* which resemble mevalovate and are competitive inhibitors of β–hydroxy-β–methylglutary or HMG CoA reductase. This inhibits cholesterol synthesis. Statins are, therefore, used in lowering blood cholesterol, e.g., lovastatin, pravastatin, simvastatin.

165. (c) Plasmids are extra-chromosomal, self replicating, usually circular, double stranded DNA molecules found naturally in many bacteria and also in some yeast. Plasmids are usually not essential for normal cell growth and division, they often confer some traits to the host organism e.g., resistance to certain antibiotics. The plasmid that is used as carrier for transferring a fragment of foreign DNA into a suitable host is called vehicle DNA or cloning vector or gene carrier.

166. (a) Primers are small, chemically synthesized oligonucleotides that are complementary to the sequences present at 3' end of the template DNA. They hybridize to the target DNA region, one to each strand of the double helix. These primers are oriented with their ends facing each other allowing synthesis of the DNA towards one another.

167. (d) Human insulin is made up of 51 amino acids arranged in two polypeptide chains, A, having 21 amino acids and B, with 30 amino acids. The two polypeptide chains are interconnected by two disulphide bridges. The hormone develops from a storage product called proinsulin. Proinsulin has three chains, A, B and C. C-chain with 33 amino acids is removed prior to insulin formation.

168. (d) Kangaroo and desert rat seldom drink water. It has a thick coat to minimise evaporative desiccation. The animal seldom comes out of its comparatively humid and cool burrow during the day time. 90% of its water requirement is met from metabolic water which is produced by respiratory breakdown of fats. 10% is obtained from food. Loss of water is minimized by producing nearly solid urine and faeces.

169. (d) *Lantana, Eichhornia* and *Parthenium* are all exotic species, which had been introduced in India. *Lantana camara* has replaced many species in forests of Uttar Pradesh and Madhya Pradesh. *Eichhornia* (water hyacinth) has clogged water bodies including wetlands resulting in death of several aquatic plants and animals. *Parthenium* has pushed out several herbs and shrubs from open places in the pains.

170. (a) Ecological diversity is of three types:

(i) Alpha diversity (Within community diversity) is species diversity in a given community or habitat. It is dependent upon species richness and evenness.

(ii) Beta diversity (Between community diversity) is biodiversity in a range of communities due to replacement of species with the change in community/habitat because of presence of different microhabitats, niches, etc.

(iii) Gamma biodiversity is diversity of habitats/ecosystems over a total landscape or geographical area.

171. (a) Archegoniates are bryophytes, pteridophytes & gymnosperms.

172. (a) The quasi-fluid nature of lipid enables lateral movement of proteins within the overall bilayer.

173. (c) Recombination nodule appears during pachytene of meiosis.

174. (b) Fats are absorbed in lacteals of small intestine by coating with proteins, before absorption and then they enter in the lymphatic circulation.

175. (b) Cardiac output = Stroke volume × Heart rate
$= 0.07 \times 75 = 5.25$ L/min

176. (a) Prolactin is secreted by anterior pituitary and is responsible for beginning the production of milk by maumary glands.

177. (a) Width of I-band decreases during muscle contraction.

178. (a) Loading and unloading of sugars is an active process as well as transport of sugar is not unidirectional but bidirectional.

179. (b) Mn is a micronutrient and thus, can be come toxic at higher concentrations

180. (b) On substrate level phosphorylation, one molecule of PGAL produces only 3 ATP [2 Glycolysis + 1 TCA cycle.